CLINICAL ORTHOPAEDIC REHABILITATION

A Team Approach

Fourth Edition

CLINICAL ORTHOPAEDIC REHABILITATION

A Team Approach

Charles E. Giangarra, MD
Professor, Chief
Division of Sports Medicine
Department of Orthopedic Surgery
Marshall University
Joan C. Edwards School of Medicine
Huntington, West Virginia;
Head, Team Physician
Department of Athletics
Marshall University,
Assistant Team Physician, Orthopaedic Consultant
Kentucky Christian University
Grayson, Kentucky

Robert C. Manske, PT, DPT, MEd,
SCS, ATC, CSCS
Professor and Chair
Department of Physical Therapy
Wichita State University
Via Christi Sports and Orthopedic Physical
    Therapy
Via Christi Sports Medicine,
Teaching Associate
Department of Community Medicine Sciences
University of Kansas Medical Center
Via Christi Family Practice Sports Medicine
    Residency Program
Wichita, Kansas;
Teaching Associate
Department of Rehabilitation
Sciences University of Kansas Medical Center
Kansas City, Kansas

ELSEVIER

ELSEVIER

1600 John F. Kennedy Blvd.
Ste 1800
Philadelphia, PA 19103-2899

CLINICAL ORTHOPAEDIC REHABILITATION: A TEAM APPROACH,
FOURTH EDITION

ISBN: 978-0-323393706

Notices

Knowledge and best practice in this field are constantly changing. As new research and experience broaden our understanding, changes in research methods, professional practices, or medical treatment may become necessary.

Practitioners and researchers must always rely on their own experience and knowledge in evaluating and using any information, methods, compounds, or experiments described herein. In using such information or methods they should be mindful of their own safety and the safety of others, including parties for whom they have a professional responsibility.

With respect to any drug or pharmaceutical products identified, readers are advised to check the most current information provided (i) on procedures featured or (ii) by the manufacturer of each product to be administered, to verify the recommended dose or formula, the method and duration of administration, and contraindications. It is the responsibility of practitioners, relying on their own experience and knowledge of their patients, to make diagnoses, to determine dosages and the best treatment for each individual patient, and to take all appropriate safety precautions.

To the fullest extent of the law, neither the Publisher nor the authors, contributors, or editors, assume any liability for any injury and/or damage to persons or property as a matter of products liability, negligence or otherwise, or from any use or operation of any methods, products, instructions, or ideas contained in the material herein.

Previous editions copyrighted 2011, 2003, and 1996.

Library of Congress Cataloging-in-Publication Data

Names: Giangarra, Charles E., editor. | Manske, Robert C., editor.
Title: Clinical orthopaedic rehabilitation : a team approach / [edited by]
   Charles E. Giangarra, Robert C. Manske.
Description: Fourth edition. | Philadelphia, PA : Elsevier, [2018] | Includes
   bibliographical references and index.
Identifiers: LCCN 2016049212| ISBN 9780323393706 (pbk. : alk. paper) | ISBN
   9780323477901 (eBook)
Subjects: | MESH: Orthopedic Procedures--methods | Musculoskeletal
   Diseases--rehabilitation | Musculoskeletal System--injuries | Wounds and
   Injuries--rehabilitation | Rehabilitation--standards | Evidence-Based
   Medicine--methods
Classification: LCC RD797 | NLM WE 168 | DDC 616.7/06515--dc23 LC record available at
https://lccn.loc.gov/2016049212

Executive Content Strategist: Dolores Meloni
Content Development Specialist: Lisa Barnes
Publishing Services Manager: Deepthi Unni
Senior Project Manager: Beula Christopher
Senior Book Designer: Margaret Reid

Printed in United States of America.

Last digit is the print number: 9   8   7   6   5   4

Working together
to grow libraries in
developing countries

www.elsevier.com • www.bookaid.org

David W. Altchek, MD
Co-Chief, Sports Medicine and Shoulder Service,
Attending Orthopedic Surgeon
Hospital for Special Surgery,
Professor of Clinical Orthopedic Surgery
Weill Medical College,
Medical Director, New York Mets
New York, New York

Michael Angeline, MD
Section of Orthopaedic Surgery
The University of Chicago Medical Center
Chicago, Illinois

Jeff Ashton, PT
Staff Physical Therapist
Cabell Huntington Hospital
Huntington, West Virginia

Jolene Bennett, PT, MA, OCS, ATC, Cert MDT
Spectrum Health Rehabilitation and Sports Medicine Services
Grand Rapids, Michigan

Allan Besselink, PT, Dip MDT
Director, Smart Sport International,
Director, Smart Life Institute,
Adjunct Assistant Professor
Physical Therapist Assistant Program
Austin Community College
Austin, Texas

Sanjeev Bhatia, MD
Naval Medical Center, San Diego
San Diego, California;
Department of Orthopaedic Surgery
Rush University Medical Center
Chicago, Illinois

Lori A. Bolgla, PT, PhD, MAcc, ATC
Associate Professor
Department of Physical Therapy in the College of Allied
    Health Sciences
Department of Orthopaedic Surgery at the Medical College of
    Georgia
The Graduate School
Augusta University
Augusta, Georgia

S. Brent Brotzman, MD
Assistant Clinical Professor
Department of Orthopaedic Surgery
University of Texas at San Antonio Health Sciences Center
San Antonio, Texas;
Assistant Professor
Department of Pediatrics
Texas A&M University System Health Sciences Center
College Station, Texas;
Former Division NCAA Team Physician
Department of Athletics
Texas A&M University–Corpus Christi
Corpus Christi, Texas;
Section Chief
Department of Orthopaedic Surgery
North Austin Medical Center,
Private Practice
North Austin Sports Medicine Medical Center
Austin, Texas

Jason Brumitt, PT, PhD, ATC, CSCS
Assistant Professor of Physical Therapy
School of Physical Therapy
George Fox University
Newberg, Oregon

David S. Butler, BPhty, MAppSc, EdD
Neuro Orthopaedic Institute
University of South Australia Adelaide
South Australia Australia

R. Matthew Camarillo, MD
Department of Orthopedics
University of Texas at Houston
Houston, Texas

Mark M. Casillas, MD
The Foot and Ankle Center of South Texas
San Antonio, Texas

Bridget Clark, PT, MSPT, DPT
Athletic Performance Lab, LLC
Austin, Texas

Alexander T. Caughran, MD
Chief Resident
Department of Orthopedic Surgery
Marshall University
Joan C. Edwards School of Medicine
Huntington, West Virginia

Michael D'Amato, MD
HealthPartners Specialty Center Orthopaedic
    and Sports Medicine
St. Paul, Minnesota

George J. Davies, DPT, MEd, PT, SCS, ATC, LAT, CSCS, PES, FAPTA
Professor
Department of Physical Therapy
Armstrong Atlantic State University
Savannah, Georgia

Michael Duke, PT, CSCS
North Austin Physical Therapy
Austin, Texas

Christopher J. Durall, PT, DPT, MS, SCS, LAT, CSCS
Director of Physical Therapy Unit
Student Health Center
University of Wisconsin, La Crosse
La Crosse, Wisconsin

Todd S. Ellenbecker, DPT, MS, SCS, OCS, CSCS
Group/Clinic Director
Physiotherapy Associates Scottsdale Sports Clinic,
National Director of Clinical Research
Physiotherapy Associates,
Director, Sports Medicine–ATP Tour
Scottsdale, Arizona

Brian K. Farr, MA, ATC, LAT, CSCS
Director, Athletic Training Educational Program
Department of Kinesiology and Health Education
The University of Texas at Austin
Austin, Texas

Larry D. Field, MD
Director, Upper Extremity Service
Mississippi Sports Medicine and Orthopaedic Center,
Clinical Associate Professor
Department of Orthopaedic Surgery
University of Mississippi Medical School
Jackson, Mississippi

G. Kelley Fitzgerald, PhD, PT
University of Pittsburgh
School of Health and Rehabilitation Sciences
Pittsburgh, Pennsylvania

Rachel M. Frank, BS
Department of Orthopaedic Surgery
Rush University Medical Center
Chicago, Illinois

Tigran Garabekyan, MD
Assistant Professor
Department of Orthopedic Surgery
Marshall University
Joan C. Edwards School of Medicine
Huntington, West Virginia

Neil S. Ghodadra, MD
Naval Medical Center, San Diego
San Diego, California;
Department of Orthopaedic Surgery
Rush University Medical Center
Chicago, Illinois

Charles E. Giangarra, MD
Professor, Chief
Division of Sports Medicine
Department of Orthopedic Surgery
Marshall University
Joan C. Edwards School of Medicine
Huntington, West Virginia;
Head, Team Physician
Department of Athletics
Marshall University,
Assistant Team Physician, Orthopaedic Consultant
Kentucky Christian University
Grayson, Kentucky

Charles Andrew Gilliland, BS, MD
Clinical Assistant Professor
Department of Orthopedic Surgery
Marshall University
Joan C. Edwards School of Medicine
Huntington, West Virginia

John A. Guido, Jr., PT, MHS, SCS, ATC, CSCS
Clinical Director
TMI Sports Therapy
Grand Prairie, Texas

J. Allen Hardin, PT, MS, SCS, ATC, LAT, CSCS
Intercollegiate Athletics
The University of Texas at Austin
Austin, Texas

Maureen A. Hardy, PT, MS, CHT
Director
Rehabilitation Services St. Dominic Hospital
Jackson, Mississippi

Timothy E. Hewett, PhD, FACSM
Professor, Director of Biomechanics
Sports Medicine Research and MST Core, Mayo Clinic
Mayo Clinic Biomechanics Laboratories and Sports Medicine
  Center
Departments of Orthopedics, Physical Medicine and
  Rehabilitation and Physiology and Biomedical Engineering
Mayo Clinic
Rochester and Minneapolis, Minnesota

Clayton F. Holmes, PT, EdD, MS, ATC
Professor and Founding Chair
Department of Physical Therapy
University of North Texas Health Science Center at Fort Worth
Forth Worth, Texas

Barbara J. Hoogenboom, EdD, PT, SCS, ATC
Associate Professor
Physical Therapy Associate Director
Grand Valley State University
Grand Rapids, Michigan

James J. Irrgang, PhD, PT, ATC
Director of Clinical Research
Department of Physical Therapy
University of Pittsburgh Medical Center
Pittsburgh, Pennsylvania

Margaret Jacobs, PT
Momentum Physical Therapy and Sports Rehabilitation
San Antonio, Texas

R. Jason Jadgchew, ATC, CSCS
Department of Orthopedic Surgery
Naval Medical Center
San Diego, California

David A. James, PT, DPT, OCS, CSCS
Associated Faculty
Physical Therapy Program
University of Colorado
Denver, Colorado

John J. Jasko, MD
Associate Professor
Department of Orthopedic Surgery
Marshall University
Joan C. Edwards School of Medicine
Huntington, West Virginia

Drew Jenk, PT, DPT
Regional Clinical Director
Sports Physical Therapy of New York
Liverpool, New York

W. Ben Kibler, MD
Medical Director
Shoulder Center of Kentucky
Lexington, Kentucky

Theresa M. Kidd, BA
North Austin Sports Medicine
Austin, Texas

Kyle Kiesel, PT, PhD, ATC, CSCS
Associate Professor of Physical Therapy
University of Evansville
Evansville, Indiana

Jonathan Yong Kim, CDR
University of San Diego
San Diego, California

Scott E. Lawrance, MS, PT, ATC, CSCS
Assistant Professor
Department of Athletic Training
University of Indianapolis
Indianapolis, Indiana

Michael Levinson, PT, CSCS
Clinical Supervisor
Sports Rehabilitation and Performance Center,
Rehabilitation Department
Hospital for Special Surgery,
Physical Therapist
New York Mets,
Faculty
Columbia University Physical Therapy School
New York, New York

Sameer Lodha, MD
Department of Orthopaedic Surgery
Rush University Medical Center
Chicago, Illinois

Janice K. Loudon, PT, PhD, SCS, ATC, CSCS
Associate Professor
Department of Physical Therapy Education
Rockhurst University
Kansas City, Missouri

Adriaan Louw, PT, MAppSc (Physio), CSMT
Instructor
International Spine and Pain Institute,
Instructor
Neuro Orthopaedic Institute,
Associate Instructor
Rockhurst University
Story City, Iowa

Joseph R. Lynch, MD
Associate Professor
Uniformed Services University of the Health Sciences
Bethesda, Maryland;
The Shoulder Clinic of Idaho
Boise, Idaho

Robert C. Manske, PT, DPT, MEd, SCS, ATC, CSCS
Professor and Chair
Department of Physical Therapy
Wichita State University
Via Christi Sports and Orthopedic Physical Therapy
Via Christi Sports Medicine,
Teaching Associate
Department of Community Medicine Sciences
University of Kansas Medical Center
Via Christi Family Practice Sports Medicine Residency
    Program
Wichita, Kansas;
Teaching Associate
Department of Rehabilitation
Sciences University of Kansas Medical Center
Kansas City, Kansas

Matthew J. Matava, MD
Washington University
Department of Orthopedic Surgery
St. Louis, Missouri

Sean Mazloom, MS
Medical Student
Chicago Medical School
Chicago, Illinois

John McMullen, MS, ATC
Director of Orthopedics-Sports Medicine
Lexington Clinic/Shoulder Center of Kentucky
Lexington, Kentucky

Morteza Meftah, MD
Ranawat Orthopaedic Center
New York, New York

Erik P. Meira, PT, SCS, CSCS
Clinical Director
Black Diamond Physical Therapy
Portland, Oregon

Keith Meister, MD
Director, TMI Sports Medicine
Head Team Physician, Texas Rangers
Arlington, Texas

Scott T. Miller, PT, MS, SCS, CSCS
Agility Physical Therapy and Sports Performance, LLC
Portage, Michigan

Josef H. Moore, PT, PhD
Professor
Army-Baylor DPT Program
Waco, Texas

Donald Nguyen, PT, MSPT, ATC, LAT
ATEP Clinical Coordinator and Assistant Athletic Trainer for Rowing
University of Texas at Austin
Austin, Texas

Cullen M. Nigrini, MSPT, MEd, PT, ATC, LAT
Elite Athletic Therapy
Austin, Texas

Steven R. Novotny, MD
Associate Professor
Department of Orthopedic Surgery
Marshall University
Joan C. Edwards School of Medicine
Huntington, West Virginia

Michael J. O'Brien, MD
Assistant Professor of Clinical Orthopaedics
Division of Sports Medicine
Department of Orthopaedics
Tulane University School of Medicine
New Orleans, Louisiana

Sinan Emre Ozgur, MD
Chief Resident
Department of Orthopedic Surgery
Marshall University
Joan C. Edwards School of Medicine
Huntington, West Virginia

Mark V. Paterno, PhD, PT, MS, SCS, ATC
Coordinator of Orthopaedic and Sports Physical Therapy
Sports Medicine Biodynamics Center
Division of Occupational and Physical Therapy
Cincinnati Children's Hospital Medical Center,
Assistant Professor
Division of Sports Medicine
Department of Pediatrics
University of Cincinnati Medical Center
Cincinnati, Ohio

Ryan T. Pitts, MD
Metropolitan Orthopedics
St. Louis, Missouri

Marisa Pontillo, PT, DPT, SCS
Penn Therapy and Fitness Weightman Hall
Philadelphia, Pennsylvania

Andrew S.T. Porter, DO, FAAFP
Director
Sports Medicine Fellowship Program
University of Kansas School of Medicine- Wichita at Via Christi,
Director
Osteopathic Family Medicine Residency Program
Kansas City University at Via Christi
Wichita, Kansas

Christie C.P. Powell, PT, MSPT, STS, USSF "D"
Co-Owner and Director
CATZ Sports Performance and Physical Therapy,
Director of Physical Therapy
Lonestar Soccer Club,
Director of Physical Therapy
Austin Huns Rugby Team
Austin, Texas

Daniel Prohaska, MD
Advanced Orthopedic Associates
Wichita, Kansas

Matthew T. Provencher, MD, CDR, MC, USN
Associate Professor of Surgery
Uniformed Services University of the Health Sciences,
Director of Orthopaedic Shoulder, Knee, and Sports Surgery
Department of Orthopaedic Surgery
Naval Medical Center, San Diego
San Diego, California

Emilio "Louie" Puentedura, PT, DPT, GDMT, OCS, FAAOMPT
Assistant Professor
Department of Physical Therapy
University of Nevada, Las Vegas
Las Vegas, Nevada

Amar S. Ranawat, MD
Associate Professor of Orthopaedic Surgery
Weill Cornell Medical College,
Associate Attending Orthopaedic Surgeon
New York-Presbyterian Hospital,
Associate Attending Orthopaedic Surgeon
Hospital for Special Surgery
Ranawat Orthopaedic Center
New York, New York

Anil S. Ranawat, MD
Assistant Professor of Orthopaedic Surgery
Weill Cornell Medical College,
Assistant Attending Orthopaedic Surgeon
New York-Presbyterian Hospital,
Assistant Attending Orthopaedic Surgeon
Hospital for Special Surgery
Ranawat Orthopedic Center
New York, New York

James T. Reagan, MD
Senior Resident
Department of Orthopedic Surgery
Marshall University
Joan C. Edwards School of Medicine
Huntington, West Virginia

Bruce Reider, MD
Professor Emeritus, Surgery
Section of Orthopaedic Surgery and Rehabilitation Medicine
University of Chicago
Chicago, Illinois

Michael P. Reiman, PT, DPT, OCS, SCS, ATC, FAAOMPT, CSCS
Assistant Professor
Department of Orthopedic Surgery
Duke University Medical Center
Durham, North Carolina

Amy G. Resler, DPT, CMP, CSCS
Department of Physical Therapy
Naval Medical Center, San Diego
San Diego, California

Bryan Riemann, PhD, ATC, FNATA
Associate Professor of Sports Medicine
Coordinator Master of Science in Sports Medicine
Director, Biodynamics and Human Performance Center
Armstrong State University
Savannah, Georgia

Toby Rogers, PhD, MPT
Associate Professor of Sports Medicine
Coordinator Master of Science in Sports Medicine
Director, Biodynamics and Human Performance Center
Armstrong State University
Savannah, Georgia

Anthony A. Romeo, MD
Associate Professor and Director
Section of Shoulder and Elbow
Department of Orthopaedic Surgery
Rush University Medical Center
Chicago, Illinois

Richard Romeyn, MD
Southeast Minnesota Sports Medicine and Orthopaedic
    Surgery Specialists
Winona, Minnesota

Michael D. Rosenthal, PT, DSc, SCS, ECS, ATC, CSCS
Assistant Professor
Doctor of Physical Therapy program
San Diego State University
San Diego, California

Felix H. Savoie III, MD
Lee C. Schlesinger Professor
Department of Orthopaedics
Tulane University School of Medicine
New Orleans, Louisiana

Suzanne Zadra Schroeder, PT, ATC
Physical Therapist
Barnes Jewish West County Hospital
STAR Center
St. Louis, Missouri

Aaron Sciascia, MS, ATC, NASM-PES
Coordinator
Shoulder Center of Kentucky
Lexington, Kentucky

K. Donald Shelbourne, MD
Shelbourne Knee Center at Methodist Hospital
Indianapolis, Indiana

Jace R. Smith, MD
Senior Resident
Department of Orthopedic Surgery
Marshall University
Joan C. Edwards School of Medicine
Huntington, West Virginia

Damien Southard, MPT
Staff Physical Therapist
Cabell Huntington Hospital
Huntington, West Virginia

Ken Stephenson, MD
Orthopaedic Foot and Ankle Specialist,
Attending Surgeon
Northstar Surgery Center,
Associate Professor
Texas Tech Health Sciences Center
Lubbock, Texas

Faustin R. Stevens, MD
Orthopaedic Surgery
Texas Tech Health Sciences Center
Lubbock, Texas

Mark Stovak, MD, FACSM, FAAFP, CAQSM
Professor
Department of Family and Community Medicine
University of Nevada, Reno School of Medicine
Reno, Nevada

Timothy F. Tyler, MS, PT, ATC
Nicholas Institute of Sports Medicine and Athletic Trauma
Lenox Hill Hospital
New York, New York

Geoffrey S. Van Thiel, MD, MBA
Division of Sports Medicine
Rush University Medical Center
Chicago, Illinois

Mark Wagner, MD
Orthopaedic Specialists, PC
Portland, Oregon

Reg B. Wilcox III, PT, DPT, MS, OCS
Clinical Supervisor
Outpatient Service
Department of Rehabilitation Services
Brigham and Women's Hospital,
Adjunct Clinical Assistant Professor
Department of Physical Therapy
School of Health and Rehabilitation Services
MGH Institute of Health Professions
Boston, Massachusetts

Daniel Woods, MD
Senior Resident
Department Orthopaedic Surgery
Marshall University
Joan C. Edwards School of Medicine
Huntington, West Virginia

FOREWORD BY GEORGE J. DAVIES

It is indeed an honor and a privilege to be invited to write the forward for the Fourth Edition of *Clinical Orthopaedic Rehabilitation*. For a book to be revised into a fourth edition is a testimonial to the quality and longevity of the contribution to the literature. *Clinical Orthopaedic Rehabilitation* is an excellent addition to the literature that provides current state of the art information for rehabilitation.

I have personally had the opportunity to work with and had the opportunity to learn from both of the editors: Charles "Chuck" Giangarra, MD, and Robert Manske, DPT. I had the privilege to work with Dr. Chuck and publish some other works with him. Dr. Chuck did his fellowship at the Kerlan-Jobe Clinic and had the opportunity to work directly with Dr. Frank Jobe as well as publish some research papers with Dr. Jobe. Dr. Chuck is an experienced surgeon with 30 years of experience and is a tremendous physician. I had the opportunity to work with Dr. Chuck for approximately 5 years before he moved on to become the head team physician at Marshall University. Dr. Chuck always had the patients' interest foremost and understood the importance of the team approach when patients had injuries or surgeries. He was always a strong proponent of the physicians and rehabilitation specialists working closely together to provide the optimum quality care for their patients. Consequently, this book reinforces many examples of the team approach to treating patients and the importance of rehabilitation to return the patients to their optimum level of performance safely.

I had the privilege to meet and work with Rob when he was selected as the second resident at Gundersen Lutheran Sports Medicine (GLSM) (GLSM was the first APTA credential public Sports Physical Therapy Residency program in the USA). Rob was a hard worker and an accomplished clinician and earned his SCS, ATC, and CSCS credentials during that year and the subsequent years. Rob has worked his way through academia from an assistant professor to a full professor and chair at Wichita State University. Since his residency program, Rob and I have collaborated on many articles, research projects, and presentations at numerous meetings during the last 20 years. Rob has excelled as a clinician, teacher, professional, and administrator and has edited or written seven textbooks that have made significant contributions to the literature. *Clinical Orthopaedic Rehabilitation* is another example of Rob's continued pursuit of excellence in contributing to the literature and educating clinicians as to the optimum evidence-based rehabilitation for orthopedic conditions.

The quality of any book is predicated on the quality and conscientiousness of its editors. So, by combining the multiple talents of these editors, the Fourth Edition of the book has maintained its past format and updated approximately eight to ten new chapters to reflect the most current evidence and research. The focus of the book is on examination, surgeries, and rehabilitation of numerous orthopedic conditions to provide state of the art treatment protocols. This new edition also includes links to videos to reinforce the content within the book. This fourth edition is an outstanding contribution to the literature and is a must read for those who are interested in utilizing the best current evidence in rehabilitation for their patients.

This book is highly recommended for physical therapists, physical therapy assistants, athletic trainers, and physicians involved in treatment of orthopedic conditions where rehabilitation is a critical component of getting the patient safely and effectively for performance enhancement back to activity.

Respectfully,

George J. Davies, DPT, MEd, PT, SCS, ATC, LAT, CSCS, PES, FAPTA
Professor-Armstrong State University, 2004–present,
Professor Emeritus, University of Wisconsin-LaCrosse, 2003,
Founder and Co-Editor, 1979
Journal of Orthopaedic and Sports Physical Therapy,
Founder and Associate Editor, 2009
Sports Health: A Multidisciplinary Approach,
Sports Physical Therapist:
Coastal Therapy, Savannah, GA, 2004–present,
Gundersen Health System, LaCrosse, WI, 1991–present

FOREWORD BY EDWARD G. MCFARLAND

It is an honor to be asked to write a foreword to this incredible book put together by two of the stars of the orthopedic community—Dr. Manske, a physical therapist, and Dr. Giangarra, an orthopedic surgeon. I have to admit that I was unfamiliar with this text until this invitation, and it was my loss. This is an incredible book that has several attributes that make it a valuable addition to the practice of physical therapists, hand therapists, and orthopedic practioners of any level: student, resident, or surgeon in practice. One important quality of this book is that for each area of the body it has a concise and informative summary of the most common conditions and injuries that affect that area. This assures that everyone in the team treating the patient has as much knowledge as possible about the injury and the rationale for the treatment and rehabilitation. I am unaware of any other text that makes the important link between the condition and the subsequent rehabilitation. Each chapter provides rehabilitation protocols for the injuries discussed in the chapter so that the rationale of the protocol is provided and readily available. These rehabilitation protocols are excellent and I wish I'd had access to them many years ago. Another strength of this book is the ability to access videos of the rehabilitation techniques. It is one thing to read about rehabilitation techniques and another to have videos that help a practitioner to get it right. Lastly, one of the best features for me as a practitioner is that I can use their rehabilitation protocols in my orthopedic practice; they are a quick reference to how the experts approach the rehabilitation of these important orthopedic conditions. I plan to use these protocols in my practice.

Drs. Manske and Giangarra not only bring their vast experience to this book, they also have recruited some of the leaders in each orthopedic topic discussed. This book has been written by the best and most visible leaders in the fields of orthopedic surgery and rehabilitation. The information has been updated and provides the latest and most up-to-date approach to clinical orthopedic rehabilitation. I would recommend this textbook to all orthopedic practitioners.

Edward G. McFarland, MD
Wayne H. Lewis Professor of Orthopaedic and Shoulder Surgery
Professor, Department of Orthopaedic Surgery
Johns Hopkins University
Baltimore, Maryland

Our goal in preparing the 4th edition of *Clinical Orthopaedic Rehabilitation: A Team Approach* was to continue to widen the breadth of the content and orthopedic and sports information to mimic that of the everyday practicing surgeon, physician, physical therapist, and athletic trainer who work in orthopedics. In increasing the breadth of content we have made this text more useful to clinicians and student clinicians. Several areas of content that are rarely seen in orthopedics except very rare special cases have been removed and other more pertinent pathologies have been included. For example, several chapters have been included in the expanded shoulder, elbow, knee, and hip sections. Dr. Charles Giangarra, a well-published author, already has brought a wealth of knowledge to many sections of the 4th edition. We have done our best to use a team approach so often seen and needed between physicians and rehabilitation specialists. The chapter authors are an exceptional group of clinicians who have presented the best available evidence regarding contemporary rehabilitation of orthopedic conditions. This dedicated multidisciplinary team of authors has added an incredible value to the foundation of this already strong book.

In the third edition Dr. Brotzman and I took tremendous steps forward to improve the overall quality and content of the information provided within the pages of this comprehensive text. Dr. Giangarra and I have continued this forward momentum with the 4th edition. Updated and new evidence-based literature covering sound examination techniques, classification systems, differential diagnosis, treatment options, and updated criteria-based rehabilitation protocols have been included. Videos of some of the most commonly used exercises are included within the text. New all-color images have been included to update the over 800 images to help the visual learner better see and appreciate injuries and exercises used to treat those injuries.

The treatment of orthopedic conditions is not static. The process of treating conditions of the muscles, bones, and nerves is and has always been dynamic. Textbooks about examination, evaluation, prognosis, and treatment of these conditions must be just as dynamic and ever changing. We hope that the readers of this text continue to feel that *Clinical Orthopaedic Rehabilitation* is the definitive reference for achieving success with the management of orthopedic conditions.

Robert C. Manske, PT, DPT, MEd, SCS, ATC, CSCS
Charles E. Giangarra, MD

ACKNOWLEDGMENTS

To my fabulous wife, Jean, and my three wonderful children, Nick, Jenna, and Cristen, who I am so very proud of and who put up with me and made the best of my multiple moves across the country until I found the right opportunity. I could not have made it this far without their love and support and for that I am eternally grateful.

To my mentor, chairman, and friend, Dr. Oliashirazi, who believed in me and has encouraged me to excel more times than I can count.

To the orthopedic residents of Marshall University who have revitalized not only my career but my enthusiasm for learning.

I would also like to thank Ashley Belmaggio MA, Meagan Bevins ATC, Tom Garton MPT, and Michael Bonar PTA for their help with this project especially in preparing many of the new photographs for publication. I could not have done it without them.

Charles E. Giangarra, MD

To Dr. Brent Brotzman and Dr. Charles E. Giangarra.

Dr. Brotzman, I want to personally thank you for taking the chance by allowing me to work with you on COR3. It was an incredible experience and I am forever indebted to you for your partnership. It is such a great resource for all health care professionals in rehabilitation and will go down as one of the best orthopedic textbooks of the last several decades.

Dr. Chuck, I appreciate your willingness to jump on this fast-moving train we call COR4 and take over for Dr. Brotzman. Your insight, mentorship, guidance, and willingness to always lend a hand have been an invaluable gift to me throughout the last 20 years. I would have never thought that when we first met back in LaCrosse in 1998 that either of us would end up with such a great project that will impact so many great rehabilitation professionals in a positive way.

Lastly a special thanks to B.J. Lehecka for reviewing and editing the spinal chapter section of this text. His insight was extremely valuable in this addition.

Robert C. Manske, PT, DPT, MEd, SCS, ATC, CSCS

CONTENTS

SECTION 4 Foot and Ankle Injuries

SECTION 5 Knee Injuries

SECTION **6** Hip Injuries

SECTION **7** Spinal Disorders

SECTION 8 Special Topics

VIDEO CONTENTS

SECTION 1

Hand and Wrist Injuries

Flexor Tendon Injuries

S. Brent Brotzman, MD | Steven R. Novotny, MD

IMPORTANT POINTS FOR REHABILITATION AFTER FLEXOR TENDON LACERATION AND REPAIR

- The goal of the tendon repair is to coapt the severed ends without bunching or leaving a gap (Fig. 1.1).
- Repaired tendons subjected to *appropriate* early motion stress will increase in strength more rapidly and develop fewer adhesions than immobilized repairs.
- Flexor rehabilitation protocols must take into account the typical tensile stresses on normally repaired flexor tendon tendons (Bezuhly et al. 2007).
  Passive motion: 500–750 g (4.9–13 N)
  Light grip: 1500–2250 g (14.7–22 N)
  Strong grip: 5000–7500 g (49–73.5 N)
  Tip pinch, index flexor digitorum profundus (FDP): 9000–13,500 g (88.2–132.3 N)
- Initially rather strong, the flexor tendon repair strength decreases significantly between days 5 and 21 (Bezuhly et al. 2007).
- The tendon is weakest during this time period because of minimal tensile strength. Strength increases quickly when controlled stress is applied in proportion to increasing tensile strength. Stressed tendons heal faster, gain strength faster, and have fewer adhesions. Tensile strength generally begins gradually increasing at 3 weeks. Generally, **blocking exercises** are initiated 1 week after active range of motion (ROM) excursion (5 weeks postoperative) (Baskies 2008).
- The **A2** and **A4** pulleys are the most important to the mechanical function of the finger. Loss of a substantial portion of either may diminish digital motion and power or lead to flexion contractures of the interphalangeal (IP) joints.
- The flexor digitorum superficialis (FDS) tendons lie on the palmar side of the FDP until they enter the A1 entrance of the digital sheath. The FDS then splits (at Champer's chiasma) and terminates into the proximal half of the middle phalanx.
- Flexor tendon excursion of as much as 9 cm is required to produce composite wrist and digital flexion. Excursion of only 2.5 cm is required for full digital flexion when the wrist is stabilized in the neutral position.
- Tendons in the hand have both intrinsic and extrinsic capabilities for healing.
- Factors that influence the formation of excursion-restricting adhesions around repaired flexor tendons include the following:
  Amount of initial trauma to the tendon and its sheath
  Tendon ischemia
  Tendon immobilization
  Gapping at the repair site
  Disruption of the vincula (blood supply), which decreases the recovery of the tendon (Fig. 1.2)
- Delayed primary repair results (within the first 10 days) are equal to or better than immediate repair of the flexor tendon.

- Immediate (primary) repair is **contraindicated** in patients with any of the following:
  Severe multiple tissue injuries to the fingers or palm
  Wound contamination
  Significant skin loss over the flexor tendons

REHABILITATION RATIONALE AND BASIC PRINCIPLES OF TREATMENT AFTER FLEXOR TENDON REPAIR

Timing

The timing of flexor tendon repair influences the rehabilitation and outcome of flexor tendon injuries.

- *Primary repair* is done within the first 12 to 24 hours after injury.
- *Delayed primary repair* is done within the first 10 days after injury.
- *If primary repair is not done, delayed primary repair should be done as soon as there is evidence of wound healing without infection.*
- *Secondary repair* is done 10 and 14 days after injury.
- *Late secondary repair* is done more than 4 weeks after injury.

After 4 weeks it is extremely difficult to deliver the flexor tendon through the digital sheath, which usually becomes extensively scarred. However, clinical situations in which the tendon repair is of secondary importance often make late repair necessary, especially for patients with massive crush injuries, inadequate soft tissue coverage, grossly contaminated or infected wounds, multiple fractures, or untreated injuries. If the sheath is not scarred or destroyed, single-stage tendon grafting, direct repair, or tendon transfer can be done. If extensive disturbance and scarring have occurred, two-stage tendon grafting with a silicone (Hunter) rod should be performed.

Before tendons can be secondarily repaired, these requirements must be met:

- Joints must be supple and have useful passive range of motion (PROM) (Boyes grade 1 or 2, Table 1.1). Restoration of PROM is aggressively obtained with rehabilitation before secondary repair is done.
- Skin coverage must be adequate.
- The surrounding tissue in which the tendon is expected to glide must be relatively free of scar tissue.
- Wound erythema and swelling must be minimal or absent.
- Fractures must have been securely fixed or healed with adequate alignment.
- Sensation in the involved digit must be undamaged or restored, or it should be possible to repair damaged nerves at the time of tendon repair directly or with nerve grafts.
- The critical A2 and A4 pulleys must be present or have been reconstructed. Secondary repair is delayed until these are reconstructed. During reconstruction, Hunter (silicone) rods are useful to maintain the lumen of the tendon sheath while the grafted pulleys are healing.

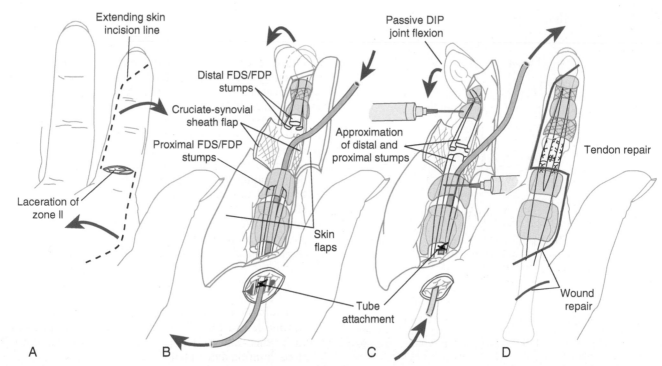

Fig. 1.1 Author's technique of flexor tendon repair in zone 2. **A,** Knife laceration through zone 2 with the digit in full flexion. The distal stumps retract distal to the skin incision with digital extension. **B,** Radial and ulnar extending incisions are used to allow wide exposure of the flexor tendon system. Note appearance of the flexor tendon system of the involved fingers after the reflection of skin flaps. The laceration occurred through the C1 cruciate area. Note the proximal and distal position of the flexor tendon stumps. Reflection of small flaps ("windows") in the cruciate-synovial sheath allows the distal flexor tendon stumps to be delivered into the wound by passive flexion of the distal interphalangeal (DIP) joint. The profundus and the superficialis stumps are retrieved proximal to the wound by passive flexion of the DIP joint. The profundus and superficialis stumps are retrieved proximal to the sheath by the use of a small catheter or infant feeding gastrostomy tube. **C,** The proximal flexor tendon stumps are maintained at the repair site by means of a transversely placed small-gauge hypodermic needle, allowing repair of the FDS slips without extension. **D,** Completed repair of both FDS and FDP tendons is shown with the DIP joint in full flexion. Extension of the DIP joint delivers the repair under the intact distal flexor tendon sheath. Wound repair is done at the conclusion of the procedure.

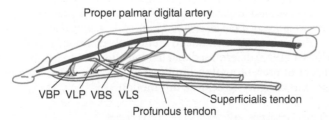

Fig. 1.2 Blood supply to the flexor tendons within the digital sheath. The segmental vascular supply to the flexor tendons is by means of the long and short vincular connections. The vinculum brevis superficialis (VBS) and the vinculum brevis profundus (VBP) consist of small triangular mesenteries near the insertion of the FDS and FDP tendons, respectively. The vinculum longum to the superficialis tendon (VLS) arises from the floor of the digital sheath of the proximal phalanx. The vinculum longum to the profundus tendon (VLP) arises from the superficialis at the level of the proximal interphalangeal (PIP) joint. The cut-away view depicts the relative avascularity of the palmar side of the flexor tendons in zones 1 and 2 as compared with the richer blood supply on the dorsal side, which connects with the vincula.

Anatomy

The anatomic zone of injury of the flexor tendons influences the outcome and rehabilitation of these injuries. The hand is divided into five distinct flexor zones (Fig. 1.3):
- *Zone 1*—from the insertion of the profundus tendon at the distal phalanx to just distal to the insertion of the sublimus
- *Zone 2*—Bunnell's "no-man's land": the critical area of pulleys between the insertion of the sublimus and the distal palmar crease

TABLE 1.1	Boyes' Preoperative Classification
Grade	**Preoperative Condition**
1	Good: minimal scar with mobile joints and no trophic changes
2	Cicatrix: heavy skin scarring from injury or previous surgery; deep scarring from failed primary repair or infection
3	Joint damage: injury to the joint with restricted range of motion
4	Nerve damage: injury to the digital nerves resulting in trophic changes in the finger
5	Multiple damage: involvement of multiple fingers with a combination of the above problems

- *Zone 3*—"area of lumbrical origin": from the beginning of the pulleys (A1) to the distal margin of the transverse carpal ligament
- *Zone 4*—area covered by the transverse carpal ligament
- *Zone 5*—area proximal to the transverse carpal ligament

As a rule, repairs to tendons injured outside the flexor sheath have much better results than repairs to tendons injured inside the sheath (zone 2).

It is essential that the A2 and A4 pulleys (Fig. 1.4) be preserved to prevent bowstringing. In the thumb, the A1 and oblique pulleys are the most important. The thumb lacks vincula for blood supply.

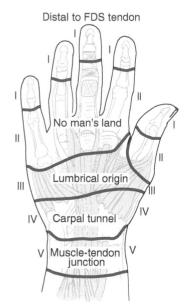

Fig. 1.3 The flexor system has been divided into five zones or levels for the purpose of discussion and treatment. Zone 2, which lies within the fibro-osseous sheath, has been called "no man's land" because it was once believed that primary repair should not be done in this zone.

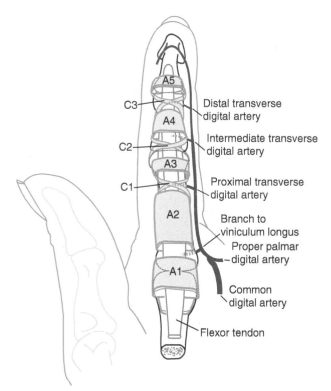

Fig. 1.4 The fibrous retinacular sheath starts at the neck of the metacarpal and ends at the distal phalanx. Condensations of the sheath form the flexor pulleys, which can be identified as five heavier annular bands and three filmy cruciform ligaments (see text).

Tendon Healing

The exact mechanism of tendon healing is still unknown. Healing probably occurs through a combination of extrinsic and intrinsic processes. *Extrinsic* healing depends on the formation of adhesions between the tendon and the surrounding tissue, providing a blood supply and fibroblasts, but unfortunately it

also prevents the tendon from gliding. *Intrinsic* healing relies on synovial fluid for nutrition and occurs only between the tendon ends.

Flexor tendons in the distal sheath have a dual source of nutrition via the vincular system and synovial diffusion. Diffusion appears to be more important than perfusion in the digital sheath (Green 1993).

Several factors have been reported to affect tendon healing:
- Age—The number of vincula (blood supply) decreases with age.
- General health—Cigarettes, caffeine, and poor general health delay healing. The patient should refrain from ingesting caffeine and smoking cigarettes during the first 4 to 6 weeks after repair.
- Scar formation—The remodeling phase is not as effective in patients who produce heavy keloid or scar.
- Motivation and compliance—Motivation and the ability to follow the postoperative rehabilitation regimen are critical factors in outcome.
- Level of injury—Zone 2 injuries are more apt to form limiting adhesions from the tendon to the surrounding tissue. In zone 4, where the flexor tendons lie in close proximity to each other, injuries tend to form tendon-to-tendon adhesions, limiting differential glide.
- Trauma and extent of injury—Crushing or blunt injuries promote more scar formation and cause more vascular trauma, impairing function and healing. Infection also impedes the healing process.
- Pulley integrity—Pulley repair is important in restoring mechanical advantage (especially A2 and A4) and maintaining tendon nutrition through synovial diffusion.
- Surgical technique—Improper handling of tissues (such as forceps marks on the tendon) and excessive postoperative hematoma formation trigger adhesion formation.

The two most frequent causes for failure of primary tendon repairs are formation of adhesions and rupture of the repaired tendon.

Through experimental and clinical observation, Duran and Houser (1975) determined that tendon glide of 3 to 5 mm is sufficient to prevent motion-limiting tendon adhesions. Exercises are thus designed to achieve this motion.

Treatment of Flexor Tendon Lacerations

Partial laceration involving ***less than 25%*** of the tendon substance can be treated by beveling the cut edges. Lacerations ***between 25% and 50%*** can be repaired with 6-0 running nylon suture in the epitenon. Lacerations involving ***more than 50%*** should be considered complete and should be repaired with a core suture and an epitenon suture.

No level 1 studies have determined superiority of one suture method or material, although a number of studies have compared different suture configurations and materials. Most studies indicate that the number of strands crossing the repair site and the number of locking loops directly affect the strength of the repair, with six- and eight-strand repairs generally shown to be stronger than four-strand or two-strand repairs; however, the increased number of strands also increases bulk and resistance to glide. Several four-strand repair techniques appear to provide adequate strength for early motion.

The following discussion is mainly for zone 2 flexor tendon lacerations. The other zones are repaired similarly, but the peculiarities of zone 2 tendon repairs will be emphasized. I still prefer a standard Brunner type incision instead of a midaxial. My exposure and opening of the tendon sheath depends on the location of its laceration and the quality of the traumatized sheath. If the laceration is through the A2 pulley, I will make controlled sheath incisions distal or proximal to the pulley. If the pulley is cut asymmetrically, I have vented the pulley for a better exposure. I prefer to work through distally based triangular openings if possible, believing the repaired sheath apex will allow enhanced gliding for the tendon anastomosis, as opposed to the transversely sutured sheath flap. Rectangular flaps for larger exposure are sometimes needed. When retrieving a tendon from the palm, I have no qualms about excising the A1 pulley for enhanced visualization. I place my core sutures approximately 1 cm from the laceration (Cao et al. 2006). The proximal core sutures are captured with a 26-gauge looped steel wire as a passer, causing minimal trauma to the native sheath.

I try not to use hypodermic needles, Keith needles, or a manufactured tendon approximator unless needed, to minimize epitendon trauma. A skilled assistant can often tension the proximal stump with traction on one set of core sutures. The core sutures should be placed dorsal as opposed to volar (Aoki et al. 1996), the running epitendon suture must have reasonable depth (Daio et al. 1996), and I repair the sheath whenever possible (Tang and Xie 2001).

Tendons lacerated sharply without need of débridement are repaired as described in Pike, Boyer and Gelberman's 2010 publication. Not surprisingly, many patients have significantly traumatized tendon edges in need of débridement. I use the ASSI Peripheral Nerve and Tendon Cutting Set (ASSI, Westbury, NY) to restore quality tendon edges. In this scenario I am more likely to use basic science principles (Zhao et al. 2002; Paillard et al. 2002; Xu and Tang 2003) and débride one slip of the superficialis tendon.

Teno Fix Repair

A stainless-steel tendon repair device (**Teno Fix,** Ortheon Medical, Columbus, OH) was reported to result in lower flexor tendon rupture rates after repair and similar functional outcomes when compared with conventional repair in a randomized, multicenter study, particularly in patients who were noncompliant with the rehabilitation protocol (Su et al. 2005, 2006). Active flexion was allowed at 4 weeks postoperatively. Solomon et al. (unpublished research) developed an "accelerated active" rehabilitation program to be used after Teno Fix repairs: Active digital flexion and extension maximum-attainable to the palm are started on the first day with the goal of full flexion at 2 weeks postoperatively. The anticipated risks with this protocol are forced passive extension, especially of the wrist and finger (e.g., fall on outstretched hand), and resisted flexion, potentially causing gapping or rupture of the repair.

The possibility of a more rapid return of function, or at least being more forgiving of rehabilitation mistakes, adds some potential attractiveness to the use of Teno Fix for flexor tendon repairs. At least one research group (Wolfe 2007) noted no benefit of using the Teno Fix system compared to the sutures techniques they used. What one doesn't know is the cost to the consumer of the product. Is the product cost worth the benefit? Kubat (2010) describes a case report with multiple tendon involvement and proposes that, at least with his patient, the savings of operative time and its associated expense may make using this product more palatable.

FDP lacerations can be repaired directly or advanced and reinserted into the distal phalanx with a pull-out wire, but they should not be advanced more than 1 cm to avoid the quadregia effect (a complication of a single digit with limited motion causing limitation of excursion and, thus, the motion of the uninvolved digits). Citing complications in 15 of 23 patients with pull-out wire (button-over-nail) repairs, 10 of which were directly related to the technique, Kang et al. (2008) questioned its continued use. Complications of the pull-out wire technique included nail deformities, fixed flexion deformities of the distal interphalangeal (DIP) joint, infection, and prolonged hypersensitivity.

A more recent technique for FDP lacerations is the use of braided polyester/monofilament polyethylene composite (Fiber-Wire, Arthrex, Naples, FL) and suture anchors rather than pull-out wires (Matsuzaki et al. 2008; McCallister et al. 2006). Reports of outcomes currently are too few to determine if this technique will allow earlier active motion than standard techniques.

Bloodless Surgery

A current topic of interest is bloodless awake surgery for more complex hand problems. I refer the reader to a recent publication by Lalonde and Martin (2013). I firmly believe in the science and employ it when appropriate. However, some patients refuse to proceed under local anesthesia. Vasculopaths, such as those with Buerger's disease, may not be appropriate candidates. Lastly, repairing extensor tendons, an easier proposition, can still be challenging when the patient involuntarily contracts muscles as the proximal tendon stump is pulled distally for repair. A posterior interosseous nerve block is easy to perform to prevent inadvertent muscle pull; a proximal median nerve block in the antecubital fossa is a little different. Gaining the skill to use an ultrasound or having an anesthesiologist perform the block if needed could be difficult.

Rehabilitation After Flexor Tendon Repair

The rehabilitation protocol chosen (Rehabilitation Protocols 1.1 and 1.2) depends on the *timing* of the repair (delayed primary or secondary), the *location* of the injury (zones 1 through 5), and the *compliance* of the patient (early mobilization for patients who are compliant and delayed mobilization for patients who are noncompliant and children younger than 7 years of age). A survey of 80 patients with flexor and extensor tendon repairs determined that **two thirds were nonadherent to their splinting regimen**, removing their splints for bathing and dressing (Sandford et al. 2008).

In a comparison of early active mobilization and standard Kleinert splintage, Yen et al. 2008 found at an average 4-month follow-up (3 to 7 months) that those in the early active mobilization group had 90% of normal grip strength, pinch, and range of motion compared to 50%, 40%, and 40%, respectively, in those with Kleinert splinting.

Sueoka and LaStayo (2008) devised an algorithm for zone 2 flexor tendon rehabilitation that uses a single clinical sign—the lag sign—to determine the progression of therapy and the need to modify existing protocols for individual patients. They defined "lag" as PROM—AROM (active ROM) ≥15 degrees and consider it a sign of tendon adherence and impairment of gliding. Rehabilitation begins with an established passive ROM Protocol (Duran), which is followed for 3.5 weeks before the presence or absence of a lag is evaluated. The presence or absence of lag is then evaluated at the patient's weekly or twice-weekly visits, and progression of therapy is modified if a lag sign is present (Rehabilitation Protocol 1.3).

REHABILITATION PROTOCOL 1.1 ■ **Rehabilitation Protocol After Immediate or Delayed Primary Repair of Flexor Tendon Injury: Modified Duran Protocol**

Marissa Pontillo, PT, DPT, SCS

Postoperative Day 1 to Week 4.5

- Keep dressing on until Day 5 postoperative.
- At Day 5: replace with light dressing and edema control prn.
- Patient is fitted with dorsal blocking splint (DBS) fashioned in:
- 20 degrees wrist flexion.
- 45 degrees MCP flexion.
- Full PIP, DIP in neutral
- Hood of splint extends to fingertips
- Controlled passive motion twice daily within constraints of splint:
  - 8 repetitions of passive flexion and active extension of the PIP joint

- Active wrist extension to neutral only
- Functional electrical stimulation (FES) with the splint on

5.5 Weeks

- Continue passive exercises.
- Discontinue use of DBS.
- Exercises are performed hourly: 12 repetitions of PIP blocking
- 12 repetitions of DIP blocking
- 12 repetitions of composite active flexion and extension
- May start PROM into flexion with overpressure

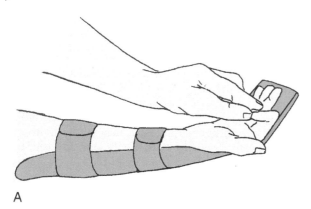 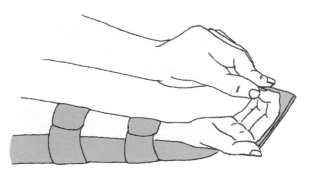

Passive flexion and extension exercises of the proximal interphalangeal (PIP) joint in a dorsal blocking splint (DBS). A, Passive flexion of PIP joint. B, The finger being extended from flexed position.

- 8 repetitions of passive flexion and active extension of the DIP joint
- 8 repetitions of active composite flexion and extension of the DIP and PIP joints with the wrist and MCP joints supported in flexion

4.5 Weeks

- Continue passive exercises as needed.
- Removal of DBS every 2 hours to perform 10 repetitions of each active flexion and extension of the wrist and of the digits
- May start intrinsic minus (hook fist) position and/or tendon gliding exercises

6 Weeks

- Initiate passive extension for the wrist and digits.

8 Weeks

- Initiate gentle strengthening.
- Putty, ball squeezes
- Towel walking with fingers
- No lifting or heavy use of the hand

10–12 Weeks

- Return to previous level of activity, including work and sport activities.

REHABILITATION PROTOCOL 1.2 ■ **Indianapolis Protocol ("Active Hold Program")**

- Indicated for patients with four-strand Tajima and horizontal mattress repair with peripheral epitendinous suture
- Patient who is motivated and compliant
- Two splints are used: the traditional dorsal blocking splint (with the wrist at 20 to 30 degrees of flexion, MCP joints in 50 degrees of flexion, and IP joints in neutral) and the Strickland tenodesis splint. The latter splint allows full wrist flexion and 30 degrees of dorsiflexion, while digits have full ROM, and MCP joints are restricted to a 60-degree extension.
- For the first 1 to 3 weeks, the modified Duran protocol is used. The patient performs repetitions of flexion and extension to the PIP and DIP joints and to the whole finger 15 times per hour. Exercise is restrained by the dorsal splint. Then, the Strickland hinged wrist splint is applied. The patient passively flexes the digits while extending the wrist. The patient then gently contracts the digits in the palm and holds for 5 seconds.

- At 4 weeks, the patient exercises 25 times every 2 hours without any splint. A dorsal blocking splint is worn between exercises until the sixth week. The digits are passively flexed while the wrist extends. Light muscle contraction is held for 5 seconds, and the wrist drops into flexion, causing digit extension through tenodesis. The patient begins active flexion and extension of the digits and wrist. Simultaneous digit and wrist extension is not allowed.
- After 5 to 14 weeks, the IP joints are flexed while the MCP joints are extended, and then the IP is extended.
- After 6 weeks, blocking exercises commence if digital flexion is more than 3 cm from the distal palmar flexion crease. No blocking is applied to the small finger FDP tendon.
- At 7 weeks, passive extension exercises are begun.
- After 8 weeks, progressive gradual strengthening is begun.
- After 14 weeks, activity is unrestricted.

(From Neumeister M, Wilhelmi BJ, Bueno Jr, RA: Flexor tendon lacerations: Treatment. http://emedicine.medscape.com/orthopedic_surgery)

REHABILITATION PROTOCOL 1.3 ● **Zone 2 Lag Sign Algorithm**

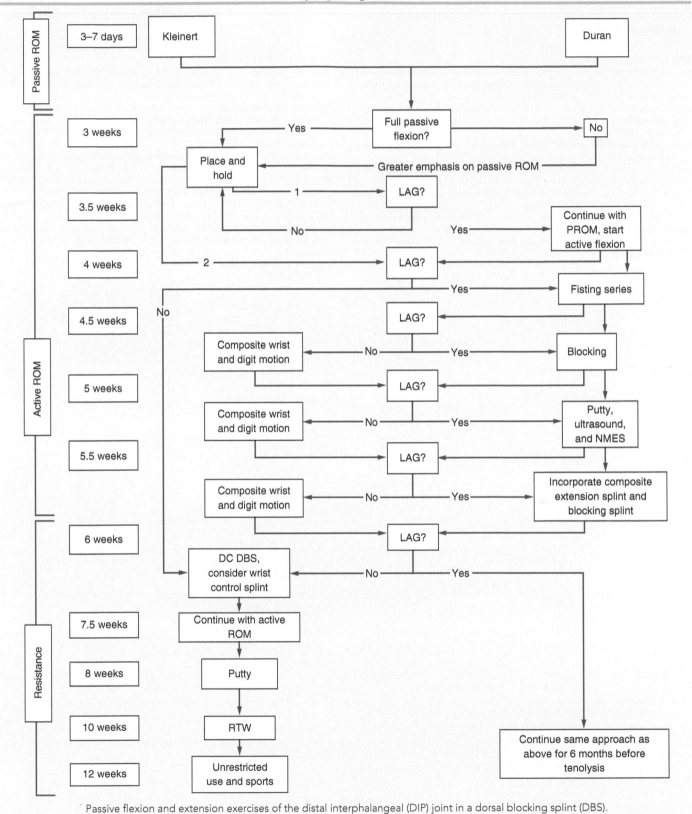

Passive flexion and extension exercises of the distal interphalangeal (DIP) joint in a dorsal blocking splint (DBS).

REFERENCES

A complete reference list is available at https://expertconsult .inkling.com/.

FURTHER READING

Amadio PC. Friction of the gliding surface. Implications for tendon surgery and rehabilitation. *J Hand Ther.* 2005;18:112–119.

Boyer MI, Goldfarb CA, Gelberman RH. Recent progress in flexor tendon healing. The modulation of tendon healing with rehabilitation variables. *J Hand Ther.* 2005;18:80–85.

Boyer MI, Strickland JW, Engles D, et al. Flexor tendon repair and rehabilitation: state of the art in 2002. *Instr Course Lect.* 2003;52:137–161.

Elliott D, Southgate CM. New concepts in managing the long tendons of the thumb after primary repair. *J Hand Ther.* 2005;18:141–156.

Evans RB. Zone I flexor tendon rehabilitation with limited extension and active flexion. *J Hand Ther.* 2005;18:128–140.

Groth GN. Clinical decision making and therapists' anatomy in the context of flexor tendon rehabilitation. *J Hand Ther.* 2008;21:254–259.

Groth GN. Current practice patterns of flexor tendon rehabilitation. *J Hand Ther.* 2005;18:169–174.

Lilly SI, Messer TM. Complications after treatment of flexor tendon injuries. *J Am Acad Orthop Surg.* 2006;14:387–396.

Pettengill KM. The evolution of early mobilization of the repaired flexor tendon. *J Hand Ther.* 2005;18:157–168.

Powell ES, Trail I. Forces transmitted along human flexor tendons—the effect of extending the fingers against the resistance provided by rubber bands. *J Hand Surg Eur.* 2009;34:186–189.

Savage R, Pritchard MG, Thomas M, et al. Differential splintage for flexor tendon rehabilitation: an experimental study of its effect on finger flexion strength. *J Hand Surg Br.* 2005;30:168–174.

Strickland JW. Development of flexor tendon surgery: twenty-five years of progress. *J Hand Surg Am.* 2000;25:214–235.

Tang JB. Clinical outcomes associated with flexor tendon repair. *Hand Clin.* 2005;21:199–210.

Tang JB. Indications, methods, postoperative motion and outcome evaluation of primary flexor tendon repairs in zone 2. *J Hand Surg Eur.* 2007;32:118–129.

Thien TB, Becker JH, Theis JC. Rehabilitation after surgery for flexor tendon injuries in the hand. *Cochrane Database Syst Rev.* 2004;(4):CD003979.

Vucekovich K, Gallardo G, Fiala K. Rehabilitation after flexor tendon repair, reconstruction, and tenolysis. *Hand Clin.* 2005;21:257–265.

Waitayawinyu T, Martineau PA, Luria S, et al. Comparative biomechanical study of flexor tendon repair using FiberWire. *J Hand Surg Am.* 2008;33:701–708.

2

Flexor Digitorum Profundus Avulsion ("Jersey Finger")

S. Brent Brotzman, MD | Steven R. Novotny, MD

BACKGROUND

Avulsion of the flexor digitorum profundus (**"jersey finger"**) can occur in any digit, but it is most common in the ring finger. This injury usually occurs when an athlete grabs an opponent's jersey and feels sudden pain as the distal phalanx of the finger is forcibly extended as it is concomitantly actively flexed (hyperextension stress applied to a flexed finger).

The resultant lack of active flexion of the DIP joint (FDP function loss) must be specifically checked to make the diagnosis (Fig. 2.1). Often the swollen finger assumes a position of extension relative to the other, more flexed fingers. The level of retraction of the FDP tendon back into the palm generally denotes the force of the avulsion.

Leddy and Packer (1977) described three types of FDP avulsions based on where the avulsed tendon retracts: type I, retraction of the FDP to the palm; type II, retraction to the proximal interphalangeal (PIP) joint; and type III, bony fragment distal to the A4 pulley. Smith's (1981) case report described a type III lesion associated with a simultaneous avulsion of the FDP from the fracture fragment. He suggested adding this pattern as a type IV, though he was not the first surgeon to comment on this anomaly. Al-Qattan (2001) reported a case series of type IV fracture with other significant concomitant distal phalanx fractures. He offers an extension of the classification to type V. As the complexity of the bony involvement increases, priorities shift to maintaining articular congruency, pilon fractures, bony mallet, and osseous stability such as shaft fractures, over early tendon excursion. This is logical and then allows extrapolation to treat such anomalies as FDP avulsions through enchondromas (Froimson and Shall 1984).

TREATMENT

The treatment of FDP avulsion is primarily surgical. The success of the treatment depends on the acuteness of diagnosis, rapidity of surgical intervention, and level of tendon retraction. Tendons with minimal retraction usually have significant attached avulsion bone fragments, which may be reattached bone-to-bone as late as 6 weeks. Tendons with a large amount of retraction often have no bone fragment and have disruption of the vascular supply (vinculum), making surgical repair more than 10 days after injury difficult because of retraction and the longer healing time of the weaker nonbone-to-bone fixation and limited blood supply to the repair. Based on a review of the literature and their clinical experience, Henry et al. (2009) listed four essentials for successful treatment of type IV extensor tendon injuries: (1) a high index of suspicion for this injury, with the use of magnetic resonance imaging (MRI) or ultrasound for confirmation if needed, (2) rigid bony fixation that prevents dorsal subluxation of the distal phalanx, (3) tendon repair that is independent of the bony fixation, and (4) early range of motion therapy (Rehabilitation Protocol 2.1).

Surgical salvage procedures for late presentation include DIP joint arthrodesis, tenodesis, and staged tendon reconstructions. Not all cases of early presentation result in tendon repair. Patient health issues may dictate a nonoperative course as being the most prudent. Patients with preexisting joint disease such as rheumatoid arthritis, osteoarthritis, and gout may be better served by a salvage procedure.

Fixation of the simple bone fragments is best achieved via lag screw fixation with appropriate-sized screws and standard AO technique. Power and Rajaratnam (2006) describe modifying an AO/Synthes modular hand plate by cutting through a hole and bending the resultant prongs to create a hook plate, thereby stabilizing the fracture.

TENDON-TO-BONE REPAIR CONSIDERATIONS

Silva et al. (1998) showed that Bunnell and Kleinert suture techniques had better load characteristics than modified Kessler using 3-0 Prolene (Ethicon, Sommerville, NJ) suture over a button. However, gapping of 8 mm occurred across suture patterns at 20 N, bringing into question the choice of suture material or number of strands. Later work demonstrated improved load to failure with more strands, yet gapping was still a problem. Brustein et al. (2001), in a cadaveric model, showed a 50% improvement in mean load to failure with a four-strand

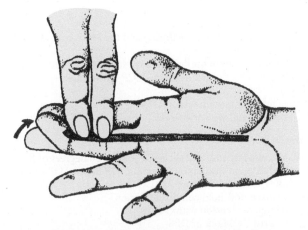

Fig. 2.1 With avulsion of the flexor digitorum profundus, the patient would be unable to flex the distal interphalangeal (DIP) joint, shown here. (From Regional Review Course in Hand Surgery. Rosemont, Illinois, American Society of Surgery of the Hand, 1991, Fig. 7).

modified Becker, two micro Mitek (Mitek Pruducts, Norwood, MA) anchor compared to monofilament Bunnell pull-out or single mini Mitek Bunnell. Boyer et al. (2002) compared 3-0 and 4-0 braided suture four-strand through bone modified Kessler and modified Becker in a load to failure model. The 3-0 modified Becker proved a significantly higher load to failure; however, the strain at 20 N load did not differ among the groups. The described models were static load to failure.

Latendresse et al. (2005) performed cyclic load testing of Prolene versus braided polyester, pull-out button extraosseous versus mini Mitek. Gap formation was 2 mm or less for the braided suture, significantly better than the monofilament groups. Load to failure was better in the extraosseous repairs, though all were greater than 20 N. Abboud et al. (2002) colinearly load tested pronged and threaded commercially available anchors in cadaveric carpal bones. They report dramatic failure of the pronged anchors compared to the threaded anchors. There are many potential confounding factors: anchor angle collinear with load, dense cortical and subchondral bone for screw purchase as opposed to cancellous, and size of the implant. This may not prove that threaded anchors will hold similarly in a distal phalanx with thinner cortex and smaller diameter. The Biomet JuggerKnot 1.4-mm suture anchor (Biomet, Warsaw, IN) reports 90 N pull-out force with a 3-0 braided suture and 115 N with a 2-0 braided suture. I have not seen cyclic loading data on this construct; however, its compact structure should be kept in mind as an option for the smaller bones.

McCallister et al. (2006) reported on clinical follow-up on 26 consecutive zone I injuries. Thirteen patients were repaired via extraosseous pull-out button and 2-0 braided polyester modified Kessler suture. The remaining 13 were repaired with 2 micro Mitek 3-0 braided polyester hemi-modified Kessler sutures tied deep to the tendon. The only significant difference between the groups was that the time to return to full-duty work was shorter in the anchor group than the pull-out suture group. Chu et al.'s (2013) cadaveric research failed to show a significant difference between standard anchor, pull-out, and a new technique of tying the suture over the distal phalanx buried proximal to the germinal matrix. This gives another option in the surgeon's arsenal, one that doesn't require further expense.

SURGEON'S PREFERENCE

I currently use mini JuggerKnot with a 3-0 braided modified Becker, two anchors side by side if bone size allows. If I feel any concern about the quality of the anchor placement or holding power, I have been adjusting to an extraosseous pull-out technique. With Chu's 2013 publication, I may consider this as my primary repair and certainly my bail-out for anchor difficulties. I only débride the tendon minimally with tenotomy scissors. I am concerned that using a tendon cutter to produce a tidy tendon end has already functionally advanced the tendon. Given Chepla et al.'s (2015) anatomic analysis of the FDP footprint and the length of many suture anchors, we may have been unintentionally advancing the tendon distally to seat the metallic anchors. Using the JuggerKnot can minimize this bias. I personally do not mind attached periosteum or frayed tendon edges because I use a 4-0 absorbable, hug the radial and ulnar distal phalanx edges, and suture the material down. I believe the scarring down of this material can only support the repair.

REHABILITATION PROTOCOL 2.1 ● **Rehabilitation Protocol After Surgical Repair of Jersey Finger With Secure Bony Repair**

S. Brent Brotzman, MD

0–10 Days

- DBS the wrist at 30 degrees flexion, the MCP joint 70 degrees flexion, and the PIP and DIP joints in full extension
- Gentle passive DIP and PIP joint flexion to 40 degrees within DBS
- Suture removal at 10 days

10 Days–3 Weeks

- Place into a removable DBS with the wrist at neutral and the MCP joint at 50 degrees of flexion.
- Gentle passive DIP joint flexion to 40 degrees, PIP joint flexion to 90 degrees within DBS
- Active MCP joint flexion to 90 degrees
- Active finger extension of IP joints within DBS, 10 repetitions per hour

3–5 Weeks

- Discontinue DBS (5–6 weeks).
- Active/assisted MCP/PIP/DIP joint ROM exercises
- Begin place-and-hold exercises.

5 Weeks +

- Strengthening/power grasping
- Progress activities
- Begin tendon gliding exercises.
- Continue PROM, scar massage.
- Begin active wrist flexion/extension.
- Composite fist and flex wrist, then extend wrist and fingers

With Purely Tendinous Repair or Poor Bony Repair (Weaker Surgical Construct)

0–10 Days

- DBS the wrist at 30 degrees flexion and the MCP joint at 70 degrees flexion
- Gentle passive DIP and PIP joint flexion to 40 degrees within DBS
- Suture removal at 10 days

10 Days–4 Weeks

- DBS the wrist at 30 degrees flexion and the MCP joint at 70 degrees flexion
- Gentle passive DIP joint flexion to 40 degrees, PIP joint flexion to 90 degrees within DBS, passive MCP joint flexion to 90 degrees
- Active finger extension within DBS
- Remove pull-out wire at 4 weeks.

4–6 Weeks

- DBS the wrist neutral and the MCP joint at 50 degrees of flexion
- Passive DIP joint flexion to 60 degrees, PIP joint to 110 degrees, and MCP joint to 90 degrees
- Gentle place-and-hold composite flexion
- Active finger extension within DBS
- Active wrist ROM out of DBS

6–8 Weeks

- Discontinue daytime splinting; night splinting only
- Active MCP/PIP/DIP joint flexion and full extension

REHABILITATION PROTOCOL 2.1 ■ **Rehabilitation Protocol After Surgical Repair of Jersey Finger With Secure Bony Repair—cont'd**

8–10 Weeks	*10 Weeks +*
• Discontinue night splinting.	• More aggressive ROM
• Assisted MCP/PIP/DIP joint ROM	• Strengthening/power grasping
• Gentle strengthening	• Unrestricted activities

REFERENCES

A complete reference list is available at https://expertconsult.inkling.com/.

FURTHER READING

Chepla K, Goitz R, Fowler J. Anatomy of the flexor digitorum profundus insertion. *J Hand Surg Am*. 2015;40:240–244.

Extensor Tendon Injuries

S. Brent Brotzman, MD | Theresa M. Kidd, BA

ANATOMY

Extensor mechanism injuries are grouped into eight anatomic zones, according to Kleinert and Verdan (1983). Odd-number zones overlie the joint levels so that zones 1, 3, 5, and 7 correspond to the DIP, PIP, metacarpal phalangeal (MCP), and wrist joint regions, respectively (Figs. 3.1 and 3.2; Table 3.1).

Normal extensor mechanism activity relies on concerted function between the intrinsic muscles of the hand and the extrinsic extensor tendons. Although PIP and DIP joint extension is normally controlled by the intrinsic muscles of the hand (interossei and lumbricals), the extrinsic tendons may provide satisfactory digital extension when MCP joint hyperextension is prevented.

An injury at one zone typically produces compensatory imbalance in neighboring zones; for example, a mallet finger deformity at the DIP joint may be accompanied by a more striking secondary swan-neck deformity at the PIP joint.

Disruption of the terminal slip of the extensor tendon allows the extensor mechanism to migrate proximally and exert a hyperextension force to the PIP joint by the central slip attachment. Thus, extensor tendon injuries cannot be considered simply static disorders.

EXTENSOR TENDON INJURIES IN ZONES 1 AND 2

Extensor tendon injuries in zones 1 and 2 **in children** should be considered Salter-Harris type II or III physeal injuries. Splinting of extremely small digits is difficult, and fixing the joint in full extension for 4 weeks produces satisfactory results. Open injuries are especially difficult to splint, and the DIP joint may be transarticularly fixed with a 22-gauge needle in the emergency department or K-wire in surgery (see Mallet Finger section). A study of 53 extensor tendon injuries in children, all of which were treated with primary repair within 24 hours of injury, reported that 98% had good or excellent results, although 22% had extension lag or loss of flexion at latest follow-up (Fitoussi et al. 2007). Factors predictive of a less successful outcome were injuries in zones 1, 2, and 3; age younger than 5 years; and complete tendon laceration.

A literature review by Soni et al. (2009) found that traditional postoperative static splinting was equivalent to early motion protocols for all uncomplicated thumb injuries and zone 1 to 3 injuries of the second through fifth digits. The only benefit of early motion therapy compared with static splinting was a quicker return to final function for proximal zones of injury in the second through fifth digits. At 6 months after surgery, results of static splinting were comparable to those with early active and passive motion (Saldana 1990, Evans 1990). Static splinting also was associated with a lower rupture rate than early active

motion and a lower cost than early active and passive motion. An earlier meta-analysis (Talsma et al. 2008) found that short-term outcomes (4 weeks postoperative) after immobilization were significantly inferior to outcomes after early controlled mobilization, but at 3 months postoperatively no significant differences were found (Rehabilitation Protocol 3.1).

EXTENSOR TENDON INJURIES IN ZONE 3

These acute closed injuries are treated similarly to zone 1 injury, with full-time extension splinting for 6 weeks, then active motion with nighttime splinting for 6 more weeks. The proximal interphalangeal joint (PIP) is extended and the distal interphalangeal joint (DIP) is left free. The important anatomic difference lies with the lateral bands. It is important to work on passive or active-assisted DIP joint flexion, which keeps the lateral bands mobile and dorsal to the axis of rotation of the PIP. Occasionally, splinting for 3 months is required before considering it a treatment failure. If the injury is open, reattachment of the central slip via bone anchor is the simplest treatment. Retrograde oblique transarticular pinning volar to the lateral bands for 4 weeks protects the repair. The DIP joint is ranged as for a closed injury. It is important that the triangular ligament be repaired if injured, helping to prevent lateral band subluxation in the recovery phase.

Chronic boutonnière injuries within months of original injury still can be treated conservatively. These patients require close follow-up and guidance. The PIP joint needs to be fully extended before it can be treated. It is common to employ wire foam extension splints or joint jacks to accomplish this. The program then resorts to a standard closed treatment program. Various surgical techniques for correction have been described. None have produced perfect results. Having an understanding of multiple techniques, anatomy at the time of surgery, and surgeons' individual strengths may allow individual treatment or an ease of changing plans on the fly.

Matev (1964) step cut the lateral bands over the middle phalanx, fed the shorter limb through the central slip stump, and attached it to the tissue middle phalanx base. Litter and Eaton (1967) transected the lateral bands distally and attached them to the middle phalanx base. The lumbrical tendon was left to its attachment to the distal phalanx for extension. Urbaniak and Hayes (1981) lifted the triangular ligament in a proximally based flap, careful to preserve the capsule. The central capsular slip was left attached on the middle phalanx base and sutured through the central slip, then repairing the triangular ligament. Ohshio et al. (1990) removed the transverse ligaments off the volar plate and sutured them over the PIP joint. The lateral bands are more dorsal and can still move. Snow (1976) used a central slip of the extensor tendon as a turn-down flap

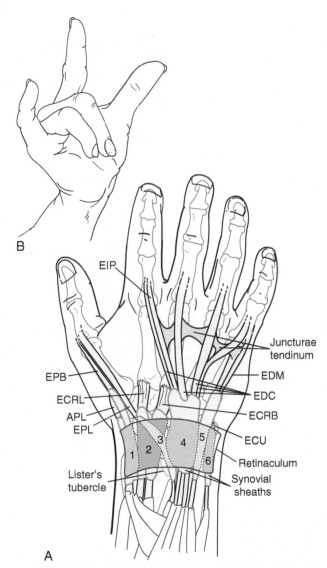

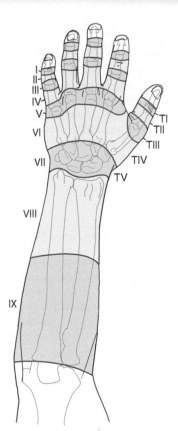

Fig. 3.2 Extensor tendon zones of injury as described by Kleinart and Verdan and by Doyle.

Fig. 3.1 A, The extensor tendons gain entrance to the hand from the forearm through the series of six canals, five fibro-osseous and one fibrous (the fifth dorsal compartment, which contains the extensor digiti minimi [EDM]). The first compartment contains the abductor pollicis longus (APL) and extensor pollicis brevis (EPB); the second, the radial wrist extensors; the third, the extensor pollicis longus (EPL), which angles around Lister's tubercle; the fourth, the extensor digitorum communis (EDC) to the fingers and the extensor indicis proprius (EIP); the fifth, the EDM; and the sixth, the extensor carpi ulnaris (ECU). The communis tendons are joined distally near the MR (metacarpophalangeal) joints by fibrous interconnections called juncturae tendinum. These juncturae are found only between the communis tendons and may aid in surgical recognition of the proprius tendon of the index finger. The proprius tendons are usually positioned to the ulnar side of the adjacent communis tendons, but variations may be present that alter this arrangement (see text). Beneath the retinaculum, the extensor tendons are covered with a synovial sheath. B, The proprius tendons to the index and little fingers are capable of independent extension, and their function may be evaluated as depicted. With the middle and ring fingers flexed into the palm, the proprius tendons can extend the little and ring fingers. Independent extension of the index finger, however, is not always lost after transfer of the indicis proprius and is less likely to be lost if the extensor hood is not injured and is probably never lost if the hood is preserved and the juncturae tendinum between the index and middle fingers is excised (see text). This figure represents the usual anatomic arrangement found over the wrist and hand, but variations are common, and the reader is referred to the section on Anatomic Variations. *ECRB*, extensor carpi radialis brevis; *ECRL*, extensor carpi radialis longus.

Zone	Finger	Thumb
I	Distal interphalangeal joint	Interphalangeal joint
II	Middle phalanx	Proximal phalanx
III	Proximal interphalangeal joint	Metacarpophalangeal joint
IV	Proximal phalanx	Metacarpal
V	MP joint	Carpometacarpal joint/radial styloid
VI	Metacarpal	
VII	Dorsal retinaculum	
VIII	Distal forearm	
IX	Mid and proximal forearm	

to graft across the defect. Ahmad and Pickford (2009) used a slip of the FDS through a drill hole exiting dorsally, weaving this into the central tendon stump as a case report, with encouraging results. Li et al. (2014) published a comparison of free grafting versus turn-down flap showing turn-down flap to be superior to free grafting. There are undoubtedly many other unique repair patterns or combinations that may work. Individual surgical experience may dictate ultimate technique choice.

EXTENSOR TENDON INJURIES IN ZONES 4, 5, AND 6

Normal function is usually possible after unilateral injuries to the dorsal apparatus, and splinting and immobilization are not recommended. Complete disruptions of the dorsal expansion and central slip lacerations are repaired (Rehabilitation Protocol 3.2). Tendon repair technique depends on the geometry of the tendon. If flatter and unable to accept core sutures, multiple nonabsorbable figure-of-eight sutures with knots placed subtendinous are utilized. If the tendon accepts core sutures with epitendinous running sutures, repair is the same as a flexor tendon.

Zone 5 Extensor Tendon Subluxations

Zone 5 extensor tendon subluxations rarely respond to a splinting program. The affected MCP joint can be splinted in full extension and radial deviation for 4 weeks, with the understanding that surgical intervention will probably be required. Painful popping and swelling, in addition to a problematic extensor lag with radial deviation of the involved digit, usually require reconstruction.

Acute closed radial sagittal band injuries if treated conservatively within three weeks of injury produce satisfactory results. Rayan and Murry (1994) reported on 28 nonrheumatoid patients classified into injury without instability (Type I), injury with subluxation (Type II), and injury with dislocation (Type III). Good results were obtained if conservative treatment was initiated by three weeks post injury. In a biomechanical study out of the same group, Young and Rayan (2000) showed that with ulnar sagittal band disruption the tendon was not unstable. The serial sectioning of the radial sagittal band showed proximal disruption produced subluxation, distal disruption showed no instability, and complete disruption caused dislocation. Wrist flexion exacerbated further destabilizing forces on the tendon. A 2006 retrospective study (Catalano et al. 2006) with a hand-based sling splint keeping the injured digit extended at the MCP relative to its neighbors and immediate active interphalangeal joint motion had 7 of 10 patients with good or excellent results (8 of 11 sagittal band disruptions). Three patients had moderate subluxation with the treatment and one underwent surgical repair.

Acute open injuries should be repaired directly, and chronic symptomatic injuries can be reconstructed with local tissue. Most reconstructive procedures use portions of the juncturae tendinum (ElMaraghy and Pennings 2013) *or extensor tendon slips (Watson et al. 1997) anchored to the deep transverse metacarpal ligament or looped around the lumbrical tendon (Rehabilitation Protocol 3.3).* Kang and Carlson (2010) reported a centralization technique with a tendon graft through a bone tunnel in the metacarpal neck looped around the extensor tendon. The drill holes are asymetric in that the ulnar bone hole is just ulnar to the extensor tendon and buttresses the ulnarly directed subluxation forces, and the radial hole is more radial and slightly volar. This contruct may allow earlier mobilization more aggressively.

EXTENSOR TENDON INJURIES IN ZONES 7 AND 8

Extensor tendon injuries in zones 7 and 8 are usually from lacerations, but attritional ruptures secondary to remote distal radial fractures and rheumatoid synovitis may occur at the wrist level. These may require tendon transfers, free tendon grafts, or side-by-side transfers rather than direct repair. The splinting program for these, however, is identical to that for penetrating trauma.

Repairs done 3 weeks or more after the injury may weaken the extensor pollicis longus (EPL) muscle sufficiently for electrical stimulation to become necessary for tendon glide. The EPL is selectively strengthened by thumb retropulsion exercises done against resistance with the palm held on a flat surface (Rehabilitation Protocol 3.4).

Extensor Tenolysis

Indications

- Digital active or passive motion has reached a plateau after injury
- Restricted, isolated, or composite active or passive flexion of the PIP or DIP joint
- Otherwise passively supple digit that exhibits an extensor lag (Fig. 3.3)

Surgical intervention for extension contractures frequently follows an extensive period of presurgical therapy. Patients who have been active in their rehabilitation are more apt to appreciate that an early postsurgical program is vital to their final outcome. Presurgical patient counseling should always be attempted to delineate and establish the patient's responsibility in the immediate postsurgical tenolysis program.

The quality of the extensor tendon, bone, and joint encountered at surgery may alter the intended program, and the

TABLE 3.1	Zones of Extensor Mechanism Injury	
Zone	**Finger**	**Thumb**
1	DIP joint	IP joint
2	Middle phalanx	Proximal phalanx
3	Apex PIP joint	MCP joint
4	Proximal phalanx	Metacarpal
5	Apex MCP joint	—
6	Dorsal hand	—
7	Dorsal retinaculum	Dorsal retinaculum
8	Distal forearm	Distal forearm

DIP, distal interphalangeal; IP, interphalangeal; PIP, proximal interphalangeal; MCP, metacarpophalangeal.
From Kleinert HE, Verdan C. Report of the committee on tendon injuries. J Hand Surg 1983;8:794.

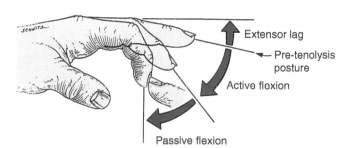

Fig. 3.3 Passive supple digit with an extensor lag is an indication for possible extensor tenolysis. (From Strickland JW: The Hand: Master Techniques in Orthopaedic Surgery. Philadelphia, Lippincott-Raven, 1998.)

surgeon relays this information to the therapist and the patient. Ideally, the surgical procedures are done with the patient under local anesthesia or awakened from the general anesthesia near the end of the procedure to allow active digit movement by the patient at the surgeon's request. The patient can then see the gains achieved, and the surgeon can evaluate active motion, tendon glide, and the need for additional releases. Unusual circumstances may be well served by having the therapist observe the operative procedure.

Frequently, MCP and PIP joint capsular and ligament releases are necessary to obtain the desired joint motion. Complete collateral ligament resection may be required, and special attention may be necessary in the early postoperative period for resultant instability. Extensive tenolyses may require analgesic dosing before and during therapy sessions. Indwelling catheters also may be needed for instillation of local anesthetics for this purpose (Rehabilitation Protocol 3.5).

MALLET FINGER (EXTENSOR INJURY—ZONE 1)
Background

Avulsion of the extensor tendon from its distal insertion at the dorsum of the DIP joint produces an **extensor lag** at the DIP joint. The avulsion may occur with or without a bony fragment avulsion from the dorsum of the distal phalanx. **This is termed a mallet finger of bony origin or mallet finger of tendinous origin** (Fig. 3.4). The hallmark finding of a mallet finger is a

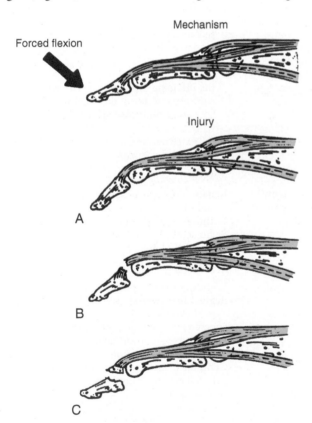

Fig. 3.4 **A,** Stretching of the common extensor mechanism. **B,** Mallet finger of tendinous origin (complete disruption of the extensor tendon). **C,** Mallet finger of bony origin. (From Delee J, Drez D [eds]: Orthopaedic Sports Medicine. Philadelphia, WB Saunders, 1994, p. 1011.)

flexed or dropped posture of the DIP joint and an inability to actively extend or straighten the DIP joint. The mechanism is typically forced flexion of the fingertip, often from the impact of a thrown ball, though a surprising number of patients have innocuous histories such as cleaning a spot off fabric and reaching between cushions on a couch.

Classification of Mallet Finger

Doyle (1993) described four types of mallet injury:
- Type I—extensor tendon avulsion from the distal phalanx
- Type II—laceration of the extensor tendon
- Type III—deep avulsion injuring the skin and tendon
- Type IV—fracture of the distal phalanx with three subtypes:
    Type IV A—transepiphyseal fracture in a child
    Type IV B—less than half of the articular surface of the joint involved with no subluxation
    Type IV C—more than half of the articular surface involved and may involve volar subluxation

Treatment

Abound and Brown (1968) found that several factors are likely to lead to a **poor prognosis** after mallet finger injury:
- Age older than 60 years
- Delay in treatment of more than 4 weeks
- Initial extensor lag of more than 50 degrees
- Too short a period of immobilization (<4 weeks)
- Short, stubby fingers
- Peripheral vascular disease or associated arthritis

No treatment regimen exists that guarantees a return to preinjury status. When the choices are to treat or not treat, or to open or to not open, good results are generally obtained by following certain principles.

Continuous extension splinting of the DIP joint, leaving the PIP free for 6 to 10 weeks, is the typical treatment for mallet fingers of **tendinous origin** (Fig. 3.5). A variety of splints has been developed for treatment of mallet finger. Most commonly used are the Stack splint, the perforated thermoplastic splint,

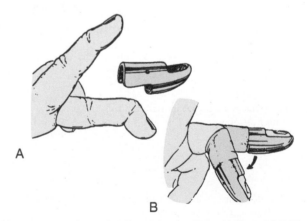

Fig. 3.5 **A,** Use of a stack splint at the distal interphalangeal (DIP) joint for closed treatment of mallet finger (note extension lag). The splint is held in place with paper or adhesive tape. **B,** Active range of motion exercises of the proximal interphalangeal (PIP) joint used to keep the joint from stiffening during DIP joint immobilization. (A and B, From Regional Review Course in Hand Surgery. Memphis, American Society of Surgery of the Hand, 1991, Fig. 13.)

and the aluminum-foam splint for 6 weeks. If the joint lags at this time, another 4 weeks of continuous extension splinting is recommended. If **no extensor lag exists at 6 weeks the splint is discontinued during the day and range of motion is started. Night splinting for 6 weeks is continued and splinting during sports activities or heavy labor for an additional 6 weeks is recommended.** My patients are advised that if the splint comes off and the finger droops they should record that day. On the next visit we will adjust our splint starting date to correspond to this mishap date. I evaluate compliance in my patients at 2 weeks of splinting. If an alternative program appears to be better for the patient, a change can be made early in the treatment process instead of 6 to 10 weeks down the road. Transarticular pinning is the most common secondary treatment.

The patient must work on active ROM of the MCP and PIP joints to avoid stiffening of these uninvolved joints. At no point during the healing process is the DIP joint allowed to drop into flexion or the treatment must be repeated from the beginning. During skin care or washing, the finger must be held continuously in extension with the other hand while the splint is off.

Although splinting is the treatment of choice for most acute and chronic mallet finger injuries, surgery may be indicated for individuals who are unable to comply with a splinting regimen or for patients who would have difficulty performing their jobs with an external splint. Surgical options for acute mallet fractures include transarticular pinning of the DIP joint, compression pinning, and extension block pinning for mallet fractures. For chronic tendinous injuries (more than 4 weeks after injury) a trial of conservative care should be instituted because similar results with acute treatment have been obtained after an 8-week average delay in treatment (Garberman et al. 1994). Compliance is always of concern. Facca et al. (2007) use a splint temporarily glued to the nail plate. Their large series and good results provide validity to their concept. Surgical options include terminal extensor tendon shortening, tenodermodesis, reconstruction of the oblique retinacular ligament, and central slip tenotomy (see Rehabilitation Protocol 3.1). Arthrodesis may be required as a salvage procedure for mallet fingers caused by arthritis, infection, or failed surgery.

REHABILITATION PROTOCOL 3.1 ● Treatment and Rehabilitation of Chronic Extensor Tendon Injuries in Zones 1 and 2

Tenodermodesis	Central Slip Tenotomy (Fowler)	Oblique Retinacular Ligament Reconstruction
Tenodermodesis is a simple procedure used in relatively young patients who are unable to accept the mallet finger disability. With the use of a local anesthetic, the DIP joint is fully extended and the redundant pseudotendon is excised so that the edges of the tendon coapt. A Kirschner wire may be used temporarily to fix the DIP joint in full extension.	With the use of a local anesthetic, the insertion of the central slip is sectioned where it blends with the PIP joint dorsal capsule. The combined lateral band and the extrinsic contribution should be left undisturbed. Proximal migration of the dorsal apparatus improves the extensor force at the DIP joint. A 10- to 15-degree extensor lag at the PIP joint may occur.	Reconstruction of the oblique retinacular ligament is done for correction of a chronic mallet finger deformity and secondary swan-neck deformity. A free tendon graft, such as the palmaris longus tendon, is passed from the dorsal base of the distal phalanx and volar to the axis of the PIP joint. The graft is anchored to the contralateral side of the proximal phalanx at the fibro-osseous rim. Kirschner wires temporarily fix the DIP joint in full extension and the PIP joint in 10 to 15 degrees of flexion.
3–5 Days	**0–2 Weeks**	**3 Weeks**
Remove the postoperative splint and fit the DIP joint with an extension splint. A pin protection splint may be necessary if the pin is left exposed; however, some patients have their pins buried to allow unsplinted use of the finger. PIP joint exercises are begun to maintain full PIP joint motion.	The postoperative dressing maintains the PIP joint at 45 degrees of flexion and the DIP joint at 0 degrees.	Remove the bulky postoperative dressing and sutures. Withdraw the PIP joint pin. Begin active flexion and extension exercises of the PIP joint.
	2–4 Weeks	**4–5 Weeks**
	Allow active DIP joint extension and flexion. Allow full extension of the PIP joint from 45 degrees of flexion.	Withdraw the DIP joint K-wire. Begin full active and passive PIP and DIP joint exercises. Supplement home exercises with a supervised program over the next 2 to 3 weeks to achieve full motion. Continue internal splinting of the DIP joint in full extension until 6 weeks after the operation.
5 Weeks	**4 Weeks**	
Remove the Kirschner wire and begin active DIP motion with interval splinting. Continue nightly splinting for an additional 3 weeks.	Begin full finger motion exercises.	

REHABILITATION PROTOCOL 3.2 ■ After Surgical Repair of Extensor Tendon Injuries in Zones 4, 5, and 6

0–2 Weeks

- Allow active and passive PIP joint exercises, and keep the MCP joint in full extension and the wrist in 40 degrees of extension.

2 Weeks

- Remove the sutures and fit the patient with a removable splint.
- Keep the MCP joints in full extension and the wrist in neutral position.
- Continue PIP joint exercises and remove the splint for scar massage and hygienic purposes only.

4–6 Weeks

- Begin MCP and wrist joint active flexion exercises with interval and night splinting with the wrist in neutral position.
- Over the next 2 weeks, begin active-assisted and gentle passive flexion exercises.

6 Weeks

- Discontinue splinting unless an extensor lag develops at the MCP joint.
- Use passive wrist flexion exercises as necessary.

REHABILITATION PROTOCOL 3.3 ■ After Surgical Repair of Zone 5 Extensor Tendon Subluxation

2 Weeks

- Remove the postoperative dressing and sutures.
- Keep the MCP joints in full extension.
- Fashion a removable volar short arm splint to maintain the operated finger MCP joint in full extension and radial deviation.
- Allow periodic splint removal for hygienic purposes and scar massage.
- Allow full PIP and DIP joint motion.

4 Weeks

- Begin MCP joint active and active-assisted exercises hourly with interval daily and full-time night splinting.
- At week 5, begin gentle passive MCP joint motion if necessary to gain full MCP joint flexion.

6 Weeks

- Discontinue splinting during the day and allow full activity.

REHABILITATION PROTOCOL 3.4 ■ After Surgical Repair of Extensor Tendon Injuries in Zones 7 and 8

0–2 Weeks

- Maintain the wrist in 30 to 40 degrees of extension with postoperative splint.
- Encourage hand elevation and full PIP and DIP joint motion to reduce swelling and edema.
- Treat any significant swelling by loosening the dressing and elevating the extremity.

2–4 Weeks

- At 2 weeks remove the postoperative dressing and sutures.
- Fashion a volar splint to keep the wrist in 20 degrees of extension and the MCP joints of the affected finger(s) in full extension.
- Continue full PIP and DIP joint motion exercises and initiate scar massage to improve skin-tendon glide during the next 2 weeks.

4–6 Weeks

- Begin hourly wrist and MCP joint exercises, with interval and nightly splinting over the next 2 weeks.
- From week 4 to 5, hold the wrist in extension during the MCP joint flexion exercises and extend the MCP joints during the wrist flexion exercises.
- Composite wrist and finger flexion from the fifth week forward. An MCP joint extension lag of more than 10 to 20 degrees requires interval daily splinting.
- Splinting program can be discontinued at 6 weeks.

6–7 Weeks

- Begin gentle passive ROM.
- Begin resistive extension exercises.

REHABILITATION PROTOCOL 3.5 ■ After Extensor Tenolysis

0–24 Hours

- Apply a light compressive postoperative dressing to allow as much digital motion as possible. Anticipate bleeding through the dressing, and implement exercises hourly in 10-minute sessions to achieve as much of the motion noted intraoperatively as possible.

1 Day–4 Weeks

- Remove the surgical dressings and drains at the first therapy visit. Apply light compressive sterile dressings.
- Edema control measures are critical at this stage.
- Continue active and passive ROM exercises hourly for 10- to 15-minute sessions. Poor IP joint flexion during the first session is an indication for flexor FES. Extensor FES should be used initially with the wrist, MCP, PIP, and DIP joints passively extended to promote maximal proximal tendon excursion. After several stimulations in this position, place the wrist, MCP, and PIP joints into more flexion and continue FES.
- Remove the sutures at 2 weeks; dynamic flexion splints and taping may be required.
- Use splints to keep the joint in question in full extension between exercises and at night for the first 4 weeks. Extensor lags of 5 to 10 degrees are acceptable and are not indications to continue splint wear after this period.

4–6 Weeks

- Continue hourly exercise sessions during the day for 10-minute sessions. Emphasis is on achieving MCP and IP joint flexion.

Continued

REHABILITATION PROTOCOL 3.5 ▪ After Extensor Tenolysis—cont'd

- Continue passive motion with greater emphasis during this period, especially for the MCP and IP joints.
- Continue extension night splinting until the sixth week.

6 Weeks

- Encourage the patient to resume normal activity.
- Edema control measures may be required. Intermittent Coban wrapping of the digits may be useful in conjunction with an oral inflammatory agent.
- Banana splints (foam cylindrical digital sheaths) also can be effective for edema control.

The therapist must have acquired some critical information regarding the patient's tenolysis. Specific therapeutic program and anticipated outcomes depend on the following:

- The quality of the tendon(s) undergoing tenolysis.
- The condition of the joint the tendon acts about.
- The stability of the joint the tendon acts about.
- The joint motions achieved during the surgical procedure. Passive motions are easily obtained; however, active motions in both extension and flexion are even more beneficial to guiding patient therapy goals.

Achieving maximal MCP and PIP joint flexion during the first 3 weeks is essential. Significant gains after this period are uncommon.

REFERENCES

A complete reference list is available at https://expertconsult.inkling.com/.

FURTHER READING

Mallet Finger

Bendre AA, Hartigan BJ, Kalainov DM. Mallet finger. *J Am Acad Orthop Surg.* 2005;13:336–344.

Bowers WH, Hurst LC. Chronic mallet finger: the use of Fowler's central slip release. *J Hand Surg.* 1978;3:373.

Crosby CA, Wehbé MA. Early protected motion after extensor tendon repair. *J Hand Surg Am.* 1999;24:1061–1070.

Geyman JP, Fink K, Sullivan SD. Conservative versus surgical treatment of mallet finger: a pooled quantitative literature evaluation. *J Am Board Fam Pract.* 1998;11:382–390.

Handoll HH, Vaghela MV. Interventions for treating mallet finger injuries. *Cochrane Database Syst Rev.* 2004;3:CD004574.

Kalainov DM, Hoepfner PE, Hartigan BJ, et al. Nonsurgical treatment of closed mallet finger fractures. *J Hand Surg Am.* 2005;30:580–586.

Kardestuncer T, Bae DS, Waters PM. The results of tenodermodesis for severe chronic mallet finger deformity in children. *J Pediatr Orthop.* 2008;28:81–85.

King HJ, Shin SJ, Kang ES. Complications of operative treatment for mallet fractures of the distal phalanx. *J Hand Surg Br.* 2001;26:28–31.

Peterson JJ, Bancroft LW. Injuries of the fingers and thumb in the athlete. *Clin Sports Med.* 2006;25:527–542.

Simpson D, McQueen MM, Kumar P. Mallet deformity in sport. *J Hand Surg Br.* 2001;26:32–33.

Sorene ED, Goodwin DR. Tenodermodesis for established mallet finger deformity. *Scand J Plast Reconstr Surg Hand Surg.* 2004;38:43–45.

Stark HH, Gainor BJ, Ashworth CR, et al. Operative treatment of intraarticular fractures of the dorsal aspect of the distal phalanx of digits. *J Bone Joint Surg.* 1987;69A:892.

Stern PJ, Kastrup JJ. Complications and prognosis of treatment of mallet finger. *J Hand Surg.* 1988;13A:329.

Tuttle HG, Olvey SP, Stern PJ. Tendon avulsion injuries of the distal phalanx. *Clin Orthop Rel Res.* 2006;445:157–168.

Wehbe MA, Schneider LH. Mallet fractures. *J Bone Joint Surg.* 1984;66A:658.

Wood VE. Fractures of the hand in children. *Orthop Clin North Am.* 1976;7:527.

Boutonnière Deformity

Lin JD, Strauch RJ. Closed soft tissue extensor mechanism injuries (mallet, boutonniere, and sagittal band). *J Hand Surg Am.* 2014;39:1005–1011.

Matson JL, Bozentka DJ. Extensor tendon injuries. *J Hand Surg Am.* 2010;35:854–861.

To P, Watson JT. Boutonniere deformity. *J Hand Surg Am.* 2011;36:139–141.

Fractures and Dislocations of the Hand

Maureen A. Hardy, PT, MS, CHT | S. Brent Brotzman, MD | Steven R. Novotny, MD

Fractures and dislocations involving the hand are classified as stable or unstable injuries to determine the appropriate treatment. *Stable* fractures are those that would not displace if some degree of early digital motion were allowed. *Unstable* fractures are those that displace to an unacceptable degree if early digital motion is allowed. Although some unstable fractures can be converted to stable fractures with closed reduction, it is difficult to predict which of these will maintain their stability throughout the early treatment phase. *For this reason, most unstable fractures should undergo closed reduction and percutaneous pinning or open reduction internal fixation (ORIF) to allow early protected digital motion and thus prevent stiffness.*

Fractures that often require surgical intervention include the following:

- Open fractures
- Comminuted displaced fractures
- Fractures associated with joint dislocation or subluxation
- Displaced or angulated or malrotated spiral fractures
- Displaced intra-articular fractures, especially around the PIP joint
- Fractures in which there is loss of bone
- Multiple fractures

Because of the hand's propensity to quickly form a permanently stiffening scar, unstable fractures must be surgically converted to stable fractures (e.g., pinning) to allow early ROM exercises. Failure to use early ROM will result in a stiff hand with poor function regardless of radiographic bony healing.

METACARPAL AND PHALANGEAL FRACTURES

General Principles

- General rehabilitation principles for hand fractures include early active ROM and tendon gliding using synergistic wrist positions and blocking techniques, including blocking splints.
- **Radiographic evidence of healing in hand fractures almost always lags behind clinical healing.** At 6 weeks, with a nontender clinically healed fracture the radiograph typically still shows the original fracture line. The clinician must go by clinical examination (presence or absence of point tenderness) when making treatment decisions.
- Most metacarpal and phalangeal fractures can be treated nonoperatively using closed methods that emphasize alignment and early protected motion.
- All splinting programs for metacarpal or phalangeal fractures recognize the need to position the metacarpophalangeal joints in flexion to avoid extension contractures.

- The thumb metacarpophalangeal is not exempt from this rule, and many stiff thumbs result from hyperextended thumb spica immobilization.
- The interphalangeal joints typically are rested in full extension.
- Greer's principles of splinting (REDUCE) should be incorporated in casting or splinting of these fractures.
  R: Reduction of the fracture is maintained.
  E: Eliminate contractures through proper positioning.
  D: Don't immobilize any of these fractures for more than 3 weeks.
  U: Uninvolved joint should not be splinted in stable fractures.
  C: Creases of the skin should not be obstructed by the splint.
  E: Early active tendon gliding is encouraged. Edema is poorly tolerated by the hand. RICE (rest, ice, compression, elevation) is emphasized for edema control. Distended, edematous joints predictably move into positions that permit the greatest expansion of the joint capsule and collateral ligaments. Edema postures the hand into wrist flexion, metacarpophalangeal joint extension, interphalangeal joint flexion, and thumb adduction: a "dropped claw hand." Functional splinting seeks to place the hand in a position that avoids this deformed posturing.
- The most important tendon gliding exercises (Fig. 4.1) to initiate early rehab are for the flexor digitorum superficialis (FDS), FDP, extensor digitorum communis (EDC), and central slip to prevent tendon adherence to fracture callus.

METACARPAL FRACTURES

- The metacarpals typically have a good blood supply, with rapid healing at 6 weeks.
- As a result of the volar pull of the interosseous muscles, the bone in a metacarpal neck or shaft fracture will tend to angulate with the fracture apex directed dorsally (i.e., the distal fragment is volar).
- The most important rehabilitation considerations with metacarpal fracture are preservation of metacarpophalangeal joint flexion and maintenance of EDC glide.
- Table 4.1 lists the potential problems with metacarpal fractures and therapeutic interventions.

Nondisplaced metacarpal fractures are stable injuries and are treated with application of an anteroposterior splint in the **position of function**: the wrist in 30 to 60 degrees of extension, the MCP joints in 70 degrees of flexion, and the IP joints in 0 to 10 degrees of flexion. In this position the important ligaments of the wrist and hand are maintained in maximal tension to prevent contractures (Fig. 4.2). **Exceptions to splinting for metacarpal fractures may include treatment of boxer's fractures** (see page 25 in Chapter 5).

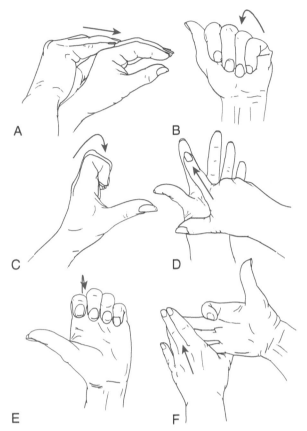

Fig. 4.1 Tendon glide exercises. **A,** Intrinsic plus posture to achieve central slip/lateral bands glide over proximal phalanx (P1). **B,** Sublimis fist posture to promote selective FDS tendon glide. **C,** Claw posture to achieve extensor digitorum communis (EDC) tendon glide over metacarpal bone. **D,** Flexor digitorum profundus (FDP) blocking exercises to glide FDP tendon over P1. **E,** Hook fist posture to promote selective FDP tendon glide. **F,** Flexor digitorum sublimis (FDS) blocking exercise to glide FDS tendon over middle phalanx.

Allowing early PIP and DIP joint motion is essential. Motion prevents adhesions between the tendons and the underlying fracture and controls edema.

PHALANGEAL FRACTURES OF THE HAND

- Phalangeal fractures lack intrinsic muscle support, are more unstable than metacarpal fractures, and are adversely affected by the tension in the long tendons of the fingers.
- Because of the pull of the FDS insertion into the middle phalanx, a proximal fracture of the middle phalanx will angulate with the fracture apex dorsal and a distal fracture will involve angulation with the apex volar (Fig. 5.3). Because of the deforming tendon forces, fractures in these areas that present initially as displaced are unlikely to remain reduced after reduction and typically require operative fixation.
- Phalangeal fractures respond less favorably to immobilization than metacarpal fractures, with a predicted 84% return of motion compared with 96% return of motion in the metacarpals (Shehadi 1991).
- If phalangeal immobilization is continued for longer than 4 weeks, the motion drops to 66%.
- Reasons cited for poor results in the literature typically are comminuted fractures, open fractures, and multiple fractures.

TABLE 4.1	Potential Problems With Phalangeal Fractures and Strategies for Therapeutic Intervention
	Maureen A. Hardy PT, MS CHT

Potential Problems	Prevention and Treatment
Loss of MP flexion	Circumferential PIP and DIP extension splint to concentrate flexor power at MP joint; NMES to interossei
Loss of PIP extension	Central slip blocking exercises; during the day MP extension block splint to concentrate extensor power at PIP joint; at night PIP extension gutter splint; NMES to EDC and interossei with dual-channel setup
Loss of PIP flexion	Isolated FDP tendon glide exercises; during the day MP flexion blocking splint to concentrate flexor power at PIP joint; at night flexion glove; NMES to FDS
Loss of DIP extension	Resume night extension splinting; NMES to interossei
Loss of DIP flexion	Isolated FDP tendon glide exercises; PIP flexion blocking splint to concentrate flexor power at DIP joint; stretch ORL tightness; NMES to FDP
Lateral instability, any joint	Buddy strap or finger-hinged splint that prevents lateral stress
Impending boutonnière deformity	Early DIP active flexion to maintain length of lateral bands
Impending swan-neck deformity	FDS tendon glide at PIP joint and terminal extensor tendon glide at the DIP joint
Pseudo claw deformity	Splint to hold MP joint in flexion with PIP joint full extensor glide
Pain	Resume protective splinting until healing is ascertained; address edema, desensitization program

MP, metacarpophalangeal; PIP, proximal interphalangeal; DIP, distal interphalangeal; NMES, neuromuscular electrical stimulation; EDC, extensor digitorum communis; FDP, flexor digitorum profundus; FDS, flexor digitorum superficialis; ORL, oblique retinacular ligament.

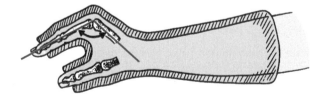

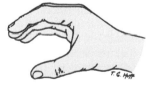

Fig. 4.2 Position of immobilization of the hand involves splinting the wrist in approximately 30 degrees of extension, the metacarpophalangeal (MCP) joints in 60 to 80 degrees of flexion, and the interphalangeal (IP) joints in full extension. (From Delee J, Drez D [eds]: Orthopaedic Sports Medicine. Philadelphia, WB Saunders, 1994.)

TABLE 4.2	Managing Proximal Interphalangeal Joint Injuries of the Hand	
Injury	**Clinical Manifestations or Special Considerations**	**Treatment**
Sprain	Stable joint with active and passive motion; negative radiographs; pain and swelling only	Buddy tape for comfort; begin early ROM exercises, ice, NSAIDs
Open dislocation	Dislocated exposed joint	Irrigation, débridement, and antibiotics; treat as any open fracture or dislocation
DORSAL PIP DISLOCATION		
Type 1	Hyperextension, volar plate avulsion, minor collateral ligament tear	Reduction; very brief immobilization (3–5 days) followed by ROM exercises with buddy taping and close x-ray follow-up
Type 2	Dorsal dislocation, volar plate avulsion, major collateral ligament tear	Same as type 1
Type 3	Stable fracture-dislocation: <40% of articular arc on fracture fragment	Extension block splint; refer to hand surgeon
	Unstable fracture-dislocation: >40% of articular arc on fracture fragment	Extension block splint; open reduction with internal fixation if closed treatment impossible; refer to hand surgeon
Lateral dislocation	Secondary to collateral ligament injury and avulsion and/or rupture of volar plate; angulation >20 degrees indicates complete rupture	Same as dorsal dislocation types 1 and 2 if joint is stable and congruous through active ROM
VOLAR PIP DISLOCATION		
Straight volar dislocation	Proximal condyle causes significant injury to central extensor slip (may reduce easily, but extensor tendon may be seriously injured; requires careful examination)	Refer to a hand surgeon experienced in these rare injuries; closed reduction with traction with metatarsophalangeal and PIP flexed and extended wrist; full-extension immobilization of PIP joint if postreduction x-rays show no subluxation; if closed reduction is not achieved or subluxation persists, surgery recommended
Ulnar or radial volar displacement	Condyle often buttonholes through central slip and lateral band; reduction often extremely difficult	Same as straight volar PIP dislocation

ROM, range of motion; NSAIDs, nonsteroidal anti-inflammatory drugs; PIP, proximal interphalangeal.
From Laimore JR, Engber WD. Serious, but often subtle finger injuries. Phys Sports Med 1998;l26(6):226.

- Weiss and Hastings (1993) investigated initiation of motion in patients with proximal phalangeal fractures treated with Kirschner-wire fixation and found no long-term differences in finger range of motion when motion was initiated between 1 and 21 days; however, if motion was delayed more than 21 days, there was a significant loss of motion.
- Table 4.2 lists potential problems and interventions for phalangeal fractures.

Comminuted phalangeal fractures, especially those that involve diaphyseal segments with thick cortices, may be slow to heal and may require fixation for up to 6 weeks.

PROXIMAL INTERPHALANGEAL JOINT INJURIES

Three types of proximal interphalangeal joint dislocations (Fig. 5.4; Table 4.2) or fracture-dislocations have been described: lateral, volar (rotatory), and dorsal (Fig. 5.5). Each results from a different mechanism of injury and has specific associated complications. The treatment of PIP injuries is dictated by the stability of the injury.

Stable lesions are treated with buddy taping of the injured digit to the noninjured digit adjacent to the torn or compromised collateral ligament. **Unstable injuries** are often associated with an intra-articular fracture of the middle phalanx (usually affecting more than 20% of the joint surface). However, even very tiny volar avulsion fractures may be associated with dorsal subluxation of the middle phalanx and be unstable. This is best assessed with fluoroscopy where the point of reduction can be accurately ascertained by sequential flexion of the PIP joint (Morgan and Slowman 2001).

Unstable injuries often are treated by dorsal extension block splinting (Fig. 5.6) with the initial digit flexion at the point where the stable reduction was obtained fluoroscopically. Incremental increase of extension of the splint and digit is done on a weekly basis for 4 weeks or until full extension at the joint has been obtained. Buddy taping is continued for 3 months during sports participation.

If reduction cannot be obtained or easily held by closed methods, then operative intervention is a must.

Early edema management and early active and passive ROM (within the confines of the extension block splint) are paramount to minimize scar adhesion formation and subsequent contractures.

Volar PIP joint dislocations are less common than dorsal dislocations and are often difficult to reduce by closed techniques because of entrapment of the lateral bands around the flare of the proximal phalangeal head. If not treated properly, these injuries may result in a boutonnière deformity (combined PIP joint flexion and DIP joint extension contracture). Usually, the joint is stable after closed or open reduction; however, static PIP joint extension splinting is recommended for 6 weeks to allow healing of the central slip (Rehabilitation Protocol 4.1).

Avulsion fractures involving the dorsal margin of the middle phalanx occur at the insertion of the central slip. These fractures may be treated by closed technique; however, if the fragment is displaced more than 2 mm proximally with the finger splinted in extension, ORIF of the fragment is indicated.

Dorsal fracture-dislocations of the PIP joint are much more common than volar dislocations. If less than 50% of the articular surface is involved, these injuries usually are stable after closed reduction and protective splinting (Rehabilitation Protocol 4.2).

Dorsal fracture-dislocations involving more than 40% of the articular surface may be unstable, even with the digit in flexion, and may require surgical intervention. The Eaton volar plate advancement is probably the most common procedure used (Fig. 5.7). The fracture fragments are excised, and the volar plate is advanced into the remaining portion of the middle phalanx. A key point is the resection of both collateral ligaments and the pull-out sutures are placed as far apart as possible through the middle phalanx to keep the volar plate maximally wide (Eaton and Malerich 1980). The PIP joint usually is pinned in 30 degrees of flexion (Rehabilitation Protocol 4.3). Other means of treating this fracture pattern have been reported, and should be reviewed. Hemi-hamate arthroplasty (McAuliffe 2009), dynamic distraction external fixation (Rutland et al. 2008), percutaneous fixation (Vitale et al. 2011, Waris and Alanen 2010), open reduction and volar fixation (Cheah et al. 2012), circlage wiring, and dynamic distraction fixation are multiple options. The bag of surgical options must have more than one tool.

Dorsal dislocations of the PIP joint without associated fractures are usually stable after closed reduction. Stability is tested after reduction under digital block, and, if the joint is believed to be stable, buddy taping for 3 to 6 weeks, early active ROM exercises, and edema control are necessary. If instability is present with passive extension of the joint, a dorsal blocking splint (DBS) similar to that used in fracture-dislocations should be used.

REHABILITATION PROTOCOL 4.1 ● After Volar Proximal Interphalangeal Joint Dislocation or Avulsion Fracture

After Closed Reduction

- An extension gutter splint is fitted for continuous wear with the PIP joint in neutral position.
- The patient should perform active and passive ROM exercises of the MCP and DIP joints approximately six times a day.
- PIP joint motion is not allowed for 6 weeks.
- Begin active ROM exercises at 6 weeks in combination with intermittent daytime splinting and continuous night splinting for an additional 2 weeks.

After ORIF

- The transarticular pin is removed 2 to 4 weeks after the wound has healed.
- Continuous splinting in an extension gutter splint is continued for a total of 6 weeks.
- The remainder of the protocol is similar to that after closed reduction.
- Extension splinting is continued as long as an extensor lag is present, and passive flexion exercises are avoided as long as an extension lag of 30 degrees or more is present.

REHABILITATION PROTOCOL 4.2 ● Rehabilitation Protocol After Dorsal Fracture-Dislocation of the Proximal Interphalangeal Joint

- If the injury is believed to be stable after closed reduction, a dorsal blocking splint (DBS) is applied with the PIP joint in 30 degrees of flexion. This allows full flexion but prevents the terminal 30 degrees of PIP joint extension.
- After 3 weeks, the DBS is adjusted at weekly intervals to increase PIP joint extension by about 10 degrees each week.
- The splint should be in neutral position by the sixth week, then discontinued.
- An active ROM program is begun, and dynamic extension splinting is used as needed.
- Progressive strengthening exercises are begun at 6 weeks.

REHABILITATION PROTOCOL 4.3 ● Rehabilitation Protocol After Dorsal Fracture-Dislocation of the Proximal Interphalangeal Joint Involving More Than 40% of the Articular Surface

- At 3 weeks after surgery, the pin is removed from the PIP joint and a DBS is fitted with the PIP joint in 30 degrees of flexion for continuous wear.
- Active and active-assisted ROM exercises are begun within the restraints of the DBS.
- At 5 weeks, the DBS is discontinued and active and passive extension exercises are continued.
- At 6 weeks, dynamic extension splinting may be necessary if full passive extension has not been regained.

REFERENCES

A complete reference list is available at https://expertconsult.inkling.com/.

FURTHER READING

Agee JM. Unstable fracture-dislocations of the proximal interphalangeal joint: treatment with the force couple splint. *Clin Orthop.* 1987;214:101.

Aitken S, Court-Brown CM. The epidemiology of sports-related fractures of the hand. *Injury.* 2008;39:1377–1383.

Ali A, Hamman J, Mass, DP. The biomechanical effects of angulated boxer's fractures. *J Hand Surg Am.* 1999;24:835–844.

Bernstein ML, Chung KC. Hand fractures and their management: an international view. *Injury.* 2006;37:1043–1048.

Bushnell BD, Draeger RW, Crosby CG, et al. Management of intra-articular metacarpal base fractures of the second through fifth metacarpals. *J Hand Surg Am.* 2008;33:573–583.

Calfee RP, Sommerkamp TG. Fracture-dislocation about the finger joints. *J Hand Surg Am.* 2009;34:1140–1147.

Carlsen BT, Moran SL. Thumb trauma: Bennett fractures, Rolando fractures, and ulnar collateral ligament injuries. *J Hand Surg Am.* 2009;34:945–952.

Dailiana Z, Agorastakis D, Varitimidis S, et al. Use of a mini-external fixator for the treatment of hand fractures. *J Hand Surg Am.* 2009;34:630–636.

Feehan LM, Basset K. Is there evidence for early mobilization following an extraarticular hand fracture? *J Hand Ther.* 2004;17:300–308.

Freeland AE, Orbay JL. Extraarticular hand fractures in adults: a review of new developments. *Clin Orthop Rel Res.* 2006;445:133–145.

Geissler WB. Operative fixation of metacarpal and phalangeal fractures in athletes. *Hand Clin.* 2009;25:409–421.

Hardy MA. Principles of metacarpal and phalangeal fracture management: a review of rehabilitation concepts. *J Orthop Sports Phys Ther.* 2004;34:781–799.

Harris AR, Beckbenbaugh RD, Nettrour JF, et al. Metacarpal neck fractures: results of treatment with traction reduction and cast immobilization. *Hand (N Y).* 2009;4:161–164.

Henry MH. Fractures of the proximal phalanx and metacarpals in the hand: preferred methods of stabilization. *J Am Acad Orthop Surg.* 2008; 16:586–595.

Hofmeister EP, Kim J, Shin AY. Comparison of 2 methods of immobilization of fifth metacarpal neck fractures: a prospective randomized study. *J Hand Surg Am.* 2008;33:1362–1368.

Jobe MT. Fractures and dislocations of the hand. In: Gustilo RB, Kyle RK, Templeman D, eds. *Fractures and Dislocations.* St. Louis: Mosby; 1993.

Kawamura K, Chung KC. Fixation choices for closed simple unstable oblique phalangeal and metacarpal fingers. *Hand Clin.* 2006;22:278–295.

Kozin SH, Thoder JJ, Lieberman G. Operative treatment of metacarpal and phalangeal shaft fractures. *J Am Acad Orthop Surg.* 2000;8:111–121.

Lee SG, Jupiter JB. Phalangeal and metacarpal fractures of the hand. *Hand Clin.* 2000;16:323–332.

Mall NA, Carlisle JC, Matava MJ, et al. Upper extremity injuries in the National Football League: part I: hand and digital injuries. *Am J Sports Med.* 2008;36:1938–1944.

Ozer K, Gillani S, Williams A, et al. Comparison of intramedullary nailing versus plate-screw fixation of extra-articular metacarpal fractures. *J Hand Surg Am.* 2008;33:1724–1731.

Peterson JJ, Bancroft LW. Injuries of the fingers and thumb in the athlete. *Clin Sports Med.* 2006;25:527–542.

Ring D. Malunion and nonunion of the metacarpals and phalanges. *Instr Course Lect.* 2006;55:121–128.

Singletary S, Freeland AE, Jarrett CA. Metacarpal fractures in athletes: treatment, rehabilitation, and safe early return to play. *J Hand Ther.* 2003; 16:171–179.

Sohn RC, Jahng KH, Curtiss SB, et al. Comparison of metacarpal plating methods. *J Hand Surg Am.* 2008;33:316–321.

Tavassoli J, Ruland RT, Hogan CJ, et al. Three cast techniques for the treatment of extra-articular metacarpal fractures. Comparison of short-term outcomes and final fracture alignments. *J Bone Joint Surg Am.* 2005; 87:2196–2201.

Wong TC, Ip FK, Yeung SH. Comparison between percutaneous transverse fixation and intramedullary K-wires in treating closed fractures of the metacarpal neck of the little finger. *J Hand Surg Br.* 2006;31:61–65.

5

Fifth Metacarpal Neck Fracture (Boxer's Fracture)

S. Brent Brotzman, MD | Theresa M. Kidd, BA | Maureen A. Hardy, PT, MS, CHT | Steven R. Novotny, MD

BACKGROUND

Metacarpal neck fractures are among the most common fractures in the hand. Fracture of the fifth metacarpal is by far the most frequent and has been termed a *boxer's fracture.* Trained pugilists will strike on the second and third metacarpal heads. These bones are larger and can resist a greater load to failure. The second and third metacarpals have less of a longitudinal bow, thus less natural bending moment when loaded. And finally, the second and third CMC joints are relatively immobile, keeping the metacarpals in the same spatial orientation when loaded. Alas, the fifth metacarpal is smaller, has a greater natural bow, and the CMC joints are flexible. When the fifth metacarpal is loaded, the CMC joint flexes, functionally increasing the bow of the bone and increasing its bending moment arm. All of these factors contribute to the relative frequency of this injury.

CLINICAL HISTORY AND EXAMINATION

Patients usually have pain, swelling, and loss of motion about the MCP joint. Occasionally a rotational deformity is present. Careful examination is performed to evaluate for malrotation of the fifth digit when the patient makes a fist (Fig. 5.1), palpation of the palm for prominence of the distal fragment (palmarly angulated) in the palm, and extensor lag of the involved finger. Unfortunately, pain inhibition can prevent the patient from demonstrating full motion or tendon excursion. An ulnar nerve block at the wrist will eliminate the pain component; however, intrinsic muscle paralysis could cause clawing. This could be mistaken for pseudoclawing. Pseudoclawing results from extrinsic tendon imbalance. The extensor tendon force is increased by passive tenodesis effect with the tendon is

stretched over the flexed metacarpal fracture. The flexor tendon pull is weakened from the functional shortening of the metacarpal. This can weaken lumbrical pull to extend the IP joints. The fracture angle also functionally lengthens the interossei, weakening their contribution to IP extension.

Measuring the fracture apex angulation can be subjective because we are measuring the change in angle of a curved bone. The neck region of the fifth metacarpal is naturally curved at least 15 degrees. Thus, the significance of the measured angle must reflect this natural curve. I use the distal third of the metacarpal when making this measurement. Besides the longitudinal arc of the metacarpals, the hand has a transverse arc. A lateral view of the hand does not give a true lateral view of each metacarpal. A lateral of the fifth and fourth metacarpals is best achieved with a 20- to 45-degree pronated lateral (20–45 degrees pronated oblique) of the hand. A lateral of the second and third is best seen on a 20- to 45-degree supinated lateral (20–45 degree supinated oblique).

TREATMENT

Treatment is based on the degree of angulation or displacement, as measured on the appropriate radiograph of the hand. Metacarpal neck fractures are usually impacted and angulated with the distal fragment angled palmarly by the mechanics causing the fracture. Loss of bony support via volar neck comminution, intrinsic muscle spasm or increased muscle tone, and splint inefficiency once hematoma resorbs contribute to loss of reduction during the healing process. Excessive angulation causes cosmetic loss of the MCP joint knuckle and may cause the palmar metacarpal head to be prominent in the palm.

Ali et al. (1999) report that 30 degrees of metacarpal angulation resulted in a loss of 22% of MCP ROM. This report uses the flexor digiti minimi and its effect on MCP motion and its calculated strength loss based on other physiologic studies and their conclusions (Jacobson 1992, Elftman 1996). Ali's study doesn't include potential contributions from the abductor digiti minimi, the third palmar interossei, or the lumbrical to the little finger in flexion of the MCP joint. Skeletal muscle recruitment patterns have been shown to vary depending on the length of the muscle when stimulated and the applied force (McNulty and Cresswell 2004). Howell et al. also have shown that changes in the type or distribution of synaptic inputs to motoneurons during movement can override pre- and postsynaptic factors that shape recruitment order in isometric conditions (Howell 1995). These may be factors in why the theoretical degree of acceptable fracture angulation when healed has not completely matched some clinical outcomes reported (Hunter 1970, Lowdon 1986, Konradson 1990, Theeuwen 1991, Staius 2003). Pace et al. (2015) published their results of patients treated without and

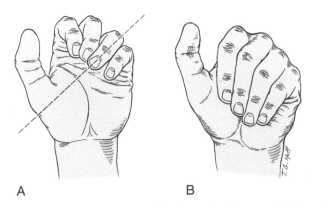

Fig. 5.1 A, To determine rotational and angular alignment of the hand skeleton, the nails should be parallel with the digits in extension. B, In flexion, the digits should all point to the scaphoid tuberosity.

with reduction. At follow-up the two groups displayed no difference in angulation. They conclude surgery is indicated when maintenance is desired.

If angulation or displacement is unacceptable, closed reduction can be attempted with wrist block anesthesia using the maneuver credited to Jahss (1938), in which the proximal phalanx is flexed to 90 degrees and used to apply a dorsally directed force to the metacarpal head (Fig. 5.2). The hand is then splinted in an ulnar gutter splint for about 3 weeks with the MCP joint at 80 degrees of flexion, the PIP joint straight, and the DIP joint free. Clinically I have found the Jahss technique very unpredictable. Having the luxury of a mini c-arm at my disposal, I frequently find the MCP joint cannot be flexed to 90 degrees. Placing the proximal phalanx perpendicular to the long axis of the hand has the MCP joint flexed 90 degrees minus the degree of fracture dorsal angulation. With the Jahss technique the total force applied during reduction can be broken down into a component vector force applied dorsalward to reduce the fracture and a component force axially loading the fracture.

My treatment paradigm is to buddy tape stable fractures, with elastic bandage for comfort and edema control. We offer a removable gutter splint for the patient to wear in environments where safety is an issue and for comfort. If rotational deformity is present we recommend reduction. If after discussing expectations on fracture healing the patient expresses concern about deformity cosmetics, a reduction is offered. A wrist ulnar nerve block is utilized, and an ulnar gutter splint with the fourth and

fifth digits are used. I cross the MCP and leave the interphalangeal joints free. Three point molding is applied (Harris et al. 2009). Splinting is discontinued at 3 weeks and range of motion pursued.

Rapid mobilization of the fingers is required to avoid scarring, adhesions, and stiffness unrelated to the fracture itself but rather to the propensity of an immobilized hand to quickly stiffen.

Statius Muller et al. (2003) prospectively treated 35 patients with boxer's fractures with a mean fracture angulation of 39 degrees (range 15 to 70 degrees). Patients were randomly allocated to treatment with either an ulnar gutter plaster cast for a period of 3 weeks followed by mobilization or a **pressure bandage for only 1 week and immediate mobilization within limits imposed by pain**. Between the two groups, no statistical differences were found with respect to ROM, satisfaction, pain perception, return to work and hobby, or need for physical therapy. In our clinic we employ the pressure bandage technique for our boxer's fractures with good result.

Bansal and Craigen (2007) treated 40 boxer's fractures with reduction and casting and 40 with buddy taping and range of motion only with instructions to return only if problems were experienced. The Disabilities of the Arm, Shoulder, and Hand (DASH) scores for the two groups were identical at 12 weeks, and the untreated group returned to work 2 weeks earlier and had a significantly higher satisfaction rate on their "care."

Operative treatment of boxer's fractures is indicated if the following occur:

- Fracture alignment remains unacceptable (authors' recommendations vary, but >40 degrees displacement).
- Late redisplacement beyond acceptable parameters occurs in a previously reduced fracture.
- Malrotation of the finger that cannot be controlled by static splinting techniques

Operative fixation usually involves percutaneous pinning of the fracture; however, open reduction and internal fixation (ORIF) may be required. Fractures treated percutaneously require about 3 weeks of protective splinting and ROM exercises. Those undergoing open reduction and internal fixation can proceed with immediate motion if a stable construct is achieved. Numerous papers have been published on various techniques.

Retrograde intramedullary screws have been reported by Boulton et al. (2010) and Ruchelsman et al. (2014). A minimal tendon splitting incision is utilized, reaming over guide wire, small cannulated screws, appropriate closure, and immediate motion.

Antegrade intramedullary pinning is a proven concept (Kim and Kim 2015). At 3 months antegrade proved superior to retrograde; however, the two groups eventually normalized at 6 months.

Facca et al. (2010) compared locked plating for boxer's fractures versus antegrade K-wires and demonstrated higher expense and poorer motion with plating. The authors recommend antegrade K-wires as their treatment of choice.

Page and Stern (1998) retrospectively reviewed their institution's series of metacarpal and phalangeal ORIF. They report 36% major complications despite stable fixation and early mobilization. They do not condemn plate fixation and attribute the results to frequent use of plates in open and phalangeal fractures.

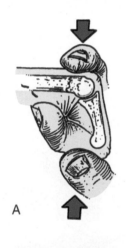

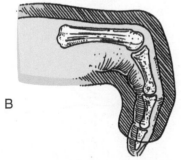

Fig. 5.2 Maneuver of Jahss. **A,** The proximal interphalangeal (PIP) joint is flexed 90 degrees, and the examiner stabilizes the metacarpal proximal to the neck fracture, then pushes the finger to dorsally displace the volar angulated boxer's fracture to "straight." **B,** Splint is molded in reduced position with the ulnar gutter in the position of function. (From Regional Review Course in Hand Surgery. Rosemont, Illinois, American Society for Surgery of the Hand, 1991.)

Phalangeal Fractures of the Hand

- Phalangeal fractures lack intrinsic muscle support, are more unstable than metacarpal fractures, and are adversely affected by the tension in the long tendons of the fingers.
- Because of the pull of the FDS insertion into the middle phalanx, a proximal fracture of the middle phalanx will angulate with the fracture apex dorsal and a distal fracture will involve angulation with the apex volar (Fig. 5.3). Because of the deforming tendon forces, fractures in these areas that present initially as displaced are unlikely to remain reduced after reduction and typically require operative fixation.
- Phalangeal fractures respond less favorably to immobilization than metacarpal fractures, with a predicted 84% return of motion compared with 96% return of motion in the metacarpals (Shehadi 1991).
- If phalangeal immobilization is continued for longer than 4 weeks, the motion drops to 66%.
- Reasons cited for poor results in the literature typically are comminuted fractures, open fractures, and multiple fractures.
- Weiss and Hastings (1993) investigated initiation of motion in patients with proximal phalangeal fractures treated with Kirschner-wire fixation and found no long-term differences in finger range of motion when motion was initiated between 1 and 21 days; however, if motion was delayed more than 21 days, there was a significant loss of motion.
- Table 4.1 lists potential problems and interventions for phalangeal fractures.

Comminuted phalangeal fractures, especially those that involve diaphyseal segments with thick cortices, may be slow to heal and may require fixation for up to 6 weeks.

Proximal Interphalangeal Joint Injuries

Three types of proximal interphalangeal joint dislocations (Fig. 5.4; Table 4.2) or fracture-dislocations have been described: lateral, volar (rotatory), and dorsal (Fig. 5.5). Each results from a different mechanism of injury and has specific associated complications. The treatment of PIP injuries is dictated by the stability of the injury.

Stable lesions are treated with buddy taping of the injured digit to the noninjured digit adjacent to the torn or compromised collateral ligament. **Unstable injuries** are often associated with an intra-articular fracture of the middle phalanx (usually affecting more than 20% of the joint surface). However, even very tiny volar avulsion fractures may be associated with dorsal subluxation of the middle phalanx and be unstable. This is best assessed with fluoroscopy where the point of reduction can be accurately ascertained by sequential flexion of the PIP joint (Morgan and Slowman 2001).

Unstable injuries often are treated by dorsal extension block splinting (Fig. 5.6) with the initial digit flexion at the point

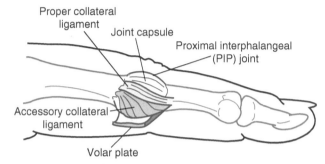

Fig. 5.4 Anatomy of the volar plate and collateral ligaments of the proximal interphalangeal (PIP) joint. (Adapted with permission from Breen TF: Sports-related injuries of the hand, in Pappas AM, Walzer J [eds]: Upper Extremity Injuries in the Athlete. New York, Churchill Livingston, 1995, p. 459.)

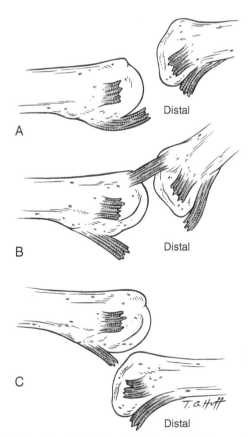

Fig. 5.5 Dislocations in the hand are classified by the position of the distal skeletal unit in relation to its proximal counterpart. **A,** Dorsal proximal interphalangeal (PIP) joint dislocation. **B,** Lateral PIP joint dislocation. **C,** Palmar PIP joint dislocation. (From Browner B, Skeletal Trauma, 4 Ed. Philadelphia, Saunders, 2009. Fig 38-132.)

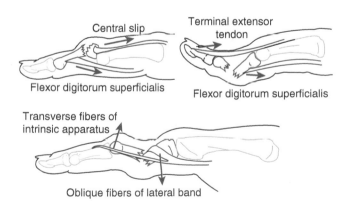

Fig. 5.3 Deforming forces on phalangeal fractures. (Adapted with permission from Breen TF: Sports-related injuries of the hand, in Pappas AM, Walzer J [eds]: Upper Extremity Injuries in the Athlete. New York, Churchill Livingston, 1995, p. 475.)

where the stable reduction was obtained fluoroscopically. Incremental increase of extension of the splint and digit is done on a weekly basis for 4 weeks or until full extension at the joint has

been obtained. Buddy taping is continued for 3 months during sports participation.

If reduction cannot be obtained or easily held by closed methods, then operative intervention is a must.

Early edema management and early active and passive ROM (within the confines of the extension block splint) are paramount to minimize scar adhesion formation and subsequent contractures.

Volar PIP joint dislocations are less common than dorsal dislocations and are often difficult to reduce by closed techniques because of entrapment of the lateral bands around the flare of the proximal phalangeal head. If not treated properly, these injuries may result in a boutonnière deformity (combined PIP joint flexion and DIP joint extension contracture). Usually, the joint is stable after closed or open reduction; however, static PIP joint extension splinting is recommended for 6 weeks to allow healing of the central slip (see Rehabilitation Protocol 4.1).

Avulsion fractures involving the dorsal margin of the middle phalanx occur at the insertion of the central slip. These fractures may be treated by closed technique; however, if the fragment is displaced more than 2 mm proximally with the finger splinted in extension, ORIF of the fragment is indicated.

Dorsal fracture-dislocations of the PIP joint are much more common than volar dislocations. If less than 50% of the articular surface is involved, these injuries usually are stable after

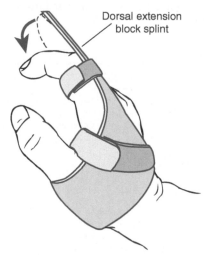

Fig. 5.6   Dorsal extension block splint. (Adapted with permission from Breen TF: Sports-related injuries of the hand, in Pappas AM, Walzer J [eds]: Upper Extremity Injuries in the Athlete. New York, Churchill Livingston, 1995, p. 461.)

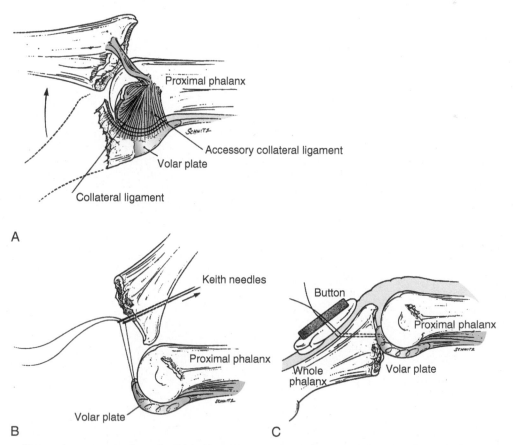

Fig. 5.7   **A,** Pathology of injury demonstrating loss of collateral ligament support to the joint, producing marked instability. Eaton volar plate arthroplasty is commonly used when more than 40% comminution or impaction of the inferior aspect of the middle phalanx of the proximal interphalangeal (PIP) joint is present. **B,** Sutures are passed through the lateral margins of the defect, exiting dorsally. The comminuted fragment has been excised, and the volar plate is being advanced. **C,** Sutures are tied over a padded button, drawing the volar plate into the defect and simultaneously reducing the PIP joint. (From Strickland JW: The Hand: Master Techniques in Orthopaedic Surgery. Philadelphia, Lippincott-Raven, f1999.)

closed reduction and protective splinting (see Rehabilitation Protocol 4.2).

Dorsal fracture-dislocations involving more than 40% of the articular surface may be unstable, even with the digit in flexion, and may require surgical intervention. The Eaton volar plate advancement is probably the most common procedure used (Fig. 5.7). The fracture fragments are excised, and the volar plate is advanced into the remaining portion of the middle phalanx. The PIP joint usually is pinned in 30 degrees of flexion (see Rehabilitation Protocol 4.3).

Dorsal dislocations of the PIP joint without associated fractures are usually stable after closed reduction. Stability is tested after reduction under digital block, and, if the joint is believed to be stable, buddy taping for 3 to 6 weeks, early active ROM exercises, and edema control are necessary. If instability is present with passive extension of the joint, a dorsal blocking splint (DBS) similar to that used in fracture-dislocations should be used.

REFERENCES

A complete reference list is available at https://expertconsult .inkling.com/.

FURTHER READING

Kollitz KM, Hammert WC, Vedder NC, et al. Metacarpal fractures: treatments and complications. *Hand.* 2014;9:16–23.

Porter ML, Hodgkinson JP, Hirst P. The boxer's fracture: a prospective study of functional recovery. *Arch Emer Med.* 1988;5:212–215.

Van Aaken J, Kampfen S, Berli M, et al. Outcome of boxer's fractures treated by a soft wrap and buddy taping: a prospective study. *Hand.* 2007;2:212–217.

Injuries to the Ulnar Collateral Ligament of the Thumb Metacarpophalangeal Joint (Gamekeeper's Thumb)

S. Brent Brotzman, MD | Steven R. Novotny, MD

BACKGROUND

The classic **"gamekeeper's thumb"** was first described in Scottish gamekeepers as a chronic instability of the thumb MCP joint ulnar collateral ligament. Stener in 1962 reported the non-healing lesion of the UCL outside the adductor aponeurosis, not specifically an acute injury. **"Skier's thumb"** was coined by Schultz, Brown, and Fox in 1973, with skiing being the most common cause of acute ulnar collateral ligament (UCL) rupture (e.g., after a fall causing the ski pole to stress and tear the ulnar collateral ligament of the thumb MCP joint). Even though these eponyms exist, most injuries do not involve sports.

Static lateral pinch stability is provided by a strong collateral ligament complex: Proper UCL runs from the metacarpal lateral condyle to the proximal phalanx and the accessory collateral ligaments, which attach more volarly on the metacarpal and insert on the volar plate and sesamoids. The proper collateral ligaments are taut in flexion while the accessories are in taut extension. The tendinous attachments of the thenar muscles—especially the adductor pollicis attaching into the ulnar sesamoid—contribute some dynamic stability. The UCL provides resistance to radially applied forces (e.g., pinching or holding large objects). A torn UCL weakens the key pinch grip strength and allows volar subluxation of the proximal phalanx. With prolonged instability, the MCP joint frequently degenerates.

The amount of valgus laxity of normal thumbs varies widely. In full MCP joint extension, valgus laxity averages 6 degrees, and in 15 degrees of MCP joint flexion it increases to an average of 12 degrees. It has been shown that the valgus laxity may vary if the joint is tested in supination and pronation (Mayer et al. 2014). It is recommended to standardize the stress examination in neutral rotation. The adductor aponeurosis (when torn or pulled distally) frequently entraps the UCL, preventing anatomic ligament reduction and healing of the UCL (**Stener lesion**) (Fig. 6.1). The typical **mechanism of injury** is an extreme valgus stress to the thumb (e.g., falling on an abducted thumb).

EVALUATION

Patients typically have a history of a valgus injury to the thumb followed by pain, swelling, and frequently ecchymosis at the ulnar aspect of the thumb MCP joint. Palpation of the ulnar aspect of the MCP joint may reveal a small lump, which may be indicative of a Stener lesion or avulsion fracture. Radiographs are necessary to evaluate for fractures, which may have significant ramifications on management. Dinowitz et al. (1997) reported a series of 9 patients with avulsion fractures with <2.0 mm displacement who all did poorly after at least 6 weeks of immobilization and rehab. Rotation of the fragment was felt to limit healing. All were salvaged with subsequent surgery. Kaplan reported on two patients with well-aligned fractures with displaced ligaments (Kaplan 1998). Shear fractures can occur after the ligament has been avulsed.

In addition to plain films (three views of the thumb and carpus), valgus stress testing radiographs should be obtained. Because patients who are acutely injured will guard from pain, 1% lidocaine should be injected into the joint before stress testing. Many patients are seen days or weeks after the injury and the intra-articular lidocaine may not be adequate. Performing wrist median and radial nerve blocks provides complete anesthesia and allows multiple examinations if needed. Also an

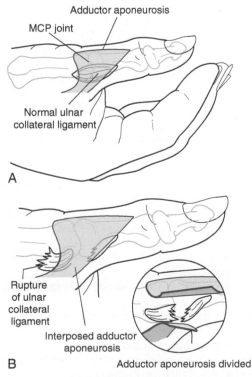

Fig. 6.1 Complete rupture of the ulnar collateral ligament resulting in a Stener lesion. The distal attachment has been avulsed from the bone. AB, The interposed adductor aponeurosis prevents the ligament from being reduced. Therefore, leaving joint potentially unstable.

MCP joint anesthetic injection insufflates tissue, which could influence the fit of a brace or cast, especially once the fluid absorbs. The integrity of the proper (ulnar collateral) ligament is **assessed by valgus stress testing with the MCP joint of the thumb in 30 degrees of joint flexion.** This test can be done clinically or with radiographic documentation. Some concern exists as to whether an exuberant exam can precipitate a Stener lesion. Adler et al. demonstrated on cadavers that serial ligament sectioning and stressing a Stener lesion could not be provoked (Adler et al. 2012). The literature varies as to the degree of angulation on valgus stressing that is compatible with complete rupture of the UCL. **Thirty to 35 degrees of radial deviation of the thumb on valgus stressing or 15 degrees greater than the uninjured side indicates a complete UCL rupture and is an indication for surgical correction.** With complete ruptures (>30 degrees of opening) the likelihood of a UCL ligament displacement (Stener lesion) is greater than 80%.

The question of need or utility of advanced imaging should be discussed because they could be part of the evaluation. No advanced imaging technique has 100% sensitivity or specificity, and there is a cost involved. We are finding longer times for insurance companies to authorize or deny a study, which could turn an acute injury to a chronic injury before the special imaging is complete, then requiring another wait for surgical authorization. Papandrea and Fowler in 2008 reviewed current literature on ultrasound and MRI for evaluation of this injury. Given the structural and time constraints of MRI, ultrasound (possibly office-based ultrasound) could lead to a conclusion sooner. Looking at just two articles on ultrasound diagnosis of UCL Stener lesions shows there may be uncertainty in ultrasound conclusions. O'Callaghan et al. report 48 patients studied by ultrasound per protocol. All 13 patients with positive tests were explored (O'Callaghan et al. 1994). Ten of 13 positive tests showed true Stener lesions; the remainder at surgery were labeled partial Stener lesions. In Susic et al.'s publication 14 patients with clinically unstable UCL underwent US (Susic et al. 1999). At surgery all were ruptured, 5 were Stener lesions, yet only two of the five were identified on ultrasound. That means 60% of the dislocated lesions were missed on ultrasound.

TREATMENT

Stable Thumb on Valgus Stressing (No Stener Lesion)

- The ligament is only partially torn, and healing will occur with nonoperative treatment.
- The thumb is immobilized for 4 weeks in a short arm spica cast or thermoplastic splint (molded), usually with the thumb IP joint free.
- Active and passive thumb motion is begun at 3 to 4 weeks, but valgus is avoided.
- If ROM is painful at 3 to 4 weeks, re-evaluation by a physician is indicated.
- The thermoplastic splint is removed several times a day for active ROM exercises.
- Grip-strengthening exercises are begun at 6 weeks after injury. A brace is worn for protection in contact situations for 2 months (Rehabilitation Protocol 6.1).
- If one has access to reliable hand therapy, comparable results have been achieved with a fabricated forearm-based spica splint hinged at the MCP (Sollerman et al. 1991).

- The MCP is allowed an arc of 50 degrees motion. Other authors express satisfaction with a hand-based hinged MCP splint allowing a 35-degree arc of motion (Michaud et al. 2010). These rehab studies discuss the monitoring and individual modifications rationale during the healing period. Biomechanical modeling of strains on repaired UCL has shown load to failure three times higher than loads expected with flexion and extension (Harley et al. 2004). This study supports the clinical findings of the early motion rehab protocol post surgery.

Unstable Thumb on Valgus Stressing (>30 Degrees)

- Because 80% of patients with a complete rupture are found to have a Stener lesion (thus obtaining a poor healing result if treated nonoperatively), it is critical to make the correct diagnosis of stable versus unstable gamekeeper's thumb. As we've seen, it isn't possible to be 100% accurate with advanced imaging. Physical exam is excellent at diagnosing instability; absent fractures, bony excrescences, or concomitant soft tissue tumors, a palpable enlargement ulnar to the metacarpal head, can be considered diagnostic. Without other evidence one needs to discuss risks and benefits of the three treatment paths—surgery, imaging, conservative care—and encourage patient involvement in the decision.
- Operative repair requires direct visualization of the local anatomy. Results can be improved by re-creation of normal anatomy. Carlson has demonstrated the anatomic origins and insertions of both the UCL and RCL of the thumb MCP joint (Carlson et al. 2012). They determined the center of the ulnar collateral ligament origin to be 4.2 mm volar to the dorsal surface of the metacarpal head, 5.3 mm proximal to the articular surface, and 7 mm from the volar cortex. The phalangeal insertion center was 9.2 mm from the dorsal surface, 3.4 mm distal to the articular surface and 2.8 mm dorsal to the volar cortex. This work provides context to the deliberateness with which placement of anchors or drill holes is undertaken. Lee et al.'s biomechanical simulation study to determine optimal tunnel placement for UCL reconstruction used four constructs: cruciate, two parallel, proximal apex V, and distal apex V (Lee et al. 2005). All constructs restored valgus load stability. The proximal apex V restored range of motion not significantly different from the native state. The other 3 constructs resulted in significantly decreased range of motion.
- Numerous published reports exist demonstrating effective surgical repair of avulsed ulnar collateral ligaments and repair of bony involvement. Weiland et al. (1997) reported anchored repairs in acute injury with excellent functional results. Tip, chuck, key, and pinch strengths and laxity were almost indistinguishable comparing operative and noninjured sides. Grip strength was slightly decreased. Range of motion loss was approximately 10 degrees at the MPJ and IPJ. Twenty percent of patients had self-reported minor symptoms at maximum exertion. Glickel et al. reported results for UCL replacement for chronic instability. A tendon graft was passed intraosseously and tied extracutaneously (Glickel et al. 1993). Twenty-four of 26 patients had good or excellent results with significantly improved function and few complications. Osterman et al. (1981) reported their results using acute repair, reconstruction with graft, and reconstruction

REHABILITATION PROTOCOL 6.1 ● Rehabilitation Protocol After Repair or Reconstruction of the Ulnar Collateral Ligament of the Thumb Metacarpophalangeal Joint

The early motion protocol allows 35–50 degree motion with hinged splint protecting the MCP from radial or ulnar deviation. Static splint with ADLs if pain at 2 to 3 weeks. If no pain at 6 weeks, brace not necessary at night or light activities. Protected repair from aggressive activity. If pain continues at 6 weeks, brace for a total of 12 weeks.

3 Weeks

- Remove bulky dressing.
- Remove MCP joint pin (K-wire) if used for joint stabilization.
- Fit with wrist and thumb static splint for continual wear.

6 Weeks

- Begin active and gentle passive ROM exercises of the thumb for 10 minutes each hour.

- *Avoid any lateral stress to the MCP joint of the thumb.*
- Begin dynamic splinting if necessary to increase passive ROM of the thumb.

8 Weeks

- Discontinue splinting. Wrist and thumb static splint or short opponens splint may be useful during sports-related activities or heavy lifting.
- Begin progressive strengthening.

12 Weeks

- Allow the patient to return to unrestricted activity.

---

with adductor advancement. Acute repair had the best results with 92% pinch strength and 84% normal motion. Both types of reconstruction gave adequate function. Adductor advancement resulted in a slight strength advantage (85% vs 81%), however, the graft reconstruction had a significantly improved range of motion over advancement (78% vs 65%). They reported that repair within two weeks produces the best result, and reconstruction in chronic injury demonstrates significant functional improvement.

- Most surgeons feel more comfortable with an open procedure. Ryu and Fagan (1995) with soft tissue Stener and Badia (2006) with bony injury demonstrated successful treatment in their patients via arthroscopic treatment.

REFERENCES

A complete reference list is available at https://expertconsult.inkling.com/.

FURTHER READING

Bean HG, Tencher AF, Trumble TE. The effect of thumb metacarpophalangeal ulnar collateral ligament attachment site of joint range of motion: an in vivo study. *J Hand Surg Am*. 1999;24:283–287.

Chuter GS, Muwanga CL, Irwin LR. Ulnar collateral ligament injuries of the thumb: 10 years of surgical experience. *Injury*. 2009;40:652–656.

Heyman P. Injuries to the ulnar collateral ligament of the thumb metacarpophalangeal joint. *J Am Acad Orth Surg*. 1997;5:224–229.

Nerve Compression Syndromes

S. Brent Brotzman, MD | Steven R. Novotny, MD

NERVE COMPRESSION PHYSIOLOGY

The microanatomic, physiologic, and biochemical changes occurring intraneurally upon compression ultimately determine the symptoms patients manifest and eventually the surgical results when treated. Though we can't know exactly what impact compression had on the neural tissue in each patient, one can start understanding at a basic level the anatomy and physiology as a primer to more advanced knowledge. This information then can be interpreted for patients, helping them understand the rationale for treatment and expectations with management.

Lundborg (1979) has long studied nerve physiology and microanatomy. Using freshly amputated human extremities, he showed that the microvascular anatomy is arranged similarly to multiple animal models studied. This infers the transportability of information gained from previous studies. The microvascular anatomy is of segmental fascicle vascularization by epineurial vessels. Each fascicle presents a well-defined combination vascular system of endoneurial and perineurial microcirculation. Intraneurial dissection could disrupt valuable blood supply. Rydevik et al. (1980), using a rabbit vagus nerve, demonstrated that 50 mm Hg pressure for 2 hours produced axoplasmic protein transport blockage at the site of compression. Though the block was reversible within a day, pressures of 200 and 400 mm Hg similarly applied resulted in axoplasmic blocks for 1 and 3 days respectively. They demonstrated that axons may survive without undergoing Wallerian degeneration; however, fast axonal transport is blocked for at least a day. Rydevik et al. (1981) in a different model demonstrated progressive microvascular dysfunction with progressive pressure. Interference in venular flow occurred between 20 to 30 mm Hg, and arteriolar and intrafascicular capillary flow changed at 40 to 50 mm Hg. At 60 to 80 mm Hg complete neural blood flow block is observed. No or very slow stagnant blood flow was seen for 7 days after 400 mm Hg pressure for 2 hours.

Lundborg et al. (1983) measured increases in intraneurial fluid with compression. Endoneurial tissue fluid pressure was still elevated at 24 hours. They expressed concern for capillary occlusion with this pressure and possible resultant dysfunction. O'Brien et al. (1987) used a chronic compression rat nerve model and demonstrated progressive perineural thickening at 5 months with peripheral demyelination. This progressed with time to marked thinning of myelin and Wallerian degeneration at 8 months. This continued until the study end at 12 months. Conduction velocities decreased progressively after 5 months. Mackinnon et al. (1985) used the chronic compression model in primates measuring histologic and morphometric parameters. There was no difference between those treated with decompression and decompression with internal neurolysis.

Nemoto et al. (1987) in a canine model reported incomplete conduction blocks and mild axonal degeneration with single compression and complete block and severe axonal degeneration in half the animals with double compression. The loss of nerve function was greater in the double compression than the sum of a single proximal and distal compression combined. Good therapeutic effects were obtained with release of both compression sites while incomplete effect was noted with release of only one block.

Fullerton (1963) reported serial EMG/NCV studies during 30 minutes of ischemia. In the control subjects variable changes were noted with time; however, by 30 minutes all subjects had 50% reduction in amplitude and area of the evoked potential. When the median nerve was stimulated at the elbow, action potential started to decrease between 10 and 18 minutes, and no potentials were recorded at 30 minutes. Subjects diagnosed with carpal tunnel syndrome tested similarly showed a trend of ischemia changes earlier than controls, though some patients seemed to be protected from ischemia. All showed proximal nerve changes even if the carpal tunnel segment hadn't been affected yet.

CARPAL TUNNEL SYNDROME
Background

Carpal tunnel syndrome (CTS) is relatively common (the most common peripheral neuropathy), affecting 1% of the general population. It occurs most frequently during middle or advanced age, with 83% of 1215 study patients older than 40 years, with a mean age of 54 years (Madison 1992). Women are affected twice as frequently as men. A more recent review (Bickel, 2010) estimates one to three cases per 1000 subjects per year, with a prevalence of 50 cases per 1000 subjects per year.

The carpal tunnel is a rigid, confined fibro-osseous space that physiologically acts as a "closed compartment." Tung (2010) measured compliance of the evacuated carpal tunnel in various animal systems in comparison to human cadaveric specimens to propose an animal model for future research avenues. Holmes et al. (2012) measured modulus of elasticity in six zones, proximal, and mid-distal on the radial and ulnar sides. The proximal and radial sections were stiffer compared to the opposing zones. Adding this knowledge may contribute to the understanding of carpal tunnel mechanics. Li (Li et al. 2011, Gabra and Li 2013) in companion articles has shown that the size of the carpal tunnel increases when balloon loads are applied at 9% and 14% when pressures of 100 mm Hg and 200 mm Hg are utilized. They also show that the soft tissue coating the osseous tunnel is 24% of the measures bony canal. This reinforces the concept that any condition that adds to the soft tissue decreases the area available for structures traversing the canal. These contents include the median nerve, nine tendons, and a variable amount of tenosynovium. CTS is caused by compression of the median nerve at the wrist (Fig. 7.1). The clinical syndrome is characterized by pain, numbness, or tingling in the distribution of the median nerve: the palmar aspect of the thumb, index, long finger, and radial side of the ring finger. These symptoms may affect all or a combination of the thumb, index, long, and ring fingers to a variable degree. Pain and **paresthesias at night** in the median nerve distribution are common symptoms (Table 7.1); activity-related symptoms may be the only history if nocturnal symptoms are not significant enough to awake the patient or not present upon awakening. Pain complaints proximally are more of a deep ache when present.

The posturing with prolonged flexion or extension of the wrists during sleep is believed to contribute to the progression of nocturnal symptoms via carpal tunnel pressure changes (Gelbermann et al. 1981, Rojviroj et al. 1990). Conditions that alter fluid balance such as pregnancy and use of oral contraceptives and chronic conditions such as diabetes (Vinik 2004) and hemodialysis may predispose to CTS (Ono et al. 1994, Shinohara et al. 2011). CTS associated with **pregnancy** usually is transitory and typically resolves spontaneously. However, those affected during pregnancy have a high rate of recurrence later in life. Sex hormones (Toesca et al. 2008, Kim et al. 2010) have been shown to alter the histology in idiopathic CTS patients' transverse ligament and tenosynovium, and the assumption from this would be that pregnancy-related changes may not reverse completely postpartum. Surgery should be avoided during pregnancy. Nocturnal bracing, activity reduction, and steroidal injection control symptoms until parturition, which is usually curative.

Biochemical and immunohistologic studies reveal a deeper layer of complexity in CTS. Freeland et al. (2002) collected serum and biopsy specimens from 41 consecutive idiopathic carpal tunnel patients with abnormal electrodiagnostic tests and compared them to controls. In the study subjects, the serum and synovial malondialdehyde, along with synovial IL-6, prostaglandin PGE2 were elevated. This pattern with the absence of IL-1 supports a noninflammatory ischemia-reperfusion etiology. Ettema et al. (2004) analyzed tenosynovial biopsies from idiopathic CTS patients and volunteers. They demonstrated increased type 3 collagen content in the tissue and TGF-B expression in the fibroblasts of the patient specimens. A biochemical treatise is impractical in this manuscript. To be aware of the coming research in this field is appropriate. If in the future this arm of research produces blood tests determining who should have early surgery, who can wait, who should never have surgery; who should be re-explored and who should be left alone; and who should be held responsible when causality is questioned, it will be a major leap in patient care.

Typical Clinical Presentation

Paresthesia, pain, and numbness or tingling in the palmar surface of the hand in the distribution of the median nerve (Fig. 7.2) (i.e., the palmar aspect of the three and one-half radial

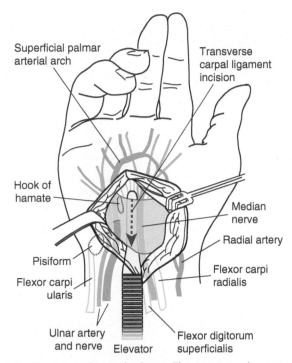

Fig. 7.1 Open carpal tunnel release. The transverse ligament is divided in a distal to proximal direction near the hook of the hamate. A Carroll or Lorenz elevator may be placed beneath the transverse carpal ligament to protect the median nerve.

TABLE 7.1	Interpreting Findings in Patients With Carpal Tunnel Syndrome
Degree of CTS	**Findings**
Dynamic	Symptoms primarily activity induced; patient otherwise asymptomatic; no detectable physical findings
Mild	Patient has intermittent symptoms; decreased light-touch sensibility; digital compression test usually positive but Tinel sign and positive result on Phalen maneuver may or may not be present
Moderate	Frequent symptoms; decreased vibratory perception in median nerve distribution; positive Phalen maneuver and digital compression test; Tinel sign present; increased two-point discrimination; weakness of thenar muscles
Severe	Symptoms are persistent; marked increase in or absence of two-point discrimination; thenar muscle atrophy

CTS, carpal tunnel syndrome.

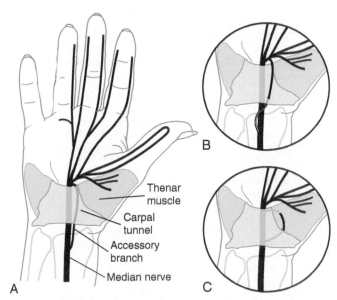

Fig. 7.2 Variation in median nerve anatomy in the carpal tunnel. Group IV variations include those rare instances in which the thenar branch leaves the median nerve proximal to the carpal tunnel. **A,** Accessory branch. **B,** Accessory branch from the ulnar aspect of the median nerve. **C,** Accessory branch running directly into the thenar musculature.

digits) are the most common symptoms. Nocturnal pain is also common. Activities of daily living (such as driving a car, holding a cup, and typing) often aggravate pain. Pain and paresthesia are sometimes relieved by the patient massaging, shaking the hand, or placing it in a dependent position.

Several provocative tests should be considered to aid in the evaluation and diagnosis of CTS. No one test has been identified as a gold standard for identifying CTS. In a meta-analysis of the literature (Keith et al. 2009) **Phalen test** results ranged in sensitivity from 46% to 80% and in specificity from 51% to 91%. The **Tinel sign** ranged in sensitivity from 28% to 73% and in specificity from 44% to 95%. The **median nerve compression test, Durkan test** (Durkan 1991), ranged in sensitivity from 4% to

79% and in specificity from 25% to 96%. Combining the results of more than one provocative test might increase the sensitivities and specificities. For example, combined results of the Phalen and median nerve compression tests yielded a sensitivity of 92% and a specificity of 92%.

Provocative Testing Maneuvers (Table 7.2)

Phalen Maneuver (Fig. 7.3, A)
- The patient's wrists are placed in complete (but not forced) flexion.
- If paresthesias in the median nerve distribution occur within the 60-second test, the test is positive for CTS.

TABLE 7.2	Available Tests Used to Diagnose Carpal Tunnel Syndrome				
N	Test	Method	Condition Measured	Positive Result	Interpretation of Positive Result
1*	Phalen maneuver	Patient holds wrist in marked flexion for 30–60 sec	Paresthesia in response to position	Numbness or tingling on radial side digits	Probable CTS (sensitivity, 0.75; specificity, 0.47); Gellman found best sensitivity of provocative tests
2*	Percussion test (Tinel sign)	Examiner lightly taps along median nerve at the wrist, proximal to distal	Site of nerve lesion	Tingling response in fingers	Probable CTS if response is at the wrist (sensitivity, 0.60; specificity 0.67)
3*	Carpal tunnel compression	Direct compression of median nerve by examiner	Paresthesias in response to pressure	Paresthesias within 30 sec	Probable CTS (sensitivity, 0.87; specificity, 0.90)
4	Hand diagram	Patient marks sites of pain or altered sensation on outline	Patient's perception of site of nerve deficit	Pain depiction on palmar side of radial digits without depiction of the palm	Probable CTS (sensitivity, 0.96; specificity, 0.73), negative predictive value of a negative test, 0.91
5	Hand volume stress test	Measure hand volume by water displacement; repeat after 7-min stress test and 10-min rest	Hand volume	Hand volume increased by ≥10 mL	Probable dynamic CTS
6	Static two-point discrimination	Determine minimum separation of two points perceived as distinct when lightly touched on palmar surface of digit	Innervation density of slowly adapting fibers	Failure to discriminate points <6 mm apart	Advanced nerve dysfunction (late finding)
7	Moving two-point discrimination	As above, but with points moving	Innervation density of slowly adapting fibers	Failure to discriminate points <5 mm apart	Advanced nerve dysfunction (late finding)
8	Vibrometry	Vibrometer head is placed on palmar side of digit; amplitude at 120 Hz increased to threshold of perception; compare median and ulnar nerves in both hands	Threshold of quickly adapting fibers	Asymmetry in contralateral hand or between radial and ulnar digits	Probable CTS (sensitivity, 0.87)
9*	Semmes-Weinstein monofilament test	Monofilaments of increasing diameter touched to palmar side of digit until patient can tell which digit is untouched	Threshold of slowly adapting fibers	Value >2.83 in radial digits	Median nerve impairment (sensitivity, 0.83)
10*	Distal sensory latency and conduction velocity	Orthodromic stimulus and recording across the wrist	Latency and conduction velocity of sensory fibers	Latency >3.5 ms or asymmetry >0.5 ms compared with contralateral hand	Probable CTS
11*	Distal sensory latency and conduction velocity	Orthodromic stimulus and recording across wrist	Latency and conduction velocity of motor fibers of median nerve	Latency >4.5 ms or asymmetry >1 ms	Probable CTS
12	Electromyography	Needle electrodes placed in muscle	Denervation of thenar muscles	Fibrillation potentials, sharp waves, increased insertional activity	Very advanced motor median nerve compression

CTS, carpal tunnel syndrome.
*Most common tests/methods used in our practice.
Adapted from Szabo RM, Madison M. Carpal tunnel syndrome. Orthop Clin North Am 1992;1:103.

- Gellman and associates (1986) found this to be the most sensitive (sensitivity, 75%) of the provocative maneuvers in their study of CTS.

Tinel Sign (Median Nerve Percussion) (Fig. 7.3, *B*)
- The Tinel sign may be elicited by lightly tapping the patient's median nerve at the wrist, moving from proximal to distal.
- The sign is positive if the patient complains of tingling or electric shock–like sensation in the distribution of the median nerve.

Sensory Testing of the Median Nerve Distribution. Decreased sensation may be tested by the following:
- *Threshold tests:* Semmes-Weinstein monofilament 2.83 gm; vibrometry perception of a 256-cps tuning fork.
- *Innervation density tests:* two-point discrimination.
- Sensory loss and thenar muscle weakness often are *late findings.*

Additional Special Tests for Evaluation

- Durkan's carpal tunnel direct compression (30 seconds)
- Palpation of pronator teres/Tinel test at pronator teres, palpation of leading edge of the active pronator resisted in a supinated position
- Spurling maneuver for foraminal neuritis
- Motor, sensory, and reflex testing in suspected radiculopathy
- Inspection for weakness or atrophy of thenar eminence (a late finding of CTS)
- Detailed history and physical exam for concomitant neurologic pathology or metabolic effectors of nerves: diabetes, thyroid disease, history of chemotherapy, renal disease, hereditary motor and sensory neuropathies
- If gray area, electromyographic/nerve conduction velocity (EMG/NCV) testing of *entire* involved upper extremity to exclude cervical radiculopathy versus CTS versus pronator syndrome, possible mononeuritis multiplex

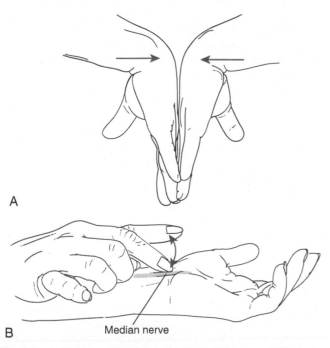

Fig. 7.3 A, Diagram of Phalen test (Miller). B, Diagram of Tinel test.

Electrodiagnostic Evaluation

Electrodiagnostic studies are a useful adjunct to clinical evaluation, but they do not supplant the need for a careful history and physical examination. These tests are indicated when the clinical picture is ambiguous or there is suspicion of other entrapments or neuropathies. Clinical guidelines formulated by the American Academy of Orthopaedic Surgeons (Keith et al. 2009) suggest that electrodiagnostic testing may be appropriate in the presence of thenar atrophy and/or persistent numbness (level V evidence) and definitely should be used if clinical or provocative tests are positive and surgical management is being considered (levels II and III evidence).

A myriad of papers can be reviewed as to whether electodiagnostic studies contribute to patient treatment. Glowacki et al. (1996) reviewed their institution's CTS treatment outcomes with respect to electrodiagnostic findings. The treatment success rates were equivalent between the groups of positive electrical tests, negative tests, and those without testing. Clinical presentation and physical examination proved the most reliable predictor. Graham (2008) has shown that in the majority of patients who by history and physical exam demonstrate CTS, electrodiagnostic studies do not add to the probability of diagnosing CTS in any clinically relevant extent.

- Patients with **systemic peripheral neuropathies** (e.g., diabetes, alcoholism, hypothyroidism) may have abnormal sensory distribution not unique to the median nerve distribution.
- More proximal compressive neuropathies (e.g., C6 **cervical radiculopathy**) will produce sensory deficits in the C6 distribution (well beyond median nerve distribution), weakness in the C6 innervated muscles (biceps), and an abnormal biceps reflex.
- Electrodiagnostic tests are helpful in distinguishing local compressive neuropathies (such as CTS) from peripheral systemic neuropathies (such as diabetic neuropathy). Usually they confirm the presence of both.
- The criterion for a positive electrodiagnostic test is a motor latency greater than 4.0 M/sec and a sensory latency of greater than 3.5 M/sec or a 0.4 ms difference between the median and ulnar sensory latencies.

The interpretation of findings in patients with CTS is classified in Table 7.2.

BOX 7.1 DIFFERENTIAL DIAGNOSIS OF CARPAL TUNNEL SYNDROME

Thoracic outlet syndrome (TOS)
TOS exam includes Adson's test, Wright's costoclavicular maneuver, Roos test, etc. Palpation for masses in the supraclavicular and infraclavicular fossa is performed.
Cervical radiculopathy (CR)
CR has a positive Spurling test of the neck, proximal arm/neck symptoms, dermatomal distribution. Neck pain is a negative result.
Brachial plexopathy
Pronator teres syndrome (PTS)
Median nerve compression in the proximal forearm (PTS) rather than the wrist (CTS) has similar median nerve symptoms. PTS is usually associated with activity-induced daytime paresthesias rather than nighttime paresthesias (CTS).

Tenderness and Tinel palpable at pronator teres in the forearm, not at the carpal tunnel

PTS (more proximal) involves the median nerve innervated extrinsic forearm motors and the palmar cutaneous nerve branch of the median nerve (unlike CTS).

Digital nerve compression (bowler's thumb)

Caused by direct pressure applied to the palm or digits (base of the thumb in bowler's thumb)

Tenderness and Tinel sign localized to the thumb digit rather than carpal tunnel

Neuropathy (systemic)

Alcohol, diabetes, hypothyroidism—more diffuse neuropathy findings noted

Tenosynovitis (RA)

Complex Regional Pain Syndrome

Type 1 sympathetically mediated—pain out of proportion, hyperalgia to allodynia, vascular dysautonomia, can migrate from the original injury site

Type 2 nonsympathetically mediated—burning is hallmark, does not migrate. Often indistinguishable from type 1 in early phases

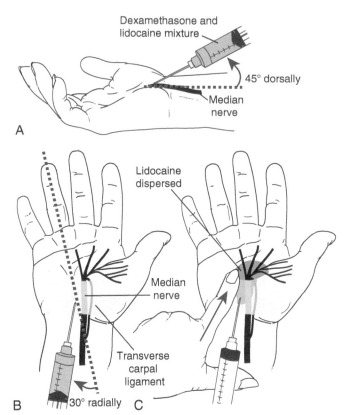

Fig. 7.4 **A,** During carpal tunnel injection, a 25- or 27-gauge needle is used to introduce a mixture of dexamethasone and lidocaine into the carpal canal. **B,** Needle is aligned with the ring finger and directed 45 degrees dorsally and 30 degrees radially as it is advanced slowly beneath the transverse carpal ligament into the tunnel. **C,** After injection, lidocaine is dispersed. Injection into the nerve should be avoided. If any paresthesias occur during injection, the needle is immediately withdrawn and redirected.

Treatment

- All patients should undergo **initial conservative management** unless the presentation is acute and associated with trauma (such as CTS associated with acute distal radius fracture).
- All patients with **acute CTS** should have the wrist taken out of flexion in the cast and placed in neutral (see section on distal radial fractures).
- Circumferential casts should be removed or bivalved or converted to splints, and icing and elevation above the heart should be initiated.
- Close serial observation should check for possible "emergent" carpal tunnel release if symptoms do not improve.
- Some authors recommend measurement of wrist compartment pressure.

Nonoperative Management

Nonoperative treatment may include the following:

- A **prefabricated wrist splint,** which places the wrist in a neutral position, may be worn at night; daytime splinting may be done if the patient's job allows.
- Pressure in the carpal tunnel is lowest with the wrist in 2 ± 9 degrees of extension and 2 ± 6 degrees of ulnar deviation. Prefabricated splints typically align the wrist in 20 to 30 degrees of extension; however, CTS is treated more effectively with the wrist in neutral.
- In a study of 45 patients treated for severe CTS in a tertiary referral center, the authors concluded that patients with more severe initial symptoms are unlikely to respond to night-splint therapy (12 weeks of splinting in this study), but those with less severe symptoms should be offered a trial of nighttime splinting before surgery (Boyd et al. 2005).
- **Activity modification** (discontinuing use of vibratory machinery or placing a support under unsupported arms at the computer) may be tried.
- Studies have shown that fewer than 25% of patients who had **cortisone injection** into the carpal tunnel (not into the ac-

tual median nerve) were symptom free at 18 months after injection. As many as 80% of patients do derive *temporary relief* with cortisone injection and splinting. Green (1993) found that symptoms typically recurred 2 to 4 months after cortisone injection, leading to operative treatment in 46% of patients. The technique for injection is shown in Fig. 7.4. If injection creates paresthesias in the hand, the needle should be immediately withdrawn and redirected from its location in the median nerve; injection ***should not*** be into the median nerve.

- Vitamin B₆ has not been shown in clinical trials to have any therapeutic effect on CTS, but it may help "missed" neuropathies (pyridoxine deficiency).
- Nonsteroidal anti-inflammatory drugs (NSAIDs) can be used for control of inflammation, but they are not as effective as steroid injections.
- Any underlying systemic disease (such as diabetes, rheumatoid arthritis, or hypothyroidism) must be controlled.

Surgical Treatment

Carpal tunnel release was given a grade A recommendation (level I evidence) in the CTS treatment guidelines formulated by the American Academy of Orthopaedic Surgeons (Keith et al. 2009). These guidelines recommend surgical treatment of CTS

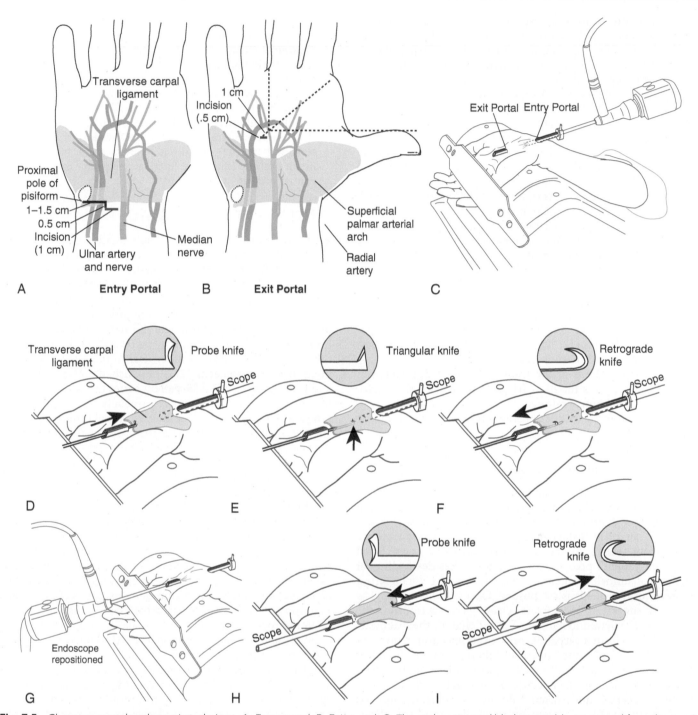

Fig. 7.5 Chow two-portal endoscopic technique. **A,** Entry portal. **B,** Exit portal. **C,** The endoscope and blade assembly are passed from the proximal incision through the distal incision, deep to the transverse carpal ligament (TCL). **D,** The distal edge of the TCL is released using a probe knife. **E,** A second cut is made in the midsection of the TCL with a triangular knife. **F,** The first and second cuts are connected with a retrograde knife. **G,** The endoscope is repositioned beneath the TCL through the distal portal. **H,** A probe knife is inserted to release the proximal edge of the TCL. **I,** A retrograde knife is inserted into the midsection of the TCL and drawn proximally to complete the release.

by complete division of the flexor retinaculum, regardless of the specific surgical technique.

Indications for surgical treatment of CTS include the following:

- Thenar atrophy or weakness
- Sensation loss on objective measures
- Fibrillation potentials on electromyelograms
- Symptoms that persist more than a year despite appropriate conservative measures

The goals of carpal tunnel release are as follows:

- Decompression of the nerve
- Improvement of nerve excursion
- Prevention of progressive nerve damage

Although endoscopic and minimal-incision techniques have been described, our preferred technique has been **open carpal tunnel release** (complication rate of 10% to 18%) rather than endoscopic release (complication rate up to 35% in some studies) (Figs. 7.1 and 7.5). In our experience, the times to return to work and sporting activities have not been different enough between the two procedures to warrant the differences in complication rates (increased frequency of digital nerve lacerations, higher incidence of incomplete release with endoscopic technique). Several comparative studies have shown faster functional recovery and faster relief of pain after endoscopic release at short-term follow-up, but longer follow-up showed equivalent results of open and endoscopic methods (Vasiliadis et al. 2010) in a level VI retrospective study, (Atroshi et al. 2009) level I evidence, (Scholten et al. 2007) and meta-analysis. Lengthy immobilization of the wrist should be avoided after routine carpal tunnel release. Several level II studies indicate no benefits of immobilization for longer than 2 weeks (Bury et al. 1995, Cook et al. 1995, Finsen et al. 1999, Martins et al. 2006). Detrimental effects of immobilization include adhesion formation, stiffness, and prevention of nerve and tendon movement, which can compromise carpal tunnel release (Rehabilitation Protocol 7.1).

Complications After Carpal Tunnel Release

- The most common complication after open carpal tunnel release is *pillar pain* (25%), with symptom resolution in most patients within 3 months (Ludlow et al. 1997).
- Incomplete release of the transverse carpal ligament with persistent CTS is the most frequent complication of endoscopic carpal tunnel release.
- CTS recurs in 7% to 20% of patients treated surgically during their lifetime.

Failed Carpal Tunnel Release

My algorithm for working up and treating patients with failure to improve, worsening, limited improvement, or worsening after limited improvement subsequent to CTR is straightforward. A complete history and physical exam and neurologic exam from neck to fingertips are performed. This is correlated with the patient's preoperative symptoms. Besides findings at the carpal tunnel, frequently a site of potential double crush or secondary neuritis is established. Occasionally the surgical scar will suggest an incomplete release. Past electrodiagnostic studies are reviewed looking for missed clues in the diagnostic process. I perform a carpal tunnel steroid injection in hopes of mitigating patient symptoms. Hand therapy for nerve-gliding techniques and scar modification is instituted. I find those who respond favorably to the injection have a higher success rate if further surgery is undertaken. I do order a contrast-enhanced MRI looking for intact ligament, mass effect, and scar tissue. Workers' compensation cases undergo a new electrodiagnostic study if conservative care fails; in this scenario, improvement in the nerve study warrants a cautious approach if the MRI fails to show entrapment.

BOWLER'S THUMB (DIGITAL NEURITIS)

Digital nerve compression, or bowler's thumb, is a compression neuropathy of the ulnar digital nerve of the thumb. Repetitive pressure of the thumb hole of the bowling ball to this area results in formation of a perineural fibrosis or neuroma-type formation of the ulnar digital nerve.

Patients present with a painful mass at the base of the thumb and paresthesia. A Tinel sign is usually elicited, and the mass is tender to palpation. Differential diagnoses include ganglion, inclusion cyst, and painful callous.

Treatment includes the following:
- A protective thumb shell
- Relative rest from bowling or offending activity
- Backsetting the thumbhole of the bowling ball to increase thumb extension and abduction
- Avoiding full insertion of the thumb into the thumbhole
- If conservative measures fail, consideration of decompression and internal neurolysis, translocation of the digital nerve dorsally (Swanson 2009), or neuroma resection with primary repair

PRONATOR SYNDROME

Pronator syndrome is used to denote median nerve compressive symptoms in and around the pronator muscle. Beaton and Anson (Beaton 1939) and a follow-up report by Jameson and Anson (1952) showed in 83% of specimens the median nerve ran between the two heads of the pronator and in 9% the nerve ran deep to the humeral head of the pronator, with an absent ulnar head. In 6% of specimens the nerve was deep to both heads and in the least common pattern (2%) the nerve split the humeral head and ran superficial to the remainder of the ulnar head. Johnson et al. (1979) published a 71-patient series and Hartz et al. (1981) a 39-patient series that similarly report overall good results. The patients clinically exhibit neurogenic symptoms usually not well defined as carpal tunnel and physical examination of tenderness in the pronator region and varying symptom exacerbation while activating the three common structures responsible: pronator, lacertus fibrosis, and superficialis arcade. The offending location of the pronator can be at the proximal origin of its humeral head; thus the nerve must be visualized free and clear of the proximal muscle edge before considering it decompressed. Supracondylar processes are relatively rare anatomic variants and even rarer cause for proximal median nerve or brachial artery compression. The bone itself or Struther's ligament could compress the structures. The process is palpable proximal to the medial epicondyle and palpation of the region often exacerbates symptoms. Extension of the elbow can exacerbate symptoms while flexion often improves symptoms.

Acute anterior interosseous nerve (AIN) palsy is a separate entity from pronator syndrome. Miller-Breslow et al. (1990) reported on nine patients with 10 cases of complete or partial acute AIN paralysis. The eight treated by observation showed spontaneous recovery starting in 6 months and complete by one year. The two cases that underwent surgery also recovered in one year. All cases had an episode of sudden pain preceding the paralysis without trauma. Electrodiagnostic tests confirmed AIN involvement. They suggest this entity is neuritis, rather than a compressive neuropathy, and thus recommend observation.

The standard open pronator decompression involves a 6-cm oblique incision along the leading edge of the pronator muscle. Cutaneous nerves are protected and large veins are ligated only if needed. The soft tissue envelope is elevated proximally and distally as far as can be visualized and retracted with two Army-Navy retractors 90 degrees from each other. Nested Scofields having longer shoes may provide greater visibility. The lacertus and fascia are opened the whole length. Distally, the radial artery is protected and mobilized radially if needed. Gentle retraction of the pronator medially usually exposes the medial nerve at some level. This provides the depth at which the tissue should be dissected to completely expose and decompress the nerve. Once the nerve is visualized all material is lysed anteriorly, protecting the motor branches. Distally, the superficialis arcade is split and I elevate the muscle with a retractor to visualize as distally as possible. Usually there is an artery with two veins crossing the distal extent of the exposure; frequently the color of the nerve looks more normal at this level. Proximally, if I find the nerve intramuscular, I extend the incision proximally to the ligament of Struthers region to safely decompress the nerve as it exits the pronator. If a large collateral artery travels with the nerve I frequently find a structure proximally that could contribute to compression. If the nerve stays radial to the proximal pronator and with the brachial artery proximally, I only lyse the perineural sheeting anteriorly on the nerve in this region as far as can be seen. I finger dissect on top of the nerve and use the blunt end of a DeBakey forceps as a probe proximally. If any concerns exist the incision is extended.

RADIAL NERVE COMPRESSION
Radial Sensory Neuritis

For this discussion we will exclude radial nerve pathology proximal to the elbow. Wartenberg's syndrome is the eponym of distal radial sensory neuralgia. The irritation of the radial sensory nerve distal to the brachioradialis (BR) musculotendinous junction to where it penetrates the forearm fascia from deep to superficial produces paresthesia and pain. Tinel sign can localize the level of the nerve injury; however, confounding factors can exist. Patients with previous surgical scars can have neuroma or multiple locations for nerve traction. Regeneration of nerve fibers can produce an advancing Tinel in addition to the primary area of findings. Unless Tinel is performed over time, the advancing nerve regeneration could be noted as static. Concomitant tendinopathies, de Quervain's or intersection syndrome, can influence the clinical picture. Wartenberg (1932) wasn't the first to report radial sensory neuralgia, but he did report on five cases in 1932. Common histories include crushing or compressive injuries, repetitive forceful pronation and extension activity, and metabolic disturbances such as diabetes and dialysis.

Braidwood (1975) reported a small series of radial sensory neuritis. Two thirds responded well to conservative means. The four treated by resection of the nerve and allowing it to retract under the BR muscle belly for protection had good results. Dellon and Mackinnon (1986) reported on 51 patients, in which 37% responded to conservative means. Of those undergoing surgery 86% were considered good to excellent results. Only 43% returned to their regular jobs; 22% were in vocational rehabilitation. Some patients had multiple conditions or injuries that precluded a return to their previous occupation. Lanzetta and Foucher (1993) published a series of 52 cases, in which 71% responded nonoperatively with good or excellent results. Of the 15 cases treated operatively, 74% rated good or excellent at follow-up. They report a high incidence (50%) of associated de Quervain's in their population—a cautionary tale.

Mackinnon and Dellon's surgical approach is a 6- to 8-cm incision centered on the Tinel area longitudinally but volar to place the scar away from the nerve. The dorsal fascia is opened, retracting the BR volarly and continuing the lysis of fascia between the BR and ECRL 6 cm proximally. Neurolysis is performed allowing the nerve mobility, and it is continued distally until the nerve is loose in the subcutaneous tissue. An internal neurolysis is considered or performed in patients with chronic sensory deficits. The internal neurolysis continues until internal fibrosis is lysed and a normal fascicular pattern is found. Consideration should be given to using a nerve wrap technique to prevent adhesions in this scenario. Severe nerve trauma warrants considering resecting and burying the radial sensory nerve stump.

Zoch and Aigner (1997) reported 10 patients, nine women, treated over a 2-year period with freeing the nerve and longitudinally cutting and repairing the BR tendon to transpose the nerve dorsally. Their 10 patients were free of symptoms at 6 weeks.

Proximal Radial Nerve and Posterior Interosseous Nerve Compression

The radial tunnel originates close to the radiocapitellar joint. The medial border is the brachialis muscle and more distally the biceps tendon and associated fibrous structures. The extensor carpi radialis longus (ECRL) and extensor carpi radialis brevis (ECRB) form the roof and lateral margins. The distal supinator marks the furthest extent. The posterior interosseous nerve (PIN) diverges from the proper radial nerve before the arcade of Froshe. The areas of anatomic compressions include fascial tissue superficial to the radiocapitellar joint, ECRB fibrous bands (often connected to the arcade of Froshe), leash of Henry (radial recurrent vessels), arcade of Froshe, and the distal fibrous border of the supinator. Fuss and Wurzl (1991), Prasartritha et al. (1993), and Hazani et al. (2008) performed human anatomic dissection studies of this region. Overall their observations corroborated each other and portray a fairly uniform construct of this region.

Prasartritha's 31 cadaveric specimens showed no evidence of compressive lesions. Their specimens had a tendinous arcade of Froshe in 57%, membranous in 43%. The distal supinator was tendinous in 65% and membranous in 35%. In only 2% of their specimens did the PIN send motor branches to the ECRB. In Fuss and Wurzl's 50 dissection specimens the innervation to the BR and ECRL lay proximal to Hueter's line (intercondylar axis). The ECRB received one branch at 4 cm distal to Hueter's line. The ECRB had a fibrous band contribution to the arcade region 0.5 to 1 cm proximal to the arcade. Hazani's 18 cadaveric specimens demonstrated a stable PIN course 3.5 cm distal to the radial head coursing 7.4 cm intramuscularly in the supinator. The line of travel is from the radial head to mid-dorsal wrist consistently. This information could allow a greater ease and increased safety during surgery.

Roles and Maudsley (1972), in a follow-up to the senior author's 1956 report of treating recurrent lateral epicondylitis as a nerve entrapment, reported 35 of 38 patients with good to excellent results. They used a BR muscle splitting incision, decompressed all fascial material on top of the nerve as could be seen proximal through the arcade, and lysed the leading part of the supinator muscle. The leash of Henry was divided. Lister et al. (1979) reported 19 of 20 patients with complete relief with the same surgical exposure as Maudsley. Sponseller and Engber (1983) reported a case of a patient with arcade of Froshe and distal supinator compression. Since there are multiple potential sites of compression, this comes as no surprise.

Sotereanos et al. (1999) report overall poor results in their institution's treatment of radial nerve compression patients. Their group was dominated by workers' compensation patients, 28 of 35 cases. Seven cases had more than one nerve decompressed at the same time and seven patients were lost to follow-up. The authors rated 11 of 28 (39%) good or excellent results while the patients rated themselves 18 of 28 (64%) good or excellent. Twelve patients had concomitant lateral epicondyle release or revision lateral epicondyle release. Interestingly 15 of 17 patients with poor to fair results were receiving workers' compensation benefits. Only 12 patients in this study returned to work. Atroshi et al. (1995) also report relatively poor outcomes in their group. Of 37 consecutive cases 13 reported substantial pain relief, 15 were satisfied with the outcome, and 16 returned to previous level of employment. Atroshi questions the validity of diagnostic criteria with this diagnosis. One concern would be the lack of complete supinator decompression given reports of distal PIN compression in the era of double crush. Also some reports fail to provide information on duration of symptoms and length of conservative treatment before proceeding with surgery. Given the basic science of nerve physiology, biochemistry and microanatomic changes documented with prolonged nerve compression, the nerve may not revert to normal after decompression, and given secondary gain issues, it may be impossible to produce a uniform surgical result across all patient subgroups.

My surgical approach is a dorsal incision opening the interval between the mobile wad and the extensor digitorum communis (EDC). It's easiest to find the interval distally and to work proximally. Occasionally a branch of the lateral antebrachial cutaneous nerve is in the field and is preserved. Proximally the ECRB and EDC share a septum. I take the ECRB fibers sharply off the septum and continue to the lateral epicondyle region, and I cross it if a lateral release is also needed. Deeper, there is thin fascia connecting the ECRB to the arcade of Froshe and proximally to the capsule region that is released. There is a fascia binding the EDC to the supinator region; it is opened, which then allows exposure of the whole supinator. By bending the elbow, extending the wrist, and anteriorly retracting the mobile wad, your field of vison extends centimeters proximal to the arcade. I first open the arcade on top of the PIN and continue distally. You can palpate the PIN in the supinator and I incrementally divide the superficial head on top of the nerve from proximal to distal. The distal edge of the supinator usually is a thick myotendinous structure and must be lysed. The PIN motor branches turn acutely from deep to superficial here and can be easily injured without due care. Retractors must be placed carefully in this area under direct vision to not damage the motor branches. The assistant cannot retract exuberantly. Once the PIN is released a longitudinal neurolysis is performed. The PIN is usually tortuous in thickened fibrofatty tissue just outside the arcade. I dissect off this tissue, having identified the correct plane at the arcade region, and follow it proximally. I do repair the EDC ECRB interval.

ULNAR NERVE COMPRESSION
Proximal Ulnar Nerve Compression

Cubital tunnel syndrome is a constellation of symptoms referable to ulnar nerve dysfunction in the elbow region, more often around the cubital tunnel. Internal nerve physiology has been discussed in the median nerve section. Patients that do the best are those with the least amount of preoperative "damage" to the nerve (Adelaar 1984). Physical examination is the gold standard at localizing the disease process; electrodiagnostic studies often sort out secondary issues. A metabolic polyperipheral neuropathy upon evidence of focal nerve slowing could portend a delayed recovery postsurgery or even result in a lessened result. Electrodiagnostic findings of a chronic C8 root dysfunction upon a progressive cubital tunnel syndrome could explain an inferior result. Those with chronic sensory deficits, intrinsic atrophy,

clawing, Froment's sign, or Wartenberg's sign are not diagnostic dilemmas. The question remains if a possible double crush phenomenon exists, affecting the intensity of the symptoms and the potential outcome. Electrodiagnostic studies can help sort out cervical spine disease from Guyon's canal compression.

Classic physical examination of the cubital tunnel includes an elbow flexion test and Tinel's along the course of the nerve. Depending on body habitus and whether the nerve is regenerating, Tinel's may be unreliable. Control subjects have a 24% positive response to Tinel's. The elbow flexion test is performed in maximum flexion for at least 1 minute and up to 3 minutes. Symptoms occurring early may indicate true cubital tunnel. Ochi et al. (2012) assessed the sensitivity and specificity of a 5-second shoulder abduction internal rotation combined with elbow flexion in control patients and suspected cubital tunnel patients. The sensitivities/specificities of the 5-second elbow flexion were 25%/100%, shoulder internal rotation 58%/100%, and the combined shoulder internal rotation and elbow flexion 87%/98%.

Pseudo thoracic outlet syndrome (TOS) is far more common than true TOS; any nerve tension can contribute to true entrapment symptoms. An index of suspicion, the nonspecific generalization of symptom location and description, and body habitus may increase concern for this nerve tension problem. Wright's maneuver, Adson's test, costoclavicular maneuver, Roos test, and percussion of the supraclavicular and infraclavicular fossa all have been described with meaning; Nord et al. (2008) showed a high false positive rate in normal subjects and even higher in those with peripheral nerve entrapment.

Nerve testing can neither tell us how a patient feels, nor can it tell us if an individual patient will respond to treatment. The amount of change seen does correlate with outcome. Anderton et al. (2011) reported on 75 patients who underwent cubital tunnel surgery for symptoms. Those with a negative nerve conduction test had 100% resolution, those with a positive test had 81% resolution, and those without a test had 89% resolution. They feel the patients can be treated safely with decompression alone without a preceding electrodiagnostic test. There are legitimate reasons for diagnostic testing for perplexing symptoms that could be upper motor neuron disease, demyelinating conditions, and hereditary conditions.

Research using high resolution ultrasound in evaluating peripheral nerve entrapment has shown a significantly enlarged ulnar nerve in cubital tunnel patients compared to control subjects (Wiesler 2006). The same technique has been applied to patients clinically diagnosed with cubital tunnel syndrome with normal electrodiagnostic studies. Yoon et al. (2010) showed the same increased diameter of ulnar nerves in patients with clinically diagnosed cubital tunnel syndrome as in those with positive electrodiagnostic studies. Due to legal concerns, testing for the foreseeable future will remain with us.

The question isn't whether symptomatic cubital tunnel that fails conservative care be treated surgically or not, but is decompression in situ or decompression and transposition the question? Two meta-analyses (Zlowodzki et al. 2007, Macadam et al. 2008) have shown no difference in outcomes with either technique, decompression in situ or decompression and anterior transposition. This may not completely answer the question scientifically because endoscopically assisted and medial epicondylectomy were not included. Thus at this point, surgical technique may be personal preference of the surgeon in primary surgical cases. In patients who have had previous elbow trauma or nearby surgical incisions, congenital anatomic variations may dictate a change from the surgeon's regular practice pattern.

Guyon's Canal

The canal anatomy starts at the proximal extent of the transverse carpal ligament and ends at the aponeurotic arch of the hypothenar muscles. The floor is made of the transverse carpal ligament and hypothenar muscles. The roof is the volar carpal ligament. The ulnar border is the pisiform, pisohamate ligament, and abductor digiti minimi muscle belly. The radial border is the hook of the hamate. The contents are the ulnar nerve, ulnar artery, and venae commitantae. If there is a focal lesion the symptoms may denote the location. Zone 1 compression is proximal to the bifurcation and the symptoms are mixed motor and sensory. Zone 2 involves the deep motor branch and classically is painless motor dysfunction. Zone 3 is distal to the bifurcation and is a sensory disturbance or pain in the nerve distribution. The etiologies are straightforward: chronic compression as in cyclist's palsy, pseudoaneurysm, aneurysm, thrombosed ulnar artery, ganglion cyst, foreign body, hamate fracture, or infection. Others may not come to mind immediately such as rheumatoid mass, chronic calcinosis, tophi, benign neoplasias, and very rarely malignancies. If radiographs are normal and trauma has occurred, a CT scan for hook of the hamate fracture would be needed. An Allen's test would rule out a thrombosed ulnar artery. Oral steroids would be utilized in history of autoimmune disease to try to decompress the inflammatory mass. An MRI would be obtained to make a final diagnosis and plan ultimate treatment and possible surgical approach.

REHABILITATION PROTOCOL 7.1 ▪ **Rehabilitation Protocol After Open Release of Carpal Tunnel Syndrome**

0–7 Days
- Encourage gentle wrist extension and flexion exercises and full finger flexion and extension exercises immediately after surgery in the postsurgical dressing.

7 Days
- Remove the dressing.
- Prohibit the patient from submerging the hand in liquids, but permit showering.
- Discontinue the wrist splint if the patient is comfortable.

7–14 Days
- Permit the patient to use the hand in activities of daily living as pain allows.

2 Weeks
- Remove the sutures and begin ROM and gradual strengthening exercises.

- Achieve initial scar remodeling by using Elastomer or silicon gel-sheet scar pad at night and deep scar massage.
- If scar tenderness is intense, use desensitization techniques such as applying various textures to the area using light pressure and progressing to deep pressure. Textures include cotton, velour, wool, and Velcro.
- Control pain and edema with the use of Isotoner gloves or electrical stimulation.

2–4 Weeks
- Advance the patient to more rigorous activities; allow the patient to return to work if pain permits. The patient can use a padded glove for tasks that require pressure to be applied over the tender palmar scars.
- Begin pinch/grip strengthening with Baltimore Therapeutic Equipment work-simulator activities.

REFERENCES

A complete reference list is available at https://expertconsult.inkling.com/.

FURTHER READING

Botte MJ. Controversies in carpal tunnel syndrome. *Instr Course Lect.* 2008;57:199–212.

Dang AC, Rodner CM. Unusual compression neuropathies of the forearm, part 1: radial nerve. *J Hand Surg Am.* 2009;34:1906–1914.

Dang AC, Rodner CM. Unusual compression neuropathies of the forearm, part II: median nerve. *J Hand Surg Am.* 2009;34:1915–1920.

Elhassan B, Steinmann S. Entrapment neuropathy of the ulnar nerve. *J Am Acad Orthop Surg.* 2007;15:672–681.

Henry SL, Hubbard BA, Concanno MJ. Splinting after carpal tunnel release: current practice, scientific evidence, and trends. *Plast Reconstr Surg.* 2008;122:1095–1099.

Ibrahim T, Majid I, Clarke M, et al. Outcome of carpal tunnel decompression: the influence of age, gender, and occupation. *Int Orthop.* 2009;33:1305–1309.

Koo JT, Szabo RM. Compression neuropathies of the median nerve. *J Am Soc Surg Hand.* 2004;4:156–175.

Medina McKeon JM, Yancosek KE. Neural gliding techniques for the treatment of carpal tunnel syndrome: a systematic review. *J Sport Rehabil.* 2008;17:324–341.

Plate AM, Green SM. Compressive radial neuropathies. *Instr Course Lect.* 2000;49:295–304.

Pomerance J, Zurakowski D, Fine I. The cost-effectiveness of nonsurgical versus surgical treatment of carpal tunnel syndrome. *J Hand Surg Am.* 2009;34:1193–1200.

8 Scaphoid Fractures

S. Brent Brotzman, MD | Steven R. Novotny, MD

BACKGROUND

The scaphoid (carpal navicular) is the most commonly fractured of the carpal bones, and carpal fractures often are difficult to diagnose and treat. Complications include nonunion and malunion, which alter wrist kinematics. This can lead to pain, decreased ROM, decrease in strength, and early radiocarpal arthrosis.

The **scaphoid blood supply is precarious.** The radial artery branches enter the scaphoid on the dorsal ridge, distal third, and lateral-volar surfaces. The **proximal third** of the scaphoid receives its blood supply from intraosseous circulation in about one-third of scaphoids and thus is **at high risk of osteonecrosis (ON).**

Scaphoid fractures usually are **classified by location of fracture: proximal third, middle third (or waist), distal third, or tuberosity.** Fractures of the middle third are most common, and distal third fractures are rare. Besides the location of the fracture, comminution and displacement have a dramatic impact on the healing rate.

CLINICAL HISTORY AND EXAMINATION

Scaphoid fractures usually occur with hyperextension and radial flexion of the wrist, most often in young active male patients. Patients usually have tenderness in the anatomic snuffbox (between the first and the second dorsal compartments), less commonly on the distal scaphoid tuberosity volarly, and may have increased pain with axial compression of the thumb metacarpal and decreased grip strength. Nondisplaced scaphoid fractures are often difficult to evaluate radiographically because of the bone's oblique orientation in the wrist and the minimal calcific disruption seen.

Initial radiographs should include posteroanterior (PA), oblique, lateral, and ulnar deviation PA. If there is any question clinically, an MRI is extremely sensitive in detecting scaphoid fractures as early as 2 days after injury. A comparison of MRI and bone scintigraphy found a sensitivity of 80% and specificity of 100% for MRI done within 24 hours of injury and 100% and 90%, respectively, for bone scintigraphy done 3 to 5 days after injury (Beeres et al. 2008). Bone contusion and micro fractures will produce edematous changes that will be seen on the MRI at this time, which could lead to an overcautious diagnosis and unnecessarily prolonged treatment.

If an MRI is unavailable, patients with snuffbox tenderness should be immobilized for 10 to 14 days and then return for repeat radiographs out of the splint. If follow-up radiographs are positive the diagnosis is certain; however if negative, clinical exam should dictate further imaging (Low 2005). If the diagnosis is still questionable, a bone scan is indicated (Tiel-van Buul 1993).

Assessment of **scaphoid fracture displacement** is crucial for treatment and is often best assessed with thin section (1-mm) computed tomography (CT) scans. Displacement is defined as a fracture gap of more than 1 mm, a lateral scapholunate angle greater than 60 degrees, lateral radiolunate angle greater than 15 degrees, or intrascaphoid angle greater than 35 degrees.

Most clinically diagnosed scaphoid fractures turn out to be nonfactual fractures. Sjolin and Andersen (1988) reported on 108 patients with clinically diagnosed scaphoid fractures. They report 14 days of sick time with plaster and 4 days with a soft wrap. Two fractures were suspected radiographically, and four had avulsion fragments from the tuberosity; however, none had verifiable complete fractures. They conclude that since these fractures almost always heal irrespective of treatment, soft dressing should be used. Jacobsen (1995) provides a more complete thought on this clinical question. Of their 231 patients with clinical scaphoid fracture, only three were proven on subsequent radiographs; if four to five quality radiographs are taken and viewed by an experienced radiologist almost 100% of factual fractures can be seen on the initial radiographs. They recommend supportive bandage during the observation period if the initial radiographs are negative.

The question of long arm cast versus short arm cast and thumb spica or not hasn't been completely answered. Gellman (1989) published a small series of long arm thumb spica versus short arm thumb spica treated scaphoid fractures. Those treated initially with a long system healed radiographically faster without nonunion. Those treated with a short system healed slower, with some delayed and nonunions. They recommend initial long arm treatment. Clay (1991) randomized 392 fresh fractures to short arm thumb spica or short arm cast treatment. Of the 292 followed for 6 months, the incidence of nonunion was independent of which cast was used. Patients were followed every 2 weeks for cast change as needed and immobilized for 8 weeks. Unfortunately almost 25% of enrolled patients didn't complete follow-up, and only 60% of proximal pole fractures were definitely healed. The small number of proximal pole fractures followed (12, and only six definitely healed) still doesn't answer the question if all nondisplaced scaphoid fractures should be treated equally. One common theme when authors report good results with cast immobilization is frequent evaluation for cast loosening, molding the cast into the palm, and discussion of compliance issues.

Two meta-analysis studies with different inclusion criteria recently were published. Doornberg (2011) looked mainly at types of immobilization and functional outcome from randomized trials and didn't detect a clinical difference between the types of treatment. Alshryda (2012) showed that the type of immobilization wasn't a factor as long as the wrist was not placed in flexion, operative treatment did not produce a higher union rate in nondisplaced fractures, and open repair trended superior to percutaneous treatment.

TREATMENT

Truly nondisplaced fractures can be treated closed and nearly always heal with well molded cast immobilization. Above- or below-elbow casting is still a subject of controversy. In proximal fractures we prefer 6 weeks of long arm thumb spica casting, followed by a minimum of 3 weeks of short arm thumb spica casting. If radiographs do not demonstrate healing we immobilize for another 3 weeks. Scaphoid union can be verified with thin section CT scan if needed at this time. The expense would only be warranted for very few. Most are continued with immobilization until radiographic union. Waist and distal fractures are treated with a short arm system. If on follow-up radiographs the fracture displaces or fracture line significantly widens we revert to screw fixation.

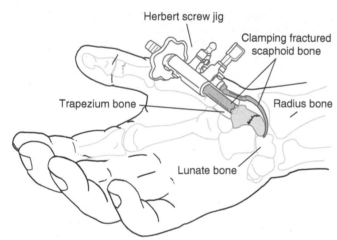

Fig. 8.1 Combined passive flexion and extension exercises of the metacarpophalangeal (MCP), proximal interphalangeal (PIP), and distal interphalangeal (DIP) joints.

Surgical treatment is indicated for the following:
• Nondisplaced fractures in which the complications of prolonged immobilization (wrist stiffness, thenar atrophy, and delayed return to heavy labor or sports) would be intolerable
• Scaphoid fractures previously unrecognized or untreated
• Displaced scaphoid fractures (see previous for criteria for displacement)
• Scaphoid nonunions

For nondisplaced or minimally displaced fractures, percutaneous fixation with cannulated screws has become accepted treatment. A recent meta-analysis reported that percutaneous fixation may result in union 5 weeks earlier than cast treatment and return to sport or work about 7 weeks earlier than with cast treatment (Modi et al. 2009). For fractures with **marked** displacement, ORIF is mandatory (Fig. 8.1) (Rehabilitation Protocol 8.1). Huene (Huene 1979) reported a small series of scaphoid repairs including four athletes. All athletes were returned to their sport within 6 to 8 weeks unprotected. Rettig (Rettig 1994) retrospectively reviewed 30 athletes injured preseason or early season and those who planned on participating in a subsequent season sport. Those who could play in a cast were allowed to; those whose sport didn't allow a playing cast had screw fixation. After surgery return to sports was allowed once range of motion was within 10% of the opposite side and the fracture wasn't tender. Both had comparable results.

REHABILITATION

Once released from the cast, a standard mobilization protocol such as with a distal radius fracture is undertaken. Active-assisted range of motion and progressive strengthening are the therapy mainstays. Heat as an adjunct for joint mobilization or cold for new rounds of swelling can be employed at home in addition to massage and tendon and nerve glides. The overall emphasis is on patient accountability. The therapist needs to ensure that clients understand their home program responsibilities completely. Most personal activities can be resumed once protective range of motion is restored. Safety issues may dictate a graduated return to previous level of function due to workplace safety concerns.

REHABILITATION PROTOCOL 8.1 ▪ **Rehabilitation Protocol After Treatment and Rehabilitation for Scaphoid Fractures**

For Fractures Treated Closed (Nonoperative), Treatment in Thumb Spica Cast

0–6 Weeks
• Above elbow thumb spica cast for proximal pole, short arm thumb spica for mid and distal poles
• Active shoulder ROM
• Active second through fifth MCP/PIP/DIP joint ROM

6–12 Weeks
• Short arm thumb spica cast
• Continue shoulder and finger exercises.
• Begin active elbow flexion/extension/supination/ pronation.

12 Weeks or Bony Union
• CT scan to confirm union if radiographs in doubt. If not united, continue short arm thumb spica cast.
• If cysts are forming intramedullary, reverting to screw fixation and possible bone grafting should be considered.

12–14 Weeks
• Assuming union at 12 weeks, removable thumb spica splint
• Begin home exercise program.
• Active/gentle-assisted wrist flexion/extension ROM
• Active/gentle-assisted wrist radial/ulnar flexion ROM
• Active/gentle-assisted thumb MCP/IP joint ROM
• Active/gentle-assisted thenar cone exercise

14–18 Weeks
• Discontinue all splinting.
• Formalized physical/occupational therapy
• Active/aggressive-assisted wrist flexion/extension ROM
• Active/aggressive-assisted wrist radial/ulnar flexion ROM
• Active/aggressive-assisted thumb MCP/IP joint ROM
• Active/aggressive-assisted thenar cone exercise

Continued

REHABILITATION PROTOCOL 8.1 ● **Rehabilitation Protocol After Treatment and Rehabilitation for Scaphoid Fractures—cont'd**

18 Weeks +

- Grip strengthening, aggressive ROM
- Unrestricted activities

For Scaphoid Fractures Treated With ORIF

0–10 Days

- Elevate sugar-tong thumb spica splint, ice
- Shoulder ROM
- MCP/PIP/DIP joint active ROM exercises

10 Days–4 Weeks

- Suture removal
- Exos forearm-based thumb spica rigid splint to allow washing and scar modification, or casting for a total of 3 to 4 weeks after surgery
- Continue hand/elbow/shoulder ROM.

4–7 Weeks

- Removeable short arm thumb spica splint system
- Elbow active/assisted extension, flexion/supination/pronation; continue fingers 2 through 5 active ROM and shoulder active ROM
- Wrist motion is initiated active only, not passive.

8–10 Weeks (Assuming Union)

- Emphasis on home exercise program
- Active/gentle-assisted wrist flexion and extension ROM
- Active/gentle-assisted wrist radial/ulnar flexion ROM
- Active/gentle-assisted thumb MCP/IP joint ROM
- Active/gentle-assisted thenar cone exercise
- Once fracture union present, progressive strengthening can be instituted

10–14 Weeks

- Discontinue all splinting.
- Formalized physical/occupational therapy can be discontinued with patient understanding of his or her responsibility and good early recovery. Continue formal office program if poor progress
- Active/aggressive-assisted wrist flexion/extension ROM
- Active/aggressive-assisted wrist radial/ulnar flexion ROM
- Active/aggressive-assisted thumb MCP/IP joint ROM
- Active/aggressive-assisted thenar cone exercise

14 Weeks +

- Aggressive ROM if still needed
- Unrestricted activities

REFERENCES

A complete reference list is available at https://expertconsult .inkling.com/.

FURTHER READING

Beeres FJ, Rhemrey SJ, den Hollander P, et al. Early magnetic resonance imaging compared with bone scintigraphy in suspected scaphoid fractures. *J Bone Joint Surg Br*. 2009;90:1250.

Martineau PA, Berry GK, Harvey EJ. Plating for distal radius fractures. *Hand Clin*. 2010;26:61.

Yin ZG, Zhang JB, Kan SL, et al. Diagnosing suspected scaphoid fractures: a systematic review and meta-analysis. *Clin Orthop Rel Res*. 2009;468(3):723–734.

9

Triangular Fibrocartilage Complex Injury

Felix H. Savoie III, MD | Michael J. O'Brien, MD | Larry D. Field, MD

CLINICAL BACKGROUND

The triangular fibrocartilage complex is an arrangement of several structures. The primary structure is the triangular fibrocartilage or meniscal disc that is a relatively avascular disclike structure that provides a cushion effect between the distal articular surface of the ulna and the proximal carpal row, primarily the triquetrum.

Much like the menisci in the knee, vascular studies have demonstrated poor central vascularity, whereas the peripheral 15% to 20% has the arterial inflow required for healing. In addition, there is no vascular contribution from the radial base of the TFCC. **Thus, central defects or tears tend to have difficulty healing and more peripheral injuries heal at a much higher rate.**

The disc is a biconcave structure with a radial attachment that blends with the articular cartilage of the radius. The ulnar attachment lies at the base of the ulnar styloid (Fig. 9.1). The anterior and posterior thickenings of the TFCC are confluent with the anterior and posterior radioulnar capsule and are called the *palmar* and *dorsal radioulnar ligaments*. These structures develop tension as the forearm is pronated and supinated and provide the primary stabilization to the DRUJ (Fig. 9.2). The TFCC itself is under maximal tension in neutral rotation. Additional attachments to the lunate, triquetrum, hamate, and the base of the fifth metacarpal have been described. These structures, combined with the extensor carpi ulnaris subsheath, make up the TFCC. Normal function of the DRUJ requires the normal relationship of these anatomic structures. Tear, injury, or degeneration of any one structure leads to pathophysiology of the DRUJ and abnormal kinesis of the wrist and forearm. When evaluating *ulnar-sided wrist pain* or painful forearm rotation, several entities should be considered.

CLASSIFICATION

The most widely accepted classification system of TFCC injuries is that developed by Palmer (1989) (Fig. 9.3). *TFCC tears are divided into two categories: traumatic and degenerative.* The system uses clinical, radiographic, anatomic, and biomechanical data to define each tear. Rehabilitation of these lesions is based on the type of procedure performed. In **Class 1A or 2A lesions** the central portion of the disc is débrided, and in this case, the rehabilitation is a return to activities as tolerated after wound healing has taken place. For most other TFCC lesions, a more extensive immobilization period followed by aggressive physical therapy is required.

DIAGNOSIS

A thorough history is critical to the diagnosis of TFCC lesions. Factors such as onset and duration of symptoms, type and force of trauma, eliciting activities, recent changes in symptoms, and past treatment attempts should be noted. Most TFCC injuries are caused by a fall on an outstretched hand, rotational injuries, or repetitive axial loading. *Patients complain of ulnar-sided wrist pain; clicking; and often crepitation with forearm rotation, gripping, or ulnar deviation of the wrist.* Tenderness often is present on either the dorsal or the palmar side of the TFCC. Instability of the DRUJ or clicking may or may not be elicited. Care should be taken to rule out extensor carpi ulnaris (ECU) tendon subluxation and radial-sided wrist injuries.

Provocative maneuvers are often helpful in differentiating TFCC injuries from lunotriquetral pathology.
- First, the pisotriquetral joint should be tested to rule out disease at this joint. With the wrist in neutral rotation, the triquetrum is firmly compressed against the lunate.
- The **"shuck test"** (Reagan et al. 1984) may be a more sensitive test of the lunotriquetral joint. The lunotriquetral joint is grasped between the thumb and the index finger while the wrist is stabilized with the other hand and the lunotriquetral joint is "shucked" in a dorsal-to-palmar direction.
- The **shear test** has been described as the most sensitive test to elicit lunotriquetral pathology. In this test, one thumb is placed against the pisiform and the other thumb stabilizes the lunate on its dorsal surface. As the examiner's thumbs are forced toward the carpus, a shear force is created in the lunotriquetral joint.
- The **press test** has been reported to be 100% sensitive for TFFC tears (Lester et al. 1995). In the press test, the patient grasps both sides of a chair seat while sitting in the chair. The patient then presses the body weight directly upward, and if the pain replicates the ulnar-sided pain, the test is considered positive.

Once a normal lunotriquetral joint is established, the TFCC is then evaluated.
- The **TFCC grind test** is very sensitive in eliciting tears in the TFCC and DRUJ instability. With the wrist in neutral rotation and ulnarly deviated, it is rolled palmarly then dorsally. Pain or a click suggests a TFCC tear. When done with the forearm fully pronated, the dorsal radioulnar ligaments are

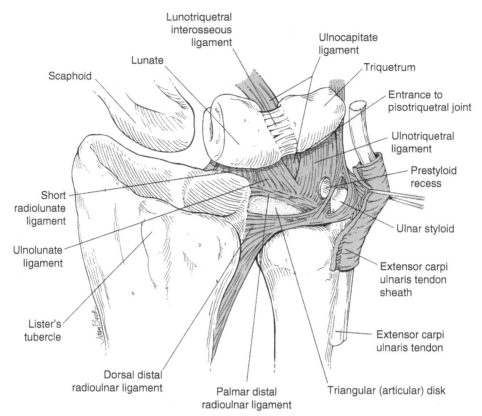

Fig. 9.1   Anatomy of the triangular fibrocartilage complex. (From Cooney WP, Linscheid RL, Dobyns JH: The Wrist Diagnosis and Operative Treatment. St. Louis, Mosby, 1998.)

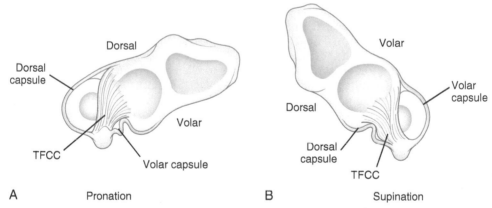

Fig. 9.2   **A,** Right wrist in pronation. The dorsal capsule is tight, and the volar margin of the triangular fibrocartilage complex (TFCC; the volar radioulnar ligament) is tight. **B,** Right wrist in supination. The volar distal radioulnar joint capsule is tight, and the dorsal margin of the TFCC (dorsal radioulnar ligament) is tight as the dorsal margin of the radius moves farther away from the base of the ulnar styloid.

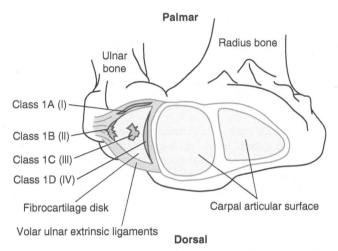

Fig. 9.3 The Palmer classification of acute tears of the triangular fibrocartilage complex. Class 1A, central tear of the fibrocartilage disk tissue (I). Class 1B, ulnar-sided peripheral detachment (II). Class 1C, tear of the volar ulnar extrinsic ligaments (III). Class 1D, radial-sided peripheral attachment (IV).

tested. With the forearm fully supinated, the volar radioulnar ligaments are assessed.

- The **piano key test** evaluates DRUJ stability. With the forearm fully pronated, the distal ulna is balloted from dorsal to volar. This test correlates with the "piano key sign" seen on lateral wrist radiographs.
- Another more recently described physical sign is the **"fovea sign,"** which consists of tenderness that replicates the patient's pain when pressure is applied to the region of the fovea. In a series of 272 patients who had wrist arthroscopy, the fovea sign had a sensitivity of 95% and a specificity of 86% (Tay et al. 2007).

IMAGING STUDIES

Radiographs of the wrist include PA, lateral, and oblique views taken with the shoulder abducted to 90 degrees, the elbow flexed to 90 degrees, and the forearm flat on the table. When indicated, specialty views such as a supination–pronation, a clenched-fist PA, and a 30-degree supination view to assess the pisotriquetral joint may be obtained.

Arthrography may be used as a confirmatory test. Radiopaque contrast material is injected directly into the radiocarpal joint. If a tear is present, the dye will extravasate into the region of the tear. Some reports suggest that three-compartment (radiocarpal, DRUJ, and midcarpal) injections are a more accurate method of assessing TFCC lesions. Care must be taken when interpreting wrist arthrograms because a high occurrence of false-negative readings has been reported. Asymptomatic TFCC, interosseous ligament tears, and details of the exact tear location may also appear on wrist arthrography, although adjacent soft tissue structures or articular surfaces are not well delineated. Plain arthrography has largely been supplanted by MRI.

MRI of the wrist has evolved into a useful resource in diagnosing TFCC lesions. Although an experienced radiologist is imperative, the coils and techniques are now approaching arthroscopy in sensitivity and predictive value of TFCC tears. *Potter et al. (1997) reported that MRI had a sensitivity of 100%, specificity of 90%, and accuracy of 97% in 57 wrists with arthroscopically verified*

BOX 9.1 DIFFERENTIAL DIAGNOSIS OF ULNAR-SIDED WRIST PAIN

Radial shortening (e.g., comminuted distal radial fracture) relative to the ulna
Triangular fibrocartilage complex tear (central versus peripheral)
Degenerative joint disease
Lunotriquetral arthritis
Extensor carpi ulnaris (ECU) instability or tendinitis
Fracture of the hook of the hamate
Flexor carpi ulnaris (FCU) calcific tendinitis
Pisotriquetral arthritis
Ulnar artery stenosis
Guyon's canal syndrome
Ulnar styloid fracture
Congenital positive ulnar variance
Ulnar nerve disease

BOX 9.2 CLASSIFICATION OF TRIANGULAR FIBROCARTILAGE COMPLEX (TFCC) LESIONS (PALMER)

CLASS 1: TRAUMATIC

A. Central perforation
B. Ulnar avulsion
   With ulnar styloid fracture
   Without ulnar styloid fracture
C. Distal avulsion
D. Radial avulsion
   With sigmoid notch fracture
   Without sigmoid notch fracture

CLASS 2: DEGENERATIVE (ULNOCARPAL ABUTMENT SYNDROME)

A. TFCC wear
B. TFCC wear
   With lunate or ulnar chondromalacia
C. TFCC perforation
   With lunate or ulnar chondromalacia
D. TFCC perforation
   With lunate or ulnar chondromalacia
   With lunotriquetral ligament perforation
E. TFCC perforation
   With lunate or ulnar chondromalacia
   With lunotriquetral ligament perforation
   With ulnocarpal arthritis

TFCC lesions. More recent studies indicate lower accuracy rates (≈70% to 80%) and only approximately 40% for lesion localization with MRI. The advantage of MRI over arthrography lies in the ability to identify the location of the lesion.

The "gold standard" in diagnosing wrist injuries is arthroscopy. No other technique is as accurate or reliable in locating the lesion. In addition, arthroscopy allows the surgeon to palpate and observe every structure in the wrist, making it easier to treat all possible components of the injury. Arthroscopy also avoids the complications associated with open wrist surgery and allows a speedier rehabilitation after immobilization.

TREATMENT

Surgical intervention for TFCC injuries is indicated only after a full course of nonoperative measures.

Initially, the wrist is *braced* for 4 to 6 weeks. NSAIDs are used, and occasionally a *corticosteroid injection* may be beneficial. After *immobilization, physical therapy* is initiated. First, active-assisted and passive ROM exercises are begun. Then, aggressive motion exercises and resisted strengthening rehabilitation are added, followed by plyometric and sports-specific therapy. Most patients with TFCC tears respond well to bracing and therapy.

If nonoperative care fails and symptoms persist, surgery is indicated. In athletes, surgery may be done earlier because of competitive and seasonal considerations. Although a controversial issue, delaying surgical treatment of TFCC tears may adversely affect the outcome.

Surgical intervention is predicated on the type of TFCC tear (Fig. 9.3). Treatment of some tears remains controversial, whereas treatment of others is more widely accepted.

Arthroscopic débridement and repair have been shown to achieve results similar to those obtained with open procedures (Anderson et al. 2008, McAdams et al. 2009). In one retrospective series of 16 high-level competitive athletes, return to play averaged 3.3 months after arthroscopic débridement or repair. Return to play was delayed in athletes with concomitant ulnar-sided wrist injuries (McAdams et al. 2009).

- For **Type 1A** tears, débridement of the central tear is usually preferred if there is no DRUJ instability. Up to two thirds of the central disc can be removed without significantly altering the biomechanics of the wrist. Care must be taken to avoid violating the volar or dorsal radioulnar ligaments to prevent DRUJ instability.
- **Type 1B** tears affect the periphery of the TFCC. This is recognized by the loss of the "trampoline" effect of the central

BOX 9.3   EVALUATION AND MANAGEMENT OF ACUTE ULNAR-SIDED WRIST TRAUMA

DRUJ Manual Stress Examination	Focal Tenderness Examination (positive ulnocarpal stress test plus)	Radiographic Examination	Treatment
Stable DRUJ Check amplitude and end-point compared with contralateral side in supination, neutral, and pronation.	Tender over disc radial to ECU, or tender over ulnar sling but not tender at fovea precisely	No fracture of radius near the sigmoid notch Distal tip of ulnar styloid may or may not have a small fracture fragment	Initial: cortisone steroid injection of ulnocarpal joint up to 2 times at 3-week intervals Final: arthroscopic débridement of loose fibrocartilage tissue fragments that prove mechanically unstable to direct probe manipulation Supplemental: ulnar shortening osteotomy if preexisting ulnocarpal impaction
Unstable DRUJ	Tender specifically at fovea (i.e., positive "fovea sign")	No fracture of ulna near fovea	Open repair of purely ligamentous avulsion of ulnar attachment of radioulnar ligaments, arthroscopic repair, or immobilization of the DRUJ in supination. Palmaris longus tendon graft augmentation may be required with late presentation (after 6 weeks).
Unstable DRUJ	Tender at ulnar styloid	Displaced fracture of ulnar styloid involving its base and containing the foveal region	Tension band wiring of styloid fragment. Make sure that radioulnar ligaments actually attach to styloid fragment.
Unstable DRUJ	Tender radially over disc and margin of sigmoid notch	Displaced fracture of distal radius involving the margin of the sigmoid notch	Open or arthroscopic reduction and fixation of displaced sigmoid notch marginal fragments with Kirschner wire or screw

DRUJ, distal radioulnar joint; ECU, extensor carpi ulnaris.

REHABILITATION PROTOCOL 9.1 ■ Rehabilitation Protocol After TFCC Débridement

Felix H. Savoie III, MD, Michael O'Brien, MD, Larry D. Field, MD

The protocol initially focuses on tissue healing and early immobilization. When TFCC repair is performed, the wrist is immobilized for 6 weeks and forearm pronation/supination is prevented for the same period of time with the use of a Muenster cast.

Phase 1: 0–7 Days
- Soft dressing to encourage wound healing and decrease soft tissue edema

Phase 2: 7 Days Variable
- ROM exercises are encouraged.
- Return to normal activities as tolerated

Phase 3: When Pain Free
- Resisted strengthening exercises, plyometrics, and sports-specific rehabilitation (see later)

disc. Repairs of these tears usually heal because of the adequate blood supply.

- **Type 1D** tears fall in the controversial category. Traditional treatment has been débridement of the tear followed by early motion. Several authors, however, have reported improved results with surgical repair of these tears. In our clinic, repair of radial-sided tears to the sigmoid notch of the radius is preferred (Rehabilitation Protocols 9.1 and 9.2).

Type 2 tears are degenerative by definition and often occur in athletes who stress their wrists (gymnastics,

---

REHABILITATION PROTOCOL 9.2 ● **Rehabilitation Protocol After Repair of TFCC Tear (With OR Without Lunotriquetral Pinning)**

Felix H. Savoie III, MD, Michael O'Brien, MD, Larry D. Field, MD

Phase 1: 0–7 Days

- The immediate postoperative period focuses on decreasing the soft tissue edema and the joint effusion. Maintaining an immobilized wrist and elbow is important, and a combination of ice or cold therapy and elevation are desired. The upper extremity is placed in a sling.
- Finger flexion/extension exercises are initiated to prevent possible tenodesis and decrease soft tissue edema.
- Active-assisted and passive shoulder ROM exercises are instituted to prevent loss of motion in the glenohumeral joint. These are performed at home.

7 Days–2 Weeks

- During the first office visit, the sutures are removed and a Münster cast is applied. Once again, the wrist is completely immobilized and elbow flexion/extension is encouraged.
- Hand and shoulder ROM exercises are continued.
- Sling is removed.

2–4 Weeks

- The hard cast is removed and a removable Münster cast or brace applied.
- Cast is removed for gentle wrist flexion and extension twice a day.

4–6 Weeks

- The Münster cast is replaced to account for decreased swelling. Elbow flexion and extension are continued, but forearm rotation is avoided.
- Gentle wrist flexion/extension exercises are initiated.
- Progression to a strongly resistive squeeze ball is begun.
- Hand and shoulder exercises are continued.

6 Weeks

- The Münster cast is removed and a neutral wrist splint is used as needed.
- Lunotriquetral wires (if used) are removed in the office.
- Active pain-free pronation and supination are allowed.

8 Weeks

- Progressive active and passive ROM exercises are instituted in the six planes of wrist motion (see section on distal radius fractures).
- Once pain-free ROM exercises are accomplished, strengthening exercises are begun.
1. Weighted wrist curls in six planes of wrist motion using small dumbbells or elastic tubing. This includes the volar, dorsal, ulnar, radial, pronation, and supination directions. Once strength returns, the Cybex machine may be used to further develop pronation–supination strength.
2. Four-way diagonal upper extremity patterns utilizing dumbbells, cable weights, or elastic tubing
3. Flexor–pronator forearm exercises. Wrist begins in extension, supination, and radial deviation, and utilizing a dumbbell as resistance, the wrist is brought into flexion, pronation, and ulnar deviation.
4. Resisted finger extension/flexion exercise with hand grips and elastic tubing

5. Upper extremity plyometrics are instituted. Once wall-falling/push-off is accomplished (see 6A), weighted medicine ball exercises are begun. Initially, a 1-pound ball is used; then the weight of the ball is progressed as indicated.
6. The plyometrics exercises are tailored to the patient's activity interests. If the patient is an athlete, sports-specific exercises are added.
   A. Wall-falling in which a patient stands 3 to 4 feet from a wall. Patient falls into the wall, catching on hands, and rebounds to starting position.
   B. Medicine ball throw in which a medicine ball is grasped with both hands in chest position. Ball is push-passed to a partner or trampoline. On return, the ball is taken into the overhead position.
   C. Medicine ball throw in which a medicine ball is grasped with both hands in the chest position. Ball is push-passed to a partner or trampoline. On return, the ball is taken into the chest position.
   D. Medicine ball throw in which a medicine ball is push-passed off a wall and rebounded in the chest position.
   E. Medicine ball throw in which the ball is grasped in one hand in the diagonal position and thrown to a partner or trampoline. Rebound is taken in the diagonal position over the shoulder. This may be performed across the body or with both hands.
   F. Medicine ball throw in which the patient is lying supine with upper extremity unsupported abducted to 90 degrees and externally rotated to 90 degrees. A medicine ball weighing 8 ounces to 2 pounds is dropped by a partner from a height of 2 to 3 feet. When the ball is caught, it is returned to a partner in a throwing motion as rapidly as possible.
   G. Medicine ball push-up with wrist in palmar flexion, dorsiflexion, radial deviation, and ulna deviation. This may be performed with the knees on the ground to begin with and progress to weight on toes as strength returns.
- Sports-specific exercises are designed to emulate the biomechanical activity encountered during play. With overhead and throwing athletes, the following program should be instituted:
   - Initially, ROM exercises establish pain-free motion. All aforementioned exercises are instituted and developed.
   - A weighted baton is used to recreate the motion of throwing, shooting, or racquet sport. This is progressed to elastic resistance. Ball-free batting practice is likewise begun.
   - Finally, actual throwing, shooting, or overhead racquet activities are begun.
   - Contact athletes, such as football linemen, will begin bench presses and bench flies. Initially, the bars are unweighted. Painless weight progression and repetition progression as tolerated are performed.
   - Work-hardening tasks such as using a wrench and pliers to tighten nuts and bolts are done. A screwdriver may be used to tighten/loosen screws.

3 Months

- Minimum time for splint-free return to sports

throwing and racquet sports, wheelchair sports). Nonoperative treatment should be continued for at least 3 months before arthroscopy. Most of these lesions are in patients with an ulna neutral or positive wrist. In these patients, débridement of the central degenerative disc tear is followed by an extra-articular ulnar shortening procedure such as the wafer procedure.

REFERENCES

A complete reference list is available at https://expertconsult.inkling.com/.

FURTHER READING

Adams BD. Partial excision of the triangular fibrocartilage complex articular disc: biomechanical study. *J Hand Surg.* 1993;18A:919.

Ahn AK, Chang D, Plate AM. Triangular fibrocartilage complex tears: a review. *Bull NYU Hosp Jt Dis.* 2007;64:114–118.

Atzel A. New trends in arthroscopic management of type 1-B TFCC injuries with DRUJ instability. *J Hand Surg Eur.* 2009;34:582–591.

Byrk FS, Savoie FHIII, Field LD. The role of arthroscopy in the diagnosis and management of cartilaginous lesions of the wrist. *Hand Clin.* 1999;15(3):423.

Cooney WP, Linscheid RL, Dobyns JH. Triangular fibrocartilage tears. *J Hand Surg.* 1994;19A:143.

Corso SJ, Savoie FH, Geissler WB, et al. Arthroscopic repair of peripheral avulsions of the triangular fibrocartilage complex of the wrist: a multicenter study. *Arthroscopy.* 1997;13:78.

Estrella EP, Hung LK, Ho PC, et al. Arthroscopic repair of triangular fibrocartilage complex tears. *Arthroscopy.* 2007;23:729–737.

Feldon P, Terrono AL, Belsky MR. Wafer distal ulna resection for triangular fibrocartilage tears and/or ulna impaction syndrome. *J Hand Surg.* 1992;17A:731.

Fellinger M, Peicha G, Seibert FJ, et al. Radial avulsion of the triangular fibrocartilage complex in acute wrist trauma: a new technique for arthroscopic repair. *Arthroscopy.* 1997;13:370.

Henry MH. Management of acute triangular fibrocartilage complex injury of the wrist. *J Am Acad Orthop Surg.* 2008;16:320–329.

Jantea CL, Baltzer A, Ruther W. Arthroscopic repair of radial-sided lesions of the fibrocartilage complex. *Hand Clin.* 1995;11:31.

Johnstone DJ, Thorogood S, Smith WH, et al. A comparison of magnetic resonance imaging and arthroscopy in the investigation of chronic wrist pain. *J Hand Surg.* 1997;22B(6):714.

Levinsohn EM, Rosen ID, Palmer AK. Wrist arthrography: value of the three-compartment injection method. *Radiology.* 1991;179:231.

Loftus JB, Palmer AK. Disorders of the distal radioulnar joint and triangular fibrocartilage complex: an overview. In: Lichtman DM, Alexander AH, eds. *The Wrist and Its Disorders.* 2nd ed. Philadelphia: WB Saunders; 1997:385–414.

Nagle DJ. Triangular fibrocartilage complex tears in the athlete. *Clin Sports Med.* 2001;20:155–166.

Palmer AK, Glisson RR, Werner FW. Ulnar variance determination. *J Hand Surg.* 1982;7A:376.

Palmer AK, Werner FW. The triangular fibrocartilage complex of the wrist: anatomy and function. *J Hand Surg.* 1981;6A:153.

Palmer AK, Werner FW, Glisson RR, et al. Partial excision of the triangular fibrocartilage complex. *J Hand Surg.* 1988;13A:403.

Papapetropoulos PA, Ruch DS. Arthroscopic repair of triangular fibrocartilage complex tears in athletes. *Hand Clin.* 2009;25:389–394.

Pederzini L, Luchetti R, Soragni O, et al. Evaluation of the triangular fibrocartilage complex tears by arthroscopy, arthrography and magnetic resonance imaging. *Arthroscopy.* 1992;8:191.

Peterson RK, Savoie FH, Field LD. Arthroscopic treatment of sports injuries to the triangular fibrocartilage. *Sports Med Artho Rev.* 1998;6:262.

Reiter MB, Wolf U, Schmid, et al. Arthroscopic repair of Palmer 1B triangular fibrocartilage complex tears. *Arthroscopy.* 2008;24:1244–1250.

Roth JH, Haddad RG. Radiocarpal arthroscopy and arthrography in the diagnosis of ulnar wrist pain. *Arthroscopy.* 1986;2:234.

Sagerman SD, Short W. Arthroscopic repair of radial-sided triangular fibrocartilage complex tears. *Arthroscopy.* 1996;12:339.

Savoie FH. The role of arthroscopy in the diagnosis and management of cartilaginous lesions of the wrist. *Hand Clin.* 1995;11:1.

Trumble TE, Gilbert M, Bedder N. Arthroscopic repair of the triangular fibrocartilage complex. *Arthroscopy.* 1996;12:588.

Viegas SF, Patterson RM, Hokanson JA, et al. Wrist anatomy: incidence, distribution and correlation of anatomic variations, tears and arthrosis. *J Hand Surg.* 1993;18A:463.

Metacarpal Phalangeal Joint Arthroplasty

Steven R. Novotny, MD

Arthroplasty of the metacarpal phalangeal joints of the hand has been around for decades, and yet the debate as to which type of arthroplasty to use in which patients still hasn't been settled. The FDA has limited the newer implants—Ascension PyroCarbon, Avanta Polyethylene resurfacing, and others—to humanitarian use only. Thus organizations with certain relationships to the federal government, such as medical schools, residencies with salaries supported by the government, and Veteran Affairs facilities, must review each patient for consideration of compassionate use or have a research protocol fully vetted and approved by the IRB committee to enroll patients in these research studies. Those in private practice can utilize these products just by discussing this with their patients along with the risks and benefits of the surgery.

A complete history of MCP arthroplasty is impractical for our purposes, though knowing some of the past may put the present in perspective and shed light on the future (Berger 1989). Capsulectomy and various MCP débridement without interposition have been tried with reasonable results on selected, often highly motivated patients with reasonable outcomes. The results were never good enough to recommend the wholesale advocacy of these procedures.

In the 1950s and early 1960s a series of solid metal stem hinge implants were developed. Brannon and Klein (1959), Flatt (1961), and Richards are names associated with these. None of them lasted long. Brannon published last on this in 1959, noting it as a salvage procedure, and all his patients returned to military function. No further mention is made of this enterprise. Richards' prosthesis had short intramedullary stems, limited fixation, and short joint lifespan. Flatt's prosthesis had tuning fork–like duel stems instead of solid shanks. Zachariae (1967) reported on 6 patients with 11 Flatt prosthesis. Two became infected with one removed, all prostheses subsided if the joints continued articulating, and rheumatoid patients on steroids showed some resorption by 6 months. Overall function was maintained and pain relief persisted over the 4-year review. The authors still considered the procedure valuable, especially for pain control in the elderly. Flatt and Ellison's (1972) review of 167 MCP showed a 10% complication rate including prosthetic failure, severe soft tissue erosion, fracture, and severe resorption. Others (Blair et al. 1984) have independently confirmed the results and have affirmed patient satisfaction in the face of significant complications.

Resection arthroplasty and resection interposition arthroplasty of the MCP joint were formalized as an acceptable treatment by Fowler (1962) in 1962, Vainio (1974), and Tupper (1989) in 1989. Their techniques varied, with Fowler resecting the head in a "V" shaped fashion and the extensor tendon tenodesed to the proximal phalanx to prevent swan neck deformity. Vainio transversely resected the metacarpal head and cut the extensor tendon at the resection level, inserting the distal stump as an interposition sutured to the volar proximal phalanx base. The proximal tendon end was then repaired to the extensor tendon at the dorsal proximal phalanx level restoring extensor function. Tupper attached the volar plate to the dorsal metacarpal neck. He rebalanced the joint deforming forces in a fashion now considered standard when rebalancing a rheumatoid MCP joint during arthroplasty.

Riordan and Fowler (1989) reviewed resection arthroplasty techniques, including surgeons not mentioned in the preceding paragraphs. They report all techniques result in resorption of bone and eventual tendency toward instability of the MCP joint and deformity. This does not always diminish function or patient satisfaction.

Silicone rubber arthroplasties are most associated with Alfred Swanson (Swanson 1972, Manerfelt and Andersson 1975), though other names and relatively similar prostheses are available (NeuFlex, Sutter). The painful arthritic joint is resected and the stemmed silicone spacer is initially held in place intramedullary while encapsulation around the joint occurs. The new functionally adaptive fibrous capsule develops around the joint spacer component. The immediate postoperative position and control of joint motion during the first 6 to 8 weeks by dynamic brace therapy are critical to this process. Slight pistoning of the prosthesis is normal and is felt to increase the life of the prosthesis by distributing stresses over a larger volume of the prosthesis. Repair or reconstruction (Swanson 1972, Kleinert and Sunil 2005) of the radial collateral ligament of the MCP along with extensor tendon realignment are critical to outcome.

Ferlic et al. (1975) reported their experience and overall good results with silicone rubber implants as Swanson had in 1972. Escott et al. (2010) in a randomized controlled level 1 study showed no statistical difference in functional outcomes between Swanson and NeuFlex prostheses. NeuFlex prostheses tended toward greater range of motion while the Swanson prostheses patients reported greater function and esthetics, though functional improvement could not be quantified. Parkkila and colleagues (2005) in a level 2 study of Swanson and Sutter MCP prostheses showed no significant difference except in index finger motion.

Waljee and Chung (2012) followed 46 patients for 2 years after silicone MCP arthroplasty. Patients were satisfied if pain was reduced, the extension lag was less than 30 degrees, the ulnar drift improved to less than 9 degrees, and the flexion improved an average of 10 degrees.

The trend is to replace osteoarthritic MCP joints with a more rigid prosthesis, metal-backed high molecular weight polyethylene (HMWPE), metal metacarpal head and plastic phalangeal component, or pyro carbon. Rettig et al. (2005) reported pain relief and motion sparing with silicone arthroplasty of the MCP joints at intermediate follow-up averaging 40 months. Dickson et al. (2015) in a published study utilizing pyrocarbon MCP prostheses demonstrated overall satisfaction and function; lucency developed around all prostheses without reduction in outcome. Failures leading to revision occurred within 18 months. Stern (Wall and Stern 2013) two years previously reported a very similar experience.

REHABILITATION

Nicola Massy-Westropp (2008, 2012) has published on the lack of consistent reporting of rehabilitation protocols in the literature. Most published reports on MCP arthroplasty do not report their rehab protocol precisely enough to be implemented by the readers. The only conclusion they can agree on is that therapy does improve MCP motion. Randomized controlled studies are lacking in this research arena; given the low numbers of patients it may not be practical unless matched studies are undertaken. Problems will always be present such as the inherent amount of disease, potential for tissue recovery, comorbidities, and medical management before and after the index procedure and how this could influence the eventual outcome (Rehabilitation protocols 10.1 and 10.2).

REHABILITATION PROTOCOL 10.1 ● Standard Rheumatoid Arthritis Protocol

In rheumatoid patients multiple joints—most likely all MCPs—have been replaced, in distinction to osteoarthritic patients in whom mainly the long and/or index are involved.

3–5 Days Postoperative

Bulky dressing removed, light compressive dressing utilized
Digital edema instituted, not hand until wound solidly healed
Modified long dorsal outrigger fabricated for continuous wear during day
- Wrist 15 degrees extension
- Slings under proximal phalanx, the outrigger is radial to the MCP, rubber bands angle 60 degrees to phalanx, to retard natural tendency to drift ulnarly, MCPs too neutral—AVOID HYPEREXTENSION
- Supinator attachment to index finger worn between dynamic sessions
Resting pan splint for nighttime
- Wrist 15 degrees extension and digits full extension, dividers to maintain linear alignment, index supinator strap if needed
AROM exercises initiated 10 minutes each hour in dynamic splint. Emphasize MCP flexion followed by IP motion into fist position, ending in full extension.
PROM twice a day, 15-minute reps each digit. Small finger often has the greatest difficulty. If difficulty with the joint, PROM may increase the number of passive sessions as long as the extensor lag <30 degrees. If the patient can obtain 70 to 80 degrees of active flexion, passive exercises are eliminated.

10–21 Days Postoperative

Scar modification is initiated once sutures are out and the tissue appears healthy to accept; all scar modification is performed gently.
Dynamic flexion splinting and/or frequency of passive flexion is increased if passive flexion >50 degrees

3–4 Weeks Postoperative

Light compressive dressing changed to elastic bandage
If difficultly achieving active MCP extension, reduce extension component of the brace to utilize wrist tenodesis effect on the MCPs
Wrist can be returned to slight extension after each session.

6 Weeks Postoperative

30 minutes light prehensile activity out of splint 3 to 4 times a day, no forceful or sustained grip. A soft ulnar drift splint can be used if indicated. Radial deviation activity while hand placed on flat surface is encouraged. Supinator tab is removed.

10–12 Weeks Postoperative

The dorsal outrigger can be discontinued at the surgeon's discretion. The pan splint is continued nightly for one year. Some company literature recommends pan splint for life.
Dynamic flexion splinting is discontinued once desired passive flexion is achieved.
Strengthening is encouraged by squeezing a cylinder of putty **unless** ulnar drift is present. If ulnar deviation is present, strengthening will increase the ulnar drift and is not indicated.

REHABILITATION PROTOCOL 10.2 ● Standard Osteoarthritic and Post-Traumatic Protocol

With an inherent greater level of soft tissue stability, the rehabilitation is slightly more aggressive with respect to eventual strengthening and potential return to a more aggressive lifestyle. If significant joint rebalancing, ligament reconstruction, or tendon grafting is needed, these factors may change the rehabilitation protocol.

1–3 Days Postoperative

- Light compressive dressing and outrigger initiated
- Dynamic flexion splinting can be initiated in one week if passive flexion >70 degrees. It may be necessary to use up to 6 hours of interval dynamic splinting per day.
- If difficulty in obtaining flexion and the extensor lag <15 degrees, reposition the pan splint to 15 degrees MCP flexion

6 Weeks Postoperative

- Progressive strengthening may be initiated.
- Outrigger discontinued between 6–8 weeks
- Dynamic flexion splint continued typically up to 12 weeks

8–10 Weeks Postoperative

- A more aggressive strengthening program may be initiated. Simulated job tasks and increased loading exercises to ensure a return to employment are appropriate.

10–12 Weeks Postoperative

- Dynamic flexion splint is discontinued.

12–16 Weeks Postoperative

- Resting night splint can be discontinued.

REFERENCES

A complete reference list is available at https://expertconsult.inkling.com/.

Rehabilitation After Total Elbow Arthroplasty

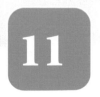
The Total Elbow

Sinan Emre Ozgur, MD | Charles E. Giangarra, MD

Total elbow arthroplasty (TEA) is a procedure that replaces the ulnohumeral articulation with a prosthetic device. The primary goal of TEA is to provide pain relief from a variety of conditions that result in destruction of the native ulnohumeral joint, causing pain and dysfunction refractory to conservative measures. A wide variety of conditions can cause destruction of the native joint including but not limited to: osteoarthritis, inflammatory arthritis, septic arthritis, post-traumatic arthritis, and acute fractures. Depending on the chronicity and etiology of disruption to the native joint, the surrounding soft tissue and motion are affected in a variety of ways. Chronic conditions such as osteoarthritis and inflammatory arthritis generally cause their damage to the joint over a period of time. Pain or mechanical blocks to motion such as contractures or osteophytes may limit the native joint from a normal arc of motion that may or may not be corrected at the time of surgery. Certain acute fractures, especially in the elderly population, are treated with TEA (Cobb 1997, Garcia 2002, McKee 2009).

Fig. 11.1 demonstrates the treatment of a comminuted intra-articular distal humerus fracture in a 61-year-old female status post fall from standing height. The associated injuries with these acute fractures must be communicated between the surgeon and therapist. The surrounding integrity of soft tissue dictates the type of prosthesis used: constrained (linked) versus nonconstrained (unlinked). In a nonconstrained implant, the collateral ligaments of the elbow are left intact. In the constrained implant, the collateral ligaments are resected in addition to the bony articulations. The type of prosthesis used dictates the postoperative therapy. It is important to note that varus and valgus stresses to the elbow should be protected in the early phase of nonconstrained devices. The ulnar nerve is decompressed at the time of surgery. Perhaps the most critical aspect in dictating postoperative therapy is the type of approach used to replace the elbow joint; what is done with the triceps and whether it was temporarily reflected, peeled back, or the overall integrity was left intact largely dictate postoperative instructions. The surgeon's preference regarding incision healing will also dictate timing of motion. Generally, a weight limit is placed on the extremity after surgery.

Communication between the surgeon and therapist is crucial in maintaining surgeon preferences and ultimately optimizing patient outcomes. Ultimately, specifics regarding when to start motion, incision concerns, and whether passive motion may be used are often surgeon specific. An anterior extension splint instead of a posterior splint may be applied by the surgeon if there is concern regarding pressure against the incision. The following protocol (Rehabilitation protocols 11.1 and 11.2) is used for a triceps sparing approach using a constrained type device.

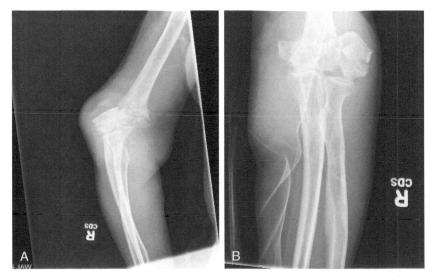

Fig. 11.1 61-year-old female with comminuted fracture of the distal humerus extending into the articular surface. Images **A-C** show injury radiographs and images **D-F** were taken after total elbow arthroplasty.

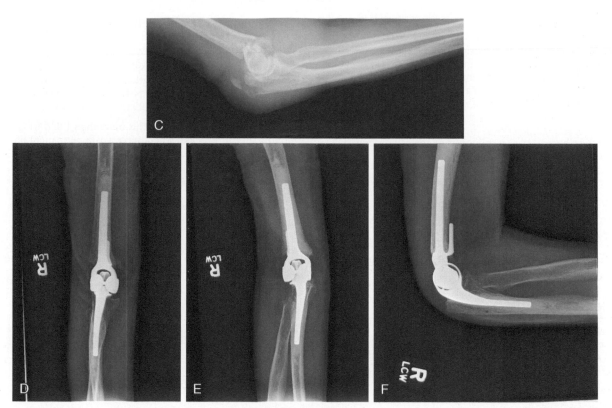

Fig. 11.1, cont'd

REHABILITATION PROTOCOL 11.1 ■ After Total Elbow Replacement (Triceps Sparing)

Week 1

- Hand and shoulder function encouraged immediately or as soon as the brachial plexus block has dissipated.
- At 3 days, postsurgical splint and dressings are removed and replaced with a removable posterior extension splint to allow for gentle active range of motion.
- Active range of motion exercises for the elbow and forearm are performed six times a day for 10 to 15 minutes. Posterior extension splint should be worn between exercise sessions and at night.

Week 2

- Passive and active ROM exercises may be initiated to the elbow.
- Range of motion is progressed as a home program, emphasizing extension and flexion.

Week 6

- Discontinue elbow extension splint during the day if elbow stability is adequate.

Week 8

- Discontinue elbow extension splint at night.
- Initiate gradual, gentle strengthening exercises for the hand and forearm. Light resistance may be begun to the elbow.
- Perform therapy within the patient's comfort level.

   The patient is advised not to lift more than 1 lb during the first 3 months after surgery and will observe a 5-lb permanent lifetime lifting restriction for the extremity.

Some surgeons prefer to reflect the triceps attachment during surgery. In this instance the therapy must also protect the triceps as it heals back to its insertion. The following protocol is a general guideline for therapy instructions when the triceps has been reflected and repaired back to its insertion during surgery.

Due to the release of the extensor mechanism, active extension against resistance is delayed until at least six weeks post-surgery. The following protocol is for a triceps reflecting approach with a constrained prosthesis.

REHABILITATION PROTOCOL 11.2 ■ After Total Elbow Replacement (Triceps Reflecting)

(Dachs et al 2015)

Week 1

- Hand and shoulder function encouraged immediately or as soon as the brachial plexus block has dissipated.
- An anterior or posterior extension splint is applied

Week 2

- Post surgical splint is removed. Staple and sutures removed at initial postoperative visit
- Active range of motion for flexion, pronation, supination exercises for the elbow and forearm are performed six times a day for 10 to

Continued

REHABILITATION PROTOCOL 11.2 ● After Total Elbow Replacement (Triceps Reflecting)—cont'd

15 minutes. Gravity assisted extension may be used. Active extension should be avoided for at least six weeks. Posterior extension splint should be worn between exercise sessions and at night.
- Range of motion is progressed as a home program, emphasizing extension and flexion.

Week 6
- Discontinue elbow extension splint during the day if elbow stability is adequate.
- Initiation of active elbow extension without resistance

Week 8
- Discontinue elbow extension splint at night.
- Initiate gradual, gentle strengthening exercises for the hand and forearm. Light resistance may be begun to the elbow.
- Perform therapy within the patient's comfort level.

The patient is advised not to lift more than 1 lb during the first 3 months after surgery and will observe a 5-lb permanent lifetime lifting restriction for the extremity.

REFERENCES

A complete reference list is available at https://expertconsult.inkling.com/.

McKee MD, Veillette CJ, Hall JA, et al. A multicenter, prospective, randomized, controlled trial of open reduction-internal fixation versus total elbow arthroplasty for displaced intra-articular distal humeral fractures in elderly patients. *J Shoulder Elbow Surg.* 2009;18(1):3–12.

FURTHER READING

Choo A, Ramsey ML. Total elbow arthroplasty: current options. *J Am Acad Orthop Surg.* 2013;21:427–437.
Dachs RP, et al. Total elbow arthroplasty: outcomes after triceps-detaching and triceps-sparing approaches. *J Shoulder Elbow Surg.* 2015;24:339–347.

12

Rehabilitation After Fractures of the Forearm and Elbow

Sinan Emre Ozgur, MD | Charles E. Giangarra, MD

FRACTURES OF THE RADIUS AND ULNAR SHAFT

The radius and ulna make up the bones of the forearm and the movement and articulation changes moving from the wrist to the elbow. The ulna can mostly be considered to be a straight bone while the radius has a curvature to it called the radial bow. A strong interosseous membrane holds the two bones together. Some fractures of the forearm are coupled with a dislocation of the joint proximal or distal to the fracture. A fracture of the ulna with a dislocation of the radial head is called a Monteggia fracture dislocation. A fracture of the radius with a disruption/dislocation of the distal radioulnar joint is called a Galeazzi fracture dislocation. In adults fractures of the radius and ulna are rarely treated nonoperatively, and no current study has compared the outcomes of nonoperative versus operative treatment of nondisplaced fractures of the forearm (Schutle 2014).

Generally fractures of the radius and ulna are fixed via direct methods such as open reduction internal fixation (ORIF) with plates and screws or indirect methods such as intramedullary (IM) devices. An example of a 24-year-old male with radial and ulnar shaft fractures treated with ORIF is shown in Fig. 12.1. With significant soft tissue disruption an external fixator may be placed where threaded pins are inserted bicortically into the bone with external rods connecting the pin to stabilize the fracture. After surgery the forearm may be immobilized until sutures are removed. The patient is instructed to be nonweight bearing on that extremity until the bones heal, generally six to eight weeks. Range of motion of the fingers, wrist, and elbow is encouraged throughout the postoperative course. Edema control is important early. After the bone has sufficiently healed, strengthening exercise may be initiated to regain the lost strength secondary to activity restrictions. Ultimately the patient should regain motion and strength after the bones have united. Significant loss of motion should be evaluated by the surgeon for possible complications such as malunion or radioulnar synostosis.

BOTH BONE FOREARM FRACTURE REHABILITATION (BOLAND 2011)
Phase I: (Weeks 0–2)

- Patient is placed into a splint and surgical incisions are protected
- Sutures or staples are removed at week two.
- Elevation of extremity encouraged
- Edema control and ROM of fingers

Phase II: (Weeks 2–6)

- Active and active-assisted ROM of elbow, forearm, and wrist
- No repetitive forearm twisting
- 5-pound weight restriction though some surgeons prefer strict nonweight bearing

Phase III: (Weeks 6 and Beyond)

- Lifting and twisting restrictions lifted once union has been achieved
- Work on regaining preoperative motion if not already achieved.
- It is crucial to communicate with the treating surgeon regarding when union has been achieved and when restrictions may be removed or surgeon preference regarding weight lifting limits despite lack of full union.

FRACTURES OF THE ELBOW

The elbow is an articulation of the distal humerus and the proximal ulna and radius. The most distal portion of the humerus laterally is made up of the capitellum, which is covered with articular cartilage as it articulates with the radial head. Moving proximally up the lateral distal humerus is the lateral epicondyle and lateral condyle before the distal flare of the humerus starts to narrow as it makes up the humeral shaft. The most distal aspect of the medial humerus is the trochlea, which is covered with articular cartilage as it articulates with the proximal aspect of the ulna: the olecranon. Like the medial side, the proximal aspect of the medial distal humerus is the medial epicondyle and medial condyle as it narrows to the humeral shaft. The bony articulation of the elbow helps maintain the stability of the elbow. The ulnohumeral articulation is considered a hinge type joint. The radiocapitellar joint is considered a pivot joint. The third articulation is between the radial head and proximal ulna. Collectively the different types of joints of the elbow allow for flexion and extension as well as pronation and supination. The normal full motion of the elbow in women aged 20 to 44 is 150.0 degrees of flexion and 4.7 degrees of extension (www.cdc.gov/ncbddd/jointrom/). In men the normal motion is 144.6 degrees of flexion and 0.8 degrees of extension (www.cdc.gov/ncbddd/jointrom/). The normal pronation and supination in women are 82.0 degrees and 90.6 respectively (www.cdc.gov/ncbddd/jointrom/). In men the normal pronation is 76.9 degrees and 85.0 degrees of supination (www.cdc.gov/ncbddd/jointrom/). As one would expect, this motion decreases with age (www.cdc.gov/ncbddd/jointrom/).

The surrounding ligaments and capsule of the elbow are critical in the inherent stability of the elbow. The medial collateral

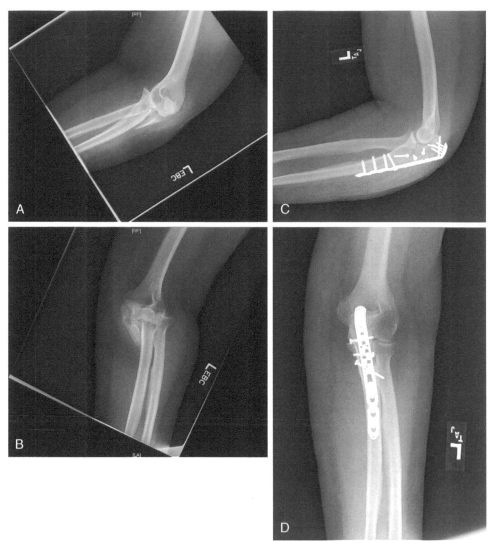

Fig. 12.1   24-year-old male with radius and ulnar shaft fractures. Images **A** and **B** are preoperative radiographs and images **C** and **D** are postoperative images after ORIF.

ligament (MCL) and lateral collateral ligament (LCL) are critical in the stability of the elbow with regards to valgus and varus stresses (Morrey 1983). The annular ligament is an important stabilizer to keep the radial head reduced and the radial head itself is an important secondary stabilizer to valgus stress of the elbow (Morrey 1983). The anterior capsule is also important in elbow stability (Morrey 1983).

RADIAL NECK AND HEAD FRACTURES

The radial head articulates with the capitellum at the elbow and may be injured in isolated radial head or neck fractures or in association with fractures of the forearm or elbow dislocations. A large majority of these fractures in isolation may be treated nonoperatively if there is not a block to motion or less than 2 mm of articular step-off. Initially these patients are placed into a simple sling for comfort and are encouraged to start motion immediately to prevent stiffness. Motion may be inhibited early due to the hemarthrosis that develops from the fracture, and the treating physician may aspirate the joint to reduce the volume to help facilitate early motion. Active

and passive motion are encouraged early on and restricted weight bearing for the first six to eight weeks until bony union is achieved. Keys for successful rehabilitation include maintaining preinjury motion.

For those fractures that require operative treatment, the type of treatment depends on the extent of the injury. Operative treatment includes open reduction internal fixation (ORIF), resection of the radial head, or replacement of the radial head with a prosthetic device. Resection of the radial head without replacement is an option when the surrounding MCL and interosseous membrane are competent, though long-term outcomes studies have shown conflicting results regarding success (Tejwani 2007). For the younger population the choice of fixation with screws versus replacement is dependent on the amount of comminution. Fig. 12.2 demonstrates a 39-year-old male who sustained trauma to his outstretched hand resulting in a displaced and comminuted radial head fracture treated with radial head arthroplasty. In isolated radial head fractures that are not associated with elbow ligamentous injuries, the surgical approach preserves the inherent soft tissue stability of the elbow. Postoperative therapy is based on surgeon preference regarding incision

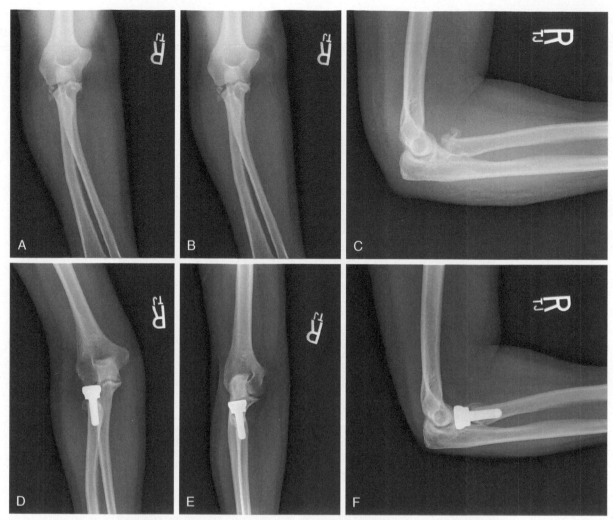

Fig. 12.2 39-year-old male who fell down a flight of stairs and sustained a comminuted radial head fracture treated with radial head arthroplasty. Images A-C are preoperative images and images D-F demonstrate the radial head component.

healing but generally consists of active and active-assisted ROM exercises. Passive exercises are discouraged. Non-weight bearing occurs for six to eight weeks until bony union is achieved but ultimately initiation of weight bearing is left to the discretion of the surgeon. The posterior interosseous nerve (PIN) may be injured or stretched during surgery and the therapist must inform the surgeon if PIN symptoms are present. The rehab protocol is changed with associated ligamentous disruptions.

SIMPLE OR COMPLEX ELBOW DISLOCATIONS

Elbow dislocations can be broken up into simple and complex patterns. Simple dislocations of the elbow are those in which the injury is only ligamentous without any associated fractures. Complex dislocations are elbow dislocations with associated fractures.

For the majority of simple dislocations, the treatment is nonoperative with initiation of early ROM. Conscious sedation is generally all that is required to reduce the elbow back into place. When the elbow is reduced the treating physician will place the elbow through a ROM with varus and valgus stress. As long as the elbow is stable throughout the arc of motion the patient is generally placed in a splint with the elbow flexed to 90 degrees for a week. Early ROM with a therapist is encouraged. If the elbow is unstable throughout an arc of motion the physician will splint the elbow in a reduced position and may elect for ligamentous repair. The therapy initiated after repair should follow that in the ligamentous repair protocol chapter (Rehabilitation protocols 12.1 and 12.2).

Complex elbow dislocations are elbow dislocations that include associated fractures. The most common associated fractures include the radial head, coronoid process of the ulna, and the olecranon. The "terrible triad" elbow dislocation commonly mentioned is an elbow dislocation with injuries to the coronoid process, radial head, and lateral collateral ligament. Complex elbow dislocations may be divided further into the particular mechanism: axial, valgus posterolateral rotatory, and varus posteromedial rotatory injuries (Wyrick 2015). The majority of complex fracture dislocations are treated with surgery. The postoperative guidelines generally are dictated by what bony structures are repaired. If any ligamentous structures are concomitantly repaired, then the postoperative protocol will also protect any stress to the repaired collateral ligament.

In the axial complex elbow dislocation the collateral ligaments are often intact whereas the olecranon is fractured with an associated radial head dislocation (Wyrick 2015). In the valgus posterolateral rotatory injury pattern the lateral collateral ligament, radial head, coronoid process, and, in extreme injuries, the medial collateral ligament are injured (Wyrick 2015). In the varus posteromedial rotatory injury pattern the lateral collateral ligament and coronoid process are injured (Wyrick 2015).

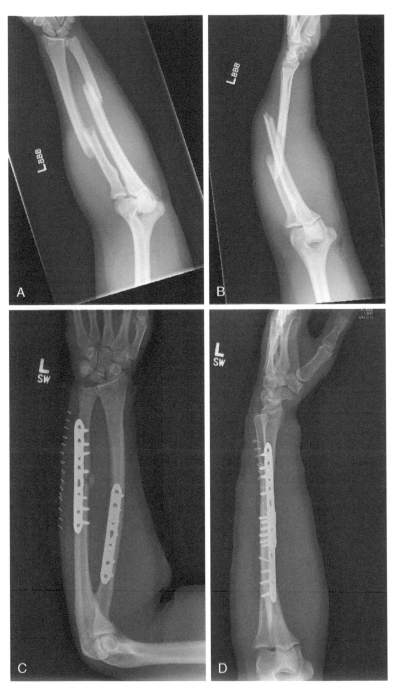

Fig. 12.3   57-year-old female with a fracture of her olecranon with radial head dislocation. Images **A** and **B** are preoperative radiographs of her injury. Images **C** and **D** are postoperative images after ORIF.

REHABILITATION PROTOCOL 12.1 ▪ **Radial Head Fracture Rehab Protocol Without Associated Ligamentous Injury or Repair**

Phase I (0–2 Weeks)

- Radial head ORIF immobilized in splint for 1 to 2 weeks
- Radial head replacement without associated ligamentous injury may start ROM if tolerable the first postoperative day
- A sling for comfort may be used in early postoperative period
- Elbow active and active-assisted ROM for flexion and extension
- Stress in the coronal plane (varus/valgus) should be avoided by performing ROM with arm close to body.
- Avoid flexion in pronation.
- An extension splint may be used with subsequent increase in extension parameters per surgeon discretion in radial head replacement.
- Maintain motion of adjacent joints.

Phase II (2–6 Weeks)

- Sutures or staples removed at two weeks
- Continue Phase I exercises.
- Active and active-assisted supination and pronation are initiated.
- By end of 6 weeks full ROM of elbow in flexion and extension should be obtained
- Maintain motion of adjacent joints.
- Check with surgeon regarding bony healing in ORIF group but should generally be achieved by 6 weeks
- Weight restriction limitations decreased per surgeon discretion.

Phase III (6 Weeks and Beyond)

- Continue previous exercise.
- By 8 weeks full preoperative motion should be obtained, including supination and pronation.

Olecranon Fractures

The proximal ulna articulation with the distal humerus is a hinge type joint. It forms a semilunar shape as it articulates with the trochlea of the distal humerus. The most proximal aspect of the olecranon articulates with the olecranon fossa of the distal humerus posteriorly and the coronoid process articulates with the coronoid fossa of the humerus anteriorly. Fractures of the olecranon can occur in isolation or with other structures such as the radial head, coronoid process, or collateral ligaments of the elbow. Isolated fractures of the ulna are classified by the Mayo classification (Morrey 1995).

The classification helps dictate treatment as it classifies based on the amount of displacement, comminution, and stability of the elbow.

Olecranon fractures that are minimally displaced and stable may be treated with nonoperative measures. Generally the elbow is splinted or casted in 90 degrees of flexion for three to four weeks with gentle active motion initiated (Ring 2010).

The degree of extension and flexion and when to start active-assisted ROM are at the discretion of the surgeon and are dependent on healing and initial fracture characteristics.

Olecranon fractures in the elderly not amenable to repair may be treated with excision and advancement of the triceps (Newman 2009). In this instance the postoperative therapy mirrors that of a triceps repair. Resistant exercise should not be initiated until 12 weeks after surgery (Newman 2009).

Operative fixation of the olecranon includes tension band wiring, intramedullary fixation, or fixation with plates and screws. Tension band wiring and intramedullary screw fixation are generally reserved for the simpler, noncomminuted fractures, and plate and screw fixation are used for the more complex and comminuted fractures. An example of a 57-year-old female with an olecranon fracture treated with ORIF is shown in Fig. 12.3. Depending on surgeon's preference for soft tissue, healing therapy may be initiated a week after surgery. Gentle active ROM is encouraged. Active ROM against resistance is generally reserved until six to eight weeks after surgery or once bony union is evident (Newman 2009).

Postoperative Care for Olecranon Fractures (Newman 2009, Ring 2011)

Phase I (0–2 Weeks)

- Posterior splint placed for 1 to 2 weeks
- Gentle passive and active-assisted ROM are started after splint removal.
- For highly comminuted fractures where direction compression cannot be achieved a splint may be placed for longer than two weeks with motion delayed per surgeon discretion.

Phase II (2–6 Weeks)

- Sutures or staples removed at week two
- Continue gentle movements of elbow, no resistance exercises
- Maintain ROM of shoulder, wrist, and fingers.

Phase III (6 Weeks and Beyond)

- Once confirmation of bony union has been achieved, gentle and progressive resistance exercises may be initiated.
- Weight bearing restrictions decreased as bony union is achieved
- Work on regaining preoperative ROM.

(http://www.eorif.com/Elbowforearm/Radial%20head%20Rehab.html, Singh et al. 2011, Rosenblatt 2011.)

REHABILITATION PROTOCOL 12.2

Simple Elbow Dislocation Rehab Protocol (Cohen 1998)

Phase I (0–1 Week)

- Elbow splinted in 90 degrees flexion for 5 to 10 days

Phase II (1–6 Weeks)

- Splint removed and ROM initiated
- A sling or splint may be used in early phase for comfort
- Extension gradually increased over 3 to 6 weeks
- A hinged brace may be used blocking certain degrees of extension if continued instability occurs at certain motions of movement. Extension blocking parameters and progression per treating physician discretion
- Avoid passive ROM.

Complex Elbow Dislocation: Axial Mechanism With Olecranon Fracture and Radial Head Dislocation (Wyrick 2015)

Phase I (0–1 Week)

- Elbow is splinted for one week

Phase II (1–6 Weeks)

- Sutures or staples removed at two weeks
- Postoperative splint removed
- Flexion, extension, pronation, and supination ROM exercises started after splint removal
- Hinged elbow brace may be used by treating surgeon to help with stability
- Full, unprotected ROM delayed up to 4 weeks in elderly or severely comminuted fractures per surgeon preference

Phase III (6–8 Weeks and Beyond)

- Resistive exercises are initiated.

Complex Elbow Dislocation: Valgus Posterolateral Rotatory Injury With Lateral Collateral Ligament Tear, Radial Head, and Coronoid Fractures (Wyrick 2015)

Phase I (0–1 Week)

- Extremity splinted according to ligaments repaired

Phase II (1–4 Weeks)

- Sutures or staples removed at two weeks
- Splint removed after one week
- Hinged elbow brace placed with terminal extension limited to 30 degrees for 4 weeks
- Gentle active ROM
- No passive ROM of elbow
- Forearm pronation and supination exercises with elbow at 90 degrees and done with elbow at side to avoid varus or valgus stress

Phase III (6–8 Weeks and Beyond)

- Resistive exercises initiated and progressed if bony union is evident

Complex Elbow Dislocation: Varus Posteromedial Rotatory Injury With Lateral Collateral Ligament Tear and Coronoid Fracture (Wyrick 2015)

Phase I (0–1 Week)

- Elbow placed in postoperative splint

Phase II (1-6 Weeks)

- Sutures or staples removed at two weeks
- Splint removed and hinged elbow brace placed
- Gentle active ROM
- Avoid varus stress by performing exercises with elbow close to the body
- Stability of coronoid fixation dictates degree of extension
- Terminal 30 degrees of extension blocked for 4 weeks for coronoid fixation concerns

Phase III (6–8 Weeks and Beyond)

- Resistive exercises initiated and progressed if bony union is evident

REFERENCES

A complete reference list is available at https://expertconsult.inkling.com/.

FURTHER READING

Cohen MS, Hastings II H. Acute elbow dislocation: evaluation and management. *J Am Acad Orthop Surg.* 1998;6:15–23.

Newman SDS, Mauffrey C, Krikler S. Olecranon fractures. *Injury.* 2009;40(6): 575–581.

Schutle LM, Meals CG, Neviaser RJ. Management of adult diaphyseal both-bone forearm fractures. *J Am Acad Orthop Surg.* 2014;22:437–446.

Tejwani NC, Mehta H. Fractures of the radial head and neck: current concepts in management. *J Am Acad Orthop Surg.* 2007;15:380–387.

Wyrick JD, Dailey SK, Gunzenhaeuser JM, et al. Management of complex elbow dislocations: a mechanistic approach. *J Am Acad Orthop Surg.* 2015;23: 297–306.

Pediatric Elbow Injuries in the Throwing Athlete: Emphasis on Prevention

Robert C. Manske, PT, DPT, MEd, SCS, ATC, CSCS | Mark Stovak, MD, FACSM, FAAFP, CAQSM

INTRODUCTION

Approximately 30 million children and teenagers participate in organized sports in the United States (Adirim and Cheng 2003). Every year in the United States, approximately 15 million children and adults play organized baseball including 5.7 million children in eighth grade or lower (Fleisig and Andrews 2012). Despite the fact that sports are the leading cause of injury in adolescent athletes, it is estimated that more than half of those injuries are preventable (Emery 2003). Pain in the elbow is a common occurrence in young baseball players, especially pitchers. Table 13.1 lists possible differential diagnoses in adolescents with elbow pain. Studies have found that, during a season, 26% to 35% of youth baseball players have either shoulder or elbow pain, with self-reported shoulder pain in more than 30% of pitchers and elbow pain in more than 25% immediately following a game (Lyman et al. 2001, Lyman et al. 2002). In 2010, the incidence of serious elbow or shoulder injury for pitchers was 5% (serious injury was defined as surgery or retirement from baseball). The risk factor with the strongest correlation of injury is pitching. Specifically, increased pitches per game, innings pitched per season, and months pitched per year are all associated with increased risk of elbow injury. Additional risk factors included playing for concurrent teams, pitching with arm fatigue, and pitchers that also played catcher (Fleisig and Andrews 2012).

LITTLE LEAGUER'S ELBOW

The simple act of throwing is violent because of the stresses it places on the elbow. Because ligaments and muscles are attached to the bone at the medial elbow at a time when the secondary ossification centers are not fused, a **traction apophysitis** can occur when this growth plate is not able to withstand the forces placed on it. Little Leaguer's elbow includes a host of elbow pathologies in a young throwing athlete. The various types of injuries that can be considered Little Leaguer's elbow are listed in Table 13.2.

MEDIAL TENSION INJURIES

Medial tension injuries most commonly include medial epicondylar apophysitis. With repetitive stress to the medial elbow in the throwing adolescent, the flexor pronator mass and the ulnar collateral ligament apply tensile forces that cause medial epicondyle apophysitis (Pappas 1982, Rudzki and Paletta 2004). This apophysitis is thought to occur rather than rupture of the ulnar collateral ligament (Joyce et al. 1995). Chronic attritional tears of the ulnar collateral ligament are fairly rare in adolescent athletes (Ireland and Andrews 1988). Despite this rarity, it appears that ulnar collateral injuries are increasing in high school athletes. Petty et al. (2004) reported that the percentage of high school athletes who required ulnar collateral ligament reconstruction in their center jumped from 8% between 1988 and 1994 to 13% between 1995 and mid-2003. Injuries to the ulnar collateral ligament in adolescent athletes generally occur as acute events, rather than through attrition as in older, more skeletally mature athletes.

LATERAL COMPRESSION INJURIES

Several conditions caused by compression of the lateral side of the elbow can occur in younger throwers. Two of the more common are osteochondritis dissecans (OCD) and Panner's disease. Although traditionally these have been thought to be the same condition by some, they are separate entities. Osteochondritis is a localized condition involving articular cartilage that has separated from the underlying subchondral bone and is caused by repetitive trauma (Yadao et al. 2004). Panner's disease is a focal osteonecrosis of the entire capitellum seen primarily in boys aged 7 to 12 years old and is not associated with trauma (Yadao et al. 2004).

POSTERIOR COMPRESSION INJURIES

Whereas medial and lateral elbow pain occur as a result of "valgus extension overload" during the late cocking–early acceleration phase of throwing, posterior pain occurs during the terminal phase of throwing as the elbow is locked into full extension. The synovium can be pinched in the olecranon when the elbow is in full extension, resulting in posterior impingement syndrome, or the posterior apophysis can be stressed by triceps traction, causing olecranon apophysitis (Crowther 2009).

PREVENTION

Parents and coaches need to be more proactive to protect players, especially those who are at risk. Unfortunately, these are most commonly the "better players," which is why they may develop these problems to begin with. Fleisig and Andrews (2012) suggest that the risk of elbow problems in younger athletes can be reduced by following these guidelines (Little League Baseball—The Learning Curve):

1. Watch and respond to signs of fatigue (e.g., decreased ball velocity, decreased accuracy, changing mechanics (posture or elbow position), or increased time between pitches). If a thrower looks fatigued or complains of fatigue, rest is recommended.

TABLE 13.1	Adolescent Elbow Pain Differential Diagnosis	
Locale	**Possible Diagnosis**	**Age (years)**
Lateral	Avascular necrosis of capitellum (Panner's)	7–12
	Osteochondritis dissecans	12–16
Medial	Medial apophysitis (Little Leaguer's elbow)	9–12
	Medial collateral ligament strain/sprain	All
	Flexor/pronator strain	All
	Medial epicondyle avulsion	<18
	Ulnar neuritis	All
Posterior	Olecranon apophysitis	9–14
	Olecranon (posterior) impingement	All
	Olecranon osteochondrosis	9–14
	Triceps/olecranon tip avulsions	9–14
Other	Stress fracture	All
	Loose bodies	>18
	Synovitis	All

TABLE 13.2	Forms of Little Leaguer's Elbow

Medial epicondyle fragmentation
Medial epicondyle avulsion
Delayed apophyseal growth of medial epicondyle
Accelerated apophyseal growth of medial epicondyle
Delayed closure of the medial epicondylar apophysis
Delayed closure of the olecranon apophysis
Osteochondrosis of the capitellum
Osteochondritis of the capitellum
Osteochondrosis of the radial head
Osteochondritis of the radial head
Hypertrophy of the ulna
Olecranon apophysitis

2. No overhead throwing of any kind for at least 2 to 3 months (preferably 4 months) with no competitive baseball pitching for at least 4 months per year.
3. Do not pitch more than 100 innings in games in any calendar year.
4. Follow limits for pitch counts and days rest.
5. Avoid pitching on multiple teams with overlapping seasons.
6. Learn good throwing biomechanics as soon as possible. The first step should be basic throwing technique for fastballs and change-ups.
7. Avoid radar guns.
8. A pitcher should not also be a catcher for his team. The pitcher-catcher combination results in added throws and may increase the risk of injury.
9. If a pitcher complains of elbow or shoulder pain, discontinue throwing until evaluated by a sports medicine physician.
10. Inspire youth throwers to have fun playing baseball and other sports. Participation and enjoyment of various physical activities will increase athleticism and interest in sports.

Several associations have provided recommendations regarding adolescent athletes and prevention of both elbow and shoulder problems. The American Academy of Pediatrics (American Academy of Pediatricians Policy statement: baseball and softball 2012) and USA Baseball each have guidelines regarding pitch counts. The American Academy of Pediatrics recommends limits of 200 pitches per week or 90 per outing, while the USA Baseball Medical and Safety Advisory Committee recommends a more

TABLE 13.3	Pitch Count Limits and Required Rest Recommendations					

It is important for each league to set workload limits for their pitchers to limit the likelihood of pitching with fatigue. Research has shown that pitch counts are the most accurate and effective means of doing so.

Age	Daily Max (Pitches in Game)	Required Rest (Pitches)				
		0 Days	1 Days	2 Days	3 Days	4 Days
7-8	50	1-20	21-35	36-50	N/A	N/A
9-10	75	1-20	21-35	36-50	51-65	66+
11-12	85	1-20	21-35	36-50	51-65	66+
13-14	95	1-20	21-35	36-50	51-65	66+
15-16	95	1-30	31-45	46-60	61-75	76+
17-18	105	1-30	31-45	46-60	61-75	76+
19-22	120	1-30	31-45	46-60	61-75	76+

From Pitch Smart USA Baseball. http://m.mlb.com/pitchsmart/pitching-guidelines/.

stringent 75 to 125 pitches per week or 50 to 75 pitches per outing depending on age (Committee on Sports Medicine and Fitness, USA Baseball Medical and Safety Advisory Committee 2001).

USA BASEBALL GUIDELINES

USA Baseball has developed guidelines and recommendations in an effort to decrease the risk of elbow or shoulder injury in vulnerable adolescent athletes.

Pitch Counts

Pitch counts should be carefully monitored and regulated in adolescents. Recommended limits vary depending on age of the pitcher (Table 13.3).

Pitch Types

Previously various recommendations were made for ages in which certain types of pitches were recommended. Although ages for pitch counts are no longer recommended, it is strongly suggested that younger pitchers (ages 9-12) avoid throwing pitches other than fastballs and change-ups. After the age of 13-14, players can begin using breaking pitches after development of a consistent fastball and change-up.

Lyman et al. (2002) evaluated the association between pitch counts, pitch types, and pitching mechanics with shoulder and elbow pain in young pitchers. They found that more than half of 476 pitchers between the ages of 9 and 14 years of age had shoulder or elbow pain during a single season. Throwing a curveball was associated with a 52% increased risk of developing shoulder pain, and throwing a slider was associated with an 86% increased risk of elbow pain. They also found a significant relationship between the number of pitches thrown during a game and during a season and the rate of elbow pain and shoulder pain.

Although improper throwing biomechanics continues to be a risk factor for injury, Fleisig and Andrews' 2012 article describes several studies comparing curveball and fastball biomechanical elbow varus torque stresses and most showed the curveball stresses to be less than those of the fastball. They concluded that clinical, epidemiologic, and biomechanical data do not support the claim that throwing curveballs at a young age is a risk factor for elbow injury. However, despite this information, many organizations and leading clinicians believe this is a risk factor and they still discourage curveballs before skeletal maturity (Fleisig and Andrews 2012).

Multiple Appearances

Although youth pitchers normally remain in the game at another position after being relieved from pitching, having a player return without a proper warmup may be deleterious to the athlete's shoulder and elbow. Soft tissues around the shoulder and elbow must be slowly and progressively warmed up, especially when already fatigued from previous high-level activity. Youth pitchers should be discouraged from returning to the mound in a game once they have been removed as a pitcher.

Showcases

Showcases give young players greater opportunities to display their baseball skills to scouts at higher levels. This may be fine for position players, but for pitchers, this may have a dramatic negative effect on throwing health. These showcases are typically near the end of the season, when the pitcher is probably already fatigued and in desperate need of rest and recovery. If the season ended abruptly, this young player may be out of throwing shape and may try to compensate by throwing harder on a deconditioned arm. Overthrowing in an attempt to impress higher-level coaches is most certainly a way to produce shoulder and elbow injuries. Recommendations are for pitchers not to participate in showcases because of the risk of injury. The importance of showcases should be de-emphasized, and pitchers should be given adequate rest and recovery time to appropriately prepare.

Year-Round Baseball

To maintain a high level of competition, some young athletes play baseball year round. It appears that multisport athletes may be becoming a thing of the past. This is especially true in southern states that typically have relatively warm weather all year. Year-round throwing dramatically increases the risk of injury to the elbow and shoulder. Youth baseball pitchers are encouraged to throw at most 9 months in a given year. For at least 3 months adolescent pitchers should not play baseball or participate in other sporting activities that involve overhead activity, such as football, track and field, and swimming.

REFERENCES

A complete reference list is available at https://expertconsult.inkling.com/.

FURTHER READING

Cassas KJ, Cassettari-Wayhs A. Childhood and adolescent sports-related overuse injuries. *Am Fam Physician.* 2006;73:1014–1033.

Cox K, Manske RC, Stovak M. Unpublished research. *Do high school coaches follow the recommendations of USA Baseball Medical and Safety Advisory Committee?* 2009.

Dun S, et al. A biomechanical comparison of youth baseball pitches: is the curveball potentially harmful? *Am J Sports Med.* 2009;36:686–692.

Jones G. Pitch counts, pitch types, and prevention ptrategies in the adolescent/Little League baseball player. *Sports Medicine Update.* July/August 2011:2–6.

Nissen CW, et al. A biomechanical comparison of the fastball and curveball in adolescent baseball pitchers. *Am J Sports Med.* 2009;37:1492–1498.

14

Medial Collateral Ligament and Ulnar Nerve Injury at the Elbow

Michael Levinson, PT, CSCS | David W. Altchek, MD

The prevalence of medial collateral ligament (MCL) reconstruction is increasing in professional and high school athletes. Common misconceptions exist regarding MCL reconstruction within media covering professional sports. Media typically overestimate the ability of a professional pitcher to return and many believe the return will be within one year (Conte et al. 2015). The MCL and ulnar nerve of the elbow are frequently injured in throwing athletes. Injuries occur most frequently in baseball players, especially pitchers; however, injuries in other throwing athletes such as quarterbacks and javelin throwers have been documented. Pitching generates a large valgus torque at the elbow. The angular velocity of the elbow from flexion to extension has been documented to reach 3000 degrees/second. Conservative treatment of these injuries has been poorly documented and without satisfactory results. Improved surgical techniques and greater understanding of rehabilitation principles have made surgery a more successful option for return to throwing.

ANATOMY AND BIOMECHANICS

The MCL is composed of two primary bundles. The anterior bundle runs from the sublime tubercle of the ulna and inserts on the inferior surface of the medial epicondyle. The anterior bundle tightens in extension and loosens in flexion. The posterior band runs from the posterior portion of the medial epicondyle and inserts at the ulna proximal and posterior to the sublime tubercle (Fig. 14.1). The posterior bundle tightens in flexion and loosens in extension. The anterior bundle is the prime focus of the MCL reconstruction. The ulnar nerve runs in the cubital tunnel, the space posterior to the medial epicondyle. The nerve is significantly exposed at the roof of the tunnel, which is referred to as the cubital tunnel retinaculum.

MECHANISM OF INJURY

Injury to the MCL is a result of the repetitive, extreme valgus loads to the elbow while throwing. The MCL is the primary restraint to valgus stress at the elbow. Dillman et al. (1995) demonstrated that a fastball thrown by an elite baseball pitcher produces a load that approaches the actual tensile strength of the MCL. The MCL attempts to withstand these forces during the late cocking and acceleration phases of throwing. Repetitive overloading can result in inflammation and microtears of the ligament, which can eventually lead to failure. Continuing to throw with instability can lead to degenerative changes in the elbow.

Repetitive valgus stresses can also result in ulnar nerve injury, which may be exacerbated by ligamentous insufficiency.

These stresses may lead to medial traction on the ulnar nerve, resulting in chronic subluxation or dislocation of the nerve outside the ulnar groove. In addition, throwers often have a hypertrophied flexor–pronator mass, which may compress the nerve during muscle contraction. Injuries to the ulnar nerve may be isolated or associated with an MCL injury.

EVALUATION

Diagnosis of MCL insufficiency is based on the history, physical examination, magnetic resonance imaging (MRI), and arthroscopy. History is often chronic medial elbow pain with throwing, especially during the late cocking and early acceleration phases. It often prevents throwing completely. Physical examination includes a valgus stress test that reproduces the symptoms of increased valgus laxity. MRI findings clearly consistent with an MCL injury assist in making the diagnosis. Finally, a positive arthroscopic test, which is defined as more than 1 mm of opening between the coronoid and the medial humerus, is often used.

SURGICAL TREATMENT
Medial Collateral Ligament Reconstruction

Reconstruction of the MCL has been proven to be a very effective method to return athletes to their prior level of competition. Cain et al. (2010) found that 83% of their athletes returned to previous level of competition or higher, including 83% after reconstruction. Reconstruction of the medial collateral ligament is performed using the "docking technique" described by Altchek et al. (2000). The anterior bundle is the

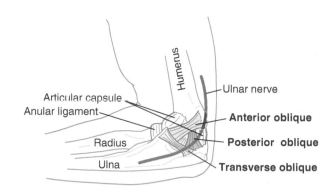

Fig. 14.1 MCL complex of the elbow, consisting of three bundles: anterior, posterior, and transverse oblique.

primary focus of the reconstruction. The ipsilateral palmaris longus is the graft of choice. In the absence of this muscle, the gracilus is used. Our rehabilitation guidelines are not affected by graft choice; however, when using the gracilis, the affected lower extremity must be considered.

This procedure includes a routine arthroscopic evaluation of the elbow through a muscle-splitting approach that preserves the flexor–pronator origin (Fig. 14.2). Bone tunnels are created in the humerus and ulna. The graft is "docked" securely in the tunnels with sutures (Fig. 14.3). This technique minimizes the number of tunnels and reduces the size of the drill holes, while also avoiding an obligatory ulnar nerve transposition.

Ulnar Nerve Transposition

Anterior transposition is the most common surgical treatment for compression of the ulnar nerve. By transferring the nerve

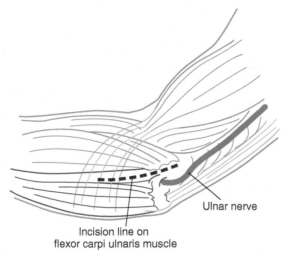

Fig. 14.2 Exposure is created by splitting the flexor carpi ulnaris muscle. (Redrawn from Levinson M: Ulnar Collateral Reconstruction in Postsurgical Rehabilitation Guidelines for the Orthopedic Clinician. 1st edition, St. Louis, Elsevier, 2006.)

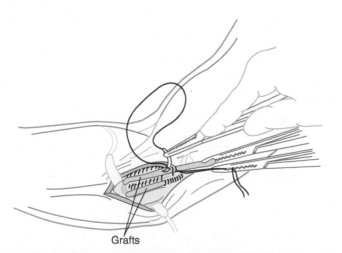

Fig. 14.3 Docking technique: The graft is "docked" securely into the bone tunnels using sutures. (Redrawn from Levinson M: Ulnar Collateral Reconstruction in Postsurgical Rehabilitation Guidelines for the Orthopedic Clinician. 1st edition, St. Louis, Elsevier, 2006.)

anteriorly, the nerve is effectively lengthened, decreasing tension during flexion. The ulnar nerve is removed from the cubital tunnel and transferred anteriorly to the medial epicondyle. It is then secured with a fascial sling to avoid ulnar subluxation back over the medial epicondyle.

Rehabilitation Overview and Principles

The rehabilitation program following MCL reconstruction is based on the healing restraints and functional demands of the graft (Rehabilitation Protocol 14.1). Time frames for returning to certain activities are based on allowing the graft to both strengthen adequately and regain adequate flexibility. The program features early, safe range of motion (ROM) to allow optimal tissue healing and minimize the effects of immobilization. Elbow ROM in a hinged brace is initiated after 1 week to prevent contracture, provide pain control, enhance collagen formation, and nourish articular cartilage. Range of motion is increased gradually in the brace over the initial 6-week postoperative period. Aggressive, passive stretching should be avoided throughout rehabilitation. Elbow extension is restored using a low-load, long-duration stretch, which has been demonstrated to be an effective method for restoring ROM. Soft tissue mobilization may be needed to decrease muscle guarding, pain, and swelling and can help facilitate a faster return to full motion.

Strengthening is initiated at 6 weeks and, following kinetic chain principles, the focus of the rehabilitation program is on the scapula and glenohumeral joint. Rotator cuff strengthening is avoided until 8 to 9 weeks to avoid any excessive, early valgus stress on the elbow. As the program is progressed, a full upper extremity strengthening program is incorporated. Exercises and drills are incorporated to reproduce the functional demands of the throwing athlete. This includes eccentric training, overhead training, endurance training, and speed training. With a normal strength base, plyometric activities are introduced prior to throwing and hitting.

A recent alteration to the rehabilitation program involves the forearm musculature. Aggressive strengthening of the flexor–pronator group can result in tendinitis or further injury. Most throwers have adequate strength of these muscles secondary to throwing and other upper extremity exercises they perform. Therefore isolated exercises for the flexor–pronator group are minimized or avoided.

Normal flexibility of the entire upper extremity should be restored. Specific emphasis is placed on restoring glenohumeral internal rotation. Glenohumeral internal rotation has been demonstrated to form the physiologic counter to the valgus torque generated during the late cocking phase of throwing. In addition, internal rotation deficits have been associated with valgus instability of the elbow.

Neuromuscular dynamic stability exercises include the trunk and lower extremities. Hannon and colleagues (2014) assessed lower extremity balance in baseball players with MCL injuries prior to surgery and at three months postoperatively. They found balance deficits on the stance and lead limbs prior to surgery compared to a three month follow-up. Exercises such as single leg balance, BOSU squats, tilt board squats, or the star excursion exercise help to develop hip and trunk stability. Core stabilization can be done with well arm side planks and rhythmic stabilization trunk drills.

REHABILITATION PROTOCOL 14.1   ■   **Medial Collateral Ligament Reconstruction Guidelines**

Postoperative Phase 1 (Weeks 1–4)

Goals

- Promote healing.
- Decrease pain and inflammation.
- Begin to restore range of motion (ROM) to 30 to 105 degrees.

Treatment

- Splint at 50 to 60 degrees for 1 week.
- Active ROM in brace (Weeks 1–3: 45 to 90 degrees, Week 4: 30 to 105 degrees)
- Scapula isometrics
- Gripping exercises

Postoperative Phase 2 (Weeks 4–6)

Goals

- Active ROM: 15 to 115 degrees
- Minimal pain and swelling

Treatment

- Continue active ROM in brace.
- Pain-free isometrics (forward flexion, shoulder extension, elbow flexion–extension)
- Manual scapula stabilization
- Modalities as needed

Postoperative Phase 3 (Weeks 6–12)

Goals

- Restore full ROM.
- Restore upper extremity strength to 5/5.
- Begin to restore upper extremity endurance.

Treatment

- Continue active ROM.

- Low-intensity/long-duration stretch for extension
- Begin isotonics for scapula, shoulder, and elbow.
- Begin internal rotation (IR)/external rotation (ER) strengthening at 8 weeks.
- Upper body ergometer
- Begin neuromuscular drills.
- Proprioceptive neuromuscular facilitation (PNF) patterns when strength is adequate
- Modalities as needed

Postoperative Phase 4 (Weeks 12–16)

Goals

- Restore full strength and flexibility.
- Restore normal neuromuscular function.
- Prepare for return to activity.

Treatment

- Advance IR/ER to 90/90 position.
- Begin light forearm/wrist strengthening (MD directed).
- Continue endurance training.
- Begin plyometrics program.
- Full upper extremity flexibility program
- Address trunk and lower extremities.

Postoperative Phase 5 (Months 4–9)

Goals

- Return to activity.
- Prevent re-injury.

Treatment

- Begin interval throwing program at 4 months.
- Begin interval hitting program at 5 months.
- Continue strengthening and flexibility exercises.

Interval programs are crucial to assist the athlete to return to competition. A consistent, methodical approach to warm-up, stretching, and gradual progression of activity can help guide a more successful return to activity. When upper extremity strength and flexibility have been normalized, an interval throwing program is usually initiated at 4 months. An interval hitting program can begin at 5 months. This can be progressed from dry swings to hitting off a tee to live pitching. Pitchers who have completed a long toss program can throw off the mound at 9 months and not expect to pitch competitively until about 1 year.

Rehabilitation following ulnar nerve transposition follows the same progression as the MCL reconstruction; however, the progression is generally shorter (Rehabilitation Protocol 14.2). The brace is discontinued after 3 weeks, at which time a formal strengthening program is begun. A throwing program normally can be initiated at 10 to 12 weeks.

Conservative Treatment of Medial Collateral Ligament Injuries

Little scientific data exist to support conservative treatment, especially in competitive throwers, for return to pre-injury activity level. However, at times conservative treatment may be an option (Rehabilitation Protocol 14.3).

The goals of the initial phase of treatment are to reduce pain and inflammation, promote soft tissue healing, and avoid loss of ROM. Acute, traumatic injuries are sometimes braced; however, chronic, throwing injuries are not. The elbow has a tendency to become stiff. Reasons for stiffness include the high degree of congruency of the ulnohumeral joint, the inflammatory response of the anterior capsule to trauma, fibrosis of the flexor–pronator, and the fact that the joint is traversed by muscle rather than tendons. Care is taken to avoid or minimize valgus stress to the elbow during the early phases of rehabilitation.

During the intermediate and advanced phases of rehabilitation, the goal is to restore full ROM, strength, and flexibility of the entire upper extremity. Functional progressions are similar to those of postsurgical guidelines with internal and external rotation exercises incorporated into the program later to avoid excessive valgus stress to the elbow. Time frames for these phases tend to be more individual, based on the patient's symptoms and functional demands. For example, a throwing athlete must be able to perform overhead activities and complete a plyometric exercise program before beginning a throwing program.

REHABILITATION PROTOCOL 14.2 ▪ Ulnar Nerve Transposition Guidelines

Postoperative Phase 1 (Weeks 1–4)

Goals

- Promote healing.
- Decrease pain and inflammation.
- Begin to restore ROM to 15 to 100 degrees.

Treatment

- Splint at 60 degrees for 1 week.
- Elbow active ROM in brace (Weeks 1–3: 15 to 100 degrees)
- Wrist active ROM
- Gripping exercises
- Scapula isometrics
- Manual scapula stabilization exercises

Postoperative Phase 2 (Weeks 4–6)

Goals

- Minimal pain and swelling
- Restore full ROM.
- Begin to restore upper extremity strength.

Treatment

- Discontinue brace.
- Continue active ROM (no passive ROM by clinician).
- Begin isotonics for scapula, shoulder, and elbow.
- Begin IR/ER strengthening at 6 weeks.
- Upper body ergometry (when adequate ROM)

Postoperative Phase 3 (Weeks 6–8)

Goals

- Restore upper extremity strength to 5/5.
- Restore upper extremity endurance.
- Restore upper extremity flexibility.

Treatment

- Progress isotonics for scapula, shoulder, and elbow
- Advance shoulder strengthening to overhead (PNF, 90/90).
- Begin upper extremity flexibility.
- Begin light forearm/wrist strengthening (MD directed).
- Begin neuromuscular drills.

Postoperative Phase 4 (Weeks 8–12)

Goals

- Return to activity.
- Prevent re-injury.

Treatment

- Continue full upper extremity strengthening program.
- Continue full upper extremity flexibility program.
- Begin plyometrics program.
- Advance to interval throwing program (if plyometrics are tolerated well).

REHABILITATION PROTOCOL 14.3 ▪ Conservative Medial Collateral Ligament Injury Guidelines

Acute Phase

Goals

- Promote healing.
- Decrease pain and inflammation.
- Begin to restore ROM.

Treatment

- Brace (optional per MD)
- Active ROM (AROM)
- Isometrics (scapula, deltoid)
- Gripping exercises

Intermediate Phase

Goals

- Restore full ROM.
- Minimal pain and swelling
- Begin to restore strength.

Treatment

- D/C brace
- Continue AROM.
- Begin isotonics for scapula, shoulder, and elbow (no IR/ER).

Advanced Strengthening Phase

Goals

- Restore upper extremity strength to 5/5.
- Begin to restore upper extremity endurance.
- Begin to restore upper extremity flexibility.

Treatment

- Progress strengthening of scapula, shoulder, and elbow
- Begin IR/ER strengthening.
- Begin light forearm/wrist strengthening (MD directed).
- Neuromuscular drills
- Begin upper extremity flexibility (emphasis on posterior shoulder).

Return to Sport Phase

Goals

- Return to sport.
- Prevent re-injury.

Treatment

- Continue aggressive upper extremity strength and flexibility.
- Progress to overhead activities.
- Begin plyometrics.
- Begin sport-specific interval program.

REFERENCES

A complete reference list is available at https://expertconsult .inkling.com/.

FURTHER READING

Altchek DW, Andrews JR. *The Athlete's Elbow.* 1st ed. Philadelphia: Lippincott Williams & Wilkins; 2001.

Altchek DW, Levinson M. Rehab after MCL reconstruction. *Biomech.* 2001;5:22–28.

Dines JS, Frank JB, Akerman M, et al. Glenohumeral internal rotation deficits in baseball players with ulnar collateral ligament insufficiency. *Am J Sports Med.* 2009;37:566–570.

Dodson CC, Thomas A, Dines JS, et al. Medial ulnar collateral reconstruction of the elbow in throwing athletes. *Am J Sports Med.* 2006;34:1926–1933.

Keefe DT, Lintner DM. Nerve injuries in the throwing elbow. *Clin Sports Med.* 2004;23:723–742.

Levinson M. Ulnar collateral ligament reconstruction. In: Cioppa-Mosca J, Cahill J, Young Tucker C, eds. *Postsurgical Rehabilitation Guidelines for the Orthopedic Clinician.* 1st ed. St. Louis: Elsevier; 2006.

Rettig AC, Sherill C, Dale S, et al. Nonoperative treatment of ulnar collateral ligament injuries in throwing athletes. *Am J Sports Med.* 2001;29:15–17.

Rouhrbough JT, Altchek DW, Hyman J, et al. Medial collateral ligament reconstruction of the elbow using the docking technique. *Am J Sports Med.* 2002;30:541–548.

Wilk KE, Levinson M. Rehabilitation of the athlete's elbow. In: Altchek DA, Andrews JR, eds. *The Athlete's Elbow.* 1st ed. Philadelphia: Lippincott Williams & Wilkins; 2001.

15

Treating Flexion Contracture (Loss of Extension) in Throwing Athletes

Tigran Garabekyan, MD | Charles E. Giangarra, MD

- Flexion contracture (loss of extension) in throwing athletes is most often a result of **valgus extension overload syndrome.** Repetitive near-tensile failure loads sustained by the anterior bundle of the ulnar collateral ligament in late cocking/early acceleration result in attenuation or rupture and subsequent valgus instability. This results in increased contact stress between the radial head and capitellum in addition to the medial olecranon fossa and the olecranon. In response to supraphysiologic loads, reactive osteophytes develop on the proximal olecranon and corresponding olecranon fossa (kissing osteophytes), which subsequently impinge and limit terminal extension. Occasionally, hypertrophic osteophytes may fracture and form loose bodies, further limiting extension (O'Holleran et al, 2006).
- Elbow contracture can affect all aspects of elbow and forearm motion including flexion, extension, supination, and pronation.
- Gelinas et al. (2000) reported that 50% of professional baseball pitchers tested had an elbow flexion contracture. Typically, a loss of up to 10 degrees of extension is unnoticed by the athlete and is not required for "functional" elbow range of motion (ROM).
- Nonoperative treatment remains the initial means of treatment and prevention of elbow contracture. Early elbow ROM and supervised therapy are advocated to prevent motion loss.
- **Low-load, long-duration stretching** (LLLDS) (Fig. 15.1) is advocated for restoration of extension. High-intensity, short-duration stretching is **contraindicated** for limited elbow ROM (may produce heterotopic ossification).
- Initial treatment includes moist heat and ultrasound, dynamic splinting at night during sleep (LLLD), joint mobilizations, and ROM exercises at end ranges done several times a day.
- Joint mobilization techniques to the humeroulnar, radiohumeral, and ulnohumeral joint can be performed conservatively to try to increase elbow ROM in all planes. To improve elbow extension ROM a physical therapist can perform humeral ulnar distraction (Fig. 15.2), or a dorsal glide of the radius at the radioulnar joint (Fig. 15.3) or radiohumeral joint (Fig. 15.4).
- If nonoperative measures fail in an athlete who wishes to return to the same level of competition or in the rare patient with loss of functional motion, arthroscopic surgery can be performed to remove loose bodies, débride impinging osteophytes, and treat articular cartilage lesions.
- Accelerated rehabilitation after this surgery is required, but overly aggressive rehabilitation must be avoided to help prevent inflammation (and thus reflex splinting and stiffness) of the elbow.
- Timmerman and Andrews (1994) followed 19 cases of posttraumatic arthrofibrosis of the elbow treated with arthroscopic débridement and manipulation. At a 29-month follow-up, extension improved from 29 to 11 degrees and flexion from 123 to 134 degrees.
- Bionna et al. (2010) followed 26 athletes with chief complaint of limited elbow extension following arthroscopic contracture release. All 26 elbows improved both subjectively and objectively. Twenty-two of the athletes returned to sport at their prior level.
- Araghi et al. (2010) followed 20 patients who underwent surgery for release of a stiff elbow. Fifty-one required examination under anesthesia a mean of 40 days after surgery. Forty-four patients by one year had increased elbow motion by 40 degrees.
- The fundamental goal of physical therapy after arthroscopy period is the restoration of joint ROM and flexibility within the healing parameters of the structures involved.
  Recommended criteria for a safe return to sports include
  - Painless and full ROM
  - No tenderness
  - Satisfactory isokinetic muscular strength testing
  - Satisfactory clinical examination
  See Rehabilitation Protocol 15.1 for the treatment protocol following elbow arthroscopy.

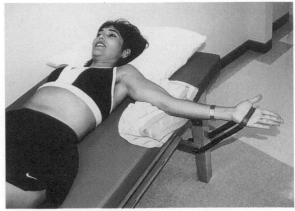

Fig. 15.1 Low-load, long-duration stretching of the elbow for restoration of full elbow extension.

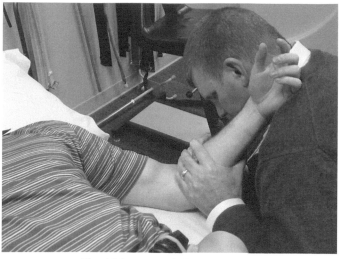

Fig. 15.2   Humeral ulnar distraction.

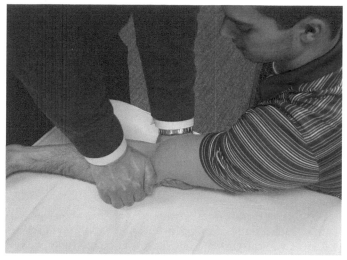

Fig. 15.3   Dorsal glide of radius at radioulnar joint.

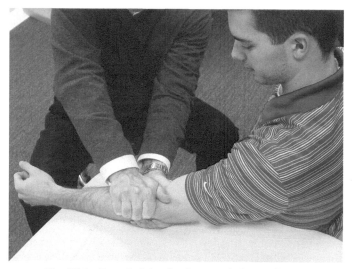

Fig. 15.4   Dorsal glide of radius at radiohumeral joint.

REHABILITATION PROTOCOL 15.1 ▪ After Elbow Arthroscopy

Phase 1: Immediate Motion Phase

Goals

- Restore motion (with emphasis on terminal extension).
- Diminish pain and inflammation.
- Retard muscle atrophy.
- Criteria allowing progression to phase 2:
  - Full ROM, minimal pain/tenderness, at least grade 4/5 manual muscle testing

Days 1–3

- ROM to tolerance (elbow passive/active flexion/extension) (two sets of 10/hour)
- Overpressure into extension (at least 10 degrees)
- Isometric exercises for wrist and elbow (flexion/extension/pronation/supination)
- Compression and ice hourly
- May use aqua therapy, pulsed galvanic stimulation, ultrasound, and transcutaneous neuromuscular stimulation.

Days 4–9

- ROM extension–flexion (at least 5 to 120 degrees)
- Overpressure into extension: 5-lb weight, elbow in full extension (four to five times daily)
- Continue isometrics and gripping exercises.
- Continue use of ice.

Days 10–14

- Full passive ROM
- ROM exercises (two sets of 10/hour)
- Stretch into extension.
- Continue isometrics.

Phase 2: Intermediate Phase

Goals

- Maintain full ROM.
- Gradually improve strength and endurance.
- Resume neuromuscular control of the elbow.

REHABILITATION PROTOCOL 15.1 ■ After Elbow Arthroscopy—cont'd

- Criteria allowing progression to phase 3:
  - Full and painless ROM, no tenderness about elbow, and strength that is 70% of the opposite side

Weeks 2–4

- Upper extremity muscle strengthening utilizing isotonic contraction (including rotator cuff and periscapular muscles)
- Dumbbell progressive resistance exercises and elastic band exercises
- ROM exercises (address internal rotation deficit in glenohumeral joint)
- Overpressure into extension: stretch for 2 minutes (three to four times daily)
- Continue use of ice postexercise.

Phase 3: Advanced Strengthening Phase

Goals

- Increase total arm strength, power, endurance, and neuromuscular control.
- Criteria allowing return to competitive sport:
  - Full and painless ROM, no tenderness about elbow, an isokinetic strength test that fulfills established criteria, and a satisfactory clinical examination

Weeks 4–8

- Advanced strengthening exercises
- Plyometrics
- Sport-related activities
- Interval throwing program (usually initiated at 4–6 weeks)

REFERENCES

A complete reference list is available at https://expertconsult.inkling.com/.

FURTHER READING

Bennett JB, Mehlhoff TL. Total elbow arthroplasty: surgical technique. *J Hand Surg Am.* 2009;34(5):933–939.

Bruno RJ, Lee ML, Strauch RJ, et al. Posttraumatic elbow stiffness: evaluation and management. *J Am Acad Orthop Surg.* 2002;10(2):106–116.

Cain Jr EL, Dugas JR, Wolf RS, et al. Elbow injuries in throwing athletes: a current concepts review. *Am J Sports Med.* 2003;31(4):621–635.

Chen FS, Rokito AS, Jobe FW. Medial elbow problems in the overhead-throwing athlete. *J Am Acad Orthop Surg.* 2001;9(2):99–113.

Cheung EV, Adams R, Morrey BF. Primary osteoarthritis of the elbow: current treatment options. *J Am Acad Orthop Surg.* 2008;16(2):77–87.

Evans PJ, Nandi S, Maschke S, et al. Prevention and treatment of elbow stiffness. *J Hand Surg Am.* 2009;34(4):769–778.

Gramstad GD, Galatz LM. Management of elbow osteoarthritis. *J Bone Joint Surg Am.* 2006;88(2):421–430.

Kauffman JI, Chen AL, Stuchin S, et al. Surgical management of the rheumatoid elbow. *J Am Acad Orthop Surg.* 2003;11(2):100–108.

Kokkalis ZT, Schmidt CC, Sotereanos DG. Elbow arthritis: current concepts. *J Hand Surg Am.* 2009;34(4):761–768.

Lindenhovius AL, Jupiter JB. The posttraumatic stiff elbow: a review of the literature. *J Hand Surg Am.* 2007;32(10):1605–1623.

Morrey BF. Post-traumatic contracture of the elbow. Operative treatment, including distraction arthroplasty. *J Bone Joint Surg Am.* 1990;72(4):601–618.

O'Holleran JD, Altchek DW. The thrower's elbow: arthroscopic treatment of valgus extension overload syndrome. *HSS J.* 2006;2(1):83–93.

van der Lugt JC, Rozing PM. Systematic review of primary total elbow prostheses used for the rheumatoid elbow. *Clin Rheumatol.* 2004;23(4):291–298.

Post-Traumatic Elbow Stiffness

Daniel Woods, MD | Charles E. Giangarra, MD

DEFINITION

The elbow contains three major articulating surfaces. The articulation of the humeral trochlea and the trochlear notch of the ulna is the major facilitator of flexion and extension about the elbow. The radiocapitellar articulation supports motion in both the flexion and extension of the elbow in addition to supination and pronation of the forearm. The proximal radioulnar joint allows supination and pronation movements of the forearm.

The physiologic range of motion has been defined by the American Academy of Orthopaedic Surgeons to be 0 to 146 degrees with respect to extension and flexion, 71 degrees of forearm pronation, and 84 degrees of forearm supination. More important, the functional arc of motion as defined by Morrey et al. (1981) is elbow flexion from 30 to 130 degrees and 100 degrees of forearm rotation, including 50 degrees of supination and 50 degrees of pronation. The functional impairment caused by elbow stiffness is delineated by the individual needs of each patient.

CLASSIFICATION

The etiology of elbow stiffness has been classified by various authors. Kay (1998) based his scheme on the anatomic components involved. Type I involves soft tissue contractures; type II involves soft tissue contractures with ossification; type III involves nondisplaced articular fracture with soft tissue contracture; type IV involves displaced intra-articular fractures with soft tissue contracture; and type V involves post-traumatic bony bars blocking elbow motion.

Morrey (1990) classified elbow stiffness into intrinsic, extrinsic, and mixed causes (Table 16.1). Intrinsic causes are related to intra-articular pathology resulting from deformities or malalignment of the articular surface, intra-articular adhesions, loose bodies, impinging osteophytes, and fibrosis within the olecranon or coronoid fossa. Extrinsic causes are related to all entities aside from the articular surface. Examples include skin contracture from scars or burns, capsular and collateral ligament contracture, and heterotopic ossification. Another important extrinsic cause is injury to brachialis or triceps resulting in a hemarthrosis, which may cause scarring, fibrosis, and limitation of motion. Entrapment of the ulnar nerve can lead to pain resulting in loss of motion and eventual capsular contracture. Mixed etiologies are defined as extrinsic contractures resulting from intrinsic pathology.

HETEROTOPIC OSSIFICATION

Heterotopic ossification (HO) is an important cause of post-traumatic stiffness of the elbow. Direct trauma, neural axis injury, surgical intervention, and forceful passive manipulation may cause HO, which is directly related to the severity of the initial injury. Noted radiographically approximately 4 to 6 weeks following the event, HO presents with swelling, hyperemia, and loss of motion of the affected joint. HO in the upper extremity has been classified by Hastings and Graham (1994) into three types: I, without functional limitation; II, subtotal limitation; and III, complete bony ankylosis (Table 16.2). Treatment consists of physical therapy and indomethacin or a diphosphonate to begin shortly after the insult. If HO continues to progress, surgical excision of the heterotopic bone when the hyperemia and swelling begin to diminish is indicated. When the HO matures, prompt surgical treatment is important to avoid soft-tissue contractures that may result from prolonged loss of motion.

EVALUATION OF THE STIFF ELBOW
History

The history of a patient presenting with a stiff elbow should include onset, duration, character, and progression of symptoms. Pain is an infrequent finding in post-traumatic elbow stiffness and implies arthrosis of the joint, entrapment neuropathy,

TABLE 16.1	Morrey's Causes of Elbow Stiffness by Location of Pathology

EXTRINSIC
Skin, subcutaneous tissue
Capsule (posterior/anterior)
Collateral ligament contracture
Myostatic contracture (posterior/anterior)
Heterotopic ossification

INTRINSIC
Articular deformity
Articular adhesions
Impinging osteophytes
• Coronoid
• Olecranon
Impinging fibrosis
• Coronoid fossa
• Olecranon fossa
Loose bodies

TABLE 16.2	Heterotopic Ossification Classification: Upper Extremity	
Class		**Description**
I		Without functional limitation
II		Subtotal limitation
IIA		Limitation in flexion/extension
IIB		Limitation in pronation/supination
IIC		Limitation in both planes of motion
III		Complete bony ankylosis

infection, or instability. Important findings with regard to the elbow include history of a traumatic event, previous surgery, and septic arthritis. Comorbid conditions such as hemophilia, which causes hemarthroses, or a spastic neuropathy, which may result in neuropathic joint degeneration, are also important. Finally, the functional demands of the patient with respect to vocation and leisure-time activity have important implications on the treatment regimen.

Physical Examination

The physical examination should consist of a thorough neurovascular examination with particular attention to the ulnar and median nerves, which may be involved in trauma to the elbow or encompassed by HO around the elbow joint. The presence of burns, scars, or areas of fibrosis on the skin surrounding the joint should be noted. The active and passive range of motion in flexion and extension and supination and pronation should be recorded. It is important to understand that deficits in the flexion–extension plane are a result of ulnohumeral pathology, whereas deficits in forearm supination and pronation imply a radiocapitellar or proximal radioulnar etiology. Attention to a soft or hard end point at the extremes of each motion is paramount to determining whether a soft tissue or bony constraint is hindering motion. The appreciation of crepitus through range of motion may indicate loose body, fracture, or degenerative changes.

Radiographic Evaluation

Radiographic evaluation should consist of anteroposterior, lateral, and oblique views of the elbow. Fractures, bony blocks to motion, articular loose bodies, degenerative changes, and HO may be noted on the initial radiographs. Computed tomography with three-dimensional reconstructions is helpful in defining the articular anatomy and surgical planning in the presence of HO. Magnetic resonance imaging is not routinely used in the evaluation of elbow stiffness.

NONSURGICAL TREATMENT

The goal of nonsurgical therapy is a functional, painless, and stable range of motion. Initial treatment of post-traumatic elbow stiffness consists of gradual passive manipulation progressing to active-assisted stretching of the elbow controlled by the patient or a physical therapist. Adjuncts to this therapy may include nonsteroidal anti-inflammatory drugs (NSAIDs), heat or ice application, and therapy modalities such as massage, iontophoresis, ultrasound, and electrical stimulation.

The next line of treatment for the stiff elbow is the use of splinting. Dynamic splinting in which a constant prolonged force is supplied through spring or rubber band tension has been used in patients with deficits in flexion and extension. Although positive outcomes have been reported by Søjbjerg (1996) and others, patient compliance is a problem because of the continuous strain and resultant painful muscle spasm of the antagonistic muscle groups.

Static progressive adjustable splints such as the turnbuckle splint—used for flexion–extension deficits—supination–pronation splints, and even serial casting are options. These splints sequentially increase as more motion is allowed by the soft tissues. Twenty-five to 43-degree increases in flexion–extension have been noted with turnbuckle casting, and similar results have been noted with serial casting. Both progressive static splints and dynamic splinting are most effective when used for patients with symptoms of less than 6 months to 1 year with little articular involvement.

Custom-molded orthoses with the capability of 0 to 140 degrees of flexion have been used in 20-minute intervals to provide distraction at the extremes of flexion and extension. These have been combined with static interval splints to reinforce gains in motion with limited success. Continuous passive motion machines also have been used, but their benefit is questionable because of the lack of stress at the extremes of motion. They have been useful in the prevention of postoperative elbow stiffness.

Closed manipulation under anesthesia has been used to treat elbow stiffness. This procedure is not without complications, including iatrogenic fracture, articular cartilage damage, and soft tissue damage leading to hemarthrosis and fibrosis. Postmanipulation swelling and pain may actually limit elbow range of motion. Heterotopic ossification has been noted to form following vigorous closed manipulation.

SURGICAL TREATMENT

Patients who continue to experience pain and limitation to a functional range of motion despite nonsurgical therapy are candidates for surgical treatment. It is important to select patients with realistic expectations who are motivated to withstand the rigorous postsurgical rehabilitation protocol. The choice of procedure depends on the extent of damage to the articular cartilage, whether the loss of motion occurs in flexion or extension, and if bony blocks or HO contributes to the elbow stiffness.

Surgical candidates with absent or minimal articular cartilage defects should undergo soft tissue release and removal of bony blocks to motion. Soft tissue releases include brachialis muscle slide, anterior or posterior capsulectomy, removal of any soft tissue hindering motion in the olecranon fossa, and removal of any bony blockades when encountered intraoperatively. Those with moderate articular cartilage lesions in whom conservative therapy fails are treated with débridement arthroplasty or the Outerbridge-Kashiwagi ulnohumeral arthroplasty of the olecranon, olecranon fossa, coronoid, coronoid fossa, and the radial head. For severe degenerative arthritic changes, surgical treatment options are based on the age and demands of the patient. Individuals older than 60 years or younger than 60 years with low functional demands are candidates for total elbow arthroplasty, whereas active individuals younger than age 60 are more likely to benefit from fascial interpositional arthroplasty using autologous fascia lata, autologous skin, or allograft Achilles tendon placed between the resected bony ends.

POSTSURGICAL PROTOCOL

Rehabilitation after surgery differs according to the specific procedure but adheres to three basic principles: restoring a functional range of motion, strengthening the surrounding musculature, and re-establishing motions needed for functional activity in the affected elbow. Mobilization of the elbow is aided by sufficient pain control and should begin 2 days following surgery. This can be accomplished through gentle manipulation by physical therapists or through a continuous passive motion machine. Early forceful manipulation is contraindicated because of the possibility of causing heterotopic ossification. Extended rehabilitation similar to the preoperative rehabilitation, using dynamic or static splinting along with progressive manual stretching, should be continued until no further motion is gained. Some authors advocate the use of perioperative radiation to decrease the risk of postoperative heterotopic ossification. Current radiation regimens include 1000 centigray (cGy) over five treatments or a single 700- to 800-cGy dosage within 2 days of the surgery.

REFERENCES

A complete reference list is available at https://expertconsult .inkling.com/.

FURTHER READING

Bennett JB, Mehlhoff TL. Total elbow arthroplasty: surgical technique. *J Hand Surg Am.* 2009;34(5):933–939.

Bruno RJ, Lee ML, Strauch RJ, et al. Posttraumatic elbow stiffness: evaluation and management. *J Am Acad Orthop Surg.* 2002;10(2):106–116.

Cain Jr EL, Dugas JR, Wolf RS, et al. Elbow injuries in throwing athletes: a current concepts review. *Am J Sports Med.* 2003;31(4):621–635.

Chen FS, Rokito AS, Jobe FW. Medial elbow problems in the overhead-throwing athlete. *J Am Acad Orthop Surg.* 2001;9(2):99–113.

Cheung EV, Adams R, Morrey BF. Primary osteoarthritis of the elbow: current treatment options. *J Am Acad Orthop Surg.* 2008;16(2):77–87.

Evans PJ, Nandi S, Maschke S, et al. Prevention and treatment of elbow stiffness. *J Hand Surg Am.* 2009;34(4):769–778.

Gramstad GD, Galatz LM. Management of elbow osteoarthritis. *J Bone Joint Surg Am.* 2006;88(2):421–430.

Kauffman JI, Chen AL, Stuchin S, et al. Surgical management of the rheumatoid elbow. *J Am Acad Orthop Surg.* 2003;11(2):100–108.

Kokkalis ZT, Schmidt CC, Sotereanos DG. Elbow arthritis: current concepts. *J Hand Surg Am.* 2009;34(4):761–768.

Lindenhovius AL, Jupiter JB. The posttraumatic stiff elbow: a review of the literature. *J Hand Surg Am.* 2007;32(10):1605–1623.

Morrey BF. Post-traumatic contracture of the elbow. Operative treatment, including distraction arthroplasty. *J Bone Joint Surg Am.* 1990;72(4):601–618.

Morrey BF. 2009 Total elbow arthroplasty did not differ from open reduction and internal fixation with regard to reoperation rates. *J Bone Joint Surg Am.* 2010;91(8).

O'Holleran JD, Altchek DW. The thrower's elbow: arthroscopic treatment of valgus extension overload syndrome. *HSS J.* 2006;2(1):83–93.

van der Lugt JC, Rozing PM. Systematic review of primary total elbow prostheses used for the rheumatoid elbow. *Clin Rheumatol.* 2004;23(4):291–298.

Treatment and Rehabilitation of Elbow Dislocations

Michael J. O'Brien, MD | Felix H. Savoie III, MD

REHABILITATION CONSIDERATIONS

- Elbow dislocations constitute 11% to 28% of all injuries to the elbow (Mehloff et al. 1988).
- It is the most common dislocation in children younger than age 10 and the second most common dislocation in adults behind the shoulder (Morrey 1993).
- The annual incidence of acute dislocation is 6 per 100,000 persons (Linscheid and Wheeler 1965).
- Of all elbow dislocations, 90% are posterior or posterolateral.
- **Loss of terminal extension** is the most common complication, with contractures reported in up to 60% of cases (Mehloff et al. 1988).
- Immobilization for more than 3 weeks has been associated with persistent stiffness and joint contractures (Mehloff et al. 1988, Broberg and Morrey 1987).
- These complications highlight the need for rehabilitation with early initiation of active range of motion (ROM) of the elbow.

ANATOMY AND BIOMECHANICS

The elbow joint consists of two types of articulations and thus allows two types of motion. The ulnohumeral articulation resembles a hinge joint, allowing flexion and extension, whereas the radiohumeral and proximal radioulnar joint allows axial rotation (Morrey 1986). Stability of the elbow joint is provided by the osseous articulations, medial and lateral collateral ligaments, and traversing muscles.

- The medial collateral ligament (see Fig. 14.1), or ulnar collateral ligament, consists of three parts: anterior, posterior, and transverse segments. The anterior bundle is the strongest and most distinct component, whereas the posterior bundle exists as a thickening of the posterior capsule and provides stability at 90 degrees of flexion.
- The lateral ligament complex (Fig. 17.1) consists of the radial collateral ligament, the annular ligament, and the lateral ulnar collateral ligament. The lateral ulnar collateral ligament contributes the most to stability on the lateral side of the elbow. Injury to this structure can lead to posterolateral rotatory instability.
- Primary stabilizers of the elbow joint include the ulnohumeral articulation, the anterior band of the medial collateral ligament, and the lateral ulnar collateral ligament.
- Secondary stabilizers include the radial head, the coronoid, and the anterior joint capsule (Fig. 17.2). Dynamic stability is provided by the muscles traversing the joint, including the brachialis and the triceps (An and Morrey 2000, Funk et al. 1987), the common extensor musculature origin, and the flexor–pronator musculature origin.

MECHANISM OF INJURY

- The mechanism of injury producing elbow dislocation is usually a fall on an outstretched hand with the arm abducted.
- Motor vehicle accidents, direct trauma, sports injuries, and other high-energy mechanisms account for a minority of dislocations in young individuals.
- The median age for elbow dislocation is 30 years (Josefsson and Nilsson 1986).

EVALUATION AND RADIOGRAPHS

- The diagnosis of acute elbow dislocation is relatively straightforward.
- Soft tissue swelling and an obvious deformity are noted on inspection.
- A thorough neurovascular examination of the upper extremity is mandatory before and after reduction.
- The wrist and shoulder must be palpated and examined to rule out concomitant injury, which can be present in 10% to 15% of cases (Morrey 1995).
- The forearm should be examined after reduction for tenderness over the distal radioulnar joint and interosseous membrane to identify a variant of the Essex-Lopresti injury.
- Appropriate radiographs (**anterior–posterior, lateral, and oblique views**) must be obtained prior to reduction maneuvers to identify the direction of the dislocation and any associated periarticular fractures. Oblique radiographs may be particularly helpful in identifying fractures of the radial head or coronoid.
- If comminuted fractures are present, computed tomography may help identify the fracture pattern.
- Postreduction films must be obtained to verify concentric reduction and to identify any loose bodies in the joint. A true lateral film of the elbow is paramount to assess congruency of the ulnohumeral joint.

CLASSIFICATION

- Instability can be categorized anatomically as *simple* (with no associated fracture) or *complex* (with associated fracture).
- Simple dislocations are classified as anterior or posterior. **Posterior dislocation is the most common** (Mezera and Hotchkiss 2001) (Fig. 17.2) and is further subdivided by the direction of the dislocated ulna (**posterior, posteromedial, posterolateral, direct lateral**).
- **Complex dislocations most frequently involve fracture of the radial head, the coronoid process, or the olecranon.** Radial head fractures occur in approximately 10% of elbow

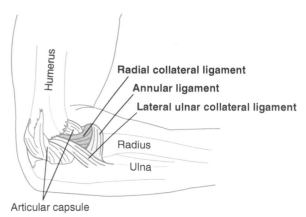

Fig. 17.1 The lateral ligament complex consists of the radial collateral ligament, the annular ligament, and the lateral ulnar collateral ligament. The lateral ulnar collateral ligament contributes the most to stability on the lateral side of the elbow. Injury to this structure can lead to posterolateral rotatory instability.

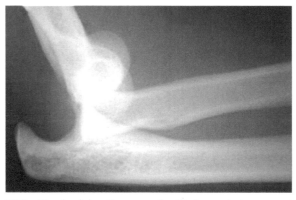

Fig. 17.2 Simple dislocations are classified as anterior or posterior. Posterior dislocation is by far the most common and is further subdivided by the direction of the dislocated ulna (posterior, posteromedial, posterolateral, direct lateral).

dislocations, whereas coronoid fractures occur in 2% to 18% (Morrey 1995).

- The risk of post-traumatic arthrosis is increased significantly with complex dislocations (Broberg and Morrey 1987).
- The constellation of elbow dislocation with concurrent fractures of the radial head and the coronoid process has been termed "the terrible triad," suggesting the poor outcomes associated with its treatment.
- Recurrent dislocations also are uncommon and usually result from failure of the capsular and ligamentous constraints to heal sufficiently.
- Unrecognized fractures or chondral injuries may be discovered at the time of surgery. Durig et al. (1979) reported unrecognized osteochondral injuries in nearly 100% of acute elbow dislocations at the time of operative exploration.

TREATMENT

The initial treatment of an elbow dislocation is reduction of the dislocation. Reduction requires adequate analgesia and muscle relaxation and usually can be done in the emergency department.

Reduction of a posterior dislocation uses application of longitudinal traction to the forearm beginning with the elbow in extension. One hand is placed on the forearm, pulling longitudinal traction, while the examiner's other hand is placed around the elbow joint. With traction applied, correcting for varus or valgus alignment, the elbow is gently brought into a flexed position. The fingers of the hand around the elbow joint apply an anterior pressure on the olecranon, while the thumb is placed in the antecubital fossa applying a counter posterior force, gently levering the olecranon anteriorly and distally around the trochlea of the distal humerus. A palpable reduction "clunk" may be felt and is a favorable sign for improved joint stability.

Once reduction has been achieved, the elbow should be taken through a gentle ROM, including flexion, extension, and rotation. The examiner should pay particular attention to recurrent posterior instability and the degree of extension at which the olecranon begins to subluxate.

Final radiographs should be obtained to confirm concentric reduction and again look for associated periarticular fractures.

If the reduction is concentric and the elbow joint is stable, a posterior splint is applied with the elbow in 90 degrees of flexion for 5 to 7 days.

Operative Treatment

- Surgery for acute elbow dislocations is rare and is indicated for only a few situations:
  - Nonconcentric reductions, representing interposition of bone or soft tissue in the joint
  - Instability that requires splinting the elbow in more than 50 to 60 degrees of flexion
  - When associated with unstable fractures about the joint
- Posterolateral dislocations can be managed without surgical treatment because they usually remain stable after closed reduction (Hobgood et al. 2008, O'Driscoll et al. 2001, Sheps et al. 2004).
- Complete elbow dislocations cause rupture of both the medial and lateral ligamentous structures. Josefsson et al. (1987) surgically explored 31 pure elbow dislocations and found complete rupture of the medial and lateral ligaments in every case, usually from the humeral origin.
- The elbow can be approached through two separate medial and lateral incisions or through a posterior utilitarian incision with large, full-thickness skin flaps. Repairing deep structures first and working superficially have been advocated (Pugh et al. 2004).
- External fixators may be required as a last resort to gain stability of the joint.
- Prospective studies have shown no advantage of early collateral ligament repair over early ROM for simple elbow dislocations (Josefsson et al. 1987).
- If therapeutic modalities are ineffective after 6 months and an elbow contracture of more than 30 to 40 degrees remains, then a capsular release can be considered (Husband and Hastings 1990).

COMPLICATIONS

- Residual post-traumatic stiffness is by far the most common and is much more common than instability following dislocation.

- Many patients lose the terminal 10 to 15 degrees of extension (Morrey 1993).
- Complication rates increase with complex dislocations and those that require operative intervention.
- Insufficiency of the lateral collateral ligament complex can lead to subtle instability after elbow dislocation. In this condition, described as **posterolateral rotatory instability (PLRI)**, the ulnohumeral joint does not dislocate but rather pivots, opening up laterally in supination (O'Driscoll et al. 1991) (Fig. 17.3).
- Brachial artery disruptions rarely occur; fewer than 30 cases have been reported in the literature. Pulses may be diminished while the elbow is dislocated but rapidly return once the elbow is reduced.
- Nerve injury also is uncommon. The ulnar nerve is most often involved with a stretch neuropraxia.
- Calcification of the soft tissues is relatively common following elbow dislocation. This has been reported in up to 75% of cases (Josefsson et al. 1984) but rarely limits motion.
- True heterotopic ossification (with mature bone in nonosseous soft tissue) that limits motion is rare, occurring in fewer than 5% of cases. In patients at high risk, such as those with a closed head injury, prophylaxis with NSAIDs or low-dose irradiation should be considered. If resection of ectopic bone is necessary, it is best done when the bone appears mature on plain radiographs. This usually occurs at least 6 months after the initial trauma (Hastings and Graham 1994).

REHABILITATION CONSIDERATIONS

- Most agree that extended casting and prolonged immobilization lead to elbow post-traumatic stiffness and should be avoided (O'Driscoll 1999, Pennig et al. 2000, Stavlas et al. 2004)
- For simple elbow dislocations, early *active ROM* is the key to preventing post-traumatic stiffness and obtaining a favorable result.
- The elbow is splinted for 5 to 7 days to allow soft tissue rest.
- Soft tissue swelling can be controlled with compressive dressings and application of ice.
- Beginning at day 5 to 7, a hinged elbow brace from 30 to 90 degrees is applied and *active ROM* is initiated. Active ROM requires muscle activation and assists with elbow stability and compression across the joint.
- ROM is increased in the hinged elbow brace 10 to 15 degrees per week.
- Passive ROM should be avoided because it increases swelling and inflammation.
- Valgus stress to the elbow should be avoided because it may disrupt healing of the MCL and lead to instability or recurrent dislocation.
- During this time, no strengthening or resistive exercises should be prescribed because this may place tension on the healing ligamentous structures.
- Dynamic splints or progressive static splints may be initiated if ROM is not steadily improving by 6 weeks.
- Elbow flexion returns first, with full flexion obtained by 6 to 12 weeks. Extension returns more slowly and may continue to improve for 3 to 5 months.
- Forced terminal extension should be avoided.
- At 6 to 8 weeks, strengthening can begin (Rehabilitation Protocol 17.1).

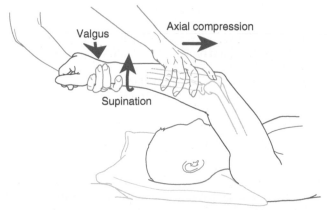

Fig. 17.3 Posterolateral rotatory instability (PLRI) of the elbow is assessed with axial compression, valgus stress, and forced supination.

REHABILITATION PROTOCOL 17.1 ◾
Rehabilitation Protocol After Elbow Dislocation

Phase 1 (Days 1–5)
- Immobilize elbow in well-padded posterior long-arm splint with elbow at 90 degrees of flexion and neutral rotation.
- Avoid passive ROM of the elbow.
- Avoid valgus stress to elbow, such as shoulder abduction and external rotation.
- Begin active ROM of hand and fingers with putty or squeeze ball.
- Use ice or cryo-compression sleeve liberally.

Phase 2 (Days 6–14)
- Remove posterior long-arm splint and place in hinged elbow brace, locked from 30 to 90 degrees of flexion.
- Repeat radiographs to confirm reduction.
- Begin active ROM from 30 to 90 degrees, full pronation/supination.
- Avoid passive ROM of the elbow.
- Avoid valgus stress to the elbow.
- Begin full active ROM of wrist and hand in all planes.
- Begin flexion and extension isometrics.
- Begin shoulder active ROM in all planes, and avoid abduction and external rotation.

Phase 3 (Weeks 2–6)
- Maintain hinged elbow brace. Increase elbow extension 5 degrees per week and elbow flexion 10 degrees per week.
- Goal is full extension to full flexion by 6 weeks postinjury.
- Begin gentle stretching at 5 to 6 weeks if stiffness persists.
- Add progressive resistive exercises to elbow and wrist.
- At 6 weeks shoulder internal/external rotation exercises may be initiated.
- When full elbow motion is obtained, initiate sports-specific exercises and drills.
- Athlete may return to play when strength reaches 90% of contralateral arm.

RESULTS

- Good to excellent results have been reported in 75% to 100% of simple dislocations (Lansinger et al. 1984).
- Fractures and operative treatment may negatively affect results (Broberg and Morrey 1987, Lansinger et al. 1984).

- A minor loss of terminal extension of 10 to 15 degrees may occur (Josefsson et al. 1984).
- Long-term follow-up reveals that up to 50% of patients complain of residual pain or discomfort following elbow dislocation (Mehloff et al. 1988).
- Approximately 60% of patients believe that the injured elbow does not function as well as the contralateral side (Josefsson et al. 1987).
- Mechanical testing has confirmed a 15% average loss of elbow strength (Broberg and Morrey 1987).

REFERENCES

A complete reference list is available at https://expertconsult
.inkling.com/.

FURTHER READING

Cohen MS, Hastings HH. Rotatory instability of the elbow: the role of the lateral stabilizers. *J Bone Joint Surg Am.* 1997;79:225–233.

Josefsson PO, Gentz CF, Johnell O, et al. Surgical versus non-surgical treatment of ligamentous injuries following dislocation of the elbow joint: a prospective randomized study. *J Bone Joint Surg Am.* 1987;69:605–608.

Josefsson PO, Gentz CF, Johnell O, et al. Surgical versus non-surgical treatment of ligamentous injuries following dislocation of the elbow joint. *Clin Orthop.* 1987;214:165–169.

Osborne G, Cotterill P. Recurrent dislocation of the elbow. *J Bone Joint Surg Br.* 1966;48B:340–346.

Lateral and Medial Humeral Epicondylitis

Todd S. Ellenbecker, DPT, MS, SCS, OCS, CSCS | George J. Davies, DPT, MEd, PT, SCS, ATC, LAT, CSCS, PES, FAPTA

INTRODUCTION

Injuries to the elbow, specifically humeral epicondylitis, occur frequently as a result of the repetitive loads encountered in athletes from both repetitive and forceful muscular activations inherent in throwing, hitting, serving, and spiking. Management involves early diagnosis and treatment coupled with a total arm strengthening or kinetic chain rehabilitation emphasis.

EPIDEMIOLOGY AND ETIOLOGY

One of the most common repetitive overuse injuries of the elbow is humeral epicondylitis. Epidemiologic incidences of humeral epicondylitis range from 35% to 50% in adult tennis players, far greater than that reported in elite junior players (11% to 12%).

Tennis elbow was originally described by Runge in 1873. Cyriax (1983) listed 26 causes of tennis elbow, whereas Goldie (1964) reported hypervascularization of the extensor aponeurosis and an increased quantity of free nerve endings in the subtendinous space. Leadbetter (1992) described humeral epicondylitis as a degenerative condition consisting of a time-dependent process including vascular, chemical, and cellular events that lead to a failure of the cell-matrix healing response in human tendon. This description of tendon injury differs from earlier theories where an inflammatory response was considered as a primary factor; hence, the term "tendinitis" was used as opposed to the term recommended by Leadbetter (1992) and Nirschl (1992).

Nirschl and Ashman (2003) defined humeral epicondylitis as an extra-articular tendinous injury characterized by excessive vascular granulation and an impaired tendon healing response termed "angiofibroblastic hyperplasia." Kraushaar and Nirschl (1999) studied specimens of injured tendon obtained from areas of chronic overuse and reported a lack of large numbers of lymphocytes, macrophages, and neutrophils. Instead, tendinosis appears to be a degenerative process characterized by large populations of fibroblasts, disorganized collagen, and vascular hyperplasia. It is not clear why tendinosis is painful, given the lack of inflammatory cells, and why the collagen does not mature.

Nirschl (1992) described the primary structure involved in lateral humeral epicondylitis as the tendon of the extensor carpi radialis brevis. One third of cases involve the extensor communis tendon. Additionally, the extensor carpi radialis longus and extensor carpi ulnaris can be involved. The primary site of medial humeral epicondylitis is the flexor carpi radialis, pronator teres, and flexor carpi ulnaris tendons. Finally, Nirschl (1992) reported the incidence of lateral humeral epicondylitis

is far greater than that of medial humeral epicondylitis in recreational tennis players and in the leading arm (left arm in a right-handed golfer), whereas medial humeral epicondylitis is far more common in elite tennis players and throwing athletes because of the powerful loading of the flexor and pronator muscle–tendon units during the valgus extension overload inherent in the acceleration phase of those overhead movement patterns. Additionally, the trailing arm of the golfer (right arm in a right-handed golfer) is reportedly more likely to have medial symptoms than lateral.

CLINICAL EXAMINATION OF THE ELBOW

Structural inspection must also include a complete and thorough inspection of the entire upper extremity and trunk. The heavy reliance on the kinetic chain for power generation in sports and daily activities and the important role of the elbow as a link in the kinetic chain necessitate examination of the entire upper extremity and trunk. Because many overuse injuries occur in athletic individuals, structural inspection of the athlete with an injured elbow can be complicated by a lack of bilateral symmetry in the upper extremities. Adaptive changes are commonly encountered during clinical examination of the athletic elbow, particularly in the unilaterally dominant upper extremity athlete. Use of the contralateral extremity as a baseline is particularly important in athletes to determine the degree of actual adaptation that may be a contributing factor in the injury presentation. A brief overview of the common adaptations can provide valuable information to assist the clinician during the structural inspection of the injured athlete with elbow pain.

ANATOMIC ADAPTATIONS IN THE ATHLETIC ELBOW

Several classic studies have reported on elbow range of motion (ROM) adaptations.

- King et al. (1969) initially reported on elbow ROM in professional baseball pitchers. Fifty percent of the pitchers have a flexion contracture of the dominant elbow, with 30% of subjects demonstrating a cubitus valgus deformity.
- Chinn et al. (1974) measured world-class professional adult tennis players and reported significant dominant arm elbow flexion contractures.
- More recently Ellenbecker et al. (2002) measured elbow flexion contractures averaging 5 degrees in a population of 40 healthy professional baseball pitchers. Directly related to

elbow function was wrist flexibility, which was significantly less in extension on the dominant arm as a result of tightness of the wrist flexor musculature, with no difference in wrist flexion ROM between extremities.

- Wright et al. (2006) reported on 33 throwing athletes prior to the competitive season. The average loss of elbow extension was 7 degrees, and the average loss of flexion was 5.5 degrees.
- Ellenbecker and Roetert (1994) examined senior tennis players 55 years of age and older and found flexion contractures averaging 10 degrees in the dominant elbow and significantly less wrist flexion ROM. The higher utilization of the wrist extensor musculature is likely the cause of limited wrist flexor ROM among the senior tennis players, as opposed to the reduced wrist extension ROM from excessive overuse of the wrist flexor muscles inherent in baseball pitching.

Although beyond the scope of this chapter, glenohumeral joint rotational ROM should be measured because of the role of glenohumeral internal rotation deficiency in valgus loading of the throwing elbow (Dines et al. 2009). Identification of a loss of glenohumeral joint internal rotation and, more importantly, loss of total rotation ROM with internal rotation ROM loss should lead the clinician to interventions to correct the proximal rotational deficiency in addition to providing proximal stabilization of the scapulothoracic and glenohumeral joints.

Several studies have also been cited regarding osseous adaptations in the athletic elbow.

- Priest et al. (1974 and 1977) studied 84 world-ranked tennis players using radiography. An average of 6.5 bony changes were found on the dominant elbow of each player. Additionally, two times as many bony adaptations, such as spurs, were seen on the medial aspect of the elbow as compared to the lateral. The coronoid process of the ulna was the number-one site of osseous adaptation or spurring. An average of 44% increase in thickness of the anterior humeral cortex was found on the dominant arm with an 11% increase in cortical thickness reported in the radius of the dominant tennis-playing extremity.
- In an magnetic resonance imaging (MRI) study, Waslewski et al. (2002) found osteophytes at the proximal or distal insertion of the ulnar collateral ligament in 5 of 20 asymptomatic professional baseball pitchers and posterior osteophytes in 2 of 20 pitchers.
- In addition to the ROM and osseous adaptations, muscular adaptations occur. Isometric grip strength revealed unilateral increases in strength in elite junior, adult, and senior tennis players ranging from 10% to 30%.
- Ellenbecker (1991) and Ellenbecker and Roetert (2003) measured isokinetic wrist and forearm strength in highly skilled mature adult tennis players and in elite junior tennis players and found 10% to 25% greater wrist flexion and extension and forearm pronation strength on the dominant extremity as compared to the nondominant extremity. No differences between extremities in forearm supination strength were measured. No difference between extremities was found in elbow flexion strength, but dominant arm elbow extension strength was significantly stronger than the non-tennis-playing extremity.
- Research on professional throwing athletes has identified significantly greater wrist flexion and forearm pronation strength on the dominant arm by as much as 15% to 35% compared to the nondominant extremity, with no difference in wrist extension or forearm supination strength between extremities.

- Wilk, Arrigo, and Andrews (1993) reported 10% to 20% greater elbow flexion strength in professional baseball pitchers on the dominant arm and 5% to 15% greater elbow extension strength as compared to the nondominant extremity.

These data help to portray the chronic muscular adaptations that can be present in the overhead athlete and active individual who presents with an elbow injury. These findings help to determine realistic and accurate discharge strength levels following rehabilitation. Failure to return the stabilizing musculature in the dominant extremity to its status (10% to as much as 35%) in these athletes may represent an incomplete rehabilitation and prohibit the return to full activity.

ELBOW EXAMINATION SPECIAL TESTS

In addition to accurate measurement of both distal and proximal upper extremity joint ROM, radiographic screening, and muscular strength assessment, several other tests should be included in the comprehensive elbow examination. Several common tests are highlighted based on their overall importance. The reader is referred to Morrey (1993), Ellenbecker and Mattalino (1997), and Magee (2013) for more complete information on examination of the elbow.

Clinical testing of the joints proximal and distal to the elbow allows ruling out referred symptoms and ensures that elbow pain is from a local musculoskeletal origin. Overpressure of the cervical spine in the motions of flexion–extension and lateral flexion–rotation and the quadrant or *Spurling test* combining extension with ipsilateral lateral flexion and rotation are used to clear the cervical spine and rule out radicular symptoms. Tong et al. (2002) found diagnostic accuracy to be a sensitivity of 30% and specificity of 93% for the Spurling maneuver. As this test is not sensitive but specific for cervical radiculopathy, caution must be used when basing the clinical diagnosis on this examination maneuver alone.

In addition to clearing the cervical spine centrally, clearing the glenohumeral joint is important. Determining the presence of concomitant impingement or instability is recommended. Use of the *sulcus sign* to determine the presence of multidirectional instability of the glenohumeral joint, along with the *subluxation–relocation sign* and *load and shift test,* can provide valuable insight into the status of the glenohumeral joint stability. The *impingement signs* of Neer (1983) and Hawkins and Kennedy (1980) are helpful to rule out proximal tendon pathology.

Full inspection of the scapulothoracic joint also is recommended. Our clinical experience suggests a high association of scapular and rotator cuff weakness with elbow overuse. Thus a thorough inspection of the proximal joint is extremely important in the comprehensive management of elbow pathology.

Therefore, removal of the patient's shirt or examination of the patient in a gown with full exposure of the upper back is highly recommended. Kibler et al. (2002) devised a classification system for scapular pathology. Careful observation of the patient at rest and with the hands placed on the hips, and during active overhead movements, is recommended to identify prominence of particular borders of the scapula and a lack of close association with the thoracic wall during movement. Bilateral comparison forms the primary basis for identifying scapular pathology; however, in many athletes, bilateral scapular pathology can be observed.

Several tests specific for the elbow should be performed to assist in the diagnosis of humeral epicondylitis and, more importantly, rule out other types of elbow dysfunction. These include Tinel test, varus and valgus stress tests, milking test, valgus extension overpressure test, bounce home test, provocation tests, and the moving valgus test.

- The ***Tinel test*** involves tapping of the ulnar nerve in the medial region of the elbow, over the cubital tunnel retinaculum. Reproduction of paresthesias or tingling along the distal course of the ulnar nerve indicates ulnar nerve irritability.
- The ***valgus stress test*** evaluates integrity of the ulnar collateral ligament. The position used for testing the anterior band of the ulnar collateral ligament is characterized by 15 to 25 degrees of elbow flexion and forearm supination. The slight elbow flexed position unlocks the olecranon from the olecranon fossa and decreases the stability provided by the osseous congruity of the joint. A greater relative stress is placed on the medial ulnar collateral ligament. Reproduction of medial elbow pain, in addition to unilateral increases in ulnohumeral joint laxity, indicates a positive test. Grading typically is done using the American Academy of Orthopedic Surgeons guidelines of 0 to 5 mm grade I, 5 to 10 mm grade II, and greater than 10 mm grade III. Use of greater than 25 degrees of elbow flexion will increase the amount of humeral rotation during performance of the valgus stress test and lead to misleading information. Safran et al. (2005) studied the effect of forearm rotation during performance of the valgus stress test of the elbow. They found that laxity of the ulnohumeral joint was always greatest when the elbow was tested with the forearm in neutral rotation as compared to either the fully pronated or supinated position.
- The ***milking sign*** is a test the patient performs on himself or herself, with the elbow in approximately 90 degrees of elbow flexion. By reaching under the involved elbow with the contralateral extremity, the patient grasps the thumb of the injured extremity and pulls in a lateral direction, placing a valgus stress on the flexed elbow. Some patients may not have enough flexibility to perform this maneuver, and a valgus stress can be imparted by the examiner to mimic this movement, which stresses the posterior band of the ulnar collateral ligament.
- The ***varus stress test*** is performed using similar degrees of elbow flexion and shoulder and forearm positioning. This test assesses the integrity of the lateral ulnar collateral ligament, and should be performed along with the valgus stress test, to completely evaluate the medial–lateral stability of the ulnohumeral joint.
- The ***valgus extension overpressure test*** by Andrews et al. (1993) determines if posterior elbow pain is caused by a posteromedial osteophyte abutting the medial margin of the trochlea and the olecranon fossa. This test is performed by passively extending the elbow while maintaining a valgus stress to the elbow. This test is meant to simulate the stresses placed on the posteromedial part of the elbow during the acceleration phase of the throwing or serving motion. Reproduction of pain in the posteromedial aspect of the elbow indicates a positive test.

Some of the most useful tests for identifying humeral epicondylitis include provocation tests to screen the muscle–tendon units of the elbow. Provocation tests consist of manual muscle tests to determine pain reproduction. The specific tests used to screen the elbow joint include wrist and finger flexion and extension (Fig. 18.1) and forearm pronation and supination. These tests can be used to provoke the muscle–tendon unit at the lateral or medial epicondyle. Testing of the elbow at or near full extension can often recreate localized lateral or medial elbow pain secondary to tendon degeneration. Reproduction of lateral or medial elbow pain with resistive muscle testing (provocation testing) may indicate concomitant tendon injury at the elbow and would direct the clinician to perform a more complete elbow examination. Careful palpation of the extensor origin at the lateral epicondyle and medial epicondyle is also indicated. Careful inspection of the orientation of the tendons on the lateral epicondyle shows that the primary insertion of the extensor carpi radialis longus is actually on the lateral supracondylar ridge proximal to the lateral humeral epicondyle. Additionally, the extensor carpi radialis brevis (ECRB) can be palpated on the medial aspect of the lateral epicondyle just proximal to the extensor digitorum communis (EDC), with the extensor carpi ulnaris being just distal to the EDC.

The ***moving valgus test*** is performed with the patient's upper extremity in approximately 90 degrees of abduction (Fig. 18.2). The elbow is maximally flexed and a moderate valgus stress is imparted to the elbow to simulate the late cocking phase of the throwing motion. Maintaining the modest valgus stress on the elbow, the elbow is extended from the fully flexed position. A positive test for ulnar collateral ligament injury is confirmed when reproduction of the patient's pain occurs maximally over the medial ulnar collateral ligament between 120 and 70 degrees in what we have termed the *"shear angle"* or pain zone. O'Driscoll et al. (2005) examined 21 athletes with a primary complaint of medial elbow pain from medial collateral ligament insufficiency or other valgus overload abnormality using the moving valgus test. The test was highly sensitive (100%) and specific (75%) when compared with arthroscopic exploration of the medial ulnar collateral ligament. This test can provide valuable clinical input during the evaluation of the patient with medial elbow pain.

These special examination techniques are unique to the elbow and, when combined with a thorough examination of the upper extremity kinetic chain and cervical spine, can result in an objectively based assessment of the patient's pathology and enable the clinician to design a treatment plan based on the examination findings.

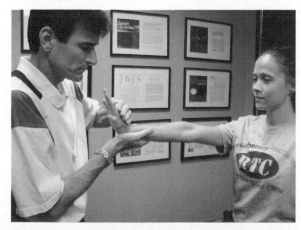

Fig. 18.1 Extension provocation test performed with the elbow near extension to provoke the muscle–tendon unit.

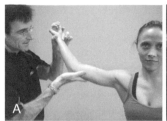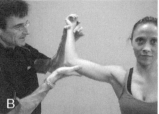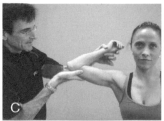

Fig. 18.2   A-C, Moving valgus test for medial ulnar collateral ligament.

TREATMENT

Initial treatments are to reduce pain and increase ROM, muscular strength, and overall function of the injured upper extremity. The entire upper extremity kinetic chain is evaluated and integrated into the treatment process. Understanding the treatment basis for tendinitis versus tendinosis is a very important distinction for the treatment of humeral epicondylitis. Additionally, the importance of rotator cuff and scapular stabilization, often viewed as only applicable for the treatment of shoulder dysfunction, is outlined because it is an extremely important base for distal upper extremity treatment. Finally, exercise progressions and return to activity guidelines are described.

Tendinitis Versus Tendinosis

Wilson and Best (2005) noted that there is a common misconception that symptomatic tendon injuries are inflammatory; because of this, these injuries often are mislabeled as "tendinitis." Acute inflammatory tendinopathies exist, but many patients have chronic symptoms, suggesting a degenerative condition that should be labeled as "tendinosis" or "tendinopathy." Many terms have been used to describe lateral humeral epicondylitis, including tennis elbow, epicondylalgia, tendinitis, tendinosis, and tendinopathy (Stasinopoulos and Johnson 2006). Lateral elbow tendinopathy seems to be the most appropriate term to use in clinical practice because other terms make reference to inappropriate etiologic, anatomic, and pathophysiologic terms.

Zeisig et al. (2006) and Riley (2008) noted that tennis elbow or ECRB tendinosis is a condition with an unknown etiology and pathogenesis that is difficult to treat. Croisier et al. (2007) reports that, in spite of the many conservative treatment procedures, prolonged symptoms and relapse are frequent. Most treatment options have been evaluated for efficacy in well-designed clinical trials, yet there is a generally favorable response to nonoperative or conservative management. Wilson and Best (2005) and Gabel (1999) indicated that about 80% of overuse tendinopathies fully recover within 3 to 6 months.

DEFINITIONS: TENDINITIS AND TENDINOSIS

Several studies have described the histopathologic findings with tennis elbow as chronic degeneration, regeneration, and microtears of the tendinous tissue called tendinosis. Neurochemicals including glutamate, substance P, and calcitonin gene-related peptides have been identified in patients with chronic tennis elbow and in animal models of tendinopathy. More recent research shows that tendons exhibit areas of degeneration and a distinct lack of inflammatory cells (Ashe

et al. 2004). Consequently, tendinosis is degeneration of the collagen tissue as a result of aging, microtrauma, or vascular compromise. Riley (2005) described the tendon matrix as being maintained by the resident tenocytes, and there is evidence of a continuous process of matrix remodeling, although the rate of turnover varies at different sites. A change in remodeling activity is associated with the onset of tendinopathy and some changes are consistent with repair, but they may also be an adaptive response to changes in mechanical loading. Additionally, repeated minor strain is thought to be the major precipitating factor in tendinopathy. Metalloproteinase enzymes have an important role in the tendon matrix; the role of these enzymes in tendon pathology is unknown, and further work is required to identify novel and specific molecular targets for therapy. Riley (2008) reported neuropeptides and other factors released by stimulated cells or nerve endings in or around the tendon might influence matrix turnover and provide novel targets for therapeutic intervention.

Alfredson and Ohberg (2005) using color Doppler examination showed structural tendon changes with hypoechoic areas and a local neovascularization, corresponding to the painful area. Treatment with sclerosing injections, targeting the area with neovessels, has the potential to eliminate pain in the tendons and allow patients to go back to full patellar tendon loading activity. Ohberg and Alfredson (2004) examined the occurrence of neovascularization in the Achilles tendon before and after eccentric training. After 12 weeks of painful eccentric calf muscle training, there was a more normal tendon structure, and in the majority of the tendons there was no remaining neovascularization.

Additionally, Ohberg et al. (2004) reported that after a 12-week eccentric calf muscle training program most patients with mid-portion painful chronic Achilles tendinosis showed a localized decrease in tendon thickness and a normalized tendon structure. Remaining structural tendon abnormalities seemed to be associated with residual pain in the tendon. Fredberg and Stengaard-Pedersen (2008) stated that newer studies using immunohistochemistry and flow cytometry have detected inflammatory cells. Consequently, the "tendinitis myth" needs continued investigation. Existing data indicate that the initiators of the tendinopathic pathway include many proinflammatory agents. Because of the complex interaction between the classic proinflammatory agents and neuropeptides, it seems impossible and somewhat irrelevant to distinguish between chemical and neurogenic inflammation. Furthermore, glucocorticoids are, at the moment, an effective treatment in tendinopathy with regard to pain reduction, tendon thickness, and neovascularization. An inflammatory process may be related not only to the development of tendinopathy, but also to chronic tendinopathy.

Wilson and Best (2005) described many of the clinical findings of tendinopathy. The natural history is gradually increasing load-related localized pain coinciding with increased activity. The examination should check for the signs of inflammation (swelling, pain, erythema, and heat), which would be indicative of a tendinitis response, asymmetry, ROM testing, palpation for tenderness, and examination maneuvers that simulate tendon loading and reproduce pain. Despite the absence of inflammation, patients with tennis elbow present with pain. Zeisig et al. (2006) suggested that the pain involves a neurogenic inflammation mediated via the neuropeptide substance P. Furthermore, the area with vascularity found in the extensor origin seems to be related to pain. Most likely, the findings correspond with the vasculo-neural in-growth that has been demonstrated in other painful tendinosis conditions.

There is no consensus regarding the optimal treatment for tendinitis or tendinosis. Paoloni et al. (2003) indicated that no treatment has been universally successful. Nirschl (1992) and Nirschl and Ashman (2004) described the primary goal of nonsurgical treatment as revitalization of the unhealthy tissue that produces pain. Revascularization and collagen repair of the pathologic tissue are keys to a successful rehabilitation program. Successful nonsurgical treatment involves rehabilitative resistance exercises and progression. A variety of treatment interventions have been reported in the literature, including hypospray, topical nitric oxide, oxygen free radicals, ice, phonophoresis and ultrasound (Klaiman et al. 1998), low-level laser, extracorporeal shock wave therapy, deep transverse friction massage (DTFM), manipulation and mobilization, acupuncture, bracing, orthotics, combined low-level laser and plyometrics, eccentric training programs, eccentric isokinetic program, and a combined exercise program.

Manias and Stasinopoulos (2006) compared an exercise program alone to the same program supplemented by icing. After 3 months follow-up no differences in the pain reduction between groups was found. Because of the confounding variables with multiple treatment interventions, it is difficult to determine the icing efficacy. Klaiman et al. (1998) demonstrated that ultrasound resulted in decreased pain and increased pressure tolerance in selected soft tissue injuries.

Bjordal et al. (2008) performed a systematic review and meta-analysis of studies reporting low-level laser therapy (LLLT) for the treatment of humeral epicondylitis. Twelve randomized controlled trials met methodologic inclusion criteria. LLLT administered with optimal doses of 904-nm and possibly 632-nm wavelengths directly to the lateral elbow tendon insertions offer short-term pain relief and less disability alone and in conjunction with exercise. Stasinopoulos and Johnson (2005) in a qualitative analysis of 9 studies found poor results with LLLT, because it is a dose-response modality and the optimal treatment dosage has not been identified.

Rompe and Maffulli (2007) performed a qualitative study-by-study assessment. In a qualitative systematic per-study analysis identifying common and diverging details of 10 randomized controlled trials (948 subjects) evidence was found for effectiveness of shockwave treatment for tennis elbow under well-defined, restrictive conditions only.

Brosseau et al. (2002) in a Cochrane review determined that DTFM combined with other physiotherapy modalities did not show consistent benefit in the control of pain or improvement of grip strength and functional status for patients with extensor carpi radialis tendinitis. LLLT and plyometrics were more effective using a variety of outcome measures than plyometrics by themselves.

ECCENTRIC TRAINING PROGRAMS

One variable commonly studied with tendon pathology is eccentric overload training (EOT). Limited research regarding the efficacy of EOT for humeral epicondylitis and treatment of other tendon overuse injuries exists. Kingma et al. (2007) performed a systematic review of EOT in those with chronic Achilles tendinopathy. Nine included trials that showed pain improvement after EOT; however, due to methodologic shortcomings of the trials, definite conclusion could be drawn concerning the effects of EOT. Although the effects of EOT in tendinopathy on pain are promising, the magnitude of effects cannot be determined. Knobloch et al. (2007) using a laser Doppler system for capillary blood flow, tissue oxygen saturation, and postcapillary venous filling pressure evaluated the tendon's microcirculation in response to a 12-week daily painful home-based eccentric training regimen (3×15 repetitions per tendon each day). Daily EOT for Achilles tendinopathy was found to be a safe and easy measure, with beneficial effects on the microcirculatory tendon levels without adverse effects in mid-portion and insertional Achilles tendinopathy. Malliaras et al. (2008), in a review of eccentric training programs for humeral epicondylitis, determined that EOT has demonstrated encouraging results.

COMBINED EXERCISE PROGRAMS

Stasinopoulos et al. (2005) described strengthening and stretching exercise programs for the treatment of humeral epicondylitis. They recommended slow progressive EOT exercises with the elbow in extension, forearm in pronation, and wrist in an extended position. The speed of loading and the details (repetitions, sets, volume) of the EOT were not defined. Static stretching exercises to the lateral muscle–tendon unit before and after the EOT for 30 to 45 seconds with a 30-second rest interval between exercises were also recommended. Details of the optimal parameters for treating humeral epicondylitis have yet to be elucidated in a well-designed trial.

ROTATOR CUFF AND SCAPULAR STABILIZATION

In addition to the use of therapeutic modalities and EOT to treat elbow tendon injuries, proximal stabilization and exercise techniques are also warranted. Several key scapular strengthening exercises are recommended to target the lower trapezius and serratus anterior force couple. Scapular stabilization exercises are emphasized and include external rotation with retraction, an exercise shown to recruit the lower trapezius at a rate 3.3 times more than the upper trapezius and utilize the important position of scapular retraction. Multiple seated rowing variations are recommended including the lawnmower and low row variations (Kibler et al. 2008) (Video 18.1).

Progression to closed-chain exercise using the "plus" position, characterized by maximal scapular protraction, has been recommended by Moesley et al. (1992) and Decker et al. (1999) for its inherent maximal serratus anterior recruitment (Video 18.2). Closed-chain step-ups, quadruped position rhythmic stabilization, and variations of the pointer position (unilateral arm and ipsilateral leg extension weight bearing) are all used in endurance-oriented formats (timed sets of 30 seconds or more) to enhance scapular stabilization. Uhl et al. (2003) demonstrated the effects of increasing weight bearing and successive decreases in the number of weight-bearing limbs on muscle activation of the rotator cuff and scapular musculature.

Strengthening the posterior rotator cuff to provide strength, fatigue resistance, and optimal muscle balance is of importance when working with athletes. Fig. 18.3 shows our recommended exercises for rotator cuff strengthening, based on EMG research showing high levels of posterior rotator cuff muscle activation (Video 18.3). Use of the prone horizontal abduction is emphasized because research has shown this position creates high levels of supraspinatus muscular activation, making it an alternative to the empty can exercise, which often may cause impingement due to the combined movements of internal rotation and elevation. Three sets of 15 to 20 repetitions are recommended to create a fatigue response and improve local muscular endurance. For those with elbow dysfunction, these can be performed using a cuff weight

1. SIDE-LYING EXTERNAL ROTATION:
Lie on uninvolved side, with involved arm at side, with a small pillow between arm and body. Keeping elbow of involved arm bent and fixed to side, raise arm into external rotation. Slowly lower to starting position and repeat.

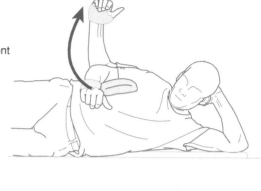

2. SHOULDER EXTENSION:
Lie on table on stomach, with involved arm hanging straight to the floor. With thumb pointed outward, raise arm straight back into extension toward your hip. Slowly lower arm and repeat.

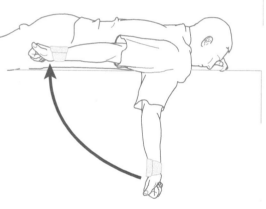

3. PRONE HORIZONTAL ABDUCTION:
Lie on table on stomach, with involved arm hanging straight to the floor. With thumb pointed outward, raise arm out to the side, parallel to the floor. Slowly lower arm, and repeat.

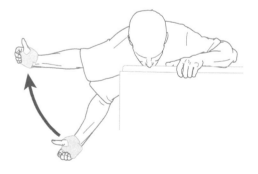

4. 90/90 EXTERNAL ROTATION:
Lie on table on stomach, with shoulder abducted to 90 degrees and arm supported on table, with elbow bent at 90 degrees. Keeping the shoulder and elbow fixed, rotate arm into external rotation, slowly lower to start position, and repeat.

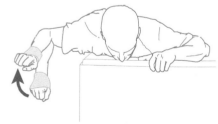

Fig. 18.3 Rotator cuff exercise movement patterns based on electromyographic (EMG) research emphasizing posterior rotator cuff activation and positions with less than 90 degrees of glenohumeral joint elevation.

attached proximal to the elbow if the distal weight attachment provokes pain or stresses the healing structures. These isotonic exercises are coupled with an external rotation with elastic resistance to strengthen the posterior rotator cuff in both neutral and 90-degree abducted positions in the scapular plane (Video 18.4).

Carter et al. (2007) studied the effects of an 8-week upper extremity plyometric program and external rotation strengthening with elastic resistance. They found increased eccentric external rotation strength, concentric internal rotation strength, and improved throwing velocity in collegiate baseball players. Fig. 18.4 shows a prone 90/90 plyometric exercise with the athlete maintaining a retracted scapular position. The plyo ball is rapidly dropped and caught over a 2- to 3-inch (3- to 6-cm) movement distance for sets of 30 to as much as 40 seconds to increase local muscular endurance. This exercise also provides a fatigue response to the wrist flexors and extensors as a result of the rapid grasping and releasing of the ball. Another exercise used is the reverse-catch plyometric exercise, performed with the glenohumeral joint in the 90/90 position. The ball is tossed from behind the patient to eccentrically load the posterior rotator cuff (external rotators) with a rapid concentric external rotation movement performed as the patient throws the ball back, keeping the 90/90 abducted position of the shoulder and elbow. These one-arm plyometric exercises can be preceded by two-arm catches over the shoulder to determine readiness for the one-arm loading. Small (0.5-kg, 1-pound) medicine balls or soft weights (Theraband, Hygenic Corporation, Akron, OH) are used initially with progression to 1 to 1.5 kg as the patient progresses in both skill and strength development.

ADVANCED DISTAL UPPER EXTREMITY EXERCISES FOR REHABILITATION OF HUMERAL EPICONDYLITIS

Exercises to improve strength and promote muscular endurance of the forearm and wrist include both traditional curls for the flexors and extensors with either light isotonic dumbbells (Videos 18.5 and 18.6) or elastic tubing or bands and forearm pronation–supination and radioulnar deviation with a counterbalanced weight. These exercises help provide additional muscular support to the distal extremity and help counter the large forces generated in this region with both throwing and overhead serving motions.

Progression to isokinetic exercise for wrist flexion–extension and forearm pronation–supination is recommended once tolerance to more basic isotonic exercises is demonstrated. Intermediate and fast contractile velocities (180 to 300 degrees per second) are used to simulate speeds used in functional activities. Three to five sets of 15 to 20 repetitions are recommended for endurance stimulus.

More advanced, ballistic-type exercises can be integrated for end-stage strengthening in patients returning to aggressive work activity or those who need high levels of muscular strength and endurance. Rapid ball dribbling in sets of 30 seconds with a basketball or small physio ball both off the ground and in an elevated position off the wall (Fig. 18.5) is recommended. Additionally, specific plyometric drills for the forearm musculature include wrist flexion flips and wrist flexion snaps (Video 18.7).

RETURN TO SPORT/INTERVAL RETURN PROGRAMS

Of the phases used in the rehabilitation process for elbow injury, the return to activity phase is most frequently ignored or cut short, resulting in risks of re-injury. Objective criteria for entry into this stage are tolerance of the resistive exercise series, objectively documented strength equal to the contralateral extremity with either manual assessment or preferably isokinetic testing and isometric strength, distal grip strength measured with a dynamometer, and a functional ROM. It is important to note that often elite athletes exhibit musculoskeletal adaptations described earlier in this section.

Characteristics of interval sport return programs include alternate-day performance and gradual intensity and repetition progressions. In the interval tennis program, for example, low-compression tennis balls such as the Pro-Penn Star Ball (Penn Racquet Sports, Phoenix, AZ) or foam balls are used during the teaching process of tennis to children. These balls are highly recommended for use during the initial phase of the return-to-tennis program and result in a decrease in impact stress and increased patient tolerance to the activity. Additionally, performing the interval program under supervision, either during therapy or with a knowledgeable teaching professional or coach, allows biomechanical evaluation of technique and guards against overzealous intensity levels, which can be a common mistake in well-intentioned, motivated patients. Using the return program on alternate days, with rest between sessions, allows for full recovery, thus decreases in re-injury.

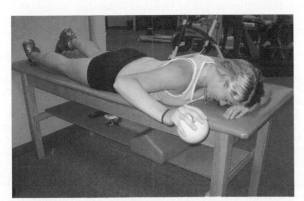

Fig. 18.4 Prone 90/90 external rotation plyometric.

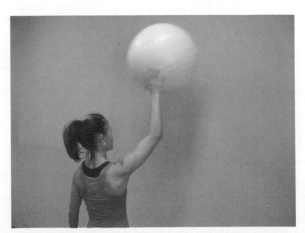

Fig. 18.5 Ball dribbling for distal upper extremity strengthening.

The reader is referred to these publications for additional discussion of this important process of interval tennis programs (Ellenbecker et al. 2006). Similar concepts are used in interval throwing programs, which have been published previously (Reinhold et al. 2002). Throwing mechanics evaluation using video and by a qualified coach or biomechanist is a very important part of the return-to-activity phase of the rehabilitation process.

Two other important aspects of the return to sport are the continued application of resistive exercise and the modification or evaluation of equipment. Continuation of the total arm strength rehabilitation exercises using elastic resistance, medicine balls, and isotonic or isokinetic resistance is important to continue to enhance not only strength but also muscular endurance. Inspection and modification of the patient's tennis racquet or golf clubs also are important. Lowering string tension several pounds and ensuring that the player uses a more resilient or softer string, such as a coreless multifilament synthetic string or gut, are widely recommended for tennis players with upper extremity injury histories. Grip size also is important, with research showing changes in muscular activity with alteration of handle or grip size. Measurement of proper grip size has been described by Nirschl and Sobel (1981) as corresponding to the distance between the distal tip of the ring finger along the radial border of the finger to the proximal palmar crease. A counterforce brace also can be used to decrease stress on the insertion of the flexor and extensor tendons during work or sport activity.

REFERENCES

A complete reference list is available at https://expertconsult.inkling.com/.

FURTHER READING

Adelsberg S. An EMG analysis of selected muscles with rackets of increasing grip size. *Am J Sports Med.* 1986;14:139–142.

Bagg SD, Forrest WJ. A biomechanical analysis of scapular rotation during arm abduction in the scapular plane. *Arch Phys Med Rehabil.* 1988:238–245.

Blackburn TA, McLeod WD, White B, et al. EMG analysis of posterior rotator cuff exercises. *Athletic Training.* 1990;25:40.

Borsa PA, Dover GC, Wilk KE, et al. Glenohumeral range of motion and stiffness in professional baseball pitchers. *Med Sci Sports Exerc.* 2006;38(1):21–26.

Boyer MI, Hastings H. Lateral tennis elbow: is there any science out there? *J Shoulder Elbow Surg.* 1999;8:481–491.

Carroll R. Tennis elbow: incidence in local league players. *Br J Sports Med.* 1981;15:250–255.

Coonrad RW, Hooper WR. Tennis elbow: its course, natural history, conservative and surgical management. *J Bone Joint Surg.* 1973;55-A:1177–1182.

Cyriax JH, Cyriax PJ. *Illustrated Manual of Orthopaedic Medicine.* London: Butterworth; 1983.

Dunn JH, Kim JJ, Davis L, et al. Ten- to 14-year follow-up on the Nirschl surgical procedure for lateral epicondylitis. *Am J Sports Med.* 2008;36(2):261–266.

Ellenbecker TS. Rehabilitation of shoulder and elbow injuries in tennis players. *Clin Sports Med.* 1995;14(1):87–110.

Ellenbecker TS, Mattalino AJ, Elam EA, et al. Medial elbow laxity in professional baseball pitchers: a bilateral comparison using stress radiography. *Am J Sports Med.* 1998;26(3):420–424.

Eygendaal D, Rahussen FT, Diercks RL. Biomechanics of the elbow joint in tennis players and relation to pathology. *Br J Sports Med.* 2007;41:820–823.

Fedorczyk JM. Tennis elbow: blending basic science with clinical practice. *J Hand Ther.* 2006;19:146–153.

Fleck SJ, Kraemer WJ. *Designing Resistance Training Programs.* Champaign, IL: Human Kinetics Publishers; 1987.

Fleisig GS, Andrews JR, Dillman CJ, et al. Kinetics of baseball pitching with implications about injury mechanisms. *Am J Sports Med.* 1995;23:233.

Glousman RE, Barron J, Jobe FW, et al. An electromyographic analysis of the elbow in normal and injured pitchers with medial collateral ligament insufficiency. *Am J Sports Med.* 1992;20:311–317.

Greenbaum B, Itamura J, Vangsness CT, et al. Extensor carpi radialis brevis. *J Bone Joint Surgery Br.* 1999;81(5):926–929.

Groppel JL, Nirschl RP. A biomechanical and electromyographical analysis of the effects of counter force braces on the tennis player. *Am J Sports Med.* 1986;14:195–200.

Hang YS, Peng SM. An epidemiological study of upper extremity injury in tennis players with particular reference to tennis elbow. *J Formos Med Assoc.* 1984;83:307–316.

Hughes GR, Currey HL. Hypospray treatment of tennis elbow. *Ann Rheum Dis.* 1969;28:58–62.

Ilfeld FW, Field SM. Treatment of tennis elbow. Use of a special brace. *JAMA.* 1966;195:67–70.

Jobe FW, Kivitne RS. Shoulder pain in the overhand or throwing athlete. *Orthop Rev.* 1989;18:963–975.

Kamien M. A rational management of tennis elbow. *Sports Med.* 1990;9:173–191.

Kibler WB. Clinical biomechanics of the elbow in tennis. Implications for evaluation and diagnosis. *Med Sci Sports Exerc.* 1994;26:1203–1206.

Kibler WB. Role of the scapula in the overhead throwing motion. *Contemp Orthop.* 1991;22(5):525–532.

Kibler WB. The role of the scapula in athletic shoulder function. *Am J Sports Med.* 1998;26(2):325–337.

Kibler WB, Chandler TJ, Livingston BP, et al. Shoulder range of motion in elite tennis players. *Am J Sports Med.* 1996;24(3):279–285.

Kulund DN, Rockwell DA, Brubaker CE. The long term effects of playing tennis. *Phys Sportsmed.* 1979;7:87–92.

Maffulli N, Wong J, Almekinders LC. Types and epidemiology of tendinopathy. *Clin Sports Med.* 2003;22:675–692.

Malanga GA, Jenp YN, Growney ES, et al. EMG analysis of shoulder positioning in testing and strengthening the supraspinatus. *Med Sci Sports Exercise.* 1996;28(6):661–664.

McCabe RA, Tyler TF, Nicholas SJ, et al. Selective activation of the lower trapezius muscle in patients with shoulder impingement. *J Orthop Sports Phys Ther.* 2001;31(1). A–45. (Abstract).

McFarland EG, Torpey BM, Carl LA. Evaluation of shoulder laxity. *Sports Med.* 1996;22:264–272.

Morrey B, An KN. Articular and ligamentous contributions to the stability of the elbow joint. *Am J Sports Med.* 1983;11:315–319.

Murrell GA. Oxygen free radicals and tendon healing. *J Shoulder Elbow Surg.* 2007;16:S208–S214.

Ollivierre CO, Nirschl RP. Tennis elbow: current concepts of treatment and rehabilitation. *Sports Med.* 1996;22(2):133–139.

Pfefer MT, Cooper SR, Uhl NL. Chiropractic management of tendinopathy: a literature synthesis. *J Manipulative Physiol Ther.* 2009;32:41–52.

Reinhold MM, Wilk KE, Fleisig GS, et al. Electromyographic analysis of the rotator cuff and deltoid musculature during common shoulder external rotation exercises. *J Orthop Sports Phys Ther.* 2004;34(7):385–394.

Roetert EP, Ellenbecker TS, Brown SW. Shoulder internal and external rotation range of motion in nationally ranked junior tennis players: a longitudinal analysis. *J Strength Cond Res.* 2000;14(2):140–143.

Rompe JD, Furia J, Maffulli N. Eccentric loading compared with shock wave treatment for chronic insertional Achilles tendinopathy. A randomized controlled trial. *J Bone Joint Surg.* 2008;90-A:52–61.

Ryu KN, McCormick J, Jobe FW, et al. An electromyographic analysis of shoulder function in tennis players. *Am J Sports Med.* 1988;16:481–485.

Seil R, Wilmes P, Nuhrenborger C. Extracorporal shock wave therapy for tendinopathies. *Expert Rev Med Devices.* 2006;3:463–470.

Sems R, Dimeff JP, Iannotti. Extracorporeal shock wave therapy in the treatment of chronic tendinopathies. *J Am Acad Orthop Surg.* 2006;14:195–204.

Stasinopoulos D, Stasinopoulos I. Comparison of effects of exercise programme, pulsed ultrasound, and transverse friction in the treatment of chronic patellar tendinopathy. *Clin Rehabil.* 2004;18:347–352.

Stergioulas A. Effects of low-level laser and plyometric exercises in the treatment of lateral epicondylitis. *Photomed Laser Surg.* 2007;25:205–213.

Stergioulas A, Stergioula M, Aarskog R, et al. Effects of low-level laser therapy and eccentric exercises in the treatment of recreational athletes with chronic Achilles tendinopathy. *Am J Sports med.* 2008;36:881–887.

Stoddard A. Manipulation of the elbow joint. *Physiother.* 1971;57:259–260.

Townsend H, Jobe FW, Pink M, et al. Electromyographic analysis of the glenohumeral muscles during a baseball rehabilitation program. *Am J Sports Med.* 1991;19:264.

United States Tennis Association: unpublished Data.

Wainstein JL, Nailor TE. Tendinitis and tendinosis of the elbow, wrist and hands. *Clin Occup Environ Med.* 2006;5:299–322.

Winge S, Jorgensen U, Nielsen AL. Epidemiology of injuries in Danish championship tennis. *Int J Sports Med.* 1989;10:368–371.

19

Forearm Upper Extremity Nerve Entrapment Injuries

Steven R. Novotny, MD

PRONATOR SYNDROME

Pronator syndrome is used to denote median nerve compressive symptoms in and around the pronator muscle. Beaton and Anson (1939) and Jamieson and Anson (1952) showed that in 83% of specimens the median nerve ran between the two heads of the pronator, and in 9% the nerve ran deep to the humeral head of the pronator, with an absent ulnar head. In 6% of specimens the nerve was deep to both heads, and in the least common pattern (2%) the nerve split the humeral head and ran superficial to the remainder of the ulnar head. Johnson et al. (1979) published a 71-patient series and Hartz et al. (1981) a 39-patient series that both reported overall good results with surgical treatment. The patients clinically exhibit neurogenic symptoms usually not well defined as carpal tunnel, physical examination of tenderness in the pronator region, and varying symptom exacerbation while activating the three common structures responsible: pronator, lacertus fibrosis, and superficialis arcade. The offending location of the pronator can be at the proximal origin of its humeral head, thus the nerve must be visualized free and clear of the proximal muscle edge before considering it decompressed. Supracondylar processes are a relatively rare anatomic variant and even rarer cause for proximal median nerve or brachial artery compression. The bone itself or Struther's ligament could compress the structures. The process is palpable proximal to the medial epicondyle and palpation often exacerbates symptoms. Extension of the elbow can exacerbate symptoms whereas flexion often improves symptoms.

Acute anterior interosseous nerve (AIN) palsy is a separate entity from pronator syndrome. Miller-Breslow and colleagues (1990) reported on nine patients with 10 cases of complete or partial acute AIN paralysis. The eight treated by observation showed spontaneous recovery starting in 6 months and complete by 1 year. The two cases that underwent surgery also recovered in 1 year. All cases had an episode of sudden pain preceding the paralysis without trauma. Electrodiagnostic tests confirmed AIN involvement. This may suggest the entity is neuritis, rather than a compressive neuropathy, and thus recommend observation.

The standard open pronator decompression involves a 6-cm oblique incision along the leading edge of the pronator muscle. Cutaneous nerves are protected and large veins are ligated only if needed. The soft tissue envelope is elevated proximally and distally as far as can be visualized and retracted with two Army-Navy retractors 90 degrees from each other. Nested Scofields having longer shoes may provide greater visibility. The lacertus and fascia are opened the whole length. Distally, the radial artery is protected and mobilized radially if needed. Gentle retraction of the pronator medially usually exposes the medial nerve at some level. This provides the depth at which the tissue needs be dissected to completely expose and decompress the nerve. Once the nerve is visualized all material is lysed anteriorly, protecting the motor branches. Distally, the superficialis arcade is split and the muscle is elevated with a retractor to visualize as far distally as possible. Usually there is an artery with two veins crossing the distal extent of the exposure; frequently the color of the nerve looks more normal at this level. Proximally, if the nerve is found intramuscular, the incision is extended proximally to the ligament of Struthers region to safely decompress the nerve as it exits the pronator. If a large collateral artery travels with the nerve, it is frequently found with a structure proximally that could contribute to compression. If the nerve stays radial to the proximal pronator and with the brachial artery proximally, lysis of the perineural sheeting is only needed anteriorly on the nerve in this region, as far as can be seen. Finger dissection on top of the nerve is performed and the blunt end of a Debakey forceps is used as a probe proximally. If any concerns exist, the incision is extended proximally.

RADIAL NERVE COMPRESSION
Radial Sensory Neuritis

This chapter excludes radial nerve pathology proximal to the elbow. Wartenberg's syndrome is the eponym of distal radial sensory neuralgia. The irritation of the radial sensory nerve distal to the brachioradialis (BR) musculotendinous junction to where it penetrates the forearm fascia from deep to superficial produces paresthesia and pain. The Tinel sign can localize the level of the nerve injury; however, confounding factors can exist. Patients with previous surgical scars can have neuroma or multiple locations for nerve traction. Regeneration of nerve fibers can produce an advancing Tinel in addition to the primary area of findings. Unless Tinel testing is performed over time the advancing nerve regeneration could be noted as static. Concomitant tendinopathies, de Quervain's or intersection syndrome, can influence the clinical picture. Wartenberg (1932) wasn't the first to report radial sensory neuralgia; however he did report on five cases in 1932. Common histories include crushing or compressive injuries, repetitive forceful pronation and extension activity, and metabolic disturbances such as diabetes and dialysis. Braidwood (1975) reported a small series of radial sensory neuritis. Two thirds responded to conservative means, the four treated by resection of the nerve, allowing it to retract under the BR muscle belly for protection, with good results. Dellon and Mackinnon (1986) reported on 51 patients, and 37% responded by conservative means. Of those undergoing surgery 86% were considered good to excellent results. Only 43% returned to their regular jobs; 22% were in vocational rehabilitation. Some patients had multiple conditions or injuries that precluded a return to their previous occupations. Lanzetta and Foucher, 1993 published a series of 52 cases in which 71% responded nonoperatively with good or excellent results. Of the 15 patients treated operatively, 74% rated good or excellent at follow-up. They report a high incidence (50%) of associated de Quervain's in their population—a cautionary tale.

Mackinnon and Dellon's surgical approach is a 6-8 cm incision centered on the Tinel area longitudinally but volar to place the scar away from the nerve. The dorsal fascia is opened retracting the BR volarly and continuing the lysis of fascia between the BR and extensor carpi radialis longus (ECRL) 6 cm proximally. Neurolysis is performed allowing the nerve mobility and is continued distally until the nerve is loose in the subcutaneous tissue. An internal neurolysis is considered or performed in patients with chronic sensory deficits. The internal neurolysis continues until internal fibrosis is lysed and a normal fascicular pattern is found. Consideration should be given to using a nerve wrap technique to prevent adhesions in this scenario. Severe nerve trauma warrants considering resecting and burying the radial sensory nerve stump.

Zoch and Aigner (1997) reported on 10 patients, nine women, treated over a 2-year period with freeing the nerve and longitudinally cutting and repairing the BR tendon to transpose the nerve dorsally. Their 10 patients were free of symptoms at 6 weeks.

Proximal Radial Nerve and Posterior Interosseous Nerve Compression

The radial tunnel originates close to the radiocapitellar joint. The medial border is the brachialis muscle and more distally the biceps tendon and associated fibrous structures. The ECRL and extensor carpi radialis brevis (ECRB) form the roof and lateral margins. The distal supinator marks the furthest extent. The posterior interosseous nerve (PIN) diverges from the proper radial nerve before the arcade of Froshe. The areas of anatomic compressions include fascial tissue superficial to the radiocapitellar joint, ECRB fibrous bands (often connected to the arcade of Froshe), leash of Henry (radial recurrent vessels), arcade of Froshe, and the distal fibrous border of the supinator. Fuss and Wurzl (1991), Prasartritha et al. (1993), and Hazani et al. (2008) performed human anatomic dissection studies of this region. Overall their observations corroborated each other and portray a fairly uniform construct of this region.

Prasartritha's 31 cadaveric specimens showed no evidence of compressive lesions. Specimens had a tendinous arcade of Froshe in 57%, membranous in 43%. The distal supinator was tendinous in 65% and membranous in 35%. In only 2% of their specimens did the PIN send motor branches to the ECRB. In Fuss and Wurzl's 50 dissection specimens the innervation to the BR and ECRL lay proximal to Hueter's line (intercondylar axis). The ECRB received one branch at 4 cm distal to Hueter's line. The ECRB had a fibrous band contribution to the arcade region .5 to 1 cm proximal to the arcade. Hazani's 18 cadaveric specimens demonstrated a stable PIN course 3.5 cm distal to the radial head coursing 7.4 cm intramuscularly in the supinator. The line of travel is consistently from the radial head to mid-dorsal wrist. This information could allow greater ease and increased safety during surgery.

Roles and Maudsley (1972) in a follow-up to the senior author's 1956 report of treating recurrent lateral epicondylitis

as a nerve entrapment reported 35 of 38 patients with good to excellent results. They used a BR muscle splitting incision, decompressed all fascial material on top of the nerve as could be seen proximal through the arcade, and lysed the leading part of the supinator muscle. The leash of Henry was divided. Lister et al. (1979) reported 19 of 20 patients had complete relief with the same surgical exposure as Roles and Maudsley. Sponseller and Engber (1983) case reported a patient with arcade of Froshe and distal supinator compression. Since there are multiple potential sites of compression, this comes as no surprise.

Sotereanos et al. (1999) reported overall poor results in their treatment of radial nerve compression patients. Their group was dominated by workers' compensation patients, 28 of 35 cases. Seven cases had more than one nerve decompressed at the same time and seven patients were lost to follow-up. The authors rated 11 of 28 (39%) good or excellent results while the patients rated themselves 18 of 28 (64%) good or excellent. Twelve patients had concomitant lateral epicondyle release or revision lateral epicondyle release. Interestingly, 15 of 17 patients with poor to fair results were receiving workers' compensation benefits. Only 12 patients in this study returned to work. Atroshi et al. (1995) also reported relatively poor outcomes in their group. Of 37 consecutive cases 13 reported substantial pain relief, 15 were satisfied with the outcome, and 16 returned to their previous level of employment. Atroshi questions the validity of diagnostic criteria with this diagnosis. One concern would be the lack of complete supinator decompression given reports of distal PIN compression in the era of double crush. Also some reports fail to provide information on duration of symptoms and length of conservative management before proceeding with surgery. Given the basic science of nerve physiology, biochemistry, and micro-anatomic changes documented with prolonged nerve compression that may not revert to normal after decompression, and given secondary gain issues, it may be impossible to produce a uniform surgical result across all patient subgroups.

My surgical approach is a dorsal incision opening the interval between the mobile wad and the extensor digitorum communis (EDC). It is easiest to find the interval distally and to work proximally. Occasionally a branch of the lateral antebrachial cutaneous nerve is in the field and is preserved. Proximally the ECRB and EDC share a septum, the ECRB fibers are taken sharply off the septum and continue to the lateral epicondyle region, and it may be crossed if a lateral release is also needed. Deeper, there is thin fascia connecting the ECRB to the arcade of Froshe and proximally to the capsule region, which is released. The fascia binding the EDC to the supinator region is opened, which allows exposure of the whole supinator. By bending the elbow, extending the wrist, and anteriorly retracting the mobile wad, the field of vision extends centimeters proximal to the arcade. The arcade is first opened on top of the PIN and continues distally. Palpation of the PIN in the supinator can be performed and incremental division of the superficial head on top of the nerve from proximal to distal. The distal edge of the supinator usually is a thick myotendinous structure and must be lysed. The PIN motor branches turn acutely from deep to superficial here and easily can be injured without due care. Retractors must be placed carefully in this area under direct vision to prevent damage to the motor branches. The assistant cannot retract exuberantly. Once the PIN is released, a longitudinal perineurolysis is performed. The PIN is usually tortuous in thickened fibrofatty tissue proximal to the arcade. Tissue is dissected off the nerve at the arcade region and followed proximally. The EDC ECRB interval is closed.

ULNAR NERVE COMPRESSION
Proximal Ulnar Nerve Compression/Cubital Tunnel

Cubital tunnel syndrome is a constellation of symptoms referable to ulnar nerve dysfunction in the elbow region, more often around the cubital tunnel. Internal nerve physiology has been discussed in the median nerve section. Patients that do the best are those with the least amount of "damage" to the nerve preoperatively (Adelaar et al. 1984). Physical examination is the gold standard for localizing the disease process, and electrodiagnostic studies often sort out secondary issues. A metabolic polyperipheral neuropathy upon evidence of focal nerve slowing could portend a delayed recovery post surgery or even result in a lessened result. Electrodiagnostic findings of a chronic C8 root dysfunction upon a progressive cubital tunnel syndrome could explain an inferior result. Those with chronic sensory deficits, intrinsic atrophy, clawing, Froment's sign, or Wartenberg's sign are not diagnostic dilemmas. The question remains if a possible double crush phenomenon exists, affecting the intensity of the symptoms and the potential outcome. Electrodiagnostic studies can help sort out cervical spine disease from Guyon's canal compression.

Classic physical examination of the cubital tunnel includes an elbow flexion test and Tinel test along the course of the nerve. Depending on body habitus and whether or not the nerve is regenerating, Tinel may be unreliable. Control subjects have a 24% positive response to Tinel. The elbow flexion test is performed in maximum hold for at least 1 minute and up to 3 minutes. Symptoms occurring early may indicate true cubital tunnel. Ochi et al. (2012) assessed the sensitivity and specificity of a 5-second shoulder abduction internal rotation combined with elbow flexion in control patients and suspected cubital tunnel patients. The sensitivities/specificities of the 5-second elbow flexion were 25%/100%, shoulder internal rotation 58%/100%, and the combined shoulder internal rotation and elbow flexion 87%/98%.

Pseudo thoracic outlet syndrome (TOS) is far more common than true TOS; any nerve tension can contribute to true entrapment symptoms. An index of suspicion, the nonspecific generalization of symptom location and description, and body habitus may increase concern for this nerve tension problem. Wright's maneuver, Adson's test, costoclavicular maneuver, Roos test, and percussion of the supraclavicular and infraclavicular fossa all have been described with meaning; Nord et al. (2008) showed a high false positive rate in normal subjects and even higher in those with peripheral nerve entrapment.

Nerve testing can neither tell us how a patient feels, nor can it tell us if an individual patient will respond to treatment. The amount of change seen does correlate with outcome. Anderton et al. (2011) reported on 75 patients who underwent cubital tunnel surgery for symptoms. Those with a negative nerve conduction test had 100% resolution, those with a positive test had 81% resolution, and those without a test had 89% resolution. Patients can be treated safely with decompression alone without a preceding electrodiagnostic test. There are legitimate reasons for diagnostic testing for perplexing symptoms that could be upper motor neuron disease, demyelinating conditions, or hereditary conditions.

Research using high resolution ultrasound in evaluating peripheral nerve entrapment has shown a significantly enlarged ulnar nerve in cubital tunnel patients compared to control subjects (Weisler 2006). In further work the same technique has been applied to patients clinically diagnosed with cubital tunnel syndrome with normal electrodiagnostic studies. Yoon et al. (2010) showed the same increased diameter of ulnar nerves in clinically diagnosed cubital tunnel syndrome as in those with positive electrodiagnostic studies. Due to legal concerns, assigning blame or avoiding blame, testing will remain with us for the foreseeable future.

The question is not should symptomatic cubital tunnel that fails conservative care be treated surgically or not; the question may be is decompression in situ or decompression and transposition best? Two meta-analysis studies (Zlowdowski et al. 2007, Macadam et al. 2008) showed no difference in outcomes with either technique, decompression in situ or decompression and anterior transposition. This may not completely answer the question scientifically because endoscopically assisted and medial epicondylectomy were not included. Thus at this point, surgical technique may be personal preference of the surgeon in primary surgical cases. In patients who have had previous elbow trauma, previous surgical interventions or congenital anatomic variations may dictate a change from the surgeon's regular practice pattern.

PERIPHERAL NERVE REHABILITATION

Neurodynamic techniques are the main conservative and postsurgical rehabilitation exercises implemented. Patient education is the key to compliance with the regimen. This education requires a discussion about simple anatomy and biological healing principles. Patients appreciate this approach rather than being given a handout.

In carpal tunnel syndrome the nerve must be able to move with the tendons when the fingers are flexed. It may also need to be moved independently of the tenosynovium to prevent increased neurotension when the hand is gripping. The median nerve is anterior to the axis of the wrist joint rotation, and any dorsiflexion of the joint passively mobilizes or stretches the nerve, a "neurodesis effect." Simultaneously, the flexor tendons travel proximally. Any connective tissue, tenosynovium, and perineural elements must allow the flexor tendons and median nerve to move independently to limit nerve tension.

The proximal forearm and elbow region are different. The median and radial neural spaces are anterior to the axis of rotation of the elbow, tenosynovial lined tendons do not travel with the nerves, and the joint only moves through varying degrees of flexion. While stretching taut soft tissue that crosses a nerve, it makes sense to flex the elbow. This "detensioning" of the nerves in elbow flexion with passive pronator and supinator stretch might minimize further nerve trauma.

The pronator must be relaxed to minimize nerve compression when mobilizing the median nerve in this region. To "pull" the nerve distally through this region the wrist is passively dorsiflexed with the fingers extended while the forearm is passively pronated and elbow flexed. To have the median nerve travel proximally, flex the wrist and fingers passively while extending the elbow in the relaxed pronated position.

For the cubital tunnel, the ulnar nerve runs posterior to the axis of elbow motion and thus is tensioned with elbow flexion. Sliding of the ulnar nerve would be accomplished with elbow extension and shoulder extension and abduction. Reversing the slide requires elbow flexion with shoulder flexion and adduction. Ten slow repetitions of all nerve slide techniques are encouraged every 2 hours during the day.

After surgery, the patients are encouraged to restart the nerve gliding techniques, joint mobilization, and active-assisted tendon glides two to three days postoperatively.

WHAT I TELL MY PATIENTS

Patients are told three major nerves in the upper extremity all run through one or more tight or potentially tight spaces that may get tighter as we get older and cause nerve compression during our lifetimes. If direct nerve pressure increases due to muscle enlargement, traumatic fibrosis, or postural contracture, these can change nerve microcirculation. Whether this leads to an anoxic environment, direct axonal compression, or venous congestive edema may not be known individually; however, it is known to be injurious.

Patients are told that nerves move as our joints and muscle move. They are not static structures. If nerves do not glide or slide appropriately, the zone of tightness directly increases nerve tension when the extremity is used, leading to nerve dysfunction. These "spaces" may have different names such as tunnel, syndrome, or canal, but it is the same nerve compressive physiology for all nerves. The relative frequency with which a nerve is involved and where it is involved is driven mainly by genetics and a small amount by the environment we inhabit.

Patients need to assess their lives—homes, hobbies, chores, passions, work environment—and change positions every 1 to 1½ hours and do 2 to 3 minutes of nerve gliding techniques during the day. They should avoid extreme positioning for long periods of time or resting the extremity on surfaces that apply direct pressure on the nerves.

FURTHER READING

Adelaar RS, Foster WC, McDowell C. The treatment of cubital tunnel. *J Hand Surg Am*. 1984;9:90–95.

Anderton M, Shah F, Webb M, et al. Nerve conduction studies and their significance in cubital tunnel syndrome. *JBJS Br*. 2011;93(Supp III):294.

Atroshi I, Johnsson R, Ornstein E. Radial tunnel release: a review of 37 consecutive cases with one to five year follow-up. *Acta Orthop Scand*. 1995;66:522–527.

Beaton LE, Anson BJ. The relation of the median nerve to the pronator teres muscle. *Anat Rec*. 1939;75:23–26.

Braidwood AS. Superficial radial neuropathy. *JBJS Br*. 1975;57:380–383.

Dellon AL, Mackinnon SE. Radial sensory entrapment in the forearm. *J Hand Surg Am*. 1986;11:199–205.

Fuss FK, Wurzl GH. Radial nerve entrapment at the elbow: surgical anatomy. *J Hand Surg Am*. 1991;16:742–747.

Hartz CR, Linscheid RL, Gramse RR, et al. The pronator teres syndrome: compression neuropathy of the median nerve. *J Hand Surg Am*. 1981;6: 885–890.

Hazani R, Engineer NJ, Mowlavi A, et al. Anatomic landmarks for the radial tunnel. *Open Acc J Plast Surg*. 2008;8:377–382.

Jamieson RW, Anson BJ. The relation of the median nerve to the heads of the origin of the pronator teres muscle, a study of 300 specimens. *Q Bull Northwest Univ Med School*. 1952;26:34–35.

Johnson RK, Spinner M, Shrewsbury MM. Median nerve entrapment syndrome in the proximal forearm. *J Hand Surg Am*. 1979;4:48–51.

Lanzetta M, Foucher G. Entrapment of the superficial branch of the radial nerve (Wartenberg's syndrome). A report of 52 cases. *Int Orthop*. 1993;17:342–345.

Lister GD, Belsole RB, Kleinert HE. The radial tunnel syndrome. *J Hand Surg Am*. 1979;4:52–59.

Macadam SA, Gandhi R, Bezuhly M, et al. Simple decompression versus anterior subcutaneous and submuscular transposition of the ulnar nerve for cubital tunnel syndrome: a meta-analysis. *J Hand Surg Am*. 2008;33:1314–1324.

Miller-Breslow A, Terrono A, Millender LH. Nonoperative treatment of anterior interosseous nerve paralysis. *J Hand Surg Am*. 1990;15:493–496.

Nord KM, Kapoor P, Fisher J, et al. False positive rate of thoracic outlet syndrome diagnostic maneuvers. *Electromyogr Clin Neurophysiol*. 2008;48:67–74.

Ochi K, Horiuchi Y, Tanabe A, et al. Shoulder internal rotation elbow flexion test for diagnosing cubital tunnel syndrome. *J Shoulder Elbow Surg*. 2012;21:777–781.

Prasartritha T, Liupolvanish P, Rojanakit A. A study of the posterior interosseous nerve (PIN) and the radial tunnel in 30 thai cadavers. *J Hand Surg Am*. 1993;18:107–112.

Roles NC, Maudsley RH. Radial tunnel syndrome resistant tennis elbow as a nerve entrapment. *JBJS Br*. 1972;3:499–508.

Sotereanos DG, Varitimidis SE, Giannakopoulos PN, et al. Results of surgical treatment for radial tunnel syndrome. *J Hand Surg Am*. 1999;24:566–570.

Sponseller PD, Engber WD. Double-entrapment radial tunnel syndrome. *J Hand Surg Am*. 1983;8,420–423.

Wartenberg R. Cheiralgia paresthetica isolierte neuritis des ramus superficialis nervi radialis. *Z Ger Neurol Psychiatry*. 1932;141:145–155.

Wiesler ER, Chloros GD, Cartwright MS, et al. Ultrasound in the diagnosis of ulnar neuropathy at the cubital tunnel. *J Hand Surg Am*. 2006;31:1088–1092.

Yoon JS, Walker FO, Cartwright MS. Ulnar neuropathy with normal electrodiagnosis and abnormal nerve ultrasound. *Arch Phys Med Rehabil*. 2010;91:318–320.

Zlowodzki M, Chan S, Bhandari M, et al. Anterior transposition compared with simple decompression for treatment of cubital tunnel syndrome. A meta-analysis of randomized, controlled trials. *JBJS Am*. 2007;89:2591–2598.

Zoch G, Aigner N. Wartenberg syndrome: a rare or rarely diagnosed compression syndrome of the radial nerve? *Handchir Mikrochir Plast Chir*. 1997;29:139–143.

SECTION 3

Shoulder Injuries

General Principles of Shoulder Rehabilitation

Robert C. Manske, PT, DPT, MEd, SCS, ATC, CSCS

BACKGROUND

Normal function of the "shoulder complex" requires the coordinated movements of the sternoclavicular (SC), acromioclavicular (AC), and glenohumeral (GH) joints; the scapulothoracic articulation; and the motion interface between the rotator cuff and the overlying coracoacromial arch. Successful elevation of the arm requires a minimum of 30 to 40 degrees of clavicular elevation, at least 45 to 60 degrees of scapula rotation, and 120 degrees of GH elevation. Motion across these articulations is accomplished by the interaction of approximately 30 muscles. Pathologic changes in any portion of the complex may disrupt the normal biomechanics of the shoulder.

The **primary goal** of the shoulder complex is to position the hand in space for activities of daily living. During overhead athletic activities such as throwing and serving, the shoulder's secondary function is as the "funnel" through which the forces from the larger, stronger muscles of the legs and trunk are passed to the muscles of the arm, forearm, and hand, which have finer motor skills (Burkhart et al. 2003a-c) The ability to execute these actions successfully comes from the inherent mobility and functional stability of the GH joint.

"Unrestricted" motion occurs at the GH joint as a result of its osseous configuration (Fig. 20.1). A large humeral head articulating with a small glenoid socket allows extremes of motion at the expense of the stability that is seen in other joints (Table 20.1). Similarly, the scapula is very mobile on the thoracic wall. This enables it to follow the humerus, positioning the glenoid appropriately while avoiding humeral impingement on the acromion. Osseous stability of the GH joint is enhanced by the fibrocartilaginous labrum, which functions to enlarge and deepen the socket while increasing the conformity of the articulating surfaces. However, the majority of the stability at the shoulder is determined by the soft tissue structures that cross it. The ligaments and capsule form the static stabilizers and function to limit translation and rotation of the humeral head on the glenoid. The **superior GH ligament** has been shown to be an important inferior stabilizer. The **middle GH ligament** imparts stability against anterior translation with the arm in external rotation and abduction less than 90 degrees. The **inferior GH ligament** is the most important anterior stabilizer with the shoulder in 90 degrees of abduction and external rotation, which represents the most unstable position of the shoulder (Fig. 20.2). A list of ligamentous and capsular structures that can limit shoulder motion can be seen in Table 20.2. The muscles make up the dynamic stabilizers of the GH joint and impart stability in a variety of ways. During muscle contraction, they provide increased capsuloligamentous stiffness, which increases joint stability. They act as dynamic ligaments when their passive elements are put on stretch. Most important, they make up the components of force couples that control the position of the humerus and scapula, helping to appropriately direct the forces crossing the GH joint (Poppen and Walker 1978) (Table 20.3). A force couple occurs when several muscles work in unison by applying differing forces to create a common motion. Force couples may include differing muscles contracting concentrically, isometrically, or eccentrically. A force couple at the shoulder occurs as the deltoid abducts the shoulder and is counterbalanced by the rotator cuff muscles that contract to compress the humeral head into the glenoid fossa (Fig. 20.3). Another shoulder force couple occurs between the serratus anterior, which is counterbalanced by the three parts of the trapezius, levator scapulae, and rhomboids (Fig. 20.4). Proper scapula motion and stability are critical for normal shoulder function. The scapula forms a stable base from which all shoulder motion occurs, and correct positioning is necessary for efficient and powerful GH joint movement. Abnormal scapula alignment and movement, or **scapulothoracic dyskinesis,** can result in clinical findings consistent with instability and/or impingement syndrome. Strengthening of the scapular stabilizers is an important component of the rehabilitation protocol after all shoulder injuries and is essential for a complete functional recovery of the shoulder complex.

In most patients, rehabilitation after a shoulder injury should initially focus on pain control and regaining the coordinated motion throughout all components of the shoulder complex. Once motion is regained, attention is shifted to strengthening and re-educating the muscles around the shoulder to perform their normal tasks. To reproduce the precision with which the shoulder complex functions, the muscles need to be re-educated through "learned motor patterns." These patterns position the shoulder complex in "predetermined" ways and activate the muscles in precise synchronization to maximize recovery of function. Associated conditioning of the lower extremities and trunk muscles is extremely important because more than 50% of the kinetic energy during throwing and serving is generated from the legs and trunk muscles. Therefore, rehabilitation of all components of the kinetic chain is required before the successful return of competitive or strenuous overhead athletic activities.

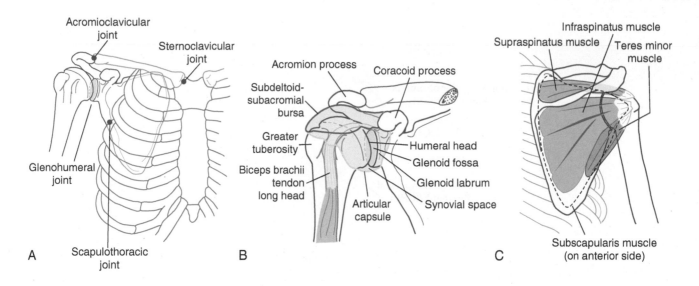

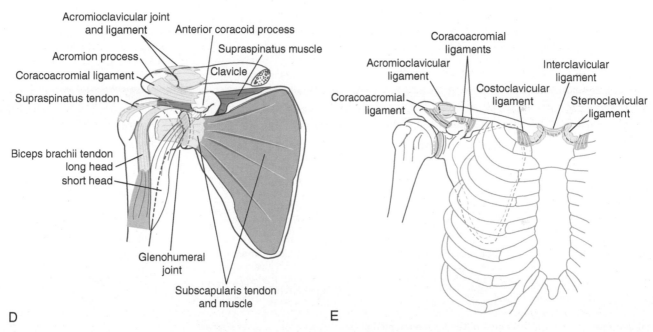

Fig. 20.1   A, Shoulder joint osteology. B, Shoulder musculature. The shallow glenohumeral (GH) joint *(anterior view)* derives some stability from the surrounding tendons and musculature, most significantly the rotator cuff (C, *posterior view*), which consists of the supraspinatus, infraspinatus, teres minor, and subscapularis tendons. The acromioclavicular (AC) articulation (D, *anterior view*) is surrounded by the AC and coracoclavicular (CC) ligaments. E, The AC ligament gives anterior–posterior and medial–lateral stability to the AC joint, and the CC ligaments provide vertical stability. The sternoclavicular joint has little bony stability but strong ligaments—primarily the costoclavicular, sternoclavicular, and interclavicular—that contribute to joint stability.

TABLE 20.1	Normal Joint Motions and Bony Positions Around the Shoulder Joint	
SCAPULA		
Rotation through arc of 65 degrees with shoulder abduction		
Translation on thorax up to 15 cm		
GLENOHUMERAL JOINT		
Abduction	140 degrees	
Internal/external rotation	90 degrees/90 degrees	
Translation		
Anterior–posterior	5–10 mm	
Inferior–superior	4–5 mm	
Total rotations		
Baseball	185 degrees	
Tennis	165 degrees	

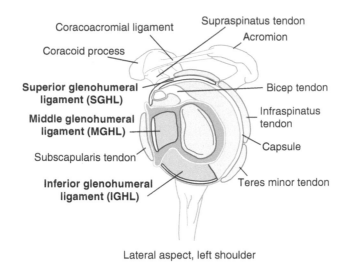

Lateral aspect, left shoulder

Fig. 20.2   Glenohumeral (GH) ligaments and the rotator cuff stabilizers of the GH joint.

TABLE 20.2	Structures Limiting Movement in Different Degrees of Abduction			
Angle of Abduction	**Lateral Rotation**	**Neutral**	**Medial Rotation**
0 degrees	Superior GH ligament Anterior capsule	Coracohumeral ligament Superior GH ligament Capsule (anterior and posterior) Supraspinatus	Posterior capsule
0 to 45 degrees (note: 30 to 45 degrees abduc- tion in scapular plane [resting position]—maximum loose- ness of shoulder)	Coracohumeral ligament Superior GH ligament Anterior capsule	Middle GH ligament Posterior capsule Subscapularis Infraspinatus Teres minor	Posterior capsule
45 to 60 degrees	Middle GH ligament Coracohumeral ligament Inferior GH ligament (anterior band) Anterior capsule	Middle GH ligament Inferior GH ligament (especially anterior portion) Subscapularis Infraspinatus Teres minor	Inferior GH ligament (posterior band) Posterior capsule
60 to 90 degrees	Inferior GH ligament (anterior band) Anterior capsule	Inferior GH ligament (especially posterior portion) Middle GH ligament	Inferior GH ligament (posterior band) Posterior capsule
90 to 120 degrees	Inferior GH ligament (anterior band) Anterior capsule	Inferior GH ligament	Inferior GH ligament (posterior band) Posterior capsule
120 to 180 degrees	Inferior GH ligament (anterior band) Anterior capsule	Inferior GH ligament	Inferior -GH ligament (posterior band) Posterior capsule

GH, glenohumeral.
Data from Curl LA, Warren RF: Glenohumeral joint stability—selective cutting studies on the static capsular restraints. Clin Orthop Relat Res 330:54–65, 1996; and Peat M, Culham E: Functional anatomy of the shoulder complex. In Andrews JR, Wilks KE, editors: The athlete's shoulder, New York, 1994, Churchill Livingstone.

TABLE 20.3	Forces and Loads on the Shoulder in Normal Athletic Activity	
ROTATIONAL VELOCITIES		
Baseball	7000 degrees/sec	
Tennis serve	1500 degrees/sec	
Tennis forehand	245 degrees/sec	
Tennis backhand	870 degrees/sec	
ANGULAR VELOCITIES		
Baseball	1150 degrees/sec	
ACCELERATION FORCES		
Internal rotation	60 Nm	
Horizontal adduction	70 Nm	
Anterior shear	400 Nm	
DECELERATION FORCES		
Horizontal abduction	80 Nm	
Posterior shear	500 Nm	
Compression	70 Nm	

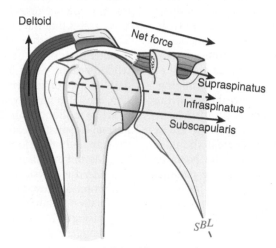

Fig. 20.3 Rotator cuff and deltoid force couple.

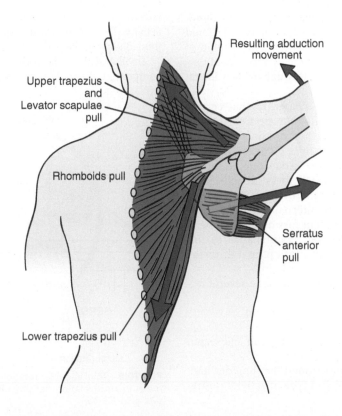

Fig. 20.4 Scapulothoracic force couple between the three parts of the trapezius and the serratus anterior.

SHOULDER REHABILITATION

MARISA PONTILLO, PT, DPT, SCS

Many pathologic conditions can affect the shoulder complex. As with other parts of the musculoskeletal system, these can be the result of either acute trauma or repetitive microtrauma. Acute or chronic injury may result in the disruption of motion, strength, kinesthesia, or dynamic stability. Rehabilitation professionals can positively influence all of these components.

All four shoulder joints work in concert and should be evaluated and impairments should subsequently be treated. On evaluation, obvious findings are easily diagnosed and may involve mechanical disruptions such as gross instability, massive muscle tears, or severe impairments such as significant loss of motion or strength. These contrast with subtle findings that are more difficult to diagnose and just as difficult to treat. Subtle findings may include, but are not limited to, increased humeral translation from a loss of glenohumeral internal rotation mobility, superior humeral head migration as a result of rotator cuff weakness, abnormal scapular static positioning, or altered movement patterns secondary to weakness of the trapezius or serratus anterior muscles. For successful rehabilitation, recognition and treatment of the pathology are as important as understanding its impact on normal shoulder function. Regardless of underlying pathology, the goals of rehabilitation are functional recovery and returning patients to their previous level of activity.

The most important factor that determines the success or failure of a particular shoulder rehabilitation protocol is establishing the correct diagnosis. In the present health care environment, patients may be referred to physical therapy by primary care physicians and self-referral. If after evaluation and treatment the patient does not progress, careful re-evaluation followed by referral to appropriate imaging (i.e., radiography, computed tomography, or magnetic resonance imaging) should be considered. For example, a locked posterior dislocation of the humeral head is missed 80% of the time by the initial treating physician and may only be apparent through axillary lateral radiographs.

On evaluation, it is important to recognize that certain "abnormalities" are in fact adaptations that are necessary to the patient's sport, especially in unilateral dominant athletes. For example, throwing athletes will acquire increased mobility in the anterior capsule and increased external rotation mobility at 90 degrees of abduction (referred to as glenohumeral external rotation gain—GERG). This increase in GERG adaptation may result in glenohumeral internal rotation deficit (GIRD) in which there is a concomitant loss of glenohumeral internal rotation (Fig. 20.5). However, maintenance of this excessive external rotation is imperative for optimal throwing mechanics.

Designing a rehabilitation program should take several factors into account:
- the degree and type of mechanical disruption,
- the chronicity of the problem,
- the strength and endurance of the rotator cuff and scapular musculature,
- the flexibility of the soft tissues around the shoulder, and
- the patient's anticipated level and type of activity postrehabilitation.

Rehabilitation should focus on the elimination of pain and the restoration of functional movement through dynamic stability of the rotator cuff and scapular musculature. With all therapeutic activities, painful arcs and positions that may exacerbate impingement or subluxation should be avoided.

Tissue irritability is a major factor in determining prognosis and goals, initial interventions, and the rate of exercise progression. Because this will reflect the patient's level of inflammation, it should be assessed at initial evaluation and throughout the course of care to guide treatment. A shoulder with high irritability needs to be treated with much more caution and may require more treatments dedicated to pain relief early. Once pain has resolved to some degree more traditional therapy such as range of motion (ROM) and strengthening can begin.

In general, rehabilitation after an injury or surgery should begin with early motion to help restore normal shoulder mechanics. This may involve active or passive ROM or joint mobilizations, respecting the biomechanical properties of healing tissue. The benefits of early mobilization, well established in the literature in other parts of the body, include decreased pain and enhanced tendon healing. Strict immobilization can be responsible for the development of further impairments through rotator cuff inhibition, muscular atrophy, and poor neuromuscular control. A lack of active motion within the shoulder complex compromises the normal kinematic relationship between the glenohumeral and the scapulothoracic joints and can lead to rotator cuff abnormalities. Motion exercises should not be performed if the clinician and referring physician believe that the surgical repair may be compromised. Low-grade joint mobilization may help with pain modulation through activation of type I mechanoreceptors without causing stretching or deformation of the capsule.

Strengthening should respect healing structures while progressing the patient to his or her functional goals. To this end, the appropriate mode of exercise should be considered: isometric, concentric, or eccentric training or open- or closed-chain activities. One must also consider the resultant amount of muscle activation with each activity. These factors will dictate the suitability of the amount of joint loading to the patient's current phase of rehabilitation.

Involving the scapulothoracic musculature is an important component of shoulder rehabilitation. Scapulothoracic muscles

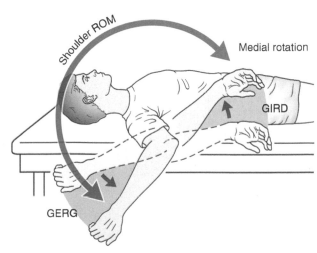

Fig. 20.5 Total shoulder rotation range of motion including glenohumeral internal rotation deficit (GIRD) and glenohumeral external rotation gain (GERG).

provide a stable base for the shoulder and are imperative for optimal shoulder function through their role as dynamic stabilizers to the scapulothoracic joint. Scapular weakness may contribute to subacromial impingement by affecting muscle firing patterns and scapulohumeral rhythm. A loss of scapular rhythm usually results in a loss of scapular motions including upward rotation, external rotation, and posterior tilting. With those important scapular motions decreased the acromion rests in a position that is more likely to create impingement with the supraspinatus and the long head of the biceps with the acromion undersurface, causing either primary or secondary impingement.

Integration of the kinetic chain has been advocated for thorough rehabilitation of the shoulder. Muscle activation of the upper extremity occurs in a proximal-to-distal sequence and reflects innate motor control patterns. The trunk and legs contribute to upper extremity motion through transferring energy and force to the upper extremity. Functional movement patterns that integrate the kinetic chain should be integrated into the rehabilitation process.

Therapeutic exercise should involve not only strengthening shoulder girdle musculature but also neuromuscular re-education. The role of the rotator cuff is to provide dynamic stability to the GH joint, working with the scapular stabilizers to move the upper extremity in a consistent, coordinated fashion. Muscle coordination patterns and kinesthesia can be enhanced through specific intervention techniques. Perturbation training, rhythmic stabilization, and/or proprioceptive neuromuscular facilitation activities may be useful components of treatment.

With the shoulder complex, it is important to work from less to more provocative positions. For example, external rotation performed with the arm by the side will potentially be less stressful than if performed at 90 degrees of abduction. However, it may be important to a patient's functional goals to perform work or a sport overhead; thus patients may need to progress to therapeutic activities in this more stressful position. In addition, although performing prone horizontal abduction with full external rotation demonstrates high electromyographic (EMG) activity of the supraspinatus, it may invoke symptoms for patients with impingement syndrome who do not yet have adequate rotator cuff or scapular strength or endurance. In the early phases of rehabilitation, substitute exercises such as standing scapular plane elevation may be more appropriate. Additionally, early on it must be remembered that the majority of the rotator cuff and scapular muscles will need only light isotonic resistance. These muscles when isolated are exercises usually using long lever arms via holding weights in the hands. Weights of 1 to 2 lbs may be enough to begin a program for most people.

Return-to-sport activities should be incorporated in the final phases of rehabilitation. Once a patient demonstrates sufficient strength and neuromuscular control, then he or she can begin plyometric exercises. Plyometric exercises improve power and encourage maximal firing of the rotator cuff and scapular muscles. Plyometric exercises provide a necessary transition to high-speed activities and will train the musculature to the specific demands of an individual's sport.

Returning to weight lifting may be a goal for many. Progressive resistive training is permissible when there is minimal to no pain, full ROM, and adequate strength to accommodate for imposed demands. Education regarding adaptations of equipment and upper extremity positioning and the avoidance of provocative positioning is mandated. For example, patients with posterior instability should avoid "locking out" the upper extremity during a bench press because of the increased posterior shear in this position. Likewise, patients with anterior instability will want to avoid positions that place the anterior capsule on stretch (90 degrees of shoulder abduction and 90 degrees of external rotation) (Durall et al. 2001).

In addition to clinical re-evaluations, upper extremity or shoulder-specific outcome forms will provide subjective information about a patient's self-reported pain, satisfaction, and functional status. These have been shown to demonstrate reliability, validity, and responsiveness to change over time. The Penn Shoulder Score; modified American Shoulder and Elbow Surgeons score; Western Ontario Shoulder Instability Index; Simple Shoulder Test; and Disabilities of the Arm, Shoulder, and Hand score are examples of outcome scores commonly used for these purposes. Outcome scores can aid in monitoring progress and provide documented information as to the effectiveness of current treatment.

REFERENCES

A complete reference list is available at https://expertconsult .inkling.com/.

FURTHER READING

Clark MG, Dewing CB, Schroder DT, et al. Normal shoulder outcome score values in the young, active adult. *J Shoulder Elbow Surg*. 2009;18:424–428.

Davies GJ, Dickoff-Hoffman S. Neuromuscular testing and rehabilitation of the shoulder complex. *J Orthop Sports Phys Ther*. 1993;18:449–458.

Engle RP, Canner GC. Posterior shoulder instability: approach to rehabilitation. *J Orthop Sports Phys Ther*. 1989;10:488–494.

Hintermeister RA, Lange GW, Schultheis, et al. Electromyographic activity and applied load during shoulder rehabilitation exercises using elastic resistance. *Am J Sports Med*. 1998;26:210–220.

Leggin BG, Michener LA, Shaffer MA, et al. The Penn Shoulder Score: reliability and validity. *J Orthop Sports Phys Ther*. 2006;36:138–151.

McMullen J, Uhl TL. A kinetic chain approach for shoulder rehabilitation. *J Athl Train*. 2000;35:329–337.

Meister K, Andrews JR. Classification and treatment of rotator cuff injuries in the overhead athlete. *J Orthop Sports Phys Ther*. 1993;12:413–421.

Rubin BD, Kibler WB. Fundamental principles of shoulder rehabilitation: conservative to postoperative management. *Arthroscopy*. 2002;18:29–39.

Schmitt L, Snyder-Mackler L. Role of scapular stabilizers in etiology and treatment of impingement syndrome. *J Orthop Sports Phys Ther*. 1999;29:31–38.

Importance of the History in the Diagnosis of Shoulder Pathology

Richard Romeyn, MD | Robert C. Manske, PT, DPT, MEd, SCS, ATC, CSCS

The patient history is the first step in the evaluation of shoulder symptoms. The possible diagnoses will be confirmed or refuted during the physical examination and radiographic evaluation. Because different pathologies may manifest themselves with similar presenting complaints, with the underlying problem producing only secondary symptoms (although these will be the ones apparent to the patient), assessment of the shoulder is uniquely challenging, and an illuminating history requires the examiner to be well organized and ask specific and focused questions because patients generally do not readily volunteer all necessary information. These questions should be asked consistently in a structured and organized format so that they can be replicated easily with each evaluation. If done in this manner, rarely will an important question be missed or forgotten.

When taking a history, the crucial elements about which one must inquire are as follows:

1. *Patient age:* Most shoulder pathologies occur characteristically within a specific age range.
2. *Presenting complaint:* Subjective complaints most frequently include pain, instability, weakness, crepitus, and stiffness, the character and location of which offer clues to the underlying diagnosis.
3. *Details of the onset of symptoms (Mechanism of injury):* Did the symptoms have a traumatic or insidious origin; did they arise subsequent to a new recreational activity or occupational demand?
4. *Duration of symptoms:* Are they acute, subacute, or chronic?
5. *Response to previous treatment:* Has the patient taken medication for the symptoms; rested or protected the shoulder; or had injections, physical therapy, or surgery? Never assume previously rendered diagnoses are correct or that previous treatment was appropriately prescribed or successfully completed. Obtain and review all treatment reports and protocols.
6. *General health:* Diabetes and hypothyroidism are associated with adhesive capsulitis; rheumatoid disease can present with shoulder pain; depression, workers' compensation and other insurance claims, and other life stresses can magnify shoulder symptoms.
7. *Hand dominance:* In some of the general population and certainly with unilaterally dominant sport athletes the dominant shoulder may sit slightly lower due to increased muscle mass or shoulder laxity. Range of motion may be different from that of the nondominant side.

Following are the most commonly encountered primary shoulder pathologies to keep in mind when evaluating a symptomatic shoulder, along with the most likely elements in the history that will suggest them. **Always keep in mind the fact that more than one pathology may be present concurrently.**

- Structural injury to the rotator cuff
- Glenohumeral instability
- Detachment of the superior glenoid labrum (i.e., SLAP lesion)
- Scapulothoracic dyskinesia, core stability deficits, and other fitness or technique-related provocations
- Adhesive capsulitis ("frozen shoulder")
- Calcific tendinitis
- Biceps tendon pathology
- Acromioclavicular degenerative joint disease
- Glenohumeral degenerative joint disease
- Cervical spine pathology
- Fractures

STRUCTURAL INJURY TO THE ROTATOR CUFF

Although traumatic tears of the rotator cuff have been reported even in children, structural injury to the cuff is most characteristic in those older than age 40 years. Rotator cuff tears are so characteristic of the elderly population that anyone older than age 60 with shoulder pain can be presumed to have a rotator cuff tear until proved otherwise. Younger patients with cuff symptoms tend to have only irritation of the rotator cuff (tendinosis) rather than structural injury, with their pathology and symptoms frequently being the secondary manifestation of occult primary pathology such as glenohumeral instability, SLAP tears, scapulothoracic dyskinesia, core stability deficits, or poor biomechanics.

Rotator cuff pathology may be of insidious onset, but it is most often produced by a traumatic event or acute overuse, particularly with an abduction/external rotation mechanism. In the elderly, rotator cuff tears frequently occur during falls. Night pain is characteristic of primary rotator cuff pathology and may be severe enough to prevent sleep or awaken the patient from sleep if she or he rolls onto the affected shoulder. Patients with cuff disease find relief by placing the affected arm overhead with the hand behind the head (the so-called Saha position). Pain is minimal with use of the arm below breast level and is maximal between 90 and 120 degrees of active elevation/abduction. Lowering the arm from the overhead position is often more painful than raising it. Patients may describe crepitus, which is associated with chronic full-thickness cuff tears or thickening of the cuff during chronic tendinosis and scarring of the subacromial space.

Pain is localized to the subacromial area or the anterior/lateral corner of the acromion, with radiation down the lateral arm to the deltoid insertion. The pain is characteristically of a dull aching quality, with the superimposition of a sharper stabbing

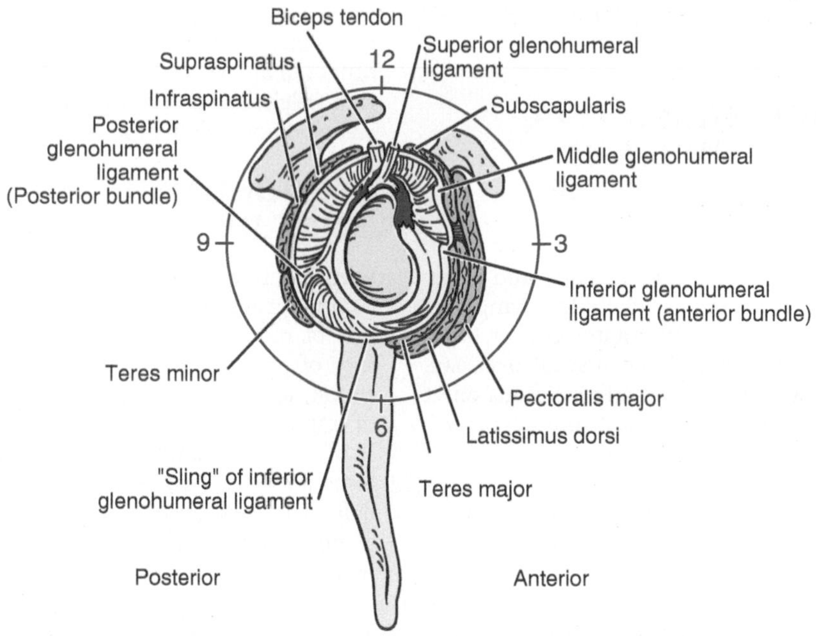

Fig. 21.1 Superior Labrum Anterior to Posterior (SLAP) tear.

pain with use of the arm in the overhead position or with internal rotation. Rotator cuff pain does not radiate distal to the elbow.

The use of medications may help relieve shoulder symptoms. Rotator cuff pain is characteristically mitigated by anti-inflammatory medications, especially subacromial corticosteroid injections, but with diminishing returns over time.

GLENOHUMERAL INSTABILITY

Glenohumeral instability is the most common underlying pathology producing shoulder symptoms in patients younger than 30 years of age. In children and teenagers, it is virtually the only likely pathology. In the elderly population, instability is associated with massive rotator cuff tears. In many instances, the symptoms reflective of glenohumeral instability had a traumatic origin of which the patient is aware. Apprehension with use of the arm in a specific position is a subjective sign of instability, but it is important to keep in mind that many patients with glenohumeral instability have no subjective awareness of that fact.

When the diagnosis of instability is suspected, an important goal when taking the history is to ascertain: (1) the degree of instability (subluxation versus dislocation), (2) the onset (traumatic versus atraumatic or overuse), (3) the direction or directions of instability (anterior, posterior, or multidirectional), and (4) whether there is a voluntary component.

The most common direction of instability, whether traumatic or occult, is anterior/inferior. The direction of instability can be determined during the history with specific questions related to the arm position that produces symptoms: external rotation, with or without abduction reflects an anterior/inferior laxity pattern (e.g., pain with the cocking position during throwing). Pain during the follow-through when throwing or during activities that position the arm in forward flexion/adduction/internal rotation suggests posterior instability. Pain that is associated with activities that apply primarily inferior distraction force to

the shoulder, such as carrying a heavy object like a suitcase or a pail of water, suggests inferior capsular laxity and multidirectional instability.

Subtle glenohumeral instability is associated with a nondescript level of discomfort and diffuse pain about the shoulder girdle. The discomfort is characteristically poorly localized and may be scapular and at the posterior joint line or anterior subacromial mimicking rotator cuff discomfort. Often patients will relate that use of the arm overhead produces numbness and tingling radiating distally without a specific dermatomal distribution. This is known as the "dead arm syndrome." A history of repetitive microtrauma, such as participation in swimming or throwing sports, without proper preparticipation conditioning is characteristically present when atraumatic glenohumeral instability produces symptoms in teenage athletes. Although labral pathology is often associated with glenohumeral instability, its presence cannot generally be predicted by specific questions during the history.

If occult glenohumeral instability was not recognized, there are associated deficits in scapulothoracic function and core stability, or poor technique was not adequately addressed during treatment, there may be a history of failed medication use, rehabilitation, or surgery.

DETACHMENT OF THE SUPERIOR GLENOID LABRUM

Tears of the superior glenoid labrum (i.e., SLAP lesion) (Fig. 21.1) do not generally produce unique primary symptoms that distinguish the pathology. Patients may describe pain generally located in the posterior shoulder or "deep inside" the joint. Large labral tears may produce "clicking" or "catching" sensations. Characteristically, they produce secondary rotator cuff symptoms or are associated with a history suggestive of glenohumeral instability. Patients often relate a history of trauma, such as a fall onto an outstretched hand, or a history of longstanding participation in an overhead throwing sport (the "peel-off" lesion associated with a tight posterior capsule).

SCAPULOTHORACIC DYSKINESIA, CORE STABILITY DEFICITS, AND OTHER FITNESS OR TECHNIQUE-RELATED PROVOCATIONS

Scapulothoracic dyskinesia, core stability deficits, and other fitness issues commonly contribute to shoulder symptoms as a result of secondary irritation of the rotator cuff or other muscle–tendon units resulting from biomechanical overload. There is frequently a history of the atraumatic insidious onset of shoulder pain associated with participation in a new recreational or occupational activity.

ADHESIVE CAPSULITIS ("FROZEN SHOULDER")

The typical "frozen shoulder" is not caused by trauma, although patients will often retrospectively recall some history of minor injury to which they ascribe the symptoms. Characteristically, patients first recognize the problem when they find it difficult to reach behind their back (secondary to an evolving internal rotation deficit). Symptoms are progressive, with "freezing," "frozen," and "thawing" stages having been defined to describe the natural history of the problem. Frequently, secondary rotator cuff pain will account for a substantial portion of the subjective symptoms. Patients may also describe posterior shoulder discomfort with a trapezius or periscapular location because those muscles become fatigued when compensating for poor glenohumeral motion. There is a significant association with diabetes and hypothyroidism, and patients should be questioned about those general health conditions. Adhesive capsulitis occurs bilaterally in this group.

CALCIFIC TENDINITIS

Calcific tendinitis is characterized by the insidious, but rapid, development of extremely severe subacromial or lateral-sided shoulder pain, characteristically in patients of middle age. Narcotics are often necessary to control the discomfort.

BICEPS TENDINOSIS

With advancing age, pathology in the long head of the biceps becomes a frequent source of shoulder pain. Biceps tendinosis is often associated with rotator cuff disease. However, pain originating in the biceps is referred to the anterior arm, as opposed to cuff disease, which is characteristically lateral. It may radiate to the elbow but not typically beyond. Because the biceps is a supinator of the forearm, patients with biceps pathology may complain of symptoms related to forearm rotation (i.e., when turning a doorknob).

ACROMIOCLAVICULAR DEGENERATIVE JOINT DISEASE

The symptom originating from the AC joint most typically is pain over the superior shoulder that increases with horizontal adduction of the arm (because that compresses the AC joint) or use of the affected arm overhead. Injury to the AC joint can occur with a fall onto the lateral shoulder, AC joint arthritis can develop insidiously over a lifetime of use or from prior trauma, and an inflammatory condition known as "osteolysis of the distal clavicle" is associated with weight lifting in young adults. AC joint disease may produce scapulothoracic dyskinesia and secondary rotator cuff discomfort.

GLENOHUMERAL DEGENERATIVE JOINT DISEASE

Glenohumeral arthritis is an uncommon condition producing generalized aching shoulder pain and progressive loss of motion. GH arthritis may be associated with a history of previous surgical procedures (open ligament stabilization, arthroscopic repair of large labral tears, and the use of implantable "pain pumps") and massive rotator cuff tears (cuff tear arthropathy), particularly in elderly women. Symptoms are often maximal at night and more tolerable during daily activities. Systemic rheumatoid arthritis may affect the glenohumeral joint, but particularly in younger individuals, it involves the AC or SC joints.

CERVICAL SPINE PATHOLOGY

Cervical spine disease typically produces pain radiating from the neck toward the posterior or superior shoulder. The pain is usually worse at the end of the day and relieved by support of the head at night. Generally, patients will experience pain and stiffness with neck motion. Especially in the elderly, a coincident association with rotator cuff disease is common. When cervical nerve root compression is present, most commonly C5 and C6 are affected, and radicular symptoms ("sharp," "stabbing," or "burning pain") involving the forearm and hand radiate distal to the elbow in a typical dermatomal distribution.

FRACTURES

Fractures about the shoulder are not uncommon in all age groups. Typically, there is a specific history of trauma, but in the osteoporotic elderly or other special situations, the injury may seem to be of minimal force. The mechanism may be direct (a fall or blow to the shoulder) or indirect (a fall on an outstretched arm). Characteristically, pain is immediate after trauma, localized to the specific point of injury, and severe enough to leave little doubt as to the nature of the problem. Diagnosis is confirmed by radiographs.

GENERAL SHOULDER REHABILITATION GOALS
Range of Motion

Once the intake evaluation is completed, the therapist should be more comfortable anticipating the patient's response to the therapeutic regimen. One of the main keys to recovery is to normalize ROM. Early professions relied on visual estimations or "quick" tests to assess shoulder motion. These tests include combined shoulder movements such as the Apley's scratch test (Fig. 21.2), reaching across the body to the other shoulder (Fig. 21.3), or reaching behind the back to palpate the highest spinous process (Fig. 21.4). These quick tests are great to observe for overall asymmetry, but they cannot give an idea of isolated losses objectively.

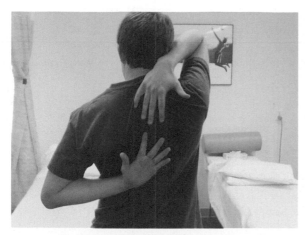

Fig. 21.2 Apley's scratch test.

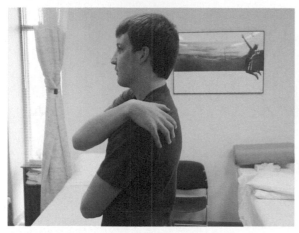

Fig. 21.3 Reaching across the body to the other shoulder to determine range of motion.

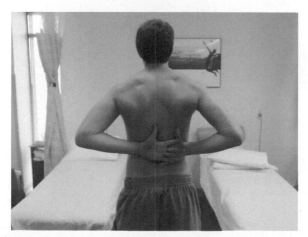

Fig. 21.4 Reaching behind the back to palpate the highest spinous process to determine range of motion.

Even more important is regaining normal arthrokinematic motions at the shoulder. Active shoulder ROM is always gathered before passive motions (Manske and Stovak 2006). Active shoulder ROM measurements are seen in Table 21.1 (Manske and Stovak 2006) and Fig. 21.5. Many times, gross overall shoulder motion may appear to be only slightly limited, whereas arthrokinematic motion is drastically dysfunctional. For example, it is not uncommon for a patient to have full glenohumeral motion yet impinge as a result of altered scapulohumeral motion from a restricted inferior or posterior shoulder capsule creating obligate humeral translations.

Therefore, it is imperative to also ensure evaluation of isolated glenohumeral motions is performed. One of the more common problematic limited motions with a variety of shoulder conditions is that of the posterior or inferior shoulder structures. Debate continues as to whether this is a result of capsular or other soft tissues. Regardless, it becomes an issue whenever elevation of the glenohumeral joint is required because it may increase the risk of impingement. Assessment of the posterior shoulder can be done by measuring isolated glenohumeral internal rotation. To perform this test the humerus is taken into passive internal rotation while the scapula is stabilized by grasping the coracoid process and the spine and monitoring for movement (Fig. 21.6). When passive slack from the posterior shoulder is taken up, the humerus will no longer internally rotate and resistance to movement will allow the scapula to tilt forward. When motion is detected or internal rotation has ceased, the examiner measures isolated glenohumeral internal rotation. Wilk et al. (2009) have shown this to be moderately reliable, whereas Manske et al. using the same technique have proved excellent test–retest reliability (Manske et al. 2015). This motion should be compared bilaterally to assess for a glenohumeral internal rotation deficit (GIRD) between involved and uninvolved shoulders. A difference of greater than 20 degrees of internal rotation is thought to be a precursor to shoulder pathology. Loss of shoulder internal rotation is not always pathologic because some of this motion may be lost as a result of bony changes in the humerus. The concept of total shoulder rotation ROM should also be mentioned. By adding the two numbers of GH internal rotation and external rotation together, a composite of total shoulder motion can be obtained (Fig. 21.7). Ellenbecker et al. (2002), measuring bilateral total rotation ROM in professional baseball and elite junior tennis players, found that although a dominant arm may show increased external rotation and less internal rotation, the total ROM was not significantly different when comparing the two shoulders. However, when Wilk and colleagues (2009) examined professional baseball pitchers, they found that those whose total ROM limitation exceeded more than a 5-degree difference were more prone to injury resulting in loss of playing time. Therefore, one needs to not only address the GIRD but also should ensure that the total ROM is not limited. Using normative data from population specific research can assist the therapist in interpreting normal ROM patterns and identifying when sport-specific adaptations or clinically significant adaptations are present (Ellenbecker 2004). Because there seems to be a threshold to determine what can be considered a clinically significant loss of internal rotation, Manske et al. (2015) have suggested two descriptions of naming GIRD—one which is pathologic and one which is a normal, nonpathologic alternation of shoulder motion in overhead athletes.

Early in rehabilitation following soft tissue shoulder repairs passive motion may predominate. These passive ROMs can be performed using Codman circumduction exercises or by therapist assistance. Passive motions can be gained in all classical directions as long as there are no soft tissue limitations. Other methods of gaining motion are through joint mobilizations.

Passive and active assistive exercises initially should begin with the patient in a supine position with the arm comfortably

TABLE 21.1	Active Shoulder Range of Motion			
	American Academy of Orthopedic Surgeons*	Kendall, McCreary, and Provance†	Hoppenfeld‡	American Medical Association§
Flexion	0–180	0–180	0–90	0–150
Extension	0–60	0–45	0–45	0–50
Abduction	0–180	0–180	0–180	0–180
Medial Rotation	0–70	0–70	0–55	0–90
Lateral Rotation	0–90	0–90	0–45	0–90

*American Academy of Orthopedic Surgeons: Joint motions: method of measuring and recording. Chicago, 1965, American Academy of Orthopedic Surgeons.
†Kendall FP, McCreary EK, Provance PG: Muscle testing and function with posture and pain, ed 4, Baltimore, 1993, Williams & Wilkins.
‡Hoppenfeld S: Physical examination of the spine and extremities, New York, 1976, Appleton-Century-Crofts.
§American Medical Association: Guide to the evaluation of permanent impairment, ed 3, Chicago, 1988, American Medical Association.
Adapted from Norkin CC, White DJ: Measurement of joint motion: a guide to goniometry, ed 2, Philadelphia, 1995, FA Davis.

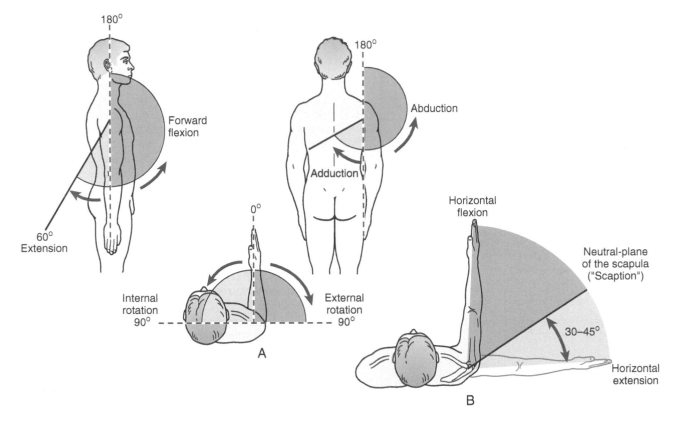

Fig. 21.5 Active shoulder range of motion measurements.

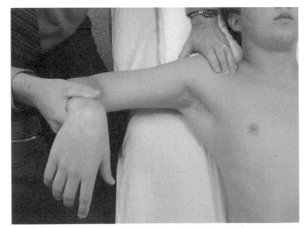

Fig. 21.6 Assessment of the posterior shoulder performed by measuring isolated glenohumeral internal rotation.

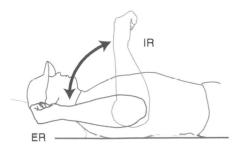

Fig. 21.7 Total rotation range of motion concept. (Redrawn from Ellenbecker TS: Clinical Examination of the Shoulder. St. Louis, Saunders, 2004, p. 54.)

at the side with a small towel roll or cushion under the elbow and the elbow flexed. This position reduces the forces crossing the shoulder joint by decreasing the effect of gravity and shortening the lever arm of the upper extremity. As the patient begins to recover pain-free motion, the exercises can be progressed to sitting or standing.

Once active motion can be initiated, the patient is encouraged to work early on pain-free ROM below 90 degrees of elevation. For most patients an early goal is 90 degrees of forward flexion and approximately 45 degrees of external rotation with the arm at the side. For surgical patients, it is the responsibility of the surgeon to obtain at least 90 degrees of stable elevation in the operating room for the therapist to be able to gain this same motion after surgery. At this point in rehabilitation, methods to gain motion include active-assisted ROM with wands or pulleys, passive joint mobilization, and passive stretching exercises (Figs. 21.8 and 21.9).

Pain Relief

Both shoulder motion and strength can be inhibited by pain and swelling, with pain being the major deterrent. Pain can be the result of the initial injury or from surgical procedures attempting to repair/replace injured tissue. Pain relief can be achieved by a variety of modalities including rest, avoidance of painful motions (e.g., immobilization; Fig. 21.10), cryotherapy, ultrasound, galvanic stimulation, and oral or injectable medications (Fig. 21.11). Previous literature substantiates effectiveness of continuous cryotherapy following surgical procedures such as open rotator cuff repairs, shoulder stabilization,

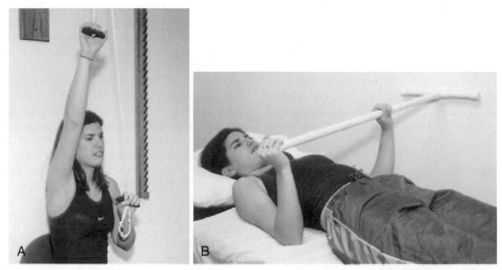

Fig. 21.8   Exercises to regain motion. Active-assisted range of motion exercises using a pulley system (*A*) and a dowel stick (*B*).

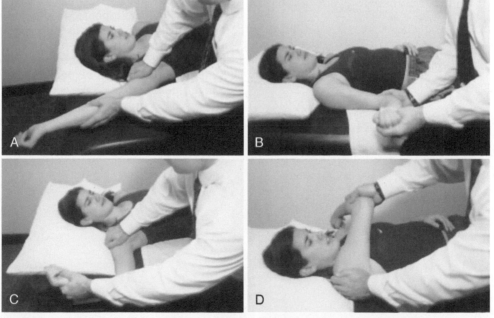

Fig. 21.9   Passive joint mobilization. **A,** Forward flexion. **B,** External rotation with the arm at the side. **C,** External rotation with the arm in 90 degrees of abduction. **D,** Cross-body adduction.

biceps tenodesis, total shoulder arthroplasty, and arthroscopic subacromial decompression (Singh et al. 2001, Speer et al. 1996) when compared to a placebo treatment. Postoperative cryotherapy results in immediate and continued cooling of both subacromial space and glenohumeral joint temperatures (Osbahr et al. 2002) and decreases the severity and frequency of pain, which allows more normal sleep patterns and increases overall postoperative shoulder surgery comfort and satisfaction (Singh et al. 2001, Speer et al. 1996). Recent evidence has shown that compressed cold therapy around the shoulder following surgery does not have any increased benefit over a standard ice wrap when outcomes were average pain, worst pain, or morphine equivalent doses of pain medication (Kraeutler et al. 2015). The theoretical mechanism behind the physiologic benefits of cryotherapy include local modulation of blood flow and oxygen utilization (White and Wells 2013) to spinal cord–mediated reflex arcs (Boyraz et al. 2009, Lee et al. 2002).

Muscle Strengthening

Appropriate timing for initiation of muscle strengthening exercises during shoulder rehabilitation is completely dependent on the diagnosis. A simple uncomplicated impingement syndrome may allow strengthening exercises

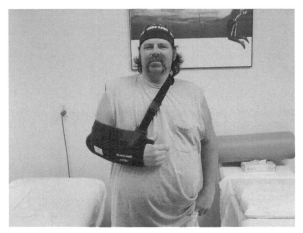

Fig. 21.10 Immobilization of the shoulder for pain relief.

to begin on day 1, whereas a postoperative rotator cuff repair may require up to 10 weeks before initiation of strengthening of the cuff, allowing the repaired tendon time to heal securely to the greater tuberosity. Strengthening of the muscles around the shoulder can be accomplished through different exercises. Early safe exercises include isometrics (Fig. 21.12) and closed kinetic chain exercises (Figs. 21.12 and 21.13). The advantage of closed chain exercises is a co-contraction of both the agonist and the antagonist muscle groups that help enhance glenohumeral stability. This co-contraction closely replicates normal physiologic motor patterns and function to help stabilize the shoulder, limiting abnormal and potentially destructive shear forces crossing the glenohumeral joint. A closed chain exercise for the upper extremity is one in which the distal segment is stabilized against a fixed object. This fixed stable object may be a wall, door, table, or floor. One example of a closed kinetic chain exercise used in an elevated, more functional position is the "clock" exercise in which the hand is stabilized against a wall or table (depending on the amount of elevation allowed) and the hand is rotated to different positions of the clock face (Fig. 21.13). This is done by creating an isometric contraction in the direction of the numbers around the clock face. Alternatively, the therapist can also give manual resistance in the same directions to the patient's arm as he or she is stabilizing it by holding on to the wall (Fig. 21.14). These motions are thought to effectively stimulate rotator cuff activity. Initially, the maneuvers are done with the shoulder in less than 90 degrees of glenohumeral abduction or flexion. As healing tissues improve and motion is recovered, strengthening progresses to greater amounts of shoulder abduction and forward flexion.

Isometric exercises can also be performed in various ranges of shoulder elevation. It is easiest to do this with the patient in supine. The "balance position" is that of 90 to 100 degrees of forward flexion of the shoulder while supine (Fig. 21.15). This position requires little activation of the deltoid so that the rotator cuff can be worked without provoking a painful shoulder response. In this position a contraction from the deltoid will result in joint compression, helping to enhance joint stability. Rhythmic stabilization or alternating isometric exercises can be performed very comfortably in the supine position and can be done for both rotator cuff and shoulder muscles.

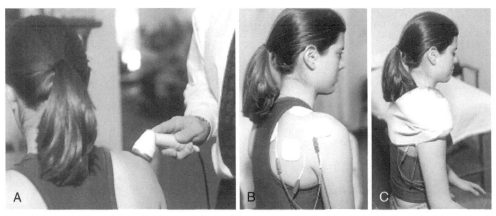

Fig. 21.11 Modalities for pain relief. **A,** Ultrasound. **B,** Galvanic stimulation. **C,** Cryotherapy.

Strengthening of scapular stabilizers is important early on in the rehabilitation program. Scapular strengthening can begin in side lying with isometric muscle contractions or isotonic contractions or even closed chain (Fig. 21.16) and progress to open kinetic chain exercises (Fig. 21.17).

Recovery can be enhanced by utilizing *proprioceptive neuromuscular facilitation* (PNF) exercises. The therapist can apply specific sensory inputs to facilitate a specific activity or movement pattern. One example of this is the D2 flexion–extension pattern for the upper extremity. During this maneuver, the therapist applies resistance as the patient moves the arm through predetermined patterns. These exercises can be done in various levels of shoulder elevation

including 30, 60, 90, and 120 degrees of elevation. These exercises are to enhance the stability of the glenohumeral joint through a given active ROM.

As the patient progresses, more progressive strengthening can be instituted by moving from isometric and closed chain exercises to those that are more isotonic and open chain in nature (Fig. 21.18). Open chain exercises are done with the distal end of the extremity no longer stabilized against a fixed object. This results in the potential for increased shear forces across the glenohumeral joint. Shoulder internal and external rotation exercises are done initially standing or seated with the shoulder in the scapular plane. The scapular plane position is recreated with the shoulder between 30 degrees and 60 degrees

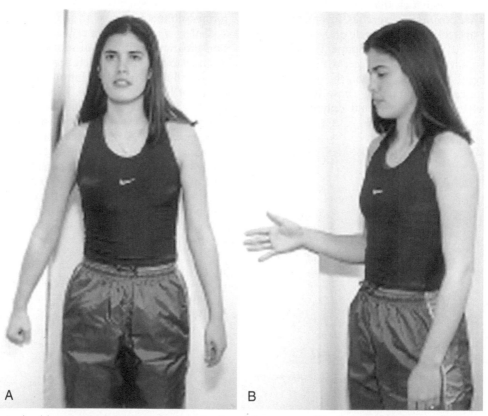

Fig. 21.12 Closed chain shoulder exercises. **A,** Isometric strengthening of the rotator cuff in abduction (pushing out against the wall). **B,** Isometric strengthening of the rotator cuff in external rotation.

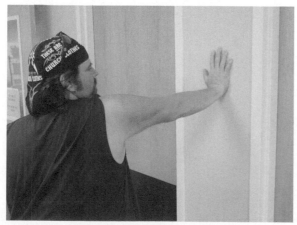

Fig. 21.13 Wall clock exercise.

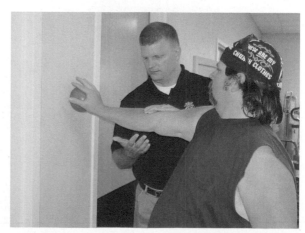

Fig. 21.14 Wall clock exercise with manual resistance.

anterior to the frontal plane of the thorax or halfway between directly in front (sagittal plane) and directly to the side (frontal plane). The scapular plane is a much more comfortable plane to exercise in because it puts less stress on the joint capsule and orients the shoulder in a position that more closely represents functional movement patterns. Rotational exercises should begin with the arm comfortably at the patient's side and advance to 90 degrees of elevation based on the patient's injury, level of discomfort, and stage of soft tissue healing. The variation in position positively stresses the dynamic stabilizers by altering the stability of the GH joint from maximum stability with the arm at the side to minimum stability with the arm in 90 degrees of abduction.

For those who participate in either competitive or recreational overhead sporting activities, the *most functional of all open chain exercises are plyometric exercises*. Plyometric activities are defined by a stretch-shortening cycle of the muscle tendon unit (Davies et al. 2015). This is a component of almost all athletic activities. Initially the muscle is eccentrically stretched and loaded. Following the stretched position the shoulder/arm quickly performs a concentric contraction. These forms of exercises are higher-level exercises that should only be included once the patient has developed an adequate strength base and achieved full ROM (Davies et al. 2015). Not all patients require plyometric training, and this should be discussed before their incorporation. Plyometric exercises are successful in development of strength and power. Tubing, medicine ball training, or free weights are all acceptable plyometric devices for the shoulder (Fig. 21.19).

Nothing is more important when rehabilitating the shoulder than remembering the musculature of the upper extremity and core. *Total arm strengthening* is a must when rehabilitating the shoulder because injuries to the shoulder that limit normal functional movement patterns and use will result in strength deficits of other upper extremity muscles. Overall conditioning including stretching, strengthening, and endurance training of the other components of the kinematic chain should be performed simultaneously with shoulder rehabilitation.

Patient motivation is a critical component of the rehabilitation program. Without self-motivation, any treatment plan is destined to fail. For complete recovery, most rehabilitation protocols will require the patient to perform some of the exercises on his or her own at home. This requires not only an understanding of the maneuvers but also the discipline for the patient to execute them on a regular basis. Patient self-motivation is even more crucial in the present medical environment with increased attention and scrutiny directed at cost containment. Many insurance carriers limit coverage for rehabilitation at the patient's expense. As a result, a comprehensive home exercise program should be outlined for the patient early in the rehabilitation process. This allows patients to augment their rehabilitation exercises at home and gives them a feeling of responsibility for their own recovery.

REFERENCES

A complete reference list is available at https://expertconsult .inkling.com/.

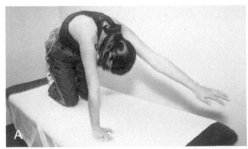

Fig. 21.15 The "balance position" is that of 90 to 100 degrees of forward flexion of the shoulder while supine.

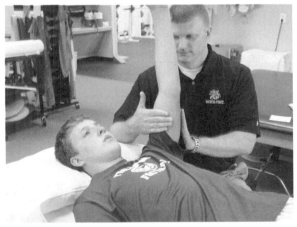
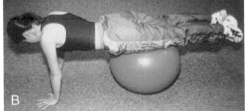
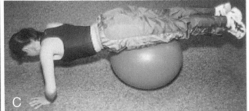

Fig. 21.16 Closed chain strengthening exercises of the scapula stabilizers. **A,** Scapular protraction. **B** and **C,** Scapular retraction.

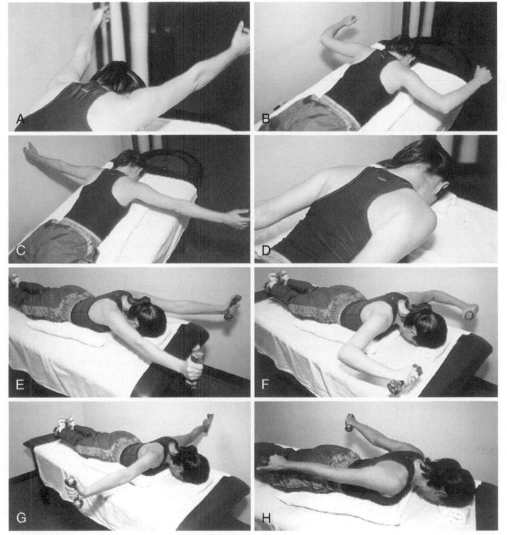

Fig. 21.17 Open chain strengthening exercises of the scapula stabilizers without (*A–D*) and with (*E–H*) lightweight dumbbells.

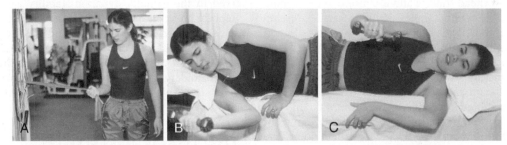

Fig. 21.18 Open chain isotonic strengthening of the rotator cuff (internal rotation) using Theraband tubing (*A*), lightweight dumbbells (*B*), and external rotation strengthening (*C*).

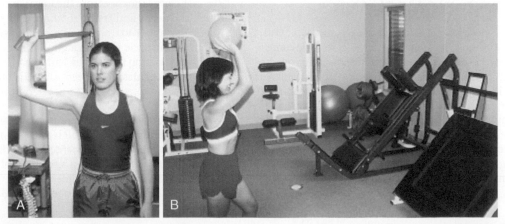

Fig. 21.19 Plyometric shoulder strengthening exercises using Theraband tubing (*A*) and an exercise ball (*B*).

Rotator Cuff Tendinitis in the Overhead Athlete

Michael J. O'Brien, MD | Felix H. Savoie III, MD

The overhead throwing motion is a complex and intricate movement that places extraordinary demands and very high stresses on the shoulder joint complex. The ability to throw a baseball over 90 miles per hour at pinpoint accuracy is the end result of a complex link in the kinetic chain that produces high-velocity overhead motion. Disruption of that kinetic chain by any means, whether by improper core strengthening, shoulder dyskinesia, poor mechanics, or poor posturing, places increased stress on the rotator cuff. Therefore, the shoulder of an overhead athlete requires special consideration. Rotator cuff tendinitis and shoulder pain in the overhead athlete represent a unique challenge for the treating clinician in terms of both diagnosis and treatment. The key to successful management hinges on a thorough evaluation, correct diagnosis, and a structured multi-phase rehabilitation protocol. Through a structured conditioning and rehabilitation program, many overhead athletes can return to play without being sidelined by surgery.

Overhead athletic activities can be classified as those movements that require repetitive motion with the arm in at least 90 degrees of forward flexion or abduction or a combination of the two. Athletes who participate in activities such as swimming, gymnastics, volleyball, or throwing sports experience this type of repetitive overhead trauma and are prone to developing injuries to the shoulder joint complex. Athletes usually develop well-described adaptations in response to stresses placed upon shoulder tissues as the result of overhead throwing activities. One such adaptation **is a degree of hyperlaxity of the glenohumeral joint, resulting from increased laxity of the anterior joint capsule with concomitant tightness of the posterior capsule.** Overhead athletes are able to function with this glenohumeral laxity by compensating with proper development of the dynamic stabilizers crossing the glenohumeral joint. The chief dynamic stabilizers are the rotator cuff, deltoid, and scapular stabilizing muscles.

ANATOMY AND BIOMECHANICS

The rotator cuff is composed of four muscles: supraspinatus, infraspinatus, teres minor, and subscapularis. These four muscles take origin on the body of the scapula and insert on the tuberosities of the proximal humerus. The rotator cuff serves several functions in glenohumeral joint motion and stability. It provides joint compression, resistance to glenohumeral translation, and some rotation in all planes of motion. It is intricately involved in powering movement of the shoulder.
- The primary role of the rotator cuff is to provide dynamic stability throughout ROM. Stability is achieved by compression of the humeral head on the glenoid by the rotator cuff tendons.

- In this way, the rotator cuff provides direct joint compression and allows the humeral head to maintain a relatively constant position in relation to the glenoid. The rotator cuff keeps the humeral head centered within the glenoid during motion and allows the deltoid to function.
- The subscapularis, infraspinatus, and teres minor depress the humeral head, counteracting the upward pull of the deltoid (Inman et al. 1944).
- The infraspinatus and teres minor are the only cuff muscles that produce external rotation.
- The subscapularis functions as a strong internal rotator of the arm but also contributes to arm abduction and humeral head depression (Otis et al. 1994). The subscapularis is the most important for extremes of internal rotation.

During overhead sports, extreme forces are placed on the rotator cuff. It is continuously challenged to keep the humeral head centered in the glenoid, preventing subluxations of the joint. If proper conditioning and sound mechanics are not used, the rotator cuff and posterior joint capsule can become inflamed and irritated. Chronic inflammation can become pathologic and lead to dysfunction of the rotator cuff. When the four cuff muscles fail to act in synchrony to keep the humeral head centered in the glenoid, dynamic stability can be compromised. Repeated microtrauma to the posterior rotator cuff and capsule leads to posterior capsule contracture. Posterior capsular tightness and loss of dynamic stability lead to increased subluxation and anterior–posterior (AP) translation of the humeral head on the glenoid, further contributing to irritation of the rotator cuff. Over time, this repetitive insult can cause tears of the rotator cuff and superior labrum.

THE THROWING CYCLE

The baseball pitch serves as the biomechanical model for many overhead throwing motions. The throwing cycle is a kinetic chain that derives energy from the lower extremities, transfers it through the pelvis and trunk rotation, and releases that energy through the upper extremity. The arm positions and motions of the throwing cycle serve as a good model for examination of rotator cuff function in overhead athletes. The throwing motion and its biomechanics have been divided into six stages: wind-up, early cocking, late cocking, acceleration, deceleration, and follow-through (Fig. 22.1).
- **Wind-Up:** Serves as the preparatory phase. Includes body rotation and ends when the ball leaves the nondominant hand. The body is raised over the center of gravity and the shoulder is placed in slight abduction and internal rotation. Minimal stress is placed on the shoulder at this position (Glousman et al. 1992, Jobe et al. 1984, Jobe et al. 1983).

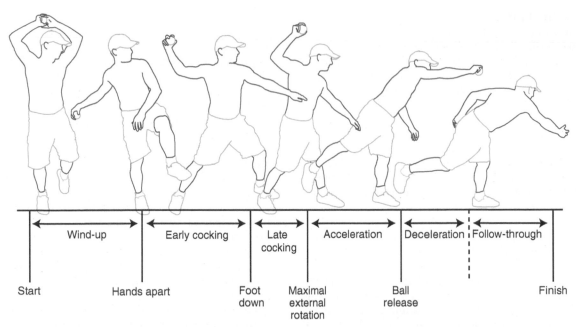

Fig. 22.1 The six phases of the throwing cycle. (Adapted with permission from DiGiovine NM, Jobe FW, Pink M, Perry J. An electromyographic analysis of the upper extremity in pitching. *J Shoulder Elbow Surg* 1:15-25, 1992.)

- **Early Cocking:** As the ball is released from the glove hand, the shoulder abducts and externally rotates. The arm starts to rotate slightly behind the body axis approximately 15 degrees. The body starts moving forward, generating momentum. Early cocking terminates as the forward foot contacts the ground and the arm has reached its top motion and does not move further backwards.
- **Late Cocking:** As the body rapidly moves forward, the dominant shoulder achieves maximal abduction and external rotation. Significant torques and forces are placed on the shoulder restraints at this extreme ROM. The scapular retracts to provide a stable glenoid surface for the humeral head. The upper arm is held in 90 to 100 degrees of abduction and the elbow moves even with the midline of the torso.
- **Acceleration:** Begins with further forward body motion and internal rotation of the shoulder leading to internal rotation of the throwing arm. Acceleration ends with ball release. Muscles become very active in this phase including triceps and the pectoralis major early and later the latissimus dorsi.
- **Deceleration:** Begins after ball release and constitutes 30% of the time required to dissipate the excess kinetic energy of the throwing motion. Tremendous forces and stress occur to the rotator cuff muscles as the arm is quickly slowed to an abrupt halt.
- **Follow-Through:** Completes the remaining 70% of the time required to dissipate the excess kinetic energy. All major muscle groups must eccentrically contract to accomplish this result. Follow-through ends when all motion is complete.

PATHOGENESIS

Injury to the shoulder during the throwing cycle is thought to occur during the late cocking phase, when the shoulder is in extreme external rotation and horizontal abduction. Abnormal motion of the humeral head relative to the glenoid can injure the superior and posterosuperior labrum and glenoid and the undersurface of the rotator cuff. Davidson and colleagues (1995) felt repetitive contact between the articular side of the rotator cuff and the posterosuperior glenoid in late cocking to be the reason for undersurface rotator cuff tears. This phenomenon has been called *internal impingement* of the shoulder or *posterior superior glenoid impingement* (Burkhart et al. 2003, Fleisig et al. 1995, Jobe 1995, Kelley and Leggin 1999, Walch et al. 1992). Several factors have been implicated in the development of internal impingement, including traction on the biceps tendon, laxity of the anterior band of the inferior glenohumeral ligament caused by excessive external rotation, posterior capsular tightness, and scapular dyskinesia.

- Pain in the late cocking phase is usually localized to the anterior aspect of the shoulder. Pain during this stage can be the result of anterior instability, as the rotator cuff attempts to counteract the excessive glenohumeral translation that results from anterior instability and posterior capsular tightness.
- Discomfort during the late cocking and early acceleration stages may be experienced posteriorly, secondary to the irritation of the posterior capsule and rotator cuff as it attempts to overcome the increased anterior laxity.
- Another potential cause is trauma to the posterior superior glenoid labrum from the repetitive stress delivered to the shoulder in these extreme positions.

Muscle imbalance and capsular tightness contribute to rotator cuff pathology by allowing excess translation at the glenohumeral joint. Weakness of the supraspinatus or subscapularis can compromise compression of the glenohumeral joint during active shoulder motion. This, in turn, leads to increased translation across the joint.

Grossman et al. (2005) quantified glenohumeral motion following external rotation capsular stretch and subsequent posterior capsular shift to simulate a posterior capsular contracture in the thrower's shoulder. In maximal external rotation in intact specimens, the humeral head moved in a posterior and inferior direction. A posterior capsular shift was performed to simulate posterior capsular contracture. Following posterior capsular shift, there was a trend toward a more superior position of the humeral head in maximal external rotation. Posterior capsular contracture causes a similar result as the head is pushed anterior–superior into the coracoacromial arch during flexion. Superior translation allows the head to migrate closer to the acromion, and an increase in the force transmitted to the rotator cuff results as the cuff is pressed between the humeral head and the overlying coracoacromial arch. The increased pressure on the cuff can lead to degradation and damage over time.

HISTORY AND PHYSICAL EXAMINATION

Evaluation of overhead athletes, particularly at higher levels, should begin prior to the season and continue intermittently throughout the season. Subjective complaints regarding performance often precede complaints of pain in the shoulder or elbow. **Common complaints include loss of command or control of the pitch, loss of pitching velocity, a subtle change in pitching mechanics, or even discomfort distant to the throwing arm.** Early identification of these problems requires open communication among players, coaches, physicians, and athletic trainers.

- The athlete must precisely define the location, onset, and duration of the discomfort.
- The timing of the discomfort during the throwing cycle can also help elucidate the pathology.
- Recent changes in the athlete's training regimen and throwing program should be ascertained.
- When evaluating the young pitcher, information about pitch counts, amount of rest between starts, and types of pitches thrown is useful because these may contribute to injury.
- Physical examination of the overhead athlete requires a global evaluation.
- Examination should include assessment of core/trunk muscle strength and lower extremities because it is integral in the transfer of energy from the lower extremities to the arm during the throwing cycle.
- Pathology or weakness of the spine, trunk, or lower extremities can ultimately affect the upper extremity and mechanics of the throwing cycle and should be diagnosed and corrected if present. These can include injury to the knee or ankle, tightness of lumbar spine muscles and those crossing the hip and knee joint, weakness of hip abductors and trunk stabilizers, and conditions affecting the mobility of the spine (lumbar degenerative disk disease).
- Provocative tests, such as a dynamic Trendelenburg test, may be useful in identifying subtle weakness of the trunk or lower extremity.

The physical examination of the shoulder and upper extremity should always begin with inspection.

- The supraspinatus and infraspinatus fossae should be inspected for muscle atrophy and compared to the contralateral side. Atrophy in these areas can be a sign of possible neurologic deficit, such as suprascapular nerve compression.

- The posterior shoulder should be carefully assessed during active arm elevation to evaluate scapular position, motion, and control. Scapular dyskinesia or winging may indicate a primary or secondary problem in the thrower's shoulder. Primary fatigue of periscapular muscles from repetitive pitching can contribute to abnormal glenohumeral motion and the development of shoulder pain. Scapular dyskinesia may also result from primary intra-articular glenohumeral pathology (Burkhart et al. 2003, Cools et al. 2007, Moseley et al. 1992).

Active and passive range of motion (PROM) should be assessed and compared to the contralateral side. The American Shoulder and Elbow Surgeons have recommended four functional ranges of motion that should be measured (Richards et al. 1994): forward elevation, internal rotation, and external rotation at the side and at 90 degrees of abduction are measured. Loss of the total arc of rotation, specifically with internal rotation, is a common finding in the glenohumeral joint of the injured pitcher (Burkhart et al. 2003). This loss is likely secondary to tightness of the posterior soft tissues, including the posterior rotator cuff and capsule.

Complete assessment of the shoulder should also include careful assessment of rotator cuff strength and glenohumeral joint laxity and provocative tests to identify intra-articular, subacromial, and acromioclavicular pathology.

- Tenderness over the greater tuberosity may indicate rotator cuff tendinitis.
- Players may demonstrate weakness in resisted external rotation and abduction in the plane of the scapula.
- Resolution of symptoms and recovery of strength after local injection of anesthetic (the so-called "impingement test") suggests rotator cuff tendinitis instead of rotator cuff tear and may aid in diagnosis.

IMAGING
Radiographs

- Imaging studies of the shoulder should always begin with plain film radiographs.
- Plain films provide visualization of the bony architecture of the shoulder. Several radiographs are important to obtain:
  - An AP view of the shoulder taken in the plane of the scapula with the arm in neutral rotation produces a perpendicular view of the glenohumeral joint.
  - The outlet view, or "scapula Y" lateral radiograph, provides a lateral view of the body of the scapula. It can identify the morphology of the acromion and the presence of subacromial spurs.
  - An axillary radiograph provides a lateral view of the glenohumeral joint with the arm fully abducted. An axillary radiograph is necessary to assess glenohumeral subluxation or dislocation.
  - Other views that may be helpful but are not needed in every case would include Stryker notch and West Point views. The Stryker notch view is done to examine for a Hill-Sachs lesion. The athlete's hand is placed on his or her head with elbow pointing straight up. The West Point view is a variation of the axillary lateral view. It is done with the athlete prone with the arm hanging off the table. The West Point view is good for examining a Bankart lesion.

Magnetic Resonance Imaging

- Magnetic resonance imaging (MRI) is the modality of choice to assess the integrity of the soft tissues about the shoulder (tendons, ligaments, and labrum).
- It can identify partial- and full-thickness cuff tears, tears of the glenoid labrum, and inflammation of the subacromial bursa.
- Magnetic resonance arthrography may assist with identification of intra-articular pathology, such as partial articular-sided rotator cuff tears, but it should be used judiciously. The examiner should take into account the discomfort that the athlete may experience following an arthrogram, which may preclude the immediate return to play.

MANAGEMENT

Frequently, rotator cuff tendinitis in the overhead athlete can be successfully treated with a well-structured and carefully implemented nonoperative rehabilitation program (Rehabilitation Protocol 22.1). Rehabilitation follows a multiphase approach with emphasis on controlling inflammation, restoring muscle

---

REHABILITATION PROTOCOL 22.1 ■ **Rehabilitation for Rotator Cuff Tendinitis in Overhead Athletes**

Phase **I**

- Passive or active-assisted range of motion (ROM) exercises are initiated in pain-free ranges to improve or maintain motion, provide gentle stress to healing collagen tissue, and optimize the subacromial gliding mechanism.
- Phase I ROM includes forward elevation and external rotation (Fig. 22.2).
  - Forward elevation is performed supine or seated with the shoulder slightly anterior to the plane of the scapula. Supine elevation allows for a more functional and comfortable stretch to the patient.

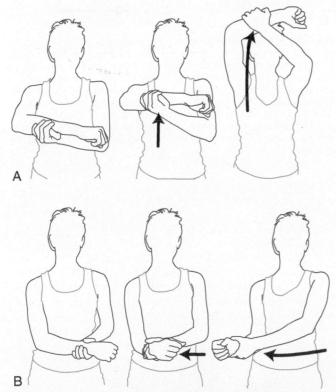

Fig. 22.2 Phase I stretching of the shoulder. Exercises to be done 10 times each, two times per day. **A,** Active-assisted forward elevation: The arm is held with the elbow straight or flexed to 90 degrees. The elbow and forearm are raised away from the body using the opposite arm to assist. The arm is raised overhead until a stretch is felt and held for 10 seconds. The arm is then gently lowered back to the side. **B,** Active-assisted external rotation: Position the hand across the stomach with the elbow tucked firmly at the side. Pivot the hand away from the body until pointing straight ahead and continue until pointing away from the body. Use the opposite arm to assist. Both exercises should remain pain free.

- External rotation is typically started with the patient supine, with the arm at 45 degrees in the plane of the scapula and supported by a pillow. This position minimizes excessive tension on the superior cuff and capsuloligamentous complex and avoids the impingement position at 90 degrees of abduction.
- If there are restrictions of external rotation with the arm in adduction or at 90 degrees of abduction, stretching can progress to these positions as long as reactivity is limited.
- Phase II ROM includes extension, internal rotation, and cross-body adduction (Fig. 22.3).
  - The athlete should be instructed to achieve a tolerable stretch and hold the position for at least 10 seconds. Each exercise is repeated 10 times, and the patient is asked to perform the exercises two to four times per day.
  - Internal rotation ROM should be approached with caution. This position places the supraspinatus in its most elongated state. Although it is typically the most limited motion, it is also the most provocative in patients with rotator cuff tendinitis.
  - Glenohumeral joint mobilization and manual stretching can be performed. Joint mobilization involves the translation of one joint surface relative to another. Oscillations are then performed at the end of the translation (Videos 22.1 and 22.2).

Phase I strengthening exercises using elastic bands, or free weights of 1 to 4 pounds, can also be initiated in this early phase. Elastic bands may be easier to use and are more portable for the patient to use at home. The patient can exercise with the bands in the erect position and better integrate the scapular muscles (Videos 22.3 and 22.4).

- These exercises include external rotation, internal rotation, flexion (protraction), and extension (retraction) (Figs. 22.4 and 22.5).
  - The patient is asked to begin in the starting position with no slack on the band. Patients are asked to "set" their scapula to integrate the scapular muscles. They are then asked to per-

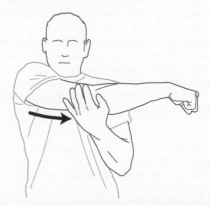

Fig. 22.3 Cross-body adduction: With the elbow straight, the affected arm is brought across the body at shoulder height. The unaffected arm can be used to pull the affected arm further across the body to stretch the posterior capsule and posterior rotator cuff.

Continued

REHABILITATION PROTOCOL 22.1 ▪ **Rehabilitation for Rotator Cuff Tendinitis in Overhead Athletes—cont'd**

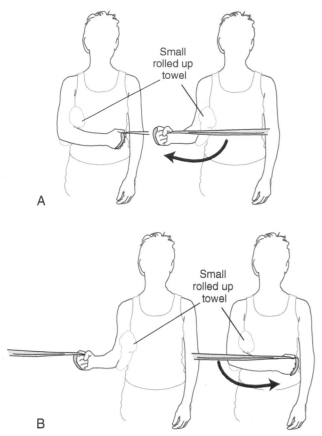

Fig. 22.4   Phase I strengthening of the shoulder. Exercises to be done 10 times each, two times per day. **A,** External rotation: With band at waist level, start with the upper arm at the side, elbow flexed to 90 degrees, and forearm across the stomach. While maintaining upper arm against the side and 90 degrees of elbow flexion, gently rotate the forearm away from the stomach and out to the side. Slowly return to starting position. **B,** Internal rotation: With band at waist level, start with the upper arm at the side, elbow flexed to 90 degrees, and forearm out to the side. While maintaining upper arm against the side and 90 degrees of elbow flexion, gently rotate the forearm in toward the stomach. Slowly return to starting position.

form 10 repetitions of the first exercise. Once they can comfortably perform three sets of an exercise without difficulty, they can progress to the next color band or add 1 pound of resistance.

- Isolated scapular strengthening exercises can be performed with elastic resistance and rowing at waist level (see Video 18.1).
- If the patient is being seen in supervised therapy, manual resistance to external and internal rotation can be used. Alternating isometrics can be performed, allowing the clinician to assess strength and reactivity.

Phase II

Patients will progress to Phase II as their pain and inflammation resolve and ROM and strength improve.
- The sleeper stretch can be used to achieve end-range internal rotation (Fig. 22.6).
- End-range forward elevation can be achieved with a wall stretch (Fig. 22.7) or a stretch behind the head (Fig. 22.8). The introduction of an overhead pulley can also achieve end-range forward elevation.

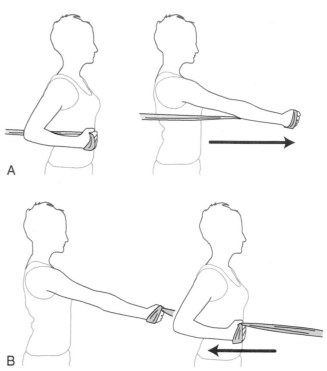

Fig. 22.5   Phase I strengthening of the shoulder. Exercises to be done 10 times each, two times per day. **A,** Shoulder flexion (protraction): Attach band to door behind patient at waist level. Begin with hand in front of shoulder with elbow bent, hand and forearm at waist level. Press hand forward until the elbow is fully extended. Slowly return to starting position. **B,** Shoulder extension (retraction): Attach band to door in front of patient at waist level. Begin with arm straight forward, elbow extended, hand at waist level. Pull the elbow back until the hand is next to the body. Slowly return to starting position.

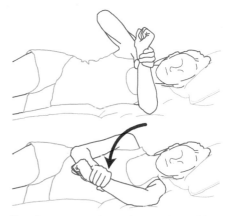

Fig. 22.6   The sleeper stretch can be used to achieve end range of internal rotation. The patient lies on the affected side, with head level and trunk straight. The shoulder is brought to 90 degrees forward flexion, and the elbow is bent to 90 degrees. Squeeze scapulas together, keeping scapulas close to the spine. Use the unaffected hand to internally rotate shoulder, pushing the affected hand down toward the bed. Hold 10 to 20 seconds and repeat five times.

REHABILITATION PROTOCOL 22.1 ● **Rehabilitation for Rotator Cuff Tendinitis in Overhead Athletes—cont'd**

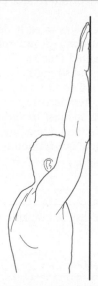

Fig. 22.7 The wall stretch can be used to achieve end-range forward elevation or forward flexion. The patient stands facing a flat wall. The affected arm is raised to full forward elevation or full forward flexion. With the palm placed flat on the wall, the patient leans forward pressing the torso into the wall. This will stretch the inferior joint capsule and inferior glenohumeral ligaments.

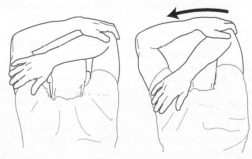

Fig. 22.8 Stretching the affected arm behind the head can also be used to achieve end-range forward elevation or forward flexion. The unaffected arm grasps the affected arm by the elbow, pulling the affected arm further behind the head to stretch the inferior joint capsule and inferior glenohumeral ligaments.

When the patient is able to achieve the third level of elastic resistance with all of the Phase I exercises, he or she can add Phase II strengthening exercises.
- Phase II consists of abduction and forward elevation to 45 degrees and external rotation at 45 degrees with the elbow supported (see Video 18.4).
- Total arm strengthening with biceps and triceps exercises can also be added at this time.

- Phase II scapular strengthening exercises include a forehand and backhand motion emphasizing protraction and retraction and combinations of movement including horizontal abduction with scapular retraction and external rotation with elastic resistance.

Phase III

At this point, ROM should be full and pain free. Athletes will progress to higher-level exercises involving functional combination movements in more provocative positions. Patients who must repetitively function with the arm at or above shoulder level should be exercised into those positions.
- Phase III exercises include prone horizontal abduction with external rotation, prone forward elevation (100 to 135 degrees) with external rotation, and standing scaption with external rotation. These exercises have all been shown to have high electromyographic (EMG) activity in the rotator cuff, deltoid, and scapular retractors.
- Athletes can begin to introduce weight-training activities using variable resistance devices. Barbells can be added for the elbow flexors and extensors and latissimus pull-downs.
- As strength and reactivity improve, exercises such as the chest press and military press using a variable resistance device can be added.
- Recommendations and instruction for proper use of gym equipment should also be done at this time. Avoid weight-training exercises with the arm behind the plane of the body or the hands behind the head. Latissimus pull-downs should be performed to the chest, not behind the head. Caution should be used when performing any type of "pushing" exercise such as chest press or shoulder press. It is best to perform these exercises with a machine to allow for greater safety.
- Patients should also be encouraged to begin with a very light weight and gradually progress to heavier weights.
- During rehabilitation, conditioning and core strengthening must be stressed.

Phase IV

Athletes should continue with the rotator cuff, deltoid, and scapular exercises with a bias toward sport-specific positions.
- Elastic resistance to sport-specific activities can be helpful for racquet sports athletes, swimmers, and throwers.
- Plyometric training using weighted balls can be used to enhance neuromuscular control, strength, and proprioception by reproducing the physiologic stretch-shortening cycle of muscle in multiple shoulder positions.
- By catching and/or throwing a weighted ball, the adductor/internal rotators are eccentrically loaded and stretched, followed by a concentric phase. This exercise can be performed by throwing to a clinician or to a mini-trampoline or rebounder.
- Other muscle groups, including the core musculature, can be targeted with various throwing motions, including chest pass, overhead two-handed throw, and overhead throw with trunk rotation (Videos 22.5 and 22.6).
- Plyometric exercises can be used to prepare the athlete for an interval sport program for throwing, tennis strokes, swimming, and so on.

balance, improving soft tissue flexibility, enhancing proprioception and neuromuscular control, and efficiently returning the athlete to competitive throwing (Wilk et al. 2002). Treatment should focus on restoration of sound mechanics during the throwing cycle, core muscle strengthening of the trunk and lower extremities, and strengthening of periscapular stabilizers.

- Early intervention is a critical component to nonoperative management of shoulder injuries in the throwing athlete.
- The quantity of rehabilitation does not always equate to quality. Each patient requires a different level of intervention, and rehabilitation programs must be individualized.
- Supervised therapy three times per week is not necessary for all patients. Many athletes need only instruction in a home program and periodic evaluation and progression of the rehabilitation program. Others may benefit from more intensive instruction and manual therapy intervention in conjunction with a home program.
- It is incumbent upon therapists, trainers, physicians, and coaches to communicate and administer the appropriate amount of structured rehabilitation to each athlete following the onset of a shoulder injury.
- The athlete needs to be educated about the healing process and the importance of rest from positions or activities that may contribute to the inflammatory process.
- Nonsteroidal anti-inflammatory medication may assist the athlete with pain control but will not expedite recovery.
- Modalities have not been shown to be very effective in the treatment of rotator cuff disease.
- Heat, cold, or both may be used to help augment treatment.
- The use of transcutaneous electrical nerve stimulation (TENS) may be beneficial as an adjunct to exercise intervention.

SUMMARY

Rotator cuff tendinitis in the overhead athlete is a pathologic and debilitating process. The extreme forces placed on the glenohumeral joint complex during the overhead throwing motion can cause anterior ligamentous laxity and posterior capsular contracture. The repetitive trauma of excessive AP translation

of the humeral head on the glenoid can lead to irritation of the dynamic stabilizers of the shoulder. If not corrected, this can ultimately lead to tears of the rotator cuff and posterior–superior labrum.

The key to treatment lies in early detection and prevention of further injury. A structured, multiphase rehabilitation protocol can be implemented focusing on stretching of posterior capsular contractures and strengthening of the rotator cuff and periscapular muscles. Conditioning and core strengthening are optimized while alterations in the mechanics of throwing are corrected. Treatment must be individualized to each athlete. Open communication among physicians, athletic trainers, coaches, and the athlete is paramount to recovery and return to play.

REFERENCES

A complete reference list is available at https://expertconsult .inkling.com/.

FURTHER READING

Fleisig GS, Andrews JR, Dillman CJ, et al. Kinetics of baseball pitching with implications about injury mechanisms. *Am J Sports Med.* 1995;23:233–239.

Jobe FW, Giangarra CE, Kvitne RS, et al. Anterior capsulolabral reconstruction of the shoulder in athletes in overhand sports. *Am J Sports Med.* 1991;19:428–434.

Kelley MJ, Leggin BG. Shoulder rehabilitation. In: Iannotti JP, Williams GR, eds. *Disorders of the Shoulder: Diagnosis and Management.* Philadelphia: Lippincott Williams & Wilkins; 1999:979–1019.

Kuhn JE. Exercise in the treatment of rotator cuff impingement: a systematic review and a synthesized evidence-based rehabilitation protocol. *J Shoulder Elbow Surg.* 2009;18:138–160.

Maitland GD. *Peripheral Manipulation.* 3rd ed. London: Butterworth; 1991.

Reinold MM, Wilk KE, Fleisig GS, et al. Electromyographic analysis of the rotator cuff and deltoid musculature during common shoulder external rotation exercises. *J Orthop Sports Phys Ther.* 2004;34(7):385–394.

Reinold MM, Macrina LC, Wilk KE, et al. Electromyographic analysis of the supraspinatus and deltoid muscles during 3 common rehabilitation exercises. *J Athl Train.* 2007;42(4):464–469.

Townsend H, Jobe FW, Pink M, et al. Electromyographic analysis of the glenohumeral muscles during a baseball rehabilitation program. *Am J Sports Med.* 1991;19:264–272.

Rotator Cuff Repair

Robert C. Manske, PT, DPT, MEd, SCS, ATC, CSCS

Rotator cuff tears and subacromial impingement are among the most common causes of shoulder pain and disability. Rotator cuff tears are among the most common conditions affecting the shoulder, accounting for 4.5 million physician visits in the United States per year (Jain et al. 2014). Up to half the population experiences at least one episode of shoulder pain per year (Luime et al. 2004). Lewis reports a lifetime risk of up to 30% and an annual risk of at least one episode to reach 50% (Lewis 2009). The frequency of rotator cuff tears increases with age and full-thickness tears are uncommon in patients younger than 40 years of age. However, the incidence of tears in the elderly dramatically increases as evidenced by rotator cuff tear in 33% of shoulders in the 50- to 60-year range and in 100% in those more than 70 years of age reported in cadavers (Lehman et al. 1995). Kibler et al. (2009) suggest that more than 50% of people over the age of 60 have at least a partial-thickness tear of their rotator cuff. Recently evidence has shown that there may also be a genetic predisposition to rotator cuff injuries because full-thickness tears in siblings have been shown to be more likely to progress over a period of 5 years compared to a control group (Gwilym et al. 2009).

The rotator cuff complex refers to the tendons of four muscles: the subscapularis, supraspinatus, infraspinatus, and teres minor. The four muscles originate on the scapula, cross the glenohumeral joint, then transition to tendons that insert onto the tuberosities of the proximal humerus (Fig. 23.1). The term "rotator cuff" may be a misnomer because the most important function of the rotator cuff may be that of compression (Chepeha 2009). Evidence suggests that the role of the rotator cuff is much more that of humeral compression than creation of an inferiorly directed force on the humerus (Soslowsky et al. 1997, Labriola et al. 2005) (Fig. 23.2). The rotator cuff has three well-recognized functions: rotation of the humeral head, stabilization of the humeral head in the glenoid socket by compressing the round head into the shallow socket, and the ability to provide "muscular balance," stabilizing the glenohumeral (GH) joint when other larger muscles crossing the shoulder contract.

Rotator cuff tears can be classified as either acute or chronic based on their timing. Additional classification can include the amount of tear as either partial (bursal or articular side tears) or complete. Most rotator cuff tears involve the supraspinatus tendon, followed closely by the infraspinatus tendon and the upper subscapularis tendon (Mehta et al. 2003, Wolf et al. 2006). Tears can also be described as either traumatic or degenerative (Box 23.1). Complete tears can be classified based on the size of the tear in square centimeters as described by Post et al. (1983) (Table 23.1). All of these factors, as well as the patient's demographic and medical background, play a role in determining a treatment plan.

Regardless of the surgical technique used, treatment goals of rotator cuff repair have not significantly changed over the years. Goals following rotator cuff repair can be seen in Box 23.2. These goals can be met using an evidence-based, progressive therapy program. For purposes of this section several different protocols are described, including those for (1) partial to small tears, (2) medium to large tears, and (3) massive tears.

Postoperative care must strike a precarious balance between restrictions that allow for tissue healing, activities that return range of motion (ROM), and gradual restoration of muscle function and strength. It is not uncommon to have residual postoperative stiffness and pain despite an excellent operative repair if the postoperative rehabilitation is not done correctly. Many variables determine the outcome following a rotator cuff repair.

TYPE OF REPAIR

Management of rotator cuff tendon tears continues to be a challenge. Few surgeons will still perform open repairs, especially in patients with anterior deltoid detachment for fear of postoperative deltoid avulsion (Gumina et al. 2008, Hata et al. 2004, Sher et al. 1997). Patients who have had a deltoid muscle detachment or release from the acromion or clavicle (e.g., traditional open rotator cuff repair) may not perform active muscle contractions of the deltoid for up to approximately 8 weeks following surgery. This is done to avoid the horrible outcome of an avulsion of the deltoid muscle. Typically three types of procedures are described with the open procedure being the oldest as it was described over 100 years ago (Codman 1911). Next in line was the advancement of the mini-open procedure that utilizes a much smaller incision. Most recently all-arthroscopic procedures have become popular. These three procedures can be thought of as an evolution or transition to newer and better techniques as biomechanics of surgery and soft tissue healing have been advanced with increasing amounts of scientific knowledge.

The open rotator cuff repair is very conservative compared to mini-open or arthroscopic repair procedures due to detachment of the deltoid. Because of the lack of use of this older procedure, a formal rehabilitation approach will not be described other than to say that active motion is not allowed until after 8 to 12 weeks depending on tissue quality and ability to reattach the required tendons. Actual gentle strengthening is not begun until after about 12 weeks at minimum. Patients are usually not even able to comfortably elevate above shoulder level before 6 months (Hawkins 1990, Hawkins et al. 1999).

The mini-open technique involves a small (less than 3 cm) vertical split with the orientation of the deltoid fibers, allowing mild, early deltoid muscle contractions. The mini-open technique is popular because it does not create the surgical morbidity of the open technique. The deltoid muscle is not taken down from the acromion, so rehabilitation is progressed somewhat faster. Additionally, with the mini-open technique, transosseous fixation, which may lead to better footprint restoration, can be used. The downfalls to the mini-open include an increased incidence of stiffness (11% to 20%) compared to an all-arthroscopic technique (Nottage 2001, Yamaguchi et al. 2001).

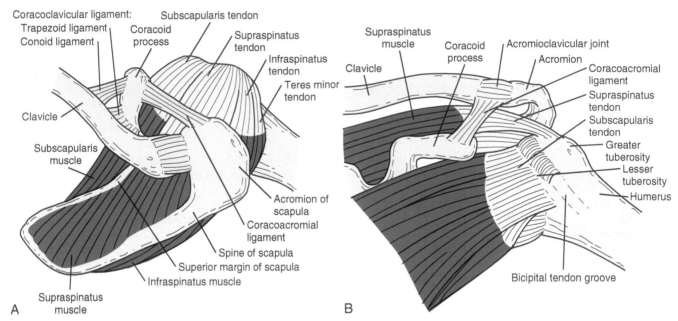

Fig. 23.1 A, superior view of rotator cuff musculature as it courses anteriorly under the coracoacromial arch to insert on the greater tuberosity. B, Anterior view of the shoulder reveals the subscapularis, which is the only anterior rotator cuff muscle that inserts onto the lesser tuberosity. (From Magee DJ, Zachazewski JE, Quillen WS, Manske RC: Pathology and Intervention in Musculoskeletal Rehabilitation. Elsevier Saunders, 2016.

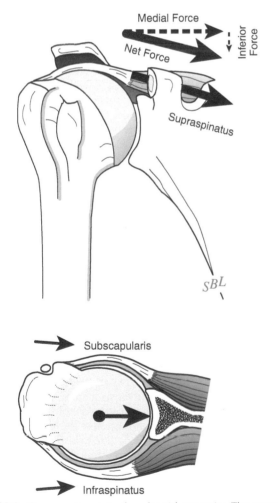

Fig. 23.2 Compressions into the glenoid concavity. The rotator cuff compresses the humeral articular convexity into the glenoid concavity. (Modified from Magee DJ, Zachazewski JE, Quillen WS, et al. Pathology and Intervention in Musculoskeletal Rehabilitation, 2nd edition, 2016, p. 244.)

TABLE 23.1	Tear Sizes
Name	**Centimeters**
Small	$(0–1\ cm^2)$
Medium	$(1–3\ cm^2)$
Large	$(3–5\ cm^2)$
Massive	$(>5\ cm^2)$

The all-arthroscopic repair of the rotator cuff actually has a slower rate of early rehabilitation progression owing to the weaker fixation of the repair as compared to that of the open procedures. This technique has to be one of the more demanding ways to operatively repair the rotator cuff. Advantages of the all-arthroscopic technique include preservation of the deltoid attachment, less postoperative pain, decreased surgical morbidity, and an earlier return of function following repair.

Regardless of the surgical approach performed, the underlying biology of healing tendons must be respected for all patients.

TEAR PATTERN

Lo and Burkhart (2003) have described four main types of tear patterns, and these include crescent-shaped tears, U-shaped tears, L-shaped and reverse L-shaped tears, and massive tears. Understanding of and recognition of the tear pattern are the first steps in determining appropriate surgical treatment.

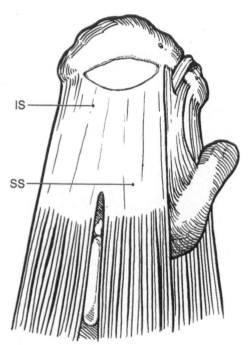

Fig. 23.3 Crescent-shaped tear. (From Miller MD, Sekiya JK: Sports Medicine. Core Knowledge in Orthopaedics. St. Louis, Mosby, 2006, p. 305, fig. 36-17A.)

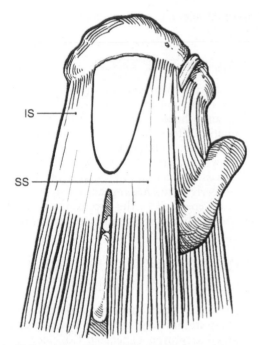

Fig. 23.4 U-shaped tear. (From Miller MD, Sekiya JK: Sports Medicine. Core Knowledge in Orthopaedics. St. Louis, Mosby, 2006, p. 306, fig. 36-17B.)

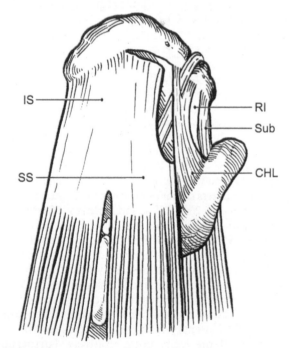

Fig. 23.5 L-shaped tear. (From Miller MD, Sekiya JK: Sports Medicine. Core Knowledge in Orthopaedics. St. Louis, Mosby, 2006, p. 307, fig. 36-17C.)

Crescent-shaped tears (Fig. 23.3). These are usually the easiest to repair. These tears rarely have a substantial amount of medial retraction; therefore, they are usually easily mobilized and able to be secured to the tuberosity without excessive tension placed upon them.

U-shaped tears (Fig. 23.4). These tears look like an extension of the crescent-shaped tear pattern that have retracted further medially. A large margin convergence is needed to secure this tear. Using a margin convergence procedure, the anterior and posterior edges of the tear are sutured back together so that the lateral edge can be more easily brought back to the greater tubercle.

L-shaped and reverse L-shaped tears (Fig. 23.5). This tear pattern involves a tendon tear from the tuberosity with an additional longitudinal split posteriorly or anteriorly involving a portion being retracted.

Massive tears. A massive tear is commonly seen in the elderly patient and involves more than one tendon. These tears tend to be problematic because of the significant amount of tendon retraction that occurs.

SIZE OF THE TEAR

Functional outcome and expectations after rotator cuff repair are directly related to the size of the tear repaired. Numerous authors have reported age and tear size to be significant factors in healing after rotator cuff repair (Bigliani et al. 1992, Boileau et al. 2005, Cole et al. 2007, Gazielly et al. 1994, Harryman et al. 1991, Nho et al. 2009).

TISSUE QUALITY

The quality of the tendon, muscular tissue, and the bone helps determine speed of rehabilitation. Thin, fatty, or weak tissue is progressed slower than excellent tissue. Of additional concern is the quality of the remaining rotator cuff muscles. The other cuff muscles (i.e., subscapularis, teres minor, and infraspinatus) play an important role in providing adequate force couples for the healthy shoulder.

LOCATION OF THE TEAR

Tears that involve posterior cuff structures require a slower progression of rehabilitation for gaining external rotation strengthening and should limit internal rotation mobility early. Rehabilitation after subscapularis repair (anterior structure) should limit resisted internal rotation for approximately 6 weeks to allow adequate soft tissue healing. Restriction of the amount of passive external rotation motion should also be restricted until early tissue healing has occurred. Most tears occur in and are confined to the supraspinatus tendon, the critical site of wear, often corresponding to the site of subacromial impingement.

ONSET OF ROTATOR CUFF TEAR AND TIMING OF THE REPAIR

Acute tears with early repair may have a slightly greater propensity to develop stiffness, and a little more aggression in early ROM programs has proven beneficial. Cofield et al. (2001) noted that patients who underwent an early repair progressed more rapidly with rehabilitation than those with a late repair. It has been shown that early intervention of a single-tendon tear may optimize healing and not allow progression to a multiple-tendon tear (Nho et al. 2009).

PATIENT VARIABLES

Several authors have reported a less successful outcome in older patients than young. This may be because of older patients typically having larger and more complex tears, probably affecting outcomes. Age and tear size are significant factors in tendon healing capabilities (Bigliani et al. 1992, Boileau et al. 2005, Cole et al. 2007, Constant and Murley 1987, Gazielly et al. 1994).

Multiple other authors agree that workers' compensations patients tend to progress slower or have less than optimal return of function (Abboud et al. 2006, Bayne and Bateman 1984, McLaughlin and Asherman 1951, Hawkins et al. 1999, Iannotti et al. 1996, Misamore et al. 1995, Paulos and Kody 1994, Shinners et al. 2002, Smith et al. 2000). Kolgonen, Chong, and Yip (Kolgonen et al. 2009) found a strong association between workers' compensation patients and poor outcomes after multiple shoulder surgeries.

Finally, researchers have noted a correlation between preoperative shoulder function and outcomes after surgical repair. Generally, patients who have an active lifestyle before surgery return to the same postoperatively. Furthermore, Henn et al. (2007) assessed preoperative expectations with an outcomes questionnaire and found that those who had a greater preoperative expectation for their recovery had better postoperative performance on several subjective outcome measures.

REHABILITATION SITUATION AND SURGEON'S PHILOSOPHIC APPROACH

Treatment with a skilled shoulder therapist rather than a home therapy program is recommended. Lastly, some physicians prefer more aggressive progression, whereas others remain conservative in their approach.

Rehabilitation after rotator cuff surgery emphasizes immediate motion, early dynamic GH joint stability, and gradual restoration of rotator cuff strength. Throughout rehabilitation, overstressing of the healing tissue is to be avoided, striking a balance between regaining shoulder mobility and promotion of soft tissue healing.

ACUTE TEARS

Patients with acute tears of the rotator cuff usually present to their physician after a traumatic injury. They have complaints of pain and sudden weakness, which may be manifested by an inability to elevate the arm. On physical examination, they have a weakness in shoulder motion of forward elevation, external rotation, or internal rotation depending on which cuff muscles are involved. Passive motion is usually intact depending on the timing of presentation. If the injury is chronic and the patient has been avoiding using the shoulder because of pain, there may be concomitant adhesive capsulitis (limitation of passive shoulder motion) and weakness of active ROM (underlying rotator cuff tear).

IMAGING

Imaging studies may be helpful in confirming the diagnosis of a chronic rotator cuff tear and may help to determine the potential success of operative treatment. A standard radiographic evaluation or "trauma shoulder series" should be obtained, including an anteroposterior (AP) view in the plane of the scapula ("true AP" of GH joint) (Fig. 23.6), a lateral view in the plane of the scapula (Fig. 23.7), and an axillary lateral view (Fig. 23.8). This may also show some proximal (superior) humeral migration, indicative of chronic rotator cuff insufficiency. Plain film radiographs can also show degenerative conditions or bone collapse consistent with a cuff tear arthropathy in which both the cuff deficiency and the arthritis contribute to the patient's symptoms. These radiographs help to eliminate other potential pathologic entities such as a fracture or dislocation.

A magnetic resonance imaging (MRI) examination of the shoulder may help to demonstrate a rotator cuff tear, its size, and degree of retraction, thus confirming the clinical diagnosis. The MRI with or without contrast can also help assess the rotator cuff musculature. Evidence of fatty or fibrous infiltration of the rotator cuff muscles is consistent with a long-standing cuff tear and is a poor prognostic indicator for a successful return of cuff function.

Ultrasound and double-contrast shoulder arthrography are additional studies that are occasionally used to diagnose rotator cuff tears, but they are less helpful for determining the age of the tear.

It is important to remember that the likelihood of an associated rotator cuff tear with a shoulder dislocation increases with age. In patients older than 40 years of age, an associated rotator cuff tear is present with shoulder dislocation in more than 30%; whereas in patients older than 60 years, it is present in more than 80%. Therefore, serial examination of the shoulder is necessary after a dislocation to evaluate the integrity of the rotator cuff. If significant symptoms of pain and weakness persist after 3 weeks, an imaging study of the rotator cuff is

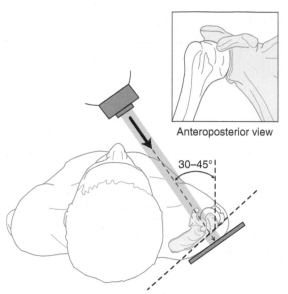

Anteroposterior view

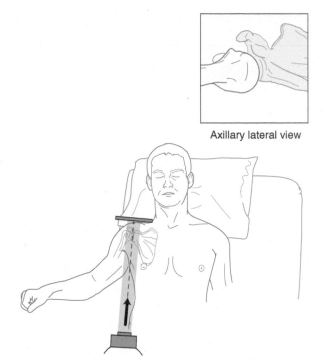

Axillary lateral view

Fig. 23.6 Radiographic evaluation of the shoulder: true anterioroposterior (AP) view. The beam must be angled 30–45 degrees. (Redrawn from Rockwood CA Jr, Matsen FA III: The Shoulder, 2nd ed. Philadelphia, WB Saunders, 1988.)

Fig. 23.8 Radiographic evaluation of the shoulder: axillary lateral view. This view is important to avoid missing acute or chronic shoulder dislocation. (Redrawn from Rockwood CA Jr, Matsen FA III: The Shoulder, 2nd ed. Philadelphia, WB Saunders, 1988.)

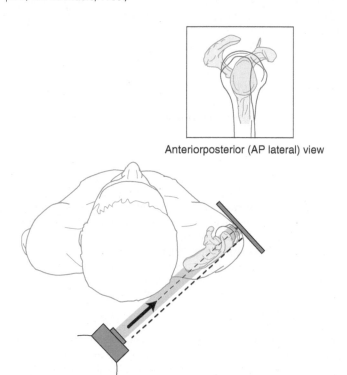

Anteriorposterior (AP lateral) view

Fig. 23.7 Radiographic evaluation of the shoulder; lateral view in the plane of the scapula. (Redrawn from Rockwood CA Jr, Matsen FA III: The Shoulder, 2nd ed. Philadelphia, WB Saunders, 1988.)

required. A torn rotator cuff after a dislocation is a surgical problem, so once the diagnosis is made, surgical repair is indicated.

EXAMINATION

On physical examination, some evidence of muscular atrophy may be seen in the supraspinatus or infraspinatus fossa. Atrophy will depend on the size and chronicity of the tear. Acute tears will rarely show signs of obvious muscle wasting. Observation looks for symmetry of shoulders. Shoulder height that is lower on the dominant side is normal and termed "handedness." This occurs due to a combination of increased muscle mass and increased shoulder laxity. A shoulder that is higher on the involved side may be held there due to protective muscle spasm. Winging or tipping of the scapula is another common finding. Winging refers to the entire medial scapular border being elevated off of the posterior thorax, whereas tipping is when just the inferior medial border is elevated away from the posterior shoulder.

Passive motion is usually maintained, but it may be associated with subacromial crepitance. Smooth active motion is diminished, and symptoms are reproduced when the arm is lowered from an overhead position. Muscle weakness is related to the size of the tear and the muscles involved. More commonly with rotator cuff tears, both elevation and external shoulder rotation will demonstrate weakness and associated pain when performing manual muscle testing.

A subacromial injection of lidocaine may help to differentiate weakness that is caused by associated painful inflammation from that caused by a cuff tendon tear. Additionally, provocative maneuvers including the Neer impingement sign (Fig. 23.9) and the Hawkins sign (Fig. 23.10) may be positive with other conditions such as rotator cuff tendinitis, bursitis, or partial-thickness rotator cuff tears.

It is important that other potential etiologies be investigated as part of the differential diagnosis. Patients with cervical radiculopathy at the C5–6 level can have an insidious onset of shoulder pain, rotator cuff weakness, and muscular atrophy in the supraspinatus and infraspinatus fossa. Atrophy in these areas can also be seen with suprascapular nerve encroachment.

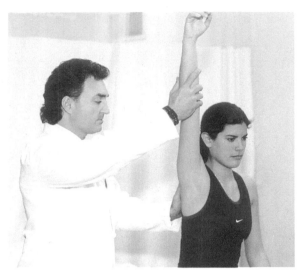

Fig. 23.9   Neer impingement test.

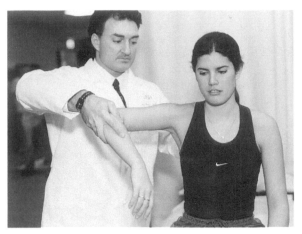

Fig. 23.10   Hawkins impingement test.

TREATMENT
Acute Tears

The recommended treatment for active patients with acute tears of the rotator cuff is surgical repair. Advantages of early operative repair include mobility of the rotator cuff, which allows technically easier repairs; good quality of the tendon, which allows a more stable repair; and in patients with cuff tears associated with a dislocation, the repair will improve GH joint stability.

Chronic Tears

Chronic rotator cuff tears may be an asymptomatic pathologic condition that has an association with the normal aging process. A variety of factors, including poor vascularity, a "hostile" environment between the coracoacromial arch and the proximal humerus, decreased use, or gradual deterioration in the tendon, contribute to the senescence of the rotator cuff, especially the supraspinatus. Lehman and colleagues (Lehman et al. 1995) found rotator cuff tears in 30% of cadavers older than 60 years and in only 6% of those younger than 60 years of age. Many patients with chronic rotator cuff tears are over the age of 50 years, have no history of shoulder trauma, and have vague complaints of intermittent shoulder pain that has become progressively more symptomatic. These patients may also have a history that is indicative of a primary impingement etiology.

Treatment of most patients with a chronic tear of the rotator cuff follows a conservative rehabilitation program. Operative intervention in this patient population is indicated for patients who are unresponsive to conservative management or demonstrate an acute tearing of a chronic injury. The primary goal of surgical management of rotator cuff tears is to obtain pain relief. Additional goals, which are easier to achieve with acute rotator cuff tears than chronic rotator cuff tears, include improved ROM, improved strength, and return of function.

Rotator cuff rehabilitation continues to evolve as the science of tendon/cuff healing continues to grow. As a result of stronger surgical fixation methods with minimal deltoid involvement, a slightly more aggressive shift has been followed for the last few years. Despite this, most protocols are based on empiric clinical experience. Because results of revision rotator cuff repairs are typically inferior to those of primary repairs, it is important to avoid active motion and resistance exercises too early (Lo and Burkhart 2004). This creates the "rotator cuff paradox" in which a too conservative approach will lead to stiffness, whereas a too aggressive approach can lead to recurrent tearing. Therefore optimal treatment, although not clearly established with high levels of evidence, requires careful judgment regarding progression and a delicate balance of motion and strengthening that must be customized to each patient.

REHABILITATION PROTOCOL

Actual protocols for various tear sizes (partial tears/small; medium/large; massive) are seen in Rehabilitation Protocols 23.1, 23.2, and 23.3. Although protocols exist for open procedures, the protocols described herein will be for all-arthroscopic rotator cuff repairs due to advancement in surgical technique. All protocols have similar outlines with four phases but are adjusted according to tear size. Clinicians should take into consideration all other comorbidities and risk factors related to postoperative stiffness.

Sling and initiation of active ROM are seen for all repairs in Table 23.2.

Immediate Postoperative Phase

Goals in the immediate postoperative phase are to (1) maintain and protect the integrity of the repair, (2) gradually increase passive range of motion, (3) diminish pain and inflammation, and (4) modify activities of daily living. The length of this phase depends upon size of repair. For partial to small tear repairs this phase may only last 3 to 4 weeks, whereas for medium and large tears it may last up to 6 weeks and for massive tears up to 8 weeks.

Because pain typically is elevated in this stage, cold therapy and electrical stimulation may be used to relieve discomfort. The initial position of immobilization is usually with the shoulder slightly abducted in the scapular plane, elbow flexed to 90 degrees, and shoulder internally rotated resting on an abduction pillow (see Fig. 21.10). Slight abduction as the immobilization placement does several things including allowing an increase in supraspinatus blood flow to decrease the "wringing out" or "watershed" effect that occurs with the arm in a completely adducted shoulder position. Secondly, it places the

REHABILITATION PROTOCOL 23.1 ■ Arthroscopic Rotator Cuff Repair Protocol for Partial-Thickness and Small Full-Thickness Tears

This protocol was developed to provide the rehabilitation professional with a guideline for a postoperative rehabilitation course for a patient who has undergone an arthroscopic rotator cuff repair of a *partial-thickness* or a *small full-thickness* rotator cuff tear. It should be stressed that this is only a protocol and should not be a substitute for clinical decision making regarding a patient's progression. Actual progression should be individualized based on your patient's physical examination, individual progress, and the presence of any postoperative complications.

The rate limiting factor in arthroscopic rotator cuff repair is the biologic healing of the cuff tendon to the humerus, which is thought to be a minimum of 8 to 12 weeks.

Progression of AROM against gravity and duration of sling use is predicated both on the size of tear and quality of tissue and should be guided by the referring physician. Refer to initial therapy referral for any specific instructions.

Phase I: Immediate Postsurgical Phase (Weeks 0–4)

Goals

- Maintain/protect integrity of repair.
- Gradually increase passive range of motion (PROM).
- Diminish pain and inflammation.
- Prevent muscular inhibition.
- Independence in modified activities of daily living

Precautions

- No active range of motion (AROM) of shoulder
- No lifting of objects, reaching behind back, excessive stretching or sudden movements
- Maintain arm in brace, sling; remove *only* for exercise.
- Sling use for 4 to 5 weeks; repaired partial to small tear size
- No support of body weight by hands
- Keep incisions clean and dry.

Days 1 to 6

- Use of abduction brace/sling (during sleep also); remove *only* for exercise
- Passive pendulum exercises (three times a day minimum)
- Finger, wrist, and elbow AROM (three times a day minimum)
- Gripping exercises (putty, handball)
- Cervical spine AROM
- Passive shoulder (PROM) done supine for more patient relaxation
- Flexion to 110 degrees
- External rotation/internal rotation (ER/IR) in scapular plane <30 degrees
- Educate patient on posture, joint protection, importance of brace/sling, pain medication use early, hygiene.
- Cryotherapy for pain and inflammation
  - Days 1 to 3: as much as possible (20 minutes/hour)
  - Days 4 to 7: postactivity, or as needed for pain

Days 7 to 35

- Continue use of abduction brace until DC from physician.
- Continue with full-time use of sling until end of week 4.
- Pendulum exercises
- Begin PROM to tolerance (supine and pain free)
- May use heat prior to ROM
- Flexion to tolerance
- ER in scapular plane ≥30 degrees
- IR in scapular plane to body/chest
- Continue elbow, hand, forearm, wrist, and finger AROM.
- Begin resisted isometrics/isotonics for elbow, hand, forearm, wrist, and fingers.
- Begin scapula muscle isometrics/sets, AROM.

- Begin GH submaximal rhythmic stabilization exercises in "balance position" (90–100 degrees of elevation) in supine position to initiate dynamic stabilization.
- Begin gentle rotator cuff submaximal isometrics (4 to 5 weeks).
- Cryotherapy as needed for pain control and inflammation
- May begin gentle general conditioning program (walking, stationary bike) with caution if unstable from pain medications
- No running or jogging
- Aquatherapy may begin approximately 3 weeks postoperatively if wounds healed.

Criteria for Progression to Next Phase (II)

- Passive forward flexion to ≥125 degrees
- Passive ER in scapular plane to ≥60 degrees (if uninvolved shoulder PROM >80 degrees)
- Passive IR in scapular plane to ≥60 degrees (if uninvolved shoulder PROM >80 degrees)
- Passive abduction in scapular plane to ≥90 degrees
- No passive pulley exercise

Phase II: Protection and Protected Active Motion Phase (Weeks 5–12)

Goals

- Allow healing of soft tissue.
- Do not overstress healing soft tissue.
- Gradually restore full passive ROM (approximately week 5).
- Decrease pain and inflammation.

Precautions

- No lifting
- No supported full body weight with hands or arms
- No sudden jerking motions
- No excessive behind back motions
- No bike or upper extremity ergometer until week 6

Weeks 5 to 6

- Continue with full-time use of sling/brace until end of week 4.
- Continue periscapular exercises.
- Gradually wean from brace starting several hours/day out, progressing as tolerated.
- Use brace/sling for comfort only until full DC by end of week 6.
- Initiate AAROM shoulder flexion from supine position
- Progressive PROM until full PROM by week 6 (should be pain free)
- May require use of heat prior to ROM exercises/joint mobilization
- Can begin passive pulley use
- May require gentle glenohumeral or scapular joint mobilization as indicated to obtain full unrestricted ROM
- Initiate prone rowing to a neutral arm position.
- Continue cryotherapy as needed post-therapy or postexercise.

Weeks 7 to 9

- Continue AROM, AAROM, and stretching as needed.
- Begin IR stretching, shoulder extension, and cross-body, sleeper stretch to mobilize posterior capsule (if needed).
- Continue periscapular exercises progressing to manual resistance to all planes.
- Seated press-ups
- Initiate AROM exercises (flexion, scapular plane, abduction, ER, IR); should be pain free; low weight; initially only weight of arm
- Do not allow shrug during AROM exercises.
- If shrug exists continue to work on cuff and do not reach/lift AROM over 90-degree elevation.
- Initiate limited strengthening program.
- Remember rotator cuff (RTC) and scapular muscles are small and need endurance more than pure strength.

Continued

REHABILITATION PROTOCOL 23.1 ■ **Arthroscopic Rotator Cuff Repair Protocol for Partial-Thickness and Small Full-Thickness Tears—cont'd**

- ER and IR with exercise bands/sport cord/tubing with adduction pillow (under axilla)
- ER isotonic exercises in side lying (low-weight, high-repetition)
- Elbow flexion and extension isotonics

Criteria for Progression to Phase III

- Full AROM

Phase III: Early Strengthening (Weeks 10–16)

Goals

- Full AROM (weeks 10–12)
- Maintain full PROM.
- Dynamic shoulder stability (GH and ST)
- Gradual restoration of GH and scapular strength, power, and endurance
- Optimize neuromuscular control.
- Gradual return to functional activities

Precautions

- No lifting objects >5 lbs, no sudden lifting or pushing
- Exercise should not be painful.

Week 10

- Continue stretching, joint mobilization, and PROM exercises as needed.
- Continue periscapular exercises.
- Dynamic strengthening exercises
- Begin light isometrics in 90/90 or higher supine, PNF D2 flexion/extension patterns against light manual resistance.
- Initiate strengthening program.
- Continue exercises as in weeks 7 to 9.
- Initiate scapular plane elevation to 90 degrees (patient must be able to elevate arm without shoulder or scapular hiking before initiating isotonic exercises. If unable, then continue cuff/scapular exercises).
- Full can (no empty can abduction exercises)
- Prone rowing
- Prone extension
- Prone horizontal abduction

Week 12

- Continue all exercises listed.
- May begin BodyBlade, Flexbar, Boing below 45 degrees
- Initiate light functional activities as tolerated.
- Initiate low-level plyometrics (two-handed, below chest level, progressing to overhead and finally one-handed drills).

Week 14

Continue all exercises listed.
Progress to fundamental exercises (bench press, shoulder press).

Criteria for Progression to Phase IV

- Ability to tolerate progression to low-level functional activities
- Demonstrate return of strength/dynamic shoulder stability.
- Re-establishment of dynamic shoulder stability
- Demonstrated adequate strength and dynamic stability for progression to more demanding work and sport-specific activities

Phase IV: Advanced Strengthening Phases (Weeks 16–22)

Goals

- Maintain full nonpainful AROM.
- Advanced conditioning exercise for enhanced functional and sports-specific use
- Improve muscular strength, power, and endurance.
- Gradual return to all functional activities

Week 16

- Continue ROM and self-capsular stretching for ROM maintenance.
- Continue periscapular exercises.
- Continue progressive strengthening.
- Advanced proprioceptive, neuromuscular activities
- Light isotonic strengthening in 90/90 position
- Initiation of light sports (golf chipping/putting, tennis ground strokes) if satisfactory clinical examination

Week 20

- Continue strengthening and stretching.
- Continue joint mobilization and stretching if motion is tight.
- Initiate interval sports program (e.g., golf, doubles tennis) if appropriate.

REHABILITATION PROTOCOL 23.2 ■ **Arthroscopic Rotator Cuff Repair Protocol: Medium to Large Tear Size**

This protocol was developed to provide the rehabilitation professional with a guideline for a postoperative rehabilitation course for a patient who has undergone an arthroscopic *medium to large* size rotator cuff tear repair. It should be stressed that this is only a protocol and should not be a substitute for clinical decision making regarding a patient's progression. Actual progression should be individualized based on your patient's physical examination, individual progress, and the presence of any postoperative complications.

The rate limiting factor in arthroscopic rotator cuff repair is the biologic healing of the cuff tendon to the humerus, which is thought to be a minimum of 8 to 12 weeks.

Progression of AROM against gravity and duration of sling use is predicated both on the size of tear and quality of tissue and should be guided by the referring physician. Refer to initial therapy referral for any specific instructions.

Phase I: Immediate Post Surgical Phase (Weeks 0–6)

Goals

- Maintain/protect integrity of repair.
- Gradually increase passive range of motion (PROM).
- Diminish pain and inflammation.
- Prevent muscular inhibition.
- Independence in modified activities of daily living
- Precautions
- No active range of motion (AROM) of shoulder
- No lifting of objects, reaching behind back, excessive stretching, or sudden movements
- Maintain arm in brace, sling; remove *only* for exercise.
- Sling use for 6 weeks; medium to large tear size
- No support of body weight by hands
- Keep incisions clean and dry.

REHABILITATION PROTOCOL 23.2 ● Arthroscopic Rotator Cuff Repair Protocol: Medium to Large Tear Size—cont'd

Days 1 to 6

- Use of abduction brace/sling (during sleep also); remove *only* for exercise
- Passive pendulum exercises (three times a day minimum)
- Finger, wrist, and elbow AROM (three times a day minimum)
- Gripping exercises (putty, handball)
- Cervical spine AROM
- Passive shoulder (PROM) done supine for more patient relaxation
- Flexion to 110 degrees
- External rotation/internal rotation (ER/IR) in scapular plane <30 degrees
- Educate patient on posture, joint protection, importance of brace/sling, pain medication use early, hygiene.
- Cryotherapy for pain and inflammation
  - Days 1 to 3: as much as possible (20 minutes/hour)
  - Days 4 to 7: postactivity or as needed for pain

Days 7 to 42

- Continue use of abduction sling/brace until the end of week 6.
- Pendulum exercises
- Begin PROM to tolerance (supine and pain free).
- May use heat prior to ROM
- Flexion to tolerance
- ER in scapular plane ≥30 degrees
- IR in scapular plane to body/chest
- Continue elbow, hand, forearm, wrist, and finger AROM.
- Begin resisted isometrics/isotonics for elbow, hand, forearm, wrist, and fingers.
- Begin scapula muscle isometrics/sets, AROM.
- Cryotherapy as needed for pain control and inflammation
- May begin gentle general conditioning program (walking, stationary bike) with caution if unstable from pain medications
- No running or jogging
- Aquatherapy may begin approximately 6 weeks postoperatively if wounds healed.

Criteria for Progression to Next Phase (II)

- Passive forward flexion to ≥125 degrees
- Passive ER in scapular plane to ≥60 degrees (if uninvolved shoulder PROM >80 degrees)
- Passive IR in scapular plane to ≥60 degrees (if uninvolved shoulder PROM >80 degrees)
- Passive abduction in scapular plane to ≥90 degrees
- No passive pulley exercise

Phase II: Protection and Protected Active Motion Phase (Weeks 7–12)

Goals

- Allow healing of soft tissue.
- Do not overstress healing soft tissue.
- Gradually restore full passive ROM (approximately week 8).
- Decrease pain and inflammation.

Precautions

- No lifting
- No supported full body weight with hands or arms
- No sudden jerking motions
- No excessive behind back motions
- No bike or upper extremity ergometer until week 8

Weeks 7 to 9

- Continue with full-time use of sling/brace until end of week 6.
- Continue periscapular exercises.
- Gradually wean from brace starting several hours a day out, progressing as tolerated.

- Use brace sling for comfort only until full DC by end of week 7.
- Initiate AAROM shoulder flexion from supine position weeks 6 to 7.
- Progressive PROM until full PROM by week 8 (should be pain free)
- May require use of heat prior to ROM exercises/joint mobilization
- Can begin passive pulley use
- May require gentle GH or scapular joint mobilization as indicated to obtain full unrestricted ROM
- Initiate prone rowing to a neutral arm position.
- Continue cryotherapy as needed post-therapy or postexercise.

Weeks 9 to 12

- Continue AROM, AAROM, and stretching as needed.
- Begin IR stretching, shoulder extension, and cross-body, sleeper stretch to mobilize posterior capsule (if needed).
- Begin gentle rotator cuff submaximal isometrics (weeks 7–8).
- Begin glenohumeral submaximal rhythmic stabilization exercises in "balance position" (90–100 degrees of elevation) in supine position to initiate dynamic stabilization.
- Continue periscapular exercises progressing to manual resistance to all planes.
- Seated press-ups
- Initiate AROM exercises (flexion, scapular plane, abduction, ER, IR); should be pain free; low weight; initially only weight of arm.
- Do not allow shrug during AROM exercises.
- If shrug exists continue to work on cuff and do not reach/lift AROM over 90-degree elevation.
- Initiate limited strengthening program.
  - *Remember rotator cuff (RTC) and scapular muscles are small and need endurance more than pure strength.
- ER and IR with exercise bands/sport cord/tubing
- ER isotonic exercises in side lying (low-weight, high-repetition) may simply start with weight of arm.
- Elbow flexion and extension isotonics

Criteria for Progression to Phase III

- Full AROM

Phase III: Early Strengthening (Weeks 12–18)

Goals

- Full AROM (weeks 12–14)
- Maintain full PROM.
- Dynamic shoulder stability (GH and ST)
- Gradual restoration of GH and scapular strength, power, and endurance
- Optimize neuromuscular control.
- Gradual return to functional activities
- Precautions
- No lifting objects >5 lbs, no sudden lifting or pushing
- Exercise should not be painful.

Week 12

- Continue stretching, joint mobilization, and PROM exercises as needed.
- Continue periscapular exercises.
- Dynamic strengthening exercises
- Initiate strengthening program.
- Continue exercises as in weeks 7 to 12.
- Scapular plane elevation to 90 degrees (patient must be able to elevate arm without shoulder or scapular hiking before initiating isotonic exercises. If unable, then continue cuff/scapular exercises.)
- Full can (no empty can abduction exercises)
- Prone rowing
- Prone extension
- Prone horizontal abduction

Continued

REHABILITATION PROTOCOL 23.2 ■ **Arthroscopic Rotator Cuff Repair Protocol: Medium to Large Tear Size—cont'd**

Week 14

- Continue all exercises listed.
- May begin BodyBlade, Flexbar, Boing below 45 degrees
- Begin light isometrics in 90/90 or higher supine, PNF D2 flexion/extension patterns against light manual resistance.
- Initiate light functional activities as tolerated.

Week 16

- Continue all exercises listed.
- Progress to fundamental exercises (bench press, shoulder press).
- Initiate low-level plyometrics (two-handed, below chest level, progressing to overhead and finally one-handed drills).

Criteria for Progression to Phase IV

- Ability to tolerate progression to low-level functional activities
- Demonstrate return of strength/dynamic shoulder stability.
- Re-establishment of dynamic shoulder stability
- Demonstrated adequate strength and dynamic stability for progression to more demanding work and sport-specific activities

Phase IV: Advanced Strengthening Phases (Weeks 18–24)

Goals

- Maintain full nonpainful AROM.

- Advanced conditioning exercise for enhanced functional and sports-specific use
- Improve muscular strength, power, and endurance.
- Gradual return to all functional activities

Week 18

- Continue ROM and self-capsular stretching for ROM maintenance.
- Continue periscapular exercises.
- Continue progressive strengthening.
- Advanced proprioceptive, neuromuscular activities
- Light isotonic strengthening in 90/90 position
- Initiation of light sports (golf chipping/putting, tennis ground strokes) if satisfactory clinical examination

Week 24

- Continue strengthening and stretching.
- Continue joint mobilization and stretching if motion is tight.
- Initiate interval sports program (e.g., golf, doubles tennis) if appropriate.

REHABILITATION PROTOCOL 23.3 ■ **Arthroscopic Rotator Cuff Repair Protocol: Massive Tear Size**

This protocol was developed to provide the rehabilitation professional with a guideline for a postoperative rehabilitation course for a patient who has undergone an arthroscopic *massive* size rotator cuff tear repair. It should be stressed that this is only a protocol and should not be a substitute for clinical decision making regarding a patient's progression. Actual progression should be individualized based on your patient's physical examination, individual progress, and the presence of any postoperative complications.

The rate limiting factor in arthroscopic rotator cuff repair is the biologic healing of the cuff tendon to the humerus, which is thought to be a minimum of 8 to 12 weeks.

Progression of active range of motion (AROM) against gravity and duration of sling use is predicated both on the size of tear and quality of tissue and should be guided by the referring physician. Refer to initial therapy referral for any specific instructions.

Phase I: Immediate Postsurgical Phase (Weeks 0–8)

Goals

- Maintain/protect integrity of repair.
- Gradually increase passive range of motion (PROM).
- Diminish pain and inflammation.
- Prevent muscular inhibition.
- Independence in modified activities of daily living
- Precautions
- No AROM of shoulder
- No lifting of objects, reaching behind back, excessive stretching, or sudden movements
- Maintain arm in brace, sling; remove *only* for exercise.
- Sling use for 8 weeks for massive tear size
- No support of body weight by hands
- Keep incisions clean and dry.

Days 1 to 14

- Use of abduction brace/sling (during sleep also); remove *only* for exercise

- Passive pendulum exercises (three times a day minimum)
- Finger, wrist, and elbow AROM (three times a day minimum)
- Gripping exercises (putty, handball)
- Cervical spine AROM
- Passive shoulder (PROM) done supine for more patient relaxation
- Flexion to 100 degrees
- External rotation/internal rotation (ER/IR) in scapular plane ≤20 degrees
- Educate patient on posture, joint protection, importance of brace/sling, pain medication use early, hygiene.
- Cryotherapy for pain and inflammation
  - Day 1 to 3: as much as possible (20 minutes/hour)
  - Day 4 to 7: post activity or as needed for pain

Weeks 2 to 8

- Continue use of abduction sling/brace until the end of week 8.
- Pendulum exercises
- Begin PROM to tolerance (supine and pain free).
- May use heat prior to ROM
- Flexion to 130 degrees
- ER in scapular plane = 30 degrees
- IR in scapular plane to body/chest at 0 degrees, abduction up to 40 degrees
- IR in scapular plane to body/chest in slight (30 degrees) abduction ≤30 degrees
- Continue elbow, hand, forearm, wrist, and finger AROM.
- Begin resisted isometrics/isotonics for elbow, hand, forearm, wrist, and fingers.
- Begin scapula muscle isometrics/sets, AROM.
- Cryotherapy as needed for pain control and inflammation
- May begin gentle general conditioning program (walking, stationary bike) with caution if unstable from pain medications
- No running or jogging
- Aquatherapy may begin approximately 10 weeks postoperatively if wounds healed.

Criteria for Progression to Next Phase (II)

- Passive forward flexion to ≥125 degrees
- Passive ER in scapular plane to ≥25 degrees (if uninvolved shoulder PROM >80 degrees)
- Passive IR in scapular plane to ≥30 degrees (if uninvolved shoulder PROM >80 degrees)
- Passive abduction in scapular plane to ≥60 degrees
- No passive pulley exercise

Phase II: Protection and Protected Active Motion Phase (Weeks 8–16)

Goals

- Allow healing of soft tissue.
- Do not overstress healing soft tissue.
- Gradually restore full passive ROM (≈weeks 12–16).
- Decrease pain and inflammation.
- Precautions
- No lifting
- No supported full body weight with hands or arms
- No sudden jerking motions
- No excessive behind back motions
- No bike or upper extremity ergometer until week 10

Weeks 8 to 10

- Continue with full-time use of sling/brace until end of week 8.
- Continue scapular exercises.
- Gradually wean from brace starting several hours a day out, progressing as tolerated.
- Use brace sling for comfort only until full DC by end of week 9.
- Initiate AAROM shoulder flexion from supine position weeks 8 to 10.
- Progressive PROM until full PROM by weeks 12 to 16 (should be pain free)
- May require use of heat prior to ROM exercises/joint mobilization
- Can begin passive pulley use
- May require gentle glenohumeral or scapular joint mobilization as indicated to obtain full unrestricted ROM
- Initiate prone rowing to a neutral arm position.
- Continue cryotherapy as needed post-therapy or postexercise.

Weeks 10 to 16

- Continue AROM, AAROM, and stretching as needed.
- Begin IR stretching, shoulder extension, and cross-body, sleeper stretch to mobilize posterior capsule (if needed).
- Begin gentle rotator cuff submaximal isometrics (10–12 weeks).
- Begin GH submaximal rhythmic stabilization exercises in "balance position" (90–100 degrees of elevation) in supine position to initiate dynamic stabilization.
- Continue periscapular exercises progressing to manual resistance to all planes.
- Seated press-ups
- Initiate AROM exercises (flexion, scapular plane, abduction, ER, IR); should be pain free; low weight; initially only weight of arm.
- Do not allow shrug during AROM exercises.
- If shrug exists continue to work on cuff and do not reach/lift AROM over 90-degree elevation.
- Initiate limited strengthening program (weeks 12–14).
  - *Remember rotator cuff (RTC) and scapular muscles are small and need endurance more than pure strength.
- ER and IR with exercise bands/sport cord/tubing
- ER isotonic exercises in side lying (low-weight, high-repetition) may simply start with weight of arm.
- Elbow flexion and extension isotonic exercises
- Full can exercise in scapular plane; no weight/load
- Prone series (extension, rowing, and horizontal abduction)

Criteria for Progression to Phase III

- Full AROM

Phase III: Early Strengthening (Weeks 16–22)

Goals

- Full AROM (weeks 12–16)
- Maintain full PROM.
- Dynamic shoulder stability (GH and ST)
- Gradual restoration of GH and scapular strength, power and endurance
- Optimize neuromuscular control.
- Gradual return to functional activities

Precautions

- No lifting objects >5 lbs; no sudden lifting or pushing
- Exercise should not be painful.

Week 16

- Continue stretching, joint mobilization, and PROM exercises as needed.
- Dynamic strengthening exercises
- Initiate strengthening program.
- Continue exercises as above weeks 9 to 16.
- Continue periscapular muscle strengthening.
- Scapular plane elevation to 90 degrees (patient must be able to elevate arm without shoulder or scapular hiking before initiating isotonic exercises. If unable then continue cuff/scapular exercises.)
- Full can (no empty can abduction exercises)
- Prone series as described earlier

Week 18

- Continue all exercises listed.
- May begin BodyBlade, Flexbar, Boing below 45 degrees
- Begin light isometrics in 90/90 or higher supine, PNF D2 flexion/extension patterns against light manual resistance.
- Initiate light functional activities as tolerated.

Week 20

- Continue all exercises listed.
- Progress to fundamental exercises (bench press, shoulder press).
- Initiate low-level plyometrics (two-handed, below chest level, progressing to overhead and finally one-handed drills).

Criteria for Progression to Phase IV

- Ability to tolerate progression to low-level functional activities
- Demonstrate return of strength/dynamic shoulder stability.
- Re-establishment of dynamic shoulder stability
- Demonstrated adequate strength and dynamic stability for progression to more demanding work and sport-specific activities

Phase IV: Advanced Strengthening Phases (Weeks 20–26)

Goals

- Maintain full nonpainful AROM.
- Advanced conditioning exercise for enhanced functional and sports-specific use
- Improve muscular strength, power, and endurance.
- Gradual return to all functional activities

Week 18

- Continue ROM and self-capsular stretching for ROM maintenance.
- Continue progressive strengthening.
- Advanced proprioceptive, neuromuscular activities
- Light isotonic strengthening in 90/90 position
- Initiation of light sports (golf chipping/putting, tennis ground strokes) if satisfactory clinical examination

Week 24

- Continue strengthening and stretching.
- Continue joint mobilization and stretching if motion is tight.
- Initiate interval sports program (e.g., golf, doubles tennis) if appropriate.

TABLE 23.2	**Sling and Initiation of Active Motion**		
Size of Tear	Sling Use	Initiation of Active Motion	
Partial to small (<1 cm)	4 weeks	4 weeks	
Medium to large (2–4 cm)	6 weeks	6 weeks	
Massive (>5 cm)	8 weeks	8 weeks	

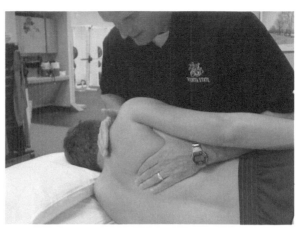

Fig. 23.11 Scapular isometrics.

supraspinatus in a position decreasing the potential of placing excessive tension across the repair due to reflex muscular contractions.

Because limited shoulder motion following rotator cuff repair is one of the biggest complications, a re-establishment of passive motion without sacrificing repair integrity is important in this phase. Depending on repair size, passive ROM predominates in this early stage. A slower rate of motion progression is warranted for those with large or massive tears. Passive motion limitations are listed in the rehabilitation protocols. Passive pendulum exercises are beneficial and cause very little active muscular activity of the cuff. Dockery et al. (1998) and Lastayo et al. (1996) found that cuff muscle activity during pendulum exercises was not different from that during continuous passive motion (CPM) or manual therapy passive motion. Recently, Ellsworth et al. (2006) found that mean supraspinatus/upper trapezius activity during the pendulum exercise in patients with shoulder pathology was activated to 25% maximum voluntary isometric contraction (MVIC), and it was slightly lower at 20% with a suspended weight. This is an EMG amount that approaches the upper level of what is considered minimal. Therapists should ensure the patient is performing a relaxed pendulum exercise with minimal muscle activity. Pendulums that are painful to perform are more than likely not creating the relaxing effect wanted and should therefore be discontinued at this early time. The remainder of the upper extremity joints can be treated with active-assisted exercises of the elbow, hand, wrist, and cervical spine.

Because of the importance of scapular stabilization and function of the rotator cuff, scapular muscle isometrics and active motion can usually begin early. Early gentle setting of the scapular muscles can be done in side-lying positions with the shoulder protected (Fig. 23.11). Motions of elevation/depression and protraction/retraction are effective to isolate scapular muscle recruitment.

Recent discussions have included use of complete removal of load to repaired tendons in an effort to improve healing. Galatz et al. (2009), using an animal model, applied botulinum toxin to paralyze the supraspinatus following rotator cuff repair. They used botulinum A and immobilized one group, allowed free range in another group, and used saline injection and casting in a control group. Complete paralysis had a negative effect on cuff healing and proved that complete removal of loads from a healing rotator cuff tendon is detrimental. A low level of controlled force is probably beneficial for tendon healing.

Passive motion predominates in this phase in an attempt to decrease adhesion formation, contractures, and limitations of periarticular structures (McCann et al. 1993, Dockery et al. 1998, Lastayo et al. 1996). These passive exercises are done to decrease the risk of forming selective hypomobilities (Harryman et al. 1990). An asymmetric tightening of the capsule with prolonged immobilization or with disuse will cause an obligate translation in the direction opposite the tight tissue constraint. After rotator cuff repairs the primary tissue that becomes tight is the posterior and anterior capsule. Furthermore, Hata et al. (2001) used arthrographic comparison between patients who had and those who did not have pain following rotator cuff repair. Patients with shoulder pain after repair had reduced capacity and motion of the GH joint. The initial postoperative treatment has a direct bearing on postoperative stiffness, and failure to begin passive ROM in the first week after the operation can lead to loss of motion.

Early rehabilitation should include both physiologic and accessory joint mobilizations. Manske et al. (2010) have determined that posterior glide accessory joint mobilization techniques with passive stretching are better than passive stretching alone for treatment of posterior shoulder tightness. Surenkok et al. (2009) recently showed that pain was decreased and shoulder motion was improved immediately following scapular mobilizations in those with painful shoulders.

An area that is oftentimes taken too lightly is the position in which to place the shoulder while performing mobilization. In cadaver studies of strain on the supraspinatus, Zuckerman et al. (1991), Muraki et al. (2007), Hatakeyama et al. (2001), and Hersche and Gerber (1998) all concluded that strains are significantly less when the humerus is placed in at least 30 to 45 degrees of elevation. This becomes most important about 3 weeks after repair because it is at this time that the repaired tendon is at its weakest (Ticker and Warner 1998).

Protection and Protected Active Motion Phase

Depending on tear size, immobilization can be discontinued from between 4 and 8 to 10 weeks. At this point gentle active assistive and active ROM can begin. Light isometric exercises predominate this phase also. These isotonic exercises should begin with the shoulder below 90 degrees of elevation or at 90 degrees in the "balance position." The balance position is used so that the deltoids will not pull the humerus superior, but rather they will generate more of a compressive force as tension generated is more horizontal at 90 degrees of elevation while supine. Exercises at this point include submaximal isometrics in multiple angles. The isometric exercises can be done initially as alternating isometrics progressing to rhythmic stabilization exercises. Initially these should be done slow and controlled, allowing the patient to watch the movement patterns in a proactive state of awareness. This can be advanced to performance in a more reactive state of awareness in which the patient does not know the direction of force or is not allowed to watch the resistance given. This increases the complexity of the isometric exercise. Heavy, more significant strengthening exercises should be avoided until the advanced strengthening phase. Gentle closed kinetic chain exercises can be done to help minimize humeral shear (Ellenbecker et al. 2006, Kibler et al. 1995). More aggressive joint mobilization techniques and passive motion can be performed if ROM is not full. Emphasis of treatment in this phase should be returning full symmetric passive ROM. Once active motion is started, the patient is not allowed to elevate the shoulder in a shrugging pattern. Starting active elevation with scapular motion rather than humeral elevation could be due to a capsular limitation or as a compensatory pattern from continued cuff weakness. If the shrug exists, exercises to regain normal scapular and glenohumeral arthrokinematics or progressive rotator cuff strengthening exercises should be continued. Motions allowed include humeral active ROM in flexion, abduction, and external and internal rotation.

Early Strengthening Phase

In the early strengthening phase, the patient should be able to tolerate low-level functional activities. Between 12 to 16 weeks of gentle isometric exercises can be progressed to isotonic exercises. All strengthening following rotator cuff repairs should not elicit a painful response. A fatigued burning sensation is desirable, but overt pain is not. Strengthening exercises at this point can include light weight isotonic exercises and use of exercise bands. Other exercises include scapular plane elevation, rowing, prone rowing, prone horizontal abduction, and resisted proprioceptive neuromuscular facilitation exercises in the D2 pattern.

Advanced Strengthening Phase

The advanced strengthening phase should be dedicated to enhancing sports or vocational activities by improving muscular strength, power, and endurance. In this phase, a gradual return to all prior functional activities should occur. Continued dynamic stabilization exercises for the rotator cuff and scapular muscles should use functional movement patterns. These include continued dumbbell exercises and those that may more closely simulate prior function. When appropriate, a gradual progression of interval sports programs can begin if warranted.

MASSIVE ROTATOR CUFF REPAIRS

Massive rotator cuff tears occur in 10% to 40% of all tears (Bedi et al. 2010). A massive rotator cuff tear will exhibit superior migration of the humeral head due to the offset forces created by the deltoid (Fig. 23.12). This chronic superior shearing can eventually result in rotator cuff arthropathy in which structural glenohumeral joint destruction occurs (Visotsky et al. 2004). Careful attention should be paid to massive rotator cuff repairs because the repaired tissue may not be as compliant as that of a smaller tear. The progression is much slower in the massive tears because the risk of retearing is increased.

Sling immobilization is continued for a full 8 weeks or more depending on tissue quality. Motion is progressed slower than

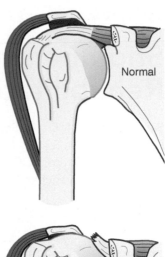
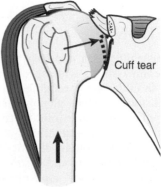

Fig. 23.12 Include description as listed: In chronic cuff deficiency, erosion of the upper glenoid may leave the shoulder with a permanent tendency toward superior subluxation that cannot be reversed by cuff repair surgery.

with smaller repairs to avoid placing excessive tension on the healing tissue. Active tension through the tissue is not allowed before 8 to 10 weeks. At this point, a gradual restoration of strength is also begun starting with the scapular muscles, progressing to the rotator cuff muscles, and finally to the deltoid. Obtaining a balance of posterior and anterior cuff musculature is the key for massive repairs. Once the normal or near normal force couples have returned, active shoulder motion can commence. A weakness of the posterior cuff muscles "uncouples" the rotator cuff force couple that allows normal arthrokinematics of normal shoulder motion. This uncoupling will allow an anterior superior translation of the humeral head with active shoulder elevation.

CONCLUSION

It should always be stressed to the patient that although he or she may be pain free and most substantial gains will be seen in the first 6 months, full unrestricted return to activity and full potential will not be achieved until about 1 full year (Matson et al. 2004, Rokito et al. 1996). Rotator cuff rehabilitation is a long and slow process!

REFERENCES

A complete reference list is available at https://expertconsult.inkling.com/.

Shoulder Instability Treatment and Rehabilitation

Sameer Lodha, MD | Sean Mazloom, MS | Amy G. Resler, DPT, CMP, CSCS |
Rachel M. Frank, BS | Neil S. Ghodadra, MD | Anthony A. Romeo, MD |
Jonathan Yong Kim, CDR | R. Jason Jadgchew, ATC, CSCS |
Matthew T. Provencher, MD, CDR, MC, USN

INTRODUCTION

Glenohumeral instability is a relatively common orthopedic problem, encompassing a wide spectrum of pathologic mobility at the shoulder joint ranging from symptomatic laxity to frank dislocation. The glenohumeral joint allows greater mobility than any other joint in the human body; however, this comes at the expense of stability. Perhaps more so than other joints, shoulder stability is predicated on adequate soft tissue (muscular and ligamentous) function and integrity, rather than bony congruity and alignment. Instability of the joint can easily result from impairments or imbalances in muscle function, ligamentous laxity, and/or bony abnormalities. Given this inherent laxity, it is not surprising that there is a relatively high incidence of instability events. A Danish registry study suggested a 1.7% overall incidence rate for the population as a whole (Hovelius et al. 1996). Young, athletic populations are at even higher risk, with a study of cadets at the United States Military Academy demonstrating an overall incidence of shoulder instability of 2.8%. In this population, trauma was identified as the most common etiology, with more than 85% of patients reporting antecedent trauma. Most concerning regarding first-time shoulder dislocations is the high recurrence rate, which has been reported as between 20% and 50% and as high as 90% in young patients. These epidemiologic findings highlight the importance of accurately identifying and appropriately treating shoulder instability. There is still, however, considerable controversy concerning appropriate treatment algorithms for shoulder instability. Prior to deciding on an appropriate treatment course, factors including patient age, type of activity/sport, activity/sport level, goals, and likelihood of compliance must be considered. In addition, the mechanism of injury and the type of damage incurred, which may include labral, capsule, biceps, and/or rotator cuff lesions, in addition to bony avulsions, will influence the most appropriate course of treatment for the patient.

Understanding these factors will permit the treating clinician to determine (1) whether nonoperative versus operative treatment is indicated, and (2) if operative intervention is required, what form this should take. In this section we briefly review the anatomy and biomechanics of the glenohumeral joint, describe the classification of instability events, discuss the available nonoperative and operative interventions for treating the spectrum of instability disorders, and provide rehabilitation protocols.

ANATOMIC CONSIDERATIONS

The range of motion (ROM) permitted at the glenohumeral joint is a consequence of minimal bony constraint provided by the humeral head and glenoid articulation. The glenoid fossa is a shallow structure, covering only 25% of the humeral head surface. Stability in the joint is therefore primarily a consequence of its static and dynamic stabilizers. The static stabilizers consist of the bony anatomy, the glenoid labrum, and capsular and ligamentous complexes and are typically only improved with surgical intervention once injured. Of note, the superior, middle, and inferior glenohumeral ligaments (SGHL, MGHL, IGHL) are especially important structures with regard to shoulder instability and thus have major implications with regard to rehabilitation following injury and/or surgery (Fig. 24.1). Specifically, the SGHL (along with the coracohumeral ligament) and MGHL are important stabilizers with regard to limiting external rotation of the adducted arm (when the arm is at the side). The IGHL is especially important in preventing anterior translation of the shoulder when in the provocative position of abduction and external rotation. The dynamic stabilizers, including the rotator cuff muscles and long head of the biceps tendon, can often be improved with an appropriate nonoperative rehabilitation program after an instability event. In fact, proper strengthening of the rotator cuff musculature and scapular stabilizers is a critical component of any rehabilitation protocol, including those for nonoperative management of shoulder instability and part of the rehabilitation following surgery.

It is particularly important to note the integrity and condition of the subscapularis with regard to rehabilitation following shoulder surgery. In many open surgical techniques, the subscapularis is detached from the lesser tuberosity of the shoulder, requiring strict limitations in the amount of permitted postoperative external rotation and internal rotation strengthening, whereas this is not as much a concern when the subscapularis is left intact (such as through a subscapularis split). Ensuring excellent communication with the surgical team and the postoperative rehabilitation team of exactly what was performed during the surgery is critical to postoperative success.

TERMINOLOGY

It is first important to differentiate **laxity** from **instability**. Instability is symptomatic laxity—as all shoulders have and require some level of laxity to move through a functional arc

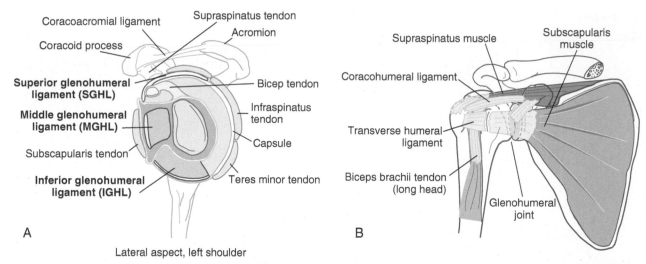

Fig. 24.1 **A,** The ligaments of the glenohumeral joint are shown, including the superior glenohumeral ligament (SGHL), inferior glenohumeral ligament (IGHL), and middle glenohumeral ligament (MGHL). **B,** An anterior (coronal) view of the rotator cuff and coracohumeral ligament (CHL) of the glenohumeral joint.

of motion. **Instability** refers to the patient experiencing symptoms of having a shoulder joint that is unstable in certain positions and is usually accompanied by increased laxity in that direction. Similar to other joints, shoulder instability varies in severity from microinstability to subluxation and ultimately to frank dislocation. **Microinstability** refers to pathologic motion of the humeral head, most often in multiple directions, secondary to generalized capsular laxity. **Subluxation** denotes translation of the humeral head beyond normal physiologic limits while still maintaining contact with the glenoid. **Dislocation** differs from subluxation in that the translation of the humeral head is significant enough to completely disassociate the articular surfaces of the humerus and the glenoid; this magnitude of instability will commonly require manual reduction.

Shoulder instability is typically described in relation to the direction of the instability event: anterior, posterior, and multidirectional. **Anterior instability** is the most common manifestation of unidirectional instability, comprising more than 90% of shoulder dislocations. However, recent evidence in young healthy active patients has shown that posterior dislocations and combined dislocations may comprise 43% of dislocations while anterior may comprise only 57% (Song et al. 2015). Regardless, dislocations most commonly occur as the result of a one-time traumatic episode to a shoulder in a vulnerable position of combined abduction and external rotation. The injury may involve an avulsion of the anteroinferior labrum from the glenoid, commonly referred to as the Bankart lesion. Occasionally a fragment of the underlying glenoid rim also may be fractured off; this lesion is referred to as a bony Bankart lesion. Other lesions can also present with symptoms of anterior instability, including subscapularis tears, humeral avulsions of the glenohumeral ligament (HAGL), superior labrum anterior to posterior (SLAP) injuries, and rotator interval lesions.

Classically, **posterior instability** is far less common than anterior instability, accounting for 2% to 10% of shoulder dislocations. Recent evidence described by Song et al. (2015) disputes this, demonstrating much higher incidences in an active young population. Posterior dislocations are often

associated with axial loads applied to the adducted arm and are classically associated with electrocution and seizures. Structural changes associated with posterior instability include avulsions of the posterior labrum (a reverse Bankart lesion), which may be associated with a posterior glenoid rim fracture. Injuries to the SGHL, the posterior band of the IGHL, the subscapularis muscle, and the coracohumeral ligament (CHL) can also be seen in posterior instability. The most common form of posterior instability is recurrent posterior instability, usually resulting in a posterior labral tear and posteroinferior capsular stretch resulting from repetitive loading with the arm in flexion and internal rotation (i.e., the bench press exercise).

Finally, **multidirectional instability (MDI)** is not typically associated with traumatic episodes. Instead, the primary dysfunction here involves either congenital or acquired capsuloligamentous laxity. As such, it may be indicative of an underlying connective tissue disorder or a result of repeated minor stretching injuries to the capsuloligamentous complex. Presenting pathology typically consists of symptomatic, abnormal humeral head translation in more than one direction, which may include recurrent subluxations or even dislocations with minimal trauma. Often multidirectional instability may be associated with general ligamentous laxity signs such as hyperextension of the thumb to wrist and hyperextension of the elbows.

DIAGNOSTIC EVALUATION: HISTORY, PHYSICAL EXAMINATION, AND IMAGING

History

A thorough history provides a foundation for accurate diagnosis of the type and magnitude of shoulder instability, which is essential for choosing appropriate treatment options. The history should identify the mechanism of the injury, previous surgical and/or nonsurgical treatment of the shoulder, and the activity level of the patient. The patient should be asked several

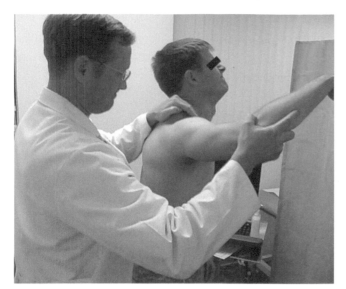

Fig. 24.2 An example of a patient with posterior shoulder instability and a positive load and shift test.

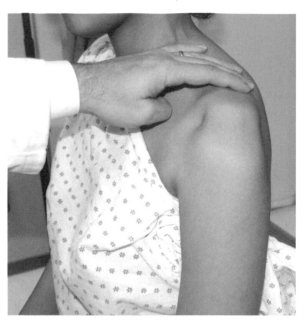

Fig. 24.3 An example of a sulcus finding demonstrating space between the acromion and the humeral head with downward traction on the arm at the side. This is not necessarily pathologic and is present in patients without documented instability and just normal laxity of the joint.

questions concerning if the injury was traumatic, if there was dislocation/subluxation and if a reduction was required, if the shoulder has been previously injured, and how the arm was positioned at the time of injury. Although these questions seem standard for any initial shoulder evaluation, the answers to these questions may rule a patient out for surgery or otherwise assist the surgeon in avoiding intraoperative and postoperative complications.

Physical Examination

Following the history, a detailed physical examination should be completed, beginning with observation.

- The clinician should examine the entire body from head to toe to determine postural alignment, scapular position, and overall core strength.
- Progressing to the shoulders, it is important to note any asymmetry, muscular atrophy, abnormal motion, edema, or scapular winging.
- The structure, function, neurologic status, and strength of the injured shoulder should be compared with the contralateral shoulder.
- Palpation will alert the clinician to specific areas of tenderness, whereas both active and passive range of motion testing will demonstrate stiffness.
- In particular, if significant stiffness is noted, range of motion must be optimized prior to any operative stabilization procedure to avoid progressive loss of motion.
- Next, strength and sensation in all planes should be evaluated because weakness in one or more planes may be significant for concomitant pathology, including rotator cuff tears.
- Shoulder stability testing should also be addressed because provocative shoulder tests and maneuvers may be used to evaluate the extent and direction of any instability.
- Anterior and posterior apprehension, relocation, load and shift (to assess for posterior instability) (Fig. 24.2), and sulcus tests (Fig. 24.3) are widely used to assess shoulder anterior and/or inferior instability.

Imaging Studies

Finally, radiographs can be extremely helpful in the evaluation of shoulder instability. Generally, a series of radiographs including a true AP, scapular Y, and axillary view will provide significant information. Additionally, a Stryker notch view is helpful for evaluating Hill-Sachs lesions (bony injury of the humeral head from anterior dislocation), whereas the West Point view may be utilized to determine glenoid bone loss. Advanced imaging may be helpful, especially in evaluating an unstable but reduced shoulder. Computed tomography (CT) scanning is useful in evaluating glenoid hypoplasia, fracture, glenoid and humeral bone loss, and retroversion. MRI is useful in visualizing the integrity of soft tissue structures, allowing an assessment of the capsulolabral structures, the rotator cuff, the rotator interval, and the tendon of the long head of the biceps (Fig. 24.4).

TREATMENT OPTIONS

Treatment options for shoulder instability include nonoperative and operative approaches. Nonoperative therapies aim to address instability symptoms by altering the pathologic mechanics of the unstable shoulder. These therapies therefore involve programs to address kinetic chain deficits, shoulder strength and flexibility, proprioception, neuromuscular control, and scapulothoracic mechanics. Surgical treatment, however, aims to directly address the structural deficiencies that may be contributing to instability through various reconstructive techniques.

Considerable controversy exists over the appropriate initial therapy for patients with instability. There is general agreement, however, on the appropriate treatment for an acute shoulder dislocation. Any unreduced dislocation must undergo closed reduction with radiographic

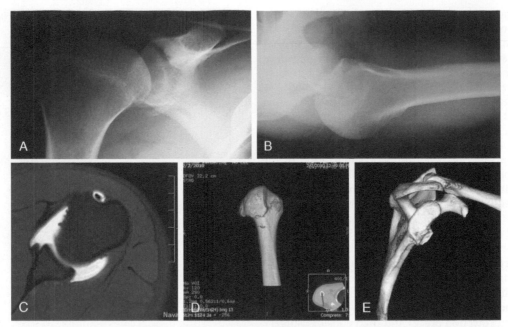

Fig. 24.4 Various imaging studies to demonstrate examples of glenohumeral instability. Anteroposterior (*A*) and axillary (*B*) radiographs that demonstrate an anterior bony Bankart injury sustained after an anterior shoulder dislocation. A magnetic resonance arthrogram that demonstrates an anterior labral tear (*C*). A computed tomography (CT) scan with three-dimensional reconstruction demonstrating a large Hill-Sachs injury (*D*). A CT scan sagittal oblique image that shows glenoid bone loss (approximately 25%) and bony Bankart injury with some attrition of the injured bone (*E*).

confirmation of reduction. It is unknown whether reduction should be performed immediately (i.e., on the field after an athlete has dislocated) or after the patient has been seen in a controlled, emergency room setting with the aid of analgesics and radiographs. Regardless, it is imperative to perform a thorough prereduction and postreduction neurovascular examination, especially with regard to anterior shoulder instability where the axillary nerve is particularly vulnerable. In general, the shoulder should be reduced as soon as possible utilizing a variety of well-described reduction techniques.

Nonoperative Treatment and Rehabilitation

Nonoperative treatment protocols typically consist of immobilization followed by rehabilitation with an experienced physical therapist. Traditionally, following anterior dislocation, the arm is most commonly immobilized in internal rotation to avoid the vulnerable and susceptible position of external rotation and abduction. However, recent studies have suggested little to no benefit to this immobilization, considering it as much a source of comfort as actual protection and stability. In fact, Itoi et al. (2007) suggested there actually may be some benefit to immobilizing the injured arm in a position of external rotation instead. The rationale for placement of the arm in external rotation centers on the fact that the Bankart lesion is forced to separate from the glenoid when the arm is placed in internal rotation, which may be detrimental to healing. In contrast, the authors describe how placing the arm in external rotation approximates the lesion to its correct anatomic position, allowing for a better healing process.

The nonoperative treatment options for anterior, posterior, and multidirectional glenohumeral instability all center on the same core issues. The immediate goals are to decrease pain and edema, protect the static stabilizers, and strengthen the dynamic stabilizers. The ultimate aim is to increase overall shoulder stability, which is facilitated via exercises designed to enhance joint proprioception and address kinetic chain deficits. With specific regard to posterior dislocations, recommendations have typically revolved around immobilization of the arm in external rotation and slight extension. More recently, however, Edwards et al. (2002) suggested that immobilization in internal rotation may be more appropriate, although this has yet to be fully studied.

Special Considerations

- First-time dislocator:
  - Overall, the nonoperative treatment options for patients following first-time shoulder dislocation are controversial, and regardless of the treatment, reported recurrence rates are high, especially for young, highly active patients. The initial results reported with immobilization in external rotation are interesting; however, larger, longer-term clinical studies are needed before any single immobilization technique can be universally recommended.
- Chronic/recurrent dislocator:
  - Nonoperative treatment has been shown to be less successful in the chronic dislocator, especially in the young athlete. Specifically, in patients younger than 20 years old with a one-time acute shoulder dislocation treated nonoperatively, recurrence rates have been reported as high as 90%.

- Consideration to level of athletics, level of patient symptoms (how often does the shoulder become unstable), and level of trauma to provoke instability (does it occur with little force such as while sleeping or lifting overhead, or with higher level sporting activities), and patient desires
- In-season athlete:
- A unique situation that requires special consideration with regard to treatment options involves the in-season athlete who wishes to continue to play. In 2004 Buss et al. studied 30 competitive in-season athletes who experienced either anterior dislocation or subluxation of the shoulder followed by treatment with rehabilitation and bracing that restricted external rotation and abduction. The authors found that 26 of the 30 patients were able to return to play and complete the season after approximately 10 days of missed time; however, 37% experienced at least one episode of recurrent instability during the season. Further, 16 athletes required surgical intervention following their competitive season. Thus, the treatment of a dislocation in an in-season athlete is generally to finish the season (possibly with the use of an external rotation protection brace) and then consider surgery once the season is finished. However, recurrences during the season after an initial dislocation require more careful discussions with the athlete for his or her desires and return-to-play capability.

POSTOPERATIVE TREATMENT AND REHABILITATION

Anterior Instability

Traumatic dislocations are often associated with significant structural injury. Despite this, studies have demonstrated that good clinical results can be obtained with nonoperative treatment in patients who are older and less active. However, the same cannot be said for patients who are young and active, particularly those involved in contact sports. In these patients, operative treatment has been shown to have a lower risk of recurrent dislocation as compared to nonoperative therapy. Patients with significant bone injury—glenoid defects (20% to 25% or more), displaced tuberosity fractures, and irreducible dislocations—should be treated with operative stabilization. Other indications for operative intervention include three or more recurrent dislocations in a year and dislocations that occur at rest or during sleep.

The open Bankart repair was once considered the gold standard in the treatment of anterior shoulder instability; however, proper patient selection combined with improvements in arthroscopic techniques and devices have allowed for postoperative results rivaling those of open stabilization. In the open procedure, the labrum is anatomically reduced and repaired to the anterior glenoid. Given the common coexistence of capsular injury and stretch, a concomitant capsular shift procedure is often performed. Various methods for the capsular shift have been described; the essential underlying goal is to repair the injured anteroinferior capsule and labral repair. Recurrence rate for open repair has been reported to be approximately 4%. As mentioned, both of these procedures are now increasingly performed arthroscopically (Figs. 24.5 and 24.6). Although initial reports described a higher recurrence rate after arthroscopic repair, recent studies have shown that recurrence rates are nearly

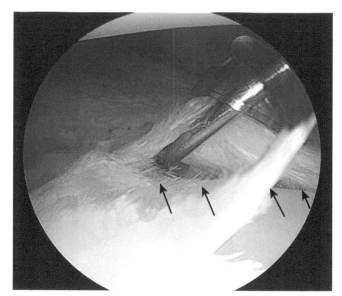

Fig. 24.5 An arthroscopic image of an anterior labral tear (soft tissue Bankart) *(black arrows)*.

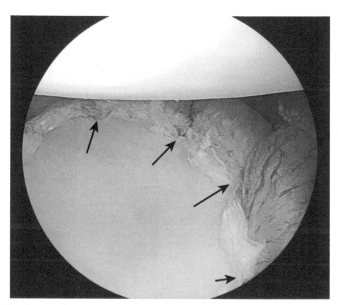

Fig. 24.6 The patient from Figure 24.5 after repair with four anchors and suture construct (capsulolabral repair). The anchors are located at the black arrows.

comparable to open repair, especially in those patients without significant glenoid bone loss or other structural abnormalities.

With the ultimate focus of regaining and then maintaining shoulder stability, the goals of postoperative rehabilitation commonly focus on avoiding common complications following anterior stabilization procedures. These complications include limited postoperative ROM related to residual stiffness; the development of recurrent instability; an inability to return to preinstability activity levels, especially in competitive overhead athletes; and, over the longer term, the development of osteoarthritis. Thus the goals of rehabilitation are to protect the surgical repair long enough to permit healing, restore full ROM, optimize stability by strengthening the dynamic stabilizers, and ultimately return to full preinjury activity.

See Rehabilitation Protocols 24.1 through 24.4 for specific rehabilitation programs.

Posterior Instability

The initial treatment for posterior instability is usually non-operative, especially in the case of an atraumatic etiology, because successful outcomes following nonoperative therapy in atraumatic subluxators have been reported. Appropriately planned strengthening programs have been shown to be effective in augmenting stability and reducing pain, especially for patients suffering from laxity secondary to repetitive microtrauma. However, the efficacy of nonoperative therapy in treating traumatic posterior dislocators is significantly lower, estimated at approximately 16%. Indications for surgical treatment therefore include the common sequelae of traumatic dislocations, including posterior glenoid rim fractures greater than 25%, displaced lesser tuberosity fractures, reverse Hill-Sachs lesions of greater than 40% of the humeral head, recurrent instability episodes, and irreducible dislocations. Patients with mechanical symptoms also often respond poorly to conservative therapy and thus may be indicated for surgical treatment. Failure of 3 to 6 months of conservative therapy is also an indication for operative repair. The most common presenting complaint in a patient with posterior shoulder instability is pain and pain with provocative exercises (the arm in flexion and internal rotation), such as bench press, push-ups, and presses.

Specific operative treatment techniques for posterior instability are similar in theory to the treatments for anterior instability. Both open and arthroscopic reverse Bankart, capsular shift and plication, and a host of bony-anatomy restorative procedures have been developed. Overall, the results of open surgical treatment of posterior instability have not been as good as those for anterior instability. This is likely a consequence both of the difficulties in obtaining adequate visualization and related to the different biomechanical properties of the posterior capsule and labrum (Figs. 24.7 and 24.8). Nevertheless, the goals of postoperative rehabilitation for posterior shoulder instability echo those of anterior stabilization procedures and include reducing pain and edema, protecting the surgical repair to allow healing, restoring full ROM, and facilitating a return to full activity.

See Rehabilitation Protocols 24.5 through 24.7 for specific rehabilitation programs.

Multidirectional Instability

Similar to anterior and posterior instability, the initial treatment for MDI is nonoperative management. Good results have been obtained in patients with generalized laxity in more than one direction, the hallmark of MDI. Operative treatment is considered only after an exhaustive course of nonoperative therapy has failed; generally, at least 6 months of therapy should be attempted.

When nonoperative treatment has failed, properly selected patients may benefit from operative interventions. Neer and Foster (1980) described an open surgical procedure to treat MDI, utilizing an inferior capsular shift permitting tensioning of both the anterior and posterior capsule. Several

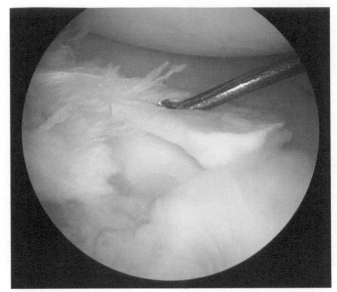

Fig. 24.7 Arthroscopic image of a posterior labral tear and associated labral flap as a result of recurrent posterior instability.

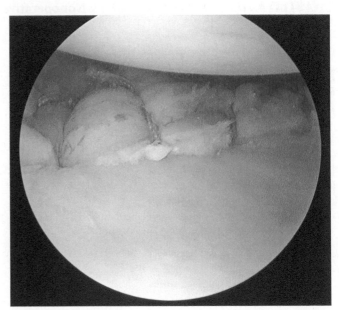

Fig. 24.8 The patient from Figure 24.7 after arthroscopic repair with suture anchors of a posterior instability injury.

other studies have reported similarly excellent results with this technique. Arthroscopic techniques have also shown excellent success rates (Figs. 24.9 and 24.10). These procedures have sought to reduce capsular redundancy through a combination of strategies, including capsular plication, closure of the rotator interval, and repair of any labral lesions. Thermal capsulorrhaphy techniques have fallen into disfavor and are no longer widely used secondary to high failure rates and numerous observations of subsequent glenohumeral chondrolysis.

See Rehabilitation Protocol 24.8 for multidirectional shoulder instability surgery (inferior capsular shift).

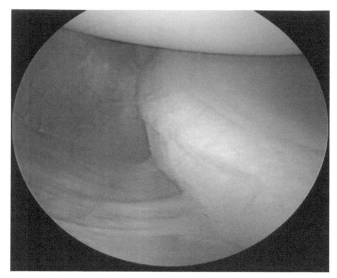

Fig. 24.9   An example of a patient with multidirectional instability with an enlarged and patulous capsule (*left side of image*) attached to the bony glenoid.

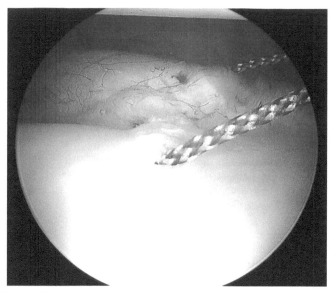

Fig. 24.10   Arthroscopic repair of a patient with multidirectional instability utilization capsular plication (repair of the capsule to the labrum without suture anchors).

REHABILITATION PROTOCOL 24.1 ● **Nonoperative Management of Anterior Shoulder Instability**

Phase I: Weeks 0–2

Goals

- Reduce pain and edema.

Restrictions

- Avoid provocative positions of the shoulder that risk recurrent instability:
  - External rotation
  - Abduction
  - Distraction

Immobilization

- Sling immobilization in neutral or external rotation
- Duration of immobilization is age-dependent based on the theoretical advantage of improved healing of the capsulolabral complex:
  - <20 years old—3–4 weeks
  - 20–30 years old—2–3 weeks
  - >30 years old—10 days–2 weeks
  - >40 years old—3–5 days

Pain Control

- Medications
  - Narcotics—for 5–7 days following a traumatic dislocation
  - Nonsteroidal anti-inflammatories (NSAIDs)—to reduce inflammation
- Therapeutic Modalities
  - Ice (Fig. 24.11), ultrasound, HVGS (high-voltage galvanic stimulation) (Fig. 24.11). Electric stimulation as shown in Fig. 24.12
  - Moist heat before therapy, ice at end of session (cryotherapy as shown in Fig. 24.11)

Exercises

1. Motion: Shoulder
   - Begins during phase I for patients 30 years and older
   - Passive range of motion (PROM) (Figure 31.6) as per the ROM guidelines outlined in phase II
   - Active-assisted ROM exercises (Fig. 24.13)

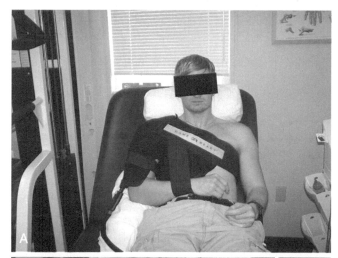

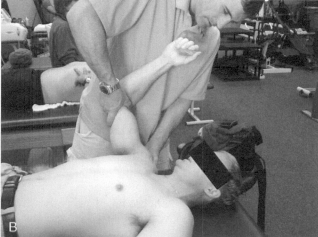

Fig. 24.11   **A,** Apply cryotherapy using shoulder cuff for pain and edema reduction. Position upper extremity with pillow, bolster, or sling for comfort. **B,** Eighty degrees day 4 picture: Therapist or athletic trainer performing passive glenohumeral joint range of motion. Above, in the scapular plane.

REHABILITATION PROTOCOL 24.1 ▪ Nonoperative Management of Anterior Shoulder Instability—cont'd

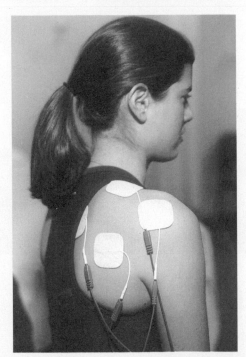

Fig. 24.12 Electric stimulation to rotator cuff and scapular musculature for pain control.

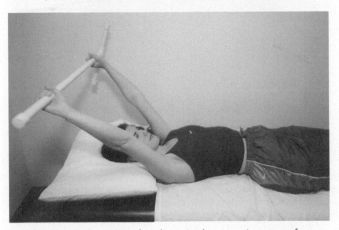

Fig. 24.13 Active-assisted and passive bar exercises are safe to perform early, especially in the supine position.

2. Motion: Elbow
   - Passive—progress to active
   - 0–130 degrees of flexion
   - Pronation and supination as tolerated
3. Muscle strengthening
   - Scapular stabilizer strengthening begins during phase I for patients 30 years and older.
   - Initiate scapular stabilization.
     - Scapular retraction or posture correction (middle trapezius and rhomboids) in seated (gravity eliminated) position with upper extremity in neutral
     - Scapular protraction (serratus anterior)
   - Grip strengthening

Phase II: Weeks 3–4

Criteria for Progression to Phase II
- Reduced pain and tenderness
- Adequate immobilization

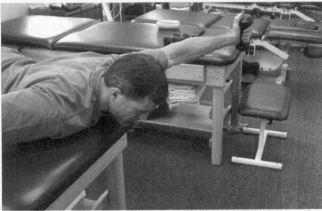

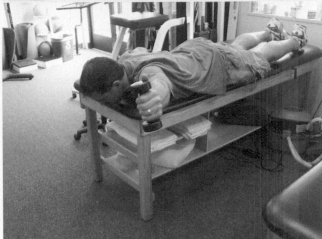

Figs. 24.14 and 24.15 Scapular stabilization, unilateral in prone with weight. Begin lying prone, shoulder in 105 degrees of abduction and externally rotated and elbow extended. Depress scapula to contract lower trapezius and follow with upper extremity movement through the entire range of motion contracting supraspinatus. Repeat as indicated without allowing compensation and progress resistance with weights.

Goals
- 90 degrees of forward flexion
- 90 degrees of abduction
- 30 degrees of external rotation with the arm at the side

Restrictions
- Avoid provocative positions of the shoulder that risk recurrent instability:
  - >140 degrees of forward flexion
  - >40 degrees of external rotation with the arm at the side
  - Avoid extension, which puts additional stress on anterior structures.

Immobilization
- Sling, as per criteria outlined in phase I

Exercises
- Proprioceptive neuromuscular facilitation (PNF) (Figs. 24.14 and 24.15):
  - Begin early rhythmic stabilization.
  - Progress from arm at side to available flexion, external rotation positions.
- Stabilization:
  - Advance scapular stabilization exercises by adding light resistance or in prone/gravity position (Figs. 24.16, 24.17, 24.18).

Continued

REHABILITATION PROTOCOL 24.1 ⬤ Nonoperative Management of Anterior Shoulder Instability—cont'd

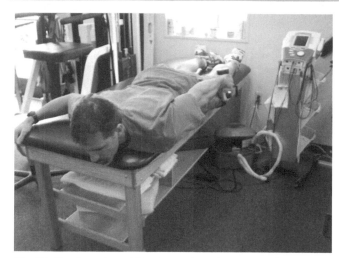

Fig. 24.16   Scapular stabilization, unilateral in prone with weight. Emphasis on lower trapezius and rhomboids. Begin lying prone, shoulder in neutral and elbow extended. Retract scapula to contract scapular stabilizers and follow with upper extremity motion. Repeat as indicated without allowing compensation and progress resistance with weights.

- Scapular retraction (rhomboids, middle trapezius)
- Scapular protraction (serratus anterior)
- Shoulder ROM:
  - Passive ROM exercises
  - Internal rotation, external rotation (only <40 degrees), forward flexion
  - Active-assisted ROM exercises
  - Active ROM exercises
- Strengthening:
  - Initiate rotator cuff strengthening with upper extremity in neutral.
  - Begin with closed chain isometric strengthening with the elbow flexed to 90 degrees and the arm comfortably at the side. Starting position is with the shoulder in the neutral position of 0 degrees of forward flexion, abduction, and external rotation. The arm should be comfortable at the patient's side.
  - Scapular depression (latissimus dorsi, lower trapezius, serratus anterior)

Phase III: Weeks 4–8

Criteria for Progression to Phase III

- Pain-free motion of 140 degrees of forward flexion and 40 degrees of external rotation with the arm at the side
- Minimal pain or tenderness with strengthening exercises
- Improvement in strength of rotator cuff and scapular stabilizers

Goals

- 160 degrees of forward flexion
- 40 degrees of external rotation with the arm in 30 to 45 degrees of abduction

Restrictions

- Avoid positions that worsen instability (e.g., abduction–external rotation):
  - >160 degrees of forward flexion
  - >40 degrees of external rotation with the arm in 30 to 45 degrees of abduction

Exercises

- Continue PNF to scapular stabilizers, GHJ stabilizers, and rotator cuff. Rhythmic stabilization, repeated contractions and slow reversals, and progressive varying speeds and resistances (Figs. 24.19 and 24.20)

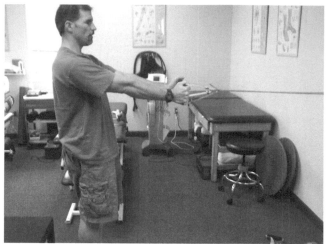

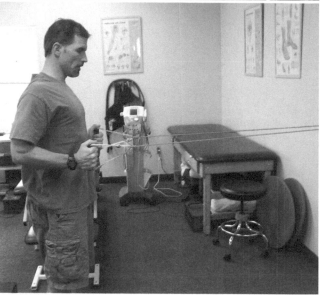

Figs. 24.17 and 24.18   Scapular rowing: Scapular stabilization with resistance band. Adduct and depress scapulae, followed by upper extremity movement. Avoid glenohumeral abduction, and keep upper extremity adjacent to thorax. Emphasize scapular stabilizers.

- Shoulder ROM:
  - Passive ROM exercises
  - Active-assisted ROM exercises
  - Active ROM exercises
- Muscle strengthening:
  - Strengthening of scapular stabilizers (as mentioned previously)
- Rotator cuff strengthening
  - Progress to advanced closed chain isometric internal and external rotation strengthening with the arm in 35 to 45 degrees of abduction.
  - Progress to strengthening with Therabands (Figs. 24.21 through 24.24). Theraband exercises permit concentric and eccentric strengthening of the shoulder muscles and are a form of isotonic exercises (characterized by variable speed and fixed resistance). Exercises are performed through an arc of 45 degrees in each of the five planes of motion.
- Six color-coded bands are available; each provides increasing resistance from 1 to 6 pounds, at increments of 1 pound.
- Progression to the next band occurs usually in 2- to 3-week intervals. Patients are instructed not to progress to the next band

REHABILITATION PROTOCOL 24.1 ● **Nonoperative Management of Anterior Shoulder Instability—cont'd**

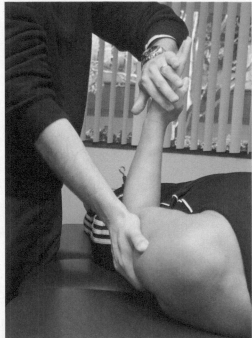

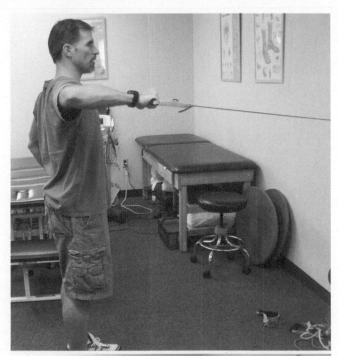

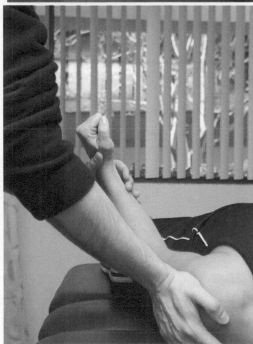

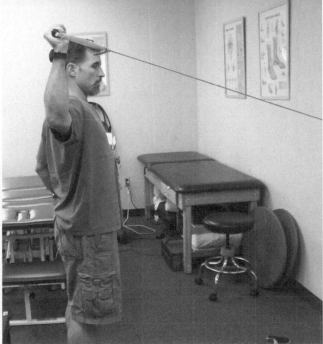

Figs. 24.19 and 24.20 Proprioceptive neuromuscular facilitation: In this example, patient or athlete is lying supine with scapular stabilizers engaged. The therapist provides manual resistance into external rotation in available and allowable range of motion. Also may begin with isometric exercise in this manner.

Figs. 24.21 and 24.22 Rotator cuff strengthening with resistance band for external rotation in 90 degrees of abduction. Stabilize scapula and pull resistance band toward 90 degrees of glenohumeral external rotation, while maintaining 90 degrees of abduction and advance resistance tubing as appropriate.

if there is any discomfort at the present level or if they are unable to perform exercise without compensatory movement strategy or scapular control.
- Progress to light isotonic dumbbell exercises.
- Advance to open chain isotonic strengthening exercises.
- Initiate deltoid strengthening in the plane of the scapula to 90 degrees of elevation.

Phase IV: Weeks 8–12

Criteria for Progression to Phase IV

- Pain-free motion of 160 degrees of forward flexion and 40 degrees of external rotation with the arm in 30 to 45 degrees of abduction
- Minimal pain or tenderness with strengthening exercises

Continued

REHABILITATION PROTOCOL 24.1 ▪ **Nonoperative Management of Anterior Shoulder Instability—cont'd**

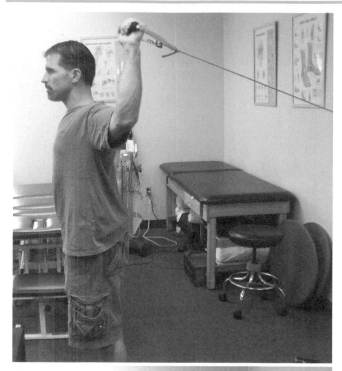

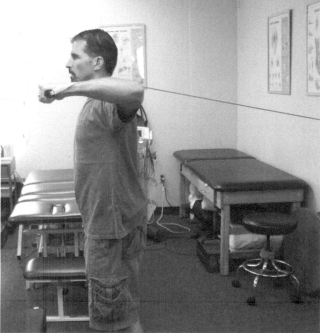

Figs. 24.23 and 24.24 Rotator cuff strengthening with resistance band for internal rotation in 90 degrees of abduction. Begin in combined ABER position. Stabilize scapula and internally rotate by 90 degrees while maintaining 90 degrees of abduction. Repeat and advance resistance tubing as appropriate.

- Continued improvement in strength of rotator cuff and scapular stabilizers
- Satisfactory physical examination

Goals

- Improve shoulder strength, power, and endurance.
- Improve neuromuscular control and shoulder proprioception.
- Restore full shoulder motion.

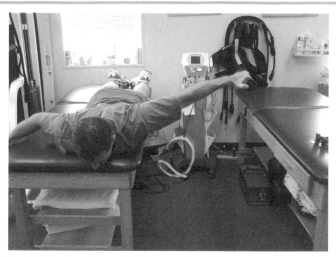

Fig. 24.25 Scapular stabilization, unilateral in prone with weight. Emphasis on middle trapezius and rhomboids. Begin lying prone, shoulder in 90 degrees of abduction and externally rotated and elbow extended. Retract scapula to contract scapular stabilizers and follow with upper extremity motion. Repeat as indicated without allowing compensation and progress resistance with weights.

Restriction

- Avoid positions that exacerbate instability (e.g., abduction–external rotation).

Exercises

- Proprioceptive training:
  - PNF patterns (Rehabilitation Protocol 24.2)
- Shoulder ROM:
  - Utilize passive, active-assisted, and active ROM exercises to obtain motion goals.
- Capsular stretching (Rehabilitation Protocol 24.1)
  - Especially posterior capsule
- Muscle strengthening:
  - Continue with rotator cuff, scapular stabilizers, and deltoid strengthening (Figs. 24.14 through 24.16, 24.25, Figs. 24.21 and 24.22). Advance dynamic shoulder stabilization (Figs. 24.26 through 24.30).
  - Eight to 12 repetitions for three sets
- Upper extremity endurance training:
  - Incorporated endurance training for the upper extremity
  - Upper body ergometer (UBE)

Phase V: Weeks 12–16

Criteria for Progression to Phase V

- Pain-free ROM
- No evidence of recurrent instability
- Recovery of 70% to 80% of shoulder strength
- Satisfactory physical examination (Fig. 24.31)

Goals

- Prepare for gradual return to functional and sporting activities.
- Establish a home exercise maintenance program that is performed at least three times per week for both stretching and strengthening.

Exercises

- Functional and sport-specific strengthening:
  - Plyometric exercises (Figure 21.6). Progress dynamic stability to end range (Fig. 24.34 in Rehabilitation Protocol 24.1).

REHABILITATION PROTOCOL 24.1 ● **Nonoperative Management of Anterior Shoulder Instability—cont'd**

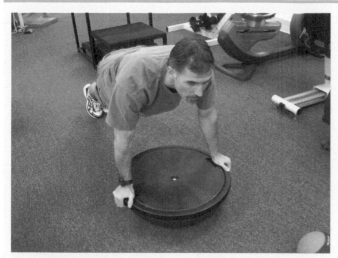

Fig. 24.26 Shoulder stabilization: isometric contraction in closed chain. Begin with 15 seconds and progress to 60 seconds. Advance to dynamic stabilization by performing a push-up on an unstable surface, (*pictured*), an inverted Bosu ball, when appropriate.

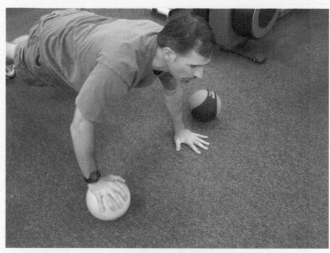

Fig. 24.27 Shoulder stabilization: isometric contraction in closed chain. Begin with 15 seconds and progress to 60 seconds. Advance to dynamic stabilization by performing a push-up on an unstable surface (*pictured*), a "plyo" or weighted ball, when appropriate.

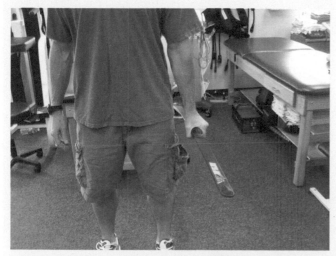

Fig. 24.28 Shoulder stabilization with Body Blade. Stabilize scapula and begin oscillating Body Blade in neutral. Begin with 30 seconds and progress to 60 seconds. Progress oscillation exercise in 45 degrees of glenohumeral joint abduction, 90 degrees of abduction, 90 degrees of flexion, and 145 degrees of scaption.

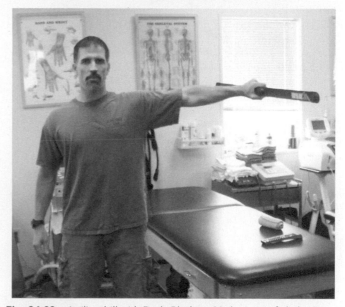

Fig. 24.29 Agility drill with Body Blade in 90 degrees of abduction.

Continued

REHABILITATION PROTOCOL 24.1 ● **Nonoperative Management of Anterior Shoulder Instability—cont'd**

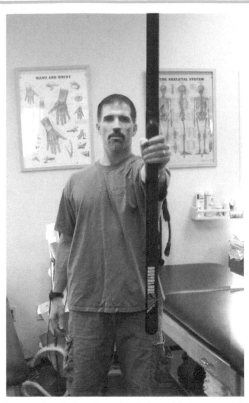

Fig. 24.30   Agility drill with Body Blade in 90 degrees of flexion.

Progressive, Systematic Interval Program for Returning to Sports
- Golfers (Table 24.1)
- Overhead athletes not before 6 months
- Throwing athletes (Tables 24.2, 24.3, and 24.4)

Warning Signs
- Persistent instability
- Loss of motion
- Lack of strength progression—especially abduction
- Continued pain

Treatment of Complications
- These patients may need to move back to earlier routines.
- May require increased utilization of pain control modalities as outlined earlier
- May require surgical intervention. Recurrent instability as defined by three or more instability events within a year, or instability that occurs at rest or during sleep, is a strong indication for surgical management.

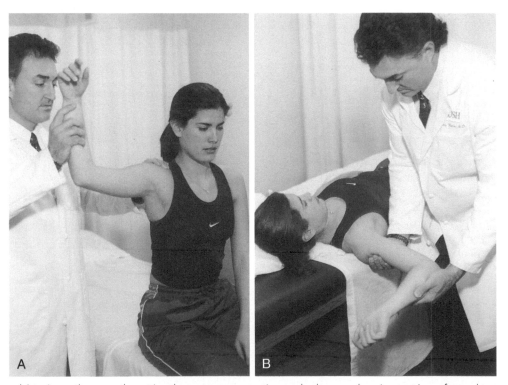

Fig. 24.31   At around 4 to 6 months, once the patient has met postoperative goals, the apprehension test is performed to ensure that there are no recurrent instability findings (*A and B*).

TABLE 24.1	Interval Golf Program		
	Monday	**Wednesday**	**Friday**
1st week	10 putts 10 chips Rest 5 min 15 chips	15 putts 15 chips Rest 5 min 25 chips	20 putts 20 chips Rest 5 min 20 putts 20 chips Rest 5 min 10 chips 10 short irons
2nd week	20 chips 10 short irons Rest 5 min 10 short irons	20 chips 15 short irons Rest 10 min 15 short irons 15 chips	15 short irons 10 medium irons Rest 10 min 20 short irons 15 chips
3rd week	15 short irons 15 medium irons Rest 10 min 5 long irons 15 short irons 15 medium irons Rest 10 min 20 chips	15 short irons 10 medium irons 10 long irons Rest 10 min 10 short irons 10 medium irons 5 long irons 5 wood	15 short irons 10 medium irons 10 long irons Rest 10 min 10 short irons 10 medium irons 10 long irons 10 wood
4th week	15 short irons 10 medium irons 10 long irons 10 drives Rest 15 min Repeat	Play 9 holes	Play 9 holes
5th week	9 holes	9 holes	18 holes

TABLE 24.2	High School, College, and Professional Baseball Pitchers' Interval Throwing Program			
Phase I	**Return to Throwing** **Throws at 50% Effort**		**Phase II**	**Return to Pitching** **Throws at Effort Level Given**
Step 1	Warmup toss to 60' 15 throws at 30'* 15 throws at 30'* 15 throws at 30'* 20 long tosses to 60'		Step 7	15 throws at 60'6" (75%)* 20 throws at 60'6" (75%)* 20 throws at 60'6" (75%)* 15 throws at 60'6" (75%)* 20 throws at 60'6" (75%)*
Step 2	Warmup toss to 75' 15 throws at 60'* 15 throws at 60'* 15 throws at 60'* 20 long tosses to 90'		Step 8	20 throws at 60'6" (75%)* 20 throws at 60'6" (75%)* 20 throws at 60'6" (75%)* 20 throws at 60'6" (75%)*
Step 3	Warmup toss to 105' 15 throws at 75'* 15 throws at 75'* 15 throws at 75'* 20 long tosses to 105'		Step 9	20 fastballs (50%)* 20 fastballs (50%)* 20 fastballs (50%)* 20 fastballs (50%)* 25 throws at 60'6" (75%)*
Step 4	Warmup toss to 120' 15 throws at 90'* 20 throws at 90'* 15 throws at 90'* 20 long tosses at 120'		Step 10	20 fastballs (50%)* 20 fastballs (75%)* 20 fastballs (50%)* 15 fastballs (75%)* 25 throws at 60'6" (75%)*
Step 5	Warmup toss to 120' 20 throws at 105'* 20 throws at 105'* 15 throws at 105'* 20 long tosses at 120'		Step 11	25 fastballs (50%)* 20 fastballs (75%)* 20 fastballs (75%)* 20 fastballs (75%)
			Phase III	**Intensified Pitching**
Step 6	Warmup toss to 120' 20 throws at 120'* 20 throws at 120'* 20 throws at 120'* 20 long tosses at 120'		Step 12	25 fastballs (75%)* 20 fastballs (100%)* 10 fastballs (75%)* 15 fastballs (100%)* 25 fastballs (75%)*

Continued

TABLE 24.2	High School, College, and Professional Baseball Pitchers' Interval Throwing Program—cont'd		
Phase III	**Intensified Pitching**	**Phase III**	**Intensified Pitching**
Step 13	(Active rest) 20 throws at 80'* 20 throws at 80'* 20 throws at 80'* 20 throws at 80'*	Step 16	15 fastballs (100%) 5 off-speed pitches* 15 fastballs (100%) 3 pickoff throws to 1st* 20 fastballs (100%) 5 off-speed pitches*
Step 14	20 fastballs (75%)* 20 fastballs (100%) 5 off-speed pitches* 15 fastballs (100%) 5 off-speed pitches* Field bunts and comebacks *(Relievers and closing pitchers can go to step 21 on the next throwing day after completing this step.)*		15 fastballs (100%) 3 pickoff throws to 2nd* 15 fastballs (100%) 5 off-speed pitches*
		Step 17	(Active rest) Repeat step 14
		Step 18	20 fastballs (100%) 5 off-speed pitches* 20 fastballs (100%) 3 pickoff throws to 1st*
Step 15	20 fastballs (100%)* 15 fastballs (100%) 5 off-speed pitches 5 pickoff throws to 1st* 20 fastballs (100%) 5 off-speed pitches* 20 fastballs (100%) 5 off-speed pitches*		20 fastballs (100%) 3 pickoff throws to 2nd* 15 fastballs (100%) 5 off-speed pitches* 15 fastballs (100%) 5 off-speed pitches*
		Step 19	Batting practice 110–120 pitches Field bunts and comebacks
		Step 20	Simulated game

*Rest 6 minutes after these sets.

TABLE 24.3	Softball Pitcher's Program	
PHASE 1: EARLY THROWING All throws are to tolerance to a maximum of 50% effort All long tosses begin with a crow-hop		**PHASE II: INITIATION OF PITCHING** All pitches are fastballs (no off-speed pitches) All pitches to tolerance or maximum effort level specified All long tosses begin with a crow-hop
Step 1	Warmup toss to 30 ft (9.14 m) 10 throws @ 30 ft (9.14 m) Rest 8 min 10 throws @ 30 ft (9.14 m) 10 long tosses to 40 ft (12.19 m)	Step 7	Warmup toss to 120 ft (36.58 m) 10 throws @ 60 ft (18.29 m) (75%) 10 throws @ 20 ft (6.10 m) (50%) Rest 8 min 10 throws @ 60 ft (18.29 m) (75%) 5 pitches @ 20 ft (6.10 m) (50%) 10 long tosses to 120 ft (36.58 m)
Step 2	Warmup toss to 45 ft (13.72 m) 10 throws @ 45 ft (13.72 m) Rest 8 min 10 throws @ 45 ft (13.72 m) 10 long tosses to 60 ft (18.29 m)	Step 8	Warmup toss to 120 ft (36.58 m) 10 throws @ 60 ft (18.29 m) (75%) 10 pitches @ 35 ft (10.67 m) (50%) Rest 8 min 10 throws @ 60 ft (18.29 m) (75%) 10 pitches @ 35 ft (10.67 m) (50%) 10 long tosses to 120 ft (36.58 m)
Step 3	Warmup toss to 60 ft (18.29 m) 10 throws @ 60 ft (18.29 m) Rest 8 min 10 throws @ 60 ft (18.29) 10 long tosses to 75 ft (22.86 m)	Step 9	Warmup toss to 120 ft (36.58 m) 10 throws @ 60 ft (18.29 m) (75%) 10 pitches @ 46 ft (14.02 m) (50%) Rest 8 min 10 throws @ 60 ft (18.29 m) (75%) 10 pitches @ 46 ft (14.02 m) (50%) 15 long tosses to 120 ft (36.58 m)
Step 4	Warmup toss to 75 ft (22.86 m) 10 throws @ 75 ft (22.86 m) Rest 8 min 10 throws @ 75 ft (22.86 m) 10 long tosses to 90 ft (27.43 m)		
Step 5	Warmup toss to 90 ft (27.43 m) 10 throws @ 90 ft (27.43 m) Rest 8 min 10 throws @ 90 ft (27.43 m) 10 long tosses to 105 ft (32.00 m)		
Step 6	Warmup toss to 105 feet (32.00 m) 10 throws @ 105 ft (32.00 m) Rest 8 min 10 throws @ 105 ft (32.00) 10 long tosses to 120 ft (36.58 m)		

TABLE 24.3	**Softball Pitcher's Program—cont'd**		
Step 10	Warmup toss to 120 ft (36.58 m) 10 throws @ 60 ft (18.29 m) (75%) 10 pitches @ 46 ft (14.02 m) (50%) Rest 8 min 10 pitches @ 46 ft (14.02 m) (50%) Rest 8 min 10 throws @ 60 ft (18.29 m) (75%) 10 pitches @ 46 ft (14.02 m) (50%) 15 long tosses to 120 ft (36.58 m)	Step 16	1 throw to each base (100%) 15 pitches (100%)* 20 pitches (75%)* 15 pitches (100%)* 20 pitches (75%)* 1 throw to each base (75%) 20 pitches (75%)*

PHASE III: INTENSIFIED PITCHING

Pitch sets 11–15 consist of 1 fastball to 1 off-speed pitch at the effort level specified

Pitch sets 16–21 consist of a percentage of pitches that match the preinjury pitch mix specific to the athlete at the effort level specified

Begin each step with warmup toss to 120 ft (36.58 m)

End each step with 20 long tosses to 120 ft (36.58 m)

Step 11	2 throws to each base (75%) 15 pitches (50%)* 15 pitches (50%)* 1 throw to each base (75%) 15 pitches (50%)*	Step 17	1 throw to each base (100%) 15 pitches (100%)* 20 pitches (75%)* 15 pitches (100%)* 15 pitches (100%)* 20 pitches (75%)* 1 throw to each base (75%) 15 pitches (75%)*
Step 12	2 throws to each base (75%) 15 pitches (50%)* 15 pitches (50%)* 15 pitches (50%)* 1 throw to each base (75%) 15 pitches (50%)*	Step 18	1 throw to each base (100%) 20 pitches (100%)* 15 pitches (100%)* 20 pitches (100%)* 15 pitches (100%)* 20 pitches (100%)* 1 throw to each base (100%) 15 pitches (100%)*
Step 13	2 throws to each base (75%) 15 pitches (50%)* 15 pitches (75%)* 15 pitches (75%)* 1 throw to each base (75%) 15 pitches (50%)*	Step 19	1 throw to each base (100%) 20 pitches (100%)* 15 pitches (100%)* 20 pitches (100%)* 15 pitches (100%)* 20 pitches (100%)* 15 pitches (100%)* 1 throw to each base (100%) 15 pitches (100%)*
Step 14	2 throws to each base (75%) 15 pitches (50%)* 15 pitches (75%)* 15 pitches (75%)* 20 pitches (50%)* 1 throw to each base (75%) 15 pitches (50%)*	Step 20	Batting practice 100–120 pitches 1 throw to each base per 25 pitches
Step 15	2 throws to each base (100%) 15 pitches (75%)* 15 pitches (75%)* 15 pitches (75%)* 15 pitches (75%)* 1 throw to each base (75%) 15 pitches (75%)*	Step 21	Simulated game 7 innings 18–20 pitches/inning 8-min rest between innings Preinjury pitch mix

TABLE 24.4	**Off-Season Program**			
ACTIVE REST AND RECOVERY				
Maintain or establish range of motion and posterior capsule flexibility	Cross-body stretch	Thumb up the back internal rotation stretch	Sleeper stretch Sleeper hang Supine posterior capsule stretch with trunk rotation	Supine passive range of motion into ER with glenohumeral stabilization
Rotator cuff and scapular strengthening and endurance program	Early cocking Scaption	Late cocking Push-up plus Tubing diagonal exercise Side-lying external rotation (ER) Prone shoulder extension with ER	Acceleration Tubing velocity	Deceleration Prone shoulder horizontal abduction and ER at 100 and 135 degrees of abduction
BIOMECHANICAL ANALYSIS				
Interval throwing programs	Long toss program		Position-specific program	

REHABILITATION PROTOCOL 24.2 ▪ **Following an Arthroscopic Anterior Surgical Stabilization Procedure**

Phase I: Weeks 0–4

Goals

- Protect healing structures.

Pain Control

- Understand management after surgical manipulation of subscapularis.
- Emphasis on assisted ROM and isometric exercises
- Gradual progress of forward flexion to 140 degrees
- 40 degrees of external rotation with arm at the side

Restrictions

- Avoid early aggressive joint mobilization and any form of ROM.
- No internal rotation strengthening for open stabilization group with removal and subsequent repair of subscapularis insertion before 6 weeks

Immobilization

- Sling immobilization: 2 to 4 weeks duration—during day and especially at night. Wean off at 2 weeks, as tolerated.

Shoulder Motion

- Restoration of ROM is the first goal of rehabilitation after surgery.
- 140 degrees of forward flexion
- 40 degrees of external rotation initially with arm at the side
- After 10 days, can progress to 40 degrees of external rotation with the arm in increasing amounts of abduction, up to 45 degrees of abduction
- If takedown of the subscapularis insertion, then restricted from active internal rotation for 4 to 6 weeks
- Avoid provocative maneuvers that recreate position of instability (e.g., abduction–external rotation).

Pain Control

- Refer to outline in phase I of Rehabilitation Protocol 24.1.

Exercises

Shoulder ROM

- After 10 days, can progress to external rotation with the arm abducted—up to 45 degrees of abduction
- No active internal rotation for patients following an open stabilization procedure with removal and subsequent repair of the subscapularis insertion for 4 to 6 weeks
- Passive ROM exercises
- Passive internal rotation to stomach for those patients restricted from active internal rotation
- Motion: Elbow
  - Passive—progress to active
  - 0–130 degrees of flexion
  - Pronation and supination as tolerated

Muscle Strengthening

- Facilitate scapulohumeral rhythm (Fig. 24.33).
- Rotator cuff strengthening (Figs. 24.21 through 24.24)
- Internal rotation (No internal rotation strengthening for open stabilization group with removal and subsequent repair of subscapularis insertion before 6 weeks)

Phase II: Weeks 4–8

Criteria for Progression to Phase II

- Minimal pain and discomfort with active ROM and closed chain strengthening exercises
- No sensation or findings of instability with previously mentioned exercises

Goals

- Continue to protect healing structures.
- Attain full ROM by week 8 except combined ABER in 90 degrees

Restrictions

- Shoulder motion: early active ROM
- 160 degrees of forward flexion
- 60 degrees of external rotation
- 70 degrees of abduction
- Avoid provocative maneuvers that recreate position of instability.
- Abduction–external rotation
- *Note*: For overhead athletes, the restrictions are less. Although there is a higher risk of recurrent instability, the need for full motion to perform overhead sports requires that most athletes regain motion to within 10 degrees of normal for the affected shoulder by 6 to 8 weeks after surgery.

Immobilization

- Sling—discontinue

Pain Control

- Refer to outline in phase I of Rehabilitation Protocol 24.1.

Shoulder Motion

- 160 degrees of forward flexion
- 50 degrees of external rotation
- 70 degrees of abduction

Exercises

- Exercises performed with the elbow flexed to 90 degrees
- Starting position is with the shoulder in the neutral position of 0 degrees of forward flexion, abduction, and external rotation.
- Exercises are performed through an arc of at least 45 degrees in each of the five planes of motion—within the guidelines of allowed motion.
  - Six color-coded bands are available; each provides increasing resistance from 1 to 6 pounds, at increments of 1 pound.
  - Progression to the next band occurs usually in 2- to 3-week intervals. Patients are instructed not to progress to the next band if there is any discomfort at the present level.
  - *Note*: For overhead athletes, the motion goals should be within 10 degrees of normal for the affected shoulder.
  - Rotator cuff (Figs. 24.21 through 24.24) and scapular stabilizers strengthening (Figs. 24.14 through 24.16 and 24.25) and Theraband exercises

Phase III: Weeks 8–12

Criteria for Progression to Phase III

- Minimal pain or discomfort with active ROM and muscle strengthening exercises
- Improved strength of rotator cuff and scapular stabilizers
- No sensation or findings of instability with previously mentioned exercises

Goals

- Improve shoulder strength, power, and endurance.
- Improve neuromuscular control and shoulder proprioception (PNF).
- Restore full shoulder motion.
- Obtain full ABER 90 degrees by week 12.
- Restore proper scapulohumeral rhythm and eliminate faulty arthrokinematics.
- Establish a home exercise maintenance program that is performed at least three times per week for both stretching and strengthening.

REHABILITATION PROTOCOL 24.2 ▪ Following an Arthroscopic Anterior Surgical Stabilization Procedure—cont'd

Pain Control

- Refer to outline in phase I of Rehabilitation Protocol 24.1.

Exercises

- Proprioceptive training: PNF patterns
- Shoulder ROM
- Active-assisted ROM exercises
- Active ROM exercises
- Passive ROM exercises
- Capsular stretching (especially posterior capsule)
- Facilitate scapulohumeral rhythm.

Muscle Strengthening

- Scapular stabilizer strengthening (Figs. 24.14 through 24.16 and 24.25)
- Rotator cuff strengthening—three times per week, 8 to 12 repetitions for three sets
- Continue with closed chain strengthening (Figs. 24.17 and 24.27).
- Continue with advancing Theraband strengthening (Figs. 24.21 through 24.24).

- Progress to light isotonic dumbbell exercises.
- Progress to open chain strengthening.

Upper Extremity Endurance Training

- Incorporated endurance training for the upper extremity
- Upper body ergometer

Functional Strengthening

- Plyometric exercises (Fig. 24.36)
- Progressive, systematic interval program for returning to sports: same as Rehabilitation Protocol 24.1
- Maximum improvement is expected by 12 months; most patients can return to sports and full-duty work status by 6 months.
- Terminal testing demonstrating resolution of apprehension testing (Fig. 24.31).

Warning Signs

- Refer to outline in phase V of Rehabilitation Protocol 24.1.

Treatment of Complications

- Refer to outline in phase V of Rehabilitation Protocol 24.1.

REHABILITATION PROTOCOL 24.3 ▪ Postoperative Rehabilitation After Open (Bankart) Anterior Capsulolabral Reconstruction

Phase I: Weeks 0–4

Goals

- Protect healing structures.
- Reduce pain and edema.
- Avoid early "overly aggressive" PROM, AROM, and joint mobilization.
- Understand how the subscapularis was managed during the repair.
- Minimize effects of immobilization.

Restrictions

- 140 degrees forward flexion
- 45 degrees external rotation (ER) in neutral position

Immobilization

- Sling immobilization: 0 to 4 weeks duration—during day and especially at night. Wean at week 2 as tolerated but should be worn during sleep for minimum of 2 weeks.

Pain Control

- Refer to outline in phase I of Rehabilitation Protocol 24.1.

Exercises

- Elbow, hand, wrist, and grip ROM (progress from PROM to AAROM to AROM)
- Elbow ROM
  - 0 to 130 degrees
  - Pronation–supination
- Shoulder ROM
  - Passive internal rotation to stomach only (**No active internal rotation** strengthening for open stabilization group with removal and subsequent repair of subscapularis insertion before 4 to 6 weeks)
  - PROM to AAROM flexion

- to 90 degrees week 1
- to 100 degrees week 2
- to 120 degrees week 3
- to 140 degrees by week 4
- ER at 45 degrees of abduction in scapular plane:
  - 15 degrees week 1 to 2
  - 30 to 45 degrees week 3
  - 45 to 60 degrees week 4
- Proprioceptive neuromuscular facilitation (PNF) (Figs. 24.19 and 24.20)
  - Begin early rhythmic stabilization.
  - Progress from arm at side to available flexion, ER positions
  - Facilitate scapular stabilizers.

Strength

- Submaximal isometrics in neutral
- Begin light Theraband resistance ER (in neutral to allowable ROM), scapular rows, and scapular depression week 3
- PROM forward flexion, scaption (full can) minimal resistance to 90 degrees
- Begin protraction closed chain.
- Prone scapular stabilizer strengthening (Fig. 24.16)
- Side-lying external rotation not >45 degrees

Phase II: Weeks 4–8

Criteria for Progression to Phase II

- Minimal pain and discomfort with active ROM and closed chain strengthening exercises
- No sensation or findings of instability with aforementioned exercises

Goals

- Continue to protect healing structures.
- Discontinue immobilization.

Continued

REHABILITATION PROTOCOL 24.3 ■ Postoperative Rehabilitation After Open (Bankart) Anterior Capsulolabral Reconstruction—cont'd

- Facilitate full PROM in all planes (full external rotation by 8 weeks).
- Normalize arthrokinematics and scapulohumeral rhythm.

Pain Control

- Refer to outline in phase I of Rehabilitation Protocol 24.1.

Restrictions

- Avoid maneuvers that recreate position of instability.
- No forceful combined abduction–external rotation
- No active internal rotation for patients following an open stabilization procedure with removal and subsequent repair of the subscapularis insertion for 4 to 6 weeks
- Immobilization
- Sling—discontinue

Exercises

- ROM
  - Flexion to 160 degrees
  - External rotation/internal rotation (ER/IR) at 90 degrees of abduction; IR to 75 degrees; ER to 75 degrees by week 6 and 90 degrees by week 8
  - PROM into combined motions, progress scaption to abduction plane
  - Rotator cuff and scapular stabilizers strengthening and Theraband exercises (no resisted IR until week 6) (Figs. 24.21 through 24.24, 24.17 and 24.18)
- Strength
- Initiate IR strength (PNF, light Therabands) at week 6.
  - Progress all strength (Therabands) of rotator cuff, deltoid, biceps, and scapular muscles (Figs. 24.14 through 24.18, 24.21, 24.24, and 24.25)
  - Closed chain (wall push-ups)
  - Dynamic stabilization exercises
  - Start light weights in open chain for deltoid, biceps, and ER side-lying.
  - Progress closed chain weight bearing (isometric and push-up position) (Figs. 24.26).
  - PNF diagonal patterns

Phase III: Weeks 8–12

Criteria for Progression to Phase III

- Minimal pain or discomfort with strengthening through full ROM

Goals

- Improve neuromuscular control and shoulder proprioception (PNF).
- Restore full combined AB/ER.
- Orient for sport-specific functional training.

Restrictions

- No throwing

Exercises

- ROM
  - Combined AB/EF passive "doorway" stretch
  - Combined AB/IR passive "doorway" stretch
- Joint mobilization
  - Posterior–inferior glenohumeral (GH) mobilization
  - Anterior GH mobilization as needed after week 10
  - Capsular stretching (especially posterior capsule)
  - Scapular mobilization
  - Facilitate scapulohumeral rhythm (Fig. 24.33).

Muscle Strengthening

- Light isotonic dumbbell exercises
- Rotator cuff strengthening—exchange Therabands with weights
- "Thrower's 10" for overhead athletes
- Begin push-up progression starting week 10.
- Lat pulls to front
- Body blade in neutral
- Begin agility drills.

Endurance Training

- Upper body ergometer and cardiac endurance

Phase IV: Weeks 12–16

Goals

- Optimize throwing mechanics and overhead function.

Restrictions

- No full throwing

Exercises

- ROM
- "Sleeper stretch" if limited IR or posterior capsule restrictions
- Functional strengthening: Plyometric exercises
- Progress Body Blade to 45 to 90 degrees of abduction (Figs. 24.28 through 24.30).
- Two-handed plyometrics (chest pass)
- Progress plyometrics to one handed (dribble).
- Begin one-handed toss (NO overhead throw).

Phase V: Weeks 16–20

Goal

- Restore overhead/serve/swing/throw by week 20.

Exercises

ROM
- Continue flexibility and full ROM exercises.
- Strength
  - Start throwing progression.
  - Plyometrics/rebounder
  - Swimming
  - Full push-ups
  - Sports-specific training
  - Progress overhead/serve/swing/throw by week 20.

REHABILITATION PROTOCOL 24.4 ● Arthroscopic Anterior Shoulder Instability Protocol

Phase I: Weeks 0–2

Goals

- Pain-free passive range of motion to limits mentioned in the following sections

Restrictions

- Ultra sling to be warn at all times for 4 to 6 weeks
- NO active biceps for 2 weeks
- Limit ER to 30 degrees, passive flexion to 90 to 120 degrees, and abduction to 45 degrees.

Exercises

- Aerobic
- Stationary bike for 30 minutes
- Easy walking on level surface for 30 minutes
- Strength
- Wrist and gripping exercises

Range of Motion

- Passive forward flexion to 120 degrees
- Passive motion in scapular plane to 120 degrees
- Passive external rotation to 30 degrees at side
- Passive abduction to 90 degrees
- Active wrist and elbow range of motion
- Passive ROM for 4 weeks

Modalities

- IFC and ice for 20 minutes

Phase II: Weeks 2–4

Goals

- Passive ROM to aforementioned limits and AAROM

Restrictions

- Limit ER to 45 and to 100 degrees and flexion to 150 degrees.
- Avoid anterior scapular stress.

Exercises

- Aerobic
- Progress passive ER to 45 degrees.
- Strength
- Start gentle isometric exercises for extension, ER, IR, and abduction.
- Start scapula proprioceptive neuromuscular facilitation.
- Same aerobic as mentioned earlier; progress to 45 to 60 minutes

Range of Motion

- Progress passive forward flexion 150 degrees, scapular 150 degrees, and abduction 100 degrees

Phase III: Weeks 4–6

Goals

- ROM in all planes

Restrictions

- Limit ER to 45 degrees, abduction to 160 degrees, and flexion to 160 degrees.

Exercises

- Aerobic
- Start treadmill.
- Strength
- Start rotator cuff in scapula plane to include internal and external rotation at low angles.

- Deltoid isometrics
- Shoulder pinches/shoulder shrugs
- PNF (Figs. 24.19 and 24.20)

ROM

- Passive ROM forward flexion to 160 degrees, scapular plane to 160 degrees, abduction to 140 degrees, and ER to 45 degrees (at side)

Phase IV: Weeks 6–12

Goals

- Progress to active ROM.
- Normal scapulothoracic motion
- Discontinue ultra sling.

Exercises

- Aerobic
- Elliptical
- Incline treadmill
- PNF (Figs. 24.19 and 24.20)
- UBE
- Strength and endurance
- Start progressive resisted Theraband exercises in various planes.
- Start Body Blade at neutral position (Fig. 24.28).

ROM

- Start active-assisted ROM (AAROM) to active ROM (AROM).
- Work on more abduction ER and abduction IR.

Phase V: Weeks 12–16

Goals

- Restore strength.

Exercise

- Aerobic: Using any of the climber machines (e.g., Versaclimber, Stairmaster)
- Strength
- Diagonal rotator cuff exercises
- External and internal rotation at 90 degrees with cable
- Push-up progression
- Plyometric exercises
- Progress Body Blade (forward flexion to 90 degrees, abduction to 90 degrees diagonal) (Figs. 24.28 through 24.30 and 24.32).

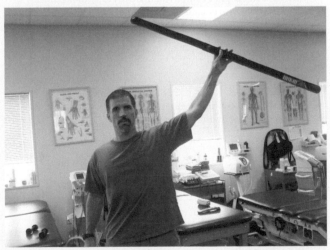

Fig. 24.32 Agility drill with Body Blade in 145 degrees of scaption.

REHABILITATION PROTOCOL 24.4 ■ Arthroscopic Anterior Shoulder Instability Protocol—cont'd

ROM

- Joint mobility grade 3 or 4

Phase VI: >16 Weeks

Goals

- Ability to perform push-ups, pull-ups, and swim

Exercises

- Aerobic
- Rowing
- May start swimming
- Strength
- Start throwing progression (short to long).
- Military press
- Lat pull-downs

REHABILITATION PROTOCOL 24.5 ■ Nonoperative Posterior Instability Protocol

Phase I: Weeks 0–2

Goal

- Control pain and reduce edema.
- Passive shoulder ROM

Precautions/Restrictions

- Flexion 90 degrees
- Abduction 60 degrees
- IR/ER 0 degrees
- NO INTERNAL ROTATION FOR 6 WEEKS
- Ultra sling at all times in neutral rotation (including sleep)

Pain Control

- Per phase I of Rehabilitation Protocol 24.1

Exercises

- Stationary bike
- Walking on level surface
- Hand gripping exercises, active wrist flexion/extension ROM
- Codman's/pendulums PASSIVE only
- PROM elbow and hand
- PROM shoulder within precautions
- PROM scapula

Modalities

- IFC stimulation for pain PRN
- Cryotherapy as needed for pain and edema reduction
- Hi-Volt stimulation for edema control

Phase II: Weeks 3–4

Goals

- Increase ROM per below, avoiding positions of instability.
- Continue to control pain.

Precautions

- Flexion 90 degrees
- Abduction 60 degrees
- ER 30 degrees
- NO INTERNAL ROTATION FOR 6 WEEKS
- Ultra sling at all times in neutral rotation (including sleep)
- Avoid posterior capsular stress by avoiding active ER or passive IR.

Exercises

- NO PULLEYS!
- Table slides abduction/flexion
- Scapular clocks
- Wrist flexion/extension
- PROM elbow flexion/extension/supination/pronation
- PROM shoulder within precautions
- PROM scapula

Modalities

- IFC stimulation for pain PRN
- Cryotherapy as needed for pain and edema reduction
- Hi-Volt stimulation for edema control

Phase III: Weeks 5–6

Goals

- Progress to AAROMs.
- Isometric exercises

Precautions

- Flexion 90 degrees
- Abduction 60 degrees
- IR neutral
- Discontinue sling until 5 weeks unless otherwise recommended by MD.

Exercises

- Table slides
- Isometrics for flexion/abduction/extension at less than 30 degrees of abduction
- AAROM flexion/abduction and progress to AROM, wall walks, and standing two way
- Scaption squeezes, foam roll squeezes no resistance
- PROM within precautions
- Scapula PROM/mobilization
- PNF (Figs. 24.19 and 24.20)

Modalities

- Cryotherapy following physical therapy or athletic training session
- Ice after PT session and REP.

Phase IVa: Weeks 7–9

Goals

- May progress PROM to full within pain limits

Precautions

- Avoid end-range resistance.

Exercises

- UBE
- Pulleys (only if full ROM not achieved)
- Ball on wall
- Prone two way
- Standing two way
- Prone row
- Side-lying ER with resistance as tolerated
- Scapular squeeze with resistance
- Bilateral (B) ER with Theraband (TB). Glenohumeral Joint (GHJ) propriceptive Neuromuscular Facilitation (PNF) D1/D2 (Diagonal 1/Diagonal 2)

REHABILITATION PROTOCOL 24.5 ■ Nonoperative Posterior Instability Protocol—cont'd

- Begin Thrower's 10 program: minimal resistance, ER/IR at neutral, and progressing to 45 degrees abduction by week 10.
- Abduction/scaption with IR limited to 30 degrees of abduction, elbow/bicep flexion, triceps extension
- Seated cable row
- Manual PROM to full flexion/abduction and ER/IR at 45 degrees abduction, GH mobs inferior and posterior capsule
- Pectoral stretching/lat stretching

Modalities

- Cryotherapy following physical therapy or athletic training session

Phase IVb: Weeks 10–12

Goals

- Increased scapular stabilizer and rotator cuff strength
- Restore full AROM.

Restrictions

- Avoid aggressive IR strengthening.
- Close observation for joint hypomobility and loss of end-range flexion, IR

Exercises

- As per phase IV weeks 7 to 9 but may progress ER/IR resistance to 90 degrees of abduction
- Cardio: may begin running on treadmill and elliptical machine
- May begin push-up progression

- Lat pull-downs in front of body
- Joint mobilization and low load prolonged duration capsular stretch PRN to restore pain-free full AROM

Modalities

- Ice after PT session.

Phase V: Weeks 13–16

Goals and Precautions

- Initiate sports-specific training exercises.

Exercises

- Thrower's 10: progress resistance as tolerated
- Begin plyometics: shot toss and progress to shot throw and overhead toss.
- Dynamic wall push-ups
- Progress push-ups to floor as tolerated.
- Rhythmic stabilization in quadruped
- Sport-specific training exercises as tolerated (no full throwing until 16 weeks)
- Phase VI: Weeks 16–20
- Exercises
- Sport-specific training
- Gentle overhead motions and may progress to full overhead serve/swing/throw at 20 weeks

REHABILITATION PROTOCOL 24.6 ■ Arthroscopic Posterior Instability Rehabilitation Protocol

Phase I: Weeks 0–2

Goals

- Pain control
- Passive ROM of shoulder, elbow, and wrist

Restrictions

- Flexion 90 degrees
- Abduction 60 degrees
- IR/ER 0 degrees
- NO INTERNAL ROTATION FOR 6 WEEKS
- Ultra sling at all times in neutral rotation (including sleep)

Pain Control

- Per phase I Rehabilitation Protocol 24.1

Exercises

- Stationary bike
- Walking on level surface
- Hand gripping exercises, active wrist flexion/extension ROM
- PROM elbow and hand
- PROM shoulder within precautions
- PROM scapula

Modalities

- IFC stimulation for pain PRN
- Ice 10 minutes every hour as necessary.
- Hi-Volt stimulation for edema control

Phase II: Weeks 3–4

Goals

- ROM exercises
- PNF
- Scapular stabilizing

Restrictions

- Flexion 90 degrees
- Abduction 60 degrees
- ER 30 degrees
- NO INTERNAL ROTATION
- Ultra sling at all times (including sleep)
- Avoid posterior capsule stretch by avoiding active ER or passive IR.

Exercises

- NO PULLEYS!
- Table slides abduction/flexion
- Scapular stabilization (Figs. 24.14 through 24.16 and 24.25)
- Wrist flexion/extension
- PROM elbow (flexion/extension/supination/pronation)
- PROM shoulder within precautions
- PROM scapula

Modalities

- IFC stimulator for pain PRN
- Ice 10 minutes every hour as necessary.
- Hi-Volt stimulator for edema control

Phase III: Weeks 5–6

Goals

- Progress to AROM.

Precautions

- Flexion 90 degrees
- Abduction 60 degrees
- IR neutral
- Discontinue sling until 5 weeks unless otherwise recommended by MD.

Continued

REHABILITATION PROTOCOL 24.6 ▪ **Arthroscopic Posterior Instability Rehabilitation Protocol—cont'd**

Exercises

- NO PULLEYS!
- Table slides
- Isometrics for flexion/abduction/extension at less than 30 degrees abduction
- AAROM flexion/abduction and progress to AROM, wall walks, and standing two way
- Scapular squeezes, foam roll squeezes, no resistance
- PROM within precautions
- Scapular PROM/mobs
- PNF (Figs. 24.19 and 24.20)

Modalities

- IFC PRN for pain
- Ice after PT session and HEP.

Phase IVa: Weeks 7–9

Goals

- May progress PROM to full within pain limits

Precautions

- Avoid end-range resistance.

Exercises

- UBE
- Pulleys (only if full ROM not achieved)
- Ball on wall
- Prone two way
- Standing two way
- Prone row
- Side-lying ER with resistance as tolerated
- Scaption squeeze with resistance
- Begin Thrower's 10 program: PNF D1/D2, ER/IR at neutral and progress to 45 degrees abduction/scaption with IR limited to 30 degrees abduction, seated press-ups, elbow/bicep flexion, triceps extension.
- Seated cable row
- Manual PROM to full flexion/abduction and ER/IR at 45 degrees abduction GH mobs inferior and posterior capsule
- Pectoral stretching/lat stretching

Modalities

- Heat with UBE for warmup.
- Ice after PT session.

Phase IVb: Weeks 10–12

Precautions

- Progress to full AROM/PROM/RROM.

Exercises

- As per phase IV weeks 7 to 9 but may progress ER/IR resistance to 90 degrees of abduction
- Cardio: may begin running on treadmill and elliptical machine
- May begin push-up progression
- Lat pull-downs in front of body
- PNF

Modalities

- Heat with UBE for warmup
- Ice after PT session.

Phase V: Weeks 13–16

Precautions

- None

Exercises

- Thrower's 10: progress resistance as tolerated
- Begin plyometics: shot toss and progress to shot throw and overhead toss.
- Dynamic wall push-ups
- Progress push-ups to floor as tolerated.
- Rhythmic stabilization in quadruped
- Sport-specific training exercises as tolerated (no full throwing until 16 weeks)
- Manual capsular mobs for full mobility

Phase VI: Weeks 16–20

Exercises

- Sport-specific training
- Gentle overhead motions and may progress to full overhead serve/swing/throw at 20 weeks

---

REHABILITATION PROTOCOL 24.7 ▪ **After Posterior Shoulder Stabilization**

Phase I: Weeks 0–4

Goals

- Pain control and immobilization

Restrictions

- No shoulder motion
- No IR for 6 weeks
- Immobilization
- Use of a gunslinger orthosis for 4 weeks

Pain Control

- Refer to outline in phase I of Rehabilitation Protocol 24.1.

Exercises

- ROM
  - Shoulder: none.
  - Elbow:
    - Passive—progress to active
    - 0 to 130 degrees of flexion
    - Pronation and supination as tolerated
- Muscle strengthening
  - Grip strengthening only

Phase II: Weeks 4–8

Criteria for Progression to Phase II

- Adequate immobilization

Restrictions

- Shoulder motion: active ROM
- Forward flexion 120 degrees
- Abduction 45 degrees
- External rotation as tolerated
- Internal rotation and adduction to stomach
- Avoid offensive maneuvers that recreate position of instability.
- Avoid excessive internal rotation.

Immobilization

- Gunslinger—discontinue

REHABILITATION PROTOCOL 24.7 ■ After Posterior Shoulder Stabilization—cont'd

Pain Control

- Refer to outline in phase I of Rehabilitation Protocol 24.1.

Exercises

- ROM
- Shoulder: passive and AAROM only:
  - Forward flexion 120 degrees
  - Abduction 45 degrees
  - External rotation as tolerated
  - Internal rotation and adduction to stomach
- RC exercises per phase II of Rehabilitation Protocol 24.1
- PNF (Figs. 24.19 and 24.20)
- Muscle strengthening
  - Closed chain strengthening exercises (Figs. 24.27 and 24.17)

Phase III: Weeks 8–12

Criteria for Progression to Phase III

- Minimal pain and discomfort with AAROM and closed chain strengthening exercises
- No sensation or findings of instability with aforementioned exercises

Goals

- 160 degrees of forward flexion
- Full external rotation
- 70 degrees of abduction
- Internal rotation and adduction to stomach

Restrictions

- Shoulder motion: active and active-assisted motion exercises
- 160 degrees of forward flexion
- Full external rotation
- 70 degrees of abduction
- Internal rotation and adduction to stomach

Pain Control

- Refer to outline in phase I of Rehabilitation Protocol 24.1.

Exercises

- Progress to active ROM exercises.

Muscle Strengthening

- Rotator cuff strengthening three times per week, 8 to 12 repetitions for three sets per phase II of Rehabilitation Protocol 24.1 (Figs. 24.21 through 24.24)
- Progress to light isotonic dumbbell exercises.
- Internal rotation
- External rotation
- Abduction
- Forward flexion
- Strengthening of scapular stabilizers (Figs. 24.14 through 24.16 and 24.25)
- Continue with closed chain strengthening exercises (Figs. 24.27 and 24.17).
- Advance to open chain isotonic strengthening exercises.
- Joint mobilization to facilitate:
  - End-range ROM and pain-free end-range IR by week 12
  - Restore GHS kinematics.
  - Scapulohumeral rhythm (Fig. 24.33)

Phase IV: Months 3–6

Criteria for Progression to Phase IV

- Minimal pain or discomfort with active ROM and muscle strengthening exercises

- Improvement in strengthening of rotator cuff and scapular stabilizers
- Satisfactory physical examination

Goals

- Improve shoulder strength, power, and endurance.
- Improve neuromuscular control and shoulder proprioception.
- Restore full shoulder motion.
- Establish a home exercise maintenance program that is performed at least three times per week for both stretching and strengthening.

Pain Control

- Refer to outline in phase I of Rehabilitation Protocol 24.1.
- Subacromial injection: corticosteroid/local anesthetic combination for patients with findings consistent with secondary impingement
- GH joint: corticosteroid/local anesthetic combination for patients whose clinical findings are consistent with GH joint pathology

Exercises

- ROM

Goals

- Obtain motion that is equal to contralateral side.
- Active ROM exercises
- Active-assisted ROM exercises
- Passive ROM exercises
- Capsular stretching (especially posterior capsule) (Fig. 24.34)
- Muscle strengthening
- Rotator cuff and scapular stabilizer strengthening as outlined earlier (Figs. 24.21 through 24.24)
- Three times per week, 8 to 12 repetitions for three sets

Upper Extremity Endurance Training

- Incorporated endurance training for the upper extremity
- Upper body ergometer

Proprioceptive Training

- PNF patterns (Figs. 24.19, 24.33 and 24.35)

Functional Strengthening

- Plyometric exercises (Fig. 24.36)

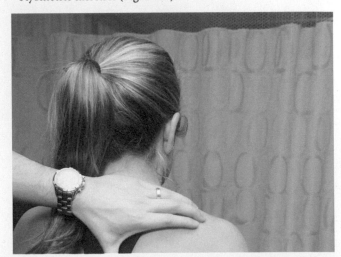

Fig. 24.33 Facilitate scapulohumeral rhythm. Therapist or athletic trainer will manually facilitate proper glenohumeral-to-scapular movement ratio.

Continued

REHABILITATION PROTOCOL 24.7 ● **After Posterior Shoulder Stabilization—cont'd**

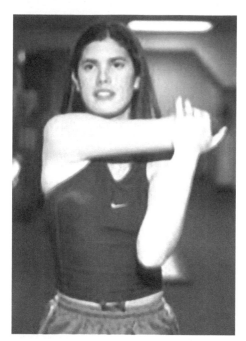

Fig. 24.34 Stretching of the posterior capsule.

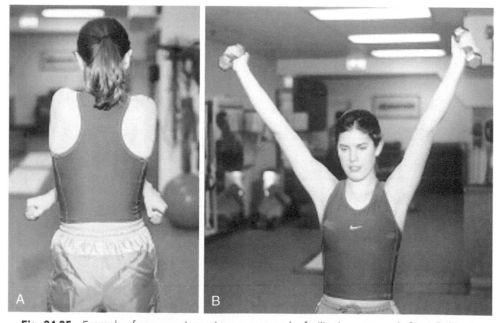

Fig. 24.35 Example of one proprioceptive neuromuscular facilitation pattern. **A,** Start. **B,** Finish.

REHABILITATION PROTOCOL 24.7 ● After Posterior Shoulder Stabilization—cont'd

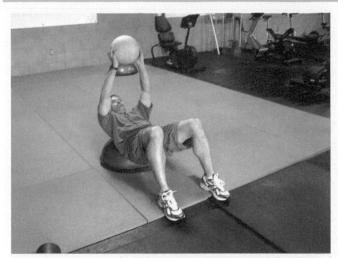

Fig. 24.36 Plyometric ball toss: lying supine, two-hand chest toss with "plyo" or weighted ball. Progress to unstable surface to increase level of difficulty. For example, lying on Bosu Ball as above.

Progressive, Systematic Interval Program for Returning to Sports
- Maximum improvement is expected by 12 months.

Warning Signs
- Refer to outline in phase V of Rehabilitation Protocol 24.1.

Treatment of Complications
- Refer to outline in phase V of Rehabilitation Protocol 24.1.

REHABILITATION PROTOCOL 24.8 ● After Open Inferior Capsular Shift for Multidirectional Instability

Phase I: Weeks 0–6

Goals
- Pain control
- PROM

Restriction
- Shoulder motion: none for 6 weeks

Immobilization
- Sling or gunslinger orthosis
- 6 weeks—during day and at night

Pain Control
- Refer to outline in phase I of Rehabilitation Protocol 24.1.

Motion: Shoulder
- None

Motion: Elbow
- Passive—progress to active
- 0 to 130 degrees of flexion
- Pronation and supination as tolerated

Muscle Strengthening
- Rotator cuff and scapular stabilizing exercises (Figs. 24.15, 24.16, 24.21 through 24.25)

Phase II: Weeks 7–12

Criteria for Progression to Phase II
- Minimal pain or discomfort with ROM and closed chain strengthening exercises
- No sensation or findings of instability with these maneuvers
- Satisfactory physical examination

Goal
- Rotator cuff strengthening

Restrictions
- Shoulder motion: active ROM only

- 140 degrees of forward flexion
- 40 degrees of external rotation
- 70 degrees of abduction
- Internal rotation to stomach
- Avoid positions that recreate instability.

Pain Control
- Refer to outline in phase I of Rehabilitation Protocol 24.1.
- Motion: Shoulder

Goals
- 140 degrees of forward flexion
- 40 degrees of external rotation
- 70 degrees of abduction
- Internal rotation to stomach

Exercises
- Active ROM exercises

Muscle Strengthening
- Rotator cuff strengthening three times per week, 8 to 12 repetitions for three sets as outlined in phase II and III of Rehabilitation Protocol 24.1 (Figs. 24.21 through 24.24)
- Progress to light isotonic dumbbell exercises.
- Internal rotation
- External rotation
- Abduction
- Forward flexion
- Strengthening of scapular stabilizers as outlined in phase II of Rehabilitation Protocol 24.1 (Figs. 24.14 through 24.16 and 24.25)
- Progress to open chain strengthening.

Phase III: Months 3–6

Criteria for Progression to Phase III
- Minimal pain or discomfort with active ROM and muscle strengthening exercises
- Improvement in strengthening of rotator cuff and scapular stabilizers
- Satisfactory physical examination

Continued

REHABILITATION PROTOCOL 24.7 ■ **After Posterior Shoulder Stabilization—cont'd**

Goals

- Improve shoulder complex strength, power, and endurance.
- Improve neuromuscular control and shoulder proprioception.
- Restore full shoulder motion.
- Establish a home exercise maintenance program that is performed at least three times per week for both stretching and strengthening.

Pain Control

- Refer to outline in phase I of Rehabilitation Protocol 24.1.
- Subacromial injection: corticosteroid/local anesthetic combination
- For patients with findings consistent with secondary impingement
- GH joint: corticosteroid/local anesthetic combination for patients whose clinical findings are consistent with GH joint pathology

Motion: Shoulder

Goals

- Obtain motion that is equal to contralateral side.
- Active ROM exercises
- Active-assisted ROM exercises
- Passive ROM exercises
- Capsular stretching for selective areas of shoulder to "balance" the laxity (do not aim for full ROM)

Muscle Strengthening

- Rotator cuff and scapular stabilizer strengthening as outlined earlier (Figs. 24.21 through 24.24)

- Three times per week, 8 to 12 repetitions for three sets
- Deltoid strengthening

Upper Extremity Endurance Training

- Incorporated endurance training for the upper extremity
- Upper body ergometer

Proprioceptive Training

- PNF patterns

Functional Strengthening

- Plyometric exercises (Fig. 24.36)

Progressive, Systematic Interval Program for Returning to Sports

- Refer to phase V of Rehabilitation Protocol 24.1.
- Maximum improvement is expected by 12 months.

Warning Signs

- Refer to outline in phase V of Rehabilitation Protocol 24.1.

Treatment of Complications

- Refer to outline in phase V of Rehabilitation Protocol 24.1.

REFERENCES

A complete reference list is available at https://expertconsult.inkling.com/.

FURTHER READING

Abrams JS, Savoie 3rd FH, Tauro JC, et al. Recent advances in the evaluation and treatment of shoulder instability: anterior, posterior, and multidirectional. *Arthroscopy*. 2002;18(9 Suppl 2):1–13.

Antoniou J, Harryman 2nd DT. Posterior instability. *Orthop Clin North Am*. 2001;32(3):463–473. ix.

Arciero RA, St Pierre P. Acute shoulder dislocation. Indications and techniques for operative management. *Clin Sports Med*. 1995;14(4):937–953.

Arciero RA, Spang JT. Complications in arthroscopic anterior shoulder stabilization: pearls and pitfalls. *Instr Course Lect*. 2008;57:113–124.

Arciero RA, Wheeler JH, Ryan JB, et al. Arthroscopic Bankart repair versus nonoperative treatment for acute, initial anterior shoulder dislocations. *Am J Sports Med*. 1994;22(5):589–594.

Aronen JG, Regan K. Decreasing the incidence of recurrence of first time anterior shoulder dislocations with rehabilitation. *Am J Sports Med*. 1984;12(4):283–291.

Bahu MJ, Trentacosta N, Vorys GC, et al. Multidirectional instability: evaluation and treatment options. *Clin Sports Med*. 2008;27(4):671–689.

Bedi A, Ryu RK. The treatment of primary anterior shoulder dislocations. *Instr Course Lect*. 2009;58:293–304.

Bey MJ, Hunter SA, Kilambi N, et al. Structural and mechanical properties of the glenohumeral joint posterior capsule. *J Shoulder Elbow Surg*. 2005;14(2):201–206.

Boileau P, Villalba M, Hery JY, et al. Risk factors for recurrence of shoulder instability after arthroscopic Bankart repair. *J Bone Joint Surg Am*. 2006;88(8):1755–1763.

Bottoni CR, Wilckens JH, DeBerardino TM, et al. A prospective, randomized evaluation of arthroscopic stabilization versus nonoperative treatment in patients with acute, traumatic, first-time shoulder dislocations. *Am J Sports Med*. 2002;30(4):576–580.

Bottoni CR. Anterior instability. In: Johnson DLMS, ed. *Clinical Sports Medicine*. Philadelphia: Elsevier; 2006:189–200.

Burkhead Jr WZ, Rockwood Jr CA. Treatment of instability of the shoulder with an exercise program. *J Bone Joint Surg Am*. 1992;74(6):890–896.

Cohen B, Romeo A, Bach B. Shoulder injuries. In: Bozeman S, Wilk K, eds. *Clinical Orthopaedic Rehabilitation*. Philadelphia: Mosby; 2003.

Cooper RA, Brems JJ. The inferior capsular-shift procedure for multidirectional instability of the shoulder. *J Bone Joint Surg Am*. 1992;74(10):1516–1521.

Finnoff JT, Doucette S, Hicken G. Glenohumeral instability and dislocation. *Phys Med Rehabil Clin N Am*. 2004;15(3):575–605.

Gibson K, Growse A, Korda L, et al. The effectiveness of rehabilitation for nonoperative management of shoulder instability: a systematic review. *J Hand Ther*. 2004;17(2):229–242.

Gill TJ, Zarins B. Open repairs for the treatment of anterior shoulder instability. *Am J Sports Med*. 2003;31(1):142–153.

Hovelius L, Eriksson K, Fredin H, et al. Recurrences after initial dislocation of the shoulder. Results of a prospective study of treatment. *J Bone Joint Surg Am*. 1983;65(3):343–349.

Hurley JA, Anderson TE, Dear W, et al. Posterior shoulder instability. Surgical versus conservative results with evaluation of glenoid version. *Am J Sports Med*. 1992;20(4):396–400.

Itoi E, Hatakeyama Y, Kido T, et al. A new method of immobilization after traumatic anterior dislocation of the shoulder: a preliminary study. *J Shoulder Elbow Surg*. 2003;12(5):413–415.

Itoi E, Hatakeyama Y, Urayama M, et al. Position of immobilization after dislocation of the shoulder. A cadaveric study. *J Bone Joint Surg Am*. 1999;81(3):385–390.

Itoi E, Sashi R, Minagawa H, et al. Position of immobilization after dislocation of the glenohumeral joint. A study with use of magnetic resonance imaging. *J Bone Joint Surg Am*. 2001;83-A(5):661–667.

Kim SH, Ha KI, Cho YB, et al. Arthroscopic anterior stabilization of the shoulder: two to six-year follow-up. *J Bone Joint Surg Am*. 2003;85-A(8):1511–1518.

Kirkley A, Werstine R, Ratjek A, et al. Prospective randomized clinical trial comparing the effectiveness of immediate arthroscopic stabilization versus immobilization and rehabilitation in first traumatic anterior dislocations of the shoulder: long-term evaluation. *Arthroscopy*. 2005;21(1):55–63.

Kralinger FS, Golser K, Wischatta R, et al. Predicting recurrence after primary anterior shoulder dislocation. *Am J Sports Med.* 2002;30(1):116–120.

Kroner K, Lind T, Jensen J. The epidemiology of shoulder dislocations. *Arch Orthop Trauma Surg.* 1989;108(5):288–290.

Kvitne RS, Jobe FW. The diagnosis and treatment of anterior instability in the throwing athlete. *Clin Orthop Relat Res.* 1993;(291):107–123.

Larrain MV, Botto GJ, Montenegro HJ, et al. Arthroscopic repair of acute traumatic anterior shoulder dislocation in young athletes. *Arthroscopy.* 2001;17(4):373–377.

Levine WN, Flatow EL. The pathophysiology of shoulder instability. *Am J Sports Med.* 2000;28(6):910–917.

Millett PJ, Clavert P, Hatch 3rd GF, et al. Recurrent posterior shoulder instability. *J Am Acad Orthop Surg.* 2006;14(8):464–476.

Owens BD, Duffey ML, Nelson BJ, et al. The incidence and characteristics of shoulder instability at the United States Military Academy. *Am J Sports Med.* 2007;35(7):1168–1173.

Provencher MT, Romeo AA. Posterior and multidirectional instability of the shoulder: challenges associated with diagnosis and management. *Instr Course Lect.* 2008;57:133–152.

Rowe CR, Sakellarides HT. Factors related to recurrences of anterior dislocations of the shoulder. *Clin Orthop.* 1961;20:40–48.

Simonet WT, Cofield RH. Prognosis in anterior shoulder dislocation. *Am J Sports Med.* 1984;12(1):19–24.

Stein DA, Jazrawi L, Bartolozzi AR. Arthroscopic stabilization of anterior shoulder instability: a review of the literature. *Arthroscopy.* 2002;18(8):912–924.

Tauber M, Resch H, Forstner R, et al. Reasons for failure after surgical repair of anterior shoulder instability. *J Shoulder Elbow Surg.* 2004;13(3):279–285.

Taylor DC, Arciero RA. Pathologic changes associated with shoulder dislocations. Arthroscopic and physical examination findings in first-time, traumatic anterior dislocations. *Am J Sports Med.* 1997;25(3):306–311.

Vermeiren J, Handelberg F, Casteleyn PP, et al. The rate of recurrence of traumatic anterior dislocation of the shoulder. A study of 154 cases and a review of the literature. *Int Orthop.* 1993;17(6):337–341.

Visser CP, Coene LN, Brand R, et al. The incidence of nerve injury in anterior dislocation of the shoulder and its influence on functional recovery. A prospective clinical and EMG study. *J Bone Joint Surg Br.* 1999;81(4):679–685.

Wang RY, Arciero RA, Mazzocca AD. The recognition and treatment of first-time shoulder dislocation in active individuals. *J Orthop Sports Phys Ther.* 2009;39(2):118–123.

Wolf EM, Cheng JC, Dickson K. Humeral avulsion of glenohumeral ligaments as a cause of anterior shoulder instability. *Arthroscopy.* 1995;11(5):600–607.

Wolf EM, Eakin CL. Arthroscopic capsular plication for posterior shoulder instability. *Arthroscopy.* 1998;14(2):153–163.

Yamaguchi K, Flatow EL. Management of multidirectional instability. *Clin Sports Med.* 1995;14(4):885–902.

Yiannakopoulos CK, Mataragas E, Antonogiannakis E. A comparison of the spectrum of intra-articular lesions in acute and chronic anterior shoulder instability. *Arthroscopy.* 2007;23(9):985–990.

25

Adhesive Capsulitis (Frozen Shoulder)

Christopher J. Durall, PT, DPT, MS, SCS, LAT, CSCS

INTRODUCTION

Adhesive capsulitis is an enigmatic condition characterized by painful, progressive, and disabling loss of active and passive glenohumeral joint range of motion in multiple planes. Approximately 2% to 5% of adults between age 40 and 70 develop adhesive capsulitis with a greater occurrence in women and in individuals with thyroid disease or diabetes. Adhesive capsulitis (also known as frozen shoulder) is commonly classified as "primary" if it occurs independent of other pathologies or "secondary" if it occurs after trauma or is associated with another condition. Secondary adhesive capsulitis has been further divided into systemic (e.g., associated with diabetes), extrinsic to the GH joint (e.g., associated with a midhumeral fracture), and intrinsic to the GH joint (e.g., associated with a rotator cuff tear) subcategories.

Adhesive capsulitis typically progresses through a series of stages that correspond to arthroscopic and histologic findings. The phases of primary frozen shoulder can be seen in Table 25.1. In the "painful" or "preadhesive" stage, patients often have mild shoulder pain and decreased glenohumeral joint ROM; however, they exhibit full ROM under anesthesia. Synovial pathology has been observed via histologic analysis during this stage, but it is not clear if this represents synovitis or synovial hyperplasia and angiogenesis without inflammation. Arthroscopic studies indicate that the synovial pathology is usually most severe in the anterosuperior capsule. The presence of multiple nerve cells in tissue samples may explain why adhesive capsulitis can be so painful.

During the "freezing" phase, synovial hyperplasia continues, accompanied by fibroblastic proliferation in the underlying GH joint capsule. ROM loss becomes more profound and sustained with or without anesthesia as a result of dense fibrotic scar formation. Elevated levels of cytokines, which regulate fibroblast proliferation and collagen synthesis, have been implicated in this process. T and B cells have been found in tissue samples, suggesting that the proliferative fibrosis is modulated by the immune system. The presence of mast cells in tissue samples supports the hypothesis that the capsular fibrosis is the result of an initial inflammatory process. High levels of tissue inhibitors of metalloproteinases (TIMPs) have also been found in individuals with adhesive capsulitis. These inhibit the enzymes that remodel the extracellular collagen matrix (matrix metalloproteinases). Of interest, the use of tissue inhibitors in the treatment of carcinomas and HIV has lead to adhesive capsulitis in several cases. Thus adhesive capsulitis appears to involve both excessive collagen synthesis and inhibited or inadequate remodeling of the collagen matrix. Of note, some authors collapse this stage and the "painful" phase into a single "painful/ freezing" stage.

In stage 3—the "stiffness" or "frozen" phase—synovial pathology begins to abate, but adhesions within the capsule decrease intra-articular volume and capsular compliance. The result is marked glenohumeral joint ROM loss, although pain during this stage tends to plateau or diminish somewhat. The glenohumeral contracture is most severe in the anterior aspect of the capsule, particularly around the rotator interval and coracohumeral ligament. The histologic appearance of the contracted glenohumeral capsule is somewhat similar to that observed with Dupuytren's disease of the palm, suggesting that the molecular biology of these disorders is similar.

During the "thawing" or "recovery" stage glenohumeral motion and shoulder function begin to improve. Painless stiffness and progressive improvement in ROM are characteristic. Although the length of each stage varies, Hannafin and Chiaia (2000) reported that the painful stage typically lasts 0 to 3 months, the freezing stage lasts 3 to 9 months, the frozen stage lasts 9 to 15 months, and the thawing stage is 15 to 24 months.

The pathogenesis of adhesive capsulitis has not been firmly established, but a number of causal factors have been reported including immune disorders, hypertension (Austin et al. 2014), autonomic neuropathy, shoulder immobilization, trauma, suprascapular-nerve compression neuropathy, psychogenic disorders, and trisomy of chromosomes 7 and/or 8. Precipitating or coinciding conditions that have been reported include Dupuytren's disease, Parkinson's disease, osteoporosis and osteopenia, cardiorespiratory disease, stroke, hyperlipidemia, ACTH deficiency, cardiac surgery, and neurosurgery.

Of interest to note is that some feel that frozen shoulders do not always possess capsular adhesions long the humerus as originally described. For that reason some have suggested that the term "adhesive capsulitis" is not an appropriate description and should not be used when describing this condition (Bunker 2009).

TYPICAL PRESENTATION

Onset of adhesive capsulitis is often insidious, although antecedent injuries or coincident medical conditions should be discussed. Symptom severity and physical findings will vary depending on the disease stage at the time of examination. As with many other glenohumeral joint pathologies, complaints of poorly localized shoulder pain with focal tenderness adjacent to the deltoid insertion and occasional pain radiation to the elbow are typical. This pain is usually aggravated by shoulder movement and alleviated by rest. Pain may be most intense at night and disrupt sleep. Difficulty with activities of daily living is common, particularly with those that require reaching behind the back, overhead, or across the body. As symptoms progress, patients have increasing difficulty finding comfortable arm positions.

Limitations of active and passive glenohumeral joint ROM are common in multiple planes. Losses greater than 50% have

TABLE 25.1	Three Phases of Primary (Idiopathic) Frozen Shoulder	
Phase	**Clinical Presentation**
Freezing phase (painful)	Duration: 10 to 36 weeks Pain and stiffness around the shoulder No history of injury Nagging, constant pain that is worse at night Little or no response to NSAIDs
Adhesive/restrictive phase	Duration: 4 to 12 weeks Pain gradually subsides but stiffness remains Pain apparent only at extremes of movement Gross reduction of glenohumeral movements with near total loss of lateral (external) rotation
Resolution phase	Duration: 12 to 42 weeks Spontaneous improvement in ROM Mean duration from onset of frozen shoulder to greatest resolution exceeds 30 weeks

NSAIDs, nonsteroidal anti-inflammatory drugs; ROM, range of motion. From Dias R, Cutts S, Massoud S: Frozen shoulder, Br Med J 2005; 2005; 331:1453-1456.

been reported. Increases in scapulothoracic joint movement are common, presumably to compensate for lost glenohumeral motion. Scapular movement aberrations may be present, including a "shrug" sign. Shoulder strength may be impaired with adhesive capsulitis, particularly in the glenohumeral internal rotators and flexors.

External rotation ROM with the arm at the side (neutral) is often significantly reduced in individuals with adhesive capsulitis. The hallmark loss of motion follows a capsular pattern of restriction, which is a characteristic pattern of motion loss, secondary to capsular involvement in synovial joints. In the glenohumeral joint a capsular pattern of restriction is seen by a loss of lateral rotation that is most affected, followed by abduction, followed by a lessor limitation of medial rotation. Other shoulder conditions that restrict external rotation in neutral (e.g., severe osteoarthritis, proximal humeral fracture, locked posterior dislocation, acute calcific bursitis/tendinitis) have specific radiographic features. Thus the diagnosis of adhesive capsulitis is often based on passive external rotation ROM loss in neutral in conjunction with normal radiographs.

Some feel that the hallmark characteristic of adhesive capsulitis is primarily the result of contracture of the rotator interval and coracohumeral ligament. Yang et al. (2009) studied the coracohumeral ligament in cadaveric specimens and found that it inserted into the rotator cuff interval and supraspinatus tendon. In 4 of the 14 cadavers the coracohumeral ligament also inserted onto the subscapularis tendon. The differing attachments may in part be the reasons for differing presentations of the limitations of motion.

Advanced imaging studies are typically reserved for recalcitrant cases or to exclude other diagnoses. MRI findings associated with adhesive capsulitis include hypertrophy and increased vascularity in the glenohumeral joint capsule. Sonographic findings associated with adhesive capsulitis include coracohumeral ligament thickening, hypoechoic vascular soft tissue in the rotator interval, and limited supraspinatus tendon sliding against the acromion. Sonography may prove increasingly useful to diagnose adhesive capsulitis because of its low cost, portability, and lack of ionizing radiation.

TREATMENT

Prior to initiating treatment, patients should be educated on the natural history and chronicity of adhesive capsulitis (Rehabilitation Protocol 25.1). This can help patients prepare for a slow progression and allay some of their concerns. Patients should also be made aware of the importance of preserving or improving motion on a symptom-limited basis. As a general rule, stretching or ROM exercises or joint mobilization techniques should be symptom-limited to avoid exacerbation. Aggressive, painful stretching is often poorly tolerated by these patients and may exacerbate the synovial pathology and subsequent fibrosis. However, low-intensity self-stretching can help reduce pain, induce muscle relaxation, and preserve or improve ROM in many patients. For many patients, pain is a more significant concern than loss of shoulder function.

Given the controversy that surrounds etiology one can clearly see that the thoughts about the treatment progression may be equally confusing to interpret. There is no universal method for management of this disorder. Systematic reviews based on low-moderate quality evidence have reported limited overall use for exercise, manual therapy, and low level laser. Most patients (Jain 2014, Maund et al. 2012, Page et al. 2014) will improve conservatively using a multimodal approach with therapeutic strategies that have been proposed to reduce pain, to elongate the contracted glenohumeral joint capsule, and/or to improve shoulder function, including oral or injected analgesics, nerve blocks, pendulum exercises, modalities (TENS, ultrasound, cold packs, diathermy, moist heat, high-voltage galvanic stimulation), stretching exercises, joint mobilization, strengthening exercises, static splinting, cortisone injection, or calcitonin injection. Surgical intervention may also be beneficial to those recalcitrant to conservative care and include capsular distension (also known as distension arthrography, brisement, or hydrodilatation), manipulation under anesthesia, and surgical contracture release. Randomized clinical trials comparing adhesive capsulitis treatment outcomes are sparse and typically involve few patients. Lack of standardization of treatment approaches makes it difficult to determine which interventions or combinations of interventions are efficacious. In many studies multiple interventions are combined. A sample rehabilitation program for adhesive capsulitis is presented at the end of the chapter.

Differences in reported success rates with various interventions may be attributable to the timing of treatment. Patients in the end stage of adhesive capsulitis may experience improvement regardless of intervention as a result of natural progression of the disease. By contrast, patients in the early stages of adhesive capsulitis are more likely to have success with GH joint intra-articular corticosteroid injections than are patients in middle or later stages. This suggests that corticosteroids have a therapeutic effect on the synovial pathology, perhaps by quelling synovitis or by inhibiting synovial angiogenesis. Immediate improvement in glenohumeral motion is common after injection, but this improvement may be attributable to the effect of anesthetics that are typically injected along with the corticosteroids. The effectiveness of corticosteroid injections in improving motion and decreasing pain seems to be most profound in the first 3 to 4 weeks in patients with adhesive capsulitis. Injections may augment the efficacy of supervised physical therapy, but this effect also appears to be short-lived. Oral steroids may also have some benefit, although data suggest that worthwhile benefits are likely to be short-lived. Still, oral or injected steroidal/nonsteroidal medications, along with stretching and mobilization techniques to increase extensibility of the glenohumeral joint capsule, should be considered for initial treatment.

The vigor of stretching and mobilization should be titrated according to patient irritability. Patients with high irritability, typified by pain that is easily aggravated with movement, may only tolerate brief bouts of low-intensity self-stretching or ROM exercise through a limited arc. Diercks and Stevens (2004) reported that patients with adhesive capsulitis who stretched below the onset of pain fared better than patients who stretched beyond their pain threshold. In the interest of patient convenience and cost containment, it may be sensible to emphasize self-ROM exercises. Moist hot packs or warm-water immersion can be utilized to promote relaxation and tissue extensibility prior to, or during, mobilization or stretching exercises.

Patients with high irritability may benefit from various analgesic physical agents (electrical stimulation, cryotherapy), although there are no evidence-based guidelines to aid clinicians. Dogru and colleagues (2008) found that patients with adhesive capsulitis treated with therapeutic ultrasound experienced improvements in ROM but not function or pain. Jewell and colleagues (2009) reported that the use of iontophoresis, phonophoresis, ultrasound, or massage *reduced* the likelihood of improvements in pain or function by 19% to 32% in patients with adhesive capsulitis, suggesting that use of these interventions should be minimized. A recent study by Russell et al. (2014) would suggest that a hospital-based exercise class can produce a rapid recovery from a frozen shoulder with a minimum number of visits to the hospital and may be more cost-effective than individualized therapy.

In the early stages of rehabilitation for frozen shoulder the patient may not be able to tolerate ROM or joint mobilization techniques due to pain. Treatment at this time may be more useful in the form of patient education and reassurance. Less stressful treatment strategies may include working on proper posture and scapular strengthening via isometric muscle "setting" until more progressive therapies can be initiated. Exercises at this time should be performed within the tolerance of pain to avoid overaggressive treatment to inflamed tissue.

Patients with moderate irritability experience pain and stiffness that are roughly equivalent. These patients are tolerant of longer bouts of stretching and/or mobilization. Griggs et al. (2002) reported satisfactory outcomes in 90% of patients in the "frozen" stage who stretched to "tolerable discomfort" in the directions of flexion, external rotation, internal rotation, and horizontal adduction. Patients in this study were instructed to exercise five times each day, but average compliance was twice daily. Other studies have also shown that daily exercise is apt to be effective in relieving symptoms with adhesive capsulitis. Of interest, 91% of patients in the Griggs study also had supervised physical therapy twice weekly. It is not clear how much therapeutic benefit was derived from the supervised sessions or even what interventions were performed. Still, numerous additional

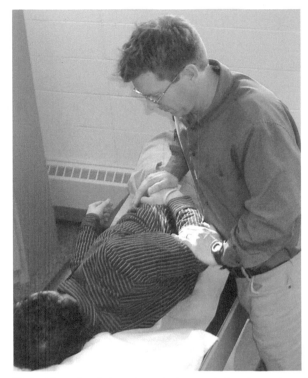

Fig. 25.1 Manual technique intended to maximize elongation of the rotator interval and coracohumeral ligament. The patient's hand remains fixed and the elbow is moved toward the table.

studies suggest that patients treated with joint mobilization, with or without concurrent interventions, tend to have better outcomes.

On the other end of the spectrum, patients with low irritability who experience stiffness more than pain should respond favorably to more aggressive mobilization and stretching, closed manipulation, or surgical release to accelerate recovery. End-range mobilization and mobilization with motion have been shown to be slightly more effective than mid-range mobilization in increasing mobility and functional ability in patients who have had adhesive capsulitis symptoms for at least 3 months. Thus patients who are too irritable for end-range mobilization may still benefit from mid-range mobilization.

Clinicians attempting to regain shoulder external rotation should perform stretching and joint mobilization techniques that target the rotator interval and coracohumeral ligament. These structures constrain inferior humeral head translation and external rotation with the arm in neutral. Anecdotally, I have found that inferior and posterior gliding mobilizations for the proximal humerus tend to be less irritating and more effective than external rotation stretching or anterior gliding mobilizations in patients with adhesive capsulitis. Johnson et al. (2007) found posterior humeral glides to be more effective in improving glenohumeral external rotation than anterior humeral glides (31.3 degrees with posterior mobilization vs. 3.0 degrees with anterior mobilization). Manual and self-stretch techniques intended to maximize elongation of the rotator interval and coracohumeral ligament are demonstrated in Figs. 25.1 and 25.2. Success with nonoperative management has been reported to be as high as 89.5%. Patients with more severe pain and functional limitations at the initiation of treatment tend to have poorer outcomes with conservative care.

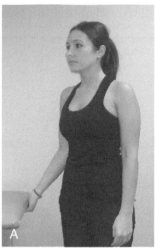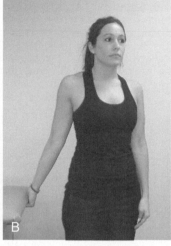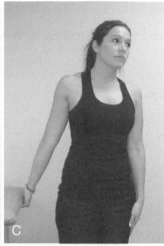

Fig. 25.2 Self-stretch technique intended to maximize elongation of the rotator interval and coracohumeral ligament. Individual grasps a heavy table or countertop with forearm supinated (*A*). The torso is rotated away from the table to externally rotate the arm (*B*). Once a tolerable level of external rotation is achieved, the individual leans torso away from the table to promote caudal glide of the humerus (*C*).

Patients who fail to respond to conservative treatment may benefit from manipulation under anesthesia, arthrographic distension, and/or arthroscopic release of the joint capsule. Arthrographic distension with saline and steroid has been shown to provide short-term pain relief and improvements in ROM and function, but it is unclear if this is superior to alternative treatments. In contrast, several studies have shown that translational (i.e., gliding) manipulation under anesthesia can be effective on a short-term and long-term basis. Success rates following manipulation under anesthesia range from 75% to 100%. Manipulation is commonly performed at end ROM abduction and internal and external rotation. Loew et al. (2005) reported that audible and palpable tissue release during manipulation are associated with a favorable treatment response. Surgical capsular release can be performed before or after manipulation with favorable results. Capsular release in patients with adhesive capsulitis is most commonly performed arthroscopically, permitting controlled, selective release of identified adhesions. Patients with severe adhesions may need to be manipulated prior to release to gain access to the GH joint. Release of the rotator interval and coracohumeral ligament has been advocated in particular because excision of these structures has been shown to substantially increase glenohumeral external rotation ROM.

Conventional wisdom holds that spontaneous resolution will occur in 1 to 3 years with adhesive capsulitis regardless of treatment. Several studies, however, report that 20% to 50% of patients with adhesive capsulitis will suffer long-term ROM deficits that may last more than 10 years. Clarke et al. (1975) reported that 42% of patients continued to have motion loss after 6 years of follow-up. Likewise, Schaffer et al. (1992) reported that 50% of patients managed nonoperatively remained symptomatic during their long-term follow-up, which occurred 2 to 11 years after their initial visit (mean = 7 years). Of these patients, 60% had a measurable restriction of shoulder motion. External rotation was the most chronically restricted movement, providing further evidence that the rotator interval and coracohumeral ligament are particularly affected by adhesive capsulitis. Hand et al. (2008) tracked outcomes in 269 shoulders affected by primary adhesive capsulitis who received no treatment (95), physical therapy (55), steroid injection (139), manipulation under anesthesia (MUA) (5), MUA and arthroscopic release (5), or MUA and arthroscopic hydrodistension (20). During the long-term follow-up (mean 52.3 months) 59% of patients reported having normal or near-normal shoulders, 35% reported persistent mild/moderate symptoms, and 6% still had severe symptoms. Persistent symptoms were reported as mild in 94% of patients, with pain being the most common complaint. Only 6% of patients complained of severe pain and/or functional loss. Patients with the most severe symptoms at condition onset had the worst long-term prognosis. In general, patients with comorbid factors, particularly diabetes, hyperthyroidism, hypothyroidism, hypoadrenalism, Parkinson's disease, cardiac disease, pulmonary disease, or cerebrovascular accident, tend to have more severe and longer lasting symptoms and tend to be more recalcitrant to treatment.

REHABILITATION PROTOCOL 25.1 ● **Frozen Shoulder (Adhesive Capsulitis) Rehabilitation Protocol**

Bernard R. Bach, MD, Mark S. Cohen, MD, Anthony A, Romeo, MD

Phase I: Weeks 0–8

Goals

- Relieve pain.
- Restore motion.

Restrictions

- None

Immobilization

- None

Pain Control

- Reduction of pain and discomfort is essential for recovery.

Medications
  - NSAIDs—first-line medications for pain control
  - GH joint injection: corticosteroid/local anesthetic combination

Continued

REHABILITATION PROTOCOL 25.1 ▣ **Frozen Shoulder (Adhesive Capsulitis) Rehabilitation Protocol—cont'd**

- Oral steroid taper—for patients with refractive or symptomatic frozen shoulder (Pearsall and Speer 1998).
- Because of potential side effects of oral steroids, patients must be thoroughly questioned about their past medical history.

Therapeutic Modalities

- Ice, ultrasound, HVGS.
- Moist heat before therapy, ice at end of session.

Motion: Shoulder

Goals

- Controlled, aggressive ROM exercises.
- Focus is on stretching at ROM limits.
- No restrictions on range, but therapist and patient have to communicate to avoid injuries.

Exercises

- Initially focus on forward flexion and external and internal rotation with the arm at the side and the elbow at 90 degrees.
- Active ROM exercises.
- Active-assisted ROM exercises (see Fig. 21.8).
- Passive ROM exercises (see Fig. 21.9).
- A home exercise program should be instituted from the beginning.
- Patients should perform ROM exercises three to five times per day.
- A sustained stretch, of 15 to 30 seconds, at the end ROMs should be part of all ROM routines.

Phase II: Weeks 8–16

Criteria for Progression to Phase II

- Improvement in shoulder discomfort.
- Improvement of shoulder motion.
- Satisfactory physical examination.

Goals

- Improve shoulder motion in all planes.
- Improve strength and endurance of rotator cuff and scapular stabilizers.

Pain Control

- Reduction of pain and discomfort is essential for recovery.

Medications

- NSAIDs—first-line medications for pain control.
- GH joint injection: corticosteroid/local anesthetic combination.
- Oral steroid taper—for patients with refractive or symptomatic frozen shoulder (Pearsall and Speer 1998).
- Because of potential side effects of oral steroids, patients must be thoroughly questioned about their past medical history.

Therapeutic Modalities

- Ice, ultrasound, HVGS.
- Moist heat before therapy, ice at end of session.

Motion: Shoulder

Goals

- 140 degrees of flexion.
- 45 degrees of external rotation.
- Internal rotation to twelfth thoracic spinous process.

Exercises

- Active ROM exercises.
- Active-assisted ROM exercises (see Fig. 21.8).
- Passive ROM exercises (see Fig. 21.9).

Muscle Strengthening

- Rotator cuff strengthening three times per week, 8 to 12 repetitions for three sets.

- Closed chain isometric strengthening with the elbow flexed to 90 degrees and the arm at the side (see Figs 21.12 to 21.14).
- Internal rotation.
- External rotation.
- Abduction.
- Flexion.
- Progress to open chain strengthening with Therabands (see Fig. 21.18, *A*).
- Exercises performed with the elbow flexed to 90 degrees.
- Starting position is with the shoulder in the neutral position of 0 degrees of flexion, abduction, and external rotation.
- Exercises are performed through an arc of 45 degrees in each of the five planes of motion.
- Six color-coded bands are available; each provides increasing resistance from 1 to 6 pounds, at increments of 1 pound.
- Progression to the next band occurs usually in 2- to 3-week intervals. Patients are instructed not to progress to the next band if there is any discomfort at the present level.
- Theraband exercises permit concentric and eccentric strengthening of the shoulder muscles and are a form of isotonic exercises (characterized by variable speed and fixed resistance).
- Internal rotation.
- External rotation.
- Abduction.
- Flexion.
- Progress to light isotonic dumbbell exercises.
- Internal rotation (see Fig. 21.18, *B*).
- External rotation (see Fig. 21.18, *C*).
- Abduction.
- Flexion.
- Strengthening of scapular stabilizers.
- Closed chain strengthening exercises (see Figs 21.16 ABC).
- Scapular retraction (rhomboideus, middle trapezius).
- Scapular protraction (serratus anterior).
- Scapular depression (latissimus dorsi, trapezius, serratus anterior).
- Shoulder shrugs (trapezius, levator scapulae).
- Progress to open chain strengthening (see Fig. 21.17).
- Deltoid strengthening.

Phase III: Months 4 and Beyond

Criteria for Progression to Phase IV

- Significant functional recovery of shoulder motion.
- Successful participation in activities of daily living.
- Resolution of painful shoulder.
- Satisfactory physical examination.

Goals

- Home maintenance exercise program.
- ROM exercises two times a day.
- Rotator cuff strengthening three times a week.
- Scapular stabilizer strengthening three times a week.
- Maximum improvement by 6 to 9 months after initiation of treatment program.

Warning Signs

- Loss of motion.
- Continued pain.

Treatment of Complications

- These patients may need to move back to earlier routines.
- May require increased utilization of pain control modalities as outlined earlier.
- If loss of motion is persistent and pain continues, patients may require surgical intervention.
- Manipulation under anesthesia.
- Arthroscopic release.

REFERENCES

A complete reference list is available at https://expertconsult
.inkling.com/.

FURTHER READING

Aydeniz A, Gursoy S, Guney E. Which musculoskeletal complications are most frequently seen in type 2 diabetes mellitus? *J Int Med Res.* 2008;36:505–511.

Bal A, Eksioglu E, Gulec B, et al. Effectiveness of corticosteroid injection in adhesive capsulitis. *Clin Rehabil.* 2008;22:503–512.

Baslund B, Thomsen BS, Jensen EM. Frozen shoulder: current concepts. *Scand J Rheumatol.* 1990;19:321–325.

Berghs BM, Sole-Molins X, Bunker TD. Arthroscopic release of adhesive capsulitis. *J Shoulder Elbow Surg.* 2004;13:180–185.

Boyle-Walker K. A profile of patients with adhesive capsulitis. *J Hand Ther.* 1997;10:222–228.

Boyles RE, Flynn TW, Whitman JM. Manipulation following regional interscalene anesthetic block for shoulder adhesive capsulitis: a case series. *Man Ther.* 2005;10:80–87.

Bruchner F. Frozen shoulder (adhesive capsulitis). *J Royal Soc Med.* 1982;75:688–689.

Buchbinder R, Green S, Youd JM, et al. Oral steroids for adhesive capsulitis. *Cochrane Database Syst Rev.* 2006:CD006189.

Bunker T, Anthony P. The pathology of frozen shoulder. *J Bone Joint Surg Br.* 1995;77-B:677–683.

Bunker TD, Esler CN. Frozen shoulder and lipids. *J Bone Joint Surg Br.* 1995;77:684–686.

Bunker TD, Reilly J, Baird KS, et al. Expression of growth factors, cytokines and matrix metalloproteinases in frozen shoulder. *J Bone Joint Surg Br.* 2000;82:768–773.

Carette S, Moffet H, Tardif J, et al. Intraarticular corticosteroids, supervised physiotherapy, or a combination of the two in the treatment of adhesive capsulitis of the shoulder: a placebo-controlled trial. *Arthritis Rheum.* 2003;48:829–838.

Choy E, Corkill M, Gibson T, et al. Isolated ACTH deficiency presenting with bilateral frozen shoulder. *Br J Rheum.* 1991;30:226–227.

Connolly JF. Unfreezing the frozen shoulder. *J Musculoskeletal Med.* 1998;15:47–57.

Dodenhoff RM, Levy O, Wilson A, et al. Manipulation under anesthesia for primary frozen shoulder: effect on early recovery and return to activity. *J Shoulder Elbow Surg.* 2000;9:23–26.

Green S, Buchbinder R, Glazier R, et al. Systematic review of randomized controlled trials of interventions for painful shoulder: selection criteria, outcome assessment, and efficacy. *BMJ.* 1998;31:354–359.

Greenberg JA, Fernandez JJ, Wang T, et al. EndoButton-assisted repair of distal biceps tendon ruptures. *J Shoulder Elbow Surg.* 2003;12:484–490.

Grubbs N. Frozen shoulder syndrome: a review of literature. *J Orthop Sports Phys Ther.* 1993;18:479–487.

Hand GC, Athanasou NA, Matthews T, et al. The pathology of frozen shoulder. *J Bone Joint Surg Br.* 2007;89:928–932.

Hannafin JA, Chiaia TA. Adhesive capsulitis: a treatment approach. *Clin Orthop Related Res.* 2000;372:95–109.

Harryman DT, Lazarus MD, Rozencwaig R. The stiff shoulder. In: Rockwood Cam Matsen FA, Wirth MA, Lippitt SB, eds. *The Shoulder.* 3rd ed. Philadephia: Saunders; 2004.

Homsi C, Bordalo-Rodrigues M, da Silva JJ, et al. Ultrasound in adhesive capsulitis of the shoulder: is assessment of the coracohumeral ligament a valuable diagnostic tool? *Skeletal Radiol.* 2006;35:673–678.

Hutchinson JW, Tierney GM, Parsons SL, et al. Dupuytren's disease and frozen shoulder induced by treatment with a matrix metalloproteinase inhibitor. *J Bone Joint Surg Br.* 1998;80:907–908.

Ide J, Takagi K. Early and long-term results of arthroscopic treatment for shoulder stiffness. *J Shoulder Elbow Surg.* 2004;13:174–179.

Jarvinen MJ, Lehto MU. The effects of early mobilisation and immobilization on the healing process following muscle injuries. *Sports Med.* 1993;15:78–89.

Jayson M. Frozen shoulder: adhesive capsulitis. *Br Med J.* 1981;283:1005–1006.

Jost B, Koch PP, Gerber C. Anatomy and functional aspects of the rotator interval. *J Shoulder Elbow Surg.* 2000;9:336–341.

Jurgel J, Rannama L, Gapeyeva H, et al. Shoulder function in patients with frozen shoulder before and after 4-week rehabilitation. *Medicina (Kaunas).* 2005;41:30–38.

Kelley MJ, McClure PW, Leggin BG. Frozen shoulder: evidence and a proposed model guiding rehabilitation. *J Orthop Sports Phys Ther.* 2009;39(2):135–148.

Kim K, Rhee K, Shin H. Adhesive capsulitis of the shoulder: dimensions of the rotator interval measured with magnetic resonance arthrography. *J Shoulder Elbow Surg.* 2009;18(3):437–442.

Lee JC, Sykes C, Saifuddin A, et al. Adhesive capsulitis: sonographic changes in the rotator cuff interval with arthroscopic correlation. *Skeletal Radiol.* 2005;34:522–527.

Levine WN, Kashyap CP, Bak SF, et al. Nonoperative management of idiopathic adhesive capsulitis. *J Shoulder Elbow Surg.* 2007;16(5):569–573.

Lundberg J. The frozen shoulder. Clinical and radiographical observations. The effect of manipulation under general anesthesia. Structure and glycosaminoglycan content of the joint capsule. Local bone metabolism. *Acta Orthop Scand.* 1969;(suppl 119):111–159.

Marx RG, Malizia RW, Kenter K, et al. Intra-articular corticosteroid injection for the treatment of idiopathic adhesive capsulitis of the shoulder. *HSS J.* 2007;3:202–207.

McClure PW, Flowers KR. Treatment of limited shoulder motion: a case study based on biomechanical considerations. *Phys Ther.* 1992;72:97–104.

Milgrom C, Novack V, Weil Y, et al. Risk factors for idiopathic frozen shoulder. *Isr Med Assoc J.* 2008;10:361–364.

Nauck M, Karakiulakis G, Perruchoud AP, et al. Corticosteroids inhibit the expression of the vascular endothelial growth factor gene in human vascular smooth muscle cells. *Eur J Pharmacol.* 1998;341:309–315.

Neer II CS, Satterlee CC, Dalsey RM, et al. The anatomy and potential effects of contracture of the coracohumeral ligament. *Clin Orthop.* 1992;280:182–185.

Neviaser RJ, Neviaser TJ. The frozen shoulder diagnosis and management. *Clin Orthop.* 1987;223:59–64.

Nicholson G. Arthroscopic capsular release for stiff shoulders. Effect of etiology on outcomes. *Arthroscopy.* 2003;19:40–49.

Okamura K, Ozaki J. Bone mineral density of the shoulder joint in frozen shoulder. *Arch Orthop Trauma Surg.* 1999;119:363–367.

Omari A, Bunker TD. Open surgical release for frozen shoulder: surgical findings and results of the release. *J Shoulder Elbow Surg.* 2001;10(4):353–357.

Ozaki J, Nakagawa Y, Sakurai G, et al. Recalcitrant chronic adhesive capsulitis of the shoulder. Role of contracture of the coracohumeral ligament and rotator interval in pathogenesis and treatment. *J Bone Joint Surg Am.* 1989;71(10):1511–1515.

Pearsall AW, Speer KP. Frozen shoulder syndrome: diagnostic and treatment strategies in the primary care setting. *Med Sci Sports Exerc.* 1998;30:s33–s39.

Reeves B. The natural history of the frozen shoulder syndrome. *Scand J Rheumatol.* 1975;14:193–196.

Riley D, Lang A, Blair R, et al. Frozen shoulder and other shoulder disturbances in Parkinson's disease. *J Neurol Neurosurg Psychiatr.* 1989;52:63–66.

Rizk TE, Pinals RS. Frozen shoulder. *Semin Arthritis Rheum.* 1982;11:440–452.

Rodeo SA, Hannafin JA, Tom J, et al. Immunolocalization of cytokines and their receptors in adhesive capsulitis of the shoulder. *J Orthop Res.* 1997;15:427–436.

Roubal PJ, Dobritt D, Placzek JD. Glenohumeral gliding manipulation following interscalene brachial plexus block in patients with adhesive capsulitis. *J Orthop Sports Phys.* 1996;24:66–77.

Ryu KN, Lee SW, Rhee YG, et al. Adhesive capsulitis of the shoulder joint: usefulness of dynamic sonography. *J Ultrasound Med.* 1993;12:445–449.

Seigel LB, Cohen NJ, Gall EP. Adhesive capsulitis: a sticky issue. *Am Fam Physician.* 1999;59:1843–1850.

Sharma R, Bajekal R, Bhan S. Frozen shoulder syndrome: a comparison of hydraulic distension and manipulation. *Int Orthop.* 1993;17:275–278.

Smith S, Devaraj V, Bunker T. The association between frozen shoulder and Dupuytren's disease. *J Shoulder Elbow Surg.* 2001;10:149–151.

Sokk J, Gapeyeva H, Ereline J, et al. Shoulder muscle strength and fatigability in patients with frozen shoulder syndrome: the effect of 4-week individualized rehabilitation. *Electromyogr Clin Neurophysiol.* 2007;47:205–213.

Stam H. Frozen shoulder: a review of current concepts. *Physiotherapy.* 1994;80:588–599.

Tuten H, Young D, Dououguih W, et al. Adhesive capsulitis of the shoulder in male cardiac surgery patients. *Orthopaedics.* 2000;23:693–696.

Uhthoff HK, Boileau P. Primary frozen shoulder: global capsular stiffness versus localized contracture. *Clin Orthop Relat Res.* 2007;456:79–84.

Van der Windt DAWM, Koes BW, Deville W, et al. Effectiveness of corticosteroid injections versus physiotherapy for treatment of painful stiff shoulder in primary care: randomized trial. *BMJ.* 1998;317:1292–1296.

Vermeulen HM, Obermann WR, Burger BJ, et al. End-range mobilization techniques in adhesive capsulitis of the shoulder joint: a multiple-subject case report. *Phys Ther.* 2000;80:1204–1213.

Winters JC, Sobel JS, Groenier KH, et al. Comparison of physiotherapy, manipulation, and corticosteroid injection for treating shoulder complaints in general practice: randomized, single blind study. *BMJ.* 1997;314:1320–1324.

Wyke B. Neurological mechanisms in spasticity: a brief review of some current concepts. *Physiotherapy.* 1976;62(10):316–319.

Yang JL, Chang CW, Chen SY, et al. Mobilization techniques in subjects with frozen shoulder syndrome: randomized multiple-treatment trial. *Phys Ther.* 2007;87:1307–1315.

Zuckerman JD. Definition and classification of frozen shoulder. *J Shoulder Elbow Surg.* 1994;3:S72.

Rehabilitation for Biceps Tendon Disorders and SLAP Lesions

Geoffrey S. Van Thiel, MD, MBA | Sanjeev Bhatia, MD | Neil S. Ghodadra, MD |
Jonathan Yong Kim, CDR | Matthew T. Provencher, MD, CDR, MC, USN

Injuries to the proximal biceps tendon, the distal biceps tendon, and the superior labrum–biceps anterior to posterior (SLAP) tendon complex have long been recognized as a potential source of pain and disability when not properly addressed. Disorders of the biceps tendon are particularly problematic in overhead athletes, throwers, and those who do activities of lifting overhead. As such, problems with the biceps may lead to significant functional disability in both the sport and work environment. Coupled with an improved understanding of anatomy and shoulder biomechanics, advances in surgical techniques have resulted in less invasive and more effective management of biceps tendon disorders and associated SLAP lesions. Recently surgical treatment for SLAP lesions has escalated astronomically and in some regions of the United States has increased by greater than 400% (Onyekwelu 2012).

It is imperative that a rehabilitation program mirror these efforts so as to optimize patient recovery both in the nonoperative and operative setting. The following section will describe the anatomy, examination, mechanism of injury, treatment, and rehabilitation for injuries to the proximal and distal biceps tendon and their associated structures.

REHABILITATION RATIONALE
Normal Anatomy

The biceps tendon is one of the few tendons in the body to span two joints: the glenohumeral complex and the elbow. Tension in the tendon, therefore, largely depends on the position of the elbow, wrist, and shoulder during muscle contraction. Proximally, the biceps has two heads, one of which originates from the coracoid process (short head) and the other that begins its course from the supraglenoid tubercle and superior labrum (long head). As the tendon travels distally in the glenohumeral joint it is encased in a synovial sheath and is considered to be intra-articular but extrasynovial. It then courses obliquely through the joint and arches over the humeral head at a 30- to 45-degree angle. As the long head exits the joint, it passes under the coracohumeral ligament and through the rotator interval into the groove between the greater and lesser tuberosities (bicipital groove). In the bicipital groove it is covered by the transverse humeral ligament with contributions from the subscapularis tendon (Fig. 26.1). Distally, the long and short heads of the biceps converge at the midshaft of the humerus then insert on the anterior aspect of the radial tuberosity. In the antecubital fossa the distal tendon blends with the bicipital aponeurosis, which helps protect the cubital fossa structures and provides an even distribution of force across the elbow. Recent cadaveric evidence has shown that the average length, width, and thickness of the external distal biceps tendon is 63.0, 6.0, and 3.0 mm (Walton et al. 2015).

Innervation of the biceps muscle is via the branches of the musculocutaneous nerve (C5). Blood supply is primarily provided by the ascending branch of the circumflex humeral artery but is augmented by the suprascapular artery proximally and the deep brachial artery distally.

Functionally, the biceps acts as a strong forearm supinator and a weak elbow flexor. However, it is more active in flexion of the supinated forearm than in flexion of the pronated forearm. Although controversial, it is also hypothesized that the long head aids in the anterosuperior stability of the humeral head by resisting torsional forces at the shoulder and preventing humeral migration; this is particularly evident during the vulnerable position of abduction and external rotation seen in overhead athletes. Furthermore, as demonstrated by electromyographic (EMG) analysis, biceps contraction plays a prominent role during the cocking and deceleration phases of overhand and underhand throwing.

HISTORY AND PHYSICAL EXAMINATION
Proximal Biceps and Superior Labrum

The proximal biceps tendon and the associated superior labral complex must be evaluated independently of the distal biceps, given the significant differences in mechanism of injury, evaluation, and treatment. In fact, pathologic lesions of the proximal biceps and superior labral complex can be extremely difficult to diagnose, with a multitude of potential sources for anterior shoulder pain confounding the clinical picture, while clinical findings upon examination are inconsistent. Numerous tests have been developed and suggested, but most have proven difficult to validate.

The most common presenting symptom of any biceps problem in the shoulder is pain. With isolated biceps pathology, this is usually localized to the anterior shoulder and the bicipital groove. However, the picture is less clear if the superior labrum is involved. In this case, pain can occur in the anterior or posterior aspect of the shoulder with the patient often complaining of "deep" pain. Diffuse discomfort can also occur if another condition also is present, such as rotator cuff disease, subacromial impingement, acromioclavicular joint arthrosis, or shoulder instability. Thus, an accurate history is essential and includes a description of the onset of symptoms, duration and progression of pain, history of a traumatic event, activities that worsen

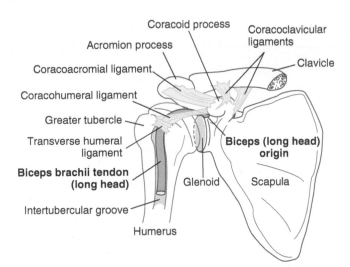

Fig. 26.1 Anterior aspect of the right shoulder showing the tendon of the long head of the biceps muscle and its relationships.

the pain, and previous treatments and outcomes. A SLAP tear is also associated with sensations of instability, popping, and other mechanical symptoms, especially with overhead or throwing activity. A decrease in throwing velocity or diminished overhead performance should also alert the examiner to a possible biceps or SLAP tear etiology.

A variety of reported clinical tests attempt to evaluate the proximal biceps complex, with no one test offering acceptable sensitivity and specificity. Due to the difficulty of diagnosing a SLAP lesion with physical examination, Kim and McFarland stated "our findings question the diagnostic value of the clinical assessment of SLAP lesions" (Kim and McFarland 2002). With regard to the biceps tendon, external and internal rotation can change the location of the pain with tendon movement. This helps differentiate from painful superficial structures, such as the anterior deltoid, which do not move with arm rotation. The **Yergason test** consists of resisted supination that causes anterior shoulder pain and is relatively specific for biceps pathology but tends to lack sensitivity. The **Speed test** is considered positive if pain is localized to the proximal biceps tendon with resisted shoulder forward flexion with the forearm supinated. This pain should be decreased if the same maneuver is done with the forearm in pronation.

SLAP lesions can be more difficult to discern. A complete examination for both rotator cuff pathology and instability must be completed first. Often the patient will have positive **Neer and Hawkins shoulder impingement signs,** which can be nonspecific indicators of shoulder pathology. The **O'Brien active compression test** is often reported to be relatively specific for superior labral lesions. For this test, the shoulder is positioned in 90 degrees of flexion, slight horizontal adduction, and internal rotation. The test is considered positive when, on resisted shoulder flexion, the patient experiences deep or anterior shoulder pain that is decreased when the maneuver is repeated with the shoulder in external rotation. Overall, physical examination findings often do not reveal a specific pain generator and other techniques must be used. Tests used for detecting SLAP tears must be performed taking into consideration the context of the clinical history and the appropriate patient demographic.

Differential diagnostic injections can be helpful in evaluating biceps tendon pathology. A subacromial lidocaine injection will relieve symptomatology if rotator cuff disease is present, but it will not relieve pain with isolated biceps pathology. A shoulder intra-articular injection can decrease pain from the superior labral complex, but bicipital groove discomfort can often persist if marked inflammation or scarring prevents infiltration of the anesthetic into the groove. In these cases, direct injection into the biceps groove and sheath can be diagnostic. Evaluation of proximal biceps pathology can be complex and the patient history, physical examination, and diagnostic injections must be combined to further clarify the pain generator.

Distal Biceps

Recent evidence has determined that distal biceps tendon ruptures may be more common than historically thought. The estimated national incidence of distal biceps tendon rupture is 2.55 per 100,000 patient-years. The local incidence is 5.35 per 100,000 patient-years. The mean and median ages of patients is 46.3 and 46.0 years. Males compose the majority of the injured population at 95% to 96% (Kelly et al. 2015). Patients with complete distal biceps tendon ruptures usually report an unexpected extension force applied to the flexed arm. Commonly, there is an associated sudden, sharp, painful tearing sensation in the antecubital region of the elbow. The intense pain subsides in a few hours and is replaced by a dull ache. Weakness in flexion is often significant in the acute rupture; however, this can dissipate with time. Weakness in supination is less pronounced and can depend on the functional demands placed on the extremity.

With an acute rupture, inspection reveals significant swelling and bruising in the antecubital fossa with associated tenderness on palpation. In fact, a defect in the biceps tendon can often be palpated if the bicipital aponeurosis has also been torn. If the tendon seems to be in continuity but is tender to palpation, a partial biceps rupture should be considered. Each of these findings should be compared to the normal side.

Several special tests are used to confirm distal biceps tendon rupture. In the hook test the examiner uses his or her index finger to palpate the patient's flexed elbow from the lateral side of the antecubital fossa in an attempt to "hook" the distal biceps tendon. On a normal flexed elbow, the finger can be inserted behind or beneath an intact tendon in an attempt to pull it forward, resulting in a negative hook test. If the tendon is torn or avulsed from the radial tuberosity, there is no structure to wrap the finger around, resulting in an abnormal or positive hook test. One hundred percent sensitivity and specificity have been reported for this test (O'Driscoll et al. 2007). The biceps aponeurosis flex test is performed by having the patient make a fist and actively flex the wrist with a supinated forearm. This will contract the flexor/pronator muscles of the forearm and put tension on the distal attachment of the biceps aponeurosis distally and ulnarly. While maintaining this position the patient is asked to flex the elbow and maintain it in a position of approximately 75 degrees of flexion. This motion tightens the tissues. If the biceps tendon and the aponeurosis are intact the examiner can then palpate the medial, lateral, and central parts of the antecubital fossa. If the aponeurosis is intact a sharp thin edge of the aponeurosis can be felt (ElMaraghy and Devereaux 2013).

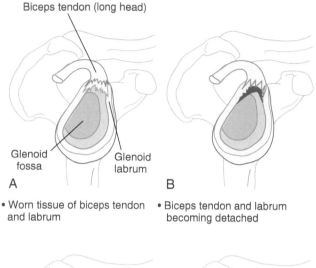

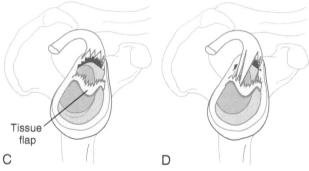

Fig. 26.2 Superior labrum anterior posterior (SLAP) lesions. **A,** Type 1. **B,** Type 2. **C,** Type 3. **D,** Type 4.

TABLE 26.1	Classification of Superior Labrum From Anterior to Posterior (SLAP) Lesions
Type	**Characteristics**
Type 1 SLAP	Degenerative fraying of the superior labrum but the biceps attachment to the labrum is intact. The biceps anchor is intact (see Fig. 36.2, A).
Type 2 SLAP	The biceps anchor has pulled away from the glenoid attachment (see Fig. 36.2, B).
Type 3 SLAP	Involve a bucket-handle tear of the superior labrum with an intact biceps anchor (see Fig. 36.2, C).
Type 4 SLAP	Similar to type 3 tears but the tear also extends into the biceps tendon (see Fig. 36.2, D). The torn biceps tendon and labrum are displaced into the joint.
Complex SLAP	A combination of two or more SLAP types, usually 2 and 3 or 2 and 4.

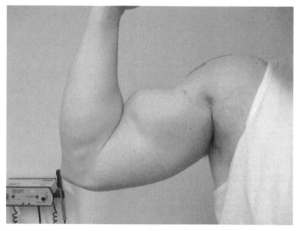

Fig. 26.3 A patient who sustained a proximal biceps tendon rupture and subsequent "Popeye" deformity of the long head of the biceps tendon (LHB), which is a result of the LHB muscle belly migrating distally.

Radiographic Evaluation

Proximal Biceps/SLAP Lesions

Imaging of patients with proximal biceps pathology is initiated with standard plain radiographs including a true anteroposterior (AP), axillary, and outlet view. Once other osseous pathology has been ruled out, additional imaging is ordered. An MRI scan allows for thorough evaluation of the proximal biceps and superior labral complex and other confounding shoulder pathology. A potential downfall is lack of reliably read MRIs. Kauffman showed that up to 35% of community-read MRI scans were interpreted as either a labral tear or a "possible labral tear" (Weber and Kauffman 2007). This is worrisome because the true incidence of labral tears is probably between 3% and 5% (Snyder et al. 1995). Ultrasound imaging has been proposed as an inexpensive and noninvasive method for evaluating bicipital tendinopathy and ruptures, but SLAP lesions are exceedingly difficult to diagnose with ultrasound. Ultrasound may help discern if the long head of the biceps (LHB), which normally resides in the bicipital groove, is subluxed or dislocated. Diagnostic arthroscopy remains the only definitive way to diagnose SLAP lesions of the shoulder (Mileski and Snyder 1998).

The diagnosis of a complete distal biceps rupture can often be made based on the physical examination (lack of distal biceps cord, decreased forearm supination strength, bruising in the antecubital fossa); however, a partial distal biceps tear can lack the pathognomonic findings. Ultrasound can again be used, but the unreliability in diagnosis and the difficulty in evaluating partial tears make MRI the study of choice for most clinicians.

Classification

Proximal Biceps/SLAP Lesions

Injuries to the superior labral and biceps complex can be categorized into four major classifications with several minor variants (Fig. 26.2 and Table 26.1).
- Type I lesions involve a degenerative fraying of the superior labrum, with the biceps anchor intact.
- Type II injuries are detachments of the biceps anchor from the superior glenoid and are the most common type.
- Type III is a bucket handle tear of the superior labrum with an intact biceps anchor.
- Type IV lesions are similar to type III, except that the tear extends into the biceps (Fig. 26.2).

Occasionally, the proximal biceps may present with an isolated rupture and is identified with a "Popeye" deformity resulting from the distal migration of the LHB portion of the biceps muscle belly (Fig. 26.3). A variety of SLAP tears and variants are demonstrated in Fig. 26.4.

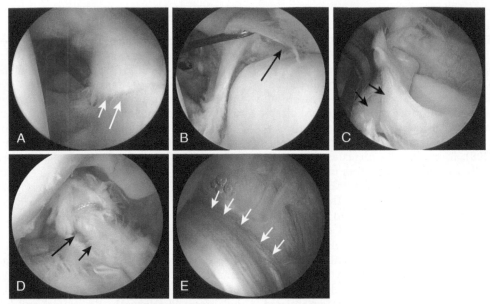

Fig. 26.4 Arthroscopic images of superior labrum anterior to posterior (SLAP) lesions. **A,** SLAP 1 (white arrows). **B,** SLAP 2 (black arrow shows detachment site). **C,** SLAP 3 (Black arrows demonstrate bucket handle tear). **D,** SLAP 4 (Black arrows demonstrate bucket handle tear with a extension into long head of biceps tendon). **E,** A lipstick biceps (white arrows mark edge of tendon), which represents inflammation of the LHB as it exits the glenohumeral joint.

TABLE 26.2	Classification of Distal Biceps Injury	
Partial Rupture	**Insertional Intrasubstance**	
Complete rupture	Acute (<4 weeks) Chronic (>4 weeks)	Intact aponeurosis Ruptured aponeurosis

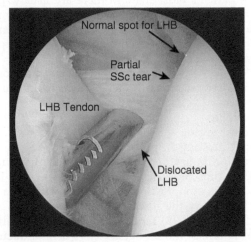

Fig. 26.5 Arthroscopic image of a dislocated long head of the biceps (LHB) medially with a concomitant subscapularis tear (superior edge). The patient was treated with a LHB tenodesis (subpectoral) and débridement of the superior edge of the partially torn subscapularis tendon.

Distal Biceps

Ramsey (1999) proposed a classification system for distal biceps ruptures (Table 26.2). Partial ruptures are defined by the location of the tear, whereas complete ruptures are characterized by their temporal relation to diagnosis and the integrity of the bicipital aponeurosis. Other variables include the location, chronicity, and integrity of the aponeurotic sheath. This classification helps dictate the available repair techniques.

Mechanism of Injury

Proximal Biceps Tendon and Superior Labrum

The proximal biceps tendon has multiple potential sites of injury including the biceps anchor, superior labrum, intraarticular tendon, and bicipital groove. Each location has a unique injury profile with different mechanisms and characteristics. These pathologic disorders can be segmented into three categories:
1. Degenerative/inflammatory
2. Instability of the tendon
3. SLAP lesions

Degeneration/inflammation: Biceps degeneration and inflammation are most likely to occur with abrasive motion as the long head of the biceps tendon runs through the bicipital groove; it is made worse with overhead and repetitive

shoulder rotation activities. Although the tendon is affected by this degeneration, histologic analysis has indicated that the sheath is where actual inflammatory changes usually take place. As the degeneration and inflammation continue, the tendon becomes thickened and irregular and may become scarred to its bed through hemorrhagic adhesions. The primary cause of these degenerative changes is thought to be mechanical irritation of the tendon by osseous spurs from the anterior acromion or coracoacromial arch. Relatively recent interests have focused on repetitive motion in overhead athletes contributing to biceps pathology. Cross-body motion, internal rotation, and forward flexion have been shown to translate the humeral head anteriorly and superiorly. Thus, while the arm is in this position during the follow-through motion of throwing and hitting, anterior structures, such as the biceps, are at increased risk of impingement on the cora-coacromial arch. Biceps tendon degeneration and inflammation often have an insidious onset with chronicity to the symptoms.

Instability: Biceps tendon instability can manifest from mild subluxation to complete dislocation. Laxity or discontinuity of the restraining structures and ligaments can result from either repetitive wear or trauma with subsequent biceps tendon instability. In almost all cases, subluxation or dislocation of the tendon occurs in the medial direction. According to Busconi et al. (2008), in overhead athletes as the arm is abducted and externally rotated, force vectors on the biceps tendon are directed medially. During the follow-through phase, force vectors are directed laterally. This displacement of the biceps tendon not only causes pain from biceps instability but also results in further wear and degenerative changes resulting in anterior shoulder pain. Finally, a tear of the subscapularis can lead to biceps instability with the compromise of soft tissue restraints overlying the bicipital groove. Subscapularis tears can occur as a natural progression of chronic or acute massive rotator cuff tears and an isolated injury. The mechanism for an isolated rupture depends on the age group encountered. In younger (<40 years) athletes, there is usually a forceful hyperextension or external rotation, whereas in patients older than 40 there are usually preceding symptoms with a lower energy injury. It is imperative to rule out a subscapularis tear if an unstable biceps tendon is detected because these are often present together (Fig. 26.5) and vice versa.

SLAP lesions: As the diagnosis and management of SLAP lesions has progressed, three distinct mechanisms of injury have been proposed.
1. Traction injury
2. Direct compression
3. Overhead throwing or "peel back" lesion

In a traction injury an eccentric firing of the long head of the biceps muscle causes injury to the superior labrum complex. With a compression mechanism, there is a shearing force caused by the impaction of the superior glenoid rim. Snyder et al. (1995) noted that this was most likely to occur during a fall onto an outstretched arm abducted and flexed slightly forward. Finally, Burkhart and Morgan (1998) proposed the existence of a biomechanical cascade in overhead athletes, resulting in a peel-back SLAP tear. Throwing athletes have increased shoulder external rotation and decreased internal rotation motion in the abducted position. These adaptations can be explained by lengthening of the anterior capsuloligamentous restraints and posterior capsular contracture and by increased proximal humeral retroversion in these athletes.

Biomechanical testing has validated each proposed mechanism. Bey et al. (1998) showed that biceps traction and inferior subluxation of the humeral head consistently created a SLAP lesion. Compression loading in cadaver shoulders has also shown that SLAP tears are more consistently created when the shoulder is forward flexed versus in an extended position. Last, the strength of the superior labrum biceps complex has been examined in multiple studies that simulate the phases of overhead throwing with a suggestion of increased stresses in late cocking and the conclusion that the position of the arm does influence the strain seen at the superior labrum.

Distal Biceps Tendon

Rupture of the distal biceps tendon is most likely to occur in the dominant extremity of men between the fourth and sixth decades of life. The average age at the time of rupture is approximately 50 years (range, 18 to 72 years). The mechanism of injury is usually a single traumatic event in which an unexpected extension force is applied to an arm flexed to 90 degrees and also supinated. Ruptures within the tendon and at the musculotendinous junction have been reported; however, most commonly the tendon will avulse from the radial tuberosity.

TREATMENT
Proximal Biceps

The initial treatment of proximal biceps pathology is nonoperative. Rest, avoidance of aggravating activities, ice, a course of anti-inflammatory medication, and formal physical rehabilitation will relieve the discomfort and increase function in most patients. Injections can also be a useful treatment and diagnostic tool and are typically used for patients with severe night pain or symptoms that fail to resolve after 6 to 8 weeks of conservative measures. The injection can be placed either in the glenohumeral joint or the biceps sheath. However, nonoperative treatment of biceps tendon instability is often unsuccessful in clinical practice. In some cases, this condition represents the natural progression of significant rotator cuff disease and the treatment must also focus on management of the rotator cuff tear.

Operative

There are no steadfast and discreet operative indications for proximal biceps pathology. However, typically surgery is considered after failure of nonsurgical treatment. An overhead throwing athlete should have undergone a period of rest followed by progressive rehabilitation. The surgical technique required to address the pathology is also not clear. It is important to consider the primary cause of the condition, location of the pathology, the integrity of the tendon, the extent of tendon involvement, related pathology, and patient activity level when planning the surgical intervention.

As stated previously, proximal biceps tendon pathology can be segmented into conditions involving degeneration/inflammation, instability, or SLAP lesions. Each subset has different treatment paradigms with corresponding surgical techniques. Degenerative or inflammatory conditions are often referred to as biceps "tendinitis" or "tenosynovitis" and require direct treatment of the diseased tendon. In contemporary shoulder surgery, the two primary options are a biceps tenotomy or tenodesis. Significant debate exists as to what the most appropriate method is and what exact technique provides the best outcomes.

Tenotomy consists of performing an intra-articular cut of the long head of the biceps tendon prior to its superior labral insertion. Tenodesis also requires a biceps tenotomy, but the long head of the biceps is then securely anchored in its resting position with a variety of fixation techniques. Each procedure effectively relieves pain; however, the benefit of performing a tenodesis is that there is a maintenance of form and possibly function in the biceps. For example, Kelly et al. (2005) showed a 70% incidence of a "Popeye" deformity with tenotomy, which is higher than that reported in the literature. A "Popeye" deformity is a prominence in the biceps muscle resulting from retraction of the tendon (Fig. 26.3). However, Gill et al. (2001) reported the results of 30 patients treated with intra-articular tenotomy as the primary procedure for biceps degeneration, instability, and recalcitrant tendinopathy. Postoperatively, only two patients complained of activity-related pain that was moderate in nature, 90% returned to their previous level of sports, and 97% returned to their previous occupation.

A biceps tenodesis can be performed with either an open or arthroscopic surgical technique. The open technique consists of a subpectoral approach to the biceps tendon with either a suture anchor or interference screw used to secure the tendon to the proximal humerus. A variety of arthroscopic techniques have been described including suturing the tendon to the conjoint tendon, interference screw fixation, and suture anchor fixation. The significant difference between the open and arthroscopic techniques is that the arthroscopic technique does not address existent pathology in the bicipital groove because the biceps is anchored proximal to the groove. In the open procedure the long head of the biceps tendon is completely removed from the groove and secured distally. The decision between tenodesis and tenotomy is made on a patient-by-patient and surgeon-by-surgeon basis. Tenotomy offers a quick return to activities, whereas the young active patient concerned with cosmesis and supination strength will often prefer tenodesis.

A chronically subluxating or dislocating biceps tendon will also often show signs of advanced inflammation or degeneration. There is usually pathology traceable to the rotator interval and rotator cuff tearing, primarily involving the subscapularis. The indications for tenotomy or tenodesis parallel those discussed previously for significant biceps tendinopathy. Additionally, coexistent pathology must be addressed. In a patient with a subscapularis rupture and unstable biceps tendon, the subscapularis can be repaired with consideration given to a biceps tenotomy/tenodesis based on the condition of the tendon. An attempt at relocation of a subluxated or dislocated tendon may be possible if the tendon is still mobile and significant degeneration has not occurred. It is extremely important to repair and tighten the rotator cuff interval in this situation to maintain the position of the tendon in the groove. Recurrent instability, with a resulting stenosed, painful tendon, is a common long-term complication following any procedure that attempts to repair the sling and stabilize the tendon in the groove.

Débridement of the intra-articular portion of the biceps tendon has been suggested for partial tears, including delamination and fraying that involves less then 25% of the tendon in young, active patients or less than 50% of the tendon in older, sedentary patients. Often, this is accompanied by a decompression of subacromial soft tissue alone in younger patients or bursectomy and acromioplasty in older patients. Many authors believe that débridement alone is not effective in eliminating symptoms or preventing eventual biceps rupture; thus biceps tenotomy or tenodesis should be undertaken in these situations.

SLAP tears represent a significant source of shoulder pathology, and the available arthroscopic treatments are based on the type and classification of the pathology. Conservative treatment of SLAP tears has seen limited success with up to 71% of total athletes returning to sports with only 66% returning to overhead sports (Edwards et al. 2010). Although initially reported to be helpful, simple débridement has shown a high rate of failure in

the athletic population unless it is for a Type I lesion (Andrews et al. 1985, Tomlinson and Glousman 1995) and some Type III lesions. Type I lesions can benefit from an arthroscopic débridement when there is substantial degeneration. Symptomatic type II lesions (Fig. 26.6) should be repaired by securing the superior labral complex to the glenoid with any of a variety of techniques; however, especially in less active patients, degenerative type II tears associated with other lesions typically do not require repair. Type III lesions are treated with resection of the unstable labral fragment and repair of the middle glenohumeral ligament if the ligament is attached to the torn fragment. Treatment of type IV tears depends on the extent of biceps tendon involvement and the age of the patient. A type IV SLAP tear includes a bucket handle portion of the labrum that extends into the biceps tendon. If the tendon is not too degenerative and the tear involves less than 30% to 40% of the tendon anchor, the tendon can simply be débrided and the superior labrum either débrided or reattached, provided the flap is large enough. If more than 40% of the tendon is involved, usually a side-to-side repair is performed, where possible, along with treatment of the labrum. Unfortunately revision SLAP repairs have postoperative outcomes that are worse than the primary repair (Park and Glousman 2011).

Distal Biceps

A trial of nonoperative treatment is advocated for patients with partial ruptures and elderly or sedentary patients with limited functional goals. Patients who opt for nonoperative treatment should be advised of a loss of 30% flexion strength and 40% supination strength and 86% decrease in supination endurance. Patients are allowed early active-assisted ROM initiated in the first week after injury. As motion returns to normal, progressive strengthening is advanced as tolerated.

Operative

Distal biceps rupture has become a more commonly recognized and treated entity, with an associated increase in the number of available repair techniques. The chosen repair technique

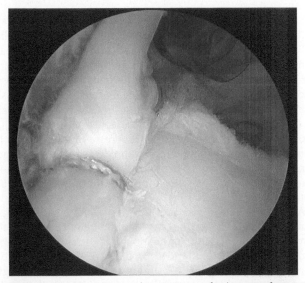

Fig. 26.6 Arthroscopic image demonstrating final repair of a superior labrum anterior posterior (SLAP) 2 lesion; an anchor is used to repair the torn superior labral complex back to the superior glenoid.

reflects specific surgeon choice and the characteristics of the tear. With an acute tear, direct repair is often possible. However, a chronic tear can require soft tissue supplementation. Boyd and Anderson (1961) first reported a two-incision repair technique of an acutely injured tendon. This has been followed by several modifications and the development of a one-incision anterior technique. In the one-incision technique the injured tendon is identified and repaired to the radial tuberosity with a suture anchor, interference screw, or an endobutton. Techniques for chronic ruptures include descriptions of tendon grafting with autogenous semitendinosus, flexor carpi radialis, or allograft Achilles tendon. Furthermore, partial ruptures that do not respond to conservative treatment are also indicated for surgery with detachment and re-repair to the tuberosity. Each method has potential complications. There is a risk of heterotopic ossification development with the two-incision technique; however, many contemporary reports have stated that this can be avoided with meticulous dissection. The anterior approach has an increased risk of radial nerve injury. Regardless, either technique can successfully restore function in a ruptured or torn tendon with high patient satisfaction.

REHABILITATION CONSIDERATIONS
Proximal Biceps

Rehabilitation for Nonoperative Management of Proximal Biceps/SLAP

Nonoperative treatment for proximal biceps pathology can be an effective treatment modality. However, it is necessary to correlate the reported physical impairments and the biceps pathology to ensure that therapy is addressing the correct underlying issue. Then, a treatment plan is developed to specifically focus on the impairments. Typically, the patient is advanced through different phases of rehabilitation, with individual modifications made based on the patient's pain, swelling, or motion.

- Phase I consists of pain management, restoration of full PROM, and restoration of normal accessory motion.
- Phase II consists of AROM exercises and early strengthening.
- Phase III entails rotator cuff and periscapular strength training, with a strong emphasis on enhancing dynamic stability.
- Finally, the return-to-sport phase focuses on power and higher speed exercises similar to sport-specific demands.

However, these phases and individual progression vary among patients. Patients who begin therapy with full passive and active shoulder ROM are able to initiate resistance training on their first visit. Conversely, patients with an acute injury or onset of pain may need to be progressed more slowly. The therapist plays an instrumental role in developing a treatment plan in which the patient is progressed efficiently through the phases of rehabilitation with minimal irritation to the healing tissue.

Any rehabilitation program for a proximal biceps or SLAP injury should also focus on restoring strength to all muscles that provide dynamic stability to the shoulder. Rotator cuff strengthening has been recommended to improve shoulder function following biceps surgery. In addition to a rotator cuff strengthening program, rhythmic stabilization exercises can be used to retrain dynamic stability of the shoulder. Rhythmic stabilization exercises (Video 26.1) should be performed at varying shoulder

and elbow positions because elbow position is thought to affect the function of the biceps at the shoulder.

Last, taking into account the injury mechanism, the therapist should avoid placing the arm in provocative positions. For example, if a compressive force caused the injury, patients should initially refrain from weight bearing. This eliminates further compressive and shear forces on the labrum. An overhead athlete who is suspected of having a "peel back" lesion should not have the arm placed in excessive external rotation, and those with traction injuries should avoid initial heavy eccentric or resisted biceps contractions.

Rehabilitation for Biceps Tenodesis/Tenotomy

Management of biceps tenotomy differs compared to tenodesis. Because there is minimal tissue healing to occur, tenotomy rehabilitation follows the same prescription as that for a tenodesis but can be more aggressive and advance quickly. The primary risk of an aggressive approach is a "Popeye" deformity (Fig. 26.3), which occurs with retraction of the biceps tendon and muscle belly, producing a prominence in the anterior arm. However, this deformity is almost exclusively cosmetic and has not been shown to have an adverse functional consequence.

For a biceps tenodesis a discussion should be had between the surgeon and the therapist with regard to postoperative protocols. As stated earlier, there are numerous techniques for the tenodesis and each may have different rehabilitation requirements. For the biceps tenodesis procedure, the patient is initially instructed on modification strategies to protect the repair, including avoidance of activities that cause contraction of the biceps muscle such as resisted elbow flexion and forearm supination. These motions are typically utilized during activities of daily living including lifting, opening door knobs, or using a screwdriver with the involved extremity.

In conjunction with activity modifications, rehabilitation after a biceps tenodesis will progress through a variety of phases based on the temporal relation to the surgical date. Rehabilitation Protocol 26.1 illustrates the protocol utilized by the senior author for rehabilitation after a subpectoral biceps tenodesis. In parallel to these phases, successful biceps recovery requires the therapist to monitor and control associated pain, swelling, and irritation. Progressively loading a healing tissue can promote soft tissue healing as long as the applied load is appropriate to the patient's stage of healing. Sharma and Maffulli (2006) stated that tendon healing occurs in three broadly overlapping stages. Patients will progress through the stages at different rates. Treatment must be individualized, based on soft tissue healing and the patient's clinical presentation.

Rehabilitation for the Operative Management of SLAP Lesions

Three variables affect the postoperative rehabilitation from a SLAP repair:
1. Type of tear
2. Type of surgical procedure
3. Surgeon preference

In general, there is a period of immobilization followed by progressive ROM exercises and strengthening. The progress through these phases is governed by the patient's response and the procedure completed; a débridement can be more aggressively rehabilitated than a repair. As mentioned earlier, this rehabilitation must be completed in the context of the patient's complete pathology. For example, rehabilitation from a SLAP repair cannot be undertaken at the expense of significant rotator cuff disease.

Débridement is the most common surgical procedure to address symptomatic SLAP lesions. In this case, rehabilitation can be divided into four general phases. The goal of phase I is to attain limited pain-free PROM. In phase II, the patient is progressed to full AROM. Then, phase III consists of the initiation of weight training followed by phase IV and the return to full activity. Specific protocols are listed in Rehabilitation Protocol 26.2.

When surgery is identified as the treatment of choice, postoperative rehabilitation will vary pending surgical findings, including the extent and location of the SLAP lesion, and other concomitant findings and procedures. Patients are led through a similar general rehabilitation as described earlier, yet at a slower pace (Rehabilitation Protocol 26.3). The senior surgeon utilizes a five-phase protocol with phases I and II focused on PROM. Phases III and IV progress through the stages of active-assisted and full AROM, followed by a return to full activities in phase V. Specific protocols are listed in Rehabilitation Protocol 26.3. A more detailed description of SLAP rehabilitation is described by Manske and Prohaska (2010). Overall, each surgeon and injury may require individualized programs, and communication between the treating surgeon and therapist is essential.

Rehabilitation After Distal Biceps Repair

Similar to SLAP repairs, a variety of operative techniques and injury patterns significantly affect the postoperative rehabilitation for distal biceps repair. Again, there are three essential considerations for the rehabilitation program:
1. Type of injury (chronic, acute, or partial rupture)
2. Type of repair (e.g., endobutton, suture anchors, bone tunnels)
3. Surgeon preference

However, all patients will progress through similar stages with different time courses. With all repairs it is necessary to balance the protection of the biceps tendon for soft tissue healing with the need for elbow motion to prevent stiffness. Thus, a chronically ruptured tendon with an allograft supplemented repair may need a more gradual return to full extension than a partial tear that has been repaired with endobutton fixation. For example, Huber (2009) proposed the following protocol as published in *DeLee and Drez's Orthopaedic Sports Medicine* for a two-incision repair with bone tunnels:
- Initial: Splint at 90 degrees
- Weeks 1–8: Active-assisted extension and passive flexion with a 10-degree increase in extension per week. Hinged elbow brace with extension limits
- Weeks 8–12: Discontinue splint with full ROM and progressive resistance training.
- Weeks 12–6 months: Strengthening
- 6 months: Return to play for the athlete

This protocol is more conservative than the procedure described by Greenberg et al. (2003) for a distal biceps tendon repair with a one-incision technique and endobutton fixation. The specifics for this program are listed in Rehabilitation Protocol 26.4, with strengthening beginning at week 6 and full return to play at week 12. These two protocols illustrate the importance of maintaining an open line of communication between the treating surgeon and the therapist.

REHABILITATION PROTOCOL 26.1 ● **Rehabilitation for an Open/Subpectoral Biceps Tenodesis**

Phase I (0–2 weeks)
- Gentle supported Codman exercises three times per day minimum.
- Passive elbow flexion, active wrist ROM, gripping exercises.
- PROM flex to 150 degrees, abduction to 150 degrees, ER to 30 degrees.
  KEY: To avoid stiffness and work on PROM of the shoulder.
  No active elbow flexion or active supination for 4 to 6 weeks.

Phase II (2–4 weeks)
- Full PROM of the shoulder. Start AAROM and AROM.
- Continue sling for up to 3 weeks total.
- Passive elbow ROM for 6 weeks.
- Gentle isometric ER/IR/abduction.
  No active elbow flexion or active supination for 4 to 6 weeks.

Phase III (4–6 weeks)
- Progressive AAROM and AROM, focus on flexion up to 160 degrees. Abduction to 160 and ER increase to 45 degrees (all with arm adducted).
- Begin work on scapular strengthening and RC strengthening program (gentle strengthening at this point)—continue to avoid active biceps exercises.

No active elbow flexion or active supination for 6 weeks.

Phase IV (6–12 weeks)
- Full ROM emphasis.
- Continue with strengthening program.
- Start focus on sport-specific strengthening exercises.
- Begin push-up progression (wall-incline-knees-standard) at 10 weeks.
- Swimming: may get in pool with kickboard only at 3 months.

Phase V (12–16 weeks)
- Continue with sport-specific strengthening exercises.
- Begin plyometrics training program for throwers.
- Advanced proprioceptive training program.
- Sports at 12 to 16 weeks except:
  - Gentle throwing at 3 months.
  - Full velocity throwing at 4 months.
  - Overhead serves (volleyball, tennis) at 4 months (gentle) and 6 months.
- Full overhead activities.
- Swimming: overhead freestyle at 4 months, breaststroke at 3 months.

REHABILITATION PROTOCOL 26.2 ● SLAP Débridement Physical Therapy Protocol

Sling for comfort for 1 to 2 weeks.

Phase I (0–2 weeks)

Aerobic

- Stationary bike for 30 minutes.
- Easy walking on level surface for 30 minutes.

Range of Motion

- Passive forward flexion to 120 degrees.
- Passive motion in scapular plane to 120 degrees.
- Passive external rotation to 20 degrees and abduction to 90 degrees.
- Active wrist range of motion.
- Codman exercises at least three times a day for 5 to 10 minutes.

Strength

- Wrist and grip only.
- Begin isometric exercises (ER/IR/abduction).

Modalities

- IFC and ice for 20 minutes.

Goals to Progress

- Pain-free passive range of motion to limits outlined earlier.

Phase II (2–4 weeks)

Aerobic

- Cross trainer and stationary bike.

Range of Motion

- Progress to active-assisted and active forward flexion to 140 degrees, scapular plane to 140 degrees, abduction to 140 degrees, and external rotation to 45 to 60 degrees.

Strength

- Start light Therabands, Body Blade, and wall push-ups.

Goal to Progress

- AROM 160 forward flexion, scaption, and abduction, 45 to 60 external rotation.

Phase III (4–6 weeks)

Aerobic

- Begin walk–run program.

Range of Motion

- Progress to full range of motion.

Strength

- Start weight training.
- Progress to push-ups, pull-ups (Gravitron).
- Sports-specific training.

Phase IV (6–12 weeks)

Aerobic

- Progress to running on treadmill.

Range of Motion

- Continue to full range of motion.

Strength

- Begin throwing /gym program.
- Posture control.

Goals

- Full range of motion.
- Full strength (rotator cuff and scapula stabilization).
- Able to perform push-up, pull-up, and run.
- Able to return to sports.

REHABILITATION PROTOCOL 26.3 ● SLAP Repair Physical Therapy Protocol

Sling to be worn at all times for 3 weeks.

Phase I (0–2 weeks)

Aerobic

- Stationary bike for 30 minutes.
- Easy walking on level surface for 30 minutes.

Range of Motion

- Passive forward flexion to 150 degrees.
- Passive motion in scapular plane to 120 degrees.
- Passive external rotation to neutral.
- Active wrist range of motion.
- Codman exercises at least three times a day for 5 to 10 minutes.

Strength

- Wrist and grip only.
- No active elbow flexion or supination for 6 weeks.

Modalities

- IFC and ice for 20 minutes.

Goals to Progress

- Pain-free passive range of motion.

Phase II (2–4 weeks)

Aerobic

- Same as previous; progress to 60 minutes.

Range of Motion

- Progress passive forward flexion to 120 to 150 degrees, scapular plane 140 degrees, and abduction 90 degrees.
- Progress passive external rotation from neutral to 20 degrees.

Strength

- Start gentle isometric exercises for extension, external rotation, internal rotation, and abduction.

Goals to Progress

- Passive ROM forward flexion to 150 degrees and external rotation to 45 degrees.
- STOP SLING AT ABOUT 4 WEEKS.

Phase III (4–6 weeks)

Aerobic

- Same as previous to include treadmill for 60 minutes.

REHABILITATION PROTOCOL 26.3 ■ SLAP Repair Physical Therapy Protocol—cont'd

Range of Motion
- Progress to active assisted with wand forward flexion 160 degrees, scapular plane 160, abduction 120 degrees, and ER 45 degrees.
- Progress to active motion.
- Discontinue sling by week 4.

Strength
- Begin gentle scapular strengthening.
- Sideline protraction and retraction of shoulder.
- Shoulder pinches.

Phase IV (6–12 weeks)
Aerobic
- May start elliptical, treadmill at incline, and progress to walk–run for 30 minutes.

Range of Motion
- Progress to full active range of motion.

Strength
- Begin rotator cuff strengthening.
- Begin light Therabands.
- Start Body Blade at neutral.

- Posture control.
- Begin push-up progression.

Goals
- Full range of motion.
- Full strength (rotator cuff and scapula stabilization).

Phase V (>12 weeks)
Aerobic
- Continue progression to running on treadmill.
- Rowing machine.
- Versaclimber.

Range of Motion
- Continue to full ROM.

Strength
- Begin throwing/gym program.
- Sport-specific exercises.

Goal by 4–6 months
- Full range of motion.
- Full strength.
- Able to perform push-up, pull-up, and run.
- Able to return to sports.

REHABILITATION PROTOCOL 26.4 ■ Distal Biceps Repair Rehabilitation

Immediate Postoperative
- Patient placed in splint at 45 degrees.

Week 1 Postoperative
- Orthoplast splint at 45 or 20 degrees depending on pain tolerance.
- Sleep and live in splint. Remove for showering but no use in shower.
- Begin active ROM against gravity only and with assist from opposite arm "within" the splint.

Week 1–4 Postoperative
- If patient has not gotten out to 20 degrees, then continue extension by 10 degrees each week.
- Continue with ROM against gravity.

Week 4 Postoperative
- Continue splint at 20 degrees. May now remove to eat/type/drive.
- Therapy can passive stretch to get to 0 degrees if stiff.
- Begin 5 pounds and advance as tolerated by pain.

Week 6 Postoperative
- Wean out of splint completely.
- Should be working now within 50% to 75% of their "max" of the opposite side.

Week 12
- Return to sport for athlete.

REFERENCES

A complete reference list is available at https://expertconsult .inkling.com/.

FURTHER READING

Bain GI, Johnson LJ, Turner PC. Treatment of partial distal biceps tendon tears. *Sports Med Arthrosc.* 2008;16:154–161.

Burkhart SS, Morgan CD, Kibler WB. The disabled throwing shoulder: spectrum of pathology: part I: pathoanatomy and biomechanics. *Arthroscopy.* 2003;19:404–420.

Clavert P, Bonnomet F, Kempf JF, et al. Contribution to the study of the pathogenesis of type II superior labrum anterior-posterior lesions: a cadaveric model of a fall on the outstretched hand. *J Shoulder Elbow Surg.* 2004;13:45–50.

Fogg QA, Hess BR, Rodgers KG, et al. Distal biceps brachii tendon anatomy revisited from a surgical perspective. *Clin Anat.* 2009;22:346–351.

Forthman CL, Zimmerman RM, Sullivan MJ, et al. Cross-sectional anatomy of the bicipital tuberosity and biceps brachii tendon insertion: relevance to anatomic tendon repair. *J Shoulder Elbow Surg.* 2008;17:522–526.

Greenberg JA, Fernandez JJ, Wang T, et al. EndoButton-assisted repair of distal biceps tendon ruptures. *J Shoulder Elbow Surg.* 2003;12:484–490.

Keener JD, Brophy RH. Superior labral tears of the shoulder: pathogenesis, evaluation, and treatment. *J Am Acad Orthop Surg.* 2009;17:627–637.

Krupp RJ, Kevern MA, Gaines MD, et al. Long head of the biceps tendon pain: differential diagnosis and treatment. *J Orthop Sports Phys Ther.* 2009;39:55–70.

Kuhn JE, Lindholm SR, Huston LJ, et al. Failure of the biceps superior labral complex: a cadaveric biomechanical investigation comparing the late cocking and early deceleration positions of throwing. *Arthroscopy.* 2003;19:373–379.

Rodosky MW, Harner CD, Fu FH. The role of the long head of the biceps muscle and superior glenoid labrum in anterior stability of the shoulder. *Am J Sports Med.* 1994;22:121–130.

Rojas IL, Provencher MT, Bhatia S, et al. Biceps activity during windmill softball pitching: injury implications and comparison with overhand throwing. *Am J Sports Med.* 2009;37:558–565.

Sethi N, Wright R, Yamaguchi K. Disorders of the long head of the biceps tendon. *J Shoulder Elbow Surg.* 1999;8:644–654.

Shepard MF, Dugas JR, Zeng N, et al. Differences in the ultimate strength of the biceps anchor and the generation of type II superior labral anterior posterior lesions in a cadaveric model. *Am J Sports Med.* 2004;32:1197–1201.

Snyder SJ, Karzel RP, Del Pizzo W, et al. SLAP lesions of the shoulder. *Arthroscopy.* 1990;6:274–279.

Verma NN, Drakos M, O'Brien SJ. Arthroscopic transfer of the long head biceps to the conjoint tendon. *Arthroscopy.* 2005;21:764.

Scapular Dyskinesis

W. Ben Kibler, MD | Aaron Sciascia, MS, ATC, NASM-PES | John McMullen, MS, ATC

BACKGROUND

Normal scapulohumeral rhythm, the coordinated movement of the scapula and humerus to achieve shoulder motion, is the key to efficient shoulder function. Scapular position and motion are closely integrated with arm motion to accomplish most shoulder functions. Scapular movement is a composite of three motions: upward/downward rotation around a horizontal axis perpendicular to the plane of the scapula, internal/external rotation around a vertical axis through the plane of the scapula, and anterior/posterior tilt around a horizontal axis in the plane of the scapula. The clavicle acts as a strut for the shoulder complex, connecting the scapula to the central portion of the body. This allows two translations to occur: upward/downward translation on the thoracic wall and retraction/protraction around the rounded thorax.

The scapula has several roles in normal shoulder function. Control of static position and control of the motions and translations allow the scapula to fulfill these roles. In addition to upward rotation, the scapula must also posteriorly tilt and externally rotate to clear the acromion from the moving arm in forward elevation or abduction. Also, the scapula must synchronously internally/externally rotate and posteriorly tilt to maintain the glenoid as a congruent socket for the moving arm and maximize concavity compression and ball and socket kinematics. The scapula must be dynamically stabilized in a position of relative retraction during arm use to maximize activation of all the muscles that originate on the scapula. Finally, it is a link in the kinetic chain of integrated segment motions that starts from the ground and ends at the hand. Because of the important but minimal bony stabilization of the scapula by the clavicle, dynamic muscle function is the major method by which the scapula is stabilized and purposefully moved to accomplish its roles. This dynamic muscle function is possible due to the seventeen muscles that have their origin or insertion onto the scapula (Moore 2010). Muscle activation is coordinated in task-specific force couple patterns to allow stabilization of position and control of dynamic coupled motion.

Alterations in scapular motion and position are termed "scapular dyskinesis" and are present in 67% to 100% of shoulder injuries. One common form of dyskinesis has been described as the "SICK scapula" (Burkhart et al. 2003). This term stands for **S**capular malposition, **I**nferior medial border prominence, **Co**racoid pain and malposition, and dys**K**inesis of scapular movement. Scapular dyskinesis is a nonspecific response to a painful condition in the shoulder rather than a specific response to certain glenohumeral pathology. Scapular dyskinesis has multiple causative factors, both proximally (muscle weakness/imbalance, nerve injury) and distally (AC joint injury, superior labral tears, rotator cuff injury) based. This dyskinesis can alter the roles of the scapula in the scapula-humeral rhythm. It can result from alterations in the bony stabilizers, alterations in muscle activation patterns, or strength in the dynamic muscle stabilizers.

TREATMENT

Scapular rehabilitation is a key component of shoulder rehabilitation and should be instituted early in shoulder rehabilitation—frequently while the shoulder injury is healing. See Rehabilitation Protocol 27.1 for a detailed rehabilitation program.

Treatment of scapular dyskinesis will be successful only if the anatomic base is optimal. The earliest assessments in patients with scapular dyskinesis should evaluate for local problems such as nerve injury or scapular muscle detachment, which will not respond to therapy until they are repaired. Similarly, bony and/or tissue derangement issues such as AC separation, fractured clavicles, labral injury, rotator cuff disease, or glenohumeral instability may require surgical repair before the dyskinesis can be addressed. The large majority of cases of dyskinesis, however, are a result of muscle weakness, inhibition, or inflexibility and can be managed with rehabilitation.

Treating Inflexibilities

Scapular dyskinesis can result from muscle or joint stiffness. Pectoralis minor inflexibility decreases scapular posterior tilt, upward rotation, and external rotation. Glenohumeral internal rotation deficit, which is related to posterior muscle stiffness and capsular tightness, creates dyskinesis by producing a "wind-up" of the scapula into protraction as the arm rotates into follow-through during overhead activities. The "wind-up" can cause impingement symptoms to occur during overhead activities such as the tennis serve and baseball pitch. The utilization of the sleeper and cross-body adduction stretches can help combat tightness of the posterior soft tissue structures. Recently the modified sleeper stretch (Fig. 27.1), modified cross-body horizontal adductions stretch (Fig. 27.2), and horizontal stretch with concomitant internal rotation (Fig. 27.3) have been performed to improve flexibility of the posterior shoulder (Wilk 2013, 2016). The corner or open book stretch can address tightness of the anterior structures. In many overhead athletes the posterior shoulder is subjected to repetitive eccentric loads resulting in capsular stiffness and loss of motion. If there is a capsular stiffness component present, joint mobilizations may be used as a means to help restore glenohumeral joint arthrokinematics. Manske and colleagues have demonstrated that the use of posterior glenohumeral joint mobilizations and cross-arm stretch provide greater gain in motion than cross-arm stretching alone (Manske et al. 2010).

Treating Weakness

In our clinical practice, rehabilitation of the scapula follows a proximal-to-distal perspective. The goal of initial therapy is to achieve the position of optimal scapular function—posterior tilt, external rotation, and upward elevation. Beckett

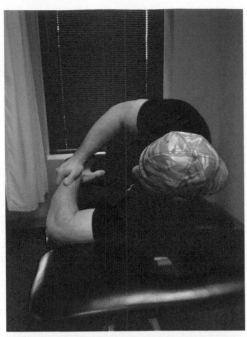

Fig. 27.1 Modified sleeper stretch.

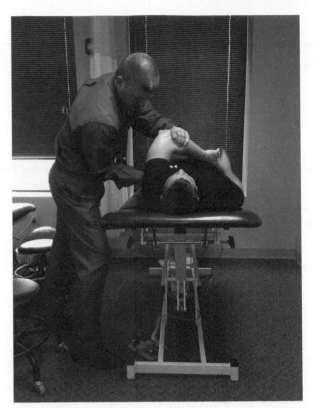

Fig. 27.3 Horizontal adduction with IR.

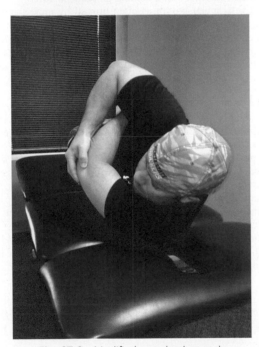

Fig. 27.2 Modified cross-body stretch.

et al. (2014) found an association between scapular dyskinesis and hip abduction weakness. When scapular position and hip strength were examined in preadolescent and adolescent baseball players, a higher rate of scapular dyskinesis was seen in the adolescent group. This same group also had poor outcomes of the single-leg squat test. The use of the single-leg squat test can be compared bilaterally. Excessive lateral trunk displacement, valgus knee collapse, excessive hip flexion, trunk flexion, lateral dropping of the pelvis, and lower extremity pain are indications that weakness or dysfunction is present. The results of Beckett et al. strongly suggest the importance of proximal control of core stability, which leads to control of three-dimensional scapular motion, which is achieved through an integrated rehabilitation regimen where the larger muscles of the lower extremity and trunk are utilized during the treatment of the scapula and shoulder. Hip and trunk flexion help facilitate scapular protraction, whereas hip and trunk extension along with trunk rotation aid in facilitating scapular retraction. It is important to note that if strength or flexibility deficits exist within the proximal segments (core, pelvis, hip, etc.), then they should be addressed prior to treating the scapula and/or shoulder.

The kinetic chain movement patterns are the framework for exercises to strengthen the scapular musculature. The serratus anterior is most important as an external rotator of the scapula, and the lower trapezius acts as a stabilizer of the acquired scapular position. Scapular stabilization protocols should focus on re-educating these muscles to act as dynamic scapula stabilizers first via the implementation of short lever, kinetic chain assisted exercises and progressing to long lever movements. Closed kinetic chain axial loading exercises begin in the early or acute phase to stimulate co-contractions of rotator cuff and scapular musculature and promote scapulohumeral control and GH joint stability. Early axial loading exercises include weight shifts, weight shifts on ball, wall push-ups, and quadruped drills. Axial loading closed kinetic chain drills are performed to stimulate the articular mechanoreceptors and aid in training proprioception (Wilk 2016). Maximal rotator cuff strength is achieved off a stabilized, retracted scapula. Rotator cuff emphasis in rehabilitation should be after scapular control is achieved and should emphasize closed chain, humeral head co-contractions. Increase in impingement pain when doing open chain rotator cuff exercises indicates the wrong emphasis at the wrong stage of the rehabilitation protocol.

A logical progression of exercises (going from isometric to dynamic) focused on strengthening the lower trapezius and serratus anterior while minimizing upper trapezius activation has been described in the literature. All of the exercises may be implemented in a preoperative therapy protocol designed to correct deficits and prepare for postoperative rehabilitation; however, in the event the anatomy needs to be protected, such as after labral or rotator cuff repair, the dynamic exercises can be started later and progressed as healing allows.

Once scapular control is achieved, integrated scapula/rotator cuff exercises that stimulate rotator cuff activation off a stabilized scapula are added. Long lever exercises such as scaption, horizontal abduction with external rotation, and 90/90 external rotation may be implemented during this stage of rehabilitation. The exercises may be done in various planes of abduction and flexion, with different amounts or types of resistance, and may be modified to be sport specific.

REHABILITATION PROTOCOL 27.1 ■ Scapular Dyskinesis

Kibler, Sciascia, and McMullen

Acute Phase (Usually 0–3 weeks)

- Initially, avoid painful arm movement and establish scapular motion.
- Begin soft tissue mobilization, electrical modalities, ultrasound, and assisted stretching, if muscular inflexibility is limiting motion. The pectoralis minor, levator scapulae, upper trapezius, latissimus dorsi, infraspinatus, and teres minor are frequently inflexible as a result of the injury process.
- Use modalities and active, active-assisted, passive, and PNF stretching techniques for these areas.
- Begin upper extremity weight shifts, wobble board exercises, rhythmic ball stabilization, and low row exercise (Figs. 27.4 and 27.5) to promote safe co-contractions.
- Use these closed kinetic chain (CKC) exercises in various planes and levels of elevation, but coordinate them with appropriate scapular positioning.
- Initiate scapular motion exercises without arm elevation.
- Use trunk flexion and forward rotation to facilitate scapular protraction and active trunk extension, backward rotation, and hip extension to facilitate scapular retraction. These postural changes

require that the patient assume a contralateral side-foot-forward stance and actively shift body weight forward for protraction and backward for retraction (Fig. 27.6). Patients who are unable to drive the trunk motion with the hips from this stance may actively stride forward and back with each reciprocal motion.

- Include arm motion with scapular motion exercises because the scapular motion improves to re-establish scapulohumeral coupling patterns. Keep the arm close to the body initially to minimize the intrinsic load.
- Emphasize lower abdominal and hip extensor exercises from the standing position. These muscle groups help stabilize the core and are instrumental in establishing thoracic posture.

Full active scapular motion is often limited by muscular inflexibility and myofascial restrictions. These soft tissue limitations must be alleviated for successful scapular rehabilitation. The pain and restriction of motion associated with these conditions limit progression through rehabilitation and lead to muscular compensation patterns, impingement, and possible GH joint injury.

Recovery Phase (3–8 weeks)

Proximal stability and muscular activation are imperative for appropriate scapular motion and strengthening. Strengthening is dependent on motion, and motion is dependent on posture.

- Continue to emphasize lower abdominal and hip extensor exercises along with flexibility exercises for the scapular stabilizers.
- Increase the loads on CKC exercises such as wall push-ups, table push-ups, and modified prone push-ups.
- Also, increase the level of arm elevation in CKC exercises as scapular control improves.

Position the patient for CKC exercises by placing the hand on a table, wall, or other object and then moving the body relative to the fixed hand to define the plane and degree of elevation. This method

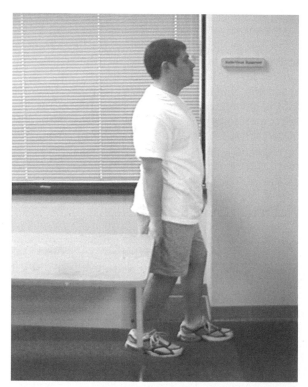

Fig. 27.4 Low row. Axial load with extension muscle activation uses thoracic extension to aid both lower trapezius and serratus anterior activation.

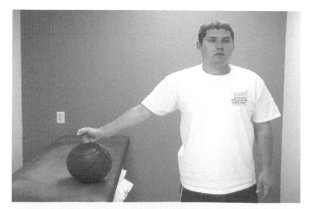

Fig. 27.5 Inferior glide. Isometric "co-contraction" increases the width of the subacromial space by depression of the scapula and humeral head.

REHABILITATION PROTOCOL 27.1 ■ Scapular Dyskinesis—cont'd

assures appropriate scapular position relative to the position of the arm. If the normal scapular positioning cannot be achieved in this manner, the arm position requires adjustment.

- Use diagonal patterns, scapular plane, and flexion to help achieve arm elevation. Progress toward active abduction. If intrinsic loads are too great with the introduction of active elevation, use axially loaded exercises as a transition to open kinetic chain (OKC) exercises. In these exercises, the patient applies a moderate load through the upper extremity, as in the CKC exercises, but also slides the arm into elevation. Wall slides (Fig. 27.7) and table slides are examples. Incorporate trunk and hip motion with these exercises.
- "Open the chain" using short lever, transverse plane movements such as during the lawnmower exercise (Fig. 27.8). The rotary motion helps facilitate scapular retraction and lessens the demand on the shoulder muscles.
- Begin tubing exercises using hip and trunk extension with retraction and hip abduction and trunk flexion with retraction (Figs. 27.9 and 27.10). Use various angles of pull and planes of motion. De-emphasize upward pull until upper trapezius dominance is eliminated.
- As scapulohumeral coupling and control are achieved, dumbbell punches may be introduced. Use complementary strides to incorporate the kinetic chain contribution and reciprocal motions (Fig. 27.11). Vary the height of punches while maintaining scapular control.

Functional Phase (6–10 weeks)

- When there is good scapular control and motion throughout the range of shoulder elevation, initiate plyometric exercises such as medicine ball toss and catch and tubing plyometrics.
- Continue to include kinetic chain activation. Move to various planes as scapular control improves.
- Slow, resisted sport-skill movements, such as the throwing motion, are good activities to promote kinetic chain stabilization while dynamically loading the scapular muscles.
- Overhead movements, in various planes, are advanced exercises requiring good scapular control through a full and loaded GH joint ROM (Figs. 27.12 and 27.13).
- Progressively add external resistance to exercises introduced earlier in the program. The volume of work becomes a progression, as do the difficulty of the exercise and the amount of resistance.
- Challenging lower extremity stability using wobble boards, trampoline, slide boards, and the like also increases the load on the scapular musculature without sacrificing the functional movements.

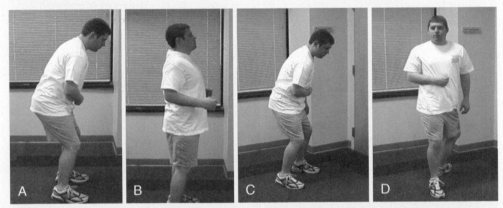

Fig. 27.6 The sternal lift and step-out exercise. In both the sternal lift (A) beginning position, (B) ending position; and the step-out exercise (C) beginning position, (D) ending position; the patient uses the lower extremity in multiple planes to help facilitate scapular retraction and depression.

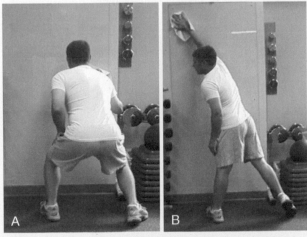

Fig. 27.7 Wall slides. While maintaining an axial load (A), the patient slides the hand in a prescribed pattern (B).

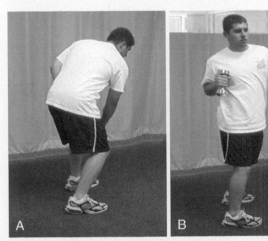

Fig. 27.8 Lawnmower. Progression from isometric exercises (not shown) to dynamic exercises that utilize the transverse plane (A) beginning position, (B) ending position.

Continued

REHABILITATION PROTOCOL 27.1 ■ **Scapular Dyskinesis—cont'd**

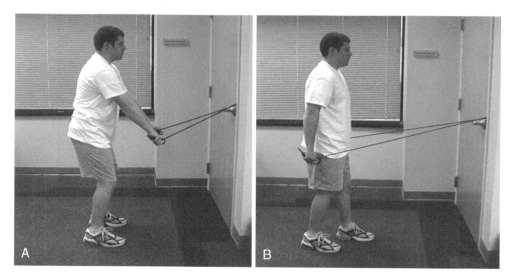

Fig. 27.9 Tubing pulls incorporating trunk and hip extension; (A) beginning position, (B) ending position.

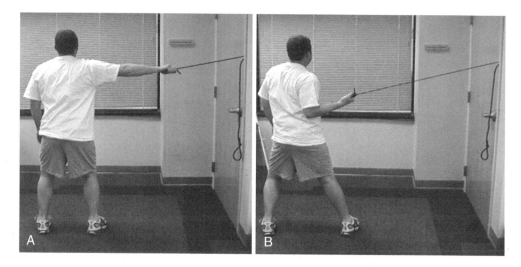

Fig. 27.10 Fencing; (A) beginning position, (B) ending position.

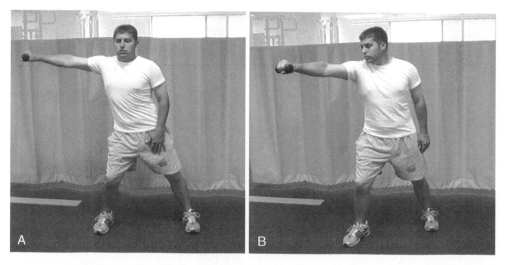

Fig. 27.11 Multidirectional punches; (A) beginning position, (B) ending position.

REHABILITATION PROTOCOL 27.1 ⬤ **Scapular Dyskinesis—cont'd**

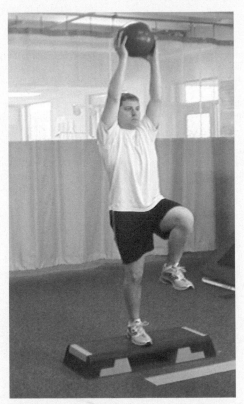

Fig. 27.12 Overhead reach with kinetic chain influence.

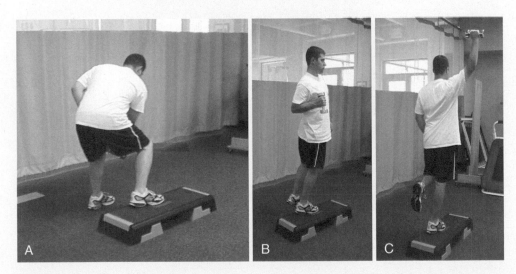

Fig. 27.13 Lawnmower with step-up; (A) beginning position, (B) intermediate position, (C) ending position.

REFERENCES

A complete reference list is available at https://expertconsult.inkling.com/.

FURTHER READING

Borstad JD, Ludewig PM. The effect of long versus short pectoralis minor resting length on scapular kinematics in healthy individuals. *J Orthop Sports Phys Ther*. 2005;35:227–238.

Burkhart SS, Morgan CD, Kibler WB. The disabled throwing shoulder: spectrum of pathology. Part I: pathoanatomy and biomechanics. *Arthroscopy*. 2003;19(4):404–420.

Burkhart SS, Morgan CD, Kibler WB. The disabled throwing shoulder: spectrum of pathology. Part III: the SICK scapula, scapular dyskinesis, the kinetic chain, and rehabilitation. *Arthroscopy*. 2003;19(6):641–661.

Kibler WB. The role of the scapula in shoulder function. *Am J Sports Med*. 1998;26(2):325–337.

Kibler WB, McMullen J, Uhl TL. Shoulder rehabilitation strategies, guidelines, and practice. *Operative Techniques in Sports Medicine*. 2000;8(4):258–267.

Kibler WB, Sciascia A, Dome D. Evaluation of apparent and absolute supraspinatus strength in patients with shoulder injury using the scapular retraction test. *Am J Sports Med*. 2006;34(10):1643–1647.

Kibler WB, Sciascia AD, Uhl TL, et al. Electromyographic analysis of specific exercises for scapular control in early phases of shoulder rehabilitation. *Am J Sports Med*. 2008;36(9):1789–1798.

Kibler WB, Sciascia AD, Wolf BR, et al. Nonacute shoulder injuries. In: Kibler WB, ed. *Orthopaedic Knowledge Update: Sports Medicine*. 4th ed. Rosemont: American Academy of Orthopaedic Surgeons; 2009:19–39.

McClure PM, Michener LA, Sennett BJ, et al. Direct 3-dimensional measurement of scapular kinematics during dynamic movements in vivo. *J Shoulder Elbow Surg*. 2001;10(3):269–277.

Moore KL. *Clinically Oriented Anatomy*. 6th ed. Lippincott Williams & Wilkins Baltimore; 2010.

Smith J, Dietrich CT, Kotajarvi BR, et al. The effect of scapular protraction on isometric shoulder rotation strength in normal subjects. *J Shoulder Elbow Surg*. 2006;15:339–343.

Rehabilitation Following Total Shoulder and Reverse Total Shoulder Arthroplasty

Todd S. Ellenbecker, DPT, MS, SCS, OCS, CSCS | Reg B. Wilcox III, PT, DPT, MS, OCS

INTRODUCTION

Shoulder arthroplasty can be indicated for degenerative and rheumatoid arthritis; fracture management; and conditions such as avascular necrosis, rotator cuff arthropathy, and chondrolysis of the glenohumeral joint. Glenohumeral arthritis results when the joint surfaces are damaged by congenital, metabolic, traumatic, degenerative, vascular, septic, or nonseptic inflammatory factors (Matsen et al. 1998). One of the most common indications for shoulder arthroplasty includes the patient with degenerative osteoarthritis. Degenerative osteoarthritis of the glenohumeral joint is less common than in the weightbearing joints (i.e., hip, knee) of the lower extremity, accounting for only 3% of all osteoarthritis lesions (Badet and Boileau 1995). Osteoarthritis of the glenohumeral joint can be classified as primary or secondary. Primary osteoarthritis usually presents with no apparent antecedent cause, whereas secondary osteoarthritis results from a preexisting problem (i.e., previous fracture, avascular necrosis, "burned-out" rheumatoid arthritis, or crystalline arthropathy).

Wear patterns in the human shoulder vary based on the type of underlying arthritic condition and causation. Characteristic wear of the subchondral bone and glenoid cartilage in the shoulder with degenerative osteoarthritis occurs posteriorly, often leaving an area anteriorly of intact cartilage (Matsen et al. 1998). The cartilage of the humeral head is typically eroded in a pattern of central baldness, the so-called Friar Tuck pattern. This differs from the pattern of humeral head wear in cuff tear arthropathy where a chronic large rotator cuff defect subjects the uncovered humeral head to abrasion against the acromion and coracoacromial arch, resulting in superior rather than central wear patterns.

Another important diagnosis for which shoulder arthroplasty is performed is capsulorrhaphy arthropathy (Parsons et al. 2005). This has resulted in a more common finding of shoulder arthritis in young active patients and often leads to early shoulder arthroplasty (Bailie et al. 2008). Neer et al. (1982) initially reported glenohumeral arthritis after anterior shoulder instability and in 1982 reported on an initial series of 26 patients who had anterior or posterior instability before arthroplasty. Many of the patients in this series had prior stabilization surgery. Samilson and Prieto (1995) later developed the term "dislocation arthropathy" after presenting a series of 74 patients with glenohumeral arthritis with prior anterior and posterior instability.

Neer et al. (1983) further reported on the association of osteoarthritis and glenohumeral instability by finding humerus subluxation in the direction opposite the initial instability as a result of excessive tightening during the initial stabilization surgery. Matsen et al. (1998) coined the term "capsulorrhaphy arthropathy" for patients developing osteoarthritis as a consequence of overly tightened soft tissue structures in the treatment of glenohumeral joint instability. Buscayret et al. (2004) reports the incidence of glenohumeral osteoarthritis to range between 12% and 62% following operative treatment of shoulder instability. Factors specific to stabilization procedures that may contribute to the development of glenohumeral arthritis include encroachment on the articular cartilage by hardware, laterally placed bone block in a Bristow or Latarjet procedure, and excessive soft tissue tensioning imparted by a Putti-Platt procedure (Matsoukis et al. 2003).

SURGICAL ASPECTS OF TOTAL SHOULDER ARTHROPLASTY

In general, surgical considerations for total shoulder arthroplasty (TSA) must first include anatomic joint reconstruction with a well-fixed, stable implant. This is done with either a cementless humeral head resurfacing implant (Fig. 28.1) or a third- or fourth-generation stemmed implant (Fig. 28.2). The ultimate goal is to match the native humeral version, inclination, offset, and height (Matsen et al. 1998). The glenoid then can be resurfaced with a prosthesis or can be managed with a number of nonimplant resurfacing techniques such as interpositional arthroplasty (Ellenbecker et al. 2008). Finally, the soft tissues must be released, balanced, and repaired to allow for adequate restoration of long-term function. The decision whether or not to resurface the glenoid, particularly in young active individuals

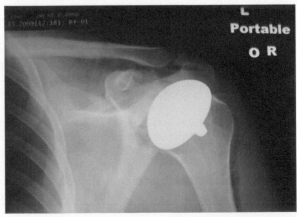

Fig. 28.1 Humeral resurfacing implant.

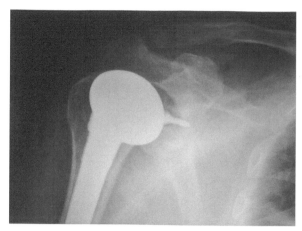

Fig. 28.2   Stemmed humeral implant.

who have early osteoarthritis or complications from chondrolysis or prior instability surgery, is difficult because one of the more common pitfalls of total shoulder arthroplasty is loosening and revision of the glenoid component (Bohsali et al. 2006). In place of a glenoid component for younger patients needing shoulder arthroplasty, other alternatives have been utilized including microfracture, reaming the glenoid to restore version, and bone graft of cysts and defects with biological covering of the glenoid surface (with either autograft or allograft tissue) (Bohsali et al. 2006, Matsen et al. 1998).

Key to the success of arthroplasty in any patient, but especially in those who desire to return to more demanding sports and functional activities, is restoring soft tissue tension. Specifically, a complete 360-degree subscapularis release is needed to increase excursion and restore external rotation. Lengthening the tendon is not needed and will ultimately weaken this structure with the potential for delayed rupture. This release will allow the humeral head to return to the center of the glenoid and permit the normal obligate translation with rotational motion (Matsen et al. 1998). This, in turn, helps to restore the normal glenohumeral forces leading to decreased pain and improved strength and function.

Rehabilitation considerations must take into account the amount of motion obtained under anesthesia after subscapularis closure. This should be communicated to the patient and the therapist. The rehabilitation goal of obtaining normal motion can be achieved in most cases. The subscapularis repair must be sound and protected for the first 6 weeks (limit external rotation to 30 to 45 degrees) (Bailie et al. 2008, Ellenbecker et al. 2008). If a larger rotator cuff repair is performed, these precautions should also be instituted according to the surgeon's confidence in the repair. Full passive motion can be performed to patient tolerance immediately after surgery in ranges of motion other than external rotation (subscapularis precautions) with rapid progression to active-assisted and active during the initial 6 weeks.

The surgical exposure used during shoulder arthroplasty has significant ramifications for the immediate postoperative management. Two approaches are typically used: the deltopectoral approach and anterior–superior or Mackenzie approach (Levy et al. 2004). The skin incision for the anterior–superior approach extends distally in a straight line from the acromioclavicular joint for a distance of 9 cm. The anterior deltoid fibers are split for a distance of not more than 6 cm to protect the axillary nerve.

The acromial attachment of the deltoid is detached to expose the anterior aspect of the acromion. The subscapularis is completely released and held by stay sutures and detached. The long head of the biceps can be dislocated posteriorly over the humeral head as the humeral head is dislocated anteriorly (Levy et al. 2004). The complete release and detachment of the subscapularis with this approach is required to gain exposure for preparation of the humeral head during hemiarthroplasty and during TSA.

SUBSCAPULARIS PRECAUTIONS

For the first 6 weeks postoperatively, subscapularis precautions must be followed. This entails limitation of passive or active external rotation ROM and no active internal rotation resistive exercise. Although gentle attempts at passive external rotation can occur to as far as 30 to 45 degrees of external rotation beyond neutral, techniques that place increased or undue tension on the anterior capsule and subscapularis are avoided. Additional precautions may be needed depending on the repair status of additional rotator cuff tendons at the time of surgery and whether long head bicep tenolysis, tenodesis, or tenotomy has been performed. Specifically, resistive exercises for the biceps brachii are not performed for the first 6 weeks postoperatively if a release of the biceps long head or tenodesis has been performed to minimize the chance of rerupture and reappearance of a "Popeye" deformity. Because it is beyond the scope of this chapter to completely discuss the entire rehabilitation process following TSA, the complete details of the authors' postoperative protocol are summarized in Rehabilitation Protocol 28.1.

KEY REHABILITATION CONCEPTS FOLLOWING TSA

The concept of obligate translation has been applied extensively in orthopedic and sports physical therapy and in orthopedics in general since the publication of Harryman et al. (1990), identifying an increase in anterior humeral head translation and shear following a controlled posterior capsular plication in cadaveric specimens. Obligate translation, defined as the translation of the humeral head in the direction opposite of the tight capsule and soft tissue structures, has been a paramount concept applied in the treatment of the overhead athlete with subtle anterior GH joint instability secondary to adaptive posterior rotator cuff and posterior capsule tightness (Grossman et al. 2005). Harryman et al. (1990) also reported the presence of obligate translation in flexion, internal and external rotation, and maximal elevation with shoulder arthroplasty following insertion of an oversized humeral head prosthesis. Shoulder arthroplasty can cause global capsular restriction as a result of the substitution of a humeral head prosthesis for a degenerative and collapsed humeral head. This overstuffing can prohibit return of optimal ROM unless adequate capsular release and early postoperative physical therapy to address capsular tightness are followed (Wirth and Rockwood 1996). Fig. 28.3 demonstrates the concept of obligate translation.

The restoration of optimal muscle balance is imperative during the rehabilitation of all shoulder injury and pathologies; however, it is particularly important following shoulder arthroplasty. Fig. 28.4 shows the effect of unbalanced muscular forces during shoulder muscular contraction and volitional movement. Unbalanced internal rotation strength or dominant anterior muscular strength development can lead to anterior

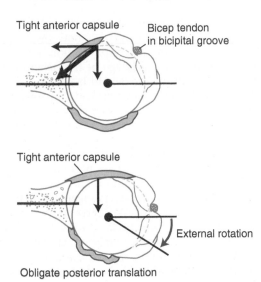

Fig. 28.3 Obligate translation. (Redrawn with permission from Rockwood C, Matsen F, Wirth M, Harryman D: The Shoulder, 2nd ed. Philadelphia, WB Saunders, 1998.)

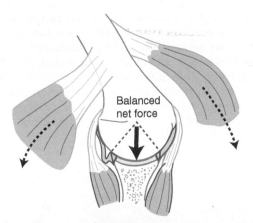

Fig. 28.4 Muscular balance. (Redrawn with permission from Rockwood C, Matsen F, Wirth M, Harryman D: The Shoulder, 2nd ed. Philadelphia, WB Saunders, 1998.)

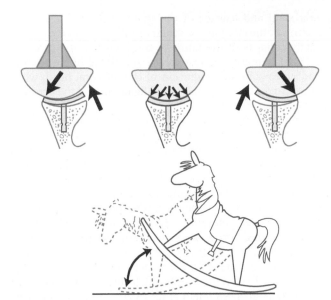

Fig. 28.5 Rocking horse phenomenon. (Redrawn with permission from Rockwood C, Matsen F, Wirth M, Harryman D: The Shoulder, 2nd ed. Philadelphia, WB Saunders, 1998.)

translation of the humeral head relative to the glenoid (Levy et al. 2004). Likewise, excessive posterior development could accentuate posterior subluxation from an eroded posterior glenoid and overly tight anterior structures (obligate translation) and produce posterior instability.

Optimal muscle balance between the external rotators (ER) and internal rotators (IR) has been reported and recommended in the range between 66% and 75% ER/IR (Ivey et al. 1984). This can be assessed with a handheld dynamometer or isometric function of an isokinetic dynamometer system to ensure proper restoration of muscle balance. Patients frequently present with overly dominant anterior muscular strength, which can jeopardize GH mechanics and lead to complications and functional impairment. Fig. 28.5 shows the "rocking horse" phenomenon, which can lead to implant loosening, one of the most frequently encountered complications following TSA (Bohsali et al. 2006, Matsen et al. 1998). Restoration of proper muscular balance via monitoring and addressing the ER/IR strength ratio and the use of ROM and GH mobilization techniques during postoperative rehabilitation ensure proper capsular excursion and minimize the effect from obligate translation and form the essential tenets of postsurgical management of the patient following shoulder arthroplasty.

OUTCOMES OF TRADITIONAL SHOULDER ARTHROPLASTY

Shoulder arthroplasty remains the definitive option for the treatment of GH arthritis. Humeral head replacement (HHR) or hemiarthroplasty and TSA are traditional options in cases of advanced arthrosis. No overall consensus has been reached regarding performance of either procedure—HHR or TSA. Both procedures have been reported to provide significant pain relief and successful outcomes (Edwards et al. 2003, Neer 1990). Several reported results favor TSA regarding pain relief and both stability and functional improvement (Bishop and Flatow 2005, Bohsali et al. 2006, Edwards et al. 2003, Gartsman et al. 2000). However, because of the possibility of glenoid loosening, leading to revision procedures in long-term TSA follow-up (Antuna et al. 2001, Bohsali et al. 2006, Sperling et al. 2002, Torchia et al. 1997), many surgeons suggest hemiarthroplasty in young patients with higher levels of physical activity with an intact rotator cuff and adequate glenoid bone stock (Bailie et al. 2008, Burkhead and Hutton 1995).

Sperling et al. (2002) reported results from patients younger than 50 with GH arthrosis undergoing HHR and Neer's TSA. The follow-up at 15 years confirmed pain relief and motion improvement in both situations. Furthermore, survival rates reached 82% at 10 years and 75% at 20 years in patients with HHR and 97% and 84% in patients with TSA. However, when using a modified Neer outcome rating system assessing patients' daily performance ability, results were not satisfactory in 60% of those who had undergone HHR nor in 48% of those who had undergone TSA. Additional information on complications and outcomes following HHR and TSA can be found in a current concepts review published by Bohsali et al. (2006).

REVERSE TSA

Cuff tear arthropathy (CTA), first described by Neer (1983, 1990), is explained as severe humeral head collapse following massive tearing of the rotator cuff (RC) with instability of the humeral head and leakage of the synovial fluid. The result is destruction of the GH joint articular cartilage, osteoporosis, and ultimately collapse of the humeral head. Hence, the centering forces of the humerus are absent, altering GH joint biomechanics, leading to superior migration of the humeral head, which over time erodes the coracoacromial ligament and the acromioclavicular joint (Fig. 28.6).

Outcomes of those with CTA having undergone a TSA have not been uniform (Arntz et al. 1991, Field et al. 1997, Levy and Copeland 2001, Sanchez-Sotelo et al. 2001, Sarris et al. 2003, Williams and Rockwood 1996, Zuckerman et al. 2000). Given that the joint mechanics are compromised, the use of a TSA prosthesis often results in suboptimal outcomes as a result of continued humeral head superior migration with glenoid loading during shoulder elevation. This glenoid loading leads to excessive shearing forces with resultant glenoid component loosening (Franklin et al. 1988). Hence, hemiarthroplasty (HA) had become the standard surgical intervention for CTA. However, outcomes have been limited in terms of pain relief and ROM (Arntz et al. 1993, Field et al. 1997, Williams and Rockwood 1996, Zuckerman et al. 2000). The inverse or reverse total shoulder arthroplasty (rTSA), first described by Grammont et al. (1993), has become the leading treatment option for those requiring a shoulder replacement for the treatment of GH arthritis with concomitant CTA, with complex fractures, or for the revision of a previously failed RC-deficient TSA (Rehabilitation Protocol 28.2). The rTSA prosthesis reverses the orientation of the shoulder joint by replacing the glenoid fossa with a glenoid base plate and glenosphere and the humeral head with a shaft and concave cup (Fig. 28.7). This prosthesis design alters the center of rotation of the shoulder joint by moving it medially and inferiorly. This subsequently increases the deltoid moment arm and deltoid tension, which enhances both the torque produced by the deltoid and the line of pull/action of the deltoid. This enhanced mechanical advantage of the deltoid compensates for the deficient RC as the deltoid becomes the primary elevator of the shoulder joint (Kontaxis and Johnson 2009, Terrier et al. 2008). In addition, it has been shown that the stability of the replaced joint is primarily maintained by compressive muscular forces (Gutierrez et al. 2008).

Outcomes regarding pain relief and functional gains for the treatment of CTA with rTSA have been good (Boileau et al. 2009, Boulahia et al. 2002, Grammont and Baulot 1993, Rittmeister and Kerschbaumer 2001, Weissinger et al. 2008). Typically patients regain in excess of 105 degrees of active shoulder elevation (Boileau et al. 2006, Boileau et al. 2005, Boulahia et al. 2002, DeButtet et al. 1997, Frankle et al. 2005, Sirveaux et al. 2004). These results are superior to those of HA for CTA (Arntz et al. 1993, Field et al. 1997, Sanchez-Sotelo et al. 2001, Williams and Rockwood 1996, Zuckerman et al. 2000). Active shoulder rotation has not been reported to improve following rTSA. Those patients with teres minor deficiency, in particular, have markedly limited active external rotation following rTSA (Boileau et al. 2005). It is critical to realize that the complication rate of this procedure varies greatly from 10% to 47% with dislocation rates between 0% to 9% (Boileau et al. 2006, Cuff et al. 2008, Deshmukh et al. 2005, Edwards et al. 2009, Frankle et al. 2005, Guery et al. 2006, Levy et al. 2007, Sirveaux et al. 2004, Werner et al. 2005). Common complications include, but are not limited to, component instability or dislocation, nerve damage, intraoperative fracture, infection, hematoma, and hardware failure.

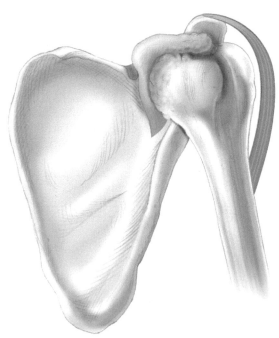

Fig. 28.6 Anterior–posterior illustration of a left shoulder with rotator cuff arthropathy. The superiorly shifted humeral head indicates rotator cuff deficiency. (Reprinted with permission of the Orthopaedic and Sports Physical Therapy Sections of the American Physical Therapy Association. Boudreau S, Boudreau E, Higgins LD, Wilcox RB: Rehabilitation following reverse total shoulder arthroplasty. *J Orthop Sports Phys Ther.* 2007;37(12):735–744. DOI: 10.2519/jospt.2007.2562.)

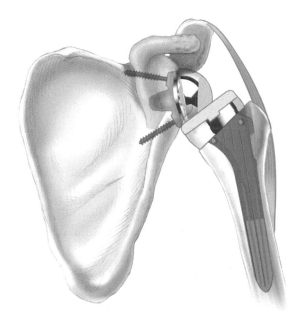

Fig. 28.7 Anterior–posterior illustration of a left shoulder after reverse total shoulder arthroplasty. The prosthesis reverses the orientation of the shoulder joint by replacing the glenoid fossa with a glenoid base plate and glenosphere and the humeral head with a shaft and concave cup. This enhances the mechanical advantage of the deltoid and compensates for the deficient rotator cuff. (Reprinted with permission of the Orthopaedic and Sports Physical Therapy Sections of the American Physical Therapy Association. Boudreau S, Boudreau E, Higgins LD, Wilcox RB: Rehabilitation following reverse total shoulder arthroplasty. *J Orthop Sports Phys Ther.* 2007;37(12):735–744. DOI: 10.2519/jospt.2007.2562.)

Collaboration between the surgeon and physical therapist is essential to ensure appropriate rehabilitation for a patient following rTSA. Therapists need to be aware of the patient's preoperative shoulder status, type of implant used, the glenoid and humeral bone quality, the integrity of the remaining or repaired RC, and the overall component stability at the time of surgical reconstruction to optimize rehabilitation. **Three key postoperative rehabilitation concepts should be considered when outlining the care for a patient following rTSA: joint protection, deltoid function, and establishing appropriate functional and ROM expectations.**

In terms of joint protection, postoperative positioning and initial activity are based on the fact that there is a higher risk of shoulder dislocation following rTSA than TSA. Patients who dislocate their rTSA do it with internal rotation and adduction in conjunction with extension. This position allows the prosthesis to escape anteriorly and inferiorly. **Functional activities such as tucking in a shirt and reaching behind one's hip and lower back are predominantly dangerous activities, particularly in the immediate postoperative phase.**

Enhancement of deltoid function following rTSA is the most important rehabilitation concept of the postoperative strengthening phase of recovery. Stability and mobility of the shoulder joint are now largely dependent on the deltoid and periscapular musculature. A number of patients demonstrate great difficulty in adequately recruiting their deltoid; the routine use of biofeedback (verbal and tactile cues, surface electromyography, and rehabilitative ultrasound imaging) to assist patients in learning recruitment strategies is beneficial. On completion of a successful rehabilitation program clinicians will likely find that the operative upper extremity will demonstrate much higher deltoid recruitment when compared to the contralateral shoulder.

The expectation for functional and ROM gains should be individually set depending on underlying pathology, the status of the ERs, and the extent to which the deltoid and periscapular musculature can be rehabilitated. There is a wide variance in functional and ROM outcomes following rTSA; therefore, patients must be reminded that their shoulder mechanics and function will have some limitations when compared to their unaffected shoulder. Patients with more active lifestyles typically will require additional education regarding their restrictions to ensure proper longevity of their new prosthesis and to minimize their risk for dislocation. Those patients who have a negative external rotation lag sign during the initial strengthening phase of rehabilitation progress quicker and tend to demonstrate better elevation ROM. Meticulous preoperative evaluation to assess the capacity of the posterior RC to actively externally rotate the humerus has a profound effect on the overall function after rTSA. Active forward elevation without external rotation may create a markedly dysfunctional upper extremity and lead to poor patient satisfaction, regardless of the intensity and effort of the patient and physical therapist postoperatively. Significant external rotation weakness should compel the surgeon to strongly consider a concomitant latissimus dorsi tendon transfer.

Because the RC is deficient and the potential for complications is higher with an rTSA, the rehabilitation course should be different from the rehabilitation following a TSA (Boudreau et al. 2007). Each rehabilitation phase is structured based on postoperative timelines that respect healing and soft tissue parameters in conjunction with intraoperative/postoperative findings, clinical presentation, and achievement of clinical goals/milestones.

PHASE I—IMMEDIATE POSTSURGICAL/JOINT PROTECTION PHASE

Goals during phase I are to maintain the integrity of the replaced joint while restoring passive ROM. Frequent cryotherapy during phase I is recommended to assist in the control of pain, minimize swelling and muscle spasm, and suppress inflammation (Singh et al. 2001). For patients having a primary rTSA with a traditional deltopectoral approach passive range of motion (PROM) may begin after the effects of the intrascalene block have resolved to ensure proper deltoid function and to make certain the patient's sensory feedback mechanisms are intact. Elevation in the plane of the scapula is gradually increased as tolerated to 90 degrees. Pure abduction is avoided because it places undue stress on the acromion. Passive external rotation should be progressed to approximately 20 to 30 degrees while in the scapular plane. In cases where the subscapularis was repaired, external rotation ROM parameters may need to be adjusted to avoid placing undue stress on the repair. Because of the complication of possible dislocation as the result of impaired shoulder stability from the deficient RC, it is recommended that no internal rotation ROM is performed for the first 6 postoperative weeks. Submaximal pain-free deltoid isometrics and periscapular isometrics with the humerus protected in the scapular plane should begin around postoperative day 4. Given that there is minimal to no intact RC following rTSA, the deltoid and periscapular musculature are the primary dynamic restraints, stabilizers, and movers of the GH joint. Beginning deltoid and periscapular isometrics will assist in restoring initial deltoid function and provide stability to the GH joint. Avoidance of shoulder hyperextension while performing posterior deltoid isometrics is critical to minimize the risk of dislocation.

During the third through the sixth postoperative weeks the initial postsurgical phase activities are advanced based on the clinical progression and presentation of the patient. As initial soft tissue healing occurs and the patient's sensory feedback improves, it allows a safer progression of passive elevation in the scapular plane to 120 degrees and then progresses to tolerance, typically up to 140 degrees by the sixth postoperative week. Based on reported outcomes of patients following rTSA, up to 138 degrees of active elevation should be expected (Boileau et al. 2005, Boulahia et al. 2002, Frankle et al. 2005, Werner et al. 2005). Passive external rotation ROM may gradually be progressed to 30 to 45 degrees, while respecting the soft tissue constraints of the subscapularis if repaired. The initiation of passive internal rotation may begin during the sixth postoperative week and should only be completed in a protected position of at least 60 degrees of abduction in the scapular plane to ensure avoidance of internal rotation with adduction.

Shoulder immobilization in an abduction-type sling, which supports the humerus in the position of the scapular plane (30 degrees of elevation and abduction) for the first 3 to 4 weeks, except during therapy, bathing, and home exercises, is recommended (Grammont and Baulot 1993). **The important concept to adhere to regarding positioning following rTSA is that the patients "should always be able to visualize their elbow regardless of what they are doing."** This positioning will assist in avoiding shoulder extension and adduction. In addition, when patients are out of the immobilizer they should be advised not to reach across their abdomen/chest wall with their operative upper extremity because this involves combined internal rotation with adduction and again increases the risk of dislocation. When the posterior cuff has been surgically repaired, its tendon quality is poor, and when the posterior capsule tissue integrity is determined to be compromised as assessed during intraoperative inspection, it is advantageous to use an external rotation immobilizer such as the Donjoy Ultrasling 15-degree ER sling (dj Orthopedics, Vista, CA) or a rigid Gunslinger Brace (Patterson Medical/Sammons Preston, Bolingbrook, IL). Having the upper extremity in 15 degrees of external rotation in the scapular plane provides an enhanced opportunity for the posterior RC to heal in a relatively shortened position during the crucial early postoperative tissue healing phase.

Patients who have required rTSA for a revision of a failed conventional TSA will generally require a longer immobilization (3–6 weeks) postoperatively. The surgical approach needs to be considered when devising the postoperative plan of care. Traditionally rTSA procedure is performed via a deltopectoral approach (Seebauer et al. 2005), which minimizes surgical trauma to the anterior deltoid; however, some surgeons will use a superior approach, retracting the anterior deltoid from the anterior lateral one-third of the clavicle. In these cases, early deltoid activity is contraindicated and patients should progress through delayed protocol to ensure adequate deltoid healing.

PHASE II—ACTIVE RANGE OF MOTION/EARLY STRENGTHENING PHASE (WEEKS 6 TO 12)

Phase II consists of the progression from PROM to active-assisted/active range of motion (AAROM/AROM) and the initiation of strengthening with the primary focus of restoring dynamic shoulder stability and enhanced mechanics. Previously stated dislocation precautions should continue to be enforced. AAROM/AROM elevation should be initiated supine where the scapula is stabilized. These activities are then progressed to more functional and dynamically challenging positions, such as inclined elevation (i.e., 30, 45, and 60 degrees of elevation), then full sitting and standing.

Close monitoring of the patient's tolerance for activity and AROM progression is crucial. One complication that some patients encounter when progressing from their immobilization phase of rehabilitation toward AROM and functional activities is a stress fracture of the acromion (Walch et al. 2009). The deltoid is tensioned as the result of the rTSA procedure, and because it is now the primary shoulder elevator, there is a high amount of force generated at the bone muscle interface of the acromion and deltoid. This factor coupled with traditional risk factors for fractures such as osteoporosis, history of steroid use, and lengthy immobilization has lead to two of our patients developing an acromial stress fracture. These fractures typically present insidiously after gaining initial AROM and functional independence, followed by a rapid decline in AROM

tolerance, pain to palpation of the acromion, no loss in PROM, pain with resisted deltoid activation, and negative radiograph imaging. Conservative management is recommended for the treatment of nondisplaced acromial stress fractures following rTSA. AROM elevation and deltoid activity should be discontinued for 4 to 6 weeks or until pain has subsided. The modified therapy program should focus on maintaining PROM and restoring IR and ER strength. It may take up to 3 months for a nondisplaced acromial stress fracture to heal. Close monitoring of the patient's status is suggested to ensure acromion displacement does not occur. If displacement occurs, surgical intervention may be indicated.

AAROM/AROM IR and ER are initiated and progressed similarly, yet rotation movements should still be completed in the scapular plane. The initiation of IR and ER submaximal isometrics is typically delayed until week 8 postoperatively to respect the soft tissue integrity of the teres minor and subscapularis if repaired. Typically the infraspinatus is irreparable and the teres minor is intact.

Initiation of isotonic strengthening should only commence in the presence of adequate mechanics and acceptable AROM of the GH and scapulothoracic joints. If isotonic strengthening is initiated before proper mechanics are established, such activity may reinforce poor mechanics and potentially lead to undue soft tissue stress. When starting isotonic strengthening, a low-weight, high-repetition program is recommended. The utilization of a deltoid strengthening lawn chair progression program, starting the patient in supine and gradually increasing the incline of the surface to ultimately perform the exercises in sitting, is a useful progression technique. Patients can progress through graduated inclines with shoulder elevation and forward reach activities.

PHASE III—MODERATE STRENGTHENING (WEEK 12+)

Phase III is initiated when the patient demonstrates appropriate PROM/AAROM/AROM and is able to isotonically activate each portion of the deltoid and periscapular musculature while demonstrating appropriate shoulder mechanics. The patient should be able to tolerate resistive strengthening of the elbow, wrist, and hand of the operative upper extremity. The primary goals of phase III are to advance strengthening and increase functional independence while maintaining appropriate pain-free shoulder mechanics. Dislocation precautions should continue to be followed for all static and dynamic activities. All strengthening exercises should be based on the principles of low weight and high repetitions to enhance shoulder endurance and minimize the risk of injury/dislocation. Most patients following rTSA have achieved functional strength gains by following progressive resisted exercises up to 1.36 kg (3 lbs) based on DeLorme's (Bayley and Kessel 1982) principles of progressive resistive exercise. Sudden lifting, pushing, and jerking motions should be avoided indefinitely to minimize the risk of injury/dislocation.

PHASE IV—CONTINUED HOME PROGRAM (TYPICALLY 4+ MONTHS)

Phase IV commences when the patient has been discharged from skilled physical therapy and is continuing with a home exercise program. To enter phase IV, the patient should be able to demonstrate functional pain-free shoulder AROM and should be independent with an appropriate strengthening program. Ultimate postoperative shoulder ROM is typically 80 to 120 degrees of elevation with functional ER up to 30 degrees. Functional use of the operative shoulder is demonstrated by a return to light household, work, and leisure activities as recommended by the patient's surgeon and physical therapist. Typically, a 4.5- to 6.8-kg (10- to 15-lb) bilateral upper extremity lifting capacity should be followed indefinitely to ensure the operative shoulder is not strained beyond its structural integrity.

SUMMARY

The role of rTSA in the management of CTA is clinically sound as it alters the mechanics of the shoulder to enhance deltoid function in the absence of a competent RC. Hence, the postoperative course for a patient following rTSA is different from the rehabilitation following a traditional TSA. The physical therapist, surgeon, and patient should work together when establishing the postoperative rehabilitation plan focused on joint protection, deltoid function, and the establishment of appropriate functional and measurable goals.

REHABILITATION PROTOCOL 28.1 ● Rehabilitation Following GH Joint Arthroplasty

General Guidelines

- Sling use and duration directed by surgeon in postoperative instructions
- Immediate postoperative passive and active-assistive ROM consisting of stomach rubs, sawing movements, and elbow ROM instructed following hospital discharge

Postoperative Weeks 1–4

- Modalities to decrease pain and inflammation
- Passive range of motion initiated with no limitation in flexion, abduction, or internal rotation. NO EXTERNAL ROTATION stretching against tension or anterior capsular mobilization in this rehabilitation phase to protect the subscapularis repair. Movement and ROM into 30 to 45 degrees of external rotation are allowed with 30 to 45 degrees of abduction by the therapist provided it is not against tension.
- Elbow, wrist, and forearm ROM/stretching
- Manually applied scapular resistive exercise for protraction/retraction and submaximal biceps/triceps manual resistance with shoulder in supported position supine
- Ball approximation (closed chain Codman's) using Swiss ball or table top

Postoperative Weeks 2–4

- Initiation of active-assistive ROM using pulley for sagittal plane flexion and scapular plane elevation

Postoperative Weeks 4–6

- Continuation of previously outlined program
- Initiation of submaximal multiple angle isometrics and manual resistive exercise for shoulder external rotation, abduction/adduction, and flexion/extension

- Upper body ergometer (UBE)
- External rotation isotonic exercise using pulley or weight/tubing with elbow supported and GH joint in scapular plane and 10 to 20 degrees of abduction (towel roll or pillow under axilla)

Postoperative Weeks 6–8

- Initiation of passive external rotation range of motion and stretching beyond neutral rotation position
- Initiation of internal rotation submaximal resistive exercise progression
- Traditional rotator cuff isotonic exercise program
  - Side-lying external rotation
  - Prone extension
  - Prone horizontal abduction (limited from neutral to scapular plane position initially with progression to coronal plane as ROM improves)
- Biceps/triceps curls in standing with GH joint in neutral resting position
- Oscillation exercise with resistance bar or Body Blade
- Rhythmic stabilization in open and closed kinetic chain environments

Postoperative Weeks 8–12

- Continuation of resistive exercise and ROM progressions
- Addition of ball dribbling and upper body plyometrics with small Swiss ball

Postoperative Weeks 12–24

- Continuation of rehabilitation
- Isometric internal/external rotation strength testing/assessment in neutral scapular plane position
- Subjective rating scale completion
- ROM assessment

REHABILITATION PROTOCOL 28.2 ● Reverse TSA Protocol

Dislocation Precautions

- NO combined shoulder adduction, internal rotation, and extension

Phase I: Immediate Postsurgical Phase/Joint Protection (Day 1–6 weeks)

Goals

- Patient and family independent with:
  - Joint protection
  - Passive range of motion (PROM)
  - Assisting with don/doff sling and clothing
- Promote healing of soft tissue/maintain the integrity of the replaced joint.
- Enhance PROM.
- Restore active range of motion (AROM) of elbow/wrist/hand.
- Independent with activities of daily living (ADLs) with modifications

Phase I Precautions

- Sling is worn for 3 to 4 weeks. May be extended longer for revision surgery
- While supine, the humerus is supported by a towel roll to avoid shoulder extension.
- No shoulder AROM. No lifting of objects with operative extremity; no supporting of body weight with involved extremity

Acute Care Therapy (Days 1–4)

- Begin PROM in supine after complete resolution of interscalene block.
  - Elevation in the scapular plane in supine to 90 degrees
  - External rotation (ER) in scapular plane to available ROM as indicated by operative findings. Typically around 20 to 30 degrees
  - NO INTERNAL ROTATION (IR) ROM

Continued

REHABILITATION PROTOCOL 28.2 ● Reverse TSA Protocol—cont'd

- Active/active-assisted ROM (A/AAROM) of cervical spine, elbow, wrist, and hand
- Begin periscapular submaximal pain-free isometrics in the scapular plane.
- Frequent cryotherapy

Days 5–21

- Continue all exercises and cryotherapy as outlined earlier.
- Begin submaximal pain-free deltoid isometrics in scapular plane (avoid shoulder extension when isolating posterior deltoid).

Weeks 3–6

- Progress with previous exercises and continue with cryotherapy.
  - Elevation in the scapular plane in supine to 120 degrees
  - ER in scapular plane to tolerance, respecting soft tissue constraints
- At 6 weeks postoperative start PROM IR to tolerance (not to exceed 50 degrees) in the scapular plane.
- Resisted exercise of elbow, wrist, and hand

Criteria for Progression to the Next Phase (Phase II)

- Tolerates shoulder PROM and AROM program for elbow, wrist, and hand
- Patient demonstrates the ability to isometrically activate all components of the deltoid and periscapular musculature.

Phase II: Active Range of Motion/Early Strengthening Phase (Weeks 6–12)

Goals

- Continue progression of PROM (full PROM is not expected).
- Gradually restore AROM.
- Control pain and inflammation.
- Allow continued healing of soft tissue/do not overstress healing tissue.

Precautions

- Continue to avoid shoulder hyperextension.
- In the presence of poor shoulder mechanics, avoid repetitive shoulder AROM.
- No lifting of objects heavier than a coffee cup or supporting of body weight with upper extremity (UE)

Weeks 6–8

- Continue with PROM program.
- Begin shoulder AAROM/AROM as appropriate.
  - Elevation in scapular plane with varying degrees of trunk elevation as appropriate (i.e., start with supine lawn chair progression with progression to sitting/standing)
  - ER and IR in the scapular plane in supine with progression to sitting/standing
- Begin GH IR and ER submaximal pain-free isometrics.
- Initiate scapulothoracic rhythmic stabilization and alternating iso-

metrics in supine as appropriate. Begin periscapular and deltoid submaximal pain-free isotonic exercises.
- Progress strengthening of elbow, wrist, and hand.
- GH and scapulothoracic joint mobilizations as indicated (Grade I and II)
- Continue use of cryotherapy as needed.
- Patient may begin to use hand of operative UE for feeding and light ADLs.

Weeks 9–12

- Continue with previous exercises and functional activity progression.
- Begin isotonic elevation in the plane of the scapula with light weights (1 to 3 pounds or 0.5 to 1.4 kg) at varying degrees of trunk elevation as appropriate (i.e., start with supine lawn chair progression with progression to sitting/standing).
- Progress to GH IR and ER isotonic strengthening exercises.

Criteria for Progression to the Next Phase (Phase III)

- Improving function of shoulder
- Patient can isotonically activate all components of the deltoid.

Phase III: Moderate Strengthening (Weeks 12+)

Goals

- Enhance functional use of operative extremity and advance functional activities.
- Enhance shoulder mechanics, muscular strength, power, and endurance.

Precautions

- No lifting of objects heavier than 6 pounds (2.7 kg) with the operative upper extremity
- No sudden lifting or pushing activities

Weeks 12–16

- Continue with the previous program as indicated.
- Progress to resisted elevation in standing as appropriate.

Phase IV: Continued Home Program (Typically 4+ months postoperative)

- Typically the patient is on a home exercise program at this stage to be performed three to four times per week with the focus on:
  - Continued strength gains.
  - Continued progression toward a return to functional and recreational activities within limits as identified by progress made during rehabilitation and outlined by surgeon and physical therapist.
- Criteria for discharge from skilled therapy:
  - Patient is able to maintain pain-free shoulder AROM demonstrating proper shoulder mechanics (typically 80 to 120 degrees of elevation with functional ER of about 30 degrees).
  - Typically able to complete light household and work activities

REFERENCES

A complete reference list is available at https://expertconsult .inkling.com/.

FURTHER READING

DeLorme T, Wilkins AL. *Progressive Resistance Exercise*. New York: Appleton-Century-Crofts; 1951.

Ellenbecker TS, Davies GJ. The application of isokinetics in testing and rehabilitation of the shoulder complex. *J Athl Train*. 2000;35(3):338–350.

Lee SB, An KN. Dynamic glenohumeral stability provided by three heads of the deltoid muscle. *Clin Orth Rel Res*. 2002;400:40–47.

Nwakama AC, Cofield RH, Kavanagh BF, et al. Semiconstrained total shoulder arthroplasty for GH arthritis and massive rotator cuff tearing. *J Shoulder Elbow Surg*. 2000;9(4):302–307.

Rockwood CA. The technique of total shoulder arthroplasty. *Instr Course Lect*. 1990;39:437–447.

Singh H, Osbahr DC, Holovacs TF, et al. The efficacy of continuous cryotherapy on the postoperative shoulder: a prospective, randomized investigation. *J Shoulder Elbow Surg*. 2001;10(6):522–525.

Upper Extremity Interval Throwing Progressions

Timothy F. Tyler, MS, PT, ATC | Drew Jenk, PT, DPT

Shoulder and elbow injuries in baseball and softball players are on the rise. Among the many reasons for this are increased participation by males and females in youth sports, increased specialization in one sport at an early age, elevated pitch counts, and poor mechanics.

Previous beliefs were that pitches such as the curveball and slider would put a young baseball player at a greater risk for injury. However, studies by Dun et al. in 2008 and Nissen et al. in 2009 provide evidence that the amount of pitches thrown, and not the type of pitch, may be more likely to cause injury. Dun et al. found that shoulder and elbow loads were greatest in the fastball and least in the change-up. Nissen and colleagues showed that the moments in the shoulder and elbow were less when throwing a curveball when compared to a fastball. Fleisig et al. (2006) provided evidence that the change-up may actually be the safest pitch to throw and that resultant joint loads were similar between the curveball and fastball. Evidence would suggest that pitch type is not likely the primary cause of shoulder and elbow injury in youth baseball players, but amount of pitching may be more likely the culprit.

Due to these findings research has moved to implicating pitch count as the cause of shoulder and elbow injury and not pitch type, as previously thought. Lyman et al. (2002) showed that youth baseball players between the ages of 9 and 14 years of age were more likely to have shoulder pain after throwing greater than 600 pitches in a season. Furthermore, it was also shown that greater than 800 pitches in a season were more likely to lead to elbow pain in the same group of athletes.

Research correlating pitch count to increased incidence of shoulder and elbow injury has led Little League Baseball to adopt more stringent pitch count guidelines as a protective mechanism for their participants. In 2007 Little League Baseball adopted a pitch count guideline based on similar recommendations. In 2008 the guidelines were further updated to include players as young as 7 years of age. Pitch limitations were adjusted based on the player's age and calendar days of rest (Table 29.1).

Davis et al. (2009) provided evidence that more improved pitching mechanics in youth baseball pitchers will likely decrease their risk for arm injury. Youth pitchers with better pitching mechanics generate lower humeral internal rotation torque, lower elbow valgus load, and more efficiency than do those with improper mechanics. Furthermore, Fleisig et al. concluded in a 1999 study that the natural progression for successful pitching is to learn proper mechanics as early as possible and to build strength as the body matures.

It seems that the preponderance of research has focused on the kinetics and kinematics of the baseball pitch, combined with the cause and effect of the biomechanics of pitching and baseball-related arm injuries. This is most often male-gender specific. However, according to the American Sports Medicine Institute, in 2008 there were approximately 2.3 million participants in Little League Baseball worldwide and another 400,000 female softball players. It is becoming increasingly important to study the effects of the softball throw relative to incidence and prevention of injury.

According to Werner et al. (2006), windmill softball pitchers are found to be at risk for overuse injuries similar to their male baseball counterparts. This is a result of excessive distraction stress at the throwing shoulder similar to baseball pitchers. There is a high amount of stress placed on the lateral aspect of the elbow in underhand throwers. However, softball pitchers have the only position on the field who consistently throw underhand. Therefore, it is important to study the similarities and differences between softball and baseball overhand throwers. Chu et al. (2009) concluded that, although many similarities exist between baseball and softball throwers, there are also some specific differences. These differences include a shorter and more open stride with less separation between the pelvis orientation and upper torso orientation, lower peak angular velocity for throwing extension and stride knee extension, lower ball velocity, lower proximal forces at the shoulder and elbow, and a longer time for the completion of the throw from foot contact to ball release. Conclusions that can be drawn from the current body of research suggest that, although female softball players have similar kinematics and kinetics compared to their male baseball counterparts, there are specific differences and there is an elevated risk of arm injury in both populations regardless of whether the athlete is throwing overhand or underhand.

Although it is important to utilize exercise such as strengthening and stretching for overhand athletes, it is also important to train specifically for their sport. One way to do this for softball and baseball throwers is to utilize the databased interval throwing programs for their respective sports. Axe et al. (1996, 2001) have studied Little League (Table 29.2), high school, collegiate, professional baseball players (Table 29.3), and collegiate softball players (Table 29.4) and have compiled data regarding number of pitches, throws, and distance per position for an entire game. They calculated respective averages per inning, per game, and

TABLE 29.1	Little League Pitching Guidelines	
League Age	**Pitches Per Day**
17–18	105
13–16	95
11–12	85
9–10	75
7–8	50

TABLE 29.2	13- to 14-Year-Old Baseball Pitchers Interval Throwing Programs

PHASE I: RETURN TO THROWING

ALL THROWS ARE AT 50% EFFORT

Step 1	Warmup toss at 60' 15 throws at 30'* 15 throws at 30'* 15 throws at 30' 20 long tosses to 60'
Step 2	Warmup toss to 75' 15 throws at 45'* 15 throws at 45'* 20 long tosses to 75'
Step 3	Warmup toss to 90' 15 throws at 60'* 15 throws at 60'* 15 throws at 60' 20 long tosses to 90'

PHASE II: RETURN TO PITCHING

FASTBALLS ARE FROM LEVEL GROUND FOLLOWING CROW-HOP

Step 4	Warmup toss to 105' 20 fastballs (50%)* 16 fastballs (50%)* 16 fastballs (50%)* 25 long tosses to 105'
Step 5	Warmup toss to 120' 20 fastballs (50%)* 16 fastballs (50%)* 16 fastballs (50%)* 25 long tosses to 105'
Step 6	Warmup toss to 120' 16 fastballs (50%)* 20 fastballs (50%)* 20 fastballs (50%)* 16 fastballs (50%)* 25 long tosses to 160'

PHASE III: INTENSIFIED PITCHING

PITCHES ARE FROM MOUND WITH NORMAL STRIDE

Step 7	Warmup toss to 120' 20 fastballs (50%)* 20 fastballs (75%)* 20 fastballs (75%)* 20 fastballs (50%)* 25 long tosses to 90'
Step 8	Warmup toss to 120' 20 fastballs (75%)* 21 fastballs (50%)* 20 fastballs (75%)* 21 fastballs (50%)* 25 long tosses to 160'

Step 9	Warmup toss to 120' 25 fastballs (50%)* 24 fastballs (75%)* 24 fastballs (75%)* 25 fastballs (50%)* 25 long tosses to 160'
Step 10	Warmup toss to 120' 25 fastballs (75%)* 25 fastballs (75%)* 25 fastballs (75%)* 20 fastballs (75%)* 25 long tosses to 160'
Step 11	(Active rest) Warmup toss to 120' 20 throws at 60' (75%) 15 throws at 80' (75%)*
Step 12	20 throws at 60' (75%) 15 throws at 80' (75%)* 20 long tosses to 160' Warmup toss to 120' 20 fastballs (100%)* 20 fastballs (75%) 6 off-speed pitches (75%)* 20 fastballs (100%)*
Step 13	20 fastballs (75%) 6 off-speed pitches (75%)* 25 long tosses to 160' Warmup toss to 120' 20 fastballs (75%) 4 throws to 1st (75%) 15 fastballs (100%) 10 off-speed pitches (100%) 20 fastballs (100%) 5 off-speed pitches (100%)* 20 fastballs (75%) 4 throws to 1st (75%)* 25 long tosses to 160'
Step 14	Warmup toss to 120' 20 fastballs (100%) Throws to 1st (100%)* 15 fastballs (100%) 10 off-speed pitches (100%)* 20 fastballs (100%) 5 off-speed pitches (100%)* 20 fastballs (75%) 5 throws to 1st (75%)* 25 long tosses to 160'
Step 15	Batting practice 100–110 pitches 10 throws to 1st field Bunts and comebacks
Step 16	Simulated game

Simulated Game
1. 10-minute warmup of 50–80 pitches with gradually increasing velocity
2. Five innings
3. 22–27 pitches per inning, including 15–20 fastballs
4. 6 minutes rest between innings
*Rest 6 minutes after these sets.

per season. After obtaining all of these data, the interval throwing program was created for Little League, college, and professional baseball players and collegiate softball players.

The databased interval throwing programs were developed based on distance and number of throws (Tables 29.2, 29.3, and 29.4). This is important because it can be used objectively to build arm strength when returning from injury or the off-season. When healthy college baseball players were asked to throw based on percentage, they could not accurately gauge the requested effort. When the pitchers were asked to throw at 50% requested effort, they actually threw at 85% of the actual speed. When the pitchers were asked to throw at 75% effort, they actually threw at 90% of the actual speed. Consequently, a throwing program based on distance and number of throws is a more objective way to build functional arm strength, as opposed to requesting different levels of effort from players at their respective positions.

As a player is progressing through the interval throwing program, it is important to recognize common throwing flaws that

TABLE 29.3	High School, College, and Professional Baseball Pitchers Interval Throwing Program		
PHASE I	**RETURN TO THROWING THROWS AT 50% EFFORT**	**PHASE III**	**INTENSIFIED PITCHING**
Step 1	Warmup toss to 60' 15 throws at 30'* 15 throws at 30'* 15 throws at 30'* 20 long tosses to 60'	Step 12	25 fastballs (75%)* 20 fastballs (100%)* 10 fastballs (75%)* 15 fastballs (100%)* 25 fastballs (75%)*
Step 2	Warmup toss to 75' 15 throws at 60'* 15 throws at 60'* 15 throws at 60'* 20 long tosses to 90'	Step 13	(Active rest) 20 throws at 80'* 20 throws at 80'* 20 throws at 80'* 20 throws at 80'*
Step 3	Warmup toss to 105' 15 throws at 75'* 15 throws at 75'* 15 throws at 75'* 20 long tosses to 105'	Step 14	20 fastballs (75%)* 20 fastballs (100%) 5 off-speed pitches* 15 fastballs (100%) 5 off-speed pitches*
Step 4	Warmup toss to 120' 15 throws at 90'* 20 throws at 90'* 15 throws at 90'* 20 long tosses at 120'		Field bunts and comebacks *(Relievers and closing pitchers can go to step 21 on the next throwing day after completing this step)*
Step 5	Warmup toss to 120' 20 throws at 105'* 20 throws at 105'* 15 throws at 105'* 20 long tosses at 120'	Step 15	20 fastballs (100%)* 15 fastballs (100%) 5 off-speed pitches 5 pickoff throws to 1st* 20 fastballs (100%) 5 off-speed pitches* 20 fastballs (100%) 5 off-speed pitches*
Step 6	Warmup toss to 120' 20 throws at 120'* 20 throws at 120'* 20 throws at 120'* 20 long tosses at 120'	Step 16	15 fastballs (100%) 5 off-speed pitches* 15 fastballs (100%) 3 pickoff throws to 1st* 20 fastballs (100%) 5 off-speed pitches* 15 fastballs (100%) 3 pickoff throws to 2nd* 15 fastballs 100%) 5 off-speed pitches*
PHASE II	**RETURN TO PITCHING THROWS AT EFFORT LEVEL GIVEN**	Step 17	(Active rest) Repeat step 14
Step 7	15 throws at 60'6" (75%)* 20 throws at 60'6" (75%)* 20 throws at 60'6" (75%)* 15 throws at 60'6" (75%)* 20 throws at 60'6" (75%)*	Step 18	20 fastballs (100%) 5 off-speed pitches* 20 fastballs (100%) 3 pickoff throws to 1st* 20 fastballs (100%) 3 pickoff throws to 2nd* 15 fastballs (100%) 5 off-speed pitches* 15 fastballs (100%) 5 off-speed pitches*
Step 8	20 throws at 60'6" (75%)* 20 throws at 60'6" (75%)* 20 throws at 60'6" (75%)*		
Step 9	20 fastballs (50%)* 20 fastballs (50%)* 20 fastballs (50%)* 20 fastballs (50%)* 25 throws at 60'6" (75%)*	Step 19	Batting practice 110–120 pitches Field bunts and comebacks
Step 10	20 fastballs (50%)* 20 fastballs (75%)* 20 fastballs (50%)* 15 fastballs (75%)* 25 throws at 60'6" (75%)*	Step 20	Simulated game
Step 11	25 fastballs (50%)* 20 fastballs (75%)* 20 fastballs (75%)* 20 fastballs (75%)* 20 fastballs (75%)		

*Rest 6 minutes after these sets.

may predispose the athlete to injury or may be indicative of current injury. It is important to note that it is not definitely known what mechanical throwing flaws will always lead to injury. However, in baseball circles, it is widely known what often leads to injury or is masking current injury. These flaws are easily noted by the naked eye or by two-dimensional video analysis. Three-dimensional video analysis is always a useful tool, but it is often cost prohibitive for many clinicians.

Throwing flaws can be broken down into eight common identifiable mechanical problems:
- loss of pelvic control at wind-up (Fig. 29.1)
- pelvis closed at foot strike (Fig. 29.2)
- strike foot planted away from home plate or the target (Fig. 29.3)
- elbow dropping below shoulder height (Fig. 29.4)
- excessive lateral trunk lean (Fig. 29.5)

- supination of the forearm at foot strike (Fig. 29.6)
- excessive shoulder internal rotation at foot strike (Fig. 29.7)
- poor finish or follow-through (Fig. 29.8)

If a clinician or coach can look for these eight common flaws, the athlete will be able to correct mechanical issues that could lead to injury in the future. Also, if the athlete is attempting to throw through an injury that has already been sustained, the clinician or coach will be able to properly address these possible injuries to return the athlete to unrestricted and pain-free levels of prior functioning.

In conclusion, baseball and softball players are predisposed to upper extremity injury in large part because of the repetitive nature of their sport. However, if the athlete builds proper strength through exercise and use of the databased interval throwing program, corrects faulty mechanics, and limits the amount of throws per season, the athlete will have an increased likelihood of completing the season without suffering upper extremity injury.

TABLE 29.4	Softball Pitcher's Program		

PHASE 1: EARLY THROWING

ALL THROWS ARE TO TOLERANCE TO A MAXIMUM OF 50% EFFORT

ALL LONG TOSSES BEGIN WITH A CROW-HOP

Step 1	Warmup toss to 30 ft 10 throws @ 30 ft Rest 8 min 10 throws @ 30 ft 10 long tosses to 40 ft	Step 9	Warmup toss to 120 ft 10 throws @ 60 ft (75%) 10 pitches @ 46 ft (50%) Rest 8 min 10 throws @ 60 ft (75%) 10 pitches @ 46 ft (50%) 15 long tosses to 120 ft
Step 2	Warmup toss to 45 ft 10 throws @ 45 ft Rest 8 min 10 throws @ 45 ft 10 long tosses to 60 ft	Step 10	Warmup toss to 120 ft 10 throws @ 60 ft (75%) 10 pitches @ 46 ft (50%) Rest 8 min 10 pitches @ 46 ft (50%) Rest 8 min 10 throws @ 60 ft (75%) 10 pitches @ 46 ft (50%) 15 long tosses to 120 ft
Step 3	Warmup toss to 60 ft 10 throws @ 60 ft Rest 8 min 10 throws @ 60 ft 10 long tosses to 75 ft		
Step 4	Warmup toss to 75 ft 10 throws @ 75 ft Rest 8 min 10 throws @ 75 ft 10 long tosses to 90 ft		**PHASE III: INTENSIFIED PITCHING**
Step 5	Warmup toss to 90 ft 10 throws @ 90 ft Rest 8 min 10 throws @ 90 ft 10 long tosses to 105 ft		**PITCH SETS 11–15 CONSIST OF 1 FASTBALL TO 1 OFF-SPEED PITCH AT THE EFFORT LEVEL SPECIFIED**
Step 6	Warmup toss to 105 ft 10 throws @ 105 ft Rest 8 min 10 throws @ 105 ft 10 long tosses to 120 ft		**PITCH SETS 16–21 CONSIST OF A PERCENTAGE OF PITCHES THAT MATCH THE PREINJURY PITCH MIX SPECIFIC TO THE ATHLETE AT THE EFFORT LEVEL SPECIFIED**

PHASE II: INITIATION OF PITCHING

ALL PITCHES ARE FASTBALLS (NO OFF-SPEED PITCHES)

ALL PITCHES TO TOLERANCE OR MAXIMUM EFFORT LEVEL SPECIFIED

ALL LONG TOSSES BEGIN WITH A CROW-HOP

BEGIN EACH STEP WITH WARMUP TOSS TO 120 FT (36.58 M)

END EACH STEP WITH 20 LONG TOSSES TO 120 FT (36.58 M)

Step 7	Warmup toss to 120 ft 10 throws @ 60 ft (75%) 10 throws @ 20 ft (50%) Rest 8 min 10 throws @ 60 ft (75%) 5 pitches @ 20 ft (50%) 10 long tosses to 120 ft	Step 11	2 throws to each base (75%) 15 pitches (50%)* 15 pitches (50%)* 1 throw to each base (75%) 15 pitches (50%)*
		Step 12	2 throws to each base (75%) 15 pitches (50%)* 15 pitches (50%)* 15 pitches (50%)* 1 throw to each base (75%) 15 pitches (50%)*
Step 8	Warmup toss to 120 ft 10 throws @ 60 ft (75%) 10 pitches @ 35 ft (50%) Rest 8 min 10 throws @ 60 ft (75%) 10 pitches @ 35 ft (50%) 10 long tosses to 120 ft	Step 13	2 throws to each base (75%) 15 pitches (50%)* 15 pitches (75%)* 15 pitches (75%)* 1 throw to each base (75%) 15 pitches (50%)*
		Step 14	2 throws to each base (75%) 15 pitches (50%)* 15 pitches (75%)* 15 pitches (75%)* 20 pitches (50%)* 1 throw to each base (75%) 15 pitches (50%)*
		Step 15	2 throws to each base (100%) 15 pitches (75%)* 15 pitches (75%)* 15 pitches (75%)* 15 pitches (75%)* 1 throw to each base (75%) 15 pitches (75%)*

TABLE 29.4	Softball Pitcher's Program—cont'd		
Step 16	1 throw to each base (100%) 15 pitches (100%)* 20 pitches (75%)* 15 pitches (100%)* 20 pitches (75%)* 1 throw to each base (75%) 20 pitches (75%)*	Step 19	1 throw to each base (100%) 20 pitches (100%)* 15 pitches (100%)* 20 pitches (100%)* 15 pitches (100%)* 20 pitches (100%)* 15 pitches (100%)*
Step 17	1 throw to each base (100%) 15 pitches (100%)* 20 pitches (75%)* 15 pitches (100%)* 15 pitches (100%)* 20 pitches (75%)* 1 throw to each base (75%) 15 pitches (75%)*		1 throw to each base (100%) 15 pitches (100%)*
		Step 20	Batting practice 100–120 pitches 1 throw to each base per 25 pitches
Step 18	1 throw to each base (100%) 20 pitches (100%)* 15 pitches (100%)* 20 pitches (100%)* 15 pitches (100%)* 20 pitches (100%)* 1 throw to each base (100%) 15 pitches (100%)*	Step 21	Simulated game 7 innings 18–20 pitches/inning 8-min rest between innings Preinjury pitch mix

*Rest 6 minutes after these sets.

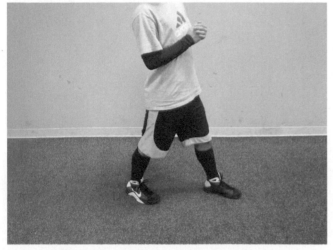

Fig. 29.1 Loss of pelvic control at wind-up.

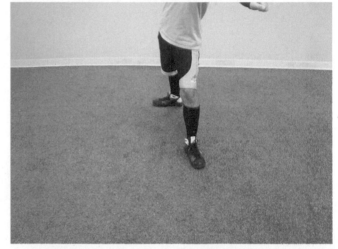

Fig. 29.3 Strike foot planted away from home plate.

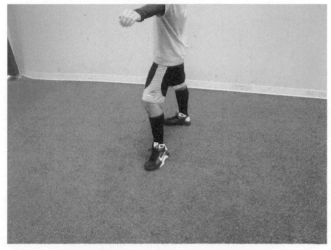

Fig. 29.2 Pelvis closed at foot strike.

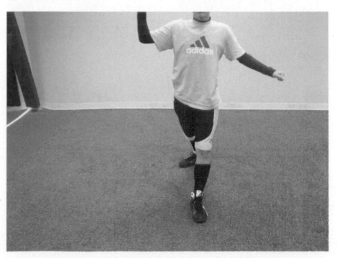

Fig. 29.4 Elbow dropping below shoulder height.

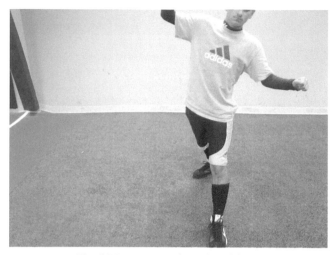

Fig. 29.5 Excessive lateral trunk lean.

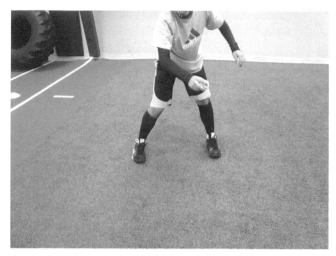

Fig. 29.8 Poor finish.

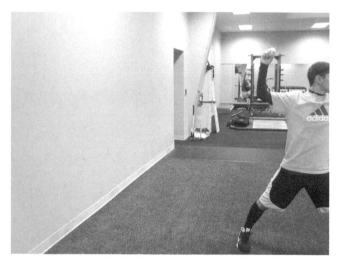

Fig. 29.6 Supination of the forearm at foot strike.

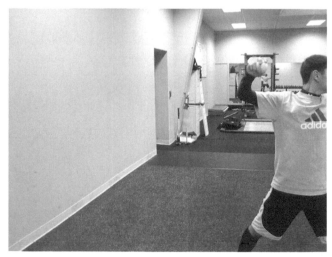

Fig. 29.7 Excessive shoulder internal rotation at foot strike.

TABLE 29.5	Interval Golf Program		
	Monday	Wednesday	Friday
1st week	10 putts 10 chips Rest 5 min 15 chips	15 putts 15 chips Rest 5 min 25 chips	20 putts 20 chips Rest 5 min 20 putts 20 chips Rest 5 min 10 chips 10 short irons
2nd week	20 chips 10 short irons Rest 5 min 10 short irons	20 chips 15 short irons Rest 10 min 15 short irons 15 chips putting	15 short irons 10 medium irons Rest 10 min 20 short irons 15 chips
3rd week	15 short irons 15 medium irons Rest 10 min 5 long irons 15 short irons 15 medium irons Rest 10 min 20 chips	15 short irons 10 medium irons 10 long irons Rest 10 min 10 short irons 10 medium irons 5 long irons 5 wood	15 short irons 10 medium irons 10 long irons Rest 10 min 10 short irons 10 medium irons 10 long irons 10 wood
4th week	15 short irons 10 medium irons 10 long irons 10 drives Rest 15 min Repeat	Play 9 holes	Play 9 holes
5th week	9 holes	9 holes	18 holes

SHOULDER INJURIES IN GOLFERS

Shoulder injuries are found to be the third most common injury in professional golfers and the fourth most common injury in amateur golfers. To effectively understand and manage a golfer's shoulder injury, it is important to recognize and understand the five phases of a proper golf swing. The swing starts with the takeaway followed by the backswing, downswing, and acceleration and ending with the follow-through. Once the patient is ready to begin the return-to-play phase, he or she may begin an interval golf program (Table 29.5). The purpose of the interval program is to allow for re-establishment of swing pace, weight transfer, and proper mechanics. It begins with chipping and putting only, followed by gradual progression to short and medium irons. When a pain-free swing is established, long irons and woods may be integrated. On returning to play, the golfer is encouraged to progress to 9 holes twice per week, then 9 holes four to five times per week, and eventually up to 18 holes several times per week.

REFERENCES

A complete reference list is available at https://expertconsult.inkling.com/.

FURTHER READING

Aguinaldo AL, Chambers H. Correlation of throwing mechanics with elbow valgus load in adult baseball pitchers. *Am J Sports Med*. 2009. Epub ahead of print 24 July.

Andrews JR, Wilk KE. *The Athlete's Shoulder*. New York: Churchill Livingstone; 1994.

Axe MJ, Windley TC, Snyder-Mackeler L. Data-based interval throwing program for collegiate softball players. *J Athl Train*. 2002;37:194–203.

Fleisig GS, Kingsley DS, Loftice JW, et al. Kinetic comparison among the fastball, curveball, change-up and slider in collegiate baseball players. *Am J Sports Med*. 2006;34:423–430.

Fleisig GS, Barrentine SW. Biomechanical aspects of the elbow in sports. *Sports Med Arthrosc*. 1995;3:149–159.

Fuss FK. The ulnar collateral ligament of the human elbow joint, anatomy function and biomechanics. *J Anat*. 1991;175:203–212.

Kim DK, Millett PJ, Warner JJ, et al. Shoulder injuries in golf. *Am J Sports Med*. 2004;32:1324–1330.

Meister K, Day T, Horodyski M, et al. Rotational motion changes in the glenohumeral joint of the adolescent/Little League baseball player. *Am J Sports Med*. 2005;33:693–698.

Shoulder Exercises for Injury Prevention in the Throwing Athlete

John A. Guido, JR., PT, MHS, SCS, ATC, CSCS | Keith Meister, MD

The goal of the off-season program for the throwing athlete is to enhance performance, prevent injury, and prepare for the upcoming season. The physical therapist can utilize the results of descriptive studies of overhand athletes documenting shoulder range of motion (ROM) and electromyographic (EMG) analysis of the shoulder musculature to create an off-season injury prevention program. Data from biomechanical studies examining kinematic and kinetic variables unique to throwing must be considered in the program design.

The focus of this section is on developing a healthy throwing shoulder and the exercises and activities that can be performed to prevent injury. The overall approach to injury prevention for the thrower's shoulder is multifaceted. Periods of rest and recovery are followed by the development of strong and explosive lower extremity and trunk musculature, establishing appropriate glenohumeral ROM, creating rotator cuff and scapular muscle strength and endurance, and ensuring that the athlete demonstrates proper throwing mechanics. Achieving this "total package" will enable the athlete to reach peak performance while decreasing injury risk.

REST AND RECOVERY

Rest and recovery are among the most important aspects of the shoulder off-season injury prevention program. Many athletes, especially in the southern half of the United States, play baseball and softball 12 months per year. Many of these athletes play on multiple teams during the same season. Many play different sports at the same time, requiring similar use of the shoulder. An example of this is the softball athlete who is also on the swim team. Windmill softball pitchers are at an even greater risk for injury when they pitch multiple games in a single tournament. High volumes of throwing in short periods of time increase the risk for overuse injuries and overtraining. Yukutake et al. (2015) developed a six-item checklist of questions that are predicative of increased risk for injuries in youth baseball players. Questions included: Have you experienced shoulder or elbow pain while throwing in the preceding 12 months?; Have you experienced a shoulder or elbow injury requiring medical treatment?; Do you participate in team training 4 days per week?; Do you participate in self-training 7 days per week?; Are you in a starting lineup?; Does your pitching arm often feel fatigued while playing baseball? If the athlete answers yes to a question, he or she gets a point. A injury risk score of >3 points increases the risk of injury to that player by 33%.

Very few of these athletes, and coaches, realize the value and importance of adequate rest and recovery. Following a periodized training schedule, athletes can participate in an organized approach to competition and strength and conditioning to maximize peak performance. Kibler and Chandler (2003) suggested that conditioning programs are increasingly oriented toward the prevention or reduction of injury, especially in the area of repetitive microtrauma or overload injuries. Athletes should play their respective sport a maximum of 9 months per year, with 2 weeks or more of rest and recovery immediately following their peak competitive phase and 6 to 8 weeks of off-season and preseason conditioning and injury prevention. The goal of this period is to create the "total package" and to prepare for the upcoming season.

CREATING A HEALTHY THROWER'S SHOULDER

Range of Motion

Evaluation of the ROM of the shoulder is essential to determine if the athlete possesses an appropriate arc of motion for throwing. Meister et al. (2005) examined rotational changes in the glenohumeral joint in 294 adolescent/Little League baseball players, ages 8 to 16 years. The results of this study demonstrated an average ROM in the dominant arm of 142.9 ± 13.1 degrees of external rotation and 35.9 ± 9.8 degrees of internal rotation, both measured at 90 degrees of abduction. Reagan et al. (2002) also examined glenohumeral ROM in 54 asymptomatic college baseball players (25 pitchers and 29 position players). These athletes presented with an average of 116.3 ± 11.4 degrees of ER and 43.0 ± 7.4 IR in the glenohumeral joint of the dominant arm. Crockett et al. (2002) assessed glenohumeral ROM in 25 professional baseball pitchers. These athletes had an average of 128 ± 9.2 degrees of ER and 62 ± 7.4 degrees of IR in the dominant arm. Werner et al. (2006) demonstrated a mean of 128 ± 16 degrees of ER and 54 ± 13 degrees of IR in the dominant arm in female softball pitchers with a mean age of 14 ± 3 years.

There are wide differences in the reported shoulder ROM for overhand athletes at various stages of their career. Table 30.1 examines the results of several studies examining ROM in the dominant and nondominant shoulder of a variety of throwing athletes. However, ROM measurements may be taken differently by different examiners. Wilk et al. (1997) recommended the following technique for measuring glenohumeral ROM: shoulder at 90 degrees of abduction and the elbow bent to 90 degrees, the shoulder itself or the coracoid process is palpated, and when scapular substitution begins ER or IR is measured. A minimal amount of external rotation and internal rotation may be needed for the shoulder to remain

TABLE 30.1	Shoulder External, Internal, and Total Arc Range of Motion Data					
	STUDY					
	DOMINANT SHOULDER			NONDOMINANT SHOULDER		
	External Rotation	Internal Rotation	Total Arc of Motion	External Rotation	Internal Rotation	Total Arc of Motion
Youth baseball (Meister et al.)	142.9 ± 13.1	35.9 ± 9.8	178.7 ± 16.5	136.6 ± 12.7	41.8 ± 8.6	178.3 ± 16.5
Youth baseball (Werner)	131 (range 116–146)	45 (range 36–55)				
College baseball (Reagan et al.)	116.3 ± 11.4	43 ± 7.4	159.5 ± 12.4	106.6 ± 11.2	51.2 ± 7.3	157.8 ± 11.5
College baseball (Werner et al.)	126 ± 1	48 ± 10				
Professional baseball (Crockett et al.)	128 ± 9.2	62 ± 7.4	189 ± 12.6	119 ± 7.2	71 ± 9.3	189 ± 12.7
Professional baseball (Reinhold et al.)	136.5 ± 9.8	54.1 ± 11.4	190.6 ± 14.6	124.2 ± 9.1	63.1 ± 14.3	187.3 ± 16.9
>3 years as a professional base-ball pitcher (Lintner et al.)	142.7	74.3	216.98			
<3 years as a professional base-ball pitcher (Lintner et al.)	139.9	55.2	194.2			
Professional baseball pitchers (Borsa et al.)	134.8 ± 10.2	68.6 ± 9.2	203.4 ± 9.7	125.8 ± 8.7	78.3 ± 10.6	204.1 ± 9.7
Professional baseball pitchers (Bigliani et al.)	118.0	Measured functional IR with thumb up the back		102.8		
Professional baseball position players (Bigliani et al.)	109.3	Measured functional IR with thumb up the back		97.1		
Professional baseball pitchers (Brown et al.)	141 ± 14.7	83 ± 13.9		132 ± 14.6	98 ± 13.2	
Professional baseball position players (Brown et al.)	132 ± 9.8	85 ± 11.9		124 ± 12.7	91 ± 13.0	
Youth softball pitch-ers (Werner et al.)	128 ± 16	54 ± 13				

healthy during throwing. This range has not been quantified at this time. Therefore, the clinician must rely on previous studies of thrower's ROM or the total arc of motion concept. For an athlete to possess appropriate thrower's ROM, his or her measurements should fall within the results of these guidelines. The total arc of motion concept describes the following: ER + IR = total arc in the glenohumeral joint of the dominant and nondominant shoulders. The total arc of motion in the dominant shoulder should be within 5 to 10 degrees of the total arc of motion in the nondominant extremity.

An athlete may not possess an appropriate thrower's ROM for several reasons. Two studies demonstrated an osseous adaptation in the thrower's shoulder related to humeral retroversion. Throwing athletes present with an increase in ER and a decrease in IR as a result of the normal bony adaptive changes that occur from repetitive throwing. Other authors have demonstrated posterior shoulder stiffness, which is believed to be related to contracture of the posterior inferior capsule and tightness in the posterior rotator cuff musculature.

Depending on age and the orientation of the glenohumeral joint, ROM may be increased if the athlete does not possess appropriate thrower's ROM. Tightness in the soft tissues surrounding the glenohumeral joint must be addressed. Loss of internal rotation has received the most attention of these two adaptations (increased ER and decreased IR) as it relates to injury in the thrower's shoulder. Athletes who present with decreased internal rotation at the 90-degree abducted position should do exercises to stretch the posterior rotator cuff and posterior joint capsule. These include the cross-body stretch (Fig. 30.1; Videos 30.1, 30.2, 30.3 and 30.4), thumb up the back towel stretch (Fig. 30.2), and sleeper stretch (Fig. 30.3), all performed for three to five repetitions with a 15-second hold. These exercises will stretch the posterior shoulder. Within-session increases in IR were observed with sleeper stretches in a population of college baseball players. However, to stretch the posterior joint capsule—a connective tissue—a low-load, long-duration stretch is performed. This can be accomplished with a 2- to 3-pound weighted hang in the sleeper stretch position, holding for 1 to 2 minutes for two repetitions. Another stretch

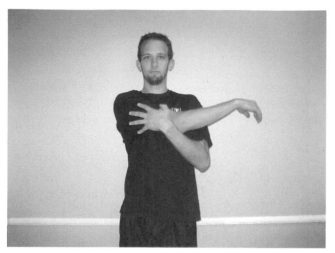

Fig. 30.1 Cross-body stretch.

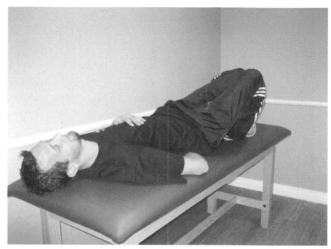

Fig. 30.4 Supine posterior capsule stretch with trunk rotation.

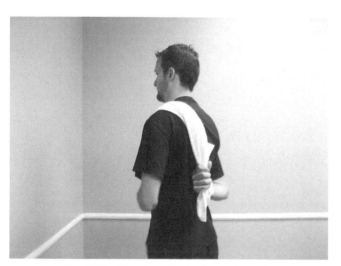

Fig. 30.2 Thumb up the back towel stretch.

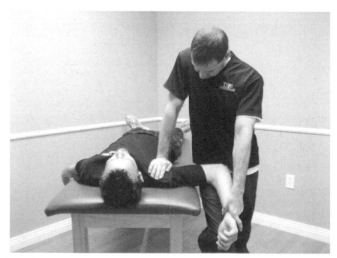

Fig. 30.5 Supine passive range of motion into external rotation with glenohumeral stabilization.

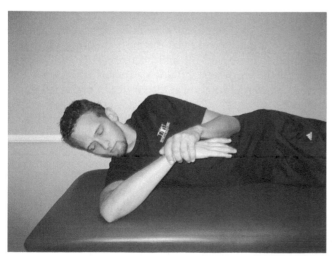

Fig. 30.3 Sleeper stretch.

can be done with the athlete supine, placing the thumb up the back and, with the lower extremities bent, letting the legs fall toward the dominant arm side to again stretch the posterior shoulder (Fig. 30.4). The athlete should hold this position for a minimum of 30 seconds and repeat for three repetitions.

If the athlete does not possess satisfactory external rotation at the 90-degree abducted position, stretching of the anterior rotator cuff and pectoral musculature should be initiated. To increase external rotation, a passive stretch in the 90-degree abducted position moving toward the maximal external rotation (late cocking) position is used. The clinician should keep the humeral head centered on the glenoid with pressure from the clinician's nonstretching hand (Fig. 30.5). Three to five repetitions of 15 seconds should be sufficient.

Stretches appropriate to each individual should be performed one time per day, even if the athlete is not throwing. The goal of the flexibility program is to bring the shoulder back into balance and restore the thrower's ROM. Once the goal is achieved, the athlete may perform these stretches only when throwing unless the shoulder starts to lose the total arc of motion.

Rotator Cuff and Scapular Muscle Strength and Endurance

Evaluation of the strength and endurance of the rotator cuff and scapular musculature may be performed using a handheld dynamometer for manual muscle testing or through the use of isokinetic testing. The shoulder external/internal rotator strength ratio, as measured isokinetically, has been reported to be 65% at 180 deg/sec and 61% at 300 deg/sec. EMG has also been used to evaluate muscle activity during commonly prescribed exercises for the shoulder of the overhand athlete and during baseball pitching. The clinician can combine the results of these EMG

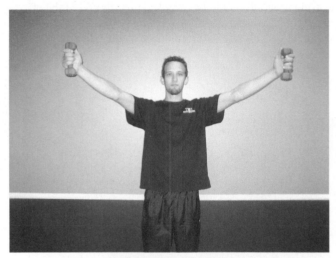

Fig. 30.6 Scaption.

studies to develop a sports-specific, evidence-based, off-season shoulder injury prevention program. Exercises should be chosen that mimic the force profiles of the rotator cuff and scapular musculature in pitching, with EMG activity that can be categorized at moderate (21% to 50% maximum voluntary contraction [MVC]) or marked (>50% MVC) levels. In the early cocking phase of the throwing motion, four muscles reach a threshold of >40% maximum voluntary isometric contraction: the deltoid, supraspinatus, trapezius, and serratus anterior (SA). Werner et al. (2006) showed that those athletes who demonstrated high ball velocity during baseball pitching reach a point of 20 degrees of horizontal adduction in the early cocking phase. This position approaches the plane of the scapula; thus, scaption is an ideal exercise to begin the injury prevention program. Scaption (Fig. 30.6) has been shown to be a qualifying exercise for the upper, middle, and lower trapezius; the supraspinatus; SA; and deltoid (Video 30.5).

The next phase of the pitching motion is the late cocking phase. During this phase, nearly all the muscles of the shoulder girdle are firing at moderate to high levels. The EMG activity demonstrates near or greater than 100% maximum voluntary isometric contraction (MVIC) for the subscapularis and SA. Forces couples are evident as the infraspinatus (IS) and levator scapulae work in conjunction with these muscles, respectively. According to Decker et al. (2003) the push-up plus and diagonal exercises (Fig. 30.7) consistently activated both the upper and lower subscapularis muscle. The push-up plus was also chosen in several other studies to generate large amplitudes in the SA (Fig. 30.8; Video 30.6). Reinold et al. (2006) reported that the exercise that elicited the most combined EMG signal for the IS and teres minor (TM) was shoulder external rotation in sidelying (IS 62% MVIC, TM 67% MVIC) (Fig. 30.9). The prone shoulder extension with ER exercise may be performed for

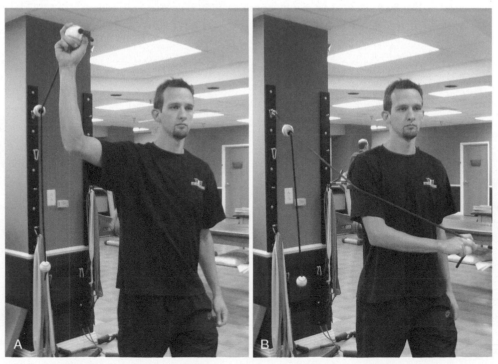

Fig. 30.7 A, Tubing diagonal start position. B, Tubing diagonal end position.

the levator scapulae (Fig. 30.10). The next phase of the throwing motion is acceleration. All of the shoulder girdle muscles, except the deltoid and biceps, are functioning at >40% MVIC. The SA accelerates the scapula, the latissimus dorsi accelerates the humerus, and the triceps accelerates the elbow. From late cocking to ball release, the athlete has less than a quarter of a second to move through this motion. Plyometric tubing exercises can be used to mimic this motion (Fig. 30.11).

Deceleration and follow-through demonstrate high EMG activity of the teres minor and trapezius with moderate activation of several other muscles. The lower trapezius and biceps slow the upper extremity, and the rotator cuff resists the high distraction forces occurring at the glenohumeral joint. The prone horizontal abduction with ER exercises, performed at 100 degrees and 135 degrees of abduction, are excellent choices to work both the lower trapezius and the rotator cuff (Figs. 30.12 and 30.13).

A similar program, with slight sports-specific variations, can be used for any overhand athlete. Table 30.2 summarizes the strengthening and endurance exercises in the rotator cuff and scapular off-season injury prevention program.

Throwing athletes perform a high number of repetitions in their respective sports. Exercise prescription should consist of a low-weight, high-repetition approach with each exercise to create strength and endurance in the rotator cuff and scapula musculature. Strength endurance is best achieved by performing 12 to 25 repetitions at 50% to 70% intensity. This is also the best repetition range to improve increased tissue vascularization and the structural integrity of the connective tissue.

Sports-specific exercise prescription and periodization are the keys to preventing injury in the thrower's shoulder. A comprehensive approach should focus on glenohumeral ROM and rotator cuff and scapular muscle strength and endurance. The athlete must develop strong and explosive trunk and lower extremity musculature. Throwing mechanics should be evaluated and an interval throwing program should be completed by the end of the off-season program. Achieving the "total package" will allow the athlete to reach peak performance while minimizing the risk for injury.

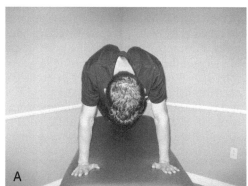 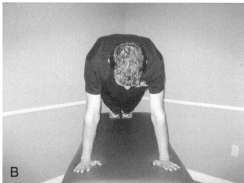

Fig. 30.8 A, Push-up plus start position. B, Push-up plus end position.

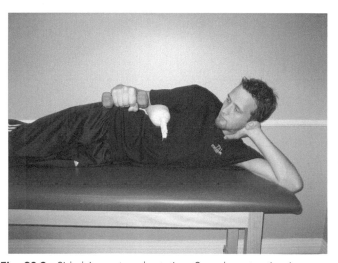

Fig. 30.9 Side-lying external rotation. Scapular retraction is encouraged throughout the exercise.

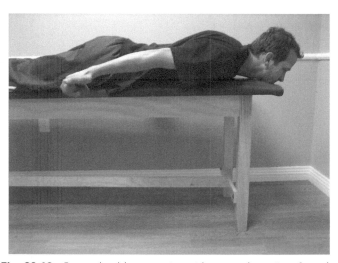

Fig. 30.10 Prone shoulder extension with external rotation. Scapular retraction is encouraged throughout the exercise.

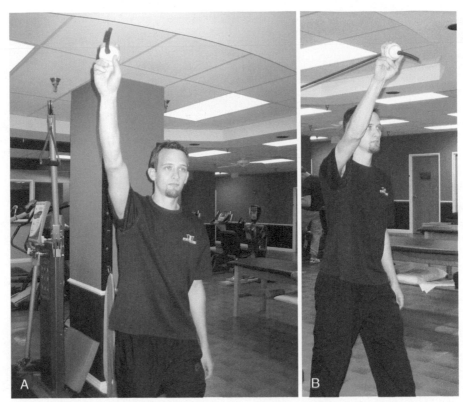

Fig. 30.11 A, Tubing velocity start position. B, Tubing velocity end position. Athlete is encouraged to move the arm through the acceleration portion of the throwing motion.

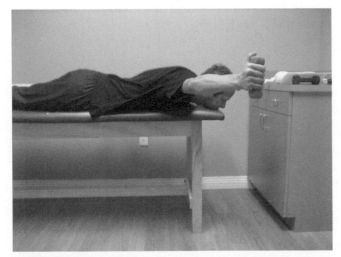

Fig. 30.12 Prone shoulder horizontal abduction and external rotation (ER) at 100 degrees of abduction. Scapular retraction is encouraged throughout the exercise.

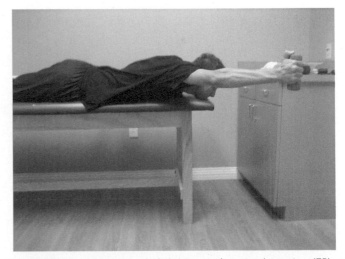

Fig. 30.13 Prone horizontal abduction and external rotation (ER) at 135 degrees of abduction. Scapular retraction is encouraged throughout the exercise.

TABLE 30.2	Off-Season Program			
ACTIVE REST AND RECOVERY				
Maintain or establish range of motion and posterior capsule flexibility	Cross-body stretch	Thumb up the back internal rotation stretch	Sleeper stretch Sleeper hang Supine posterior capsule stretch with trunk rotation	Supine passive range of motion into ER with glenohumeral stabilization
Rotator cuff and scapular strengthening and endurance program	Early cocking Scaption	Late cocking Push-up plus Tubing diagonal exercise Side-lying external rotation (ER) Prone shoulder extension with ER	Acceleration Tubing velocity	Deceleration Prone shoulder horizontal abduction and ER @ 100 and 135 degrees of abduction
BIOMECHANICAL ANALYSIS				
Interval throwing programs	Long toss program		Position-specific program	

REFERENCES

A complete reference list is available at https://expertconsult.inkling.com/.

31

Glenohumeral Internal Rotation Deficiency: Evaluation and Treatment

Todd S. Ellenbecker, DPT, MS, SCS, OCS, CSCS | W. Ben Kibler, MD | George J. Davies, DPT, MEd, PT, SCS, ATC, LAT, CSCS, PES, FAPTA

INTRODUCTION

The concept of glenohumeral internal rotation deficiency (GIRD) has been implicated as a significant factor in overuse shoulder injury and has been extensively studied in overhead athletes. This section offers an overview of the GIRD concept and the ramifications of GIRD on the athletic shoulder and covers nonoperative treatment strategies to both prevent and rehabilitate GIRD.

THE GIRD CONCEPT

Several classic papers have been published in the literature outlining both the significance and definition of GIRD. Burkhart et al. (2003) have operationally defined GIRD as a loss of internal rotation of 20 degrees or more compared to the contralateral side. This 20-degree loss of internal rotation ROM is relative to the contralateral extremities internal rotation measurement and is irrespective of the external rotation or total arc of ROM. Several other definitions of GIRD include 25 degrees of internal rotation loss relative to the contralateral extremity (Shanley et al. 2011), 18 degrees of internal rotation loss (Wilk et al. 2011), and a loss of internal rotation greater than or equal to 10% of the contralateral extremities total rotation arc (Tokish et al. 2008). Wilk and colleagues (Wilk et al. 2011) examined total range of motion in baseball players and found that those who exhibited GIRD and additionally had a loss of total rotation range of motion (TROM) greater than 5 degrees had a 2.5 times greater risk of developing shoulder problems. Despite many actual definitions of GIRD, all definitions reflect a loss of internal rotation ROM of the glenohumeral joint. One common finding present during the examination of the overhead athlete is the consistent finding of increased dominant arm external rotation (defined or referred to as external rotation gain [ERG]) and reduced dominant-arm glenohumeral joint internal rotation or GIRD (Matsen and Arntz 1990, Ellenbecker et al. 1996, 2002).

The concept of total range of motion is important to understand. Increased humeral torsion alters the arc of total motion into decreased IR ROM and increased ER ROM. The athlete will not be at risk as long as the IR loss is compensated for by a gain in ER. This normal loss of IR may be referred to as (anatomic or asymptomatic) aGIRD in which there is less than 18 degrees loss of IR with TROM within 5 degrees of uninvolved side. A (pathologic) pGIRD would be one in which the shoulder has greater than 18 degrees loss of IR and greater than 5 degrees loss of TROM (Manske R et al. 2013).

PROPOSED CAUSES OF GIRD

Several proposed mechanisms have been discussed attempting to explain this glenohumeral range of motion relationship of increased external rotation (ERG) and limited internal rotation (GIRD) (Crockett et al. 2002, Ellenbecker et al. 2002, Tokish et al. 2008). These mechanisms include tightness of the posterior capsule, tightness of the muscle tendon unit of the posterior rotator cuff (thixotropy) (Reisman et al. 2005), and changes in humeral retrotorsion (Chant et al. 2007, Crockett et al. 2002, Osbahr et al. 2002, Reagan et al. 2002). Some of the earliest proposed mechanisms for the limitation of internal rotation ROM in the dominant shoulder of the overhead athlete were offered by Pappas et al. (1985), who described thickening or capsular fibrosis, and subsequent shortening played a role in limiting internal rotation ROM. Cadaver studies have shown that experimental plication of the posterior capsule does lead to decreases in internal rotation range of motion (Gerber et al. 2003, Harryman et al. 1990).

Resiman et al. (2005) have demonstrated shortening of the muscle tendon unit following exposure to eccentric overload, a well-recognized characteristic of the follow-through phase of the throwing motion and overhead serve (Jobe et al. 1983, Ryu et al. 1988). Another study supporting the involvement of a shortened posterior rotator cuff muscle tendon unit was published by Reinold et al. (2006), who showed short-term losses in internal rotation ROM and total rotation range of motion following the performance of 60 pitches in elite-level throwers.

Finally, the humeral retroversion concept has been studied by Crockett et al. (2002) and others (Osbahr et al. 2002, Reagan et al. 2002). These studies have shown unilateral increases in humeral retroversion in throwing athletes, which would explain the increase in external rotation with accompanying internal rotation loss (GIRD).

CONSEQUENCES OF GIRD ON THE BIOMECHANICS OF THE HUMAN SHOULDER

The loss of internal rotation ROM or GIRD is significant for several biomechanical reasons with consequences affecting normal glenohumeral joint biomechanics. The relationship between internal rotation ROM loss (tightness in the posterior capsule of the shoulder) and increased anterior humeral head translation has been scientifically identified (Gerber et al. 2003, Tyler et al. 2000). The increase in anterior humeral shear force reported by

Harryman et al. (1990) was manifested by a horizontal adduction cross-body maneuver, similar to that incurred during the follow-through of the throwing motion or tennis serve. Tightness of the posterior capsule has also been linked to increased superior migration of the humeral head during shoulder elevation (Matsen and Arntz 1990). Other authors (Grossman et al. 2005, Koffler et al. 2001) studied the effects of posterior capsular tightness in a functional position of 90 degrees of abduction and 90 degrees or more of external rotation in cadaveric specimens. They found, with either imbrication of the inferior aspect of the posterior capsule or imbrication of the entire posterior capsule, that humeral head kinematics were changed or altered. In the presence of posterior capsular tightness, the humeral head will shift in an anterior superior direction, as compared to a normal shoulder with normal capsular relationships. With more extensive amounts of posterior capsular tightness, the humeral head was found to shift posterosuperiorly. These effects of altered posterior capsular tensions experimentally representing in vivo posterior glenohumeral joint capsular tightness highlight the clinical importance of utilizing a reliable and effective measurement methodology to assess internal rotation ROM during examination of the shoulder, which can lead the clinician to the selective application of treatment interventions to address a deficiency if present.

IDENTIFYING GIRD

To enhance the quality and interpretation of the measurement of glenohumeral joint rotation, several key factors should be taken into consideration. Several authors recommend measurement of glenohumeral internal and external rotation with the joint in 90 degrees of abduction in the coronal plane (Awan et al. 2002, Boon and Smith 2000, Ellenbecker et al. 1996). Care must be taken to stabilize the scapula with measurement taking place with the patient supine so that body weight can minimize scapular motion. Additionally, it is recommended that additional stabilization be provided through a posteriorly directed force by the examiner on the anterior aspect of the coracoid and shoulder during internal rotation ROM measurement (Fig. 31.1). This further serves to stabilize and limit scapular compensation, providing a more isolated internal rotation measurement. Reinold et al. (2008) showed

significant differences between different methods of stabilization and visual observation of glenohumeral internal rotation measurement. Bilateral comparison of internal rotation ROM is recommended with careful interpretation of the isolated glenohumeral motion measurements of internal rotation, external rotation, and total rotation ROM (sum of IR and ER).

PREVENTION AND TREATMENT OF GIRD

In addition to the clinical use of methods to increase internal rotation via both physiologic and accessory mobilization to address the posterior capsule and the posterior rotator cuff muscle tendon units, several stretches have been advocated for home use by patients and athletes to prevent and treat GIRD. A variety of clinical methods can be utilized and include internal rotation stretches in varying positions of abduction in the coronal and scapular plane. Formats include a prolonged static stretch and PNF contract-relax to attempt to provide an optimal load for elongation of the capsular and muscle tendon tissue. Izumi et al. (2008) tested multiple glenohumeral joint positions to determine loading on the posterior capsule in cadavers. They found the position that most optimally elongated the posterior capsule was the position of internal rotation in the scapular plane with 30 degrees of abduction. This study provides objective rationale for the use of clinical methods of internal rotation stretching to address the patient with GIRD.

Figs. 31.2 and 31.3 both show variations of stretching techniques that can be used clinically and provide scapular stabilization and containment of the humeral head by anteriorly based stabilization by the clinician's hand on the proximal humerus during the application of the internal rotation movement. It should be noted that the use of the posterior glide accessory mobilization (Fig. 31.4) can also be used to improve internal rotation ROM, but it should be used with caution and only after an assessment of posterior translation is performed with the glenohumeral joint in the scapular plane using a posterior lateral glide because of the anteverted orientation of the glenoid (Saha 1983). Patients with GIRD often may have increased posterior translation of the humeral head when properly assessed; in these patients extended applications of posterior glides would

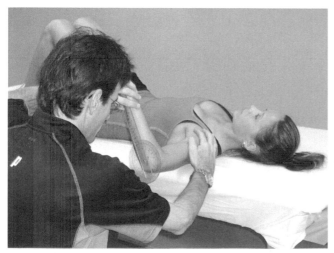

Fig. 31.1 Method of measuring glenohumeral internal rotation range of motion with scapular stabilization.

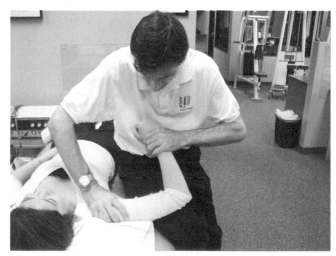

Fig. 31.2 Clinical method for stretching the posterior shoulder with internal rotation applied in the scapular plane with anterior stabilization of the proximal humerus by the clinician.

be contraindicated. Patient-specific application of this mobilization is indicated when hypomobility is effectively determined.

Several studies have been performed testing the effectiveness of home-based stretching of the shoulder to improve internal rotation ROM. Kibler and Chandler (2003) studied junior tennis players on a stretching program of internal rotation using a tennis racquet with the dominant arm placed in the lumbar region of the spine posteriorly and pulling upward. The stretch is referred to as the "up the back" stretch. Players performed a hold–relax type technique using a tennis racquet to provide overpressure. Results showed significant increases in internal rotation ROM over the 1-year training period on both the dominant and nondominant extremity.

More recent research has compared the effects of the cross-arm stretch to the sleeper stretch in a population of recreational athletes, some with significant GIRD ROM deficiency (McClure et al. 2007). The sleeper stretch (Fig. 31.5) involved internally rotating the shoulder while in a side-lying or sleeper position. The scapula is stabilized by the individual's body weight and the shoulder is internally rotated at 90 degrees of elevation. The cross-arm stretch involves arm adduction across the body at chest level and is best performed by stabilizing the lateral edge of the scapula against a wall or supportive surface to limit scapular excursion during the cross-arm movement (Fig. 31.6). In the study by McClure et al. (2007), 4 weeks of stretching produced significantly greater internal rotation gains in the group performing the cross-body stretch as compared with the sleeper stretch. The sleeper stretch group showed gains in internal rotation similar to the control group, which did not stretch during the training period. Further research is clearly needed to better define the optimal application of these stretches; however, this research does show improvement in internal rotation ROM with a home stretching program using both the sleeper and cross-body stretching techniques (McClure et al. 2007).

Manske et al. (2010) studied 39 college-aged asymptomatic individuals while performing a 4-week intervention of either a cross-body stretch or a cross-body stretch with a posterior

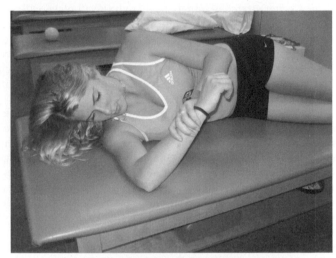

Fig. 31.5 Sleeper stretch position.

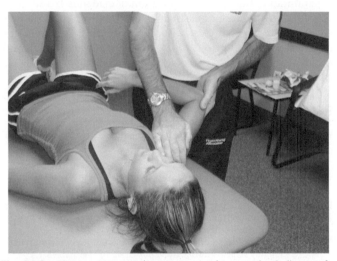

Fig. 31.3 "Figure 4" internal rotation stretching method allowing for internal rotation overpressure with stabilization.

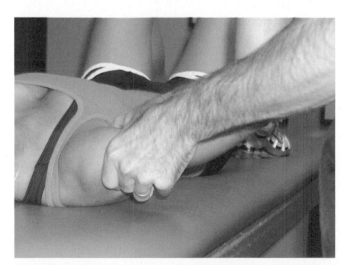

Fig. 31.4 Position for posterior glide mobilization in the scapular plane. Note: A posterior lateral direction of force application is required to allow the humerus to move along the surface of the glenoid.

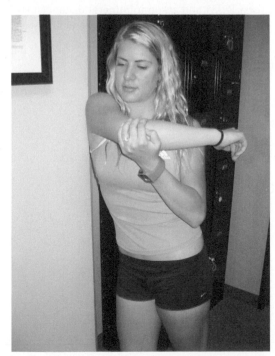

Fig. 31.6 Cross-arm stretch position.

glide mobilization. All subjects had at least a 10-degree difference in internal rotation ROM between extremities. Pretesting and post-testing using a standard inclinometer showed improved internal rotation ROM in both conditions, cross-body stretching with and without a posterior glide mobilization. The authors concluded that both methods produced increases in internal rotation ROM in individuals with a difference of at least 10 degrees of internal rotation between extremities during a 4-week stretching program. Although not significant, the addition of posterior joint mobilizations increased the internal rotation gain to a greater extent than that of stretching alone.

One final study by Laudner et al. (2008) studied the acute effects of the sleeper stretch on internal rotation ROM. Internal rotation measurements were taken before and immediately after three sets of 30-second holds of the sleeper stretch among collegiate baseball players. This study showed an increase of 3.1 degrees in internal rotation ROM immediately after the three sleeper stretches acutely in these baseball players. Based on the results of this study, acute increases in shoulder internal rotation ROM can be expected following the performance of the sleeper stretch in elite overhead athletes. Further research is needed to understand the long-term effects of this stretch and others that affect glenohumeral joint internal rotation ROM.

Maenhout and colleagues (2012) have shown that a 6-week-long daily program of sleeper stretch was able to increase acromiohumeral distance in the dominant shoulder of healthy overhead athletes with GIRD. The dominant arm showed a significant internal rotation deficit (−24.7 degrees ± 6.3 degrees) and horizontal adduction deficit (−11.8 degrees ± 7.4 degrees) and the dominant side acromiohumeral distance was significantly smaller with the arm at neutral (−0.4 ± 0.6 mm) and at 45 degrees (−0.5 ± 0.8 mm) and 60 degrees (−0.6 ± 0.7 mm) of active abduction compared with the nondominant side. After stretching, significant increase of internal rotation (+13.5 degrees ± 0.8 degrees), horizontal adduction (+10.6 degrees ± 0.9 degrees) ROM and acromiohumeral distance (+0.5 to +0.6 mm) was observed at the dominant side of the stretch group compared with prestretching measurements. No significant change of AHD was seen in the nondominant side of the stretch group and in both sides of the control group.

More recent evidence suggests that posterior rotator cuff stiffness, not glenohumeral joint mobility or humeral torsion, is associated with acute resolution in ROM deficits (Bailey et al. 2015). During examination of local mechanisms such as bony structures, glenohumeral joint mobility, and musculotendinous stiffness, it was found that posterior rotator cuff stiffness was the only tissue to respond concurrently with the gains observed in increased shoulder ROM.

SUMMARY

The concept of GIRD is an important one for any clinician treating patients with shoulder dysfunction and especially for those working with overhead athletes. Early recognition and constant monitoring of glenohumeral internal rotation ROM are needed using measurement methods that isolate glenohumeral rotation. Understanding the difference between aGIRD and pGIRD is imperative. The importance of treating pGIRD to gain ROM is paramount. The use and application of evidence-based methods to address limitations in internal rotation are indicated, with further research clearly needed to identify critical values of GIRD that have serious injury ramifications and great study of the methods used to prevent, treat, and manage internal rotation deficiency.

REFERENCES

A complete reference list is available at https://expertconsult .inkling.com/.

FURTHER READING

Brown LP, Neihues SL, Harrah A, et al. Upper extremity range of motion and isokinetic strength of the internal and external shoulder rotators in major league baseball players. *Am J Sports Med*. 1988;16:577–585.

Ellenbecker TS. Shoulder internal and external rotation strength and range of motion in highly skilled tennis players. *Isok Exerc Sci*. 1992;2:1–8.

Postural Consideration for the Female Athlete's Shoulder

Janice K. Loudon, PT, PhD, SCS, ATC, CSCS

Good posture is the key for positioning of the shoulder for activities of daily living and sporting technique. In dealing with the overhead female athlete, the clinician should pay particular attention to the athlete's posture because poor posture may lead to shoulder dysfunction. This section deals with a description of ideal posture, posture impairments, and suggested treatment.

IDEAL POSTURE

Ideal upright posture requires balance of joints and muscles in all three planes. The head should stay balanced, neither tilted nor rotated, on the neck with minimal muscle activity. The thoracic spine curves slightly posterior and serves as a base for scapula movement. Additionally, this portion of the spine needs to have sufficient mobility to allow full shoulder elevation. The scapula rests with the superior medial angle located at or near the level of the second rib and the inferior angle at the seventh to eighth rib, each located approximately 2 to 3 inches from the spine in a plane approximately 30 degrees anterior to the coronal plane. The humerus sits centered within the glenoid cavity with less than one third of the humeral head protruding in front of the acromion. Ideally, the humerus is positioned in neutral rotation with the palm of the hand facing the body. From a posterior view, the olecranon should face directly backward. Table 32.1 presents the ideal postural positions for the upper quarter.

FAULTY POSTURE

The female athlete who spends a great deal of time sitting at the computer or studying for class is more prone to postural dysfunctions. The common forward head posture with increased thoracic kyphosis leads to a chain of events that results in muscle imbalances throughout the upper quarter. This posture also places undue stress on connective tissue structures of the shoulder. Table 32.2 depicts this chain of events.

Several research articles have concluded that there is a strong relationship between faulty posture and shoulder dysfunction. Commonly the scapulae are malpositioned, which creates an environment for poor glenohumeral mechanics. Table 32.3 presents several postural faults and their associated muscle imbalances.

TREATMENT

Treatment of the female overhead athlete focuses on education, thoracic spine mobility, thoracoscapular muscle strengthening, and total body conditioning. Posture education for standing, sitting, sleeping, and sport is discussed with the athlete. Joint mobilization or manipulation to a stiff thoracic spine facilitates the normal sequencing for end-range shoulder motion. Thoracic spine mobilization techniques can be found in other sources. The athlete can be taught thoracic spine self-mobilization using a foam roller. Fig. 32.1 depicts the athlete on a foam roller while performing overhead flexion.

Thoracoscapular muscle strengthening is implemented early in the rehabilitation program prior to rotator cuff strengthening. Weakness of the scapular muscles leads to poor scapulohumeral rhythm. Additionally, the scapula serves as a link in proximal-to-distal sequencing. For throwing athletes the scapula is pivotal in transferring large forces from the legs, pelvis, and trunk to the arm and hand. These exercises should carry over to activities of daily living and posture.

The thoracoscapular muscles and the appropriate exercise selections are listed in Table 32.4. Scaption with the thumb-up position (Fig. 32.2) is an important exercise for strengthening the supraspinatus, along with the serratus anterior and rhomboids. The lower trapezius, which is commonly weak, can be strengthened with a rowing exercise (Fig. 32.3) and prone overhead arm raise (Fig. 32.4). Pink and Perry (1996) via EMG testing found that the primary thoracoscapular exercises are rows,

TABLE 32.1	Ideal Alignment of the Upper Quarter
Head	Held erect, not tilted or rotated
Shoulders	Plumb line bisects acromion; less than one-third humeral head is anterior to acromion; palms face in toward body
Scapulae	Between T2 and T7; 2 to 3 inches from spine; plane is 30 degrees anterior to frontal plane
Thoracic spine	Slightly convex posterior

TABLE 32.2	Forward Head Posture and Chain of Events

Excessive protraction occurs in the craniocervical region.
Upper cervical spine extends to maintain horizontal gaze.
Suboccipital muscles become short.
Suprahyoid shortens and the infrahyoid stretches.
Mouth remains open unless masseter and temporalis muscles contract to close mouth.
Upper trapezius and levator scapulae (attaches to first four cervical transverse processes) become short.
Upper trapezius shortening causes scapular elevation.
Thoracic kyphosis leads to abduction of the scapula (downward rotation, anterior tilt).
Scapular abduction leads to short pectoralis minor.
Rhomboids and lower trapezius lengthen.
Serratus anterior, latissimus dorsi, subscapularis, and teres major become short, leading to internal rotation of the humerus.
Internal rotation of the humerus will diminish overhead abduction.

TABLE 32.3 Postural Faults and Muscle Imbalances		
Malalignment	**Short Muscles (Tight)**	**Long Muscles (Weak)**
Thoracic kyphosis	Pectoralis major Pectoralis minor Internal obliques Shoulder adductors	Thoracic spine extensors Middle trapezius Lower trapezius
Flat thoracic spine	Thoracic spine extensors	
Anterior tilt of scapula	Pectoralis minor Biceps	Lower trapezius Middle trapezius Serratus anterior
Scapular downward rotation	Rhomboids Levator scapulae Latissimus dorsi Pectoralis minor Supraspinatus	Upper trapezius Serratus anterior Lower trapezius
Scapular abduction	Serratus anterior Pectoralis major Pectoralis minor Shoulder external rotators	Middle trapezius Lower trapezius Rhomboids
Humeral medial rotation	Pectoralis major Latissimus dorsi Shoulder internal rotators	Shoulder external rotators
Humeral anteriorly glided	Shoulder external rotators Pectoralis major	Shoulder internal rotators

TABLE 32.4 Thoracoscapular Exercise Selection	
Muscle	**Exercise**
Serratus anterior	Dynamic hug Push-up with plus Shoulder abduction (plane of scapula above 120 degrees) Flexion Serratus anterior punch Scaption Push-up with plus on knees Diagonal flexion, horizontal flexion, external rotation Wall slide
Upper trapezius	Rowing Shoulder shrug Military press Horizontal abduction (external rotation)
Middle trapezius	Horizontal abduction (neutral) Shoulder horizontal abduction Overhead arm raise in line with low trap Horizontal abduction (external rotation) Prone extension Wide grip rowing
Lower trapezius	Abduction Rowing Overhead arm raise in line with low trap Horizontal abduction (external rotation) Prone external rotation
Rhomboids	Horizontal abduction (neutral) Scaption Abduction
Levator scapula	Rowing Horizontal abduction (neutral) Shoulder shrug
Pectoralis minor	Press-up Push-up with a plus Forward punch

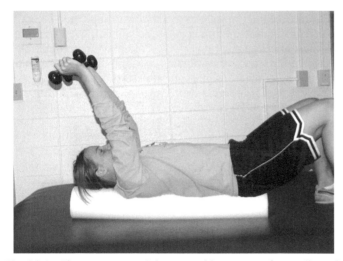

Fig. 32.1 Thoracic spine mobilization. Athlete is using foam roller with upper extremity lift.

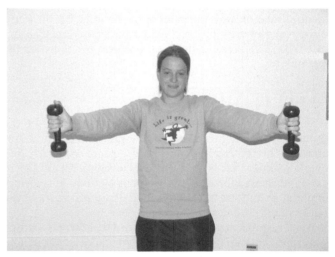

Fig. 32.2 Scaption exercise with thumbs up.

push-up with a plus, press-ups, and serratus punches. Some clinicians advocate using closed chain exercise first because it promotes stability by coactivation of muscles surrounding the shoulder. This type of exercise decreases tensile stress on shoulder ligaments and tendons and facilitates proprioceptive feedback. Examples of closed chain exercises that can be used early in the rehabilitation process include push-up with a plus, press-ups, and internal and external rotation with the elbow stabilized. All muscle strengthening exercises should begin with low weight or partial weight bearing with high repetitions (25 to 30 reps).

As the athlete carries her exercise program over to the weight room, several recommendations are worth noting. Pulling exercises should outnumber the pushing exercises by a ratio of 2:1.

Certain lifts may need to be avoided, especially in athletes with a history of shoulder impingement. These lifts include flies, military press, and bench press. It has been demonstrated that these lifts create excessive tension on the anterior capsule of the shoulder. Other lifts may need to be modified such as a pull-down coming in front of the head versus behind. Also, limiting the arm width in presses and push-ups will help minimize shoulder stress. Total body conditioning including the lower

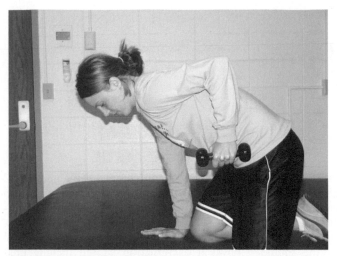

Fig. 32.3 Rowing exercise.

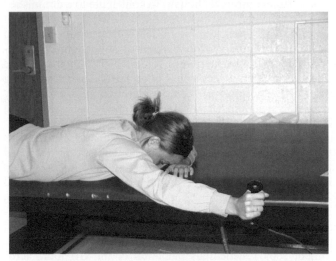

Fig. 32.4 Lower trapezius exercise: prone overhead lift.

extremities and core should also be instituted with the female athlete. Increased strength in baseball pitchers will decrease shoulder injury and improve performance.

Scapular taping may be used as an adjunct to the exercise program outlined earlier. Selkowitz and colleagues (2007) found that scapular taping decreased upper trapezius activity and increased lower trapezius activity in 21 subjects with shoulder impingement. Host (1995) used scapular taping to promote stability of the scapula in an individual with an 8-month history of shoulder impingement.

REFERENCES

A complete reference list is available at https://expertconsult.inkling.com/.

FURTHER READING

Burkhart SS, Morgan CD, Kibler WB. The disabled throwing shoulder: spectrum of pathology. Part III: the SICK scapula, scapular dyskinesis, the kinetic chain and rehabilitation. *Arthroscopy*. 2003;19(6):641–661.

Cools AM, et al. Scapular muscle recruitment patterns: trapezius muscle latency with and without impingement symptoms. *Am J Sports Med*. 2003;31(4):542–549.

Davies GJ, Ellenbecker TS. Total arm strength for shoulder and elbow overuse injuries. In: Timm K, ed. *Upper Extremity. Orthopedic Section Home Study Course*; 1993. La Crosse, WI.

Ekstrom RA, Donatelli RA, Soderberg GL. Surface electromyographic analysis of exercises for the trapezius and serratus anterior muscles. *J Orthop Sports Phys Ther*. 2003;33(5):247–358.

Gray H. *Anatomy of the Human Body*. 28th ed. Philadelphia, PA: Lea & Febiger; 1966.

Hoppenfeld S. *Physical Examination of the Spine and Extremities*. New York: Appleton-Century-Crofts; 1976:276.

Kendall FP, McCreary EK, Provance PG, et al. *Muscles Testing and Function with Posture and Pain*. 5th ed. Baltimore: Williams and Wilkins; 2005.

Kibler WB. The role of the scapula in athletic shoulder function. *Am J Sports Med*. 1998;26(2):325–337.

Ludewig PM, Cook TM. Alterations in shoulder kinematics and associated muscle activity in people with symptoms of shoulder impingement. *Phys Ther*. 2000;80(3):276–291.

Ludewig PM, Cook TM, Nawoczenski DA. Three-dimensional scapular orientation and muscle activity at selected positions of humeral elevation. *J Orthop Sports Phys Ther*. 1996;24(2):57–65.

Lukasiewicz AC, et al. Comparison of 3-dimensional scapular position and orientation between subjects with and without shoulder impingement. *J Orthop Sports Phys Ther*. 1999;29(10):574–586.

McClure PW, Michener LA, Sennett BJ, et al. Direct 3-dimensional measurement of scapular kinematics during dynamic movements in vivo. *J Shoulder Elbow Surg*. 2001;11110:269–277.

McQuade KJ, Dawson J, Smidt GL. Scapulothoracic muscle fatigue associated with alterations in scapulohumeral rhythm kinematics during maximum resistive shoulder elevation. *J Orthop Sports Phys Ther*. 1998;28:74–80.

Moseley JB, Jobe FW, Pink M, et al. EMG analysis of the scapular muscles during a shoulder rehabilitation program. *Am J Sports Med*. 1992;20(2):128–134.

Sahrmann SA. *Diagnosis and Treatment of Movement Impairment Syndromes*. St. Louis, MO: Mosby; 2002.

Stone JA, Lueken JS, Partin NB, et al. Closed kinetic chain rehabilitation for the glenohumeral joint. *J Athl Train*. 1993;28:34–37.

Voight ML, Thomson BC. The role of the scapula in the rehabilitation of shoulder injuries. *J Athl Train*. 2000;35(3):364–372.

Warner JJ, Micheli LJ, Arslanian LE, et al. Scapulothoracic motion in normal shoulders and shoulders with glenohumeral instability and impingement syndrome. *Clin Orthop. Rel Res*. 1992;285:191–199.

33

Impingement Syndrome

Michael D. Rosenthal, PT, DSc, SCS, ECS, ATC, CSCS | Josef H.
Moore, PT, PhD | Joseph R. Lynch, MD

IMPINGEMENT SYNDROME

The clinical diagnosis of "impingement syndrome" was introduced in 1972 by Dr. Charles Neer II and comprised a spectrum of disease ranging from chronic bursitis and partial tears of the supraspinatus tendon to complete tears (Neer 1972). It was hypothesized that the rotator cuff underwent progressive pathologic change due to compression against a rough undersurface of the coracoacromial arch made up of the anterior third of the acromion, the coracoacromial ligament, and the AC joint (Fig. 33.1). Since Neer's original report, greater understanding of the shoulder has led to further growth in the diagnosis and treatment of this clinical syndrome that we now understand to represent a continuum of rotator cuff pathology (Neer 1983).

Impingement syndrome—or more accurately rotator cuff pathology—can produce shoulder pain, weakness, and referred pain or paresthesias into the region of the deltoid insertion and upper lateral arm. A thorough examination of the upper extremity and axial spine is necessary to rule out other pathology that can produce similar symptoms or co-exist with impingement syndrome. The role of proximal segments (i.e., trunk and hips) should also be considered and assessed in the comprehensive evaluation of the patient with impingement syndrome. When impingement syndrome is suspected it is important to differentiate between the possible types of rotator cuff pathology: primary subacromial (coracoacromial arch), secondary subacromial (coracoacromial arch), and internal (Hayworth 2009). The majority of impingement syndrome cases are attributed to either primary or secondary (Bigliani 1997). Accurate diagnosis is necessary to guide the most appropriate course of management.

Rotator cuff impingement, regardless of the type, alters muscular function of the cuff and results in diminished dynamic control of the glenohumeral (GH) joint (Michener 2003). Until optimal strength and neuromuscular control are established, continued use of the arm at or above the level of the shoulder will produce further impingement of the rotator cuff (Manske 2013). If cuff impingement is not recognized and corrected early the problem can progress to degradation of tissue and resultant tears in the rotator cuff. The Neer classification is still widely used and described in Box 33.1.

Primary Impingement

Primary subacromial impingement is the result of an abnormal mechanical relationship between the rotator cuff and the coracoacromial arch (acromion, coracoacromial ligament, and/or coracoid process) (Bigliani 1997, Cavallo 1998). It also includes other "primary" factors that can lead to narrowing of the subacromial outlet (Table 33.1). Patients with primary impingement are usually older than 35 years and complain of anterolateral shoulder and upper lateral arm pain, with an inability to sleep on the affected side. They have complaints of shoulder weakness, which may be due to pain inhibition or true cuff pathology, and difficulty performing activities at or above the level of the shoulder. Physical examination should include postural assessment of the thoracic region, scapula, and GH joint because faulty posture is thought to contribute to a diminished subacromial outlet space (Kibler 1998, Lewis 2005). Range of motion (ROM) assessment often demonstrates limitations and pain with forward elevation (flexion or abduction) and horizontal adduction. Evaluation of rotator cuff strength with the patient's arm at his or her side is often normal, whereas testing performed in positions of shoulder elevation more consistently reproduces symptoms of pain and weakness. The Hawkin's sign, Neer impingement sign, empty can sign (Jobe's test), painful arc, external and internal rotation resistance strength tests are often positive, and the clinician should assess for localized symptom reproduction while recognizing that these tests can elicit symptoms when other shoulder pathology exists as well (Cavallo 1998, Diercks 2014, Michener 2009, Tennent 2003, Zaslav 2001). The Neer **impingement test,** performed by injecting 10 ml of 1% lidocaine (Xylocaine) into the subacromial space, can be useful in diagnosing impingement (Neer 1983, Tennent 2003). Meticulous palpation of the GH joint, acromioclavicular joint (AC), and coracoid region can also assist in determining the source of the patient's symptoms. Patients with primary impingement may have associated AC joint arthritis or a history of an AC joint sprain, which may ultimately contribute to pathologic compression of the rotator cuff. Patients often report discomfort in the anterior subacromial region and AC joint region with internal rotation maneuvers, such as scratching their back, or experience pain superiorly with shoulder abduction. Findings on physical examination that confirm AC joint pathology include localized tenderness at the AC joint with palpation, symptom reproduction (localized to the AC joint) with cross-body adduction, reproduction of pain with O'Brien's test (resisted elevation with the arm forward elevated 90 degrees, internally rotated, and horizontally adducted), and resolution of the pain with an injection of lidocaine into the AC joint. Radiologic evaluation including an anteroposterior, axillary, and supraspinatus outlet views may support the diagnosis of primary or "outlet" impingement by demonstrating bony abnormality contributing to narrowing of the subacromial space from acromial morphology, spurring, or hypertrophy of the AC joint (Balke 2013, Cavallo 1998) (Fig. 33.2).

Secondary Impingement

Secondary impingement is a clinical phenomenon that results in a "relative narrowing" of the subacromial space.

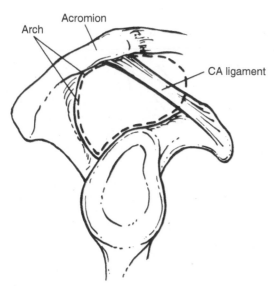

Fig. 33.1 The normal coracoacromial (CA) arch. (From F.W. Jobe, Ed: *Operative Techniques in Upper Extremity Sports Injuries.* St. Louis, Mosby, 1996.)

TABLE 33.1	Structural Factors That May Increase Subacromial Joint Impingement	
Structure	**Abnormal Characteristics**	
Acromioclavicular joint	Congenital anomaly	
	Degenerative spur formation	
Acromion	Unfused acromion (Os acromiale)	
Coracoid	Degenerative spurs on undersurface	
Rotator cuff	Malunion/nonunion of fracture	
Humerus	Congenital anomaly	
Congenital	Abnormal shape after surgery or trauma	
	Thickening of tendon from calcific deposits	
	Tendon thickening after surgery or trauma	
	Upper surface irregularities from partial or complete tears	
	Increased prominence of greater tuberosity from anomalies or malunions	

Modified from Matsen FA III, Arntz CT: Subacromial Impingement. In Rockwood CA Jr, Matsen FA III (eds): The Shoulder. Philadelphia, WB Saunders, 1990.

BOX 33.1 (NEER'S) PROGRESSIVE STAGES OF SHOULDER (PRIMARY) IMPINGEMENT

STAGE 1: EDEMA AND INFLAMMATION

Typical age: Younger than 25 yr but may occur at any age.
Clinical course: Reversible lesion.
Physical signs:
- Tenderness to palpation over the greater tuberosity of the humerus.
- Tenderness along anterior ridge or acromion.
- Painful arc of abduction between 60 and 120 degrees, increased with resistance at 90 degrees.
- Positive impingement sign.
- Shoulder ROM may be restricted with significant subacromial inflammation.

STAGE 2: FIBROSIS AND TENDINITIS

Typical age: 25–40 yr.
Clinical course: Not reversible by modification of activity.
Physical signs: Stage 1 signs plus the following:
- Greater degree of soft tissue crepitus may be felt because of scarring in the subacromial space.
- Catching sensation with lowering of arm at approximately 100 degrees.
- Limitation of active and passive ROM.

STAGE 3: BONE SPURS AND TENDON RUPTURES

Typical age: Greater than 40 yr.
Clinical course: Not reversible.
Physical signs: Stages 1 and 2 signs plus the following:
- Limitation of ROM, more pronounced with active motion.
- Atrophy of infraspinatus.
- Weakness of shoulder abduction and external rotation.
- Biceps tendon involvement.
- AC joint tenderness.

This often results from excessive GH joint mobility or scapular dyskinesis (Kibler 1998, Kibler 2013) (Fig. 33.3). In those patients who have underlying GH hypermobility, with or without instability, the symptoms of secondary rotator cuff impingement are caused by excessive demands placed on the rotator cuff to dynamically stabilize the shoulder. While the rotator cuff may effectively stabilize the hypermobile GH joint, when this requirement is coupled with repetitive overhead movement (i.e., swimming or throwing) muscular fatigue is often produced. Rotator cuff fatigue leads to the loss of the stabilizing function and allows superior migration of the humeral head (decreased depression of the humeral head during throwing and less "clearance") and is thought to result in mechanical compression of the rotator cuff on the coracoacromial arch (Chen 1999, Michener 2003, Royer 2009) (Fig. 33.4).

In patients with scapular dyskinesis (limited or excessive scapular mobility), impingement results from **improper positioning of the scapula with relation to the humerus.** This loss of neuromuscular scapular control produces insufficient retraction along with inadequate upward rotation and posterior tilting of the scapula resulting in earlier abutment of the acromion and coracoacromial arch on the underlying rotator cuff (Kibler 1998, Kibler 2013, Ludewig 2009, Michener 2003).

Patients with secondary impingement are usually younger and often participate in overhead sporting activities such as baseball, swimming, volleyball, tennis, or weight lifting. Pain and weakness with overhead motions are a common complaint and they may even describe a feeling of the arm going "dead." Physical examination should include observation of postural or soft tissue asymmetries about the shoulder girdle, ROM symmetry, strength testing of the rotator cuff and scapular stabilizing muscles, and special provocative tests such as Hawkin's test and Neer's sign. Furthermore, assessment of spinal mobility restrictions, primarily in the cervical and/or thoracic spine, should be assessed based on their potential role in impacting scapulothoracic and GH joint mobility (Kabaetse 1999, Ludewig 1996). Regional interdependence has been shown to influence shoulder symptoms and outcomes (Bergman 2004). The examiner should look for possible associated pathology, including GH joint instability, with a positive apprehension and relocation test or abnormal scapular function such as scapular winging or asymmetrical motion. Glenohumeral joint hyperlaxity, without instability, can be further assessed by the sulcus and Gagey hyperabduction tests. The scapular retraction and scapular assistance tests can effectively

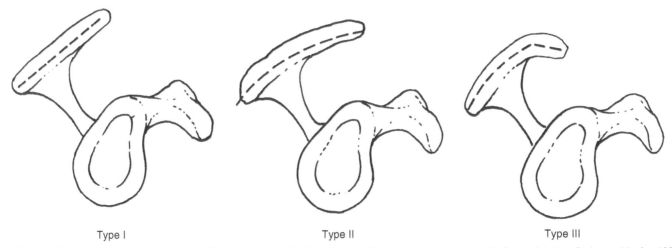

Type I   Type II   Type III

Fig. 33.2 Different acromion morphologies. (From F.W. Jobe, Ed: Operative Techniques in Upper Extremity Sports Injuries. St. Louis, Mosby, 1996.)

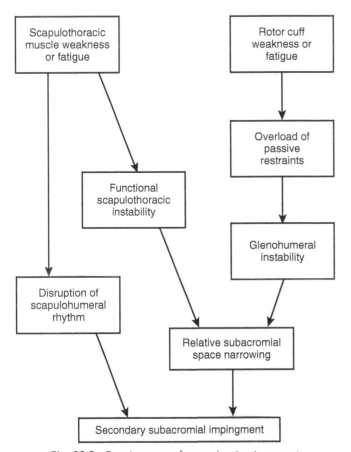

Fig. 33.3 Development of secondary impingement.

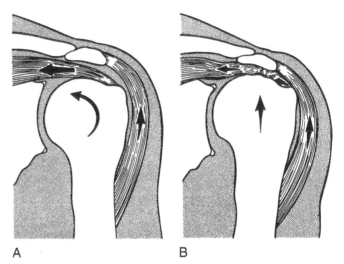

A   B

Fig. 33.4 The supraspinatus tendon (rotator cuff) helps to stabilize the head of the humerus against the upward pull of the deltoid. **A,** Subacromial impingement is prevented by the normal cuff rotator function. **B,** Deep surface tearing of the supraspinatus tendon weakens the ability of the cuff to hold the humeral head down (i.e., depress the humeral head to allow clearance under the acromion) resulting in impingement of the tendon at the acromion with overhead activities. (A and B, Redrawn from Matsen FA III, Arntz CT: Subacromial impingement. In Rockwood CA Jr, Matsen FA III, Eds.: The Shoulder. Philadelphia, WB Saunders, 1990, p. 624.)

demonstrate the impact of altered scapular neuromuscular control as a source of the patient's symptoms and indicate the potential for improved shoulder function by correcting this deficiency (Burkhart 2003, Tate 2008). **Patients with tightness in the posterior shoulder will have a loss of internal rotation. Posterior capsular tightness leads to an obligate anterosuperior translation of the humeral head and resultant diminished subacromial outlet space, which is thought to contribute to the impingement problem** (Burkhart 2003, Tyler 2000).

In patients with secondary impingement, treatment of the underlying problem should result in resolution of the "secondary impingement" symptoms. Clinicians should be aware of the potential for proximal kinetic chain deficits (i.e., lumbo-pelvic-hip complex) to contribute to secondary impingement (Kibler 1998, McMullen 2000). **Often, recognition of the underlying GH joint laxity or scapular instability is missed, and the "secondary impingement" is incorrectly treated as a "primary" impingement. A subacromial decompression may worsen the symptoms because the shoulder is rendered even more "unstable" and does not address the primary mechanical problem.**

Internal Impingement

Posterior shoulder pain produced by contact of the greater tuberosity with the posterosuperior aspect of the glenoid, when the shoulder is abducted to approximately 90 degrees and fully externally rotated, produces impingement of the posterior rotator cuff, capsule, and labrum (Gold 2007, Walch 1992). While this "internal impingement" is present in normal physiologic motion it may become pathologic with repetitive overhead activities. The pathology consists of undersurface tears of the posterior supraspinatus and/or anterior aspect of the infraspinatus tendon and often includes superior labrum anterior to posterior (SLAP) tears (Heyworth 2009). There is debate regarding causation of this syndrome (Heyworth 2009, Manske 2013). Anterior instability and inadequate neuromuscular control, enabling cuff tendon entrapment with the glenoid during excessive anterior humeral head translation, is one proposed mechanism (Cavallo 1998). Another reported mechanism is tightness within the posterior GH joint, restricting normal GH rotation and producing a posterosuperior shift in the GH contact point creating the pathologic "peel-back mechanism" (Burkhart 2003).

Patients with pathologic internal impingement are usually under 35 years of age and involved in repetitive overhead abduction and external rotation demand activities. Patient complaints often include posterior shoulder pain (specifically in the late cocking position), stiffness, and decreasing performance (i.e., loss of throwing velocity or control) (Manske 2013). Physical examination should focus on localized symptom reproduction with special tests, posterior GH joint palpation, and ROM. Posterior impingement signs and Jobe's relocation test, with specific resolution of posterior GH joint pain, are recommended (Meister 2004). Increased external rotation and decreased internal rotation are common in patients with internal impingement (Morrison 2000, Myers 2006, Tyler 2010, Tyler 2000). Concurrent shoulder pathology often exists in the presence of pathologic internal impingement so a thorough shoulder examination is important to ascertain the possibility of co-existing conditions.

TREATMENT

The key to the successful treatment of subacromial impingement is defining the underlying cause, whether it is primary or secondary to the pathologic relationship between the coracoacromial arch and the rotator cuff or due to internal impingement. Identification of the true cause is critical when conservative management fails and surgical intervention is indicated, because the operative procedures are different for these clinical entities. **For primary impingement, surgical treatment is directed toward addressing primary rotator cuff pathology such as bursitis, partial thickness or full thickness cuff tears, and abrasive or prominent surfaces of the underlying acromion and acromioclavicular joint. The surgical treatment for secondary impingement and internal impingement must address the primary mechanical abnormality, which is often not the rotator cuff or undersurface of the acromion but rather is a problem with shoulder hypermobility.** For example, if impingement symptoms develop secondary to multidirectional instability, **the surgical treatment is a stabilization surgery, not an acromioplasty.** Performing a rotator cuff procedure or acromioplasty in the setting of GH instability will not cure the shoulder problem and may serve only to make the underlying condition worse.

Nonoperative Treatment

Nonoperative treatment is frequently successful and involves a combination of treatment modalities including anti-inflammatory medications and a well-organized rehabilitation program (Box 33.2). While comprehensive rehabilitation for both primary and secondary impingement syndrome is similar, optimal outcomes are most likely to be attained with an individualized program that addresses patient-specific impairments as opposed to applying a general protocol (Bang 2000). The initial goals of the rehabilitative process are to obtain pain relief, regain motion, and promote scapulothoracic and rotator cuff neuromuscular control (Manski 2013). Along with oral medications, use of a subacromial injection with a corticosteroid may help to control the discomfort in the acute stages of the inflammatory process (Diercks 2014, Krabak 2003). Modalities such as heat and cryotherapy, while lacking in supporting research evidence, are often utilized for pain management. Research does not support the use of ultrasound or electrical stimulation, although still commonly applied, for enhancing outcomes. Improving comfort may promote more successful advances in motion and strengthening.

Because the rotator cuff tendons are intact, ROM exercises can be passive, active-assisted, and active. Initially, these are done within the patient's available pain-free range, usually below 90 degrees of abduction, to avoid reproduction of impingement symptoms. As symptoms improve, the ROM is increased. During the performance of ROM exercises it is important to ensure quality of shoulder girdle motion and avoidance of compensatory shoulder shrugging. ROM and stretching exercises should be performed at least daily (Kuhn 2009). **Selection of stretching exercises should be based on postural impairments and movement limitations.** Pectoralis minor stretching is important for both primary and secondary impingement to allow posterior tilting of the scapula and to improve subacromial outlet space (Borstad 2005, Burkhart 2003). Anterior GH joint stretching should not be performed in patients with secondary impingement. If a GH joint internal rotation deficit (GIRD) is identified, posterior capsular stretching should be initiated. Cross-chest (horizontal adduction) and "sleeper" stretches have been shown to restore normal posterior GH joint mobility (Tyler 2010). Scapular stabilization while performing these exercises is key to selectively stretching the posterior GH joint and minimizing stretch of the medial scapular stabilizers. Correction of GIRD is a key component in the treatment of both primary and internal impingement (Burkhart 2003).

Localized manual therapy techniques to address GH joint, scapulothoracic, and/or spinal mobility restrictions may also be necessary to optimize shoulder girdle complex mobility. Multiple studies have demonstrated efficacy in improving shoulder impingement symptoms by addressing spinal impairments (regional interdependence model) (Bang 2000, Bergman 2004, Boyles 2009, Rhon 2014). Soft tissue mobilization techniques can also serve as a useful adjunct in the resolution of impingement symptoms (Haahr 2005, Senbursa 2007).

Initial strength training consists of scapular control, closed chain exercises, multidirectional isometrics, and isotonics (Escamilla 2014, Kibler 2001, Kibler 1998, McMullen 2000). **Scapula stabilizing exercises** are important for patients with all types of impingement (Figures 33.5 and 33.6). The scapula forms the stable base from which the rotator cuff and scapular stabilizing muscles originate. Reciprocal motion is required between the GH and scapulothoracic joints for proper cuff function and correct positioning of the coraco-acromial arch. **Abnormal scapular movement (dyskinesis)** can be corrected, and impingement symptoms ameliorated, with manual assistance (clinician-applied scapular retraction or upward rotation) or with a scapular taping program as part of the exercise regimen (Burkhart 2003, Kibler 1998) (Fig. 33.7). Although scapular taping has become popular, further research is necessary to substantiate widespread use of this treatment technique (Hsu 2009, Thelen 2008). Restoration of normal scapular neuromuscular control should be achieved by application of a progressive dynamic strengthening program that includes coordinated movement of the trunk with the scapulothoracic and GH joints (Kibler 2001, Kibler 2013, McMullen 2000).

Closed chain exercises assist in developing proximal stability and enhancing neuromuscular control of the scapula (Fig. 33.8) while effectively strengthening the rotator cuff (Burkhart 2003, McMullen 2000, Uhl 2003). Progression of closed chain exercises from limited axial loading in kneeling or standing to greater magnitudes of axial loading will increase muscular recruitment and preparation for return to preinjury activities.

Isometric exercises begin with the arm at the side and may progress to varying angles of pain-free shoulder elevation (Escamilla 2014). Isotonic exercises, performed with the use of resistance bands, cable machines, or light dumbbells, are initially focused on rotator cuff strengthening with the arm at the side. **These exercises help restore the ability of the rotator cuff to dynamically depress and stabilize the humeral head, resulting in a relative increase in the subacromial space** (Reinold 2009, Sharkey 1995). Progression involves functional movement patterns of the shoulder (Fig. 33.9) within the available pain-free range of mobility while ensuring quality of the movement pattern. **In general, isolated flexion and abduction movements are limited in the early rehabilitation phase to avoid impingement symptoms** (McClure 2004). Isokinetic exercises may be introduced once good rotator cuff strength and scapular stability are achieved. Isokinetic training, variable resistance at a constant predetermined speed of movement, can be helpful in maximizing return of shoulder girdle power and muscular endurance (Ellenbecker 2000). Incorporation of eccentric loading training of the rotator cuff and deltoid may also contribute to functional improvements and reduction in pain for patients with nonoperative management (Jonsson 2006).

In patients with secondary impingement, strengthening is started with the arm near the patient's side and advanced through greater ranges of motion while avoiding positions that provoke symptoms of impingement or instability (i.e., combined abduction and external rotation). As dynamic stabilization (neuromuscular control) of the scapula and GH joint improves, exercises can be advanced into greater ranges of

---

BOX 33.2 CONSERVATIVE (NONOPERATIVE) TREATMENT OF SHOULDER IMPINGEMENT

Exercise progression is based on functional improvement and pain reduction, not a specific time frame. Patient education throughout all phases is important to ensure restoration of optimal shoulder girdle neuromuscular control and performance.

MODALITIES
- Heat applied before exercise may facilitate gains in ROM.
- Ice application following resistance exercises

RANGE OF MOTION (PERFORMED 1–2 TIMES DAILY)
- Active and active-assisted ROM in the scapular plane
- Posterior capsule stretching (Fig. 33.10)
- Progression to end-range stretching. End-range stretching should continue to be performed once full range of motion is achieved (i.e., through the late stage of rehabilitation).

MANUAL THERAPY
- Techniques applied by clinician to address specific GH joint capsular, scapulothoracic joint, or spinal mobility limitations. Manual therapy techniques should be initiated in the initial phase and may be necessary throughout all stages of rehabilitation.

STRENGTH TRAINING (PERFORMED ON ALTERNATING DAYS; I.E., 3 TO 4 DAYS PER WEEK)
- **Initial phase:** scapular neuromuscular control, closed chain exercises, rotator cuff isometrics, and limited range isotonics (1–3 sets of 10–15 repetitions)
- Scapular retraction, depression, PNFs, shoulder dump, scapular clocks, prone row, and low row
- Rotator cuff isometrics progressing from arm at the side to varying angles of shoulder elevation
- Begin isotonics, limited to 0 to 90 degrees of shoulder elevation, when cuff isometrics can be performed without pain.
- **Progress to intermediate phase** when normal scapulothoracic and glenohumeral motion are present through a 0- to-150 degree arc of shoulder elevation (concentric and eccentric control).

- **Intermediate phase:** Progression of strengthening and attainment of full range of motion
- Scapular retraction with horizontal abduction ("T") (Fig. 33.11), scapular "Y" (Fig. 33.12), shoulder punches, wall circles
- PNFs and rhythmic stabilization exercises
- Seated press-ups and push-up "plus" progression (wall to incline to traditional)
- Isotonics: flexion, extension, adduction, abduction, IR/ER at 45 to 90 degrees abduction, rows in standing
- Plyometric exercises (see Fig. 33.13)
- **Progress to late phase** when the patient is pain free and demonstrates normal scapulothoracic and glenohumeral mechanics throughout the full range of motion (both concentric and eccentric control) and 5/5 strength.
- **Late phase:** Focus on restoration of shoulder girdle strength, neuromuscular control, and maintenance of normal mobility.
- Individualize the rehabilitation progression to prepare the patient for specific occupational and athletic demands.
- Isokinetic exercises and testing
- Closed kinetic chain: push-up plus with diminishing support (i.e., single leg or on a physioball) and figure 8 exercises. Closed kinetic chain testing
- Strength training may include changing the stability of the base of support (i.e., double to single-leg stance and performing exercises while standing on a wobble board or foam mat). Modification of lower extremity and core support and integrated demands by performing various shoulder movements while in a split stance or athletic stance (Fig. 33.14), while squatting or lunging (Fig. 33.15), whole body diagonal movements (lift and chop) (Fig. 33.16), and unilateral lifting (dumbbells)
- Gradual return to traditional weightlifting exercises. Caution is recommended when returning to barbell pressing movements (bench, incline, and military presses) and dips because these movements can result in a return of symptoms. Behind the neck pull-downs and military press should be avoided.

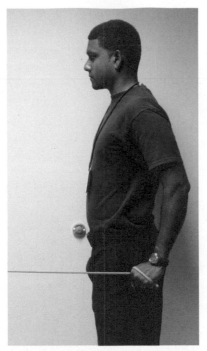

Fig. 33.5 Resistance band low row.

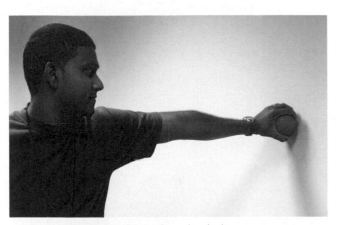

Fig. 33.6 Scapular clocks.

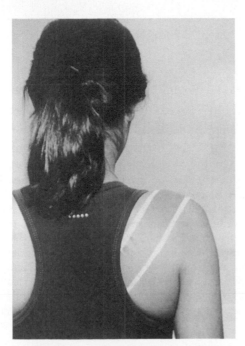

Fig. 33.7 Example of scapular taping.

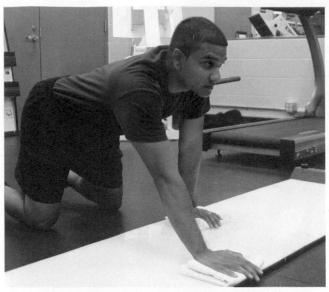

Fig. 33.8 Closed kinetic chain flexion–extension.

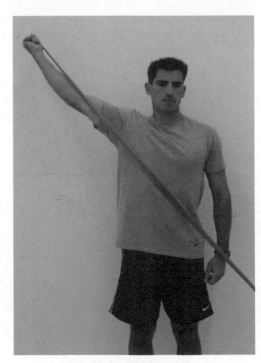

Fig. 33.9 PNF D$_2$ pattern.

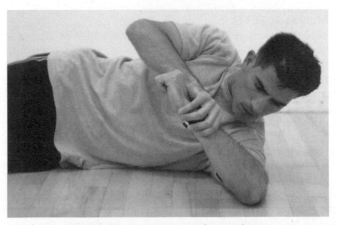

Fig. 33.10 Posterior capsule stretching.

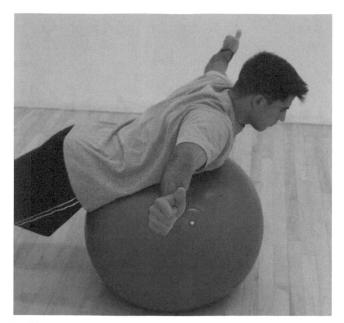

Fig. 33.11 "T" exercise, scapular retraction with horizontal abduction.

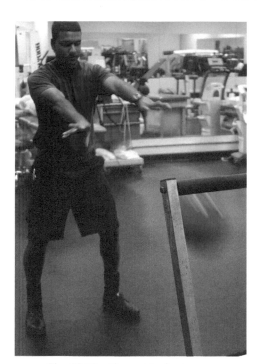

Fig. 33.13 Plyometric chest pass.

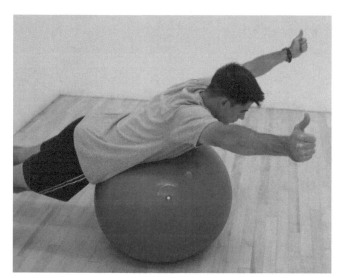

Fig. 33.12 "Y" exercise, scapular depression and retraction with shoulder flexion.

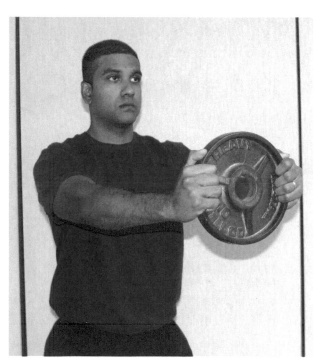

Fig. 33.14 Plate press in athletic stance.

shoulder elevation, abduction, and external rotation (Escamilla 2014, Manske 2013).

Strengthening of both the scapular musculature and rotator cuff should include increasing levels of resistance and volume of activity to improve muscular endurance. Readiness for return-to-overhead activities (sports or occupational demands) should be based on demand-specific analysis for optimal return of strength and mobility (Kibler 2001). **Return to high-demand activities based solely on absence of pain, without full return of requisite strength and mobility throughout the kinetic chain, will put the patient at risk for eventual return of impingement symptoms.**

Historically, nonoperative treatment was considered unsuccessful if no improvement occurred after a year of proper conservative management. **Today, nonoperative treatment should be considered unsuccessful if the patient shows no improvement after 3 to 6 months of a comprehensive and coordinated medical and rehabilitative program. After 6 months of appropriate conservative treatment, most patients have achieved maximal improvement from the nonoperative treatment program** (Bigliani 1997, Cavallo 1998). Adherence to nonoperative care is critical because subacromial decompression has not been shown to produce superior outcomes to nonoperative management (Gebremariam 2011, Haahr 2005, Ketola 2013, Kuhn 2009). In patients with an accurate diagnosis, failed conservative management or a plateau in recovery at

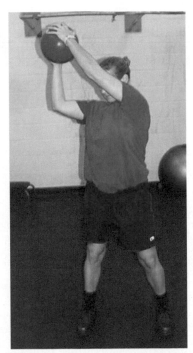

Fig. 33.15 Lift and chop, whole body PNF.

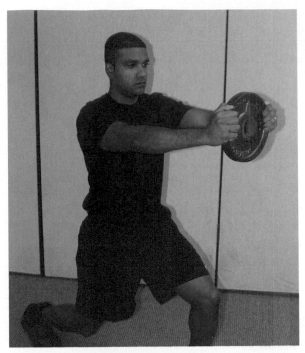

Fig. 33.16 Lunge and lift.

an undesirable level of function can be an indication for surgical intervention.

Operative Treatment

The success of operative treatment is dependent upon an accurate diagnosis, a thorough understanding of the underlying mechanical abnormality, and the technical skill of the surgeon performing the procedure designed to correct the mechanical problem. **For primary impingement syndrome,** it is believed that rotator cuff pathology is the primary problem; therefore, surgical treatment aimed at addressing the rotator cuff and surrounding anatomy is the current **procedure of choice** (Bigliani 1997). Rehabilitation after surgery focuses on pain control, improved ROM, and muscle strengthening and can be dependent on the severity of the pathology found at the time of surgery (bursitis vs. full thickness rotator cuff tear) (Box 33.3). Return to high demand sports can be limited and a comprehensive postoperative rehabilitation program must be emphasized. Outcomes from subacromial decompression have been noted to be similar in both groups that underwent arthroscopic decompression as well as those that underwent open subacromial decompression (Davis 2010, Gebremariam 2011, Husby 2003).

For secondary impingement, surgical treatment must be directed at the primary problem. For instance, if GH instability is identified as the primary problem and is associated with the development of secondary impingement type symptoms, surgical treatment should focus on addressing shoulder stability. Open or arthroscopic stabilization procedures

may be performed, with either a repair of a torn or avulsed labrum or a capsular shift (capsulorrhaphy), depending on the underlying primary etiology. The potential advantages of arthroscopic procedures include decreased operative time, less operative morbidity, less loss of motion, and a quicker recovery (Davis 2010). The rehabilitation principles after an arthroscopic stabilization procedure that includes a labral repair or suture capsulorrhaphy are similar to those after an open stabilization procedure. The biology of healing tissue is the same whether the procedure is done open or arthroscopically. The rehabilitation protocol after an open or arthroscopic Bankart repair for anterior shoulder instability is fundamentally the same (with the only notable difference of protecting the subscapularis tenotomy following a traditional open Bankart procedure).

When **internal impingement** is suspected a thorough bilateral examination under anesthesia is conducted along with diagnostic arthroscopy (Heyworth 2009). Surgical management of internal impingement may include anterior capsular plication, posterior capsular release, débridement or repair of the rotator cuff tear, and débridement or repair of the posterosuperior labral pathology (Heyworth 2009). The rehabilitation protocol implemented is pathology specific (i.e., post anterior capsulorrhaphy protocol) with special focus on maintenance of posterior capsule mobility. Clinical outcomes for surgical treatment of patients with internal impingement—particularly overhead athletes—can be guarded, particularly as it relates to return to presurgical levels of play. As such, every effort is made to correct these patients' pathology through nonsurgical means.

BOX 33.3 **PROGRESSIVE, SYSTEMATIC INTERVAL PROGRAMS FOR RETURNING TO SPORTS AFTER ARTHROSCOPIC SUBACROMIAL DECOMPRESSION (WITH MODIFICATION FOR DISTAL CLAVICLE RESECTION AND/OR ROTATOR CUFF DÉBRIDEMENT)**

PHASE 1: WEEKS 0–4

Restrictions

- ROM
- 140 degrees of forward flexion.
- 40 degrees of external rotation.
- 60 degrees of abduction.
- ROM exercises begin with the arm comfortably at the patient's side, progress to 45 degrees of abduction and eventually 90 degrees. Abduction is advanced slowly depending on patient comfort level.
- No combined abduction and rotation until 6 wk after surgery.
- No resisted motions until 4 wk postoperative.
- No cross-body adduction until 8 wk postoperatively if distal clavicle resection.

Immobilization

- Early motion is important.
- Sling immobilization for comfort only during the first 2 wk.
- Sling should be discontinued by 2 wk after surgery.
- Patients can use sling at night for comfort.

Pain Control

- Reduction of pain and discomfort is essential for recovery
- Medications
- Narcotics—10 day–2 wk following surgery.
- Nonsteroidal anti-inflammatory drugs (NSAIDs) for patients with persistent discomfort following surgery.
- Therapeutic modalities (ice, HVGS).
- Moist heat before therapy, ice at end of session.

Motion: Shoulder

Goals

- 140 degrees of forward flexion.
- 40 degrees of external rotation.
- 60 degrees of abduction.

Exercises

- Begin with Codman pendulum exercises to promote early motion.
- Passive ROM exercises (Fig. 33.17).
- Manual therapy (capsular stretching) for anterior, posterior, and inferior capsule (Fig. 33.18).
- Active-assisted ROM exercises (Fig. 33.19).
- Shoulder flexion, extension, internal and external rotation.
- Progress to active ROM exercises as comfort improves.
- Address proximal kinetic chain motion restrictions (i.e., limited thoracic extension).

Motion: Elbow

- Active
- 0 to 130 degrees.
- Pronation and supination as tolerated.

Muscle Strengthening

- Gripping exercises.
- Scapular control exercises (retraction, depression, and low row)
- Light resistance isometric IR and ER (delay until 3-4 weeks if RTC débridement is performed)

PHASE 2: WEEKS 4–8

Criteria for Progression to Phase 2

- Minimal pain and tenderness.
- Nearly complete motion.
- Scapular muscle control

Restrictions

- Progress ROM goals to
  - 160 degrees of forward flexion.
  - 45 degrees of internal rotation (vertebral level L1).
  - 60 degrees of external rotation.
  - 140 degrees of abduction.

Immobilization

- None.

Pain Control

- NSAIDs—for patients with persistent discomfort.
- Therapeutic modalities (ice, HVGS).
- Moist heat before therapy, ice at end of session.
- Subacromial injection: lidocaine/steroid—for patients with acute inflammatory symptoms that do not respond to NSAIDs.

Exercises

Motion

- Progress from active-assisted to active ROM in all directions.
- Focus on prolonged, gentle passive stretching at end ranges to increase shoulder flexibility.
- Thoracic extension to promote proximal kinetic chain function and postural awareness.
- Joint mobilizations (manual therapy) for capsular restrictions, especially the posterior capsule.

Muscle Strengthening (performed on alternating days)

- Scapular stabilizer strengthening: retraction, protraction, depression.
- Scapular proprioceptive neuromuscular facilitation (PNFs) exercises.
- Progress to open chain scapular stabilizer strengthening.
- Closed chain strengthening exercises—delay until 6 wk when RTC débridement is performed.
- Multidirectional isometric shoulder strengthening: IR, ER, extension, adduction, flexion (performed with the elbow flexed to 90 degrees).
- Open chain strengthening with resistance bands and/or dumbbells—delay until 6 to 8 wk when RTC débridement is performed.
- Starting position is with the arm at the patient's side and using a short lever arm (elbow flexed to 90 degrees) advancing to motions with a long lever arm (elbow extended).
- Exercises are performed through a pain-free arc of motion while ensuring normal GH and scapulothoracic movement patterns.
- Patients should not progress to greater level of resistance if there is any discomfort or suboptimal movement patterns at the present level.
- Progress to resistance band and light dumbbell exercises, which permit both **concentric and eccentric strengthening** of the shoulder muscles and are a form of isotonic exercises (characterized by variable speed and fixed resistance)
- IR, ER, abduction, adduction, flexion, and extension
- Note: Do not perform more than 15 repetitions for each set or more than three sets of repetitions. If this regimen is easy for the patient, then increase the resistance not the repetitions. Upper body strengthening with excessive repetitions can be counterproductive during this subacute phase of recovery.

PHASE 3: WEEKS 8–12

Criteria for Progression to Phase 3

- Full painless ROM.
- Minimal or no pain.
- At least 4/5 strength
- Absence of scapular dyskinesis

Goals

- Improve shoulder complex strength, power, and endurance.
- Improve neuromuscular control and shoulder proprioception.
- Prepare for gradual return to functional activities.

Motion

- Achieve motion equal to contralateral side.
- Utilize both ROM exercises and manual therapy to maintain motion.

BOX 33.3 PROGRESSIVE, SYSTEMATIC INTERVAL PROGRAMS FOR RETURNING TO SPORTS AFTER ARTHROSCOPIC SUBACROMIAL DECOMPRESSION (WITH MODIFICATION FOR DISTAL CLAVICLE RESECTION AND/OR ROTATOR CUFF DÉBRIDEMENT)—cont'd

Muscle Strengthening

- Advance strengthening of the shoulder complex (rotator cuff and scapular stabilizers)
- Progression should include a gradual increase in resistance and/or training volume.
- Continue strengthening on alternating days to enable neuromuscular recovery.

Functional Strengthening

- PNFs and rhythmic stabilization exercises.
- Push-up progression (wall to incline to traditional).
- Plyometric exercises.

For Patients with Concomitant Distal Clavicle Resection or RTC débridement

- Now begin cross-body adduction exercises
- First passive, advance to active motion when AC joint pain is minimal.

PHASE 4: WEEKS 12–16

Criteria for Progression to Phase 4

- Full, painless ROM.
- No pain or tenderness.
- 4+ to 5/5 strength.
- Satisfactory clinical examination.

Goals

- Progressive return to unrestricted activities.
- Maintenance of full ROM
- Advancement of strength training may include isokinetic training and gradual return to traditional weightlifting exercises. Caution is recommended when returning to barbell pressing movements (bench, incline, and military presses) and dips as these movements can result in a return of symptoms. Behind the neck pull-downs and military press should be avoided.

Progressive, Systematic Interval Program for Returning to Sports

- Throwing athletes.
- Tennis players.
- Golfers.
- Institute "Thrower's Ten" program for overhead athlete with progression to the advanced thrower's ten.
- **Maximum improvement is expected by** 4 to 6 months following an acromioplasty and 6 to 12 months following an acromioplasty combined with a distal clavicle resection.

Warning Signals

- Loss of motion—especially internal rotation.
- Lack of strength progression—especially abduction.
- Continued pain—especially at night.

Treatment of Above "Problems"

- These patients may need to move back to earlier routines.
- Return to supervised rehabilitation to address subtle losses of motion, aberrant movement patterns, and insufficient strength.
- May require increased utilization of pain control modalities as outlined above.
- If no improvement, patients may require repeat surgery
- It is important to determine that the appropriate surgical procedure was done initially.
- Issues of possible secondary gain must be evaluated.

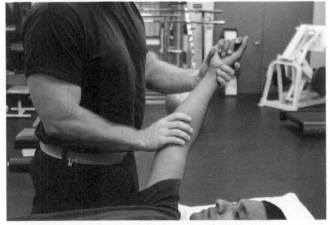

Fig. 33.17 Passive range of motion in the scapular plane.

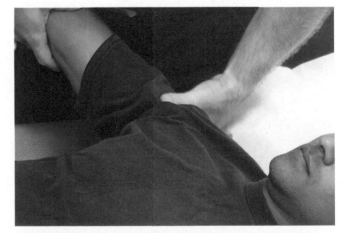

Fig. 33.18 Inferior mobilization of the glenohumeral joint.

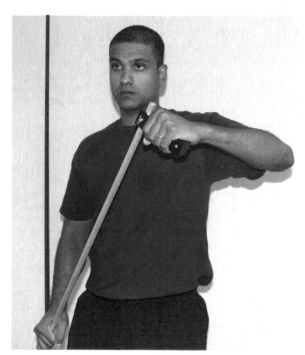

Fig. 33.19 Active-assisted range of motion.

REFERENCES

A complete reference list is available at https://expertconsult .inkling.com/.

34

Pectoralis Major Rupture Repair

Robert C. Manske, PT, DPT, MEd, SCS, ATC, CSCS | Daniel Prohaska, MD

INTRODUCTION AND OVERVIEW

The pectoralis major is a large and powerful adductor, internal rotator, and flexor of the shoulder. Rupture of the pectoralis major can be a devastating injury to an athlete. This is especially true in athletes that require powerful movements of the shoulder and arm such as weightlifters and football players. This injury can be treated conservatively, especially in the older or sedentary individual, for incomplete tears, or for the rare intramuscular crush injury (McEntire et al. 1972). However, a significant loss of strength will occur and surgery is usually recommended in those that want to continue at a high level of function (Berson 1979, Park and Espiniella 1972, Zeman et al. 1979).

Injury to the pectoralis major was first described as early as 1822 in Paris by Patissier (Patissier 1882), followed by Lettenneur in 1861 (Lettenneur 1861). Since that time through 2004 fewer than 200 cases have been reported in the literature, making this an uncommon sports injury throughout time (Aarimaa et al. 2004). Recently this injury has become more prevalent as the numbers of both professional and recreational athletes have seemed to increase (Guity et al. 2014, Quinlan et al. 2002). Another common reason for increased incidence may be the increased interest in health, fitness, and weight training combined occasionally with concomitant use of anabolic steroids (ElMaraghy and Devereaux 2012, Petilon et al. 2005).

ANATOMY

The pectoralis major muscle is a triangular muscle with origins on the clavicle, sternum, ribs, and external oblique fascia. It functions as primarily a humerus adductor and internal rotator, and the clavicular head can also assist with shoulder flexion (Provencher et al. 2010). The pectoralis major arises from a broad sheet with two heads of origin: the upper clavicular head and the lower sternocostal head. The clavicular head arises from the medial half of the clavicle, while the larger sternal head arises from the second to sixth ribs, the costal margin of the sternum, and the external oblique aponeurosis. The sternal head is significantly larger than the clavicular and accounts for greater than 80% of the total muscle volume (Fung et al. 2009). The two parts of the muscle converge laterally and insert on the lateral lip of the bicipital groove over an area of 5 cm. Fibers of the sternocostal head pass underneath the clavicular head fibers forming the deeper posterior lamina of the tendon, which rotates 180 degrees so that the inferior-most fibers are inserted at the highest or most proximal point of the humerus. The clavicular head fibers form the anterior lamina of the tendon, which inserts more distally (Kakwani et al. 2006). It is just proximal to the insertion on the lateral edge of the intertubercular sulcus that the two laminae fuse together (Fung et al. 2009). The result of this rotation of the clavicular head predisposes this inferior portion of the pectoralis major to fail first (Travis et al. 2000).

Innervation to the pectoralis major is received from the medial (C8–T1) and lateral (C5–7) pectoral nerves. The medial pectoral nerve passes through the pectoralis minor, along the lower border before it supplies the lower portion of the pectoralis major (Prakash and Saniya 2014). The medial pectoral nerve arises from the medial cord of the brachial plexus. The lateral pectoral nerve travels along the upper border of the pectoralis minor and then passes to the undersurface of the pectoralis major supplying the upper two thirds of the pectoralis major (Prakash and Saniya 2014). The lateral pectoral nerve arises from the lateral chord of the brachial plexus.

MECHANISM OF INJURY

The large majority of injuries occur in muscular young males between the ages of 20 and 40 during performance of the bench press (Butt et al. 2015). This occurs as an indirect mechanism associated with excessive tension on a maximally contracted pectoralis major muscle. This typically occurs during the eccentric phase of muscle contraction while performing the bench press when the excessively stretched fibers are unable to contract under extremely high loads. During the bench press motion this occurs as the shoulder is in an abducted, extended, and externally rotated position with maximal tension at the bottom of the repetition after the weight is lowered and the lifter is ready to return the shoulder to an adducted, flexed, and internally rotated position. Other causative injuries reported in the literature include wrestling, waterskiing, rugby, and boxing (Bak et al. 2000, Ohashi et al. 1996, Provencher et al. 2010, Wolfe et al. 1992, Zeman et al. 1979). There appears to be a correlation between the mechanism of injury and site of rupture. Tears of the muscle belly are more common with direct trauma; however, indirect trauma leads to avulsion of the humeral insertion or injury to the musculotendinous junction (Samitier et al. 2015). A pectoralis rupture is commonly accompanied by an audible "snap" or "pop" (Alho 1994, Manjarris et al. 1985, Pavlik et al. 1998, Rijnberg and van Linge 1993, Roi et al. 1990, Simonian and Morris 1996).

PHYSICAL EXAMINATION

Ecchymosis, mild swelling, and bruising can be seen over the anterior lateral chest wall or in the proximal arm (Bak et al. 2000, Butcher et al. 1996, Kretzler and Richardson 1989). In the axillary fold of the affected side, an asymmetry with loss of contour and an area of depression at the deltopectoral groove will be seen. Fig. 34.1 shows loss of contour of the pectoralis major muscle as compared to Fig. 34.2, which is the normal uninjured pectoralis major muscle. When asked to elicit an isometric contraction of the pectoralis major muscle, a classic asymmetric bulging of the chest will occur (Fig. 34.3). This clearly shows the nipple moving

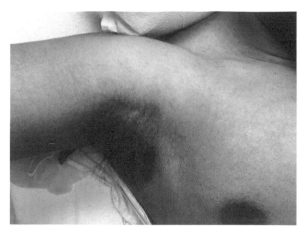

Fig. 34.1 Abnormal contour seen with a ruptured pectoralis major tendon.

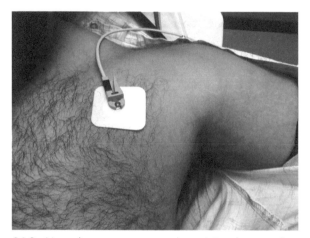

Fig. 34.2 Normal contour seen on the uninjured pectoralis major tendon.

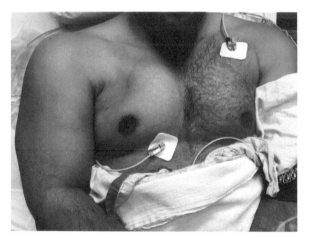

Fig. 34.3 Isometric contraction of the pectoralis major tendon shows retraction of the torn muscle tendon unit.

medially on the chest wall. Manual muscle testing will reveal a weakness in shoulder adduction and internal rotation.

Plain radiographs are usually not helpful diagnostically except in the case of bony avulsions (Butcher et al. 1996, Griffiths and Selesnick 1997, Kawashima et al. 1975, Orava et al. 1984, Verfaillie and Claes 1996). The absence of the pectoral

shadow has been described as a consistent finding for clinical diagnosis (Quinlan et al. 2002). Although ultrasound may be used to visualize tears, magnetic resonance imaging has become the imaging method of choice (Lee et al. 2000, Miller et al. 1993, Ohashi et al. 1996, Shellock et al. 1994).

INJURY CLASSIFICATION

Tietjen has proposed a functional classification for pectoralis major ruptures (Tietjen 1980). In this classification a Type I injury involves a sprain or contusion. Type II injuries include partial tears. Type III injuries were complete tears and further subclassified based on location: Type IIIA involves the sternoclavicular origin; Type IIIB the muscle belly; Type IIID the musculotendinous junction; and Type IIID the humeral insertion. Tietjen recommends that Type I and IIIB be treated nonoperatively. However, Type IIIC injuries could undergo surgical repair for a severe cosmetic deformity, whereas IIID injuries were best candidates for surgical repair.

CONSERVATIVE VERSUS SURGICAL TREATMENT

Most surgeons agree that nonoperative treatment of pectoralis major tendon tears should be reserved for tears only in older or sedentary patients and those with incomplete tears (Griffiths and Selesnick 1997). Numerous studies have demonstrated that surgical treatment of complete pectoralis major tendon tears have a defined advantage of resulting in increased strength when compared to a conservative nonsurgical approach to treatment (Alho 1994, Delport and Piper 1992, Bakalim 1965, Butters 1941, Berson 1979, Carek and Hawkins 1998, de Roguin 1992, Egan and Hall 1987, Gudmendsson 1973, Hanna et al. 2001, Hayes 1950, Krishne and Jani 1976, Lindenbaum 1975, Miller et al. 1993, Pavlik et al. 1998, Liu et al. 1992, McEntire et al. 1972, Zeman et al. 1979).

Operative Technique for Pectoralis Major Repair

The pectoralis may rupture the sternal head or both the sternal and clavicular head. Noticing the pattern of the tear can help in preoperative planning.

General anesthetic is used, with muscle relaxation. The patient is placed supine with the arm draped free. Often the back is inclined for easier visualization. The surgical approach can be made through a distal deltopectoral incision or made through the anterior axillary fold for a more cosmetic result. It is sometimes difficult to close the anterior axillary fold if the tear is chronic, and when repaired makes the arm close to the body because of pectoralis tightness, so if the situation is not acute the deltopectoral approach is used.

Dissection is carried down to the deltoid being lateral in the incision and identifying the ruptured pectoralis major. If just the sternal head is ruptured exploration must be taken under and distal to the intact clavicular head to identify the torn tendon, as the intact clavicular head will obscure the tear. Once identified, the clavicular head may be retracted superiorly to view the insertion site. If the tear is chronic, it may be necessary to identify the sternal head by developing the deltopectoral interval distally and identifying the sternal head above the clavicular head. If both heads are ruptured, dissection and identification of the tear tend to be easier. There have been explorations and failure to identify the ruptured sternal head, mistaking the intact clavicular head as an intact tendon due to failure to appreciate the insertion of the tendons on the humerus.

The tendon is freed medially of adhesions, using digital pressure, taking care on its deep surface to avoid too medial of dissection.

The pectoralis insertion site is identified just lateral to the long head of the biceps tendon and prepared using a small osteotome to make small gouges or fish scales to help heal the tendon.

Three double-loaded suture anchors are used with a tendon avulsed from the bone to repair the tendon. The tendon is repaired with a grasping stitch of choice with one limb and the second limb just through the end of the tendon and exiting 5 mm from the end so that tying the tendon pulls it tight against the bone. The tear may not be from the tendon to the bone but from tendon to tendon. Occasionally the tear is at the muscle–tendon junction. In this case suture repair only is used, and if near the muscle tendon junction, identifying layers of fascia into the muscle can give an area to suture to, but this repair pattern requires more protection postoperatively because the repair is not as secure.

The sutures are tied. The wound is irrigated. The wound is closed in layers and the skin is closed.

POSTSURGICAL REHABILITATION

Pectoralis major tendon load to failure is not currently known. Therefore, postsurgical rehabilitation soft tissue healing time frames cannot be clearly elucidated. The speed of rehabilitation progression following pectoralis major tendon repair is dependent on several surgical criteria. Direct repairs of soft tissue to tendon or tendon to tendon are more difficult due to the lack of a firm anchor for suture placement (Rijnberg and Linge 1993). Due to lack of firm anchor for tissue, greater soft tissue healing time frames have lead some authors to suggest conservative treatment time frames following a tear in the musculotendinous region (Gudmeundsson 1973, Hanna et al. 2001). Tendon-to-bone fixation is generally stronger and can be treated more progressively. Rehabilitation requires a balance of maintaining enough restriction of ROM to allow for soft tissue healing, yet still allowing enough activity and motion to restore full mobility (Manske and Prohaska 2007). Because the majority of pectoralis major ruptures are in young athletic individuals these patients must return to high levels of strength and power.

Goals for postoperative rehabilitation include (1) maintain structural integrity of the repaired tissue, (2) gradual restoration of ROM, (3) restoring and enhancing full dynamic muscle control and stability, (4) return to full unrestricted upper extremity activities including daily living and recreation and sports activities.

Immediate Postoperative Phase (0 to 2 Weeks)

Goals for the immediate postoperative phase are to (1) protect the healing tissue, (2) diminish postoperative pain and swelling, and (3) limit the effects of prolonged immobilization. As was mentioned, tendon-to-tendon repairs are more tenuous than bone-to-tendon repairs and will require longer soft tissue healing time frames (Table 34.1). The direct repairs will also require immobilization time frames to allow for adequate soft tissue healing before applying considerable stress to tissues. This immediate postoperative phase lasts for 0 to 2 weeks. Gradual initiation of PROM starts at 2 weeks. The patient maintains

TABLE 34.1	Pectoralis Tendon Repair Immobilization and Full Motion Time Frames	
Type of Repair	**Guidelines**	**Full AROM/PROM**
Tendon–tendon	Sling x 4 weeks	14–16 weeks
Bone–tendon	Sling x 3 weeks	12–14 weeks

TABLE 34.2	Range of Motion Guidelines		
Week	**ER at 0 Adduction**	**Forward Flexion**	**Abduction**
2	0	45	30
3	5	50–55	35
4	10	55–65	40
5	15	60–75	45
6	20	65–85	50
7	25	70–95	55
8	30	75–105	60
9	35	80–115	65
10	40	85–125	70
11	45	90–135	75
12	50	95–145	80

sling immobilization for 2 to 3 weeks. PROM is taken to neutral external rotation initially and allowed to increase by 5 degrees per week. Forward flexion is passively taken to 45 degrees and increasing 5 to 10 degrees every week (Table 34.2).

PROM is done to increase collagen synthesis and promote alignment of soft tissue fibers oriented parallel to the movement that is required to return full motion. No active ROM of the shoulder is allowed during this time because soft tissue healing would not tolerate this amount of stress. AROM is promoted to the elbow, forearm, hand, and wrist.

PROM is done to decrease risk of adhesion formation. Because this surgery is an extra-articular procedure, adhesions inside the joint rarely occur. Once the external incision is healed, gentle scar mobilization can occur. Scar mobilization is done parallel to the superficial incision, progressing to across the actual scar. Scar mobilization will break up collagen fibers and create a softer, flatter, paler scar that has better cosmesis (Edwards 2003).

In the immediate postoperative phase electrical modalities and cryotherapy are used to help control swelling and pain. Speer et al. (1996) demonstrated that cryotherapy is an effective adjunct following shoulder surgical procedures. Interferential electrical stimulation can be used to assist in decreasing postoperative pain, soreness, and swelling (Cameron 1999; Prentice 2002).

Intermediate Postoperative Phase (3 to 6 Weeks)

The shortest phase in the protocol is the intermediate phase, which includes postoperative weeks 3 to 6. Goals of this phase include: (1) continue progression of ROM, (2) enhance neuromuscular control, and (3) increase muscular strength. ROM progression follows Table 34.2. Full abduction and external rotation are achieved last and are not expected until 12 to 16 weeks pending type of repair (tendon–tendon versus tendon–bone). No AROM is allowed early in this phase, but near the end of the intermediate phase the patient can begin active-assisted range of motion (AAROM) through safe ranges per guidelines. ROM can be performed with therapist assistance, a cane (Fig. 34.4), or

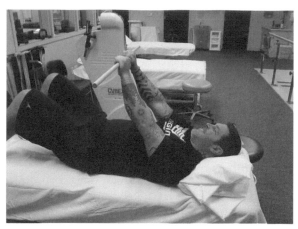

Fig. 34.4 Active-assistive range of motion performed with a cane.

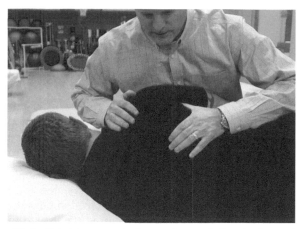

Fig. 34.6 Side-lying scapular isometric muscle "setting" exercises.

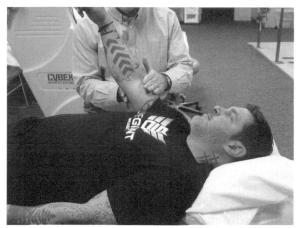

Fig. 34.5 Gentle rhythmic stabilization at low levels of shoulder elevation.

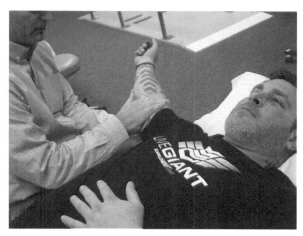

Fig. 34.7 Isometric exercises performed in a lengthened position.

a pulley. Education should be continued regarding ROM limitations at this time as overaggressive stretching can still injure repaired tissues. Painful ROM or shoulder mobility is probably detrimental to soft tissue healing and should not be allowed.

Strengthening exercises can commence by starting gentle rhythmic stabilization isometric contractions. These can be done in various shoulder and arm positions (Fig. 34.5). While supine with the arm in the balance position (90 degrees of flexion), the athlete is asked to hold the arm in this position while the clinician applies small joint perturbations in various directions. These should start by being gentle submaximal contractions (see Video 26.1). Progression of this basic isometric exercise can be done by increasing speed and altering resistance into unknown patterns. When done with the eyes open these exercises are considered proactive training, and while doing these with eyes closed they are considered reactive (Davies and Ellenbecker 1993). For optimal isometric strengthening, these contractions should be performed in 20-degree intervals. This is due to the 20-degree physiologic overflow of isometric strengthening exercises (Davies 1992). This will allow using isometric exercises to strengthen through a larger ROM than one single application of exercises.

While in the side-lying position, scapular "setting" exercises can begin (Fig. 34.6; Video 34.1). These exercises can begin to help gain scapular control. Scapular isometrics can be safely performed in all planes. Shoulder internal rotation isometrics should not be

performed early in this period, but toward the end of this phase (5 to 6 weeks) gentle submaximal exercises with the pectoralis in the shortened position can occur. All of these early isometric exercises should be very low levels, reaching a force of 2 to 4 lbs at most.

Late Strengthening Phase (6 to 12 Weeks)

The late strengthening phase lasts from 6 weeks to 12+ weeks. The goals for the late strengthening phase include: (1) achieving and maintaining full shoulder mobility with AROM and PROM and (2) gradually increasing muscular strength and endurance. By starting exercises with the shoulder adducted, minimal stress is placed on the pectoralis muscle and tendon. These activities should not be done in full horizontal adduction because this would place the pectoralis in a position of active insufficiency.

Toward the end of the late strengthening phase strengthening exercises can be performed that place the pectoralis muscle in a more lengthened position (Fig. 34.7). Placing tension on the pectoralis in a position of full horizontal abduction is not safe because this may place excessive strain on the soft tissue.

Around the 12-week period the athlete can usually begin gentle, light, isotonic tubing exercises. Near the end of this phase proprioceptive neuromuscular facilitation (PNF) techniques can begin. The PNF diagonal 2 (D2) flexion and extension patterns are helpful to gain strength and control in overhead positions

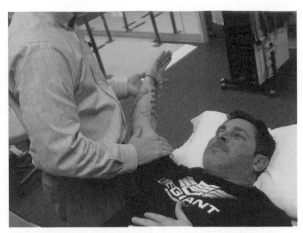

Fig. 34.8 Shoulder proprioceptive neuromuscular facilitation exercises in overhead position.

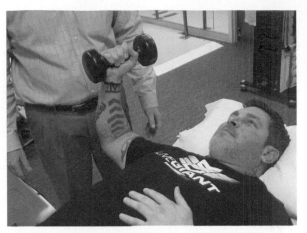

Fig. 34.9 Bench press motions

(Fig. 34.8). Initial patterns should be done with light manual resistance, progressing to greater manual or tube resistance.

By 12 weeks all AROM can be performed. Care should be taken to ensure normal glenohumeral arthrokinematics. Due to prolonged immobilization times following surgery, some limitations are common and may need to be addressed. Decreased anterior, inferior, and posterior glides should be addressed as soon as possible.

Advanced Strengthening Phase (12 to 16+ Weeks)

The final postoperative stage following pectoralis tendon repair is the advanced strengthening phase. The goals to return to full activity include: (1) achieving full AROM/PROM and (2) gradual return to full strength. When ROM is full, light higher-level activities can be performed. These activities should involve both concentric and eccentric contractions. Exercises can include bench press motions (Fig. 34.9) and plyometric activities (Fig. 34.10). For weightlifters a gradual strengthening progression can commence. No lifting greater than 50% of the athlete's previous 1 repetition max should be performed before 6 months following surgery.

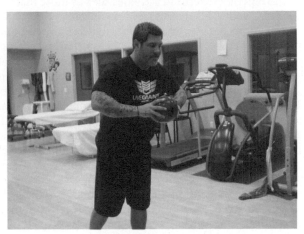

Fig. 34.10 Plyometric activity chest press motions.

REFERENCES

A complete reference list is available at https://expertconsult .inkling.com/.

35

Thoracic Outlet Syndrome in the Overhead Athlete

Robert C. Manske, PT, DPT, MEd, SCS, ATC, CSCS

INTRODUCTION

Although most upper extremity injuries in overhead athletes usually involve musculotendinous structures, lesions to nerves and blood vessels do occur. Both neurologic and vascular lesions are common in the upper extremity of overhead athletes, possibly due to repetitive overhead activities such as those that occur in pitching, volleyball, tennis, and swimming. Additionally, although rare in the overhead athlete, injuries to neurovascular structures can occur as the result of external trauma, compression, or distractive forces. These forms of lesions can cause patient complaints that are often vague and at times inconsistent, leading to frustration from health care providers attempting to treat these elusive ailments. This is troublesome because these conditions can not only cause an impediment to performance but may at times have limb-threatening consequences. Orthopedic and sports physical therapists are often the rehabilitation providers of choice for overhead athletes with upper extremity injuries and therefore must have a very high index of suspicion when evaluating neurovascular injuries. When working in a direct access marketplace, the physical therapist may be the first health care provider to be seen and subsequently may need to refer to other providers for further diagnostic procedures. The purpose of this chapter is to describe the physical examination and evaluation procedures for common neurovascular lesions and discuss both conservative and surgical treatment for these conditions.

This updated chapter will describe the clinical history, anatomic relevance, examination, evaluation, and conservative treatment of thoracic outlet syndrome (TOS).

THORACIC OUTLET SYNDROME

Thoracic outlet syndrome is a disease that involves compression of the neurovascular bundle, which courses its way from the neck to the axilla and then exits the axilla. Although Hunald originally described TOS more than 200 years ago (Tyson and Kaplan 1975), today this condition is often associated with injuries in overhead throwing athletes (Baker and Liu 1993, Nuber et al. 1990, Strukel and Garrick 1978, Rohrer JM et al. 1990, Safran 2004). Some have described two (in which venous and arterial are combined) to three categories of TOS including a neurologic compression syndrome of the brachial plexus, a vascular compression syndrome of the subclavian vein (Toby and Korman 1989), and an arterial syndrome, which is caused by compression of the subclavian artery (Freischlag and Orion 2014). The neurologic symptoms appear to be present in up to 90% to 97% of patients with TOS (DiFelice GS et al. 2002, Vogel and Jensen 1985) while arterial or venous symptoms have been thought to occur much less often in only about 2% to 5% of patients (Nemmers DW et al. 1990, Schneid K et al. 1999, Vogel and Jensen 1985). Overall it is estimated that around 90% are neurogenic origin, whereas less than 1% are arterial and 3% to 5% venous (Sanders RJ et al. 2007). This becomes very problematic because both causes tend to create similar symptoms. Because these symptoms are inconsistent and vague some even discount TOS as an actual diagnosis (Dale 1982).

Recognition of exact prevalence of TOS is difficult to track. Campbell and Landau (2008) estimated that surgeons diagnose TOS 100 times more frequently than neurologists. Cherington and Cherington (1992) imply that the diagnosis is made by surgeons according to potential reimbursement available for various procedures.

ANATOMIC RELEVANCE

The thoracic outlet consists of three passages that the brachial plexus and subclavian vessels must pass in order to supply sensation and circulation to the entire upper extremity. Commonly known as the superior thoracic outlet is the anatomic area that is bound posteriorly by the cervicothoracic spine, laterally by the first rib, and anteriorly by the manubrium (Leffert 1991).

The brachial plexus is formed by the C5 to T1 nerves. The brachial plexus exits the neck between the anterior and middle scalene muscles, which are one of the first locations of entrapment. In this area a triangle is formed by the two scalenes and the first rib, which supplies the floor (Fig. 35.1). Both the anterior and middle scalene originate from the upper cervical spine transverse processes and insert onto the first rib. Along with the brachial plexus, the subclavian artery also bisects the two scalene muscles. Together these structures then run over the first rib while maintaining a position under the inferior portion of the clavicle.

As the structures continue to course laterally they reach the costoclavicular passage, which is formed by the subclavius muscles and the clavicle, the first rib medially and posteriorly by the subscapularis. Compression at this location can be due to a overdeveloped first rib, hemorrhage, fibrosis, or congenital anomalies (Brantigan and Roos 2004, Kaminsky and Baker 2000, Pollack 1990). Any of these causes can become a space-occupying problem as the subclavian vein and axillary artery exit under the clavicle and above the first rib (Fig. 35.2). Just lateral to this area the structures run directly beneath or behind the coracoid process bordered anteriorly by the pectoralis minor muscle or tendon (Fig. 35.3).

Compression of the neurovascular triad can occur at any of the three areas described in the preceding paragraph: (1) between the middle and anterior scalene muscles, (2) between the clavicle and first rib, and (3) behind the pectoralis minor tendon.

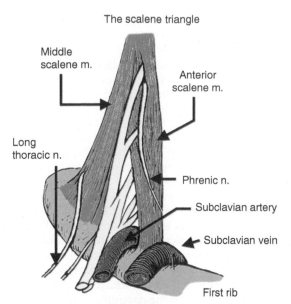

Fig. 35.1 Anatomy of the scalene triangle. The 5 nerve roots comprising the brachial plexus (C5–T1) are shown where they pass through the base of the neck within the thoracic outlet, with the scalene triangle bordered by the anterior and middle scalene muscles and the first rib. (From: Thompson RW, Driskill M. Neurovascular problems in the athletes shoulder. *Clin Sports Med.* 2008;27:789-802.)

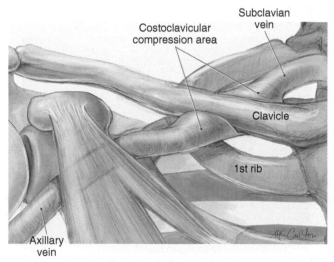

Fig. 35.2 Anatomy of the axillosubclavian vein. The subclavian vein passes under the clavicle and above the first rib as it progresses to become the axillary vein. (Image from: Baker CL, Baker CL III. Neurovascular compression syndromes of the shoulder. Fig. 27-8 page 331. In: Wilk KE, Reinold MM, Andrews JR. (eds) The Athletes Shoulder, 2nd ed. Philadelphia, PA, Churchill Livingstone, 2009.)

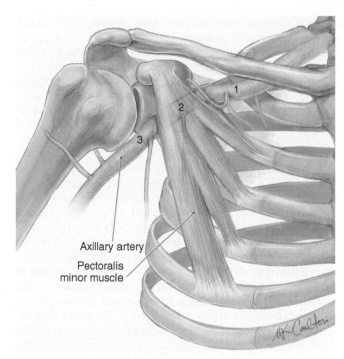

Fig. 35.3 Anatomy of the axillary artery. The axillary can be entrapped either under the clavicle between the first rib or more commonly as it exits behind the pectoralis minor muscle. (Image from: Baker CL, Baker CL III. Neurovascular compression syndromes of the shoulder. Fig. 27-8 page 331. In: Wilk KE, Reinold MM, Andrews JR. (eds) The Athletes Shoulder, 2nd ed. Philadelphia, PA, Churchill Livingstone, 2009.)

BOX 35.1 THORACIC OUTLET SYNDROME DIFFERENTIAL DIAGNOSIS

- Humeral hypertrophy
- Pectoralis minor hypertrophy
- Subtle glenohumeral instability
- Herniated cervical disk
- Cervical nerve root impingement
- Brachial neuritis
- Carpal tunnel syndrome
- Cubital tunnel syndrome
- Vascular occlusive disease
- Malignant tumors about the head, neck, and lungs
- Reflex sympathetic dystrophy
- Angina

PATHOPHYSIOLOGY

There are numerous proposed causes of TOS. Additionally, a large list of differential diagnosis will need to be thoroughly ruled out prior to determine if TOS is the actual pathology (see Box 35.1). The pathophysiology will be described based on the three areas described above. The first area is the interscalene triangle, which is bordered by the anterior scalene muscle anteriorly, the middle scalene muscle posteriorly, and the medial surface of the first rib inferiorly. Injury or trauma to the cervical spine may cause a protective spasm to the anterior or lateral neck muscles. This muscle spasm may directly or indirectly create compression at the proximal site between the anterior and middle scalene muscles (Sanders RJ & Pearce WH, 1989). Individuals required to carry heavy loads on their back such as backpacks may use accessory muscles when tired that may produce TOS type symptoms (Lain TM 1969). Although most overhead athletes are not required to carry heavy loads during their sporting activities, many are students who are required to lift an ever increasing amount of books to and from classes, which appear to be carried in backpacks a large majority of times.

A second area of concern occurs between the clavicle and the first rib. Known as the costoclavicular space it is bordered anteriorly by the middle third of the clavicle, posteromedial by the first rib, and posteriorly by the upper border of the scapula (Koknel TG 2005). Many unilaterally dominant athletes such as baseball pitchers and tennis players have substantial muscle hypertrophy in the dominant extremity. This increase in muscle mass combined with repetitive overhead activities may cause attenuation of capsular restraints resulting in increased scapular abduction and protraction. Because the entire upper extremity functions as a single kinetic chain during overhead athletic movement patterns, this increase in scapular depression may cause a concomitant increase in clavicular depression, resulting in compression on the neurovascular structures. Additionally, it is felt that any activity that causes scalene muscle spasm such as neck trauma may cause the clavicle to be elevated, thus compressing the neurovascular triad as it crosses over the first rib and under the clavicle. Numerous authors feel that the first rib in some way shape or form is the cause of TOS (Durham et al. 1995, Leffert 1991, Nehler et al. 1997).

The third area of entrapment is at the location under the pectoralis minor tendon near its attachment at the coracoid process. This area is known as the thoraco-coraco-pectoral space and is bordered by the coracoid process superiorly, the pectoralis minor anteriorly, and ribs 2 through 4 posteriorly (Richardson 1999, Remy-Jardin et al. 1997). We commonly see this in overhead athletes who have forward, or anteriorly rounded, shoulders. This is a common postural abnormality in overhead athletes in which the scapula is slightly depressed and protracted on the dominant side, possibly due to a chronically tight pectoralis minor muscle.

CLINICAL PRESENTATION WITH EXAMINATION

Because TOS can present with a wide range of symptoms the clinical presentation is often very vague. Additionally, not all patients present with similar symptoms, which commonly vary from case to case. The signs and symptoms presentation will depend on which particular nerves or vascular structures are involved and the extent of that involvement.

The common athletic patient with TOS is most often a baseball pitcher, but it has been described in multiple athletes including golfers, kayakers, weightlifters, and those involved in both tennis and volleyball (Nuber et al. 1990, Kee et al. 1995, Reekers et al. 1993, Rohrer 1990, Todd et al. 1998, Yao 1998).

All too often diagnosis of TOS is one of exclusion. Other causes such as herniated cervical disks, rotator cuff injuries, peripheral nerve entrapment, chronic pain syndromes, psychological conditions, multiple sclerosis, hypercoagulable disorders, atrial fibrillation with distal emboli, and upper extremity deep vein thrombosis all need to be considered because they can mimic the symptoms of TOS (Brooke and Freischlag 2010).

Some common complaints and symptoms include paresthesias, which can often involve the entire upper extremity rather than one specific nerve distribution. These paresthesias are usually associated with offending overhead activities. Symptom relief can range from occurring immediately following the overhead activity to not occurring for several hours after the activity has ended. These neurologic symptoms can also be seen as fatigue or heaviness in the upper extremity following overhead use in the involved upper extremity (Baker and Baker 2009).

Symptoms that are vascular in nature can also cause a feeling of heaviness and fatigue but also present with some form of distal ischemia such as cold intolerance, venous engorgement, numbness, tingling, and cyanosis of the digits. If the arterial form of TOS occurs the arm may appear paler than the uninvolved side, whereas the venous form of compromise will cause the arm to become cyanotic, blotchy, or even a purple hue (Safran 2004).

An extreme of this condition termed "effort thrombosis" should be ruled out if symptoms persist or worsen to include focal ulceration. Effort thrombosis is similar to deep venous thrombosis in the lower extremity and should be treated quickly. Effort thrombosis can be very hard to diagnosis because the symptoms may dissipate after the activity that causes it. Additionally, those that have effort thrombosis are commonly young and in relatively good health (Di Felice et al. 2002, Medler and McQueen 1993, Vogel and Jensen 1985).

Several examination tests are used to diagnose TOS. The classical Adson maneuver (Fig. 35.4) is used to implicate the scalene muscles as a site of entrapment. The athlete is asked to actively rotate his or her head toward the examined side, take a deep breath, and then hold it while the clinician extends and laterally rotates the shoulder while palpating for a decrease in pulse (Adson 1947, Adson and Coffey 1927). While rotating the head toward the side to be tested the scalenes are tightened and cause an active compression of the neurovascular bundle. With contraction of the scalenes there may also be an elevation of the first rib that could cause compression. Magee (2014) describes an alternative form of this test in which the athlete is asked to rotate the cervical spine to the opposite to the tested extremity. Either a diminished pulse or a return of the athlete's symptoms is considered a positive test for TOS.

Other tests are thought to implicate compression between the clavicle and the first rib. The costoclavicular sign (Fig. 35.5) or test attempts to compress the bundle as it runs between the clavicle and the first rib (Magee 2014). The athlete is asked to draw the shoulders into a position of retraction and depression.

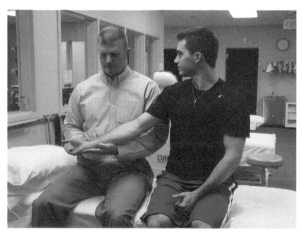

Fig. 35.4   The Adson maneuver.

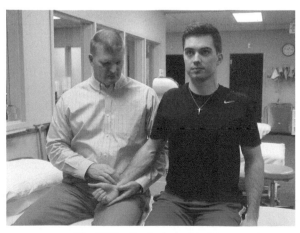

Fig. 35.5   Costoclavicular sign.

This is a position similar to that of the common military "at attention" position. Again, a diminished pulse and return of symptoms is a positive test.

Multiple tests are used to diagnose TOS due to compression behind the pectoralis minor tendon and the corocoid process. The Roos test (Fig. 35.6), which has also been known as the positive abduction and external rotation test and the elevated arm stress test, is an active test done by having the athlete abduct the shoulders 90 degrees while also flexing the elbows 90 degrees. To try to cause vascular compromise in this position, the athlete is then asked to slowly open and close his or her hands for up to three minutes (Liebenson 1988, Ribbe et al. 1984, Roos 1976).

The Wright's test, Wright's maneuver, or hyperabduction test (Fig. 35.7) is performed by taking the athlete's arm into full passive elevation and lateral rotation. While palpating for a pulse at the radial artery the athlete is asked to take a deep breath, hold it, and rotate or extend the neck to add additional effects (Wright 1984). As with all of the TOS tests, an alteration in pulse and return of symptoms are considered positive tests.

Because the symptoms and findings for TOS are not always consistent, there is not a single test that can distinctly diagnose this confusing problem. It appears better to formulate a cluster of tests or signs and symptoms together that would indicate TOS as a potential pathology. Also, many who do not have pathology or symptoms may have a decrease in radial pulse with some of these tests. The authors believe that a positive test cannot be indicated

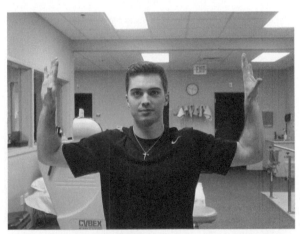

Fig. 35.6 Roos test.

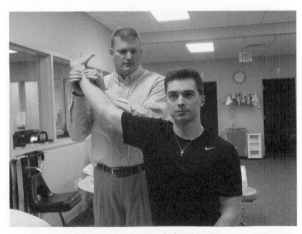

Fig. 35.7 Hyperabduction sign.

simply by a loss of pulse; rather a positive test must also include a return of symptoms (Manske and Stovak 2006). Although diagnostic tests or electrophysiologic studies are usually negative, they help to exclude other more common conditions that might cause similar symptoms (Thompson and Driskill 2008).

CONSERVATIVE AND SURGICAL MANAGEMENT

As with most orthopedic conditions, initial treatment is usually conservative. Although controversy exists regarding the optimal treatment approach for these patients, conservative measures should be attempted for patients with disputed neurogenic TOS before surgery is considered (Abe et al. 1999, Huang and Zager 2004, Landry and Moneta 2001, Novak 2003, Parziale et al. 2000, Urschel and Kourlis 2007). Good to excellent results have been seen in 76% to 100% of patients in short-term follow-up and slightly less at 59% to 88% after at least one year (Vanti et al. 2007). Poor outcome of conservative treatment of TOS has been shown to be associated with obesity, workers' compensation, and double-crush pathology involving the carpal or cubital tunnels (Novak et al. 1995).

A trial of nonsteroidal anti-inflammatory medication, injections, or medicated physical therapy modalities such as phonophoresis or iontophoresis may be beneficial in some cases. Injection of botulinum toxin into the scalenes may provide temporary relief of pain and spasm resulting from neurovascular compression in the thoracic outlet (Jordan et al. 2000, Danielson and Odderson 2008). If the patient is experiencing pain after activity that lasts for any length of time, relative rest from the offending activity is a prerequisite. Many times we see what appears to be a secondary TOS, in which the athlete has many other problems that may actually be driving the TOS that is presenting. Other factors could include impingement syndromes, subtle instabilities, scapular and rotator cuff fatigue, and strength deficits. These other conditions and pathologies must be given a chance to "calm down" before aggressive rehabilitation can begin. It must be stressed though that relative rest simply means resting enough to alleviate symptoms. For a professional athlete this may mean cutting pitching practice in half for several weeks. Other times this may mean completely stopping throwing. This depends on the activity level and irritability of the athlete.

An integral component of conservative treatment is improving posture. Leffert has reported that slouching may decrease the space available for neurovascular structures (Leffert 1994). Other causes of encroachment may be poor scapular stabilization due to fatigue or weakness of the periscapular muscles. Scapular muscle weakness and fatigue can lead to faulty scapular positioning on the posterior thorax. Kibler and Kibler and colleagues (Kibler 1998, Kibler et al. 2002) described three specific scapular dyskinesias or patterns that we commonly see occurring in the overhead athlete. In a Type I inferior angle dyskinesis the inferior medial angle of the scapula is prominent. This is sometimes known as scapular tipping. In the Kibler Type II dyskinesis the entire medial border of the scapula is elevated off the posterior thoracic wall, known commonly as scapular winging. The third type of dyskinesis is the Kibler Type III, in which the entire scapula is elevated early during initiation of shoulder movement. This is a typical pattern seen following a rotator cuff tear and is also known as the "shoulder shrug" sign.

If scapular tipping and/or winging is associated with scapular muscle fatigue or weakness, rehabilitation must commence with scapular stabilization exercises. Strengthening of the scapular stabilizers should incorporate therapeutic exercises as described by Moseley et al. (Moseley et al. 1992). The exercises that Moseley et al. found to elicit the greatest EMG activity of scapular muscles include shoulder flexion (Fig. 35.8; see Video 30.5), shoulder abduction (Fig. 35.9), shoulder abduction in the plane of the scapula, or scaption (Fig. 35.10), and the press-up plus (Fig. 35.11; see Video 30.6).

When scapular tipping and winging are due to soft tissue contracture, soft tissue manipulation or mobilization treatment may

be indicated. Common areas of inflexibility include the pectoralis minor, clavicular pectoralis muscles, and cervical muscles such as scalenes and trapezius. A recent study by Borstad and Ludewig (2006) indicated that the corner stretch (Fig. 35.12) is superior to either the sitting manual stretch or supine manual stretch when attempting to gain pectoralis minor flexibility. Because the supine manual stretch also saw increases in flexibility with the Borstad study we continue to use it also (Fig. 35.13). One final method to stretch the pectoralis and pectoralis

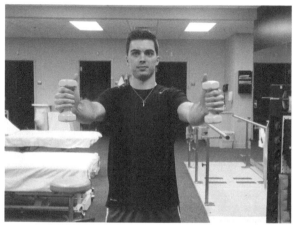

Fig. 35.8 Shoulder flexion.

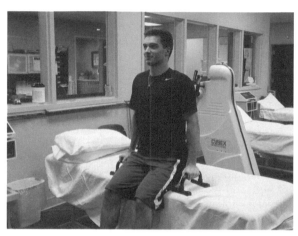

Fig. 35.11 Press-up plus.

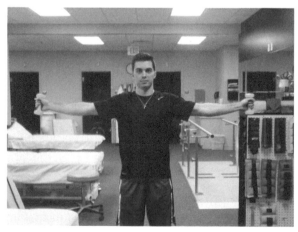

Fig. 35.9 Shoulder abduction.

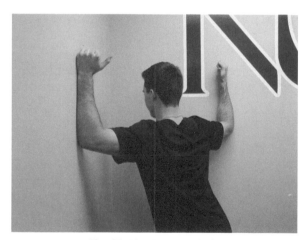

Fig. 35.12 Corner stretch.

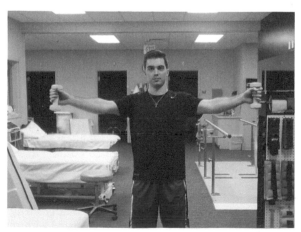

Fig. 35.10 Scapular plane elevation.

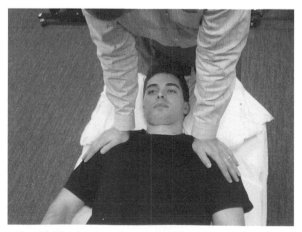

Fig. 35.13 Supine manual stretching of pectoralis minor.

minor for those athletes with glenohumeral anterior hyperlaxity or instability has been described by Durall, Manske, and Davies (Durall et al. 2001). In this method the shoulder to be stretched is placed against a corner of a wall using a towel for cushion. The stretch is initiated by retracting the shoulder blades. Further enhancement of this stretch can be done by pulling the pectoral muscles toward midline with the opposite hand. Other areas of concern may be hypomobility or faulty arthrokinematics of the acromioclavicular joint or the sternoclavicular joint. Assessment of acromioclavicular posterior to anterior glides and both elevation and depression and protraction/retraction of the sternoclavicular joint may be necessary.

It is not uncommon to use soft tissue mobilization techniques to muscles of the anterior shoulder including most commonly the pectoralis minor muscle and the subclavius. Additionally, muscles of the cervical spine can be affected due to compensatory patterns of the upper extremity. This can be done by using direct pressure, parallel deformation, or perpendicular strumming techniques to the muscle or muscle tendon unit (Fig. 35.14). Commonly when performing these techniques moist heat is applied topically to introduce muscle relaxation through dulling of the nociceptive pain fibers. Once soft tissue mobilization has been performed it is prudent to perform stretching exercises to further lengthen the affected soft tissues. Multiple methods of stretching the soft tissues can be used. Manual passive stretching of the pectoralis minor (Fig. 35.15), pectoralis major (Fig. 35.16), cervical spine (Fig. 35.17), trapezius

(Fig. 35.18), and levator scapula (Fig. 35.19) is common. If standard stretching does not appear to be beneficial, contract-relax or other proprioceptive neuromuscular facilitation techniques can be used. Using low-load long-duration stretching techniques over a foam roller is sometimes beneficial. Proper breathing techniques appear to facilitate more relaxation and thus more ease in stretching.

Because the scalene muscles attach to the first rib, when in muscle spasm they can have the propensity to create elevation of the first rib so that it approximates the lower border of the clavicle. Weakness of the shoulder and injury to the shoulder girdle can cause compression of the neurovascular bundle as it passes between the clavicle and the first rib (Leffert 1991). Restoration of first rib mobility can increase costoclavicular space and reduce imposed load on the neurovascular structures in the

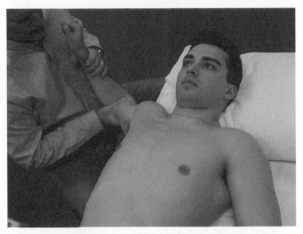

Fig. 35.16 Stretching pectoralis major.

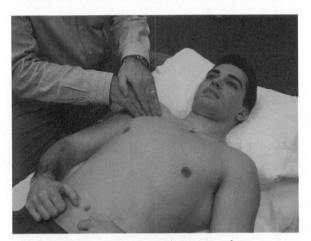

Fig. 35.14 Strumming technique to soft tissues.

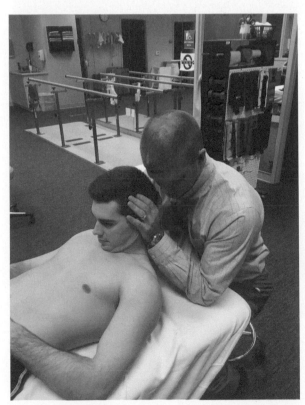

Fig. 35.17 Stretching of cervical spine.

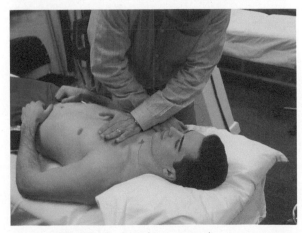

Fig. 35.15 Stretching pectoralis minor.

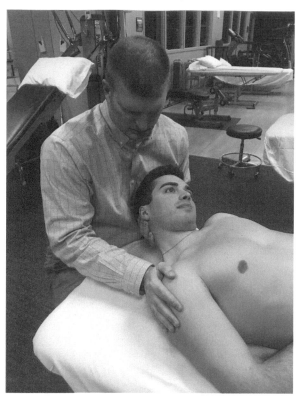

Fig. 35.18   Stretching of trapezius.

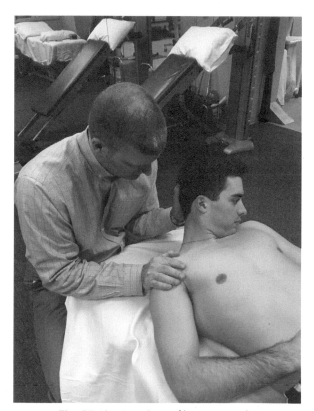

Fig. 35.19   Stretching of levator scapula.

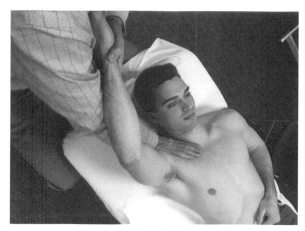

Fig. 35.20   First rib mobilization.

outlet (Hooper et al. 2010). Manual therapy techniques can be performed to mobilize the first rib (Fig. 35.20).

If a loss of neural mobility is present, neural mobilizations can be incorporated into the treatment session to improve gliding of neural tissue. Techniques can be modified to emphasize the specific region needing mobilization. These treatment techniques should be performed in a pain-free manner. Patients can also be instructed in a home program to perform initially approximately 20 repetitions gradually increasing to up to 100 repetitions as tolerated one to two times daily (Totten and Hunter 1991).

Because these conditions are commonly chronic in nature, a lengthy stint at rehabilitation should be utilized to gain the most benefit. Four to six weeks of therapy is not uncommon to try to resolve these conditions. When conservative approaches are not amenable to resolution, surgery is the next best option for symptomatic TOS. Several techniques have been described including transaxillary or supraclavicular TOS decompression with removal of the first rib, resection of the anterior and middle scalene muscles, and brachial plexus neurolysis and at times a pectoralis minor tenotomy (Thompson and Petrinec 1997, Thompson et al. 1997).

REFERENCES

A complete reference list is available at https://expertconsult .inkling.com/.

36

Proximal Humeral and Humeral Shaft Fractures

Charles E. Giangarra, MD | Jace R. Smith, MD

PROXIMAL HUMERAL FRACTURES

Introduction

Fractures of the proximal humerus are common especially in the elderly population. These injuries can be debilitating. Most orthopedic surgeons agree that the majority of these fractures are stable and can be managed conservatively; however there is a minority of these fractures that the management is controversial. There is a lack of high-level scientific evidence that would help derive a protocol for proper management. "Four recent meta-analyses of the existing literature have highlighted the paucity of Level I or II studies of these injuries" (Bucholz 2010).

There exist a variety of treatment options for these injuries, each with its own advantages and disadvantages.

Background

More than three fourths of these fractures follow low-energy domestic falls in the elderly population with low bone mineral density (Court-Brown 2001). The remainder are attributed to high-energy trauma seen in younger individuals. They represent 4% to 5% of all fractures presenting to the emergency department (Horak 1975) and approximately 5% of fractures involving the appendicular skeleton (Court-Brown 2006, Lind 1989) with a 2-to-3 to 1 female to male ratio (Court-Brown 2006, Lind 1989, Roux et al. 2012).

Anatomy and Classification

The common classification for proximal humeral fractures among orthopedic surgeons is the Neer classification because it is useful in the guidance of treatment. The classification scheme was derived from the analysis and surgical observations from 300 proximal humeral fractures Charles Neer treated while at the New York Orthopedic Hospital-Columbia Presbyterian Medical Center between 1953 and 1967 (Neer 1970). The classification system is focused around the proximal humerus fracture being composed of four major segments including the lesser tuberosity, greater tuberosity, articular surface, and humeral shaft. Neer set 45-degree angulation and 1-cm separation as the thresholds for displacement (Fig. 36.1).

The Neer classification scheme includes one-part, two-part, three-part, and four-part fractures of the proximal humerus. One-part fractures include fractures with no fragments displaced regardless of the actual number of lines seen (Fig. 36.2). In two-part fractures, one segment is displaced according to the above set criteria. This could include the greater tuberosity, lesser tuberosity, or articular surface of the anatomic or surgical neck (Fig. 36.3). In three-part fractures, either the lesser or greater tuberosity is displaced with associated displacement of the surgical neck producing a rotational deformity (Fig. 36.4). Four-part fractures occur when all four segments meet the criteria for displacement. This injury is severe and has a high rate of avascular necrosis (Fig. 36.5).

The blood supply to the humeral head is supplied predominantly by the anterior and posterior humeral circumflex artery. Historically, the anterior humeral circumflex was thought to be the main blood supply to the humeral head (Gerber 1990), but recent studies suggest that the posterior humeral circumflex artery provides 64% of the blood supply (Hettrich 2010).

The axillary nerve also needs to be evaluated during these injuries. The nerve originates off the posterior cord of the brachial plexus anterior to the subscapularis muscle. It courses through the quadrangular space along with the posterior humeral circumflex artery and vein. It divides into an anterior, posterior, and articular terminal branch. The anterior branch courses around the surgical neck of the humerus on the undersurface of the deltoid muscle. The nerve can be evaluated on physical exam through intact deltoid function and sensation over the anterolateral aspect of the shoulder.

Diagnosis and Treatment

The standard for evaluation, investigation, and diagnosis of these injuries is plain radiographs with three views of the shoulder including AP, Grashey, and axillary or scapular Y view. Additional imaging such as CT scan can be obtained for complex fracture patterns and preoperative planning. After the fracture pattern and physical exam have been established, the treating physician can decide on a treatment plan. The range of treatment options consists of nonoperative treatment, closed reduction with percutaneous pinning, open reduction with internal fixation, intramedullary nailing, hemiarthroplasty, total shoulder arthroplasty, and reverse total shoulder arthroplasty.

Most proximal humeral fractures in the elderly are stable injuries and can be successfully treated by nonoperative means (Maier 2012). Conservative treatment consists of sling immobilization initially followed by progressive rehab. Indications for conservative treatment include minimally displaced surgical neck fractures (one, two, and three part), greater tuberosity fractures displaced less than 5 mm, and fractures that are not surgical candidates.

Operative treatment of displaced, unstable fractures should be approached with the least invasive procedure providing acceptable reduction and stable fixation. To date, open reduction and internal fixation represent the standard operative

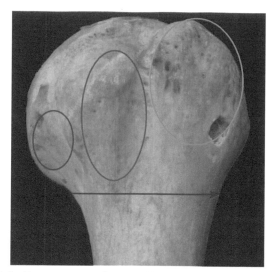

Fig. 36.1 Four segments of proximal humerus. (*Purple*, anatomic neck; *red*, lesser tuberosity; *green*, greater tuberosity; *blue*, surgical neck).

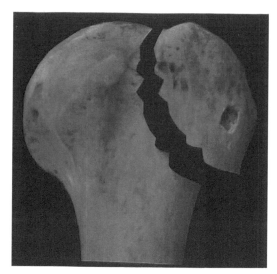

Fig. 36.3 Neer two part fracture.

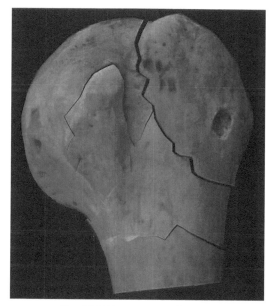

Fig. 36.2 Neer one part fracture.

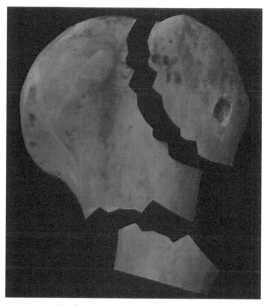

Fig. 36.4 Neer three part fracture.

procedure in two-, three-, and four-part fractures in younger patients (Maier 2014).

The outcomes associated with hemiarthroplasty relate closely to the healing of the tuberosity in an anatomic position to allow proper function of the rotator cuff (Maier 2014). Another alternative that may provide satisfactory shoulder function in the elderly patient population with preexisting rotator cuff disease or failure of first-line treatment would be a reverse total shoulder arthroplasty (Maier 2014).

Rehabilitation

The rehabilitation of these fractures is one of the most important portions of management. The goals of treatment include preventing disuse atrophy, maintaining range of motion without displacing the proximal humerus fracture, allowing gravity to assist in mobilizing the joint, avoiding exercises that reproduce

the mechanism of injury, and early intervention to begin a successful recovery. The best results seen with these injuries are typically while the patient adheres to a guided protocol, usually divided into three or four phases. Numerous protocols exist but most follow similar patterns with early passive ROM, followed by active ROM and progressive resistance, and finishing with an advanced stretching and strengthening program. Prolonged immobilization is a key factor to avoid because it leads to stiffness and decreased ROM. An example of one such protocol is seen below (Rockwood 1990).

Phase I (0 to 6 Weeks)

- Exercises started between seventh and tenth day following fracture or fixation
- Sling should not be used while performing PT

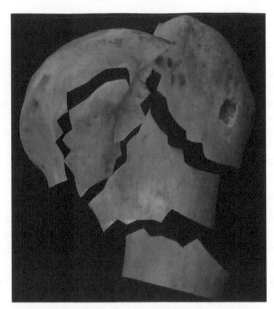

Fig. 36.5 Neer four part fracture.

- Pendulum exercises (Codman) initially
- Also should include neck, elbow, wrist, and hand ROM exercises
- Should be performing exercises 3 to 5 times per day for 30 minute sessions
- After a week, begin supine external rotation with a stick or cane with slight amount of abduction, approximately 15 to 20 degrees
- Three weeks after fracture, begin to add forward elevation exercises with pulley assistance.
- Begin isometric exercises at week 4.

Phase II (6 to 12 weeks)

- Can begin early active, resistive, and stretching exercises
- Initiate supine active forward elevation as gravity is partially eliminated.
- Eventually transition to erect position with forward elevation using a stick in the unaffected arm assisting with elevation.
- As strength progresses, can advance to active forward elevation without assistance
- Therabands can be used for progressive strengthening of internal rotators, external rotators, flexion, extension, and abduction (3 sets of 10 to 15 reps for each).
- Begin flexibility and stretching exercises to progressively increase ROM in all directions.

Phase III (>12 Weeks)

- Initiate isotonic exercises using rubber tubing and progressing to weights for strengthening.
- Concentrate on rotator cuff and scapular strengthening.
- Weights can start at 1 lb and move forward in 1-lb increments with a limit of 5 lbs. If any pain persists after exercises with weights, then discontinue the weights with the exercises.
- Progress to overhead exercises.
- Advance ROM to maximum.

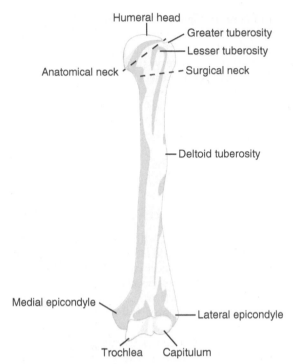

Fig. 36.6 Osteology of humerus.

HUMERAL SHAFT FRACTURES

Introduction

Humeral shaft fractures represent between 3% and 5% of all fractures (Brinker 2004), with a bimodal age distribution of young patients involved in high energy trauma or elderly patients with osteopenic bone with low energy injuries. The majority of these fractures can be treated with conservative therapy with a limited few requiring further surgical intervention for optimal outcome (Fears 1998). The extensive range of motion of the shoulder and elbow will accommodate a range of malunion and minor shortening with evidence of little functional deficit in these injuries (Sarmiento 2000).

Anatomy and Classification

The humerus is roughly cylindrical in shape and transitions to a triangular shape distally (Fig. 36.6). The fracture line typically occurs distal to the surgical neck and proximal to the supracondylar ridge. The deforming forces applied to each segment are determined by the position of the fracture line. If the fracture occurs above the level of the pectoralis major, the proximal fragment is abducted and internally rotated by the action of the rotator cuff. The pectoralis will tend to displace the distal segment medially and anteriorly. If the fracture occurs above the deltoid insertion, the deltoid will pull the lower fragment outward, while the pectoralis major, latissimus dorsi, and teres major pull the proximal fragment inward. If the fracture occurs below the deltoid insertion, the deltoid and coracobrachialis draw the proximal fragment outward and forward while the distal fragment is drawn proximal, resulting in shortening and overriding fragments. The humerus is surrounded by an anterior and posterior compartment. The median nerve, brachial artery, and musculocutaneous nerve are located in the anterior compartment for their entire course. The ulnar nerve begins in the anterior compartment and transitions to the posterior compartment at the elbow. The radial nerve begins in the posterior compartment and passes through into the anterior compartment. The most common nerve palsy associated with these fractures is the radial nerve; it is theorized that the nerve is stretched or contused in the spiral groove at the time of the fracture. Careful physical exam must include assessment for an intact radial nerve. Tingstad et al. (2000) reported a 34% incidence of radial nerve palsy in 111 fractures in polytrauma patients sustaining these injuries.

The fracture patterns can be classified either by the OTA classification or description of the fracture pattern.

Diagnosis and Treatment

Initial imaging is performed with standard radiographs of the humerus, including an AP and lateral view. If the fracture is significantly shortened, a traction view can be useful with direct axial traction to the upper extremity to assist in elucidating the fracture pattern. The majority of these fractures can be treated nonoperatively with bracing or splinting. The remainder may require further operative treatment such as open reduction and internal fixation or intramedullary nailing.

Nonoperative treatment indications include fractures that meet the criteria for acceptable alignment: <20 degrees of anterior angulation, <30 degrees varus/valgus angulation, and <3 cm of shortening. The absolute contraindications to nonoperative treatment include severe soft tissue injury or bone loss, vascular injury requiring repair, or brachial plexus injury. Initial management would consist of reduction with application of a coaptation splint followed by a Sarmiento functional brace 10 to 12 days after initial injury.

Absolute operative indications for these fracture patterns include open fracture, vascular injury requiring repair, brachial plexus injury, ipsilateral forearm fracture (floating elbow), and compartment syndrome.

Rehabilitation

The rehabilitation for humeral shaft fractures can be divided into the following three phases.

Phase I (0 to 6 Weeks)

- Sling for comfort with coaptation splint
- Transition to Sarmiento functional brace at day 10 to 12 post injury.
- Discontinue sling at two weeks.
- Encourage ROM of neck, shoulder, elbow, wrist, and hand.
- Pendulum exercises
- Exercises should be performed 3 to 5 times per day for 30-minute sessions.
- Begin passive self-assist exercises.

Phase II (6 to 12 Weeks)

- Can begin early active, resistive, and stretching exercises
- Therabands can be used for progressive strengthening of internal rotators, external rotators, flexion, extension, and abduction (3 sets of 10 to 15 reps for each).
- Begin flexibility and stretching exercises to progressively increase ROM in all directions.

Phase III (>12 Weeks)

- Initiate isotonic exercises using rubber tubing and progressing to weights for strengthening.
- Concentrate on rotator cuff and scapular strengthening.
- Weights can start at 1 lb and move forward in 1-lb increments with a limit of 5 lbs. If any pain persists after exercises with weights then discontinue the weights with the exercises.
- Progress to overhead exercises.
- Advance ROM to maximum.

REFERENCES

A complete reference list is available at https://expertconsult.inkling.com/.

The Use of a Functional Testing Algorithm (FTA) to Make Qualitative and Quantitative Decisions to Return Athletes Back to Sports Following Shoulder Injuries

George J. Davies, DPT, MEd, PT, SCS, ATC, LAT, CSCS, PES, FAPTA | Bryan Riemann, PHD, ATC, FNATA

Many clinicians need to make the decision to return athletes back to sports following a shoulder injury; however, there are (1) very few guidelines published, (2) few objective tests documented to support the clinical decision-making process, and (3) limited evidence to support this process (PubMed Search 2015, Obremskey 2005, Bhandari 2009, Sackett 2000).

So what are the very specific criteria we should use to discharge a patient from rehabilitation back to a high-risk activity like competitive sports? One method to establish criteria for return to play is to have baseline preparticipation information and following an injury have the athlete return back to "normal" for all the parameters. However, this is not always a practical solution unless comprehensive preseason screening was performed. Furthermore, being medically cleared to return to sports does not mean that the patient/athlete is functionally ready to return to sports! So what happens when an athlete returns to sports after being "cleared by us" and then gets reinjured? If a physician, physical therapist, or athletic trainer allows an athlete to return to sports, he or she may be *legally held responsible* if the athlete encounters a serious injury (Creighton 2010).

The purpose of this chapter is to describe one example of a functional testing algorithm (FTA) (criterion-based approach) for clinical decision making to return athletes back to sports following a shoulder injury. We recommend using an algorithm, defined as a process consisting of steps, with each step depending on the outcome of the previous one. In clinical medicine, an algorithm is a step-by-step protocol for management of a health care problem (Taber's Cyclopedic Medical Dictionary 1997).

We are unaware of a published FTA for parameters for returning someone back to sports following a shoulder injury, other than these publications (Davies 1998, Davies 1981).

Conceptually, an FTA can be thought of as the basic measurements being representative of impairments, strength/power testing indicating functional activity limitations, and functional testing evaluating participation restrictions or disability. Furthermore, an FTA consists of a series of tests (Box 37.1). Time and soft tissue healing from the injury or from a postsurgical condition are always considered relative to performing the FTA testing sequence.

Let's fast forward 13 years from the original FTA for the shoulder (Davies 1998) to the present time and Box 37.2 illustrates the format that can be used for clinical decision making for returning athletes back to competition following an injury to the shoulder in (Davies and Wilk 2013).

Progression during the FTA to the next higher level of testing difficulty is predicated upon passing the prior test in the series. Each successive test and its associated training regimen place increasing stress on the patient while at the same time decreasing clinical control. An example of the process of using an FTA is illustrated in Fig. 37.1. Empirically, we can rehabilitate patients faster than ever because by testing them we always know where the patient is in the rehabilitation program and can focus the interventions specifically on the patient's particular condition and status. Moreover, the patient only progresses through the level that is appropriate for him or her. Not every patient performs every test, but they progress through the level that is applicable to their functional activities. As an example, patients who are not overhead throwing athletes would not perform the overhead throwing tests, such as the Functional Throwing Performance Index. The remainder of this clinical commentary will describe the various components of the FTA for clinical decision making to return athletes back to sports following a shoulder injury using the limited research available and the empirically based clinical rationale as to why we are using some of these tests and the progressions.

FUNCTIONAL TESTING ALGORITHM METHODS

Basic Measurements

Following consideration of the time post injury and soft tissue healing, the basic measurements include: visual analog pain scales/numeric pain rating scales (0 to 10), anthropometric measurements, active range of motion (AROM), passive range of motion (PROM), lower extremity strength and balance testing, core stability testing, and quantitative and qualitative movement assessments (Davies 1981, 2013).

As a general guideline, if there is less than 10% to 15% bilateral comparison difference between the involved and uninvolved sides, the patient progresses to the next stage in the FTA. If there is a greater than 10% to 15% bilateral difference, then the patient's rehabilitation program is focused on the specific parameter (i.e., decreasing swelling, increasing ROM, etc.).

Sensorimotor Testing

Sensorimotor system testing can be performed using various methods, such as the conscious perception of proprioception testing modes: passive joint replication testing, active joint replication testing, threshold to sensation of movement (kinesthesia), end-ROM reproduction (Myers 2006), and movement screening tests. Much of the research on the shoulder sensorimotor system has focused on active angular replication testing because it is felt that active motion is a more functional method of assessing the sensorimotor system (Davies 1993, Ellenbecker 2012, Voight 1996).

Performing clinically applicable testing does not require a lot of additional or high-technology equipment. A protocol should be established as to what angles are going to be tested. Some protocols (Voight 1996) use just a few angles, whereas some of the original research (Davies 1993) used seven angles in the ROM: flexion < 90 degrees, flexion > 90 degrees, abduction < 90 degrees, abduction > 90 degrees, external rotation < 45 degrees, external rotation > 45 degrees, and then one measurement for internal rotation. The patient can be seated or supine and the shoulder joint is passively taken to a predetermined position in

the ROM, and the patient is asked to concentrate on that specific angle for 10 seconds. A measurement is performed using a goniometer or inclinometer. The patient is then returned to the starting position. The patient then performs active joint replication. The difference in degrees between the passive pre-position in the ROM and the active angular replication is calculated. The sum of the difference in degrees is divided by the number of angles measured (Davies 1993) and the difference is recorded. If the patient has deficits in this area, the focus of the rehabilitation continues to address the limitations, whereas if the values are within normal limits (WNL) the patient is progressed to the next test in the FTA.

Open Kinetic Chain Testing

The purpose of performing open kinetic chain isolated muscle testing is examining each link in the kinematic chain to determine if there are any weaknesses that may be missed if only functional testing is performed. The isolated testing is also performed for the following reasons: (1) if one does not test, then we do not know if there is a deficit; (2) if we do not test, then we do not know when a deficit is improving or resolved; (3) we can target the specific muscle that is being tested; (4) we can check for proximal or distal compensations that may also mask any weaknesses; and (5) because there is a correlation of isolated testing to functional activities (Ellenbecker 1988, Mont 1994, Treiber and Lott 1998, Davies 2011, Birke 2012).

Testing of isolated muscles can be performed with manual muscle testing (MMT), handheld dynamometry (HHD), or dynamic isokinetic muscle testing. MMT and HHD can also be thought of as field tests, whereas the isokinetic testing is considered laboratory testing. Functional testing is the key, but function is made up of individual links in the kinematic chain, therefore the importance of performing isolated testing as well.

However, some of the limitations of static MMT are that it is subjective, it only tests one point in ROM, and it does not correlate with dynamic muscle testing (Birke 2012). Handheld dynamometry allows for objective documentation of isometric muscle testing. It also has all the limitations of MMT, but at least it provides objective values from the HHD. Turner et al. (2009) performed HHD testing for the scapulothoracic muscles and rank ordered the muscles from the strongest to the weakest: upper trapezius (UT), serratus anterior (SA), middle trapezius (MT), rhomboids (R), and lower trapezius (LT). Furthermore, unilateral ratios were developed: elevation/depression (UT/LT): 2.62; protraction/retraction (SA/R): 1.45; upward rotation/downward rotation (SA/MT): 1.23. Riemann et al. (2010) performed over 2,000 HHD tests of the internal and external shoulder rotator musculature based on three selected positions to establish normative data and unilateral ratios at zero neutral degrees, 30°/30°/30° position and 90°/90° position. The results demonstrated similar findings for the zero and 30/30/30 positions; however, the forces and unilateral ratios are significantly different from the 90/90 position.

Open kinetic chain (isolated joint testing) isokinetic testing is one of the best ways to measure isolated dynamic muscle performance and is considered the gold standard for dynamic muscle performance testing. If isokinetic testing is not available, then HHD is preferred. Isokinetic testing results also correlate with functional performance tests (Wilk 1993, 1995,

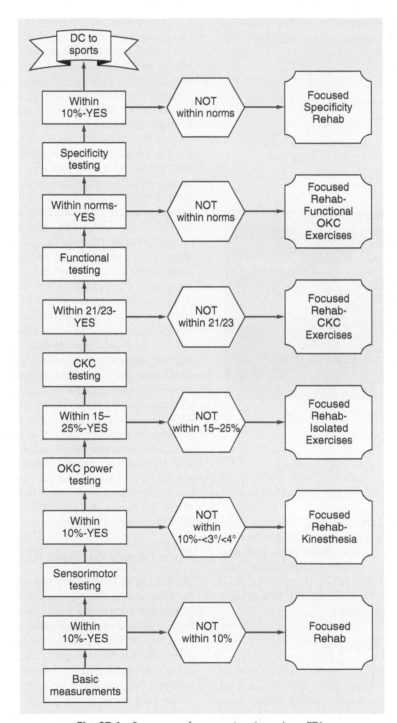

Fig. 37.1 Sequence of progression through an FTA.

Davies and Ellenbecker 2001, Ellenbecker 2000, Davies 1984, 2009, 2012).

The computerized Cybex 340 Isokinetic Dynamometer and attachments (CSMI, Stoughton, MA) using the following protocol have been used for over 40 years, but currently Biodex Medical Systems (Shirley, NY) are more commonly used. We recommend four gradient submaximal to maximal effort warmups (25%, 50%, 75%, 100%) and then 5 maximal test repetitions at 60 degrees/180 degrees/300 degrees/second. The progressive gradient warmups allow for stressing the testing motion gradually to prevent testing a patient if he or she cannot

perform the test correctly and without pain or inhibition. Furthermore, performing the gradient warmups allows for improved reliability of the testing. Descriptive norms for isokinetic testing of the shoulder are listed in numerous references (Wilk 1993, 1995, Davies and Ellenbecker 2001, Ellenbecker 2000, Davies 1984, 2009, 2012).

Codine et. al. (2005) reviewed 87 articles on isokinetics and determined that isokinetic evaluation of the shoulder revealed reliability and validity satisfactory with rigorous test methodology. Descriptive normative values (Table 37.1) are dependent on several variables, including age, gender,

TABLE 37.1	Descriptive Normative Data for the FTPI Test	
Norms	Males	Females
Throws	15	13
Accuracy	7	4
FTPI	47%	29%
Range	33–60%	17–41%
ICCs	- >	.90

Davies GJ, Hoffman SD: 1993 Neuromuscular Testing and Rehabilitation of the Shoulder Complex. J Ortho Sports Phys Ther 18(2) 449–458.

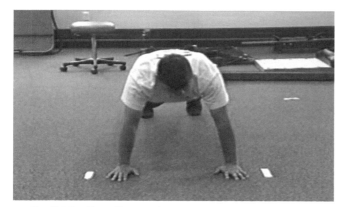

Fig. 37.2 Closed kinetic chain upper extremity stability test.

BMI, and type and intensity of activity (Wilk 1993, 1995, Davies and Ellenbecker 2001, Ellenbecker 2000, Davies 1984, 2009, 2012).

Furthermore, data analysis can include: bilateral comparison, unilateral ratio of agonist/antagonist, torque to body weight (relative/normalized data), endurance data, and normative data (Wilk 1993, 1995, Davies and Ellenbecker 2001, Ellenbecker 2000, Davies 1984, 2009, 2012). Hurd et al. (2011) demonstrated the importance of normalizing the data relative to body weight to interpret the test results.

Closed Kinetic Chain Testing

Why should closed kinetic chain (CKC) tests be performed for the upper extremity (UE) (Ellenbecker 2000, 2001)? There are numerous activities, such as gymnastics, rowing, mixed martial arts, karate, Brazilian jujitsu, wrestling, blocking in football, military training drills, and calisthenics exercises that require the use of closed kinetic chain movements. Davies developed the Closed Kinetic Chain Upper Extremity Stability Test (CKCUEST) (Goldbeck and Davies 2000). The test protocol consists of lines on the floor that are 3 feet apart (Fig. 37.2). The participant performs four gradient submaximal to maximal warmups with men in the standard push-up position and women in the push-up position from their knees. The subjects then touch both hands to each line as many times as possible in 15 seconds with 45 seconds of rest between each of the three sets. The number of touches from the three trials is then averaged for the test results; the original normative data for men was 21 touches and for women 23 touches (Sweeny et al. 2012). The Intraclass Correlational Coefficients (ICCs) for the

CKCUEST were .922. Rousch et al. (2007) tested collegiate baseball players and concluded that the CKCUEST appears to be a clinically useful test for upper extremity (UE) function. Pontillo et al. (2014) also used the CKCUEST for screening Division I football players and found the test was a good indicator of potential for injuries during the season. Using a score of 21 touches, the CKCUEST had a sensitivity of 0.83, a specificity of 0.79, and an odds ratio of 18.75 in determining whether a player sustained a shoulder injury. Pontillo et al. (2014) concluded for this sample the combination of preseason strength, fatigue, and functional testing was able to identify football players who would sustain a shoulder injury during the season. Furthermore, Sweeny et al. (2012) used the CKCUEST for rehabilitation as well as assessing a patient in a case study. Tucci et al. (2014) evaluated the CKCUEST and showed excellent inter-session reliability for scores in all samples. Results also showed excellent intra-session reliability of number of touches for all samples. Scores were greater in active compared to sedentary, with the exception of the power score. All scores were greater in active compared to sedentary and SIS males and females. SEM ranged from 1.45 to 2.76 touches (based on a 95% CI) and MDC ranged from 2.05 to 3.91(based on a 95% CI) in subjects with and without SIS. At least three touches are needed to be considered a real improvement on the CKCUEST scores. Tucci et al. (2014) concluded the CKCUEST is a reliable tool to evaluate upper extremity functional performance for sedentary, upper extremity sport-specific recreational, and sedentary males and females with SIS. Tucci et al. (2014) also studied the scapular kinematics and kinetic measures during CKCUEST for three different distances between the hands: original (36 inches), inter acromial, and 150% inter-acromial distance between hands. CKCUEST kinematic and kinetic measures were not different among three conditions based on distance between hands. However, the test might not be suitable for initial or mild level rehabilitation due to its challenging requirements.

Functional Closed Kinetic Chain Tests

The CKCUEST is considered to be a field test that requires a minimal amount of time and equipment. Riemann and Davies (2009) have started a series of CKC laboratory tests evaluating the kinetics and kinematics of the upper extremity. One of their first studies evaluated the relationship between two upper extremity functional performance tests and shoulder and trunk muscle strength, and a minimal correlation was demonstrated between the tests. The long-term goals are to correlate some of the gold standard laboratory tests (isokinetic testing, push-up ground reaction force production, etc.) with functional field tests (CKCUEST, seated shot put, etc.) to measure upper extremity power. Moreover, similar to the lower extremity performing box depth jumps, we modeled some of the original upper extremity testing to assess more aggressive and functional testing of the upper extremities. The original study by Koch et al. (2012) demonstrated the upper extremity ground reaction forces when performing clap push-ups and depth drop push-ups ranged between .69 and .78 body weights under each limb. The ground reaction forces more potently varied between the limbs (dominant slightly higher than nondominant) than on the height of the boxes from which the subject performed the drop landings. The drop landing push-ups were performed from heights of 3.8 cm, 7.6 cm, 11.4 cm (multiples of standard framing lumber). While potent differences in peak

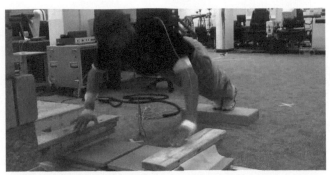

Fig. 37.3 Plyometric box drop tests for the upper extremity.

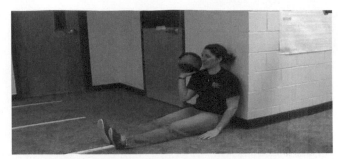

Fig. 37.4 Seated single-arm shot put test.

ground reaction forces were not revealed between the variations, as the subjects dropped from higher boxes more potent differences in rates of loading were revealed. In an attempt to determine if landing strategy changes between the variations might explain the slight peak ground reaction force variation differences, Moore et al. (2012) evaluated the elbow kinematics when performing the various push-up variations. The results did not reveal elbow kinematic differences, suggesting that perhaps shoulder kinematics were occurring. The implication of these two studies to FTA is that a hierarchy of push-ups variations, progressing from 3.8-cm drop landings to clap, can be used to assess the ability of the upper extremity to withstand large forces and rapid loading rates towards the terminal ends of rehabilitation (see Fig. 37.3).

Functional Open Kinetic Chain Testing

However, when starting to evaluate open kinetic chain (OKC) upper extremity power, there is a lack of research correlating UE strength and power assessments with sporting performance. Abernethy et al. (1995) discussed some of the controversies and challenges of power assessments. Therefore, there is a need for a device or protocol to discriminate upper extremity functional power performance within an athletic population. Rex et al. (2012) have been searching for a reliable, valid, responsive, minimal equipment needed, easy to administer UE power test that can be used as a field test. Consequently, a multicenter study between Armstrong Atlantic State University, Florida Hospital, and the University of Central Florida evaluated 180 healthy adult subjects (18 to 45 years old, 111 women, 69 men); 83 were classified as athletes and 97 were nonathletes for power tests (Ansley et al. 2009). The following upper extremity functional tests were performed by all the subjects:

- Single-arm seated shot put using dominant arm (6-pound medicine ball)
- Single-arm seated shot put using nondominant arm (6-pound medicine ball)
- Push-up tests for three sets of 15 seconds
- Modified pull-up test for three sets of 15 seconds
- Underkoeffler Overhand Softball throw for distance using the one-step (crow hop) throw approach
- Davies closed kinetic chain upper extremity stability test for three sets of 15 seconds

As a result of these tests, Negrete et al. (2011) performed a regression analysis to determine the best "field test" for predicting performance with the softball throw for distance. The

results indicated that the modified pull-up was the best predictor of functional throwing performance. Perhaps the internal rotators, which are significant muscles involved in the throwing motion, are also primary muscles involved in the modified pull-up motion.

Gillespie et al. (1988) evaluated 57 men for upper extremity power tests by using a seated shot put medicine ball throw. They compared a bench power test by moving 50 pounds through extension of the arms with distance and time measured compared to an 8-pound seated shot put distance with angle of release controlled and not controlled. All results were reliable and valid for both controlled and uncontrolled angles of release. Negrete et al. (2010) described normative data and performed a reliability test of the seated shot put (SSP) (see Fig. 37.4). A 6-pound medicine ball was placed in one hand, palm up with zero degrees of shoulder abduction. The subjects performed four gradient submaximal to maximal warmup throws followed by three maximal effort throws and the average distance was recorded to the nearest meter. Forty-six subjects were retested and ICCs were used to assess reliability. The ICC for the seated shot put tests (6 pounds) for the dominant arm was 0.988 and for the nondominant arm was 0.971. Moreover, the minimal detectable changes (MDCs) were calculated for the seated shot put tests and for the dominant arm was 17 inches and for the nondominant arm 18 inches. As the single-leg hop test is used for the limb symmetry index (LSI) of the lower extremity and has been shown to be sensitive and specific from several recent studies (Meyer et al. 2011, Arden et al. 2011, Grindem et al. 2011), we are using the SSP in a similar way for upper extremity LSI. Furthermore, we have also started normalizing the test results to the subjects' body weights and heights as illustrated in Table 37.2. Hurd et al. (2011) demonstrated the importance of normalizing the data relative to body weight to interpret the test results.

Because limited upper extremity functional performance tests (FPT) exist and FPT involving skill is complicated by UE dominance, Limbaugh et al. (2010a) tested collegiate baseball players with the standing medicine ball shot put test. The results demonstrated the combination of greater dominant arm release height, anterior displacement, anterior velocity, vertical displacement, and vertical velocity likely explains the DOM/NDOM horizontal range difference. The NDOM arm had greater lateral displacement and lateral velocity, which may represent compensatory actions. Limbaugh et al. (2010b) completed further research because athletes participating in unilateral activities were assessed to determine if the DOM/NDOM differences are skill and/ or strength/power related. The seated shot put performance

TABLE 37.2	Normative Data and Allometric Scaling for Single-arm Shot Put (SSP) Test	

Data determined for males with height of 71 in (181 cm) and weight of 180 lbs (82 kg).
Dominant arm SSP = 118 in/46 cm
Non-dominant arm SSP = 106/42 cm
Limb symmetry index is within 10%

Distance Put	Height of Subject	Score = Distance/Height
118 in	181 cm	65% +/– SD
118 in	71 cm	1.66% +/– SD
46 cm	181 cm	25% +/– SD
46 cm	71 in	65% +/– SD

Distance Put	Weight of Subject	Score = Distance/Weight
118 in	82 kg	1.44% +/– SD
118 in	180 kg	66% +/– SD
46 cm	82 kg	56% +/– SD
46 cm	180 lb	26% +/– SD

cm, centimeters; in, inches; kg, kilogram; SD, standard deviation.
Davies GJ. Personal communications, 2016.

correlates to other UE measures, such as throwing velocity, but is it sensitive to detecting bilateral or population differences? The results demonstrated the DOM arm was significantly better than NDOM in both groups. Sixty-six percent of the subjects also demonstrated bilateral asymmetry less than 10% of the time. Although our hypothesis expected baseball players, due to the unilateral overhead activity, to perform better, there were no significant differences between the baseball and non-baseball players. Perhaps baseball players' strength and conditioning programs reduced unilateral adaptations accompanying baseball activity or the seated shot put may not be sensitive enough to detect adaptations accompanying baseball activity.

Functional Throwing Tests

If the athletes are involved in an overhand throwing sport, then the patients are progressed to the overhand throwing tests. The first throwing test is a submaximal controlled throwing test performed in the clinical setting called the Functional Throwing Performance Index (FTPI) (Davies 1993). This test was developed to be performed in an indoor setting with limited space available to assess the overhand throwing motion. This can also be a variation of a quantitative and qualitative movement screening assessment for specificity of throwing performance. The dimensions for the FTPI include a line on the floor 15 feet from wall, 1 foot by 1 foot square, 4 feet from floor. The subject then performs four submaximal to maximal controlled gradient warmups (25%/50%/75%/100% effort). The player then throws a controlled maximum number of accurate throws for 30 seconds. Subjects perform three sets of throws and the results are averaged. The total number of throws is divided by the accurate number of throws and multiplied by 100 to calculate the FTPI index illustrated in Table 37.3. Malone et al. performed test-retest reliability for the FTPI test with a one-month interval between tests. This is a longer time between tests than is normally performed with reliability testing; however, the ICCs were all above 0.80.

TABLE 37.3	Functional Throwing Performance Index (FTPI)	
Norms	Males	Females
Throws	15	13
Accuracy	7	4
FTPT	47%	29%
Range	33-60%	17-41%

From Davies GJ, Dickoff-Hoffman S. Neuromuscular testing and rehabilitation of the shoulder complex. *J Orthop Sports Phys Ther.* 1993;18(2):449–458.

If the patient is an overhand throwing athlete, then the patient progresses from the FTPI, which is a controlled submaximal test, to the Underkoeffler Overhand Softball Throw for Distance, which is a maximal effort intensity test using multiple joints of the body in a functional throwing motion. This test is performed by using an overhand throw with a crow-hop. Four gradient submaximal to maximal warmup throws followed by three maximal volitional testing repetitions are performed and an average is recorded to the nearest meter. Collins et al. (1978) performed a reliability study with ICCs above 0.90.

Sports-Specific Training

The last stage of the functional testing algorithm is sports-specific tests using both quantitative and qualitative analysis. This is individualized to the patient and his/her specific recreational or competitive sports.

Other Considerations

Other considerations include psychological and emotional factors such as pain, apprehension, fear, and kinesiophobia. The presence of symptoms for longer than 3 months, average pain intensity, flexion ROM index, and fear-of-pain scores all contributed to baseline shoulder function. Lentz et al. (2009) evaluated patients with shoulder pain; however, the immediate clinical relevance of these findings is unclear in the rehabilitation of patients with shoulder dysfunctions. More recently, Baghwant et al. (2012) divided patients with shoulder dysfunctions into eight categories. Those with common musculoskeletal problems of the shoulder did demonstrate a higher kinesiophobia score.

A component of the comprehensive evaluation of the patient also includes collection of clinical outcome measures to demonstrate the effects of the functional training program. Assessment of clinical outcome should include a variety of clinician-measured outcomes that focus on measures of impaired joint and muscle function as well as limited activity, which includes many of the aforementioned performance-based measures in the FTA.

Patient-Reported Outcomes

The patients' perception of their clinical outcome is also important to assess. Patient-reported outcomes measure the patient's perception of his or her symptoms, activity, and participation. Patient-reported outcome measures can be general measures of health status that broadly measure physical, emotional, and social function or specific measures that focus primarily on the assessment of physical function. The most common general patient-reported outcome measure is the Medical Outcomes Study Short-Form 36 Item (SF-36) Health Status Measure (Ware 1992, Brazier 1992). The advantages of using a general patient-reported outcome measure are that it assesses multiple dimensions of health. As such, these measures may detect the influences of injury and rehabilitation on emotional and social function. Additionally, these measures allow for the comparison of the impact of an injury to the shoulder to a variety of other musculoskeletal and nonmusculoskeletal conditions. The disadvantages of general patient-reported outcomes are that they tend to be long and more time consuming to administer and score; they may be susceptible to ceiling effects, particularly when completed by individuals, such as athletes, who function at high levels of activity; and the content may not appear to be relevant to athletes and sports medicine clinicians.

Specific patient-reported outcome measures include region-specific measures of symptoms, activity, and participation affecting the upper extremity or specific conditions affecting the upper extremity and disease-specific measures for conditions such as rotator cuff tears or shoulder instability. Examples of region-specific patient-reported outcome measures appropriate for athletes with injuries of the upper extremity include the Disabilities of the Arm Shoulder Hand Index (DASH) (Hudak 1996), the DASH Sports Scale (Hudak 1996), the American Shoulder and Elbow Surgeons (ASES) score (Michener 2002), and the Kerlan-Jobe Orthopaedic Clinic (KJOC) Assessment for Overhead Athletes (Domb 2010). Examples of disease-specific patient-reported outcome measures that may be appropriate to assess the outcome of athletes include the Western Ontario Rotator Cuff (WORC) scale (Wessel 2005) and the Western Ontario Shoulder Instability (WOSI) scale (Kirkley 1998).

The DASH (Hudak 1996) consists of 30 items that measure upper extremity physical function (212 items), pain and symptoms (5 items), and social and emotional function (4 items) for people with disorders of the shoulder, elbow, wrist, and hand. The item scores are summed and transformed to a scale that ranges from 0 to 100 with higher scores representing greater symptoms and disability. There is good evidence for reliability, validity, and responsiveness of the DASH in a variety of populations. The DASH Sports Scale consists of four supplemental items that measure the impact of arm, shoulder, and hand conditions on playing sports. The specific questions include difficulty using normal technique, playing sport due to pain, playing sport as well as the individual would like, and spending usual time practicing or playing sport. Similar to the DASH, the item scores are summed and transformed to a scale that ranges from 0 to 100 with higher scores representing greater disability with sports. While potentially useful to assess outcome of athletes, there is little evidence for reliability, validity, and responsiveness to support interpretation and use of the DASH Sports Scale.

The ASES score (Michener 2002) is a 10-item measure of shoulder pain and function. Pain is assessed on a 10-cm visual analog scale (VAS) and accounts for 50% of the total score. The remaining 50% of the score is determined by the responses to 10 4-point Likert-scale questions related to physical function. The pain and physical function scores are summed to create a score that ranges from 0 to 100 with higher scores indicating less pain

TABLE 37.4	Psychometic Properties for Patient-Reported Outcome Measures for the Shoulder		
	DASH[1]	ASES[2]	KJOC[3]
Reliability[4]	.82–.98	.84–.96	.88
Effect Size	>.80	>.80	Not Reported
MDC[5]	2.8–5.2	.94	Not Reported
MCID[6]	10.2	6.4	Not Reported

[1]Disabilities of Arm Shoulder and Hand Index
[2]American Shoulder and Elbow Surgeons Score
[3]Kerlin Jobe Orthopaedic Clinic Functional Assessment for Overhead Athlete
[4]Values reported are intra-class correlation coefficients
[5]Minimal detectable change
[6]Minimum clinical important difference

and higher levels of physical function. There is good evidence for reliability, validity, and responsiveness of the ASES score to support its interpretation and use (Michener 2002).

The KJOC Functional Assessment for the Overhead Athlete (Domb 2010) is a 10-item scale for overhead athletes with disorders affecting the shoulder and elbow. This includes four items related to pain, one item related to interpersonal relationships related to athletic performance, and five items related to function and athletic performance. Each item is scored on a 10-cm VAS. The items are summed to create a score that ranges from 0 to 100 with higher scores representing better athletic function and fewer symptoms. Evidence for reliability, validity, and responsiveness of the KJOC Functional Assessment for the Overhead Athlete score has been provided by Alberta et al. 2010 and normative scores for overhead throwing athletes without symptoms were also provided (Cook et al. 2008).

Pyschometrically, there does not appear to be one patient-reported outcome that outperforms the others (see Table 37.4). As such, the choice of outcome measure should be determined by the patient population under consideration and the time necessary to administer and score the outcome measure.

For an athletic population, the ultimate outcome after injury and/or surgery is the ability to return to the prior level of sports in terms of intensity, frequency, duration, and absence of symptoms. Smith et al. (2012) published an article on various shoulder scales including the Shoulder Activity Scale (SAS), which is useful for measuring return to activity in athletes that participate in overhead throwing sports. The SAS consists of five questions (carrying 8 lbs., overhead objects, weightlifting with arms, swinging motion, and lifting greater than 25 lbs.), each rated in terms of frequency that the activity is performed, ranging from never/less than once per month to daily. The items are summed for a total score that ranges from 0 to 20 with higher scores indicating higher activity levels. The SAS also includes two items related to participation in contact and overhead sports that are not scored. Test–retest reliability was determined to be .92 over a 1-week period and the MDC was determined to be 3.8. The SAS is related to other activity measures but not age.

Most studies investigating return to activity measure activity retrospectively by asking individuals after the fact when they returned to activity. This is complicated by the fact that over time, an individual's participation in sports activity may change for reasons other than the status of the shoulder, such as changes in lifestyle, free time, and work and family obligations.

To improve the accuracy of measuring return to activity, pre-injury activity should be measured immediately after injury, return to activity should be measured prospectively during the course of recovery, and achievement of important milestones such as return to throwing, practice, and competition should be prospectively documented and the reasons for decreased activity should be documented.

After passing the aforementioned tests, particularly the sport-specific tests, with no residual complaints of pain, increased stiffness or effusion with a decrease in range of motion, and no functional movement quantitative or qualitative deficits, the athlete can be progressed back into activities. The athlete returns to sport-specific training programs first, practice simulations, practices, scrimmages, and then competition in his/her respective sport.

SUMMARY

The purpose of this clinical commentary describes one approach to a functional testing algorithm. Typically our clinical decision making (CDM) (based on history, subjective exam, objective physical exam, imaging, etc.) states when the athlete is ready to return to activity. However, if we also have all the functional tests to support the CDM, it provides quantitative and qualitative data to strengthen the decision to return the athlete back to activity safely.

REFERENCES

A complete reference list is available at https://expertconsult.inkling.com/.

SECTION 4

Foot and Ankle Injuries

Foot and Ankle Fractures

James T. Reagan, MD | Charles E. Giangarra, MD | John J. Jasko, MD

INTRODUCTION TO FOOT AND ANKLE TRAUMA

Foot and ankle fractures are among the more common traumatic injuries that present to emergency departments. Although rarely life threatening in isolation, these injuries can result in significant functional impairment and disability. It is the duty of the orthopedic surgeon, in concert with rehabilitation services, to maximize the functional outcome of patients after such injuries. The goal of this chapter is to provide a basic framework for the treatment of fractures of the foot and ankle that are commonly encountered. A detailed analysis of fracture types and surgical management is beyond the scope of this book. We will briefly explore etiology, mechanisms, fracture characteristics, and treatment goals to provide a background for the greater purpose of discussing rehabilitation guidelines and physical therapy goals as they pertain to different foot and ankle fractures.

ANKLE FRACTURES

Background

The incidence and severity of ankle fractures has significantly increased since the mid-20th century to approximately 187 fractures per 100,000 people each year (Egol et al. 2010c). The highest incidence occurs in elderly females and young adult males. The mechanism of injury for an ankle fracture is classically a twisting or rotational injury, and thus most are not typically regarded as high energy fractures (Davidovitch and Egol 2010). About two thirds of ankle fractures are isolated malleolar fractures; one fourth are bimalleolar, and the remaining 5% to 10% are trimalleolar (Egol et al. 2010c). Increased BMI and cigarette smoking are both considered risk factors for sustaining an ankle fracture.

Stable Versus Unstable

The ankle joint functions as a complex hinge and consists of the articulations of the distal tibia, distal fibula, and the talus. The distal tibial articular surface, termed the plafond, in concert with the medial and lateral malleoli form the ankle mortise. In addition to the bony anatomy, ligamentous structures contribute to the stability of the ankle. The deltoid ligament complex provides support to the medial aspect of the ankle. The syndesmotic ligament complex confers stability to the distal tibia-fibula articulation, and the fibular collateral ligament complex (anterior talofibular, posterior talofibular, and calcaneofibular ligaments) add lateral stability to the joint. In general, anatomic reduction and stability of the ankle mortise are the primary determinants upon which treatment decisions regarding ankle fractures are made (Davidovitch and Egol 2010).

Ankle fractures can generally be divided into avulsion fractures, isolated malleolus fractures, bimalleolar fractures, trimalleolar fractures, and those with syndesmosis disruption. Isolated avulsion fractures represent injuries where ligaments have avulsed a small piece of bone from either the medial or lateral malleoli. Thus, they often can be treated nonoperatively in a manner similar to ligamentous sprains. Isolated malleolus fractures can be treated either nonoperatively or operatively depending on the stability of the mortise and amount of displacement of the fracture. Most isolated lateral malleolus fractures at or distal to the plafond are stable injuries in which the mortise remains reduced due to the intact syndesmosis and thus may be treated nonoperatively (Davidovitch and Egol 2010). However, with lateral malleolus fractures that occur proximal to the plafond there is a higher rate of mortise instability or syndesmosis disruption, and these fracture patterns deserve further investigation with a stress radiograph to determine stability.

If a stress exam demonstrates significant lateral talar tilt or displacement or significant widening of the syndesmosis, then the fracture is unstable and thus would be appropriately treated surgically to restore the anatomy and stability of the mortise (Davidovitch and Egol 2010). Some recent literature suggests that nonoperative treatment of unstable fractures is possible if one is able to hold the mortise anatomically reduced with immobilization, but this is not the gold standard at this time. One must also consider the deleterious effects of prolonged cast immobilization that is required for nonoperative treatment of unstable fractures.

Initial treatment of displaced or unstable ankle fractures should include closed reduction and immobilization in the emergency department. Most experts would agree that bimalleolar and trimalleolar fractures are inherently unstable and therefore need to be treated with surgery (Egol et al. 2010c, Rudloff 2013). Likewise, disruption of the syndesmosis should be treated operatively to restore mortise stability (Davidovitch and Egol 2010, Rudloff 2013). Fig. 38.1, *A* is a radiograph of a trimalloelar ankle fracture with obvious syndesmosis disruption, and Fig. 38.1, *B* shows the same ankle after open reduction internal fixation (ORIF).

Rehabilitation

Stability also plays a critical role in the rehabilitation protocols used for these injuries. In the case of stable isolated malleolus fractures, including avulsion fractures, the patient can be treated with bracing and may weight bear as tolerated (WBAT) (Egol et al. 2010c). Physical therapy should initially focus on managing swelling and edema and returning ankle range of motion (ROM) to preinjury levels. Gradually, after a period of about 4 to 6 weeks, the patient may progressively wean from bracing to full weight bearing (FWB) (Davidovitch and Egol 2010). At this

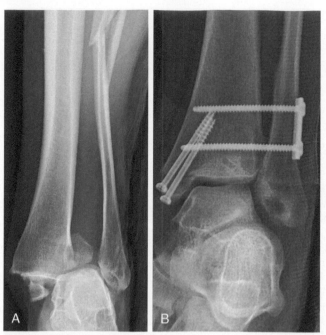

Fig. 38.1   A, AP radiograph of the ankle demonstrating a trimalleolar ankle fracture with clear syndesmosis disruption. The fibula fracture is noted to be well above the level of the syndesmosis, and the medial and posterior malleolus fragments are clearly demonstrated. **B** shows the same ankle with a mortise view after fixation of the medial malleolus and syndesmosis.

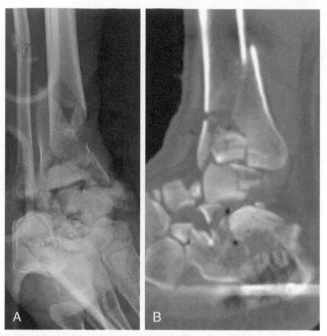

Fig. 38.2   **A**, AP radiograph of the ankle that shows a multifragmentary fracture of the distal tibia with articular involvement as well as distal fibula and talus fractures. **B** is a sagittal (lateral) CT image of the same ankle that more clearly demonstrates fracture involvement and displacement of the tibial plafond as well as associated talus and calcaneus fractures.

point, therapy should focus on strengthening of the foot and ankle musculature, in particular the lateral everters, and move on to proprioceptive training analogous to the therapy regimen used for severe ankle sprains (Chinn and Hertel 2010, Davidovitch and Egol 2010).

The final category includes unstable ankle fractures treated in an operative manner. These patients may require a period of time preoperatively to allow the swelling to decrease and provide a soft tissue envelope conducive for surgical intervention. Postoperatively, these fractures are typically held immobilized in a splint or cast for 10 to 14 days to allow wound healing. In a patient with good bone quality and stable anatomic fixation, a removable fracture boot is applied once the wound has healed so that gentle ankle active and passive ROM exercises within pain tolerance may begin (Davidovitch and Egol 2010, Egol 2011, Rudloff 2013). Studies have shown that early motion is associated with improved early functional outcomes in these fractures (Davidovitch and Egol 2010). In situations of tenuous fixation or poor bone quality and medical comorbidities, the surgeon may extend the immobilization period.

Patients are typically NWB for a period of 4 to 6 weeks postoperatively until there is radiographic evidence of healing. Exceptions to this include the neuropathic patient, which will be discussed later, and fractures requiring syndesmosis fixation, which will require about 8 weeks of NWB (Davidovitch and Egol 2010). After 6 weeks, patients may progressively WBAT and begin to work toward restoration of full ROM and strength. When FWB has been achieved, rehab progresses in a similar fashion as after an ankle sprain with functional and proprioceptive training. Studies have shown that patients return to baseline breaking function while driving about 9 weeks status post right ankle surgery (Davidovitch and Egol 2010, Egol 2011).

PILON FRACTURES

Pilon fractures are a subclass of ankle fractures that involve the weightbearing distal tibial articular surface. Pilon fractures comprise about 7% to 10% of tibial fractures, and they are most common in adult males aged 30 to 40 (Egol et al. 2010c). They are most often the result of a high-energy mechanism such as a fall from height, motor vehicle accident (MVA), motorcycle accident, or industrial accident (Baret 2010). *Pilon* is a French term that refers to a mortar and pestle; *plafond* is also a French term that refers to a ceiling. These two terms appropriately highlight the typical mechanism of injury for this fracture type, as pilon fractures are usually caused by high-energy axial loading of the ankle joint, forcing the talus into the plafond and causing an explosion fracture of the tibial plafond (Baret 2010). As such, the pilon patient will often have a severe soft tissue envelope insult associated with the fracture. However, fractures of the tibial plafond can also occur in combination with typical ankle fracture patterns as a result of a lower energy rotational mechanism, as with a sporting injury (Egol et al. 2010c, Baret 2010). Fig. 38.2, *A* is a radiograph of a pilon fracture, and Fig. 38.2, *B* shows a sagittal CT image of the same injury that clearly demonstrates fracture involving the articular surface.

Treatment

There are very limited indications for nonoperative treatment of these fractures in the general public. If the fracture is truly nondisplaced or the patient is severely debilitated or nonambulatory, then nonoperative management with immobilization in a cast may be considered (Baret 2010). However, as a general rule, pilon fractures are operative injuries in most scenarios.

Definitive surgical fixation is typically staged for pilon fractures, and the soft tissue envelope is the primary determinant with regard to timing. It is not uncommon that these fractures undergo initial stabilization with an external fixator, especially if the fracture is open or has associated severe soft tissue compromise. About 7 to 14 days after the injury, when the swelling has subsided and the soft tissue envelope has become amenable to incisions, definitive fixation may take place. The general operative goals with any pilon fracture include anatomic reduction of the articular surface, restoration of extremity length, alignment, and rotation, stable fracture fixation, bone grafting of metaphyseal defects, and early ankle motion (Baret 2010, Collinge and Prayson 2011). After surgery, the ankle is immobilized in a splint with the ankle joint in neutral position.

Rehabilitation

For nonoperative pilon fractures, patients are NWB and immobilized in a long leg cast for about 6 to 8 weeks or until radiographic evidence of fracture union is present. After the cast is discontinued, a fracture boot is used and the patient may be partial weight bearing (PWB) or WBAT depending on the treating surgeon's preference, stable fracture fixation and "degree of healing". Ankle and subtalar ROM are instituted as soon as feasibly possible; some even advocate discontinuing casting earlier than six weeks to allow earlier ROM in these fractures (Egol et al. 2010c, Baret 2010).

For the operative pilon fracture, patients will remain NWB for about 10 to 12 weeks until radiographic healing is demonstrated (Baret 2010). Postoperatively, patients are immobilized in a well-padded splint with the foot in neutral position. After 2 to 3 weeks, sutures are removed and the patient is transitioned to a removable fracture boot. Once the sutures are out and the incision has healed, ankle and subtalar ROM exercises are started, including AROM, active-assisted ROM, and gentle PROM (Baret 2010, Collinge and Prayson 2011). Early motion is critical to the success of operatively treated articular fractures, as loading of the articular cartilage with motion facilitates diffusion of nutrients and healing (Salter et al. 1980, Stover and Kellam 2007). Some gentle isometric strengthening may be instituted before weight bearing is allowed as well. After fracture union roughly 10 to 12 weeks postoperatively, patients may begin to be PWB in the fracture boot and progressively WBAT thereafter. Therapy should then focus on restoring motion, strengthening of the ankle musculature, gait training, proprioception and balance training, and progressive weaning from assistive ambulatory devices as tolerated.

TALUS FRACTURES
Background

Talus fractures rank second in frequency among the tarsal bones, with only calcaneus fractures being more common (Egol et al. 2010d). They account for about 5% to 7% of foot injuries. Chip and avulsion fractures are the most common fractures of the talus, followed by talar neck fractures (Sanders 2010). Fractures of the lateral process of the talus are common in snowboarding injuries about the foot and ankle, accounting for about 15% of snowboarding injuries in this region (Egol et al. 2010d). Most serious injuries to the talus are high energy in nature, due to MVA injuries about the foot and ankle, accounting for 0.1

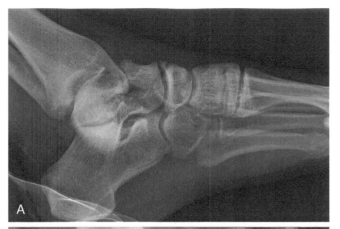

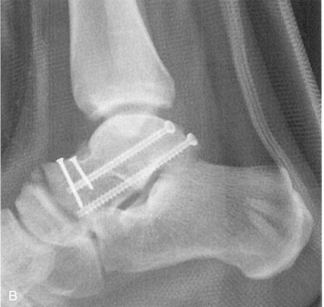

Fig. 38.3 **A,** Lateral radiograph of the foot that demonstrates a displaced talar neck fracture. **B** shows a lateral view of the same injury after reduction and screw fixation of the fracture.

to 0.85% of all fractures (Egol et al. 2010d, Sanders 2010). The most common mechanism for talar neck fractures is a hyperdorsiflexion injury (Sanders 2010). Concerning talar body fractures, which can occur in concert with talar neck fractures, the mechanism is typically an axial load to the foot and ankle (Sanders 2010). In contrast, lateral process fractures are commonly caused by lower energy inversion or eversion mechanisms (Egol et al. 2010d, Sanders 2010).

Fracture Types

There are several different types of talus fractures, including avulsions, talar neck, talar head, talar body, and lateral process fractures. Avulsion fractures for the most part are nonoperative injuries incurred in association with ankle sprains. Talar neck fractures can be treated nonoperatively if they are nondisplaced and the articular surface is congruent, but most of these require operative fixation in general. Fig. 38.3, *A* and *B* shows preoperative and postoperative radiographs of a talar neck fracture, respectively. Displacement greater than 2 mm requires operative treatment for most talar head, body, and process fractures

(Sanders 2010). Nondisplaced fractures can be managed with a trial of nonoperative immobilization. Initial treatment of displaced talus fractures, especially those associated with dislocations, consists of closed reduction and immobilization in the emergency department.

Talus fractures, especially neck and body fractures, can be problematic due to the precarious blood supply of the talus and the risk of avascular necrosis (Egol et al. 2010d, Sanders 2010). For this reason, both operative and nonoperative talus fractures are treated with longer periods of NWB than most other foot and ankle fractures. This longer immobilization may allow the blood supply to reconstitute or aid in preventing damage to any remaining blood supply to the talus (Sanders 2010).

Rehabilitation

Avulsion fractures of the talus can generally be managed, from a rehabilitation standpoint, similar to severe ankle sprains. Fractures of the lateral process, whether treated operatively or nonoperatively, can be managed with immobilization in a short leg cast or brace and NWB for about 4 to 6 weeks (Sanders 2010). Progressive mobilization on the injured extremity can then begin with a therapy focus on ankle and subtalar ROM and strengthening.

With respect to more substantial injuries to the talus, such as talar neck, body, and head fractures, the concern for vascularity of the fracture plays a role in dictating the rehabilitation timeline. Even nonoperative talar neck fractures, which are rare, require immobilization and NWB for up to 3 months or until radiographic evidence of union is present (Ishikawa 2013). Operative fractures requiring reduction and fixation methods are immobilized in a NWB splint or cast for at least 1 month. After incisions have healed and sutures are removed, gentle ROM exercises can begin. With rigid fixation, early ankle and subtalar motion are acceptable, as is gentle isometric ankle strengthening (Karges 2011). NWB is usually maintained for about 3 months postoperatively to protect the talus during the revascularization phase (Sanders 2010). Some recommend the use of a patella tendon bearing brace if there is radiographic evidence of revascularization with impending collapse to help unload the talus once weightbearing begins (Sanders 2010, Karges 2011). After evidence of union, progressive mobilization, restoration of full ROM, strengthening, gait training, and proprioceptive training may begin and progress as tolerated.

CALCANEUS FRACTURES
Background

Calcaneus fractures are often debilitating injuries that can have long-lasting effects on patient comfort and function. Overall, these fractures make up about 2% of all fractures, and the calcaneus is the most frequent tarsal bone to be fractured (Egol et al. 2010a). Displaced intra-articular fractures account for about 60% to 75% of all calcaneus fractures (Egol et al. 2010a, Sanders and Clare 2010). Ninety percent of these fractures occur in males aged 21 to 45, with most affecting industrial workers (Sanders and Clare 2010). Fractures of the calcaneus typically involve a high-energy mechanism, such as a fall from height or MVA. In addition, these fractures are most commonly caused by axial loading of the foot through the heel, with the talus being driven down into the calcaneus, causing the fracture (Sanders and Clare 2010).

Fracture Types

Fractures of the calcaneus include body fractures, anterior process fractures, and posterior tuberosity fractures. The calcaneus bone has a thin cortical shell that surrounds cancellous, well-vascularized bone. For this reason, healing of calcaneus fractures is not problematic; however, operative versus nonoperative management of these fractures remains somewhat controversial (Sanders and Clare 2010, Carr 2011). In general, displaced intra-articular fractures involving the subtalar joint (specifically the posterior facet), displaced tuberosity fractures, and fractures with greater than 25% involvement of the calcaneocuboid articulation should be treated operatively (Sanders and Clare 2010). Operative goals include restoration of normal height and width of the calcaneus, establishing neutral alignment that is not in varus, and restoration of congruent subtalar and calcaneocuboid joints (Sanders and Clare 2010, Ishikawa 2013). Fig. 38.4, A and B, shows preoperative and postoperative radiographs of a displaced intra-articular calcaneus fracture, respectively. Fig. 38.5, A and B, shows a displaced calcaneus fracture through the posterior tuberosity that was treated operatively. Initial management includes placement of a well-padded splint and edema control. Resolution of swelling will dictate operative timing, which tyically occurs 10 to 21 days after initial injury (Sanders and Clare 2010, Carr 2011).

Rehabilitation

Nonoperative calcaneus fractures, as was mentioned, are placed into a supportive well-padded splint to allow resolution of the initial fracture edema. The patient is then converted to a fracture boot or cast within 2 weeks with the ankle in neutral flexion. Early subtalar and ankle joint gentle AROM may be initiated at this point (Sanders and Clare 2010, Carr 2011). Patients are typically NWB for at least 6 to 8 weeks until radiographic evidence of fracture consolidation is present (Carr 2011).

With the operatively treated anterior process fracture, patients may be allowed to ambulate in a hard-soled inflexible shoe WBAT soon after surgery. However, regular shoe wear is not recommended for about 10 to 12 weeks to minimize the stress across the calcaneocuboid joint (Sanders and Clare 2010). Postoperatively, posterior tuberosity fractures may initially be splinted in a bit of plantarflexion to minimize the tension of the gastrocnemius–soleus complex on the fracture (Sanders and Clare 2010). At 2 weeks postoperatively, patients may be converted to a fracture boot with initiation of gentle early AROM exercises if incisions have adequately healed.

Operatively treated calcaneus fractures are placed into a short leg splint or cast in neutral position postoperatively. Because of greater concern about postoperative wound problems with calcaneus fractures, immobilization is continued until the wound is well healed, typically 2–3 weeks. The patient is then converted to a fracture boot and early subtalar and ankle ROM may be initiated (Sanders and Clare 2010, Ishikawa 2013). Isometric strengthening may begin before weight bearing, but on average these patients are kept NWB for about 8 to 10 weeks (Sanders and Clare 2010). When weight bearing begins, therapy may address restoration of full ROM, strengthening, gait training, and balance training in progressive fashion.

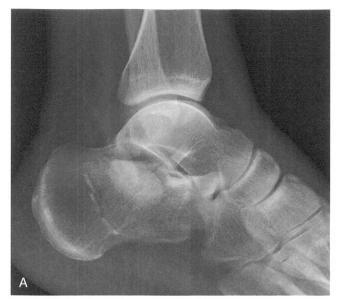

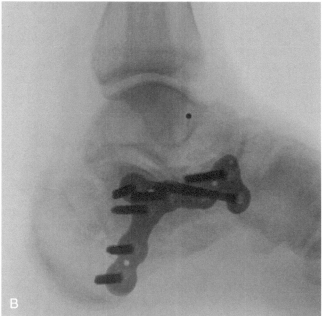

Fig. 38.4 A, Lateral radiograph demonstrating a displaced intra-articular fracture of the calcaneus, with involvement and flattening of the subtalar joint. B shows the same patient after reduction and plate and screw fixation of the fracture. Notice that the subtalar articular congruity has been largely restored.

LISFRANC FRACTURES/ DISLOCATIONS

Background

The tarsometatarsal (TMT) joint complex is commonly referred to as the Lisfranc joint, and this area is where the midfoot transitions to the forefoot. Injuries to the Lisfranc joint are fairly rare but can have debilitating consequences if not recognized and treated appropriately. It is estimated that about 20% of Lisfranc injuries are initially overlooked, especially in polytrauma patients (Egol et al. 2010b). There are a wide range of etiologies that can lead to a Lisfranc injury, including falls from a height, NVAs, and sporting injuries. Classic mechanisms include direct loading of the joint along the dorsal surface, such as a crush injury or a heavy object falling on the foot, and indirect longitudinal loading of a plantarflexed foot, which is more common in sports and falls from height. A rotational mechanism with forceful abduction of the forefoot is also described (Egol et al. 2010b, Reid and Early 2010).

Anatomy and Treatment

The anatomy of the Lisfranc joint is likened to a Roman arch, where the recessed trapezoidal second metatarsal (MT) base articulates with the middle cuneiform, forming the keystone articulation of that arch and conferring stability to the TMT joint (Egol et al. 2010b, Reid and Early 2010). There is a critical ligament, termed appropriately the Lisfranc ligament, which connects this second metatarsal base with the medial cuneiform. This ligament provides stability to the Lisfranc joint by connecting the medial column, consisting of the first MT and medial cuneiform, to the middle column, consisting of the second and third MTs and the middle and lateral cuneiforms respectively (Egol et al. 2010b, Reid and Early 2010). The lesser MTs (2–4) have strong intermetatarsal ligaments attaching them together at the bases that confer stability. However, the Lisfranc ligament performs this duty for the first and second MTs. Therefore, disruption of the Lisfranc ligament complex, in effect, destabilizes the medial portion of the TMT joint (Reid and Early 2010). In addition, instability of the Lisfranc joint can also be due to various fractures about the joint that may result in destabilization.

A critical point to emphasize here is that instability at the TMT joint, whether due to fracture or ligamentous injury, can be difficult to diagnose without stress or weightbearing radiographs (Reid and Early 2010, Clare and Sanders 2011). If no instability is noted on stress radiographs, then the injury is typically stable and better classified as a sprain. However, unstable injuries should be treated operatively to stabilize the TMT joint complex. Thus, if there is dorsal instability or greater than 2 mm displacement of the TMT joint, surgery is indicated (Reid and Early 2010). Fig. 38.6, A and B, shows orthogonal radiographic views of a Lisfranc injury, clearly demonstrating dorsal instability and incongruity at the TMT joint. Fig. 38.6, C shows the same injury after reduction and initial operative stabilization.

Rehabilitation

Postoperatively, patients with Lisfranc injuries are immobilized in a short leg splint or cast. After incisions have healed and sutures are removed at about 2 to 3 weeks, patients may transition to a removable fracture boot and begin gentle AROM exercises of the foot and ankle. Weight bearing is typically withheld until about 6 to 8 weeks postoperatively, but some authors prefer a longer period of NWB (Reid and Early 2010, Clare and Sanders 2011, Ishikawa 2013). A special consideration here is that some of these injuries are treated with primary TMT joint fusion along the medial TMT complex, especially if the injury was an isolated ligamentous injury, and these patients are immobilized and held to NWB for longer, about 10 to 12 weeks, to allow the fusion mass to solidify (Clare and Sanders 2011). After healing is demonstrated on radiographs, patients may transition to WBAT in a fracture boot and work on gaining full foot and ankle ROM and strengthening in a progressive manner. Restoring plantarflexion strength has been postulated to

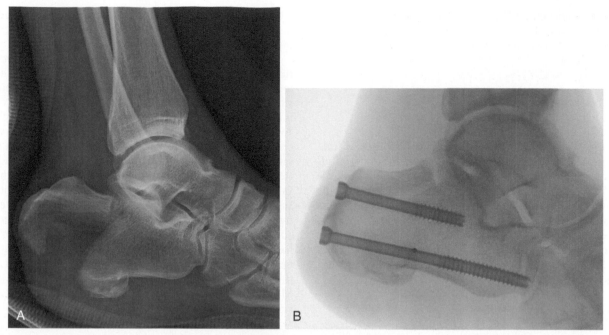

Fig. 38.5 **A,** Lateral image demonstrating a displaced calcaneus posterior tuberosity fracture known as a tongue-type fracture. The gastrocnemius–soleus complex attaches to the more proximal fragment and is responsible for the deformity observed. **B** demonstrates the postoperative result for the same patient after screw fixation of the fracture. These fractures need urgent treatment because the proximal fragment poses a risk of pressure necrosis to the posterior soft tissue structures and overlying skin.

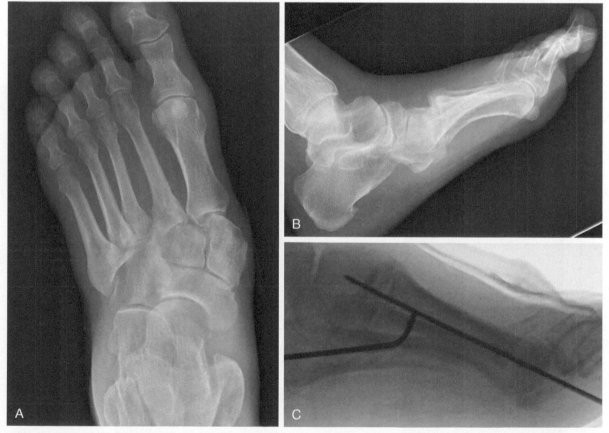

Fig. 38.6 **A and B,** AP and lateral radiographs of the same foot demonstrating dorsal and AP instability at the Lisfranc joint with a subtle fracture of the base of the second MT best seen on the AP. **C** shows a lateral projection with initial reduction and surgical stabilization with wires.

be the most important rehabilitation goal for patients with Lisfranc injuries, but gait and proprioceptive training play important roles in rehabilitation of these injuries as well (Lorenz and Beauchamp 2013).

METATARSAL FRACTURES

Background

Because the MTs play a large role in weight bearing and fractures of the MTs are relatively common, a general understanding of the treatment of these fractures is necessary for both the orthopedist and the physical therapist. These fractures can be caused by a number of different mechanisms including indirect rotational forces or direct trauma, where an object falls onto the dorsum of the forefoot (Reid and Early 2010). Stress fractures can also occur due to repetitive microtrauma and overuse, especially in the second and third MT necks and the proximal fifth MT (Egol et al. 2010b).

Fracture Location

For the most part, isolated diaphyseal fractures of the central three MTs can be treated nonoperatively with benign neglect due to strong stabilizing intermetatarsal ligaments. However, if multiple central metatarsals are fractured and displaced, then operative treatment is sometimes indicated (Reid and Early 2010). Fig. 38.7 is a radiograph showing fractures of the central 3 MTs. Fractures of the first MT lack the strong stabilizing ligamentous supports aforementioned and are therefore more likely to displace and disrupt the plantar weightbearing complex,

which includes the associated sesamoid bones. Displacement or instability of a first metatarsal fracture requires operative treatment (Egol et al. 2010b, Reid and Early 2010).

Fractures of the fifth MT are common in the athletic population. They are classified and treated according to the anatomic location of the fracture. Distal shaft fractures are treated in a similar manner to central MT shaft fractures. However, proximal fifth MT fractures are approached with a bit more caution. Avulsion fractures of the proximal lateral tuberosity are nonoperative injuries treated symptomatically. Proximal fifth metatarsal fractures occurring at the metaphyseal–diaphyseal junction (termed a Jones fracture) or in the proximal 1.5 cm of the diaphysis have a higher nonunion rate because of a tenuous blood supply (Reid and Early 2010). If treated nonoperatively, these fractures require strict NWB for 6 weeks, during which NWB A/PROM is performed. Percutaneous intramedullary screw fixation of these fractures is commonly performed in athletes or laborers to reduce the time to return to activity and to lessen the refracture rate. Figure 38.8, *A* and *B*, shows a proximal fifth MT fracture that was treated operatively with an intramedullary screw (Creevy et al. 2011).

Rehabilitation

In general, nonoperative fractures of central MT shafts and those of the mid to distal fifth MT shaft may be treated with a hard-soled shoe or fracture boot WBAT. Typically these patients can be progressed to a supportive athletic shoe within 4 to 6 weeks from the injury (Reid and Early 2010, Thordarson 2013). Similarly, nonoperative first MT fractures can be treated WBAT in a cast or fracture boot for 4 to 6 weeks, with advancement of activities and to regular shoe wear only after FWB has been

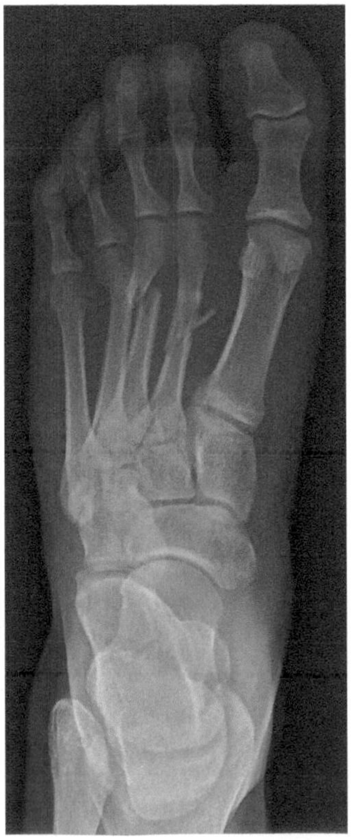

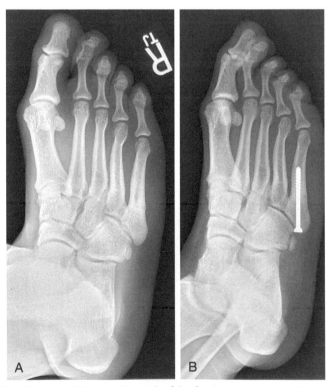

Fig. 38.7   AP radiograph of the foot demonstrating fractures of the third and fourth MT necks with a second MT shaft fracture. The third MT shows some lateral displacement of the distal fragment.

Fig. 38.8   A, Oblique radiograph of the foot demonstrating a fracture of the proximal fifth MT in an athlete. B shows the same view of the previous injury after intramedullary fixation with a screw.

comfortably achieved in the cast or boot (Egol et al. 2010b, Reid and Early 2010). Avulsion fractures of the proximal fifth MT are treated WBAT in symptomatic fashion; they may require comfort measures such as a hard-soled shoe or fracture boot for several weeks followed by a supportive athletic shoe (Thordarson 2013).

Operative fractures of the central MT are initially immobilized non weight bearing in a splint, usually for about two weeks. This is followed by a supportive athletic shoe or a hard soled shoe to support the forefoot (Reid and Early 2010, Thordarson 2013). Gentle ROM is allowed with incision healing at about two weeks postoperatively. With radiographic evidence of union, patients are progressed to WBAT in a fracture boot or hard-soled shoe for an additional 4–6 weeks (Thorvardson 2013). Operative first MT fractures are managed in a similar manner with the exception that NWB is prolonged for 8 to 10 weeks, and early ROM of the great toe is encouraged once incisions have healed. Also, full-length in-shoe orthotics can be used for medial support as needed for the first year postoperatively (Reid and Early 2010).

Nonoperative fractures of the proximal fifth MT, excluding the very proximal metaphyseal avulsion fractures, are treated with NWB immobilization for at least 6 weeks (Reid and Early 2010). After this period of NWB, patients are advanced to WBAT in a fracture boot and physical therapy may address ROM and strengthening progressively. Once asymptomatic FWB is achieved, the boot may be removed, and if there is radiographic evidence of union and the area is nontender to palpation, patients may return to sport or normal activity (Reid and Early 2010). The proper rehab protocols for proximal fifth MT fractures is more controversial. Some authors advocate very early WB and aggressive return-to-play protocol, and others advocate a 6-week NWB regimen similar to nonoperative treatment. We have adopted an intermediate plan consisting of NWB for 2 weeks postoperatively, followed by WBAT in a boot until 6 weeks, during which NWB ROM and pool therapy are begun. The patient is transferred to an athletic shoe with a custom-molded insert and WB rehab is advanced. Return to play/activity is targeted at 9 to 10 weeks if the patient has no pain and has radiographic evidence of healing. However, if any symptoms arise or persist during this process, the rehabilitation is slowed and CT scan is obtained to check for bony union prior to release to full activities.

THE NEUROPATHIC PATIENT

With regard to the neuropathic patient with a foot or ankle fracture, consideration must be given to protecting the insensate foot. Diabetics are well known to have vascular disease, and thus they typically heal at a slower rate than nondiabetics. This, in combination with the insensate foot and ankle, can lead to devastating complications, sometimes even requiring amputation. For this reason, it is recommended that neuropathic foot and ankle trauma patients be treated with slower rehab, longer immobilization, and NWB, especially operative patients. Some authors recommend doubling the periods of immobilization and NWB activity (Davidovitch and Egol 2010, Rudloff 2013). Regardless of the timeline chosen for rehabilitation, these patients must be managed cautiously and vigilantly to prevent complications.

GENERAL CONSIDERATIONS

There are several common themes with regard to foot and ankle rehabilitation. These include management of edema and swelling, appropriate instruction on mobilization and transfers for the NWB patient, prevention of the equinus contracture, and maintenance of strength and endurance in the more proximal musculature of the involved extremity. With regard to swelling and edema, the common modalities of elevation, ice, and compression play a vital role. Swelling may postpone needed operative intervention, cause problems with wound healing postoperatively, and delay rehabilitation progress. It is not uncommon that initiation of mobilization or ROM may cause an increase in foot and ankle swelling, and the patient should be educated properly to expect this swelling, and the swelling itself should be dealt with appropriately.

Transfers and mobilization with assistive devices for a NWB patient may seem intuitive to the health care professional, but this is not always the case for patients. As such, proper instruction regarding safe transfers and mobilization with crutches or a walker are critical services that rehabilitation professionals can provide to the foot and ankle trauma patient. This will minimize recumbent time in bed and allow the patient to spend more time mobilizing to help prevent blood clots and pulmonary complications. In addition, a reduction of the risk and incidence of falls is an important goal with this facet of recovery. Such training and education typically should start as early as possible and need not wait until after surgery.

Prevention of the plantarflexion contracture is also a common theme in the management of foot and ankle trauma, especially in the NWB patient. This involves routine daily stretching of the gastrocnemius–soleus complex when appropriate and also commonly involves wearing a supportive brace with the ankle held in neutral position overnight for up to a month and sometimes longer. Plantarflexion is often a more comfortable resting position for the injured ankle, and therefore one must be proactive and vigilant to prevent a contracture from occurring. The goal is to allow smooth transition through rehabilitation protocols that may be adversely affected by a contracture.

Solely focusing on the specific injury of the foot or ankle can lead to neglect of the more proximal musculature of the involved lower extremity, which can in turn lead to disuse atrophy and profound weakness of the quadriceps, hamstrings, and hip musculature. This should be avoided if at all possible, and early efforts should be made to maintain knee ROM and strength in the proximal musculature of the lower extremity. These efforts will pay dividends when the rehabilitation process approaches mobilization on and strengthening of the injured foot or ankle.

A final consideration that may prove helpful in rehabilitation of these injuries is a general protocol to aid in guiding the foot and ankle trauma patient through the recovery phases of his or her treatment. While it has been clearly demonstrated in this chapter that there are some specific key differences regarding the rehabilitation management of many of these injuries, there are far more overlapping similarities. Furthermore, most foot and ankle fracture rehabilitation schemes eventually reach a common thread, in which the treatment mirrors that of foot and ankle sprains covered elsewhere in this book. Thus, it is our contention that a general protocol detailing some of the key phases of the rehabilitation process may prove more useful than a separate protocol for each injury. After all, rehabilitation of these various fractures has a common overall objective, that is to allow optimal healing and return the patient to the maximal level of function after an injury. The following protocol is therefore meant as a loose guide for rehabilitation goals status after foot or ankle fracture operative intervention.

PHASE I: PROTECTION (WEEKS 1 TO 6)

- Note that weightbearing status and length of immobilization will depend upon the fracture, fixation strength, and treating physician preference. Assume NWB if not specified.
- Instruction in NWB ambulation and safe transfers
- Edema management
- Protection of surgical wound
- After surgical wound healing at 2 to 4 weeks, transition to removable immobilization if appropriate.
- Gentle AROM of foot and ankle within pain tolerance after surgical wound healing
- Gentle ankle isometric strengthening after surgical wound healing
- Prevention of plantarflexion contracture development with dorsiflexion stretches and removable boot worn at night
- Strengthening and conditioning of core, upper extremities, and proximal musculature of the lower extremity

PHASE II: MOBILIZATION (WEEKS 6 TO 8)

- Continued edema management and general conditioning
- Progressive AROM and PROM as tolerated
- Stretching program and stationary bike to improve ROM
- Gradual progressive weight bearing as dictated by treating physician with assistive devices as needed
- Progressive isometric and isotonic exercises for ankle
- Intrinsic foot musculature strengthening
- Initial proprioception and balance training once FWB

PHASE III: FUNCTION (WEEKS 8 TO 12)

- Progress to FWB without assistive devices.
- Restore normal gait mechanics.
- Restore full AROM and PROM.
- Agressive stretching regimen
- Progressive strengthening of foot and ankle musculature with home exercise regimen
- Increase endurance of foot and ankle musculature.
- Advance proprioception and balance training as tolerated and according to functional demands
- Sport or job specific skills training

REFERENCES

A complete reference list is available at https://expertconsult .inkling.com/.

FURTHER READING

Baret DP. Pilon fractures. In: Bucholz RW, Heckman JD, Court-Brown CM, et al., eds. *Rockwood and Green's Fractures in Adults*. Philadelphia: Lippincott Williams and Wilkins; 2010:1928–1974.

Chinn L, Hertel J. Rehabilitation of ankle and foot injuries in athletes. *Clinical Sports Medicine*. 2010;29(1):157–167.

Davidovitch RI, Egol KE. Ankle fractures. In: Bucholz RW, Heckman JD, Court-Brown CM, et al., eds. *Rockwood and Green's Fractures in Adults*. Philadelphia: Lippincott Williams and Wilkins; 2010:1975–2021.

Reid JJ, Early JS. Fractures and dislocations of the midfoot and forefoot. In: Bucholz RW, Heckman JD, Court-Brown CM, et al., eds. *Rockwood and Green's Fractures in Adults*. Philadelphia: Lippincott Williams and Wilkins; 2010:2110–2174.

Sanders DW. Talus fractures. In: Bucholz RW, Heckman JD, Court-Brown CM, et al., eds. *Rockwood and Green's Fractures in Adults*. Philadelphia: Lippincott Williams and Wilkins; 2010:2022–2063.

Sanders RW, Clare MP. Calcaneus fractures. In: Bucholz RW, Heckman JD, Court-Brown CM, et al., eds. *Rockwood and Green's Fractures in Adults*. Philadelphia: Lippincott Williams and Wilkins; 2010:2064–2109.

39

Ankle Sprains

Brian K. Farr, MA, ATC, LAT, CSCS | Donald Nguyen, PT, MSPT, ATC, LAT | Ken Stephenson, MD | Toby Rogers, PhD, MPT | Faustin R. Stevens, MD | John J. Jasko, MD

Ankle sprains are common injuries in active individuals, with an estimated incidence of 61 ankle sprains per 10,000 persons each year (Maffulli and Ferran 2008). They are the most common injury sustained by high school and collegiate athletes, accounting for up to 30% of sports injuries (Hass et al. 2010). An age of 10 to 19 years old is associated with higher rates of ankle sprains. Half of all ankle sprains occur during athletic activity. Although most of these injuries respond well to conservative therapy, chronic instability and dysfunction are known risks (Gerber et al. 1998).

In a study of 202 elite track and field athletes with lateral ankle sprains, (Malliaropoulos et al. 2009) found that 18% sustained a second sprain within 24 months; low-grade acute ankle sprains (grade I or II) resulted in a higher risk of re-injury than high-grade (grade III) sprains (Malliaropoulos et al. 2009). Because of the potential for re-injury and chronic dysfunction and the importance of a normally functioning ankle in active people, it is important that ankle sprains be managed correctly with a thorough rehabilitation and reconditioning program.

RELEVANT ANATOMY

The ankle, or talocrural joint, is a junction of the tibia, fibula, and talus (Fig. 39.1). The bony congruity confers stability to ankle joint, especially in static weight bearing in the neutral position. During motion, the anterior talofibular ligament (ATFL), calcaneofibular ligament (CFL), and posterior talofibular ligament (PTFL) provide support to the joint laterally (Fig. 39.2, *A*), whereas the deltoid ligament complex (DLC), made up of the anterior and posterior tibiotalar ligaments, the tibiocalcaneal ligament, and the tibionavicular ligament, provides medial support (Fig. 39.2, *B*). The inferior anterior and posterior tibiofibular ligaments and the interosseous membrane, collectively known as the syndesmotic complex, provide stability to the tibia-fibula articulation and thereby also support the ankle joint (Fig. 39.2, *C* and *D*).

The ATFL is the most commonly injured ligament, followed by the CFL. The CFL is usually injured in combination with the ATFL. Sprains to both the ATFL and CFL are a result of a combined inversion and plantarflexion mechanism (Fig. 39.3, *A*). The less common mechanism of eversion may cause injury to the DLC (Fig. 39.3, *B*). Injuries to the syndesmotic complex are discussed later in this chapter.

The muscle/tendon units that cross the ankle and attach to the foot provide dynamic control of the ankle. The peroneal muscle group, composed of the peroneus brevis, longus, and tertius muscles, is of significant importance because these muscles are responsible for everting the ankle and, thus, resisting inversion (Fig. 39.3, *C*). Because there are no muscles that attach directly to the talus, motion of the talus is dictated by foot and ankle position. **The most stable position of the ankle is in dorsiflexion.** As the foot moves into dorsiflexion, the talus glides posteriorly and the wider anterior portion of the talus becomes wedged into the ankle mortise. As the ankle moves into plantarflexion, the talus glides anteriorly and the ankle becomes less stable, which is why most ankle sprains involve some degree of plantarflexion as the mechanism. The ATFL is more parallel with the tibia in plantarflexion and thus more vulnerable in this position.

CLASSIFICATION OF ANKLE SPRAINS

Regardless of whether the lateral or medial ligaments are injured, the severity of an ankle sprain is typically placed into one of three grades based on the amount of ligamentous damage. The degree of tissue damage, the amount of joint laxity, and the extent of dysfunction increase with each increase in grade.

- **Grade I** ankle sprains result in a stretching of the ligamentous fibers and are considered minor sprains.
- **Grade II** ankle sprains result in a partial tearing of the ligamentous fibers and are considered to be moderate sprains.
- **Grade III** ankle sprains result in substantial tearing of the ligamentous fibers and are considered severe sprains.

DIAGNOSIS

It is only through a thorough examination that the severity of an ankle sprain can be established (Table 39.1). Detailed information on conducting a thorough examination of the ankle is beyond the scope of this text; however, common signs and

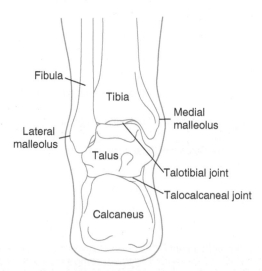

Fig. 39.1   The ankle, which is a junction of the talus, the tibia, and the fibula.

symptoms associated with each grade of lateral ankle sprain are listed in Table 39.2. The examiner must also be aware of additional injuries that can occur with ankle sprains. Such injuries include, but are not limited to, avulsion fractures, fractures, muscle and tendon strains, articular cartilage damage of the ankle mortise, and tarsal subluxations and dislocations. Although some of these injuries (such as muscle strains) can be adequately treated with the following standard treatment protocol, others (such as articular cartilage damage) may require revisions of the standard treatment protocol for ankle sprains.

The emphasis for the following standard treatment protocol is placed on treating ankle sprains in the absence of other significant injuries. It should be noted that the patient should be re-evaluated throughout the rehabilitation program for any limitations that need to be considered. For example, although it is common to include stretching of the heel cord in a rehabilitation protocol for ankle sprains, a specific patient may not have tightness of the heel cord and therefore may not need to perform the stretches. It is also important to look for signs of aggravation or re-injury (e.g., increased pain, increased tenderness, increased swelling, decreased range of motion, decreased strength). Occasionally, even the best-planned rehabilitation protocols can cause aggravation to an injury. It is important that the therapy provider know when it is time to slow down or change the protocol. Also, some patients may buy into the "no pain, no gain" philosophy and not report an increasingly painful and stiff ankle, believing it needs to be pushed harder to get better when the opposite may be true.

THE INJURY AND HEALING PROCESS

The body's healing process occurs in a natural sequence of events and can be divided into three stages: the inflammatory or acute stage; the subacute, repair, or proliferation stage; and the remodeling or maturation stage. It is important to have an understanding of what takes place during each of these stages in order to support the body's natural healing process and limit the potential for additional injury. A summary of the clinically relevant events follows.

In the **acute stage,** the cardinal signs and symptoms of inflammation (pain, edema, erythema, warmth, decreased function) are evident. This stage begins immediately after the onset of injury and typically lasts 3 to 5 days.

The **subacute stage,** which begins at about 3 days after injury and can last up to 6 weeks, is marked by a decrease in the signs and symptoms of inflammation and the beginning of tissue repair. It is during this stage that weak collagen fibers begin to develop a scar at the injured site. Approximately 7 days after injury, there is a significant amount of collagen in the area. As the subacute stage

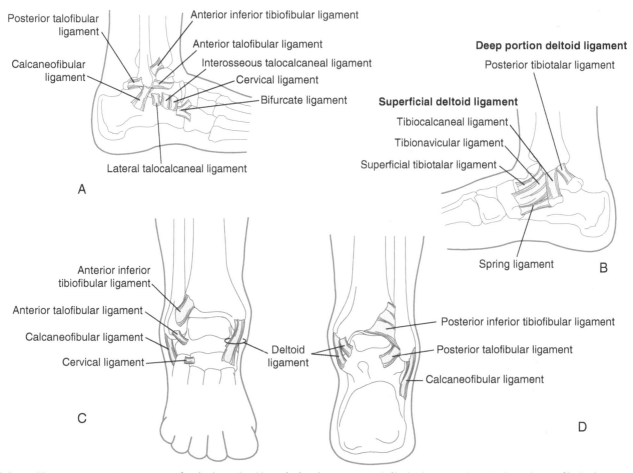

Fig. 39.2　Ankle anatomy. **A,** Static support for the lateral ankle includes the anterior talofibular ligament (ATFL), the calcaneofibular ligament (CFL), and the posterior talofibular ligament (PTFL). **B,** Static support for the medial ankle is provided by the deltoid ligament complex (DLC). **C** and **D,** An anterior (*C,* left) and posterior (*D,* right) view of the ankle showing the ATFL, CFL, PTFL, DLC, and the anterior inferior tibiofibular ligament and posterior tibiofibular ligament, which provide additional support to the joint.

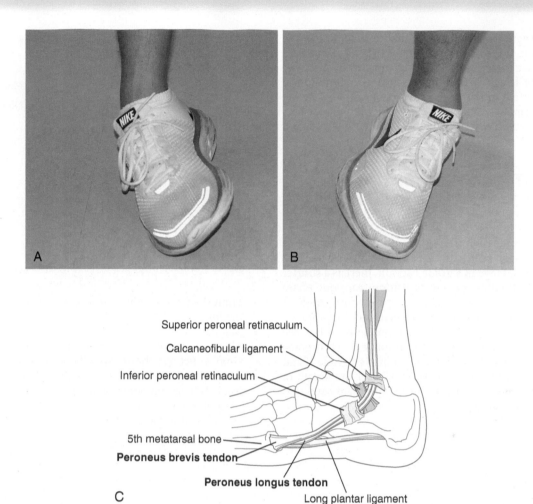

Fig. 39.3 Mechanisms of injury. **A,** Inversion with plantarflexion is the most common mechanism of injury for ankle sprains and will typically result in injury to the anterior talofibular ligament (ATFL) and possibly the calcaneofibular ligament (CFL). **B,** Although not as common as an inversion sprain, eversion is the mechanism of injury for sprains of the deltoid ligament complex (DLC). **C,** The peroneal tendons are lateral dynamic stabilizers of the ankle.

TABLE 39.1	Examination of the Ankle After an Inversion Injury

PALPATION OF THE LATERAL COLLATERALS (ANTERIOR TALOFIBULAR LIGAMENT AND CALCANEOFIBULAR LIGAMENT)

Medial palpation of the deltoid ligament

Palpation of the proximal fibula close to the knee to rule out a Maisonneuve fracture (tearing of the interosseous membrane and proximal fibula fracture)

Squeeze test to rule out ankle syndesmosis tearing with resultant ankle mortise instability

External rotation (Cotton) test to test for syndesmosis injury

Palpation of the proximal (base) fifth metatarsal to rule out avulsion fracture from peroneus brevis pull

ANTERIOR DRAWER AND INVERSION (TALAR TILT) STRESS TESTING

Motor testing of posterior tibial (inversion) and peroneal tendons (eversion)

TABLE 39.2	Clinical Signs and Symptoms Associated With Ankle Sprains	
Grade I	Grade II	Grade III
Stretching of ligaments, usually the ATFL	Partial tearing of ligaments, usually the ATFL and CFL	Substantial tearing of ligaments, may involve the PTFL in addition to the ATFL and CFL
Point tenderness	Point and diffuse tenderness	Point and diffuse tenderness
Limited dysfunction	Moderate dysfunction	Moderate to severe dysfunction
No laxity	Slight to moderate laxity	Moderate to severe laxity
Able to bear full weight	Antalgic gait and pain with FWB, may need supportive device to ambulate	Limited to no ability for FWB without supportive device
Little to no edema	Mild to moderate edema	Severe edema

ATFL, anterior talofibular ligament; CFL, calcaneofibular ligament; FWB, full weight bearing; PTFL, posterior talofibular ligament.

progresses, it is important to provide some stress to the newly forming scar tissue to minimize adherence to surrounding tissues and to encourage proper scar tissue alignment and development; however, in the early stages the collagen fibers are weak and unorganized so it is more important to avoid too much stress, which can be detrimental to the healing tissues.

Activities associated with the **maturation stage** begin approximately 1 week after injury in grade I sprains and approximately 3 weeks after injury in grade III sprains. During the maturation stage, the collagen tissues become stronger and more organized. Although nowhere near normal, the scar's tensile strength usually has increased considerably by the fifth or sixth week. It is important to stress the scar tissue adequately to decrease the potential of developing a dysfunctional scar. Appropriate levels of tissue stress will also continue to encourage proper alignment and development as the scar tissue matures. The maturation phase can last longer than a year, although patients typically return to their activity level much sooner than that.

TREATMENT AND REHABILITATION PROTOCOL FOR ACUTE ANKLE SPRAIN

It is important to remember that the duration of each stage of tissue repair depends, in part, on the extent of injury. Because there is less tissue damage in a grade I sprain, there is a shorter duration of healing with a quicker transition from one phase of tissue healing to the next when compared to a grade II sprain. This is important to consider when establishing a treatment and rehabilitation protocol because patients with grade I sprains can be progressed quicker than patients with grade II sprains. The same can be said when comparing grade II and grade III sprains. Although many factors affect the length of time before a patient can return to normal physical activities, patients with grade I sprains can often return to their normal physical activity levels within 1 to 2 weeks, whereas patients with grade II sprains can expect to return in 4 to 8 weeks. There is a greater range of expected return estimates in patients with grade III injuries, which can take as long as 12 to 16 weeks to recover.

Without ignoring where the injury is in the healing process, the clinician should progressively manage the patient's signs and symptoms, functional limitations, and impairments instead of solely focusing on the number of days since the injury. Table 39.3 lists the common signs and symptoms associated with each stage of tissue healing. Changes in the signs and symptoms, in addition to the number of days post injury, can help the clinician determine when to progress the patient's treatment and rehabilitation program.

The steps in treating and rehabilitating ankle sprains typically follow this progression:

Step 1: Protect the area from further injury.

Step 2: Decrease pain, swelling, and spasm.

Step 3: Re-establish range of motion (ROM), flexibility, and tissue mobility.

Step 4: Re-establish neuromuscular control, muscular strength, endurance, and power.

Step 5: Re-establish proprioception, coordination, and agility.

Step 6: Re-establish functional skills.

While the rehabilitation program is progressing through these steps that focus on the injured ankle, it is important to maintain overall strength and conditioning for the rest of the body. Rehabilitation Protocol 39.1 provides an outline of the ankle sprain rehabilitation protocol described here.

Acute Stage: Goals and Interventions After Ankle Sprain

During the acute phase the primary goals of the rehabilitation program are as follows:
- Protect the injured tissues from further injury.
- Encourage tissue healing.

TABLE 39.3	Clinical Signs and Symptoms Associated With the Stages of Tissue Healing	
Acute Stage	**Subacute Stage**	**Maturation Stage**
Pain at rest, ↑ w/ activity	↓ pain, TTP, swelling, heat	No s/s of inflammation
TTP	↓ spasm and guarding	↑ function
↑ swelling	↑ function	↑ ROM
Heat	↑ ROM w/↓ pain	
Protective guarding and muscle spasm	↓ laxity w/stress tests*	
Loss of function*		
Restricted and painful ROM		
Laxity w/stress tests*		

↑, increased; TTP, tenderness to palpation; ROM, range of motion; ↓, decreased; s/s, signs and symptoms.
*Presence and amount depend on severity of sprain.

- Limit the pain, swelling, and spasm associated with inflammation.
- Maintain function of the noninjured tissues.
- Maintain overall body conditioning.

Goal A: Protect the Injured Tissues From Further Injury. Although the patient should rest the injured tissues to limit additional stress and potential injury, it is important to remember that absolute rest is seldom a wise choice. Patients should be encouraged to participate in pain-free activities that do not stress the injured ligaments. The type of activities that can be safely tolerated varies with the severity of the ankle sprain. Typically with grade I ankle sprains, the patient can safely participate in light to moderate activities. Those with grade II and grade III sprains should have greater limits on their activities. Because most ankle sprains involve the lateral ligaments and are caused by plantarflexion and inversion, the patient should avoid activities that cause extremes of these motions for at least the first several days.

Protection with splinting, bracing, taping (Fig. 39.4, *A–M*), or wrapping the injured ankle may be necessary, especially in grade II or III sprains. A systematic review concluded that lace-up supports were most effective, that taping was associated with skin irritation and was no better than semi-rigid supports, and that elastic bandages were the least effective form of stabilization (Kerkhoffs et al. 2001).

Patients with grade II or III sprains also may need supportive devices such as crutches, a walking cane, or a walking boot to move about. Although there has long been debate as to whether or not to immobilize sprained ankles or omit immobilization and immediately begin a "functional treatment" plan, current practices are to use a functional treatment plan, especially when managing grades I and II sprains. A functional treatment plan limits immobilization and encourages pain-free activities that do not overstress the injured ligaments. Functional rehabilitation has been shown to be associated with more frequent return to sports and higher rates of patient satisfaction than immobilization (Kerkhoffs et al. 2001). If the patient's ankle is to be immobilized, it should be noted that long periods of immobilization may lead to prolonged joint stiffness and contractures, weakening of noninjured ligaments, and muscle atrophy.

Goal B: Encourage Tissue Healing. In a healthy patient, the body will go through its normal healing process as long as there is no additional trauma to the tissues. Rest and protection of the injured tissues are important to allow the body to progress

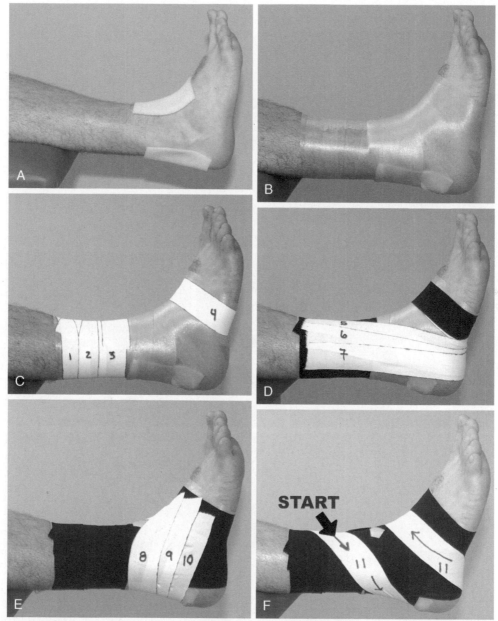

Fig. 39.4 **A,** Have the patient sit with the knee extended and the ankle dorsiflexed to a 90-degree angle. Place heel and lace pads over the Achilles tendon and the instep of the ankle. Spray the foot, ankle, and distal aspect of the lower leg with tape adhesive. **B,** Apply underwrap around the ankle from the midfoot to the midcalf. The underwrap should go up to the base of the calf muscle or approximately 5 to 6 inches above the malleoli. Efforts should be made to apply as few layers of underwrap as possible. Although no longer a common practice, the adhesive tape can be applied directly to the patient's skin without using underwrap. **C,** Apply two or three anchors to the distal aspect of the lower leg (1–3). Each strip should overlap the previous one by approximately one half of the width of the tape. Apply one anchor to the midfoot (4). **D,** Apply three stirrup strips (5–7), beginning at the medial aspect of the lower leg running inferiorly along the leg, then laterally under the rearfoot, and finishing on the lateral aspect of the lower leg. Each strip should overlap the previous one by approximately one half of the width of the tape. **E,** Apply three horse-shoe strips (8–10) running from the medial aspect of the foot to the lateral aspect beginning and ending on the distal anchor (See #4 in Part C). Note: An alternative method, called a "closed basketweave," alternates one stirrup strip with one horseshoe strip until three of each are applied. If this were to be done, strip 5 would be followed by strip 8, then strip 6 would be followed by strip 9, and strip 7 would be followed by strip 10.

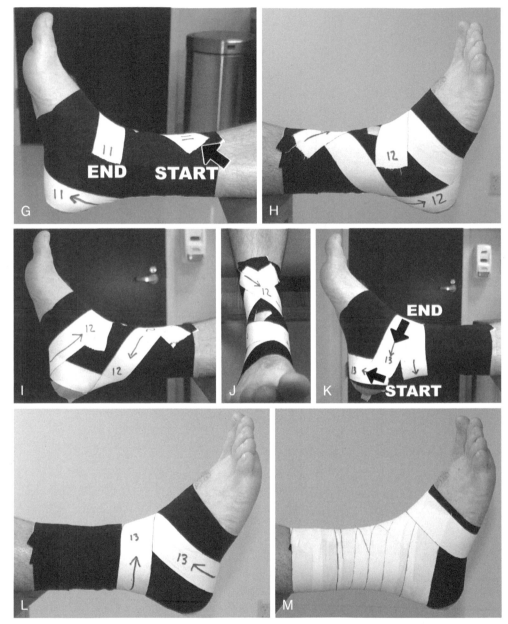

Fig. 39.4, cont'd F–J, Apply two heel locks (11,12). The first heel lock (11) begins high on the anterior aspect of the lower leg, runs posteriorly behind the calcaneus, circles along the medial aspect of the calcaneus, then finishes along the anterior–medial aspect of the midfoot. The second heel lock (12) begins high on the anterior aspect of the lower leg, runs posteriorly behind the calcaneus, circles along the lateral aspect of the calcaneus, then finishes along the anterior–lateral aspect of the midfoot. K–L, Apply a figure-eight strip (13) beginning at the medial aspect of the calcaneus and running laterally to the plantar aspect of the calcaneus, then moving medially toward the instep before moving posteriorly around the lower leg and ending up where the strip began at the medial aspect of the calcaneus. M, Finish the tape job with closing strips. Begin the strips at the superior aspect of the lower leg and work inferiorly, overlapping the previous strip by approximately one half of the width of the tape. Finish with a closing strip over the midfoot.

through its normal healing processes. Toward the end of the acute phase, pulsed ultrasound can be used to promote tissue healing while limiting undesirable thermal effects obtained with continuous ultrasound.

Goal C: Limit Pain, Swelling, and Spasm. It is important to remember that the inflammatory process is a protective mechanism and is necessary for the body to heal; however, the inflammation process needs to be controlled to minimize patient suffering and prevent chronic inflammation. The combination of rest, ice, compression, and elevation (RICE) is one of the more commonly used approaches to treat the acute inflammatory response. Ice and other forms of cryotherapy help prevent swelling, decrease pain, and limit spasm. Both elevation and compression with elastic wraps or compression stockinet assist with minimizing swelling. Electrical stimulation can also be used to minimize pain, swelling, and spasm. Therapeutic modalities that combine ice, compression, and elevation, such as an intermittent compression unit, also are beneficial.

Grade I joint mobilization techniques to the talus can also be used to minimize pain in the ankle joint. Performing a joint mobilization technique to the distal tibiofibular joint often provides pain relief when a "positional fault" is present. An anterior positional fault of the distal fibula is often seen in patients with a lateral ankle sprain. Applying a posterior mobilizing force to the distal fibula may help correct the anterior positional fault (Fig. 39.5).

Goal D: Maintain Function of Noninjured Tissues. Although rest may be needed for the injured ankle ligaments, muscles, tendons, and joint capsule, normal function of the noninjured tissues must be maintained with activity. The patient should be encouraged to engage in activities that do not stress the injured ligaments. Because most ankle sprains involve the lateral ligaments and are caused by plantarflexion and inversion, care must be taken to minimize extreme motions in those directions, especially in grade II and III sprains. With injuries that involve the deltoid ligament complex (DLC), care is taken to avoid extreme eversion. General mobility exercises are useful in preventing disuse of the noninjured tissues while minimizing stress to the injured ligaments:

- Ankle pumps
- Plantarflexion and dorsiflexion ROM progressing from passive range of motion (PROM) to active-assisted range of motion (AAROM) to active range of motion (AROM) as tolerated (Fig. 39.6)
- Heel-cord and posterior calf stretches (Fig. 39.7)
- ABCs or alphabets
- Towel curls and/or marble pick-ups (Fig. 39.8)

It is especially important to perform these types of activities if the patient is placed in a cast, splint, or walking boot or if the patient is using crutches or a cane. Prolonged use of these assistive and protective devices can result in disuse of healthy tissues around the ankle. If the patient is immobilized, placed in a walking boot, or prevented from full weight bearing (FWB) ambulation for a period, the metatarsophalangeal (MTP) joints should also be treated with some form of mobilization activities (joint mobilizations, PROM, AAROM, AROM, stretches) (Fig. 39.9). At times, patients may be hesitant to attempt partial weight bearing (PWB) or FWB, general mobility exercises, or stretching activities, even though they have been cleared to do so. In this situation, the use of cryokinetics may be warranted. One way to include cryokinetics is to place the injured ankle in a cold whirlpool bath for 15 to

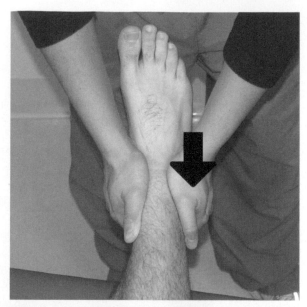

Fig. 39.5 Posterior mobilization of distal fibula to address anterior positional fault of the fibula following a lateral ankle sprain. The patient is supine on a table. The clinician places the palm of the hand on the lateral malleolus and provides a posterior force to the lateral malleolus.

20 minutes or until it becomes "numb." While the ankle is numb, the patient can begin to increase the weight bearing on the ankle, stretch, or perform general mobility exercises. This allows the patient to perform the appropriate activities in a pain-free state.

Goal E: Maintain Overall Body Conditioning. Although the injured ligaments may need to be rested, the rest of the body does not. Patients should be encouraged to engage in pain-free physical activities to maintain their overall body conditioning. Exercising on a stationary bike or upper body ergometer and nonweight bearing (NWB) running in a therapy pool can help maintain cardiovascular endurance and function without stressing the injured tissues. Strengthening exercises for the lower extremities, such as open kinetic chain knee flexion and extension and open kinetic chain hip flexion, extension, abduction, and adduction exercises, should also be performed. These exercises also help to prevent disuse issues of the noninjured body areas while minimizing stress on the injured tissues. Patients should also continue their normal strength training exercises for the trunk and upper extremities. It should be noted that many of these activities put the patient's ankle in a gravity-dependent position, which is a precaution when treating or attempting to prevent swelling. The rehabilitation provider should weigh the risks of the gravity-dependent position to the benefits of maintaining the body's overall condition. The use of a compression stockinet or elastic wrap while performing these exercises can help prevent the influx of edema to the area.

Subacute Stage: Goals and Interventions

During the subacute phase the primary goals are as follows:
- Prevent further injury.
- Minimize pain and inflammation.
- Promote tissue healing.
- Restore ROM and flexibility.
- Re-establish neuromuscular control and restore muscular strength and endurance.

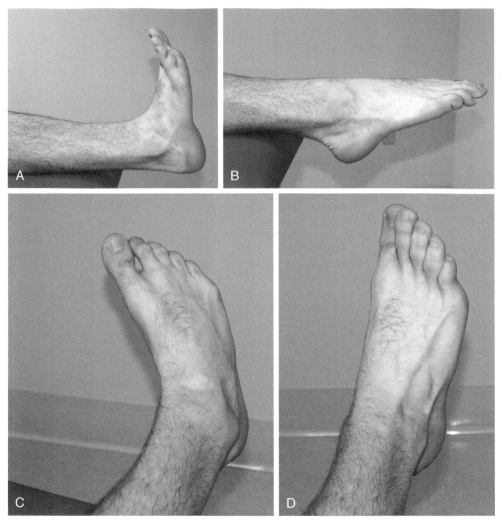

Fig. 39.6 Active range of motion (AROM). **A,** Dorsiflexion. **B,** Plantarflexion. **C,** Inversion. **D,** Eversion.

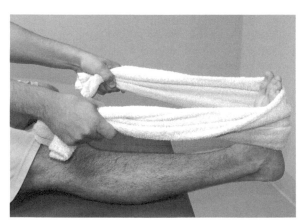

Fig. 39.7 Stretching the Achilles tendon, gastrocnemius, and soleus.

- Re-establish proprioception, agility, and coordination.
- Maintain overall body conditioning.

Goal F: Prevent Further Injury. Although the initial inflammatory response has ended and the early scar tissue is beginning to develop, it is important to remember that the scar tissue is still very weak and improper activities can easily cause re-injury. In the early days of this phase, extremes of plantarflexion and inversion should still be minimized to prevent damage to the newly formed scar tissue. Although patients who used crutches or a cane during the acute phase should be weaned from these supports as FWB becomes tolerated, other protective devices (such as brace or tape) should still be used, especially with grade II or III sprains.

Goal G: Minimize Pain and Inflammation. Continued use of therapeutic modalities is warranted at this time. As the initial signs and symptoms of acute inflammation diminish, thermotherapy techniques such as warm whirlpools and hot packs should be introduced. Thermotherapy techniques help to reduce pain, spasm, and subacute inflammation. Therapeutic ultrasound may also be used at this time, progressing from pulsed to continuous duty cycles. Continuous ultrasound also assists with pain relief, tissue healing, and reduction of subacute edema. The continued use of electrical stimulation can assist with minimizing pain and inflammation. It is still wise to continue cryotherapy, especially after activity, to reduce pain and limit inflammation. Although the goal is to minimize pain and inflammation, it should be noted that an increase in pain or inflammation, especially after the acute stage, often is a sign that the injured structures are not ready for the activity being performed. If the patient experiences an increase in pain, inflammation, or both, he or she should be re-evaluated to ensure there is no worsening of the injury and the rehabilitation

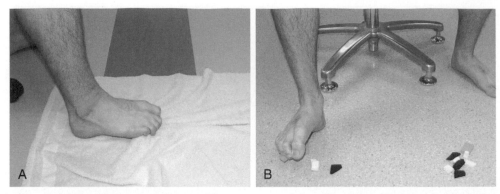

Fig. 39.8 Towel curls (**A**) and picking up objects with the toes (**B**) to maintain mobility of the foot and ankle and to strengthen the intrinsic muscles of the foot.

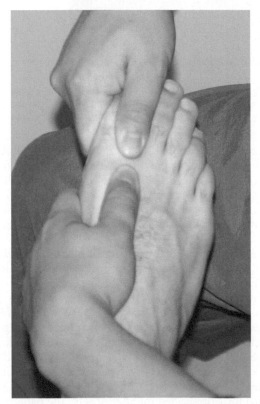

Fig. 39.9 Mobilizing the first metatarsal phalangeal (MTP) joint to maintain mobility. When patients are not able to fully weight bear (FWB) in ambulation, the MTP joints may become hypomobile.

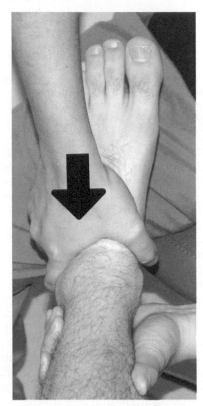

Fig. 39.10 Posterior mobilization to the talus. Grade I and II joint mobilization techniques are effective in reducing pain.

protocol should be slowed until the pain and inflammation are under control. Grades I and II joint mobilizations are also indicated at this time to assist with pain control (Fig. 39.10).

Goal H: Promote Tissue Healing. Continuing to protect the injured ligaments from re-injury will allow the body to go through its normal healing process. The continued use of therapeutic modalities such as ultrasound and thermotherapy helps promote tissue healing. The introduction of ROM and strengthening exercises will also promote proper alignment and improved strength of the scar tissue provided the activities do not produce too much stress. Therapeutic massage techniques can also be used beginning with "flushing-type" techniques such as pétrissage to promote blood flow and circulation and progressing to more aggressive techniques such as cross-friction massage to promote tissue alignment.

Goal I: Restore Range of Motion and Flexibility. The general mobility and ROM exercises that were begun in the

acute stage are continued. As the subacute stage progresses, so should the sets and reps of the exercises, the degree of motion performed, and the intensity of the stretches. The patient should be encouraged to perform ROM exercises and stretches several times throughout the day. Initially, dorsiflexion and limited plantarflexion should be emphasized. Pedaling on a stationary bike can help with both plantarflexion and dorsiflexion. If not done in the acute stage, the use of PROM or AAROM should be replaced by AROM. Use of a BAPS or wobble board can be introduced, first in a NWB position before progressing to PWB then FWB position (Fig. 39.11). The patient should be instructed to perform the motions in a slow and controlled manner at all times. The patient should begin with dorsiflexion, plantarflexion, and eversion before incorporating inversion, then progress to circling the board while touching all sides of the board in both clockwise and

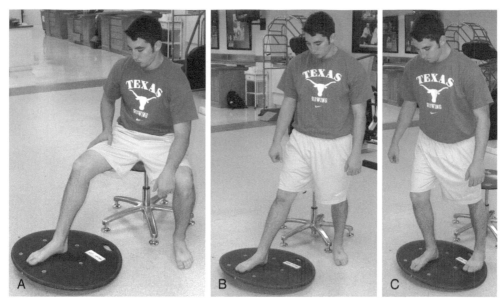

Fig. 39.11 Using a BAPS board to maintain range of motion. **A,** The patient should begin in a nonweight bearing (NWB) position and progress to a partial weight bearing position (PWB) **(B),** before moving to full weight bearing (FWB) **(C).** The patient can perform uniplanar motions in plantarflexion, dorsiflexion, inversion, and eversion or multiplanar motions by performing "circles," which require the patient to touch all of the edges of the board in both a clockwise and counterclockwise direction.

counterclockwise directions. With all of the stretches and ROM activities, the patient is instructed to gradually increase the ROM, taking extra caution with plantarflexion and inversion or other motions that cause pain. Inversion with plantarflexion should be introduced and progressed as tolerated. Cryokinetics are still indicated in the early portion of the subacute phase and can be used until the patient has little to no discomfort with the activities. Progressing from grade II to grade III joint mobilizations can be used for decreased ROM caused by altered arthrokinematics and positional faults to the fibula and talus (Fig. 39.12). Caution must be taken, however, when performing an anterior mobilization technique of the talus in a patient with a grade II or III lateral ligament sprain because an anterior movement of the talus stresses the anterior talofibular ligament and mimics the movement of the talus that occurred with the plantarflexion and inversion mechanism of injury. Because the talus subluxes anteriorly in a sprain caused by plantarflexion and inversion, a posterior mobilization to the talus may be more appropriate (see Fig. 39.10). Massage, myofascial release, and other manual therapy techniques to treat soft tissue restrictions may also help restore ROM, flexibility, and tissue mobility.

Goal J: Re-Establish Neuromuscular Control and Restore Muscular Strength and Endurance. Towel curls and marble pick-ups were included with the general mobility exercises in the acute stage; however, they also can be used to strengthen the intrinsic muscles of the foot (see Fig. 39.8). Patients can begin isometric exercises in a neutral ankle position against plantarflexion, dorsiflexion, inversion, and eversion forces. Because strength gains related to isometric exercises only strengthen the muscle at that length, it is important to progress to performing isometrics in a variety of degrees within a ROM, but painful ROM should be avoided. Isometric exercises should begin with submaximal contractions and progress to maximal contractions. Isometric exercises should be progressed to isotonic exercises as tolerated. Resistance can be provided manually, with cuff weights or elastic bands or cords (Fig. 39.13). Isotonic exercises

should begin with a limited ROM and progress to full ROM as tolerated and should progress from submaximal resistance to maximal efforts. As weight bearing becomes tolerated, heel and toe raises can be incorporated as can walking on the heels or toes (Fig. 39.14). As the patient's pain-free ROM increases, proprioceptive neuromuscular facilitation (PNF) techniques can be used.

Goal K: Re-Establish Proprioception, Agility, and Coordination. In the early phase of proprioception training, the patient may need to perform unloaded exercises such as joint repositioning if PWB or FWB is contraindicated or poorly tolerated. The patient should progress to PWB and FWB exercises as tolerated. Early exercises to encourage loading of the ankle include "weight shifts" in various directions. With weight shifts, the patient stands with his or her weight shifted to the noninjured leg, then progressively shifts the weight onto the injured leg before returning to the NWB position. This process is repeated for a prescribed number of sets. The patient should progressively shift more of his or her weight to the injured leg until equal weight is distributed on both legs. This progresses to the patient shifting more weight on the injured leg until he or she can finally bear full weight on the injured leg. These shifts should begin in a stance with the feet about shoulder-width apart and progress to a staggered stance requiring the patient to shift forward, backward, and laterally. Another exercise has the patient stepping onto a step or box and stepping down on the uninjured ankle. Once that is tolerated, the patient can step down from the box onto the injured ankle. The patient may need an assistive device such as a chair or railing in the beginning of this progression, but use of the device should be discontinued as soon as tolerated. Again, the patient should perform these step-ups and step-downs in various directions (Fig. 39.15).

The patient next progresses to activities with patient-controlled perturbations. The patient stands first in a two-foot stance with the weight evenly distributed while performing upper extremity or trunk exercises such as pulling on elastic

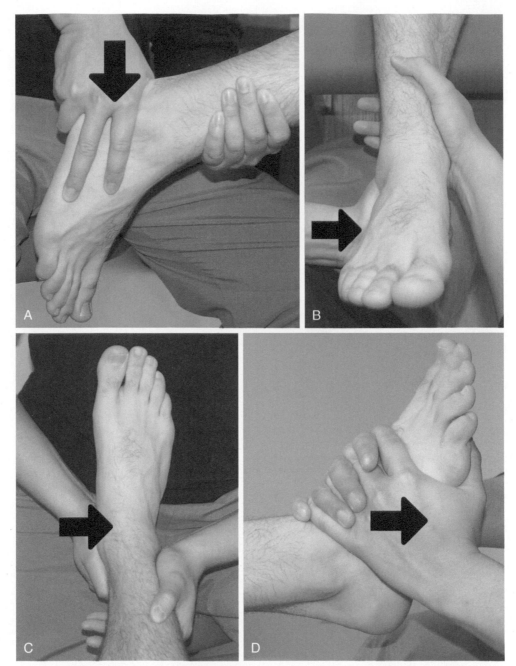

Fig. 39.12 Joint mobilization techniques to restore range of motion and arthrokinematics. **A,** Anterior mobilization to increase plantarflexion. **B,** Medial mobilization to increase eversion. **C,** Lateral mobilization to increase inversion. **D,** Distraction of the talocrural joint for pain control and general mobility.

bands in various directions, moving a weighted medicine ball in various directions, or bending over to pick up an object. The patient may also perform motions with the noninjured leg instead of, or in addition to, the upper extremity motions (Fig. 39.16). The patient should begin with uniplanar motions and progress to multiplanar motions. The patient can also perform these activities in a tandem stance (heel to toe) or a single-legged stance.

The patient then progresses to activities where he or she must react to perturbations provided by the clinician. These types of activities involve the patient standing in a two-foot stance, a tandem stance, or a single-legged stance and reacting to a perturbation caused by the clinician. These types of perturbations include pushing or pulling on the patient's body, either by direct contact or with elastic tubing or a stick, and playing catch with the patient (Fig. 39.17).

As the patient's proprioception improves, agility and coordination exercises should be introduced. Walking, walking backward, front lunges, back lunges, side lunges, step-ups, step-downs, and so on can be incorporated as tolerated. Patients can also perform lateral movement exercises on a slide board or Fitter machine (Fig. 39.18).

These exercises should progress from a two-foot stance with the feet at shoulder width, to a stance with both feet together, to a tandem stance with the feet apart, to a tandem heel to toe stance, and finally to a one-legged stance. The exercises can be

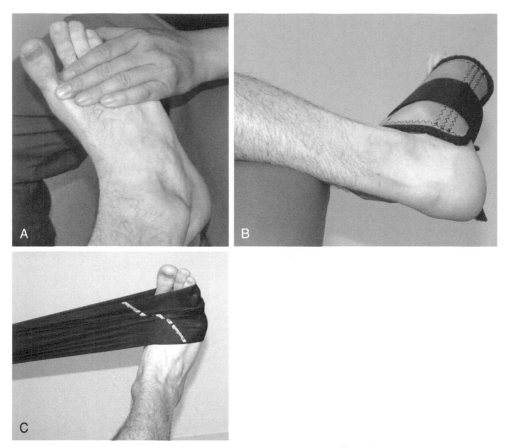

Fig. 39.13   Isotonic exercises. **A,** Eversion against manual resistance. **B,** Eversion using a cuff weight for resistance. **C,** Using an elastic band to resist eversion. Strengthening exercises should be performed in dorsiflexion, plantarflexion, inversion, and eversion.

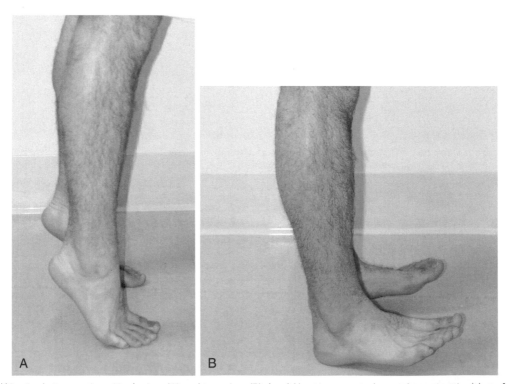

Fig. 39.14   Closed kinetic chain exercises. Heel raises (**A**) and toe raises (**B**) should be incorporated once the patient is able to fully bear weight. The patient can also walk on the toes or heels as a more functional strength training exercise.

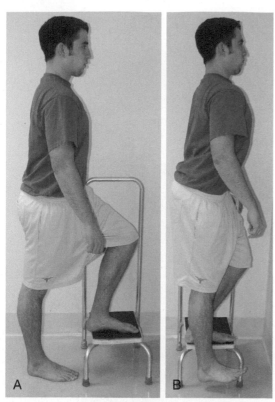

Fig. 39.15 Proprioception exercises without perturbations. A, Stepping up and down on the injured leg develops proprioception. B, Lateral step-ups increase the difficulty of the exercise.

made more difficult by having the patient perform the activities with his or her eyes closed; while shaking his or her head; or while standing on an unstable surface such as a foam pad, balance disc, or trampoline.

Goal L: Maintain Overall Body Conditioning. The same upper body and trunk exercises that were used during the acute phase can still be used in the subacute phase. As the patient better tolerates weight bearing, closed kinetic chain (CKC) lower extremity strength training exercises such as lunges, squats, leg presses, and calf raises can be added to the program (Fig. 39.19). Cardiovascular exercises such as walking, light jogging, climbing stairs (i.e., Stairmaster), and swimming can also be added.

Maturation Stage: Goals and Interventions

During the maturation phase the primary goals are as follows:
- Prevent re-injury.
- Restore ROM and flexibility.
- Improve muscular strength, endurance, and power.
- Improve proprioception, agility, and coordination.
- Improve functional (sport-specific) skills.
- Maintain overall body conditioning.

Goal M: Prevent Re-injury. While the strength of the scar tissue is increasing in this phase, patients and clinicians must still be mindful that it takes more than a year for high tensile strength to develop. Because the athlete will be performing much more functional exercises in this stage, the use of tape or a brace for additional support is warranted.

Goal N: Restore Range of Motion and Flexibility. It is important that full, functional ROM is attained, if it has not been already. Aggressive stretching techniques that focus on low-load and long-duration stretches and dynamic stretches can be used. Grades III and IV joint mobilizations may also be warranted to restore normal joint arthrokinematics. The clinician should also incorporate soft tissue techniques, such as cross-fiber massage and myofascial release techniques, to break down soft tissue adhesions.

Goal O: Improve Muscular Strength, Endurance, and Power. A solid foundation for muscular strength and endurance should have been laid throughout the subacute stage. The emphasis in the maturation stage is placed on explosive strength and power development for functional exercises. Plyometric exercises are begun at this time. The clinician must keep the demands of the patient's physical activities in mind and set up exercises that emphasize those demands. For example, if the patient is a basketball player, exercises that emphasize lateral movements, vertical jumps, and quick changes in direction should be incorporated.

Goal P: Improve Proprioception, Agility, and Coordination. In this stage of the program, work-hardening activities should be incorporated for nonathletes and sport-specific drills should be used for athletes. Exercises to improve proprioception, agility, and coordination go hand in hand with those used to improve functional skills. If not incorporated in the later days of the subacute stage, more dynamic proprioception exercises with perturbations should be included. Examples of these exercises include squatting on an unstable surface while playing catch, lunging onto an unstable surface, and jumping on a mini-trampoline. Again, the clinician should perform a needs assessment of the patient's physical activities and use that information to set up exercises that mimic the patient's normal activity levels.

Agility and coordination drills should begin with simple tasks at a slow speed in a closed environment and progress to complex tasks at faster speeds in an open environment. A closed environment is one in which the patient controls the activities. Examples of a closed environment drill are four-square hops, shuttle runs, T-shuffles, and the SEMO drill. In these activities, the patient knows what to do ahead of time. For example, run to a cone then backpedal to another cone then shuffle to another. In contrast, an open environment requires the patient to react to another person. Examples of **open environment drills** are mirroring another person's movements, guarding an offensive player in a practice drill, or trying to catch a reaction ball before it bounces twice. A good transition from closed drills to the open drills is "shadow boxing." **Shadow boxing** is similar to when a child plays a sport against a pretend opponent. Examples of this type of drill are to have a soccer player dribble down the field while avoiding "pretend" opponents or having a football wide receiver run a pattern against a pretend defender. This challenges the patient to make change of direction movements on his own without a prescribed set of movements.

Goal Q: Improve Functional/Sport-Specific Skills. Many of the drills and exercises previously listed help improve functional and sports-specific skills. Because this is the final stage of the rehabilitation program, it is important that the patient have functional ROM, strength, proprioception, agility, and coordination. This is accomplished by having the patient perform

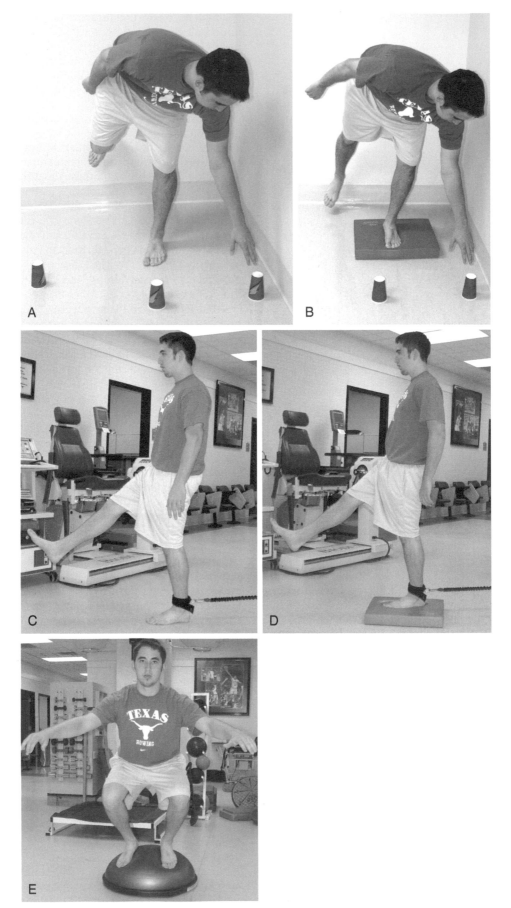

Fig. 39.16   Proprioception exercises with patient-initiated perturbations. **A,** Single-legged stance with movement. **B,** On an unstable surface. **C,** Single-legged stance with lower extremity motion. **D,** On an unstable platform. **E,** Dynamic squats on an unstable platform.

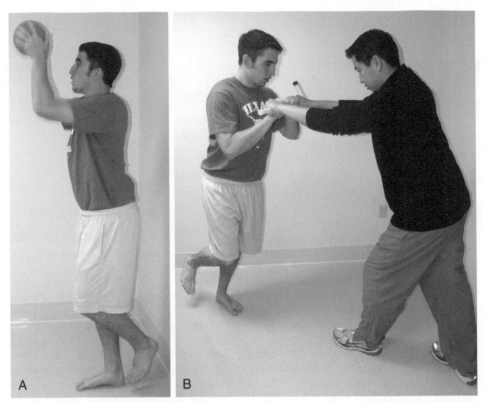

Fig. 39.17 Proprioception exercises with clinician-initiated perturbations. **A,** Single-legged stance while playing catch. **B,** "Stick fighting" drills.

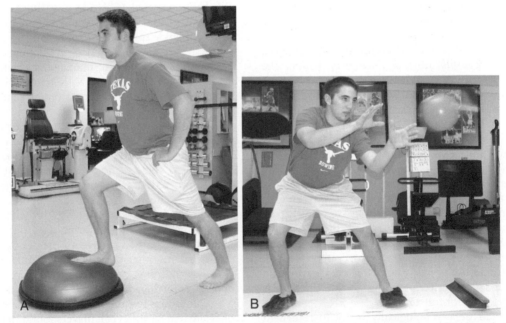

Fig. 39.18 Dynamic proprioception exercises. **A,** Lunges on an unstable surface. **B,** Lateral movements on a slide board while playing catch.

dynamic exercises or drills that are specifically related to his or her activity.

Goal R: Maintain Overall Body Conditioning. The exercises included in the subacute stage should be carried through to the maturation stage. The conditioning activities should have increased in demand and specificity as the rehabilitation program progressed. It is important that the patient have the overall conditioning that allows him or her to perform his or her activity at preinjury levels.

RETURN TO ACTIVITY CRITERIA AFTER ACUTE ANKLE SPRAIN

The goal of the rehabilitation program should be to return the patient to full activity. When making a decision regarding the patient's status and ability to return to activity, the following goals should be met.

- *The patient should be pain free* when performing his or her activity. Occasional soreness after activity is acceptable, but

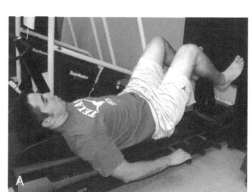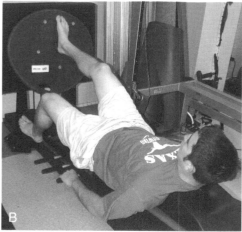

Fig. 39.19 *Closed kinetic chain exercises.* **A,** *Leg press.* **B,** *Single-leg press on an unstable platform.*

pain is not. Some patients may not be able to distinguish between the soreness that accompanies heavy exertion and pain, so a pain-scale rating system can be used. The patient rates his or her discomfort level on a scale of 0 to 10. To standardize the scale, no pain receives a score of 0, whereas a score of 10 is predetermined as the most amount of pain the patient has experienced with this ankle injury. The clinician and patient should then determine what number corresponds to the maximal discomfort level the patient can experience and still continue the activity. Clinical experience has shown a level 7 as the uppermost limit.

- *The ankle should not be swollen.* The presence of swelling indicates an inflammatory response to irritation. Continued activity on a swollen ankle can lead to chronic inflammation.
- *The ankle should have full, functional range of motion.* The key word is functional. Although the ultimate goal is to restore full ROM, there are times when a patient may not regain full ROM of the ankle. The clinician should ask himself, "Does this patient have enough ROM to safely and effectively participate in this activity?" If so, this criterion is met. If not, the patient should not be released for full activity.
- *The ankle should have full, functional muscle strength, endurance, and power.* Again, the key word is functional. The clinician should ask himself, "Does this patient have enough strength, endurance, and power to safely and effectively participate in this activity?" If so, this criterion is met. If not, the patient should not be released for full activity.
- The patient should have adequate proprioception, balance, agility, and coordination to safely and effectively participate in the activity. If so, this criterion is met. If not, the patient should not be released for full activity.
- The patient should be psychologically ready to return to activity. This is very important because many patients will undergo emotional and mental strain with an injury. The patient must have confidence that his or her ankle is able to withstand the demands of the physical activity. Educating the patient about the injury and healing process in addition to having the patient complete functional, activity-specific exercises and drills helps convince the patient that he or she is ready.

PREVENTION OF ANKLE SPRAINS

Because ankle sprains are one of the most common injuries in active individuals, it is prudent to attempt to prevent their occurrence and recurrence, especially in high-risk activities like basketball and soccer. A "prehab" program uses exercises commonly used in the rehabilitation protocol to prevent ankle sprains from occurring or recurring. Some of the more commonly used exercises include those described in the proprioception and strengthening phases in Rehabilitation Protocol 39.1. Hübscher et al. (2010) in a systematic review determined that balance training alone resulted in a significant reduction in the risk of ankle sprain, confirming the results of an earlier systematic review that found a substantially reduced risk of ankle sprains with prophylactic bracing, especially in those with a history of a previous sprain (McKeon and Hertel 2008). Special emphasis should be placed on strengthening the muscles that evert the foot.

Another common practice is the use of prophylactic ankle braces or taping techniques. Many ankle braces are on the market, ranging from slide-on neoprene sleeves to lace-up braces to semi-rigid ankle orthosis. Whereas most braces offer some form of protection, the semi-rigid type braces offer the most support. The effectiveness of bracing in preventing ankle sprain is still unclear. One recent study of prophylactic ankle bracing on the incidence of ankle injuries in a group of high school volleyball players found that overall the use of an ankle brace did not significantly alter the frequency of ankle sprains (Frey et al. 2010). In contrast, a systematic review concluded that ankle sprains were reduced by 69% with the use of ankle brace and by 71% with taping in previously injured athletes, and a study of collegiate female volleyball players found that a double-upright brace significantly reduced the rate of ankle sprain (Dizon and Reyes 2010, Pedowitz et al. 2008).

When a brace is not available or is impractical (such as in dancers), ankle taping can be used. Fig. 39.4, *A–M* demonstrates one ankle taping technique. Although the order of the specific strips can vary, the basic techniques are common with most taping protocols. One of the major drawbacks of taping is skin irritation and that the tape eventually loosens and loses its support.

REHABILITATION PROTOCOL 39.1 ■ Ankle Sprain Rehabilitation

Brian K. Farr, MA, ATC, LAT, CSCS, Donald Nguyen, PT, MSPT, ATC, LAT, Ken Stephenson, MD

Lateral Ankle Sprain

Acute Phase

Goal: Protect from further injury.
Methods:
- Rest.
- Tape (see Fig. 39.4), brace, splint, or walking boot (boot primarily for grades II–III).
- Crutches or cane as needed (primarily for grades II–III).

Goal: Encourage tissue healing
Methods:
- Rest.
- Protection (tape, brace, walking boot, etc.)
- Pulsed ultrasound (after 3 days).

Goal: Limit pain, swelling, spasm
Methods:
- Rest.
- Ice/cryotherapy.
- Compression (elastic wrap, compression stockinet, intermittent compression device).
- Electrical stimulation.
- Ankle pumps with ankle elevated.
- Grade I joint mobilizations (after 3 days) (caution with anterior mobilizations of the talus) (see Fig. 39.10).
- Manual therapy techniques to address positional fault of talus and/or fibula (see Fig. 39.5).

Goal: Maintain function of noninjured tissues
Methods:
- Pain-free passive range of motion (PROM), active-assisted range of motion (AAROM), active range of motion (AROM).
  - Ankle pumps.
  - Heel cord stretches.
  - ABCs or alphabets (can be performed in the cold whirlpool bath).
  - Towel curls (see Fig. 39.8, *A*), toe pick-ups (see Fig. 39.8, *B*).
- Partial weight bearing (PWB) or full weight bearing (FWB) as tolerated.

Goal: Maintain overall body conditioning
Methods:
- Stationary bike.
- Upper body ergometer.
- Open kinetic chain knee flexion and extension exercises.
- Open kinetic chain hip flexion, extension, abduction, adduction exercises.
- Trunk exercises.
- Upper extremity exercises (prone, supine, seated, non weight bearing (NWB), PWB).

Subacute Phase

Goal: Prevent further injury
Methods:
- Continue taping or bracing.
- Gradually progress into rehabilitation and reconditioning activities.

Goal: Promote tissue healing
Methods:
- Introduce thermotherapy (hot packs, warm whirlpool baths).
- Ultrasound (progressing to continuous cycle).
- Massage (flushing techniques in early stages, cross-friction techniques in later stages).

Goal: Minimize pain and inflammation
Methods:
- Cryotherapy (ice bags, cold whirlpool baths).
- Gradually introduce thermotherapy (hot packs, warm whirlpool baths).

- Continuous ultrasound.
- Electrical stimulation.
- Grade I to II joint mobilizations.
- Massage (flushing techniques).

Goal: Restore range of motion and flexibility
Methods:
- Progress with pain-free PROM, AAROM, AROM.
- Plantarflexion, dorsiflexion, eversion, inversion (as tolerated) (see Fig. 39.6, *A–D*).
- Ankle pumps.
- Heel cord stretches (see Fig. 39.7).
- ABCs or alphabets (can be performed in the cold whirlpool bath).
- Seated BAPS (see Fig. 39.11, *A*) or ankle disc circles (progress to PWB [see Fig. 39.1, *B1*]) and FWB [see Fig. 39.11, *C*] as tolerated).
- Joint mobilizations (progressing to grade II–III as needed) (see Fig. 39.12, *A–D*).
- Soft tissue techniques (massage, myofascial release, etc.)

Goal: Re-establish neuromuscular control and restore muscular strength and endurance
Methods:
- Towel curls.
- Marble pick-ups.
- Isometric strengthening exercises.
- Progressing to isotonic strengthening exercises.
  - Manual resistance (see Fig. 39.13, *A*), cuff weights (see Fig. 39.13, *B*), elastic bands (see Fig. 39.13, *C*), etc.
- PNF patterns.
- Progressing to PWB the FWB strengthening exercises (heel raises [see Fig. 39.14, *A*], toe raises [see Fig. 39.14, *B*], squats, lunges).

Goal: Re-establish proprioception, agility, and coordination
Methods:
- Joint repositioning (early stages).
- Progress to PWB and FWB activities as tolerated.
  - Weight shifts (forward, backward, laterally).
  - Box step-ups and step-downs (see Fig. 39.15, *A* and *B*).
  - Progress from double-legged stance to tandem stance to single legged.
  - Progress from static stances to dynamic activities (see Fig. 39.16, *A–E*, Fig. 39.17, *A* and *B*).
  - Progress from eyes open to eyes closed.
  - Progress to activities with perturbations.
  - Progress from a stable surface to an unstable surface.
  - Walking, walking backward, front lunges, backward lunges, side lunges.
  - Slide board (see Fig. 39.18, *B*), Fitter machine, BAPS board, wobble board, ankle disc, etc.
- Gradually introduce functional activities in later weeks.
  - Walking, jogging, skipping, hopping.

Goal: Maintain overall body conditioning
Methods:
- Upper body and trunk conditioning.
- Stationary biking.
- CKC exercises (squats, lunges, leg press, calf press) (Fig. 39.19, *A* and *B*).
- Swimming.
- Unloaded jogging (pool running, ZUNI unloader, antigravity treadmill).
- Progress to FWB activities (walking, stair climbing, jogging).

REHABILITATION PROTOCOL 39.1   ● Ankle Sprain Rehabilitation—cont'd

Brian K. Farr, MA, ATC, LAT, CSCS, Donald Nguyen, PT, MSPT, ATC, LAT, Ken Stephenson, MD

Maturation Phase

Goal: Prevent reinjury
Methods:
- Continue taping or bracing.

Goal: Restore ROM and flexibility
Methods:
- More aggressive stretching.
  - Low-load, long-duration static stretching.
  - Dynamic stretching activities.
- Joint mobilizations (grade III–IV as needed).
  - Talus.
  - Fibula.

Goal: Improve muscular strength, endurance, and power
Methods:
- Continue exercises from subacute stage emphasizing isotonics, proprioceptive neuromuscular facilitation (PNF), closed kinetic chain (CKC) exercises.
- Plyometrics.
- Functional exercises (jumping, running, changes of direction).

Goal: Improve proprioception, agility, and coordination
Methods:
- Emphasize advanced, dynamic exercises.
  - Stances with perturbations (i.e., playing catch).

- Single-legged stances.
- Lunges/squats on an unstable surface (Fig. 39.18, *A*).
- Exercises with eyes closed.
- Jumping rope.
- Four-square hops/side-to-side hops (Fig. 39.20).
- Shuttle runs.
- SEMO drill.
- "Shadow boxing".

Goal: Restore functional/sports-specific skills
Methods:
- Four-square hops.
- Shuttle runs.
- SEMO drill.
- "Shadow boxing".
- Forward running, backward running, lateral shuffles, carioca, figure-eight running, cutting, hopping, skipping.
- Return to sport/activity drills.

Goal: Maintain overall body conditioning
Methods:
- Upper body and trunk conditioning.
- Stationary biking.
- CKC exercises (squats, lunges, leg press, calf press).
- Walking, jogging, running, stair climbing, swimming.

Check online Videos: Hold Patterns Injured Limb On Tilt Board (Video 39.1) and Hold Patterns Uninjured Limb On Tilt Board (Video 39.2).

REFERENCES

A complete reference list is available at https://expertconsult.inkling.com/.

FURTHER READING

Ferran NA, Olivia F, Maffulli N. Ankle instability. *Sports Med Arthrosc.* 2009;17(2):139–145.

Fong DTP, Hong Y, Chan LK. A systematic review on ankle injury and ankle sprain in sports. *Sports Med.* 2007;37(1):73–94.

Kerkhoffs GM, Rowe BH, Assendelft WJ. Immobilisation for acute ankle sprain: a systematic review. *Arch Orthop Trauma Surg.* 2001;121(8):462–471.

Osborne MD, Rizzo TD. Prevention and treatment of ankle sprain in athletes. *Sports Med.* 2003;33(15):1145–1150.

Peterson W, Rembitzki IV, Koppenburg AG, et al. Treatment of acute ankle ligament injuries: a systematic review. *Arch Orthop Trauma Surg.* 2013;133:1129–1141.

Wikstrom EA, Hubbard-Turner T, McKeon PO. Understanding and treating lateral ankle sprains and their consequences. *Sports Med.* 2013;43:385–393.

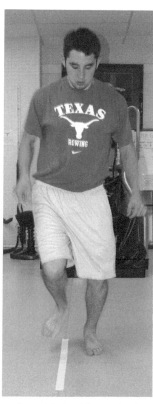

Fig. 39.20   Hopping from side to side emphasizes functional strength and power.

40

Ankle-Specific Perturbation Training

Michael Duke, PT, CSCS | S. Brent Brotzman, MD

Perturbation training has been studied and used successfully in the treatment of anterior cruciate ligament (ACL) injuries of the knee. Perturbation training involves applying destabilizing forces to the involved knee to enhance neuromuscular awareness, neuromuscular response, and dynamic stability of the knee to stabilize the knee joint. The goal of perturbation training is to educate the patient to elicit selective adaptive muscle reactions of the periarticular knee musculature in response to force administered on the platform to gain knee protective neuromuscular response (see Chapter 4).

Given the decrease in proprioception following injury to ankle ligaments, it follows that a similar system of perturbations, designed specifically for the ankle, will be equally beneficial for the patient recovering from lateral ankle sprains, especially chronic repeated ankle sprains. Those perturbation exercises described in relation to ACL rehabilitation are valid and effective ways to improve proprioception of the entire lower extremity. The addition of the following exercises will further improve stability of the ankle.

Seated tilt board perturbations (Fig. 40.1) can be implemented early in the rehabilitation process with good patient tolerance. The patient is seated in a chair, with knee bent to 90 degrees and foot on the tilt board. The therapist applies a force to the tilt board that would elicit rocking of the board, but the patient is instructed to not allow the board to move. The therapist can apply rhythmic, alternating forces; increase speed and intensity; and vary the angle of tilt. The patient can be instructed to look at the board (easier) or to look away (more difficult). Use of a BAPS board or wobble board can further increase the difficulty of the exercise. Once the patient can easily perform these challenges, the patient can then be placed in a standing position,

involved limb on the tilt board, and uninvolved limb on a block of similar height.

Standing BOSU and platform perturbations (Fig. 40.2) are performed with the involved limb on the BOSU platform, flat side up, and the uninvolved limb on a stationary platform of similar height. It is important that the patient be instructed to bear weight greater than 75% on the uninvolved limb to allow some movement of the BOSU. The patient is also instructed to not allow movement of the BOSU while the therapist applies force in varying directions, intensities, rhythms, and hold times, challenging the patient's ability to maintain stability of the ankle with these external forces. Instruct the patient to look away, toss a ball, or juggle to add difficulty to the exercise.

Other versions of ankle perturbation exercises are possible. The challenge to the therapist is to create activities that will enhance neuromuscular control and proprioception in a way that will improve functional outcomes for the patients.

CHRONIC SYMPTOMS AFTER A "SIMPLE" ANKLE SPRAIN

If chronic symptoms persist after an ankle sprain, further workup should be performed. A myriad of associated injuries may account for ongoing symptoms (Table 40.1). Of note, Gerber et al. found that the factor most predictive of residual symptoms after a lateral ankle sprain is presence of a syndesmosis sprain (Gerber et al. 1998). Therefore, in patients with ongoing ankle pain after lateral sprain, make sure there is not concomitant missed syndesmotic injury.

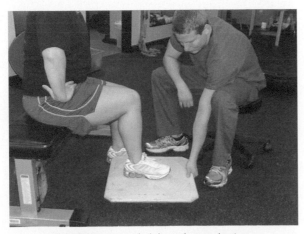

Fig. 40.1 Seated tilt board perturbations.

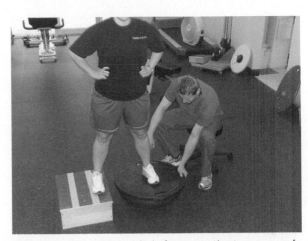

Fig. 40.2 Standing BOSU and platform perturbations are performed with the involved limb on the BOSU platform, flat side up, and the uninvolved limb on a stationary platform of similar height.

TABLE 40.1	Possible Etiologies of Recalcitrant (Chronic) Ankle Pain

Chronic ankle ligament instability (instability with minor provocation, such as stepping off a curb)
Reflex sympathetic dystrophy syndrome (RSDS)
Undetected syndesmotic sprain or diastasis
Undetected tear of the deltoid ligament (medially)
Stress fracture
Posterior tibial tendon (PTT) injury (medially)
Osteochondral fracture (very common) or osteochondritis dissecans (OCD) of the talus or tibial plafond
Os trigonum fracture (posterior pain, clicking, positive x-ray)
Subtalar joint sprain or instability
Tibiotalar synostosis (ossification of the syndesmosis impairing normal tibiofibular motion with restricted dorsiflexion on examination)
Midfoot sprain of the transverse tarsal (midtarsal), intertarsal, or tarsometatarsal joints
Bony impingement from osteophytes off the anterior tibia, with soft tissues trapped between the spur and the talus during dorsiflexion
Ankle arthritis
Undetected fractures
- Lateral, medial, or posterior malleolus
- Posterior or lateral process of the talus
- Anterior process of the calcaneus
- Fifth metatarsal
- Navicular or other midtarsal bone

Nerve injuries
- Superficial peroneal nerve stretch after ankle sprain
- Common peroneal nerve entrapment
- Tarsal tunnel syndrome (entrapment of the posterior tibia nerve)

Tumor

 Check online videos: Bosu Squats (Video 40.1) and Seated With Perturbations (Video 40.2).

REFERENCES

A complete reference list is available at https://expertconsult .inkling.com/.

FURTHER READING

Pfusterschmied J, Stöggl T, Buchecker M, et al. Effects of 4-week slackline training on lower limb joint motion and muscle activation. *J Sci Med Sport.* 2013;16(6):562–566.

Han K, Ricard MD, Fellingham GW. Effects of a 4-week exercise program on balance using elastic tubing as a perturbation force for individuals with a history of ankle sprains. *J Orthop Sports Phys Ther.* 2009;39(4):246–255.

Holmes A, Delahunt E. Treatment of common deficits associated with chronic ankle instability. *Sports Med.* 2009;39(3):207–224.

41

Chronic Ankle Instability

S. Brent Brotzman, MD | John J. Jasko, MD

Peters et al. found chronic lateral instability occurs in 10% to 30% of individuals after an acute lateral ankle sprain (Peters et al. 1991).

Persistent pain, recurrent sprains, and repeated episodes of the ankle giving way are typical symptoms of chronic instability. Chronic ankle instability can not only limit activity but also may lead to an increased risk of articular cartilage degeneration and subsequent ankle osteoarthritis.

Both mechanical and functional factors related to the initial injury have been cited as contributing to chronic ankle instability (Maffulli and Ferran 2008).

Mechanical factors include the following:
- Pathologic laxity
- Arthrokinetic restriction
- Synovial changes
- Degenerative changes

Functional factors include the following:
- Impaired proprioception/joint position sense
- Impaired neuromuscular control
- Impaired postural control
- Strength deficits

Identifying and appropriately treating chronic ankle instability are important to slow or prevent the progression of degenerative arthritis of the ankle joint. Sugimoto et al. (2009) found on ankle arthroscopy of patients with chronic ankle instability 77% of patients had chondral lesions of some degree. The duration of instability was not a factor affecting severity of chondral lesions found. The risk factors for increased severity of chondral lesions were increased age, a larger talar tilt, and varus inclination of the tibial plafond.

DIAGNOSIS

Evaluation of a patient with chronic ankle instability begins with a careful patient history to assess the presenting complaint, mechanism of injury, level of activity, and severity of disability. Clinical examination may reveal only minimal ecchymosis and swelling along the joint line. Testing for ligament laxity is easier in patients with chronic instability than in patients with acute injuries because the limb is less painful. Plain radiographs and magnetic resonance imaging (MRI) are helpful to rule out other possible causes of ankle pain and instability, such as fracture, impingement, osteochondral lesions, or peroneal tendon injury.

The usefulness of stress radiographs is controversial, with most recent studies indicating that they are of questionable value. Because of the high variability of normal ankle laxity, comparison views of the uninjured side are usually needed. Although the figures used by clinicians vary, generally 3 to 5 degrees more laxity than the uninjured side or an absolute value of 10 degrees is considered a positive finding.

An important part of the evaluation of patients with chronic ankle instability is identification of associated pathology.

Several studies have indicated that more than half of those with chronic ankle instability have associated extra-articular conditions or injuries, including articular cartilage damage, peroneal tendon injuries, impingement lesions, and associated tarsal conditions.

TREATMENT

Generally, conservative treatment is used first to treat proprioceptive deficits and any static disorders. Balance deficits have been identified in most patients with chronic ankle instability (Wikstrom et al. 2010).

A systematic analysis found that **functional rehabilitation** interventions were associated with improved ankle stability for both postural control and self-reported function in patients with chronic ankle instability (Webster and Gribble 2010), whereas a randomized controlled trial found that 4 weeks of balance training significantly improved self-reported function, static postural control, and dynamic postural control (McKeon et al. 2009).

In another group of patients with a history of ankle sprains, balance was improved after 4 weeks of elastic resistance exercise (Han and Ricard 2009).

Patients with primarily functional instability are more likely to benefit from rehabilitation than patients with primarily mechanical instability (Ajis and Maffulli 2006).

Taping and Bracing for Chronic Ankle Instability

The efficacy of bracing and taping remains undetermined, with some studies reporting no benefits and others reporting some stabilizing effects (Gribble et al. 2010, Delahunt et al. 2009).

Surgical Reconstruction for Chronic Ankle Instability

If nonsurgical management fails to alleviate symptoms, surgery is indicated. Although numerous procedures have been described for management of chronic ankle instability, they all are of two basic types: **anatomic repair (or reconstruction)** and **tenodesis stabilization (nonanatomic repair).** Anatomic repair aims to restore normal anatomy and joint mechanics and maintain ankle and subtalar motion. Waldrop showed that either bone tunnels or suture anchors can be used with equivalent initial strength and functional outcomes (Waldrop et al. 2012).

If the lateral ligaments are too badly damaged or attenuated, tenodesis stabilization historically was used. Local tendon grafts, most often a portion of the peroneal tendons, were used to restrict motion without repair of the injured ligaments. However, these tenodesing procedures were nonanatomic and

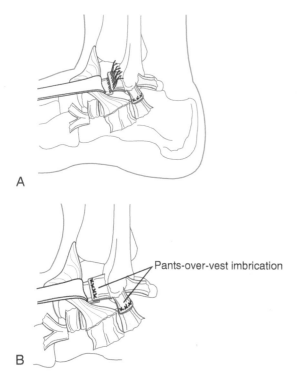

A

B

Fig. 41.1 Imbrication of the lateral ankle ligaments (Broström procedure). A, Pants over vest technique tightening ligaments. B, Completed repair.

Pants-over-vest imbrication

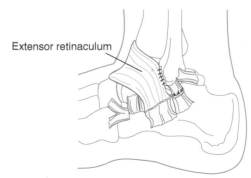

Fig. 41.2 Augmentation of the Broström repair with extensor retinaculum (Gould modification).

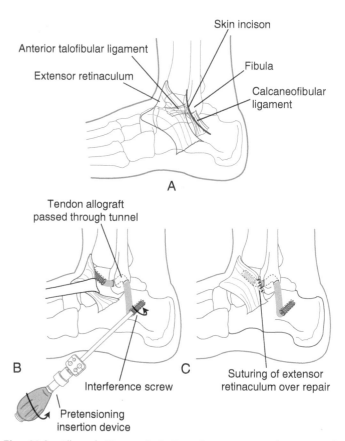

Skin incison

Anterior talofibular ligament

Extensor retinaculum

Fibula

Calcaneofibular ligament

A

Tendon allograft passed through tunnel

B

Interference screw

Pretensioning insertion device

C

Suturing of extensor retinaculum over repair

Fig. 41.3 Allograft Biotenodesis Broström-type procedure using allograft anterior tibial tendon or hamstring. A, Skin incision. B, Reconstruction using tendon graft with tenodesis interference screw to hold in place. C, Reinforcement of repair using extensor retinaculum.

disturbed ankle and hindfoot biomechanics (e.g., restricted hindfoot motion) in patients with poor remaining ligamentous tissue. A better surgical option when anatomic repair is impossible is anatomic reconstruction with fibular periosteal turn-down flaps; autogenous plantaris, gracilis, semitendinosus grafts; or allografts. We typically use allograft or autograft hamstring or tendon routed through the original origin and insertion sites of the anterior talofibular ligament (ATF) and calcaneofibular (CF) using the Biotenodesis system from Arthrex (Naples, FL, 2003). This allows an anatomic reconstruction with good isometry and no tenodesing effect. This can be augmented by a fibular periosteal flap turn-down or extensor retinaculum.

Common Surgical Techniques for Management of Chronic Lateral Ankle Instability

Anatomic repair may involve the following:

- Imbrication of the lateral ankle ligaments (Broström procedure) (Fig. 41.1)
- Augmentation of the Broström repair with extensor retinaculum (Gould modification) (Fig. 41.2)
- Allograft Biotenodesis (Arthrex, Naples, FL) Broström-type procedure using allograft anterior tibial tendon or hamstring if poor local tissue (Fig. 41.3)
- Periosteal turn-down flap off of fibula periosteum to augment the previous Broström ligament reconstruction

In general, anatomic repair techniques have produced better results than tenodesis techniques (e.g., Watson-Jones or Chrisman Snook). One comparative study reported 80% good to excellent results with anatomic reconstruction and 33% good or excellent results with the Evans procedure (Krips et al. 2002).

Arthroscopy is often performed to identify and treat intraarticular conditions such as osteochondral talar lesions, impingement, loose bodies, painful ossicles, adhesions, and osteophytes. Arthroscopic techniques have been developed for ligament repair and reconstruction (Lui 2007).

Regardless of the surgical technique, early mobilization and functional rehabilitation have been shown to produce better results than 4 to 6 weeks of immobilization (de Vries et al. 2009).

Aggressive protocols have been shown to be safe and have greatly reduced the time to return to sport (Miyamoto et al. 2104).

Rehabilitation Protocol 41.1 shows a postoperative Broström ligament rehabilitation protocol.

Extensor retinaculum

REHABILITATION PROTOCOL 41.1 ● After Modified Broström Ankle Ligament Reconstruction

Modified Hamilton Protocol

Days 0–4

- Place ankle in neutral dorsiflexion in removable walking boot and discharge patient as weight bearing as tolerated (WBAT) in boot with crutches.
- Maximally elevate and cryotherapy
- Wean crutches at 7 to 10 days to walking boot only WBAT.

Days 4–7

- Progress WBAT in removable walking boot and wean crutches at day 7 to 10.

Week 4

- Remove walking boot at 4 to 6 weeks.
- Apply air splint for protection, to be worn for 6 to 8 weeks after surgery.
- Begin gentle range of motion (ROM) exercises of the ankle.
- Begin isometric peroneal strengthening exercises.
- Avoid adduction and inversion of ankle until 6 weeks postoperative.
- Begin stationary cycling and light swimming.

Week 6

- Begin proprioception/balancing activities.
- Unilateral balancing for timed intervals
- Unilateral balancing with visual cues
- Balancing on one leg and catching #2 plyoball
- Slide board, increasing distance
- Fitter activity, catching ball
- Side-to-side bilateral hopping (progress to unilateral)
- Front-to-back bilateral hopping (progress to unilateral)
- Diagonal patterns, hopping
- Mini-tramp jogging
- Shuttle leg press and rebounding, bilateral and unilateral
- Positive deceleration, ankle everters, Kin-Com
- Complete rehabilitation of the peroneals is essential.
- Dancers should perform peroneal exercises in full plantarflexion, the position of function in these athletes.
- Early in rehabilitation, deweighted pool exercises may be beneficial.
- Dancers should perform plantarflexion/eversion exercises with a weighted belt (2–20 pounds).

Weeks 8–12

- Patient can return to dancing or sport if peroneal strength is normal and symmetric with uninvolved limb.

REFERENCES

A complete reference list is available at https://expertconsult.inkling.com/.

FURTHER READING

Hale SA, Hertel J, Olmsted-Kramer LC. The effect of a 4-week comprehensive rehabilitation program on postural control and lower extremity function in individuals with chronic ankle instability. *J Orthop Sports Phys Ther.* 2007;37:303–311.

Hamilton WG, Thompson FM, Snow SW. The modified Broström procedure for lateral instability. *Foot Ankle.* 1993;1:1.

McKeon PO, Paolini G, Ingersoll CD. Effects of balance training on gait parameters in patients with chronic ankle instability: a randomized controlled trial. *Clin Rehabil.* 2009;23:609–621.

Miyamoto W, Takao M, Yamada K, et al. Accelerated versus traditional rehabilitation after anterior talofibular ligament reconstruction for chronic lateral instability of the ankle in athletes. *Am J Sports Med.* 2014;42(6):1441–1447.

42

Syndesmotic Injuries

S. Brent Brotzman, MD | John J. Jasko, MD

Although they occur much less frequently than lateral ankle sprains, syndesmosis sprains often result in prolonged disability and lengthy recovery time. Reports from the literature indicate that between 2% and 20% of all ankle sprains involve injury to the syndesmosis. However, syndesmosis sprains are more common than lateral ankle sprains in collision sports, such as football, rugby, wrestling, and lacrosse, and in sports that involve rigid immobilization of the ankle in a boot, such as skiing and hockey (Williams et al. 2007). Some have reported that recovery from a syndesmosis injury requires almost twice the recovery time of that required for grade III lateral ankle sprains (Hopkinson et al. 1990, Taylor et al. 2007).

The most common mechanism of injury for syndesmosis sprains is external rotation of the foot relative to the tibia (Fig. 42.1). Other suggested mechanisms are eversion of the talus within the ankle mortise and excessive dorsiflexion. Syndesmosis injury may occur as a purely soft tissue injury or in association with an ankle fracture. The majority of injuries to the ankle syndesmosis occur in association with an ankle fracture. However, the purpose of this chapter is to discuss purely ligamentous syndesmosis injuries.

DIAGNOSIS

Patients with syndesmosis injuries usually complain of pain anteriorly between the distal tibia and fibular and posteromedially at the level of the ankle joint. The pain is worse when bearing weight or pushing off the ground. Physical examination begins with palpation of the limb to identify areas of tenderness. The distance the tenderness extends proximal from the distal tip of the fibula has been termed the **tenderness length** and has been shown to correlate with the severity of the injury and the time to return to sports (Nussbaum et al. 2001). Tests used for the evaluation of syndesmosis injuries include the **squeeze test, external rotation test, fibula translation test, Cotton test,** and **crossed leg test.** The squeeze test and external rotation test are useful for diagnosis of purely ligamentous injuries.

- *Squeeze test* (Fig. 42.2): Compression of the fibula to the tibia above the midpoint of the calf causes separation of the two bones distally; the test is positive if it causes pain at the area of the syndesmosis.
- *External rotation test* (Fig. 42.3): External rotation of the foot while the leg is stabilized with the knee flexed 90 degrees; the test is positive if pain is elicited over the syndesmosis.
- *Tape stabilization test:* Tightly circumferentially taping the patient's leg just above the ankle joint to stabilize syndesmosis; test is positive if toe raises; hopping and walking are less painful (Hurt 2015).
- *Crossed-leg test* (Fig. 42.4): Similar to the squeeze test, but it is self-administered. Patient sits with midtibia of affected leg resting on opposite knee and applies a gentle downward force on the medial side of the knee; the test is positive if pain is elicited in the syndesmosis area (Kiter and Bozkurt 2005).

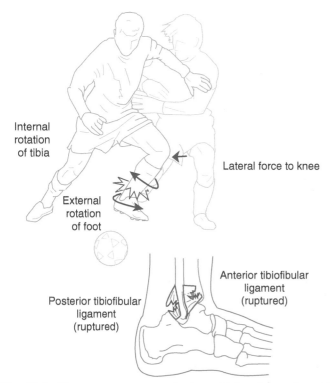

Internal rotation of tibia

Lateral force to knee

External rotation of foot

Posterior tibiofibular ligament (ruptured)

Anterior tibiofibular ligament (ruptured)

Fig. 42.1 The most common mechanism of injury for syndesmosis sprains is external rotation of the foot relative to the tibia.

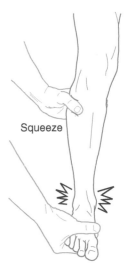

Squeeze

Fig. 42.2 Squeeze test.

- *Fibula translation (drawer) test:* Translation of the fibula from anterior to posterior; increased translation compared to the opposite side and pain with the maneuver indicate a positive test result.
- *Cotton test* (Fig. 42.5): Translation of the talus within the mortise from medial to lateral; increased translation compared to the opposite side and pain with the maneuver indicate syndesmosis injury and a deltoid ligament injury.

Routine radiographs (anteroposterior [AP], mortise, lateral) are indicated to rule out fracture of the ankle or proximal fibula and to identify disruption of the normal relationship between the distal tibia and distal fibula. Three radiographic findings are considered indications of syndesmotic injury.

- *Increased tibiofibular clear space.* The tibiofibular clear space is the distance between the medial border of the fibula and the lateral border of the posterior tibia; it is measured 1 cm proximal to the tibial plafond and should be less then 6 mm in both the AP and mortise views (Zalavras and Thordarson 2007). This is considered the most reliable indicator of syndesmosis injury (Pneumaticos et al. 2002).
- *Decreased tibiofibular overlap.* Tibiofibular overlap is the overlap of the lateral malleolus and the anterior tibial tubercle measured 1 cm proximal to the plafond. The overlap should be more than 6 mm on the AP view and more than 1 mm on the mortise view (Zalavras and Thordarson 2007).
- *Increased medial clear space.* The medial clear space is the distance between the lateral border of the medial malleolus and the medial border of the talus, measured at the level of the talar dome. On the mortise view with the ankle in neutral position, the medial clear space should be equal to or less than the superior clear space between the talar dome and the tibial plafond (Beumer et al. 2004) (see Fig. 39.1).

Other imaging methods that are useful in the diagnosis of syndesmosis injuries are stress (external rotation) radiographs, computed tomography (CT), and MRI.

CLASSIFICATION OF SYNDESMOTIC INJURY

Syndesmotic injury is typically classified based on the extent of tearing of the syndesmotic ligaments.

TREATMENT

The initial treatment of grades I and II syndesmosis sprains usually is nonoperative, consisting of a three-phase rehabilitation program individualized to each patient (Rehabilitation Protocol 42.1).

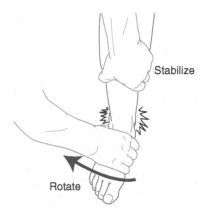

Fig. 42.3 External rotation test.

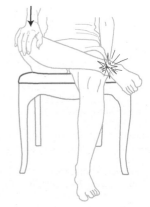

Fig. 42.4 Crossed-leg test. Patient sits with midtibia of affected leg resting on opposite knee and applies a gentle downward force on the medial side of the knee; test is positive if pain is elicited in the syndesmosis area.

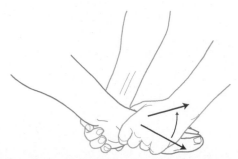

Fig. 42.5 Cotton test. Translation of the talus within the mortise from medial to lateral; increased translation compared to the opposite side and pain with the maneuver indicate syndesmosis injury and a deltoid ligament injury.

TABLE 42.1	Classification of Syndesmotic Injury		
Grade	Syndesmosis Injury	History	Examination
I	Stretch	ER injury Subacute pain and swelling Continued athletic activity	Mild swelling Mild AITFL tenderness Stable ankle ± squeeze test ± ER test
II	Partial tear	ER injury Acute pain and swelling Inability to continue athletic activity Painful gait	Moderate swelling Moderate AITFL tenderness ± squeeze test ± ER test
III	Complete tear	ER injury with associated "pop" Acute severe pain and swelling Inability to walk	Severe swelling Severe AITFL tenderness ± squeeze test ± ER test

AITFL, anterior–inferior tibiofibular ligament; ER, external rotation.

A return to play in as few as 14 days has been reported with limited immobilization followed by an aggressive rehabilitation program (Nussbaum et al. 2001). Immediate nonweight bearing with crutches or a walker is necessary to prevent further talar and fibular rotation and further disruption of the soft tissues of the syndesmosis.

Grade II sprains that fail early nonoperative treatment are candidates for surgical intervention with arthroscopy and syndesmotic fixation. The patient can undergo accelerated rehabilitation and may return to sport in 5–6 weeks. Grade III sprains with frank diastasis all need open reduction and syndesmotic fixation. Return to sport is usually 10–12 weeks, similar to ORIF of ankle fracture with syndesmotic fixation.

REHABILITATION PROTOCOL 42.1 ■ **Conservative Treatment for Syndesmosis Injury (Lin et al. 2006)**

Phase I

- Pain and swelling control: rest, ice, compression, elevation (RICE), electrical stimulation, toe curls, ankle pumps, cryotherapy
- Temporary stabilization (short leg cast, splint, brace, heel lift)
- Nonweight bearing with crutches

Criteria for Progression

- Pain and swelling subside
- Partial weight bearing possible with assistive device

Phase II

- Ambulation, partial weight bearing without pain
- Low-level balance training: bilateral standing activity; standing on balance pad or several layers of towels
- Lower-level strengthening with Theraband

Criteria for Progression

- Full ambulation with weight bearing without pain, possibly with ankle brace or heel lift

Phase III

- Unilateral balance training
- Progress from double-heel raises to single-heel raises
- Treadmill walking or overground walking
- Progression to fast walking

Criteria for Progression

- Able to perform heel raises in unilateral stance

Phase IV

- Fast pain-free walking without pain
- Jog-to-run progression
- Shuttle run and cutting maneuvers
- Sport-specific training

REFERENCES

A complete reference list is available at https://expertconsult .inkling.com/.

FURTHER READING

Amendola A, Williams G, Foster D. Evidence-based approach to treatment of acute traumatic syndesmosis (high ankle) sprains. *Sports Med Arthrosc.* 2006;14:232–236.

Beumer A. Chronic instability of the anterior syndesmosis of the ankle. *Acta Orthop Suppl.* 2007;78(327):4–36.

Clanton TO, Paul P. Syndesmosis injuries in athletes. *Foot Ankle Clin.* 2002;7:529–549.

Dattani R, Patnaik S, Kantak A, et al. Injuries to the tibiofibular syndesmosis. *J Bone Joint Surg Br.* 2008;90:405–410.

Espinosa N, Smerek JP, Myerson MS. Acute and chronic syndesmosis injuries: pathomechanisms, diagnosis and management. *Foot Ankle Clin.* 2006;11:639–657.

Hunt KJ, Phisitkul P, Pirolo J, et al. High ankle sprains and syndesmotic injuries in athletes. *J Am Acad Orthop Surg.* 2015;23(11):661–673.

Norkus SA, Floyd RT. The anatomy and mechanisms of syndesmotic ankle sprains. *J Athl Train.* 2001;36:68–73.

Rammelt S, Zwipp H, Grass R. Injuries to the distal tibiofibular syndesmosis: an evidence-based approach to acute and chronic lesions. *Foot Ankle Clin.* 2008;13:611–633.

Sikka RS, Fetzer GB, Sugarman E. Correlating MRI findings with disability in syndesmotic sprains of NFL players. *Foot Ankle Int.* 2012;33(5):371–378.

Inferior Heel Pain (Plantar Fasciitis)

S. Brent Brotzman, MD | John J. Jasko, MD

CLINICAL BACKGROUND

Plantar fasciitis is among the most common foot disorders treated by health care providers. In a survey of 500 physical therapists (Reischl 2001), all 117 who responded listed plantar fasciitis as the most common foot condition seen in their clinic. A retrospective case control study of 2002 individuals with running-related injuries (Tauton et al. 2002) found plantar fasciitis to be the most commonly reported foot condition, accounting for 8% of all injuries.

Demographic surveys indicate 2 million patients receive treatment in the United States annually, comprising 1% of visits to orthopedists. The peak population is between 40 to 60 years old.

Heel pain is best classified by anatomic location (Table 43.1). This section discusses **plantar fasciitis** (inferior heel pain). Posterior heel pain is discussed in the section on Achilles tendinitis.

ANATOMY AND PATHOMECHANICS

The plantar fascia is a dense, fibrous connective tissue structure originating from the medial tuberosity of the calcaneus (Fig. 43.1). Of its three portions—medial, lateral, and central bands—the largest is the central portion. The central portion of the fascia originates from the medial process of the calcaneal tuberosity superficial to the origin of the flexor digitorum brevis, quadratus plantae, and abductor hallucis muscle. The fascia extends through the medial longitudinal arch into individual bundles and inserts into each proximal phalanx.

The medial calcaneal nerve supplies sensation to the medial heel. The nerve to the abductor digiti minimi may rarely be compressed by the intrinsic muscles of the foot. Some studies, such as that by Baxter and Thigpen (1984), suggest that nerve entrapment (abductor digiti quinti) does on rare occasions play a role in inferior heel pain (Fig. 43.2).

The plantar fascia is an important static support for the longitudinal arch of the foot. Strain on the longitudinal arch exerts its maximal pull on the plantar fascia, especially its origin on the medial process of the calcaneal tuberosity. The plantar fascia elongates with increased loads to act as a shock absorber, but its ability to elongate is limited (especially with decreasing elasticity common with age). Passive extension of the MTP joints pulls the plantar fascia distally and also increases the height of the arch of the foot.

MYTH OF THE HEEL SPUR

The bony spur at the bottom of the heel does not cause the pain of plantar fasciitis. Rather, this is caused by the inflammation and microtears of the plantar fascia. The spur is actually the origin of the short flexors of the toes. Despite this, the misnomer persists in the lay public and the literature.

Heel spurs have been found in approximately 50% of patients with plantar fasciitis. This exceeds the 15% prevalence of radiographically visualized spurs in normal asymptomatic patients noted by Tanz (1963). However, spur formation is related to progression of age. The symptomatic loss of elasticity of the plantar fascia with the onset of middle age suggests that this subset of patients would be expected to show an increased incidence of spurs noted on radiographs.

TABLE 43.1	Differential Diagnosis of Heel Pain by Location

PLANTAR (INFERIOR) SIGNS AND SYMPTOMS
Plantar fasciitis/plantar fascia rupture/partial plantar fascia rupture
Calcaneal spur or heel spur (misnomer)
Fat pad syndrome
Calcaneal periostitis
Compression of the nerve to the abductor digiti quinti (rare)
Calcaneal apophysitis (skeletally immature patients), called Sever's disease

MEDIAL
Posterior tibial tendon disorders (insufficiency, tenosynovitis, or rupture)
Tarsal tunnel syndrome
Jogger's foot (medial plantar neuropraxia)
Medial calcaneal neuritis (very rare)

LATERAL
Peroneal tendon disorders (tendinitis, rupture)
Lateral calcaneal nerve neuritis
Posterior
Retrocalcaneal bursitis
Haglund's deformity (pump bump)
Calcaneal exostosis
Tendinoachilles tendinitis/tendinosis/partial rupture/complete rupture
Diffuse
Calcaneal stress fracture
Calcaneal fracture
Other
Systemic disorders (often bilateral heel pain present)
Reiter's syndrome
Ankylosing spondylitis
Lupus
Gouty arthropathy
Pseudogout (chondrocalcinosis)
Rheumatoid arthritis
Systemic lupus erythematosus

Modified from Doxey GE. Calcaneal pain: a review of various disorders. J Orthop Sports Phys Ther 9:925,1987.

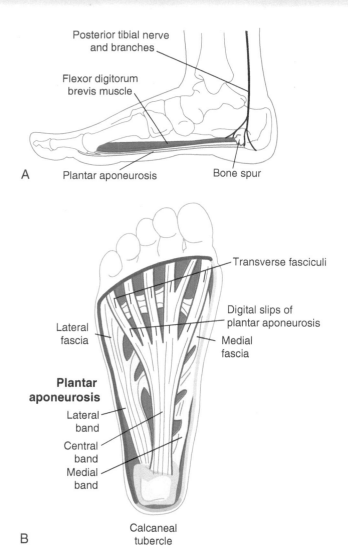

Fig. 43.1 From its origin at the calcaneal tubercle, the plantar fascia extends distally and attaches to the MTP joints and base of the toes. It is functionally divided into contiguous medial, central, and lateral bands. The fascia covers the intrinsic musculature and neurovascular anatomy of the plantar foot. A, Extent of plantar fascia from MTP joints to calcaneal tubercle. B, Medial, central and lateral bands of plantar fascia.

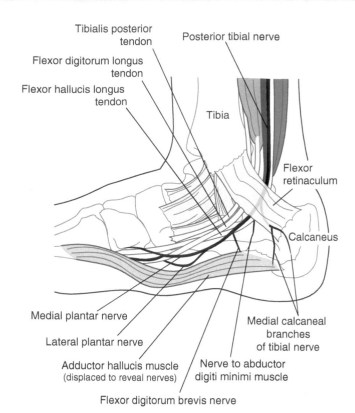

Fig. 43.2 Site of entrapment of the posterior tibial nerve and its branches. Note the nerve to the abductor digiti minimi, which on rare occasions may be entrapped with resultant inferior heel burning, neurogenic pain. (From Baxter DE, Thigpen CM. Heel pain: operative results. *Foot Ankle Int* 5:16, 1984.)

ETIOLOGY

Inferior (subcalcaneal) pain may represent a spectrum of pathologic entities including plantar fasciitis, nerve entrapment of the abductor digiti quinti nerve, periostitis, and subcalcaneal bursitis (Table 43.2).

Plantar fasciitis is more common in sports that involve running and long-distance walking and is also frequent in dancers, tennis players, basketball players, and nonathletes whose occupations require prolonged weight bearing. Direct repetitive microtrauma with heel strike to the ligamentous and nerve structures has been implicated, especially in middle-aged, overweight, nonathletic individuals who stand on hard, unyielding surfaces and in long-distance runners. The heel fat pad of the calcaneus is a honeycomb pattern of fibroelastic septa that enclose fat globules. The heel absorbs 110% of body weight at heel strike, up to 200% with running. After age 40 the fat begins to atrophy, with loss of water collagen and elastic tissue and resultant loss of shock absorption in the heel. This is a potential contributor to some sources of inferior heel pain.

Scher et al. (2009), in a study of military personnel, identified female sex, African American race, and increasing age as risk factors. Other cited risk factors for plantar fasciitis include overuse secondary to work-related prolonged weight bearing, unaccustomed running or walking, inappropriate shoe wear, and limited ankle dorsiflexion. In a case-control study, Riddle et al. (2003) determined that the risk of plantar fasciitis increased as the range of ankle dorsiflexion decreased; among independent risk factors identified, reduced ankle dorsiflexion was more important than obesity and work-related weight bearing. In a later study of disability caused by plantar fasciitis in 50 patients (Riddle et al. 2004), body mass index (BMI) was the only variable that was significantly associated with disability. Measures of pain intensity, ankle dorsiflexion, age, gender, chronicity, and time spent weight bearing were not related to disability. In a systematic review of the literature, Irving et al. (2006) found a strong association between a body mass index of 25 to 30 kg/m² and a calcaneal spur in a nonathletic population but a weak association between the development of plantar fasciitis and increased age, decreased ankle dorsiflexion, and prolonged standing.

Bone spurs may be associated with plantar fasciitis but are not believed to be the cause of it. Many studies show no clear association between spurs and plantar fasciitis. Studies of patients with plantar fasciitis report that 10% to 70% have an associated ipsilateral calcaneal spur; however, most also have a spur on the contralateral asymptomatic foot. Anatomic studies have shown the spur is located at the short flexor origin rather than at the plantar fascia origin, casting further doubt on its role in contributing to heel pain.

TABLE 43.2	Helpful Findings in Evaluating Etiologies of Heel Pain
Etiology	**Findings**
Plantar fasciitis	Pain and tenderness located inferiorly at the plantar fascia origin (not posteriorly)
	Almost all patients complain of inferior heel pain in the mornings with the first few steps and may complain of pain after prolonged walking or standing.
Plantar fascia rupture	Typically antecedent plantar fasciitis symptoms, with a pop or "crunch" during push-off or pivoting, then severe pain with subsequent inability to bear weight (or only with difficulty)
	Most commonly follows iatrogenic weakening of the fascia after cortisone injection
Calcaneal stress fracture	Much more common in athletes and runners with overuse history and repetitive high-impact activity or elderly females with osteoporosis and overuse in their walking or exercise regimen (e.g., 4 miles/day, 7 days/week). Pain is more diffuse than plantar fasciitis, with a positive squeeze test (Fig. 43.3) rather than discrete, localized inferior heel pain.
	Bone scan is positive for linear fracture rather than increased tracer uptake at plantar fascia origin as in plantar fasciitis. Unless a calcaneal stress fracture is suspected, bone scanning is not part of routine workup (Fig. 43.4).
Sever's disease (calcaneal apophysitis)	Symptoms almost identical to those of plantar fasciitis
	Occurs only in patients who are skeletally immature and have inflammation or apophysitis at the physis
	Treatment is the same as for plantar fasciitis, except a well-padded University of California at Berkeley (UCBL) orthotic is used.
Achilles tendinitis or rupture, Haglund's deformity	Pain is posterior rather than inferior. Haglund's deformity (pump bump) is tender over prominent bony deformity and often rubs or is irritated by the heel counter of the shoe.
	Patients with a complete rupture of the Achilles tendon describe a feeling of being "shot" in the tendon while pushing off, have a positive Thompson squeeze test, and have a lack of active plantar flexion except a small flicker from the long toe flexors.
Posterior tibial tendon (PTT) insufficiency	Pain is medial rather than inferior or posterior.
	Often, difficulty or inability to do a unilateral heel raise
	Often, point tender and boggy along course of PTT medially
Tarsal tunnel syndrome	Pain and numbness or tingling in medial ankle radiating into plantar aspect of foot only. No dorsal foot numbness or tingling (consider peripheral neuropathy if dorsal numbness present)
	Positive Tinel sign medially in tarsal tunnel. Electromyography is 90% accurate for identifying well-established tarsal tunnel syndrome.
	Decreased sensation in distribution of the medial plantar or lateral plantar nerve or both (plantar distribution only)
Reiter's syndrome, seronegative spondyloarthropathies	Bilateral plantar fascitis in a young male is often one of the first symptoms of an inflammatory arthritis. Consider HLA-B27 test and rheumatoid profile if other joint involvement is noted
Jogger's foot	Jogger's foot (as described by Rask) is a local nerve entrapment of the medial plantar nerve at the fibromuscular tunnel formed by the abductor hallucis muscle and its border with the navicular tuberosity.
	Most often associated with valgus hindfoot deformity (pronator) and long-distance running
	Characterized by running-induced neuritic pain (medial arch) radiating into medial toes along distribution of medial plantar nerve. This distribution is medial and on plantar aspect of the foot.

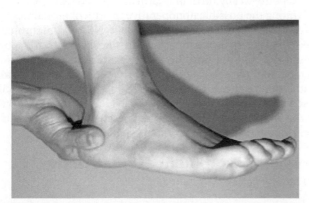

Fig. 43.3   Squeeze test of the calcaneus is positive when the patient has a stress fracture. Palpation of the calcaneal tuberosity is painful on squeeze testing.

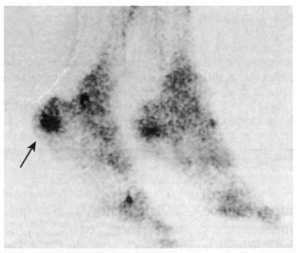

Fig. 43.4   Bone scan of the feet of a 40-year-old male runner demonstrates increased tracer uptake at the right medial calcaneal tuberosity (*arrow*) typical of acute plantar fasciitis. (From Batt T. Overuse injuries in athletes. *Phys Sports Med* 23(6):63–69, 1995.)

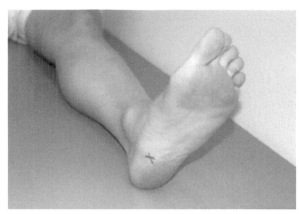

Fig. 43.5 Plantar fasciitis pain is inferior, located at the origin of the plantar fascia.

NATURAL HISTORY

Although plantar fasciitis can seem debilitating during the acute phase, it rarely causes lifelong problems. It is estimated that 90% to 95% of patients who have true plantar fasciitis recover with conservative treatment. However, it may take 6 months to 1 year, and patients often require much encouragement to continue stretching, wearing appropriate and supportive shoes, and avoiding high-impact activities or prolonged standing on hard surfaces. Operative treatment can be helpful in selected "failed" patients, but the success rate of surgery is only 50% to 85%.

BILATERAL HEEL INVOLVEMENT

Bilateral plantar fasciitis symptoms require ruling out systemic disorders such as Reiter's syndrome, ankylosing spondylitis, gouty arthropathy, and systemic lupus erythematosus. A high index of suspicion for a systemic disorder should accompany bilateral heel pain in a young male aged 15 to 35 years.

SIGNS AND SYMPTOMS

The classic presentation of plantar fasciitis includes a gradual, insidious onset of inferomedial heel pain at the insertion of the plantar fascia (Fig. 43.5). Pain and stiffness are worse with rising in the morning or after prolonged ambulation and may be exacerbated by climbing stairs or doing toe raises. **It is rare for patients with plantar fasciitis not to have pain or stiffness with the first few steps in the morning or after a prolonged rest.**

The diagnosis of plantar fasciitis is made with a reasonable level of certainty on the basis of clinical assessment alone. **History from the patient typically reports the following complaints:**

- Pain in the plantar heel region worse in morning, with the first few steps after waking or after a period of inactivity
- Insidious onset of pain in the plantar surface of the heel upon weight bearing after a period of nonweight bearing
- Some patients have an antalgic gait/limp.
- Inferior heel pain will lessen with increasing levels of activity (e.g., walking) but worsens at the end of the day.
- The history often indicates a recent increase in activity antecedent to onset of the presentation of plantar fasciitis.

EVALUATION OF PATIENTS WITH INFERIOR HEEL PAIN

- Biomechanical assessment of foot
- Pronated or pes planus foot
- Cavus-type foot (high arch)
- Assessment of fat pad (signs of atrophy)
- Presence of tight Achilles tendon
- Squeeze test of calcaneal tuberosity (medial and lateral sides of calcaneus) to evaluate for possible calcaneal stress fracture
- Evaluation for possible training errors in runners (e.g., rapid mileage increase, running on steep hills, poor running shoes, improper techniques)
- Regarding radiographic assessment Levy et al. (2006) reviewed the charts and radiographs of 157 consecutive adults (215 heels) presenting with nontraumatic heel pain and concluded that routine radiographs were of limited value in the initial evaluation of nontraumatic plantar heel pain in adults and were not necessary in the initial evaluation.
- Ultrasonography has been reported to be effective for identifying plantar fasciitis. In their meta-analysis of the literature, McMillan et al. (2009) found plantar fascia thickness as measured by ultrasonography to be the most widely reported imaging feature. The plantar fascia of individuals with chronic plantar heel pain was 2.16 mm thicker than that of control subjects, and a thickness of more than 4 mm on ultrasound examination was diagnostic of plantar fasciitis.
- Bone scan if recalcitrant pain (>6 weeks after treatment initiated) or suspected stress fracture from history
- Rheumatologic workup for patients with suspected underlying systemic process (e.g., young patients with bilateral heel pain, recalcitrant symptoms, or associated sacroiliac joint or multiple joint pain)
- Electromyographic (EMG) studies if clinical suspicion of nerve entrapment (e.g., tarsal tunnel)
- Establish correct diagnosis and rule out other possible etiologies (Tables 43.2 and 43.3).

TREATMENT OF PLANTAR FASCIITIS

A variety of treatment modalities have been described for plantar fasciitis, ranging from stretching exercises to surgery, but results have been inconsistent. Early initiation of conservative treatment (within 6 weeks of the onset of symptoms) has been shown to speed recovery; once the condition becomes chronic, the response to any form of treatment is unpredictable.

Among the possible nonoperative treatment modalities used to treat plantar fasciitis are rest, massage, NSAIDs, night splints, heel cups and pads, custom and off-the-shelf orthoses, injections, casts, and physical therapy measures such as shock wave therapy. **McPoil et al. (2008) formulated a series of clinical guidelines for the diagnosis and treatment of plantar fasciitis based on a thorough review of the available literature.** Based on the levels of evidence, they assigned levels of recommendation to several common treatment methods.

Level A Recommendation (Strong Evidence)

- Prefabricated or custom foot orthoses can provide short-term (3 months) reduction in pain and improvement in function.

TABLE 43.3	Palpatory Signs of Heel Pain Syndrome
Diagnosis	**Anatomic Location of Pain**
Plantar fasciitis	Origin of plantar aponeurosis at medial calcaneal tubercle
Fat pad syndrome	Plantar fat pad (bottom and sides)
Calcaneal periostitis	Diffuse plantar and medial and lateral calcaneal borders
Posterior tibial tendon disorders	Over medial midtarsal area at navicular, which may radiate proximally behind medial malleolus
Peroneal tendon disorders	Lateral calcaneus and peroneal tubercle
Tarsal tunnel syndrome	Diffuse plantar foot that may radiate distally with tingling, burning, and numbness in the bottom of foot only (not dorsal)
Medial calcaneal neuritis	Well-localized to anterior half of medial plantar heel pad and medial side of heel; does not radiate into distal foot
Lateral calcaneal neuritis	Heel pain that radiates laterally, more poorly localized
Calcaneal stress fracture	Diffuse pain over entire calcaneus, positive squeeze test of calcaneal tuberosity
Calcaneal apophysitis	Generalized over posterior heel, especially the sides, in patients who are skeletally immature (apophysis)
Generalized arthritis	Poorly localized but generally over entire heel pad

Modified from Doxey GE. Calcaneal pain: a review of various disorders. J Orthop Sports Phys Ther 9:30, 1987.

Level B Recommendations (Moderate Evidence)

- Calf muscle and/or plantar fascia–specific stretching can provide short-term (2 to 4 weeks) pain relief and improved function. The dose for calf stretching can be either 3 times a day or 2 times a day utilizing either a sustained (3 minute) or intermittent (20 seconds) stretching time, as neither dosage produced a statistically significant better effect.
- Night splints (1 to 3 months) should be considered for patients with symptoms lasting more than 6 months. The desired length of time for wearing the splints is 1 to 3 months. The type of night splint (posterior, anterior, or sock type) does not appear to affect outcome.
- Dexamethasone 0.4% or acetic acid delivered through iontophoresis can provide short-term (2 to 4 weeks) pain relief and improved function.

Level C Recommendations (Weak Evidence)

- Effectiveness of manual therapy and nerve mobilization to provide short-term (1 to 3 months) pain relief is supported by minimal evidence.
- Calcaneal or low-Dye taping can provide 7 to 10 days of pain relief.

Treatment

Stretching of the plantar fascia and/or the Achilles tendon has traditionally been the primary treatment of plantar fasciitis. Plantar fascia–specific stretching exercises aim to produce maximal tissue tension through a controlled stretch of the plantar fascia by reproducing the windlass mechanism. DiGiovanni et al. (2006) compared these two exercise protocols in a prospective, randomized, controlled study and found that 8 weeks of plantar fascia–specific stretching eliminated or improved pain in 52% of patients, compared to only 22% with Achilles tendon stretching. At 2-year follow-up, however, there was no difference between the two groups. Cleland et al. (2009), in a multicenter, randomized clinical trial, compared electrophysical agents and exercise to manual physical therapy and exercise and found that manual physical therapy and exercise produced better results at 4-week and 6-month follow-up evaluations.

The use of a **walking cast** for a brief period has been advocated to unload the heel and immobilize the plantar fascia to minimize repetitive microtrauma; however, the efficacy of casting has been supported only in retrospective studies, with no published prospective, controlled trials. Reported results of night splinting in large, randomized, controlled trials have been contradictory, with one reporting improvement after 1 month of night splinting (Powell et al. 1998) and another reporting no benefit (Probe et al. 1999).

Injections of corticosteroids, botulinum toxin A (BTX-A), or autologous blood into the origin of the plantar fascia have been described, mostly in small series, but there is insufficient evidence to clearly define their effectiveness. The effect of corticosteroid injection appears to be short-lived, and complications such as plantar fascia rupture and plantar fat pad atrophy have been associated with this form of treatment.

Acevedo and Beskin (1998) in a retrospective review of 765 patients treated for plantar fasciitis with steroid injection reported 36% of patients had a plantar fascial rupture as a result of the injection. **Of greater note is 50% of patients who suffered a rupture reported only a fair or poor recovery at a 27-month follow-up.** More recent studies (Genc et al. 2005, Tsai et al. 2006) have reported minimal to no risk of rupture.

One double-blind, randomized, controlled trial (Babcock et al. 2005) found a statistically significant improvement with BTX-A injection compared to saline injection, with no side effects; however, follow-up was short (8 weeks) and only 23 patients (43 feet) were included. Another prospective, randomized, controlled trial involving 64 patients compared autologous blood injection to corticosteroid injection and concluded that, although autologous blood injections were effective in reducing pain and tenderness in chronic plantar fasciitis, corticosteroid injections were superior in terms of speed of relief and extent of improvement (Lee et al. 2007); the benefits of corticosteroid injection were maintained for at least 12 months in their patients.

Platelet rich plasma (PRP) injections have shown promise in the treatment of plantar fasciitis. In a level 1 study, Monto showed a greater improvement in patients injected with PRP compared to those injected with corticosteroid. Additionally, subjective score improvement in the PRP group was maintained throughout the duration of the 2-year follow-up, whereas the corticosteroid group reverted to baseline by one year (Monto 2014).

Extracorporeal shock wave therapy (ESWT) has been shown to be effective in 60% to 80% of patients. ESWT is based on lithotripsy technology in which shock waves (acoustic impulses) are targeted to the plantar fascia origin. Currently, both high-energy (electrohydraulic) and low-energy (electromagnetic) devices are approved by the U.S. Food and Drug Administration for the treatment of chronic heel pain. A single high-energy application and multiple low-energy applications have been shown to be effective in several randomized prospective trials (Rompe et al. 2007, Ogden et al. 2001, Theodore et al. 2004, Kudo et al. 2006, Wang et al. 2006). **Current indications for ESWT are plantar fasciitis pain that has been present for 6 months or more and has not responded to at least 3 months of nonoperative treatment.** Contraindications to ESWT include hemophilia, coagulopathies, malignancies, and open physes.

Surgical Treatment of Plantar Fasciitis

Surgical treatment of plantar fasciitis generally is reserved for patients who have severe pain that interferes with work or recreation and has not responded to prolonged (12 months or more) nonsurgical treatment. Both partial and complete plantar fasciotomy have been reported in the literature; several studies have reported that fewer than 50% of patients are satisfied with their outcomes and many continue to have pain and functional limitations. Because biomechanical studies have shown that release of more than 40% of the plantar fascia has detrimental effects on other ligamentous and bony structures in the foot (Cheung et al. 2006), plantar fascia surgical release should be limited to less than 40% of the fascia.

See Rehabilitation Protocol 43.1 for a treatment algorithm for plantar fasciitis and Rehabilitation Protocol 43.2 for a home rehabilitation program.

RUPTURE OF THE PLANTAR FASCIA
Background

Although not commonly reported in the literature, partial or complete plantar fascia ruptures may occur in jumping or running sports. Often, this is missed or misdiagnosed as an acute flare-up of plantar fasciitis. Complete rupture of the plantar fascia usually results in a permanent loss of the medial (longitudinal) arch of the foot. Such collapse is typically disabling for athletes.

Examination

Patients typically complain of a pop or crunch in the inferior heel area, with immediate pain and inability to continue play. This usually occurs during push-off, jumping, or initiation of a sprint. After an antecedent cortisone injection, the trauma may be much more minor (e.g., stepping off a curb).

Weight bearing is difficult, and swelling and ecchymosis in the plantar aspect of the foot occur fairly rapidly. Palpation along the plantar fascia elicits marked point tenderness. Dorsiflexion of the toes and foot often causes pain in the plantar fascia area.

Radiographic Evaluation

Diagnosis of a plantar fascia rupture is a clinical one. Pain radiographs are taken (three views of the foot) to rule out a fracture. MRI may be used but is not necessary for diagnosis. MRI may miss the area of the actual rupture but does typically pick up the associated hemorrhage and swelling surrounding the rupture.

Treatment

Saxena and Fullem (2004) reported good results in 18 athletes with plantar fascia ruptures, all of whom were treated with 2 to 3 weeks of nonweight bearing in a below-knee or high-top boot, followed by an additional 2 to 3 weeks of weight bearing in the boot. All participated in a structured physical therapy program concomitantly. All patients returned to activity at an average of 9 weeks, and none had re-injury or sequelae that required surgery (Rehabilitation Protocol 43.3).

REHABILITATION PROTOCOL 43.1

Treatment Algorithm for Plantar Fasciitis (Neufeld and Cerrato 2008)

A. Initial Treatment

- Over-the-counter (OTC) nonsteroidal anti-inflammatories (NSAIDs) (weak evidence to support this)
- Heel pads or OTC orthosis
- Plantar fascia–specific and Achilles tendon home stretching exercises
- Night splinting

B. If No Improvement After 4–6 Weeks

- Immobilization in a cast or cam walker
- Radiographic evaluation to rule out stress fracture or other pathology
- Physical therapy with emphasis on plantar fascia stretching and Achilles stretching
- Custom orthosis
- Prescription NSAIDs (weak evidence to support this)
- Corticosteroid injection at plantar fascia origin

C. Persistent Symptoms Beyond A and B

- If some improvement has been made, treatment plan is continued
- If no improvement, MRI to confirm diagnosis, rule out stress fracture, etc.
- Consideration of alternative treatments, such as extracorporeal shock wave therapy (ESWT)
- Surgery (partial release of <40% of fascia) is considered only if all other treatments fail and the patient has pain that prevents work and recreation.

(Formulated from information in Neufeld SK, Cerrato R. Plantar Fasciitis: Evaluation and Treatment. *J Am Acad Orthop Surg* 16:338–346, 2008.)

REHABILITATION PROTOCOL 43.2 ■ **Home Rehabilitation Program for Plantar Fasciitis**

Component	Procedure	Duration and Frequency	Illustration
Stretch 1	In standing position, with involved foot farthest away from the wall, lean forward while keeping your heel on the floor and knee bent. Lean forward until you feel a stretch in the calf and/or Achilles region.	Perform this exercise at home 3 times daily for 2 repetitions, holding each for 30 seconds.	
Stretch 2	In standing position, with involved foot farthest away from the wall, lean forward while keeping your heel on the floor and the back knee straight. Lean forward until you feel a stretch in the calf and/or Achilles region.	Perform this exercise at home 3 times daily for 2 repetitions, holding each for 30 seconds.	

Continued

REHABILITATION PROTOCOL 43.2 ■ **Home Rehabilitation Program for Plantar Fasciitis—cont'd**

Component	Procedure	Duration and Frequency	Illustration
Ankle eversion self-mobilization	Stabilize your leg with your arm as shown. Your stabilizing hand should wrap around the very end of your leg, just above your ankle. Use your other hand to grasp the back part of your foot and push toward the floor.	Perform in an on–off fashion 30 times, repeat 3 times.	
Self-stretching and mobilization of plantar fascia and flexor hallucis longus	Cross the affected leg over the nonaffected leg. While placing your fingers over the base of your toes, pull the toes back toward your shin until a stretch is felt in your plantar fascia. With your other hand, mobilize the plantar fascia and flexor hallucis longus from your heel toward your toes. Start gently at first, then work deeper as tolerated.	Perform for 3 to 5 minutes.	

From Cleland JA, Abbot JH, Kidd M, Stockwell S, Cheney S, Gerard DF, Flynn TW. Manual Physical Therapy and Exercise Versus Electrophysical Agents and Exercise in the Management of Plantar Heel Pain: A Multicenter Randomized Clinical Trial. *J Orthop Sports Phys Ther* 39(8):585, 2009.

REHABILITATION PROTOCOL 43.3 ◾ After Rupture of the Plantar Fascia

S. Brent Brotzman, MD

Phase 1: Days 0–14

- Immediate nonweight bearing with crutches
- Light compression wrap changed several times a day for 2–3 days
- Ice therapy with ice massage of swollen/ecchymotic area several times a day
- Maximal elevation on four or five pillows above the level of the heart for 72 hours, then elevation for 8–12 hours a day (sleeping with pillows under the foot)
- Nonweightbearing, light, fiberglass cast on day 3, worn for 1–2 weeks, depending on resolution of pain
- NSAIDs (if not contraindicated) for 2–3 weeks
- Gentle active toe extension and flexion exercises while still in cast

Phase 2: Weeks 2–3

- Removal of fiberglass cast
- Use of 1/8-inch felt pad placed from heel to heads of metatarsals and lightly wrapped with bandage (Coban, Unna boot, Ace bandage). We use a cotton sock or Coban to keep the felt in place.
- Foot and felt wrapping are placed in a removable walking cast, which allows the foot to be taken out daily for therapy and pool exercises.
- Weight bearing is progressed from as tolerated in boot with crutches to weight bearing in boot only. Pain is the guiding factor for progression of weight bearing.

- Exercises are begun as pain allows
  - Swimming
  - Deep-water running with Aquajogger.com flotation belt
  - Stationary bicycling with no resistance
  - Gentle Achilles stretches with towel looped around foot

Phase 3: Weeks 3–8

- Proprioception exercises with BAPS board as pain allows
- Removable cast and felt typically worn for 4–6 weeks
- Active ankle strengthening exercises are progressed.
- High-impact exercises are held until patient has been completely asymptomatic (with ambulation in tennis shoe) for 2–3 weeks.
- Use of a custom orthotic layered with an overlying soft substance (such as Plastizote) is often helpful for eventual athletic participation.
- It is not uncommon to have permanent impairment in high-impact athletes who have suffered a plantar fascia rupture of more than 40%. For this reason, cortisone injections should rarely, if ever, be used in high-impact athletes.

REFERENCES

A complete reference list is available at https://expertconsult.inkling.com/.

FURTHER READING

Chuckpaiwong B, Berkson EM, Theodore GH. Extracorporeal shock wave for chronic proximal plantar fasciitis: 225 patients with results and outcome predictors. *J Foot Ankle Surg.* 2009;48:148–155.

Donley BG, Moore T, Sferra J, et al. The efficacy of oral nonsteroidal anti-inflammatory medication (NSAID) in the treatment of plantar fasciitis: a randomized, prospective, placebo-controlled study. *Foot Ankle Int.* 2007;28:20–23.

Hyland MR, Webber-Gaffney A, Cohen L, et al. Randomized controlled trial of calcaneal taping, sham taping, and plantar fascia stretching for the short-term management of plantar heel pain. *J Orthop Sports Phys Ther.* 2006;36:364–371.

Lareau CR, Sawyer GA, Wang JH, et al. Plantar and medial heel pain: diagnosis and management. *J Am Acad Orthop Surg.* 2014;22(6):372–380.

Lee SY, McKeon P, Hertel J. Does the use of orthoses improve self-reported pain and function measures in patients with plantar fasciitis? A meta-analysis. *Phys Ther Sport.* 2009;10:12–81.

Achilles Tendinopathy

S. Brent Brotzman, MD

The Achilles tendon is the largest and strongest tendon in the body. The tendon has no true synovial sheath but is encased in a **paratenon,** a single cell layer of fatty areolar tissue. The vascular supply to the tendon comes distally from intraosseous vessels from the calcaneus and proximally from intramuscular branches. There is a relative area of avascularity 2 to 6 cm from the calcaneal insertion that is more vulnerable to degeneration and injury (Fig. 44.1). Blood supply to the Achilles tendon is evident at 3 locations: the muscle tendon junction, along the course of the tendon, and at the tendon bone insertion. Vascular density is greatest proximally and least in the midportion of the tendon. Achilles tendon injuries are commonly associated with repetitive impact loading resulting from running and jumping. Pushing off the weightbearing foot with the knee extended, unexpected dorsiflexion of the ankle, and violent dorsiflexion of a plantarflexed ankle are the usual reported mechanisms for Achilles tendon rupture. Peak stress during these contractions can reach more than 2233 N or 6 to 12 times body weight (Schepsis et al. 2002, Alfredson and Lorentzon 2000, Maffulli and Ajis 2008).

The primary factors resulting in damage of the athlete's Achilles tendon (e.g., middle- and long-distance runners) are training errors such as a sudden increase in activity, a sudden increase in training intensity (distance, frequency), resuming training after a long period of inactivity, and running on uneven or loose terrain. Achilles dysfunction can also be related to postural problems (e.g., pronation), poor footwear (generally poor hindfoot support), and a tight gastrocsoleus complex.

End-organ microvasculature disease and resultant tendon degeneration appear to be the pathophysiology involved with the second subset of symptomatic Achilles patients (i.e., the elderly with degenerative Achilles tendinosis).

Achilles tendon injuries cover a spectrum of disorders (Table 44.1), and the nomenclature and classification of these injuries in the literature are confusing. Although the term "tendinitis" often is used to describe tendon pain and swelling, inflammatory cells rarely are seen in biopsy specimens of thickened and inflamed tendons unless tendon rupture has occurred. Various histopathologic entities appear to be responsible for Achilles tendon pain, and Maffulli and Kader (2002) suggested that the combination of pain, swelling, and impaired performance should be labeled **"Achilles tendinopathy."** The role of inflammation in tendinopathy remains a matter of some debate. The main argument for the inflammation theory is that injections of corticosteroids have been shown to relieve symptoms, swelling, and even ultrasound appearance of tendinopathies (Fredberg et al. 2008, Torp-Pedersen et al. 2008). However, other investigators have suggested that inflammation seems to play a minor role, citing the identification and findings of structural degeneration of the collagen matrix, intratendinous neovascularization

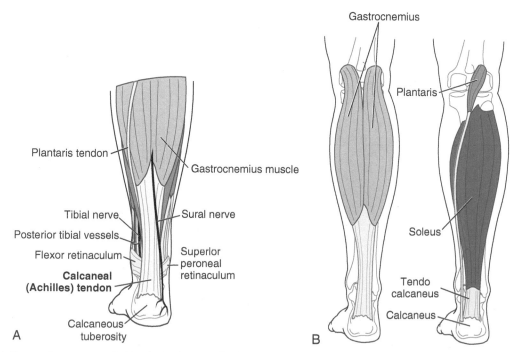

Fig. 44.1 **A,** Achilles tendon anatomy. **B,** Muscles in the superficial posterior compartment of the leg. Gastrocnemius and soleus and plantaris.

TABLE 44.1	Differential Diagnosis of Achilles Tendinitis/ Tendinosis

Partial rupture of Achilles tendon
Retrocalcaneal bursitis (or retrocalcaneal bursa)
Haglund's deformity (pump bump)
Calcaneal apophysitis (skeletally immature—Sever's apophysitis)
Calcaneal exostosis
Calcaneal stress fracture (positive squeeze test)
Calcaneal fracture (acute fall or motor vehicle accident)
Posterior tibial tendon tendinitis (medial pain)
Plantar fasciitis (inferior heel pain)

TABLE 44.2	Stages of Puddu's Noninsertional Achilles Tendon

PERITENDINITIS: INFLAMMATION INVOLVING PERITENDINOUS STRUCTURES
- Thickening of peritenon
- Fluid accumulation adjacent to tendon
- Development of adhesions

PERITENDINITIS WITH TENDINOSIS: INFLAMMATION OF PERITENDINOUS STRUCTURES + DEGENERATIVE CHANGES
- Macroscopic tendon thickening, nodularity
- Softening
- Yellowing
- Fibrillation
- Focal degeneration within tendon

TENDINOSIS: ASYMPTOMATIC DEGENERATION WITHOUT INFLAMMATION CAUSED BY ACCUMULATED MICROTRAUMA, AGING, OR BOTH
- Degenerative lesions with no evidence of peritendinitis
- Altered tendon structure
- Decreased luster
- Yellowish decoloration
- Softening

TABLE 44.3	Noninsertional Achilles Tendon Disorders		
Symptom/Sign	Peritendinitis	Peritendinitis + Tendinosis (Partial Rupture)	Tendinosis With Acute Complete Rupture
Pain	Acute	Subacute/chronic	Acute
Audible snap/pop	None	Unlikely	+
Muscle weakness	+	+	+
Antalgic gait	+	+	+
Edema	+	+	+
Pain with palpation	+	+	+
Tendon gap	-	±	+
Tendon crepitus	±	±	±
Passive dorsiflexion excursion	Decreased	Decreased	Increased
Thompson test	-	-	+
Calf atrophy	-	+	±
Single-limb toe rise	+	±	Unable to perform
Plantarflexion strength	Decreased	Decreased	Severely decreased

Modified from Coughlin MJ, Schon LC: Disorders of tendons. In Coughlin MJ, Mann RA, Saltzman CL (eds.): Surgery of the foot and ankle, 8th ed. Philadelphia: Mosby/Elsevier, 2007, p. 1224.

TABLE 44.4	Continuum of Disease in Achilles Tendon Lesions

Disorder	Pathology
Paratenonitis	Inflammation of the peritendinous structures, including the paratenon and septum
Tendinosis	Asymptomatic degeneration of tendon without inflammation, with regional focal loss of tendon structure
Paratenonitis with tendinosis	Inflammation of the peritendinous structures along with intratendinous degeneration
Retrocalcaneal bursitis	Mechanical irritation of the retrocalcaneal bursa
Insertional tendinosis	Inflammatory process within the tendinous insertion of the Achilles tendon

From Reddy SS, Pedowitz DI, Parekh SG, Omar IM, Wapner KL: Surgical treatment for chronic disease and disorders of the Achilles tendon. J Am Acad Orthop Surg 17:3-14, 2009.

(Ohberg et al. 2001), increased local concentrations of neuropeptides (Alfredson et al. 2001), and increased cell apoptosis (Pearce et al. 2009).

Two broad categories of Achilles tendon disorders may be based on location: **noninsertional and insertional.** Puddu et al. (1976) described noninsertional Achilles tendon lesions as pure peritendinitis (stage 1), peritendinitis with tendinosis (stage 2), and tendinosis (stage 3) (Tables 44.2 and 44.3). Because these distinct pathologies frequently coexist, it is helpful to consider them as a continuum of disease (Table 44.4).

Reddy et al. (2009) noted that further complicating any proposed treatment algorithm for assorted Achilles tendon pathology is that it typically presents as one of **two distinct patient populations:** the younger athlete with some component of overuse and the older community ambulatory with degenerative etiology.

Kvist et al. (1988) did note paratenonitis is commonly seen in runners, especially long- and middle-distance runners, but is uncommon in patients who are older and sedentary.

EXAMINATION

Examination is performed with the patient placed prone and the feet hanging off the edge of the table. The entire substance of the gastrocnemius–soleus myotendinous complex is palpated while the ankle is put through active and passive ROM. The leg is examined for tenderness, warmth, swelling or fullness, nodularity, or substance defect.

Decreased ankle dorsiflexion (from tightness in the gastrocnemius–soleus tendon complex) and hamstring tightness are commonly found in patients with Achilles tendon pathology (Reddy et al. 2009). While seated on the examination table, the patient's foot should be passively dorsiflexed, first with the knee flexed and then with the knee fully extended. This will tell the examiner how tight the Achilles tendon is. The **Silverskiöld test** can be used as a measure of tightness of the gastrocsoleus complex, again performed by dorsiflexing the ankle and

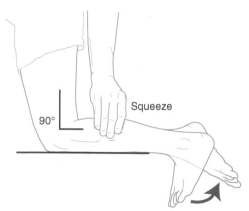

Fig. 44.2 Thompson squeeze test. This test evaluates the Achilles tendon for complete rupture. In the normal patient placed prone with the knee flexed at 90 degrees, squeezing the calf muscle will cause the foot to plantar flex (*arrow*) because the tendon is intact. In a complete rupture of the tendon, squeezing of the calf will *not* cause plantarflexion of the foot (i.e., a positive Thompson test indicates a complete rupture). This test is important because most patients with a completely ruptured Achilles tendon can still weakly plantar flex the foot, "cheating" with the long toe flexors, on request.

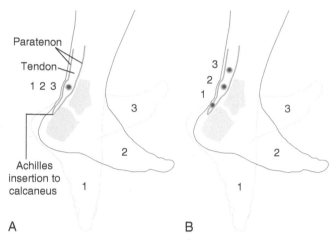

Fig. 44.3 Painful arc sign. A, In peritenonitis, the tenderness remains in one position despite moving the foot from dorsiflexion to plantarflexion. B, In the case of partial tendon rupture or tendinitis, the point of tenderness *moves* as the foot goes from dorsiflexion to plantarflexion. (*A* and *B* redrawn from Williams JG: Achilles tendon lesions in sports. Sports Med 3:114, 1986.)

alternately relaxing and then incorporating the gastroc–soleus (by flexing and extending the knee, respectively). Many females who have worn high heel shoes for years are unable to dorsiflex the foot to neutral with the knee in full extension.

Patients with paratenon involvement (paratenonitis) will exhibit a tender thickened area that does not move during active range of motion of the ankle. This differs from tendon involvement (e.g., Achilles tendinosis), which moves up and down with active range of motion of the ankle.

If Achilles rupture is suspected, the **Thompson squeeze test** is performed to evaluate the continuity of the Achilles tendon (Fig. 44.2). A positive Thompson test (no plantarflexion of the foot with squeezing of the calf muscle) usually indicates no tendon continuity and thus a complete rupture of the Achilles tendon. Calf atrophy is common in any Achilles tendon dysfunction.

IMAGING

Most Achilles problems can be diagnosed with a thorough history and physical examination. Imaging helps confirm the diagnosis, assist with surgical planning, or rule out other diagnoses.

- *Routine radiographs* are generally normal. Occasionally, calcification in the tendon or its insertion is noted. Inflammatory arthropathies (erosions) or Haglund's deformity (pump bump) can be ruled out on radiographs.
- *Ultrasound* is inexpensive and fast and allows dynamic examination, but it requires substantial interpreter experience. It is the most reliable method for determining the thickness of the Achilles tendon and the size of a gap after a complete rupture.
- *MRI* is not used for dynamic assessment, but it is superior in the detection of partial tears and the evaluation of various stages of chronic degenerative changes, such as peritendinous thickening and inflammation. MRI can be used to monitor tendon healing when recurrent partial rupture is suspected and is the best modality for surgical planning (location, size).

ACHILLES PARATENONITIS

Isolated tendinitis is especially common in middle- and long-distance runners. Diffuse tenderness and swelling usually are present on both sides of the Achilles tendon, although the medial side is more frequently involved (Heckman et al. 2009) (Rehabilitation Protocol 44.1).

Inflammation is limited to the investing paratenon without associated Achilles tendinosis. Fluid often accumulates next to the tendon; the paratenon is thickened and adherent to normal tendon tissue. Achilles paratenonitis most commonly occurs in mature athletes involved in running and jumping activities. It generally does not progress to degeneration. Histology of paratenonitis shows inflammatory cells and capillary and fibroblastic proliferation in the paratenon or peritendinous areolar tissue.

Clinical Signs and Symptoms

Pain starts with initial morning activity. The discomfort is well-localized tenderness and sharp, burning pain with activity. The discomfort is present 2 to 6 cm proximal to the insertion of the Achilles tendon into the calcaneus. Pain is primarily aggravated by activity and relieved by rest. Pain is present with single-heel raise and absent on the Thompson test. Significant heel cord contracture will exacerbate symptoms.

Swelling, local tenderness, warmth, and tendon thickening are common. Calf atrophy and weakness and tendon nodularity can be present in chronic cases. Crepitation is rare.

Painful arc sign (Fig. 44.3) is negative in paratenonitis. It is important to localize the precise area of tenderness and fullness. In paratenonitis, the area of tenderness and fullness stays fixed with active ROM of ankle. The inflammation involves only the paratenon, which is a fixed structure, unlike pathology of the Achilles tendon itself, which migrates superiorly and inferiorly with ROM of the ankle.

With acute paratenonitis, symptoms are typically transient, present only with activity, and last less than 2 weeks. Later, symptoms start at the beginning of exercising or at rest and tenderness increases. The area of tenderness is well localized and reproducible by side-to-side squeezing of the involved region.

Partial rupture may be superimposed on chronic paratenonitis and can present as an acute episode of pain and swelling.

Ultrasonography usually shows fluid surrounding the tendon in acute paratenonitis, while peritendinous adhesions, seen as thickening of the hypoechogenic paratenon, may be present in chronic paratenonitis. T1-weighted MR images show a thickened paratenon, and T2-weighted images display increased signal strength (halo sign) within the paratenon (Saxena and Cheung 2003).

ACHILLES TENDINOSIS

Tendinosis is a noninflammatory condition involving intratendinous degeneration and atrophy. The process starts with interstitial microscopic failure caused by repetitive microtrauma, aging, or a combination of these and leads to central tissue necrosis with subsequent mucoid degeneration. Achilles tendinosis most commonly occurs in mature athletes. It is associated with an increased risk of Achilles tendon rupture.

The histology generally is noninflammatory, showing decreased cellularity and fibrillation of collagen fibers within the tendon. Along with the collagen fiber disorganization, there are scattered vascular ingrowth and occasional areas of necrosis and rare calcification.

Obesity has been identified as an etiologic factor in tendinosis, as have systemic factors such as hypertension and hormone replacement therapy in women (Holmes and Lin 2006). Holmes and Lin performed an epidemiologic study of patients with MRI and examination confirmed Achilles degenerative tendinopathy. Overall, 98% of these patients had hypertension, diabetes, obesity, and steroid or estrogen exposure, suggesting probable end-organ effect causing a decrease in local microvascularity at the Achilles tendon. Again, these were the older subset of patients with degeneration of the Achilles tendon.

Increased foot pronation has been cited as a biomechanical cause of tendinosis (Järvinen et al. 2001).

Clinical Signs and Symptoms

Achilles tendinosis is often asymptomatic and remains subclinical until it presents as a rupture. It may elicit low-grade discomfort related to activities, and a palpable painless mass or nodule may be present 2 to 6 cm proximal to the insertion of the tendon. This can progress to gradual thickening of the entire tendon substance.

The painful arc sign is positive in patients with Achilles tendinosis. The thickened portion of tendon moves with active plantarflexion and dorsiflexion of the ankle (in contrast to paratenonitis, in which the area of paratenon tenderness remains in one position despite dorsiflexion and plantarflexion of the foot).

Ultrasonography may show Achilles tendinosis as a hypoechogenic area with or without intratendinous calcification (Fig. 44.4). MRI shows the thickened tendon on sagittal images, and altered signal appearance is noted within the tendon tissue (Reddy et al. 2009).

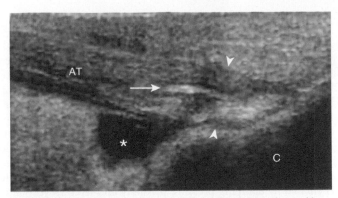

Fig. 44.4 Achilles tendon. *Arrow,* calcification; *,* retrocalcaneal bursa; *C,* calcaneus; *arrowheads,* tendinosis. (From Falsetti P, Frediani B, Acciai C, Baldi F, Filippou G, Prada EP, et al.: Ultrasonographic study of Achilles tendon and plantar fascia in chondrocalcinosis. J Rheumatol 31(11):2242–2250, 2004.)

ACHILLES PARATENONITIS WITH TENDINOSIS

Paratenonitis and tendinosis can coexist when inflammation involves both the paratenon and intratendinous focal degeneration. This gives the clinical appearance of paratenonitis because the symptoms associated with tendinosis are absent or very subtle. Most patients seek treatment for symptoms related to the paratenonitis, and usually, the tendinosis is unrecognized until both processes are noted on MRI or at surgery (most commonly after a rupture). In the acute phase, symptoms are similar to those of paratenonitis: swelling and tenderness around the middle third of the tendon. In chronic injuries, exercise-induced pain is the primary symptom. Often focal, tender nodules are the first sign of the development of tendinosis in a patient with paratenonitis.

INSERTIONAL ACHILLES TENDINITIS

Insertional Achilles tendinitis often begins as a painful inflammatory process within the tendinous insertion of the Achilles on the calcaneus. Insertional Achilles tendinitis also frequently follows the continuum outlined by Puddu: peritendonitis (stage 1), itis with osis (stage 2) and tendonosis (stage 3). It is most frequent in patients who are obese and in older or recreational athletes and often may be associated with prominent posterior calcaneal tuberosity (Haglund deformity) or retrocalcaneal bursitis (Schepsis et al. 2002). Pain may be increased by hill running, interval programs, and training errors. Patients with insertional tendinitis report morning ankle stiffness, posterior heel pain, and swelling that worsens with activity.

Examination reveals tenderness at the bone–tendon junction and limited ankle dorsiflexion (Heckman et al. 2009). Plain radiographs should be obtained to identify any prominence of the posterior calcaneal tuberosity, intratendinous calcification, or a calcaneal spur. Ultrasonography may show intratendinous calcifications or heterogeneity in the structure of the tendon fibers. T2-weighted MR images may show increased signal within the retrocalcaneal bursa and degenerative or inflammatory changes at the tendon insertion (Schepsis et al. 2002).

RETROCALCANEAL BURSITIS

Although not strictly an Achilles tendon disorder, retrocalcaneal bursitis involves inflammation of the bursa between the calcaneus and the Achilles tendon, where it is compressed by these structures during ankle dorsiflexion. The bursa can become inflamed, hypertrophied, and adherent to the Achilles tendon, which can lead to degenerative changes within the tendon (Schepsis et al. 2002). Retrocalcaneal bursitis is characterized by pain anterior to the Achilles tendon and is frequent in athletes training with uphill running.

It is diagnosed by the two-finger squeeze test, in which pain is elicited by applying pressure medially and laterally just anterior to the Achilles tendon (Heckman et al. 2009). Radiographs may show a prominence of the posterosuperior calcaneal tuberosity. MRI or ultrasonography can identify fluid within the retrocalcaneal bursa, peritendinous thickening, calcification, tendinosis, or partial tendon ruptures.

TREATMENT OF ACHILLES TENDINOPATHY

The initial treatment of all forms of Achilles tendinopathy is nonoperative, aimed to relieve symptoms, correct training errors, modify limb alignment with orthotics, and improve flexibility, and generally begins with rest, cryotherapy, and physical therapy that includes stretching and strengthening exercises. Because Achilles tendinopathy occurs in two distinct patient populations—younger athletes and older recreational athletes or nonathletes—treatment must be individualized for each patient.

For active, athletic patients with paratenonitis, conservative treatment typically involves modification of training regimens (staged cross-training), rest, ice, massage, and NSAIDs. Paratenonitis in less active, older patients (uncommon) generally is treated with immobilization with a nonarticular solid molded ankle foot orthosis, NSAIDs, and a short course of physical therapy. Corticosteroid injections are not recommended in either group because of adverse effects on the mechanical properties of the tendon and an increased risk of tendon rupture. **Brisement** (infiltration of saline or dilute local anesthetic into the paratenon sheath to break up adhesions between the paratenon and the tendon) is successful in reducing symptoms about half the time (Schepsis et al. 2002, Saltzman and Tearse, 1998, Reddy et al. 2009). See Rehabilitation Protocol 44-2 for general guidelines for Achilles tendonitis, paratenonitis, and tendinosis in high-impact athletes.

ECCENTRIC ACHILLES TRAINING FOR ACHILLES PATHOLOGY

For Achilles tendinosis physical therapy concentrates on enhancing dorsiflexion strength (**eccentric Achilles training**), which is typically limited in patients with chronic tendinopathy. Eccentric exercise programs do not involve any concentric loading, exercises are done even if painful, and load is increased until pain is present.

Multiple studies have reported good results with eccentric training in up to 90% of patients with noninsertional Achilles tendinopathy (Rompe et al. 2007 and 2008, Fahlstrom et al. 2003, Roos et al. 2004, Alfredson et al. 1998). Öhberg et al.

(2004) reported that ultrasonographic follow-up evaluation of 25 patients (26 tendons) treated with eccentric training found a localized decrease in tendon thickness and a normalized tendon structure in 19; at an average 4-year follow-up, 22 of the 25 patients were satisfied with their results.

In a randomized, prospective, multicenter comparative study, Mafi et al. (2001) reported that 18 of 22 (82%) patients treated with an eccentric exercise program returned to their previous activity levels, compared to only 8 of 22 (36%) of those who were treated with a concentric training program. Results have not been as good in nonathletic, sedentary patients: 44% of patients with an average age of 51 years (range 23 to 67) did not improve with an eccentric exercise regimen (Sayana and Maffulli 2007). Eccentric exercise also has been less effective in patients with insertional tendinosis, obtaining good results in only 32% in one study (Fahlström et al. 2003).

Several theories have been proposed to explain the effectiveness of eccentric exercise in reducing midsubstance Achilles tendon pain. *Short-term effects* include increased tendon volume and signal intensity; however, after a 12-week program, a decrease in size and a more normal tendon appearance were noted on ultrasound and MRI (Öhberg et al. 2004). Some believe that eccentric loading may lengthen the muscle–tendon unit over time and increase its capacity to bear load. Also, because vessels disappear on imaging with eccentric loading, repetitive eccentric training may reduce the area of neovascularization in this region of the tendon (Ohberg et al. 2001).

Although effective in a large percentage of patients with Achilles tendinopathy, eccentric exercise treatment may be frustrating for athletes because of the length of the treatment (typically 8 to 12 weeks). The eccentric exercises are often painful in the beginning of the treatment period, and not all patients are willing to remain compliant with the painful and lengthy exercise regimen. One randomized controlled trial involving 52 recreational athletes found that the addition of low-level laser therapy to the eccentric exercises resulted in less pain and faster recovery; results at 4 weeks in those with laser therapy were similar to those at 12 weeks in those with placebo therapy (Stergioulas et al. 2008).

ECCENTRIC EXERCISE REGIMEN

In the classic eccentric exercise regimen, the athlete stands with his or her forefoot only (both feet) close to the edge of a step, with the heels hanging off the step and the uninvolved leg providing the force to rise up onto the forefeet. The uninvolved leg is then lifted off the step so that full body weight is supported only by the involved leg (Fig. 44.5, *A*). The heel of the involved leg is then slowly lowered until it is well behind and below the edge of the step (Fig. 44.5, *B*), moving the ankle from plantarflexion to dorsiflexion. As he or she works actively to slow the descent of the heel, a strong eccentric contraction is placed on the calf muscles, and the muscles also elongate as the heel drops down. The uninvolved leg is then used to provide the force necessary to return to the starting position. Three sets of 15 repetitions are done with the knee straight and three sets are done with the knee bent to activate the soleus muscle. When the exercises can be done without pain or discomfort, weight is added by having the athlete wear a backpack (Fig. 44.5, *C*). Eventually a weight machine can be used to increase the eccentric strain. Generally, the athlete can continue training if it produces only mild

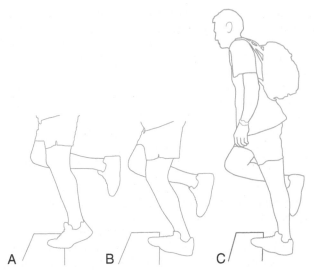

Fig. 44.5 Eccentric exercises. **A,** Starting position, where the ankle joint is in plantarflexion. The knee is slightly bent. **B,** Eccentric loading of the calf muscle with the knee slightly bent. **C,** Increasing the load by adding weight in a backpack. (Reprinted with permission from Öhberg L, Lorentzon R, Alfredson H: Eccentric training in patients with chronic Achilles tendinosis: Normalised tendon structure and decreased thickness at follow-up. Br J Sports Med 38:8–11, 2004. Figs. 1, 2, 4.)

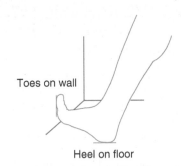

Toes on wall

Heel on floor

Fig. 44.6 Achilles "wall" calf stretch.

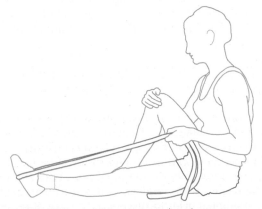

Fig. 44.7 Achilles resistance band exercises.

discomfort and no severe pain. A randomized controlled trial compared rest with eccentric training versus continued activity with eccentric training and found similar improvements in pain and function in both groups.

Other forms of eccentric exercise include wall calf stretches (Fig. 44.6), resistance band calf exercises (Fig. 44.7), and slant board stretches.

Jonsson et al. (2008) developed a modified eccentric exercise protocol for patients with insertional tendonitis in which the patient stands on the floor and performs a heel raise with the uninvolved leg, then all body weight is transferred to the involved leg. From this position, the patient slowly lowers the heel to floor level with no load with the ankle dorsiflexed. As in the standard protocol, when the exercises can be done without pain, weight is gradually added with a backpack (see Fig. 44.5). In a group of 27 patients (34 painful Achilles tendons) with an average age of 53 years (range, 25 to 77), 18 (67%) were satisfied with their results at 4-month follow-up and had returned to their previous activity levels.

Important Excerpts from Jospt Clinical Practice Guidelines for Achilles Pain, Stiffness, and Power Deficits: Achilles Tendinitis (Carcia et al. 2010)

1. Annual incidence of Achilles tendinopathy in runners has been reported to be 7% to 9%. The majority of patients suffering from Achilles tendinopathy are individuals engaged in recreational or competitive activity.
2. Athletes are more likely to become symptomatic during training rather than during competitive events.
3. There is an increased prevalence of Achilles injury as age increases. The mean age of those affected is reported to be between 30 and 50 years old.
4. The Achilles tendon undergoes morphologic and biomechanical changes with increasing age. Morphologic changes include decreased collagen diameter and density, decreased glycosaminoglycans and water content, and increased nonreducible cross-lengths. Biomechanically, the aging tendon has decreased tensile strength, linear stiffness, and ultimate load.
5. Acute irritation of healthy (nondegenerated) Achilles tendon has been associated with paratenon inflammation. More commonly, however, symptoms are chronic and associated with degenerated tendon. **Achilles tendinosis** appears to be noninflammatory and has been described as being of the lipoid or mucoid variety with regard to degeneration. *Lipoid degeneration* indicates fatty tissue deposited in the tissue. In *mucoid degeneration* the tendon takes on a grayish or brown color, which is mechanically softer. The degenerated Achilles tendon also exhibits signs of increased vascularization or neovascularization. This neovascularization has been observed to be accompanied by an ingrowth of nerve fascicles, which may in part be responsible for the pain associated with Achilles tendinopathy.
6. Level 1 studies have shown that **abnormal dorsiflexion range of motion,** either decreased or increased, has been associated with a higher incidence or risk of Achilles tendinopathy. Kaufman et al. (1999) found that less than 11.5 degrees of dorsiflexion, measured with the knee extended, increased the risk of developing Achilles tendinopathy by a factor of 3.5, when compared to those who exhibited between 11.5 degrees and 15 degrees of dorsiflexion.
7. Level 2 studies have found **abnormalities in subtalar range of motion** have been associated with Achilles tendinopathy.

Level 2 studies by McCrory et al. (1999) and Silbernagel et al. (2001) found **decreased plantarflexion strength** to be associated with Achilles pathology.

8. **Extrinsic risk factors** have been associated with Achilles tendinopathy including training errors, poor equipment, and environmental factors in several level 2 studies. Training errors in runners are cited as a sudden increase in mileage, an increase in intensity, hill training, returning from a layoff, or a combination of these factors.

9. Level 1 studies by Silbernagel et al. (2001) found a significant decrease in pain in patients treated with an **eccentric exercise regimen;** however, performance in toe raising and jumping did not improve with the eccentric group when compared to controls. The eccentric strengthening program was found to be superior **to low energy extracorporeal shock wave therapy (ESWT);** however, ESWT combined with the eccentric program was better than eccentric exercise alone.

10. Alfredson et al. (1998) had good success with a modified eccentric loading program consisting of unilateral eccentric heel raises with no concentric component. Exercises consisted of 3 sets of 15 repetitions, both with the knee extended and flexed, performed twice daily for 12 weeks. This eccentric training is thought to be beneficial because of its effect on improving microcirculation and peritendinous type I collagen synthesis (Knobloch 2007).

11. Surprisingly little evidence supports stretching to prevent or as an effective intervention for Achilles tendinopathy.

12. A recent systematic review with meta-analysis in which low-level laser therapy (LLLT) was used to treat nonregional specific tendinopathy revealed with class B evidence (moderate evidence) that clinicians should consider the use of LLLT to decrease pain and stiffness in patients with Achilles tendinopathy.

13. Carcia et al. (2010) also report class B (moderate evidence) efficacy of iontophoresis with dexamethasone to decrease pain and improve function in patients with Achilles tendinopathy.

OPERATIVE TREATMENT

Operative treatment rarely is indicated for Achilles tendinopathy unless it becomes chronic and debilitating. In patients with paratenonitis, operative treatment consists of débridement, lysis of adhesions, and excision of thickened portions of the paratenon. The thickened paratenon can be excised posteriorly, medially, and laterally around the tendon through a medial longitudinal incision. The anterior portion of the paratenon is avoided to protect the anteriorly derived blood supply to the Achilles tendon (Reddy et al. 2009). Schepsis et al. (1994) reported a satisfaction rate of 87% after operative treatment of 23 competitive or serious recreational runners with chronic paratenonitis. Endoscopic release of the constricting paratenon has been described and may reduce early postoperative morbidity (Maquirrian et al. 2002).

In approximately 25% of patients with tendinosis, nonoperative therapy fails to relieve symptoms and restore strength.

Operative treatment involves removal of the areas of degenerated tendon. Generally, if more than 50% to 75% of the tendon is involved, autogenous tendon transfer, most often the flexor hallucis longus (FHL), is recommended (Schepsis et al. 2002, Heckman et al. 2009). Older patients (>50 years of age) and those with severe degenerative tendon have worse results than younger patients with less tendon involvement. Den Hartog (2003) reported 88% good to excellent results in 26 patients with an average age of 51 years treated with FHL transfer, whereas Schepsis et al. (1994, 2002) reported only 67% satisfactory results in 66 patients, 53 of whom were competitive runners.

In patients with paratenonitis and tendinosis, earlier surgical treatment with débridement or tendon transfer may lead to earlier return of function (Nicholson et al. 2007).

For insertional tendinitis, excision of the retrocalcaneal bursa and posterior calcaneal ostectomy may be added to the operative treatment (McGarvey et al. 2002). Complete detachment and excision of the diseased Achilles insertion segment may be necessary, followed by a proximal V-Y lengthening and reattachment of the tendon with suture anchors (Wagner et al. 2006). Lengthy protection (12 weeks) is required after this procedure.

POSTOPERATIVE REHABILITATION PROGRESSION AFTER ACHILLES TENDON DÉBRIDEMENT

- Weight bearing is allowed when pain and swelling subside, usually in 7 to 10 days. In our institution we use progressively smaller felt heel lifts (Hapad, Inc., Bethel Park, PA) placed in a postoperative removable walking boot.
- Strengthening exercises are begun after 2 to 3 weeks.
- Running is begun at 6 to 10 weeks.
- Athletes usually can return to competition at 3 to 6 months.
- If tendon involvement was severe or a more complex procedure was done, return to play may take up to 12 months. After tendon transfer, immobilization is continued for 6 weeks after surgery.

OTHER TREATMENT MODALITIES FOR ACHILLES TENDINOPATHY

Other treatment modalities suggested for Achilles tendinopathy include platelet-rich plasma injection, sclerosing therapy, electrocoagulation, topical glyceryl trinitrate (GTN), aprotinin injections, extracorporeal shock wave therapy, and prolotherapy. Because of the potential morbidity and complications associated with surgical treatment, these modalities are often attempted prior to surgery in the face of recalcitrant Achilles tendinopathy. A recent Cochrane Database Review revealed inconclusive evidence and that few well-designed studies are available for review (Kearney, 2015). Larger studies with longer follow-up are needed to prove the benefits of these methods.

REHABILITATION PROTOCOL 44.1 ■ Treatment of Achilles Paratenonitis

Phase 1: 0–6 Weeks

- Rest and/or activity modification is required to reduce symptoms to a level that can achieve pain-free activity.
- If pain is severe, a walking boot or cast is worn for 3 to 8 weeks to allow pain-free activities of daily living.
- Crutch-assisted ambulation is added when there is persistent pain with boot or cast.
- Most patients have chronic pain that requires an initial period of complete rest until symptoms subside, followed by rehabilitation and gradual return to activities.
- NSAIDs and ice massage decrease pain and inflammation, particularly in the acute phase.
- A stretching program is essential. Gentle calf, Achilles, and hamstring stretching are done three to four times a day.
- Acute pain usually resolves in the first 2 weeks.
- Footwear is changed or modified if overpronation or poor hindfoot support is present.
- Athletic activity
  - Gradual return to activity
  - Adequate warmup and cooldown periods
  - Pre-exercise and postexercise stretching of gastrocnemius and soleus complex
  - Decrease duration and intensity.
  - Decrease training on hard surfaces.
  - Avoid hill and incline training.
  - Replace inadequate or worn out footwear.
- Progress to gentle strengthening using low-impact exercises.

Phase 2: 6–12 Weeks

- Indicated for failed phase 1 or recurrent symptoms after previous resolution.
- Repeat or continue phase 1 immobilization and stretching.
- Add modalities
  - Contrast baths
  - Ultrasound
- Footwear
  - Small heel lift for severe pain
  - Arch support orthotic if overpronation
- Persistent heel-cord tightness is treated with stretching exercises and use of a 5-degree dorsiflexion night ankle foot orthosis (AFO) worn for 3 months while sleeping.
- Staged cross-training program for most athletes, especially runners
- Aqua jogging and swimming, stationary cycling, exercise on stair climbing and cross-country skiing machines. Avoid repetitive impact loading (e.g., running).

Phase 3: 3 Months and Beyond

- Brisement (only for paratenonitis)
  - Dilute local anesthetic and sterile saline injected into the paratenon sheath to break up adhesion between the inflamed paratenon and the Achilles tendon (preferable to steroid injection). Can be done with ultrasound to confirm correct placement
- Corticosteroid injections
  - Generally avoided
  - Rarely indicated, only for recalcitrant cases to inhibit inflammation and prevent scar formation
  - Risk of adverse effects if injected into tendon or if overused is generally worse than any known benefit

REHABILITATION PROTOCOL 44.2 ■ General Guidelines for Achilles Tendonitis, Paratenonitis, and Tendinosis in High-Impact Athletes

S. Brent Brotzman, MD

- Establish correct diagnosis.
- **Correct underlying training and biomechanical problems.**
  - Stop rapid increase in mileage.
  - Stop hill running.
  - Correct improper intensity of training, duration, schedule, hard surface, and poor shoe wear.
  - Decrease mileage significantly and/or initiate cross-training (pool, bicycle) depending on severity of symptoms at presentation.
  - Correct functional overpronation and resultant vascular wringing of the tendon (Fig. 44.8) with a custom orthotic that usually incorporates a medial rear foot post.
  - Stop interval training.
- Soften a hard heel counter or use shoe counter heel cushions to minimize posterior "rubbing" symptoms.
- Begin a dynamic runner's stretching program before and after exercises.
- Oral anti-inflammatories (over-the-counter or COX2 inhibitors).
- **Avoid cortisone injection; this will cause weakening or rupture of the tendon.**
- Cryotherapy (ice massage) after exercise for anti-inflammatory effect.
- Correct leg-length discrepancy if noted. First try 1/4-inch heel insert for a 1/2-inch leg-length discrepancy; if not improved, go to 1/2-inch insert. "Overcorrection" (too rapid an orthotic correction of a leg-length discrepancy) may worsen symptoms.
- If symptoms persist after 4–6 weeks of conservative measures, immobilization in a removable cam boot or cast may be required for 3–6 weeks.
- Slow, painless progression to preinjury activities
  - Swimming
  - Deep-water "running" with Aquajogger.com flotation belt
  - Bicycling
  - Walking
  - Eccentric exercises for Achilles strengthening
  - Light jogging
- Eccentric strengthening of Achilles tendon should condition the tendon and make it less susceptible to overuse injuries; however, these exercises are not used until the patient is asymptomatic and pain free for 2–3 weeks; often used in the off-season
  - Heel raises in pool
  - Plantarflexion against progressively harder Therabands
  - Multiple sets of very light (20-pound) total gym or slider board exercises (Fig. 44.9; See also Figure 39-18)

Continued

REHABILITATION PROTOCOL 44.2 ■ General Guidelines for Achilles Tendonitis, Paratenonitis, and Tendinosis in High-Impact Athletes—cont'd

S. Brent Brotzman, MD

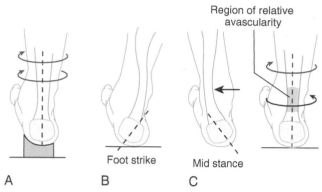

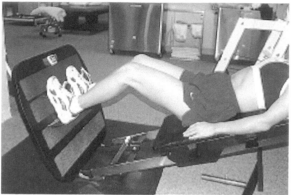

Fig. 44.8 **A,** Correction of functional overpronation by a medial rearfoot post minimizes the potential for postulated vascular wringing. **B,** Whipping action of the Achilles tendon produced by overpronation. **C,** External tibial rotation produced by knee extension conflicting with internal tibial rotation produced by prolonged pronation. This results in "wringing out" of vessels in the zone of relative avascularity. (From Clement DB, Taunton JF, Smart GW: Achilles tendinitis and peritendinitis: Etiology and treatment. Am J Sports Med 12(3):181, 1984.)

Fig. 44.9 Slider board or total gym exercises for Achilles tendon strengthening.

REFERENCES

A complete reference list is available at https://expertconsult.inkling.com/.

FURTHER READING

Freedman BR, Gordon JA, Soslowsky LJ. The Achilles tendon: fundamental properties and mechanisms governing healing. *Muscles Ligaments Tendons J. Jul 14.* 2014;4(2):245–255.

Kader D, Saxena A, Movin T, et al. Achilles tendinopathy: some aspects of basic science and clinical management. *Br J Sports Med.* 2002;36(4):239–249.

Maffulli N, Via AG, Oliva F. Chronic Achilles tendon disorders: tendinopathy and chronic rupture. *Clin Sports Med.* 2015;34(4):607–624.

Ohberg L, Alfredson H. Effects on neovascularisation behind the good results with eccentric training in chronic mid-portion Achilles tendinosis? *Knee Surg Sports Traumatol Arthrosc.* 2004;12(5):465–470.

Silbernagel KG, Gustavsson A, Thomee R, et al. Evaluation of lower leg function in patients with Achilles tendinopathy. *Knee Surg Sports Traumatol Arthrosc.* 2006;14:1207–1217.

Achilles Tendon Rupture

John J. Jasko, MD | S. Brent Brotzman, MD | Charles E. Giangarra, MD

BACKGROUND

The incidence of Achilles tendon rupture has increased dramatically in the past 50 years. The advent and popularity of recreational sports have contributed to this, because 75% of ruptures are sports related. The peak incidence occurs between 30 and 45 years of age, with a male-to-female ratio of 6:1 (Hansen et al. 2016).

The impact of these injuries in athletes is highlighted by the report of Parekh et al. in which 10 of 31 professional football players with Achilles tendon ruptures were unable to return to play in the National Football League (Parekh et al. 2009).

Acute ruptures commonly occur when pushing off with the weightbearing foot while extending the knee, but they also can be caused by a sudden or violent dorsiflexion of a plantarflexed foot (eccentric contracture). Most Achilles tendon ruptures occur approximately 2 to 6 cm proximal to its insertion on the calcaneus, in the so-called "watershed" region of reduced vascularity. Patients should also be questioned about previous steroid injection and fluoroquinolone treatment (e.g., Levaquin or ciprofloxacin) for association with tendon weakening and increased rupture risk.

CLINICAL SIGNS AND SYMPTOMS

Sharp pain and a pop heard at the time of complete rupture are commonly reported. Patients often describe a sensation of being kicked in the Achilles tendon. Most have an immediate inability to bear weight or return to activity. A palpable defect may be present in the tendon initially.

Partial rupture is associated with an acutely tender, localized swelling that occasionally involves an area of nodularity.

The Thompson test (Fig. 44.2) is positive with complete Achilles tendon rupture. The patient is placed prone, with both feet extended off the end of the table. Both calf muscles are squeezed by the examiner. If the tendon is intact, the foot will plantar flex when the calf is squeezed. If the tendon is ruptured, normal plantarflexion will not occur (a positive Thompson test).

In some patients, an accurate diagnosis of a complete rupture is difficult through physical examination alone. The tendon defect can be disguised by a large hematoma. A false-negative Thompson test result can occur because of plantarflexion of the ankle caused by extrinsic foot flexors when the accessory ankle flexors are squeezed together with the contents at the superficial posterior leg compartment. It is important to critically compare the test with results in the normal side.

Partial ruptures are also difficult to accurately diagnose, and MRI should be used to confirm the diagnosis.

TREATMENT OF ACUTE RUPTURE OF THE ACHILLES TENDON

Both nonoperative and operative treatment can be used to restore length and tension to the tendon to optimize strength and function. Both methods are reasonable, and treatment should be individualized based on operative candidacy. The patient's overall health, vascular status, and activity level are considered. Traditionally, younger patients and athletes have been treated with operative repair. A main reason for this is that studies have shown that operative repair has been associated with lower rerupture rates, more frequent return to athletic activities, quicker return to full activity, and greater plantarflexion strength (Heckman et al. 2009, Khan et al. 2005).

Khan et al., in a meta-analysis of randomized trials comparing surgical and conservative management, found rerupture rates of 3.5% in the operative group and 12.6% in the nonoperative group as well as significant weakness in the nonoperative group (Khan et al. 2005). However, many of these studies used prolonged immobilization and limited weight bearing as part of the nonoperative treatment. More recent studies have found improved function in both treatment groups when early mobilization and weight bearing have been utilized (Willits et al. 2010, Nilsson-Helander et al. 2010).

In a level 1 study, Nilsson-Helander and Silbernagel's protocol included functional bracing rather than casting in both groups (Nilsson-Helander et al. 2010). They still found a higher rerupture rate in the nonsurgical group (12% to 4%), but at 12 months the only functional difference was the heel raise in favor of the surgical group. Other recent studies, such as the randomized prospective trial by Willits et al. have shown no significant functional differences or rerupture rates between operative and nonoperative groups when early mobilization and weight bearing have been utilized in both treatment groups (Willits et al. 2010, Twaddle and Poon 2007).

Thus, there are still conflicting reports regarding surgery vs. no surgery, but after that initial decision, there is more of a consensus that accelerated rehab, early ROM, and early weight bearing are the best approaches. It is important to point out that operative treatment consistently has higher complication rates. However, complication rates have decreased with the use of smaller incisions, percutaneous techniques, and better patient selection.

NONOPERATIVE TREATMENT OF ACUTE ACHILLES TENDON RUPTURE

Nonoperative treatment requires temporary immobilization to allow hematoma consolidation. Prolonged immobilization, as mentioned above, is counterproductive to functional healing. In a meta-analysis of randomized controlled trials, Khan found that cast immobilization resulted in a rerupture rate of 12%, compared to 2% with functional bracing (Khan et al. 2005). Complications such as adhesions and infection also were more common in the cast immobilization group (36%) than in the functional bracing group (10%). Thus we use functional bracing rather than casting.

Ultrasound serial examinations can be helpful to confirm that Achilles tendon end apposition occurs with 20 degrees or less of plantarflexion of the foot. If a significant gap remains with the leg placed in 20 degrees of plantarflexion, we still favor operative treatment in young, healthy patients.

After the initial 2-week period of casting in equinus, the patient is transitioned to an articulating removable cast boot locked in 20 degrees of plantarflexion. Alternatively, a nonarticulating boot can be used with a 2-cm heel lift that approximates the 20-degree plantarflexion position. Active dorsiflexion to neutral with passive plantarflexion is begun. We previously delayed motion and weight bearing until 4 weeks for nonoperative patients. However, with the efficacy and safety shown by Willits et al. and others using accelerated protocols, we now use the same protocol for nonoperative and operative treatment of acute tears after the initial 2 weeks.

See Rehabilitation Protocol 45.1 for nonoperative management of an Achilles rupture.

OPERATIVE TREATMENT FOR ACUTE ACHILLES TENDON RUPTURE

Various operative techniques have been described for Achilles tendon repair, ranging from simple end-to-end Bunnell or Kessler suturing to more complex repairs using fascial reinforcement or tendon grafts, artificial tendon implants, and augmentation with the plantaris tendon or gastrocnemius (Fig. 45.1). In a prospective randomized study, Pajala et al. found that augmentation with a gastrocnemius turn-down technique had no advantage over simple end-to-end repair (Pajala et al. 2009).

Percutaneous, endoscopically assisted, and mini-open techniques have been developed to speed recovery and improve cosmetic results. Most studies have found lower complication rates with no increase in rerupture rates with percutaneous techniques (Deangelis et al. 2009, Gigante et al. 2008). Percutaneous repair also has been shown to be less costly than open repair (Ebinesan et al. 2008).

REHABILITATION AFTER OPERATIVE TREATMENT OF ACUTE ACHILLES TENDON RUPTURE

Historically, patients were immobilized in a rigid cast for at least 4 weeks after operative repair of Achilles tendon rupture; however, current trends emphasize minimal postoperative immobilization and early weight bearing (see Rehabilitation Protocol 45.2). A number of studies have confirmed that physical activity speeds tendon healing, and rerupture rates have not been significantly higher with early weight bearing. A meta-analysis of randomized trials comparing early weight bearing with cast immobilization found no difference in rerupture rates and better subjective outcomes with early weight bearing (Suchak et al. 2008).

Early functional treatment protocols, when compared to postoperative immobilization, led to more excellent rated subjective responses and no difference in rerupture rated in Suchak et al.'s meta-analysis.

Strom and Casillas outlined five goals of the rehabilitation program after repair of Achilles tendon rupture (Strom 2009).
1. Reduce residual pain and swelling. Modalities may include massage, ice, differential compression, graduated compression garment, contrast baths, and electrical stimulation.
2. Recover motion while preserving integrity of the repair. Clinical findings are used to guide the amount of tension placed on the repair. Warmup, including massage and deep heat, is done before and during stretching to improve dorsiflexion. Isolated stretching of the gastrocnemius muscles and the soleus–Achilles are done with the knee extended (gastrocnemius) or flexed (soleus–Achilles).
3. Strengthen the gastrocnemius–soleus–Achilles motor unit. This involves a graduated program of resistance strengthening using elastic bands and closed chain exercises (seated calf pumps, bipedal calf pumps, single-leg calf pumps, single-leg calf pumps on a balance board or trampoline).
4. Improve the strength and coordination of the entire lower extremity. Swimming, water jogging, and exercise cycling are added to the strengthening program.
5. Provide a safe and competitive return to athletic activity that avoids rerupture. Cross-training with cycle- and water-based activities are added to promote aerobic recovery and promote coordinated motor activity in both lower extremities.

Traditionally, postoperative treatment of surgically repaired Achilles tendon rupture included prolonged immobilization with the ankle in plantarflexion. This was thought to decrease the tensile stress across the repair site. However, Labib et al. measured the static tension in the Achilles tendon at varying degrees of plantarflexion before and after surgical repair (with a number 2 Krakow locking technique reinforced with 4.0

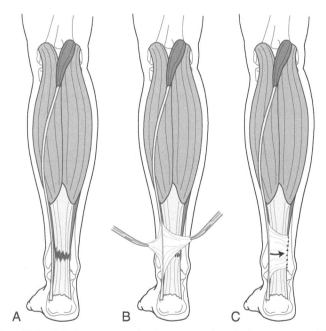

Fig. 45.1   Reinforcement with plantaris tendon. **A,** Rupture. **B,** Achilles tendon is repaired, and plantaris tendon is divided and fanned. **C,** Plantaris tendon is used to reinforce repair.

monofilament) (Labib et al. 2007). They found that static tension in the repaired Achilles tendon was equal to that of the intact tendon in all positions of plantarflexion. This study suggests that long-term positioning of the ankle in plantarflexion after secure surgical repair of a ruptured Achilles is probably not necessary.

CHRONIC ACHILLES TENDON RUPTURE

The diagnosis of chronic Achilles tendon rupture is more difficult than diagnosis of an acute rupture. The pain and swelling often have subsided and the gap between the tendon ends has filled in with fibrous tissue (Maffulli and Ajis 2008).

Weak active plantarflexion may be possible through the action of other muscles, further complicating accurate diagnosis. A limp often is present, and the calf muscles are typically atrophied. The Thompson squeeze test usually only has a flicker of plantarflexion on squeezing the calf, which is asymmetric compared to the uninvolved calf. Ultrasonography and MRI are useful to confirm the diagnosis.

Chronic Achilles tendon ruptures usually require operative reconstruction of the soft tissue defect, which may include soft tissue augmentation, V-Y advancement flaps, or local tendon transfers. The Myerson classification system provides guidelines for management (Myerson 1999) (see Table 45.1).

The chronicity and complexity of the reconstruction and repair will dictate any changes to the standard functional rehabilitation protocol that is used for acute tears. Those requiring tendon transfers, turndowns, or allograft may require a longer initial period of casting, typically 3 weeks, prior to starting ROM and weight bearing. Rehabilitation then proceeds as in acute tears/repairs. Overall progression to subsequent phases in rehab is usually prolonged with chronic tears, and full recovery can take as long as 9 to 12 months (Maffulli and Ajis 2008).

RETURN TO SPORTS RECOMMENDATIONS AFTER ACHILLES RUPTURE

Return to competitive and recreational sports is common after recovery and rehabilitation of Achilles tendon ruptures. Studies show ranges of 75% to 100% return to previous level of participation (Jallageas et al. 2013).

Time to return averages 5 to 7 months, so patience must be stressed to the athlete. The Achilles Tendon Total Rupture Score (ATRS) at 3 months can predict patients' ability to return to sport (Hansen 2016).

Most strength and functional gains occur between 3 and 6 months, but improvement can continue up until one year post injury, although some slight permanent strength deficit compared to the normal leg is not uncommon (Carmont et al. 2013).

TABLE 45.1	Myerson Classification (Chronic Achilles Rupture)	
Type	**Defect**	**Management**
I	≤1–2 cm	End-to-end repair, posterior compartment fasciotomy
II	2–5 cm	V-Y lengthening, with or without tendon transfer
III	>5 cm	Tendon transfer, with or with V-Y advancement

REHABILITATION PROTOCOL 45.1 ● **Protocol for Nonoperative Management of an Achilles Rupture**

Initial evaluation/ requirement for inclusion	Ultrasound or MRI exam showing <5-mm gap with maximal plantarflexion, <10 mm with foot in neutral, or >75% tendon apposition with foot in 20 degrees of plantarflexion
Initial management	Cast with foot in full equinus, NWB with crutches or walker
2–6 weeks	Transition to removable cast boot: If hinged, place in 20 degrees plantarflexion; not hinged (flat): 2-cm heel wedge to approximate 20 degrees plantarflexion WBAT in boot; use crutches with boot until no pain or limp Active dorsiflexion to neutral, inversion/eversion below neutral, no resistance Modalities to control swelling Hip/knee exercises as appropriate Hydrotherapy: NWB, adhere to motion restrictions Wear boot all times except for bathing (NWB) or exercises
6–8 weeks	Removable cast boot at neutral; remove heel wedge Wear boot all times except for bathing or exercises WBAT in boot, wean off crutches Dorsiflexion stretching, slowly Graduated resistance exercises (open and closed kinetic chain as well as functional activities); Dual support heel raises During supervised PT, start balance proprioceptive exercises, stationary bike, elliptical trainer in regular shoe Hydrotherapy with underwater treadmill

Continued

REHABILITATION PROTOCOL 45.1 ⬛ **Protocol for Nonoperative Management of an Achilles Rupture—cont'd**

8–12 weeks	Remove boot.
	1-cm heel lift in shoe
	Continue to progress ROM, strength, proprioception
12 weeks	Continue to progress ROM, strength, proprioception
	Retrain strength, power, endurance
	Increase dynamic weightbearing exercise, include plyometric training
	Sport-specific retraining

MRI, magnetic resonance imaging; *NWB*, nonweight bearing; *WBAT*, weight bearing as tolerated.
Adapted From: Willits K, Ammendola A, Fowler, P et al. Operative vs. Nonoperative Treatment of Acute Achilles Tendon Ruptures, *JBJS* 92:2767-75, 2010.

REHABILITATION PROTOCOL 45.2 ⬛ **Rehabilitation After Repair of Acute Achilles Tendon Rupture**

Initial management	Postoperative splint in equinus; NWB with crutches or walker
2–6 weeks	Transition to removable cast boot: If hinged, place in 20 degrees plantarflexion; not hinged (flat): 2-cm heel wedge to approximate 20 degrees plantarflexion
	WBAT in boot; use crutches with boot until no pain or limp
	Active dorsiflexion to neutral, inversion/eversion below neutral, no resistance
	Modalities to control swelling
	Hip/knee exercises as appropriate
	Hydrotherapy: NWB, adhere to motion restrictions
	Wear boot all times except for bathing (NWB) or exercises
6–8 weeks	Removable cast boot at neutral; remove heel wedge
	Wear boot all times except for bathing or exercises
	WBAT in boot, wean off crutches
	Dorsiflexion stretching, slowly
	Graduated resistance exercises (open and closed kinetic chain as well as functional activities); Dual support heel raises
	During supervised PT, start balance proprioceptive exercises, stationary bike, elliptical trainer in regular shoe
	Hydrotherapy with underwater treadmill
8–12 weeks	Remove boot.
	1-cm heel lift in shoe
	Continue to progress ROM, strength, proprioception
12 weeks	Continue to progress ROM, strength, proprioception
	Retrain strength, power, endurance
	Increase dynamic weightbearing exercise, include plyometric training
	Sport-specific retraining

MRI, magnetic resonance imaging; *NWB*, nonweight bearing; *WBAT*, weight bearing as tolerated.
Adapted From: Willits K, Ammendola A, Fowler, P et al. Operative vs. Nonoperative Treatment of Acute Achilles Tendon Ruptures. *JBJS* 92:2767-75, 2010.

REFERENCES

A complete reference list is available at https://expertconsult .inkling.com/.

FURTHER READING

Gigante A, Moschini A, Verdenelli A, et al. Open versus percutaneous repair in the treatment of acute Achilles tendon rupture: a randomized prospective study. *Knee Surg Sports Traumatol Arthrosc.* 2008;16:204–209.

Hansen MS, Christensen M, Budolfsen T, et al. Achilles tendon Total Rupture Score at 3 months can predict patients' ability to return to sport 1 year after injury. *Knee Surg Sports Traumatol Arthrosc.* 2016;24:1365–1371.

Heikkinen J, Lantto I, Flinkkilä T, et al. Augmented compared with nonaugmented surgical repair after total Achilles rupture: results of a prospective randomized trial with thirteen or more years of follow-up. *J Bone Joint Surg Am.* 2016;98(2):85–92.

Hufner TM, Brandes DB, Thermann H, et al. Long-term results after functional nonoperative treatment of Achilles tendon rupture. *Foot Ankle Int.* 2006;27:167–171.

Metz R, Verleisdonk EJ, van der Heijden GJ, et al. Acute Achilles tendon rupture: minimally invasive surgery versus nonoperative treatment with immediate full weightbearing—a randomized, controlled trial. *Am J Sports Med.* 2008;36:1688–1694.

Suchak AA, Spooner C, Reid DC, et al. Postoperative rehabilitation protocols for Achilles tendon ruptures: a meta-analysis. *Clin Orthop Relat Res.* 2006;445:216–221.

Willits K, Ammendola A, Fowler P, et al. Operative vs. nonoperative treatment of acute Achilles tendon ruptures. *JBJS.* 2010;92:2767–2775.

First Metatarsophalangeal Joint Sprain (Turf Toe)

Mark M. Casillas, MD | Margaret Jacobs, PT

Turf toe describes a range of injuries to the capsuloligamentous complex of the first MTP joint. The first MTP joint ROM is variable. The neutral position is described by 0 (or 180) degrees of angulation between a line through the first metatarsal and a line through the hallux. Dorsiflexion, the ROM above the neutral position, varies between 60 and 100 degrees. Plantarflexion, the ROM below the neutral position, varies between 10 and 40 degrees. The ROM is noncrepitant and pain free in the uninjured joint.

The power to move the MTP joint is provided by both intrinsic (flexor hallucis brevis, extensor hallucis brevis, abductor hallucis, adductor hallucis) and extrinsic (flexor hallucis longus, extensor hallucis longus) muscle groups. Two sesamoid bones—medial (or tibial) sesamoid and lateral (or fibular) sesamoid—provide mechanical advantage to the intrinsic plantar flexors by increasing the distance between the empirical center of joint rotation and the respective tendons (Fig. 46.1). The sesamoid complex articulates with facets on the plantar aspect of the first metatarsal head and is stabilized by a plantar capsule (plantar plate) and a ridge (or crista) on the metatarsal head that separates the two sesamoids.

The mechanism of the first MTP joint sprain is forced dorsiflexion of the MTP joint (Fig. 46.2). The typical football-associated injury occurs when a player firmly plants his forefoot and is then struck from behind. The continued forward motion of the leg over the fixed forefoot produces hyperdorsiflexion of the first MTP joint and increased tension on the plantar plate and capsule. Taken to an extreme, these forces may continue and produce a dorsal impaction injury to the cartilage and bone of the metatarsal head.

The extreme motion required to produce an acute injury is more likely to occur in an overly flexible shoe as opposed to a relatively stiff-soled shoe. The playing surface has also been implicated as an associated factor. The hard playing surface of an artificial turf field may result in an increased incidence of first MTP joint sprain—hence the term "turf toe." A chronic, cumulative injury mechanism is associated with similar risk factors.

The mechanism of injury for a first MTP joint sprain is by no means specific. A multitude of afflictions to the first MTP joint and its contiguous structures must be ruled out (Table 46.1).

Table 46.2 provides information on acute first metatarsophalangeal joint sprain classification.

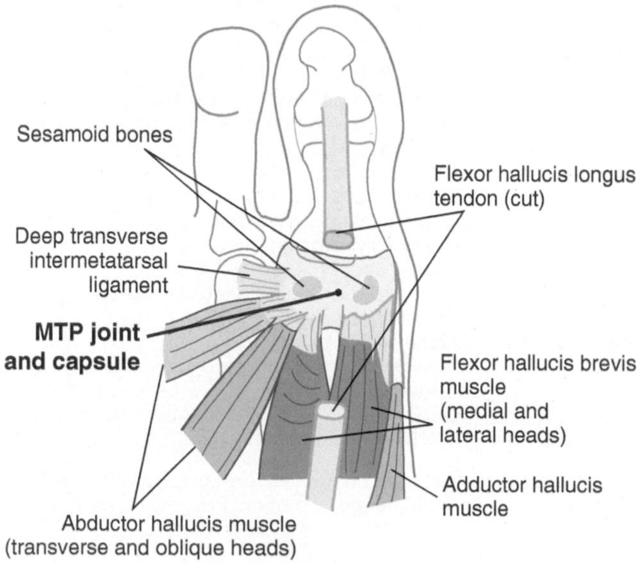

SIGNS AND SYMPTOMS

First MTP joint sprains are associated with acute localized pain, swelling, ecchymosis, and guarding. Increasing degrees of swelling, pain, and loss of joint motion are noted as the severity of the injury increases. An antalgic gait and a tendency to avoid loading of the first ray by foot supination may be present.

RADIOGRAPHIC EVALUATION

The standard radiographic evaluation includes AP and lateral views of the weightbearing foot and a sesamoid projection. The diagnosis is confirmed on the MRI when capsular tears and associated edema are demonstrated. Bone scan, CT, and MRI may be used to rule out sesamoid avascular necrosis, sesamoid fracture, sesamoid stress injury, hallux MTP joint arthrosis, metatarsal–sesamoid arthrosis, or stenosing flexor tenosynovitis.

Typical findings in patients with turf toe injuries from a physical examination include the following:
- First MTP joint swelling
- Ecchymosis adjacent to the area of capsular injury
- Plantar tenderness at the MTP joint
- Pain with passive MTP joint dorsiflexion
- Pain with joint loading (walking, push-off, crouching with the MTP joint extended)
- Decreased dorsiflexion of the MTP joint
- Vertical instability of first MTP (positive "Lachman" exam of the toe)

Fig. 46.1 Anatomy of the MTP joint, which is affected in a turf toe injury. The tendons of the flexor hallucis brevis, adductor hallucis, and abductor hallucis muscles combine with the deep transverse metatarsal ligaments to form the fibrocartilaginous plate on the plantar aspect of the MTP joint capsule. The two sesamoid bones are contained within the fibrocartilaginous plate.

Labels in figure:
Sesamoid bones
Flexor hallucis longus tendon (cut)
Deep transverse intermetatarsal ligament
MTP joint and capsule
Flexor hallucis brevis muscle (medial and lateral heads)
Adductor hallucis muscle
Abductor hallucis muscle (transverse and oblique heads)

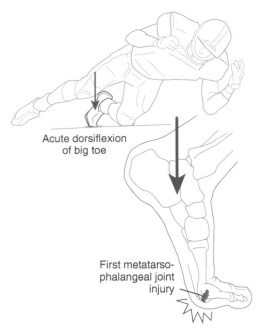

Fig. 46.2 Mechanism of injury for turf toe is acute dorsiflexion of the first metatarsophalangeal joint. (From Miller MD, Cooper DE, Warner JJP: Review of sports medicine and arthroscopy. Philadelphia, WB Saunders, 2002.)

TABLE 46.1	Pathology of the First Metatarsophalangeal Joint	
Differential Diagnosis	**Significant Findings**
First MTP joint sprain (turf toe)	Acute or chronic injury Tender MTP joint Limited motion
Hallux fracture	Acute injury Tenderness isolated to MTP or phalanx Fracture seen on radiograph, bone scan, CT, or MRI
Hallux dislocation	Acute injury Severe deformity on examination, verified by radiograph
Hallux rigidus	Chronic condition Limited dorsiflexion, painful ROM Dorsal metatarsal osteophyte on lateral radiograph
Hallux arthrosis (arthritic first MTP joint)	Chronic condition Painful and limited ROM Loss of joint space on radiograph
Sesamoid fracture	Acute injury Tenderness isolated to sesamoid Fracture seen on radiograph, bone scan, CT, or MRI
Sesamoid stress fracture	Chronic injury Tenderness isolated to sesamoid Stress fracture seen on radiograph, bone scan, CT, or MRI
Sesamoid nonunion	Acute or chronic injury Tenderness isolated to sesamoid Nonunion seen on radiograph, bone scan, CT, or MRI
Bipartite sesamoid	Congenital lack of fusion of the two ossicles of the sesamoid, leaving a radiolucent line (cartilage) between the two ossicles, often mistaken for a fracture Nontender to palpation, asymptomatic Comparison radiographs of the opposite foot may reveal a similar bipartite (bilateral) sesamoid High incidence of bilaterality with bipartite sesamoids, so take a comparison radiograph to differentiate bipartite from a sesamoid fracture
Sesamoid arthrosis	Acute or chronic injury Painful ROM Tenderness isolated to sesamoid Arthrosis seen on radiograph, bone scan, CT, or MRI
Sesamoid avascular necrosis	Acute or chronic injury Tenderness isolated to sesamoid Fragmentation seen on radiograph, CT, or MRI
Stenosing flexor tenosynovitis	Overuse syndrome Trigger phenomenon Painful flexor hallucis longus excursion Tenosynovitis seen on MRI
Gout	Acute severe pain Tenderness, erythema, and joint irritability localized to first MTP Often elevated uric acid, sodium urate crystals on aspiration of joint

MTP, metatarsophalangeal; CT, computed tomography; MRI, magnetic resonance imaging; ROM, range of motion; FHL, flexor hallucis longus.

Typical findings in patients with turf toe injuries from a radiographic examination include the following:

- Soft tissue swelling
- Small periarticular bony avulsions
- Intra-articular loose bodies
- Diastasis of bipartite sesamoid
- Sesamoid fracture
- Migration of the sesamoids*

TREATMENT

Acute injuries are treated with the RICE (rest, ice, compression, elevation) method followed by a gentle ROM program and protected weight bearing. Taping is not advised for an acute injury because it may compromise circulation. The use of a walking boot or short leg cast with toe spica extension in slight plantarflexion will help protect the hallux from extension at the MTP joint and allows the athlete to bear weight as tolerated. Gentle ROM exercises can begin as early as 3 to 5 days after injury if symptoms permit. With the toe protected with a boot or toe spica taping, low-impact exercises can be attempted, but explosive, push-off activities should not be tried until low-impact exercises and jogging can be done pain free and 50 to 60 degrees of painless passive dorsiflexion of the hallux MTP is possible.

Chronic injuries are treated with a ROM program and protected weight bearing. The hallux MTP joint is supported by a variety of methods including walking cast, removable walking cast, rigid shoe modifications, rigid shoe inserts, stiff-soled shoes, and various taping methods (Fig. 46.3). The joint is also protected by reducing activity levels, increasing rest intervals and duration, and avoiding rigid playing surfaces. NSAIDs and ice are used as adjuncts to reduce inflammation. Intra-articular steroids are of no benefit and may be detrimental to the joint.

Operative treatment is rare for most isolated first MTP joint sprains. A grade 3 injury with plantar plate disruption and

*Adapted from Klein SE. Conditions of the forefoot. In: DeLee JC, Drez D Jr, Miller MD (eds.). *DeLee & Drez's Orthopaedic Sports Medicine: Principles and Practice*, 3rd ed. Philadelphia: Elsevier, 2010, pp. 2081–2087.

TABLE 46.2	Acute First Metatarsophalangeal (MTP) Joint Sprain Classification		
Grade	Description/Findings	Treatment	Return to Play
I	Attenuation of plantar structures Localized swelling Minimal ecchymosis	Symptomatic	Return as tolerated
II	Partial tear of plantar structures Moderate swelling Restricted motion because of pain	Walking boot Crutches as needed	Up to 2 weeks May need taping on return to play
III	Complete disruption of plantar structures Significant swelling/ecchymosis Hallux flexion weakness Frank instability of hallux MTP	Long-term immobilization in boot or cast OR Surgical reconstruction	6 to 10 weeks depending on sport and position Likely to need taping on return to play

Adapted from Anderson RB, Shawen SB: Great-toe disorders. In Porter DA, Schon LC (eds.). Baxter's the foot and ankle in sport, 2nd edition. Philadelphia, 2007, Elsevier Health Sciences, pp. 411–433.

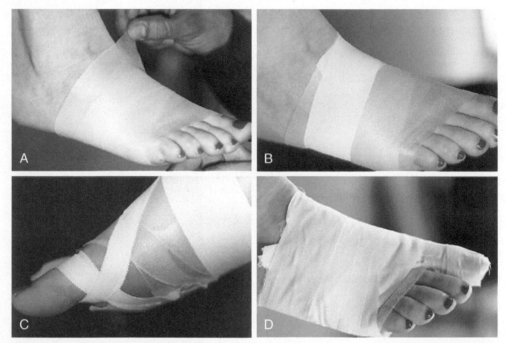

Fig. 46.3 Dorsiflexion-limiting taping method: underwrap (*A*), base or foundation (*B*), 1-inch strips crossing on the plantar side of the joint (*C*), and the circumferential cover to complete and secure the tape (*D*).

proximal migration of the sesamoids may warrant surgical intervention.

Prevention of turf toe includes the use of supportive footwear (with avoidance of overly flexible shoe forefoot) and firm inserts and avoidance of hard playing surfaces (e.g., Astroturf) when possible.

REHABILITATION FOR TURF TOE

Fundamental to the protocol (Rehabilitation Protocol 46.1) is the prevention of recurrent injury by limiting hallux MTP dorsiflexion with appropriate shoe wear, taping, or rigid shoe inserts. Taping is useful but is limited by time-related failure and the poor results associated with self-application. Off-the-shelf devices, such as steel leaf plates and low-profile carbon fiber inserts, are readily available. Custom devices may be used for difficult sizes or specialty shoe wear. The phases of rehabilitation are variable in length and depend completely on the re-establishment of ROM and resolution of pain. Flexibility is emphasized throughout the protocol.

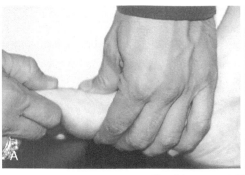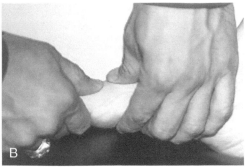

Fig. 46.4 First MTP joint mobilization.

REHABILITATION PROTOCOL 46.1 ▪ Treatment of Turf Toe

Phase 1: Acute Phase—Days 0–5

- Rest, ice bath, contrast bath, whirlpool bath, and ultrasound for pain, inflammation, and joint stiffness
- Joint mobilization (Fig. 46.4) followed by gentle, passive, and active range of motion (ROM)
- Isometrics around the metatarsophalangeal joint as pain allows
- Cross-training activities, such as water activities and cycling, for aerobic fitness
- Protective taping and shoe modifications for continued weight-bearing activities

Phase 2: Subacute Phase—Weeks 1–6

- Modalities to decrease inflammation and joint stiffness
- Emphasis on increasing flexibility and ROM, with both passive and active methods and joint mobilization
- Progressive strengthening
- Towel scrunches
- Toe pick-up activities
  - Manual resistive hallux MTP dorsiflexion and plantarflexion
  - Seated toe and ankle dorsiflexion with progression to standing
  - Seated isolated toe dorsiflexion with progression to standing
  - Seated supination–pronation with progression to standing
- Balance activities, with progression of difficulty to include biomechanical ankle platform system (BAPS) (Fig. 46.5)
- Cross-training activities (slide board, water running, cycling) to maintain aerobic fitness

Phase 3: Return-to-Sport Phase—Week 7

- Continued use of protective inserts or taping
- Continued ROM and strength exercises
- Running, to progress within limits of a pain-free schedule
- Monitored plyometric and cutting program, with progression of difficulty

Care should be taken to avoid re-injury during these activities.

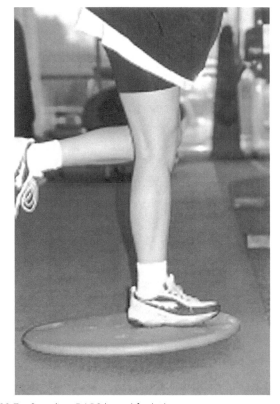

Fig. 46.5 Standing BAPS board for balance.

FURTHER READING

Bowers Jr KD, Martin RB. Turf-toe: a shoe-surface related football injury. *Med Sci Sports Exerc.* 1976;8:81.

Faltus J, Mullenix K, Moorman 3rd CT, et al. Case series of first metatarsophalangeal joint injuries in division 1 college athletes. *Sports Health.* 2014;6(6):519–526.

Mason LW, Molloy AP. Turf toe and disorders of the sesamoid complex. *Clin Sports Med.* 2015;34(4):725–739.

McCormick JJ, Anderson RB. Rehabilitation following turf toe injury and plantar plate repair. *Clin Sports Med.* 2009;29:313–334.

SECTION 5

Knee Injuries

47

Anterior Cruciate Ligament Injuries

S. Brent Brotzman, MD

BACKGROUND

The anterior cruciate ligament (ACL) is the most frequently completely disrupted ligament in the knee; most of these injuries occur in athletes (Fig. 47.1). More than 100,000 ACL reconstructions are done each year in the United States.

About 80% of sports-related ACL tears are noncontact injuries, occurring during pivoting maneuvers or landing from a jump. Noncontact ACL injuries are more common in females than in males (see section on ACL injuries in female athletes). *Only 60,000 individuals with ACL deficiency actually undergo reconstruction annually.*

Hewett et al. (2005) in a level II study found that prescreened female athletes with subsequent ACL injury demonstrated increased **dynamic knee valgus** (Fig. 47.2) and high knee abduction loads on **landing from a jump.** Knee abduction moments, which directly contribute to lower extremity dynamic valgus and joint knee load, had a sensitivity of 78% and specificity of 73% for predicting future ACL injury. Neuromuscular training has been shown to decrease knee adduction moments at the knee (Hewitt et al. 1996), and this will be addressed at great length in the ensuing chapter.

Although the natural history of the **ACL-deficient knee** has not been clearly defined, it is known that ACL injury often results in long-term problems, such as subsequent meniscal injuries, failure of secondary stabilizers, and development of **osteoarthritis** (OA).

Although a number of studies have suggested that OA eventually develops in 60% to 90% of individuals with ACL injuries (Beynnon 2005 Part 1, Andersson et al. 2009), a recent systematic review of the literature (Øiestad et al. 2009) concerning OA of the tibiofemoral joint more than 10 years after ACL injury suggests that these estimates are too high. The lack of a universal methodologic radiographic classification made it difficult to draw firm conclusions, but these investigators determined that in the highest-rated studies the reported prevalence of knee OA after isolated ACL injury was between 0% and 13%, and with meniscal injury, it was between 21% and 48% (level II evidence).

Associated meniscal injury is the most commonly cited factor contributing to the development of OA after ACL injury, followed by articular cartilage injuries. A 7-year prospective study of patients with reconstruction of an acute ACL injury found that 66% of those with concomitant meniscectomy developed OA, compared to only 11% of those without meniscal injury (Jomha et al. 1999). Subjective follow-up of 928 patients 5 to 15 years after ACL reconstruction found normal or nearly normal knees in 87% of patients with both menisci present, compared to 63% of those with partial or total meniscectomies (Shelbourne and Gray 2000). Of 54 National Football League players who had meniscectomy or ACL reconstruction or both, those with both procedures had shorter careers (fewer games started, fewer games played, and fewer years in the sport) than those with either procedure alone (Brophy et al. 2009).

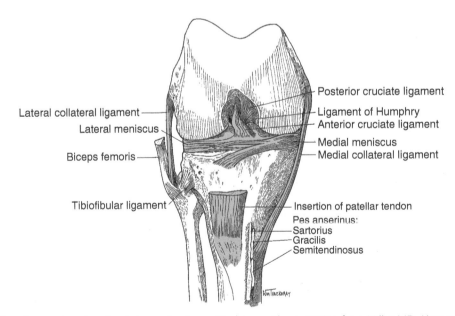

Fig. 47.1 Anterior cruciate ligament and anatomic knee structures. (Redrawn with permission from Miller MD, Howard RF, Planchar KD: Surgical Atlas of Sports Medicine. Philadelphia, Saunders, 2003, p. 74, Fig. 10-3.)

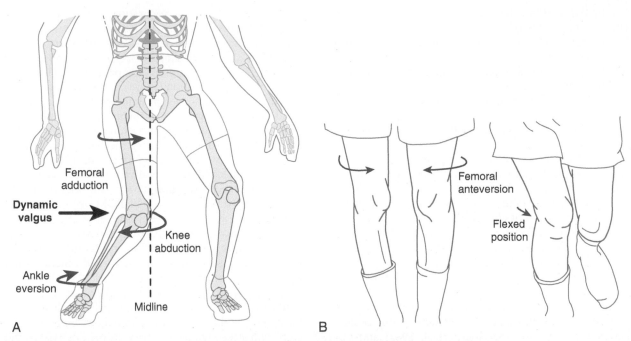

Fig. 47.2 **A,** Dynamic valgus is defined as the position or motion, measured in three dimensions, of the distal femur toward the distal tibia away from the midline of the body. Dynamic valgus includes the indicated motions and moments. **B,** In individuals with anterior knee pain the alignment may appear rather straight—no excessive genu valgum or valgus—but there is significant internal rotation of the femors, indicating femoral anteversion. The patellae are pointing toward one another *(left)*. This is accentuated when the individual gets in a flexed position: The femur goes into further adduction and internal rotation *(right)*. (Redrawn with permission from Hewett TE, Myer GD, Ford KR, Heidt RS Jr, Colosimo AJ, McLean SG, van den Bogert AJ, et al.: Biomechanical measures of neuromuscular control and valgus loading of the knee predict anterior cruciate ligament injury risk in female athletes. *Am J Sports Med* 33:4, 2005.)

Successful reconstruction of the ACL has been proven to improve short-term function and perhaps decrease the risk of subsequent meniscal injury, but it may not decrease the likelihood of OA (Lohmander and Roos 1994), particularly in patients with concomitant meniscal or articular cartilage injuries.

TREATMENT OF ACL INJURIES
Nonoperative Treatment (ACL-Deficient Knee)

- Levy and Meier (2003) reported the incidence of subsequent meniscal tears in ACL-deficient knees is 40% at year 1, 60% at year 5, and 80% by 10 years after the initial untreated ACL disruption.
- Lohmander and Roos (1994) in a meta-analysis of 33 studies found that the efficacy of ACL reconstruction in retarding the progression of OA was not substantiated. Presence of meniscal injury at time of ACL injury has a high correlation with eventual development of arthritis.
- Some patients who are ACL-deficient, however, have physiologic responses and motor control strategies that allow successful compensation for their ACL absence (copers). Copers are defined as patients who have returned to full sports and preinjury activity without instability for at least 1 year.
- Nakayama and Beard have similiarly demonstrated much improved dynamic knee stability and function in patients with ACL deficiency after rehabilitation that included perturbation training. Perturbation training for nonoperatively treated and postoperative ACL reconstruction in addition to traditional strengthening should be advocated.

Despite the success of current ACL reconstruction methods, not all patients require surgical reconstruction. Currently, there are no firm criteria for determining which patients are candidates for ACL reconstruction versus nonoperative management.

Several authors have suggested criteria for nonoperative treatment in ACL tears: Fitzgerald et al. (2000) developed guidelines for selecting appropriate candidates for nonoperative ACL deficiency management (e.g., initiation of perturbation and strengthening program). The *primary criteria* were no concomitant ligament (e.g., medial collateral ligament) or meniscal damage and a unilateral ACL injury. Other criteria include the following:

1. Timed hop test score of 80% of the uninjured limb
2. Knee Outcome Survey Activities of Daily Living Scale score of 80% or more
3. Global rating of knee function of 60% or more
4. No more than one episode of giving way in the time from injury to testing

The success rate in Fitzgerald's perturbation ACL rehabilitation group was 92% (11/12 patients). The likelihood ratio calculated for this study suggested patients would be five times more likely to successfully return to high-level physical activity if they receive the perturbation training than if they receive only a standard ACL rehabilitation strength training program.

Moksnes et al. (2008) in a level Ib study found that 70% of patients classified as potential noncopers in Fitzgerald's original screening examination were true copers after 1 year of nonoperative treatment.

1. These authors' observation was that the development of knee function in subjects with nonoperatively treated ACL injuries simply took time.
2. At 1-year follow-up, 70% of the subjects initially classi-

fied by Fitzgerald's criteria as noncopers were true copers (Beynnon et al. 2005).

Other possible criteria for nonoperative ACL treatment include the following:

- Minimal exposure to high-risk activities such as sports and heavy work activities
- Willingness to avoid high-risk activity
- Age older than 40 years
- Success in prolonged coping with or adaptation to ACL deficiency
- Advanced arthritis of the involved joint
- Inability or unwillingness to comply to postoperative rehabilitation

Most reports of successful nonoperative treatment of ACL injuries come from case series (level IV evidence). One prospective cohort study (level II evidence) of 100 consecutive patients with nonoperatively treated (early activity modification and neuromuscular knee rehabilitation) ACL injuries found that at 15-year follow-up 68% had asymptomatic knees (Neuman et al. 2008).

Of four randomized controlled studies comparing nonoperative to operative treatment (level I evidence), one reported no difference in outcomes (Sandberg et al. 1987) and three reported superior results with operative treatment (Andersson et al. 1989 and 1991, Odensten et al. 1985).

Although age of more than 40 years has been considered a relative indication for nonoperative treatment, several studies have reported results in older patients similar to those in younger patients, and age alone is not an absolute indicator for nonoperative treatment. Many individuals aged 40 years and older remain athletically active and are not willing to accept the limitations knee instability places on their activities.

Operative ACL Reconstruction

ACL reconstruction is almost universally recommended for patients with high-risk lifestyles that require heavy work or who participate in certain sports or recreational activities. Other indications for ACL reconstruction include repeated episodes of giving way despite rehabilitation, meniscal tears, severe injuries to other knee ligaments, generalized ligamentous laxity, and recurrent instability with activities of daily living (Beynnon et al. 2005 Part 1). Once operative reconstruction is chosen, a number of controversial areas must be considered: timing of surgery; choice of graft, autograft, or allograft; one- or two-bundle technique; fixation method; and rehabilitation protocol (accelerated or nonaccelerated).

A study of National Basketball Association players with ACL injuries and subsequent reconstruction by sports medicine physicians found that 22% did not return to competition and 44% of those who did return had decreases in their levels of performance despite reconstruction (Busfield et al. 2009, level IV evidence).

Timing of surgery. Because many patients had difficulty regaining full knee motion after acute or early reconstruction, delayed reconstruction has been suggested to minimize the possibility of postoperative arthrofibrosis. Good results have been reported after both acute and delayed reconstruction, mostly in retrospective case series. A prospective study compared outcomes in patients who had ACL reconstruction at four time points after injury (Hunter et al. 1996): within 48 hours, between 3 and 7 days, between 1 and 3 weeks, and qr534 more than 3

weeks. They found that restoration of knee motion and ACL integrity after ACL reconstruction was independent of the timing of surgery. Shelbourne and Patel (1995) suggested that the timing of ACL surgery should not be based on absolute time limits from injury. They reported that patients who had obtained an excellent range of motion (ROM), little swelling, good leg control, and an excellent mental state before surgery generally had good outcomes, regardless of the timing of surgery. Mayr et al. (2004) confirmed these observations in a retrospective review of 223 patients with ACL reconstructions: 70% of patients with a swollen, inflamed knee at the time of undergoing ACL reconstruction developed postoperative arthrofibrosis. It appears that the timing of reconstruction is not as important as the condition of the knee before surgery: Full ROM, minimal effusion, and minimal pain are required (Beynnon et al. 2005, Part 1).

Graft choice. Bone-patellar tendon-bone (BPTB) autografts (Fig. 47.3) have been historically considered the "gold standard" for ACL reconstructions, although good outcomes have been reported with other graft choices, particularly hamstring grafts (Fig. 47.4, *A–H*). A number of studies have compared BPTB grafts with four-strand hamstring grafts, with most reporting no significant difference in functional outcomes, although difficulty with kneeling was more commonly reported by those with BPTB grafts.

A meta-analysis by Yunes et al. (2001) found that patients with BPTB grafts had anteroposterior knee laxity values that were closer to normal than did those with four-strand hamstring grafts, and a later meta-analysis by Goldblatt et al. (2005) found that more patients with BPTB grafts had KT-1000 manual-maximum side-to-side laxity differences of less than 3 mm than did those with four-strand hamstring grafts; fewer of those with BPTB grafts had significant flexion loss. Those with hamstring grafts had less patellofemoral crepitance, anterior knee pain, and extension loss.

Autograft versus allograft. Suggested advantages of allografts over autografts include decreased morbidity, preservation of the extensor or flexor mechanisms, decreased operative time, availability of larger grafts, lower incidence of arthrofibrosis, and improved cosmetic result. Disadvantages of allografts include risk of infection, slow or incomplete graft incorporation and remodeling, higher costs, availability, tunnel enlargement, and alteration of the structural properties of the graft by sterilization and storage procedures. Two meta-analyses comparing autografts and allografts found no significant differences in short-term clinical outcomes (Foster et al. 2010, Carey et al. 2009); however, Mehta et al. (2010) found higher revision rates with BPTB allografts than with autografts and higher IKDC (International Knee Documentation Committee) scores in those with autografts.

A prospective comparison (level II evidence) of outcomes of 37 patients with autografts and 47 with allografts found similar clinical outcome scores at 3 to 6 years after surgery (Edgar et al. 2008). A retrospective review of 3126 ACL reconstructions (1777 with autografts and 1349 with allografts) found that the use of an allograft did not increase the risk of infection (less than 1% in both groups); hamstring tendon autografts had a higher frequency of infection than either BPTB autografts or allografts (Barker et al. 2010).

Single- or double-bundle reconstruction. The rationale for two-bundle reconstruction is based on the identification of two distinct ACL bundles: the anteromedial (AM) and the posterolateral (PL) bundle (Fig. 47.5). The femoral insertion sites of

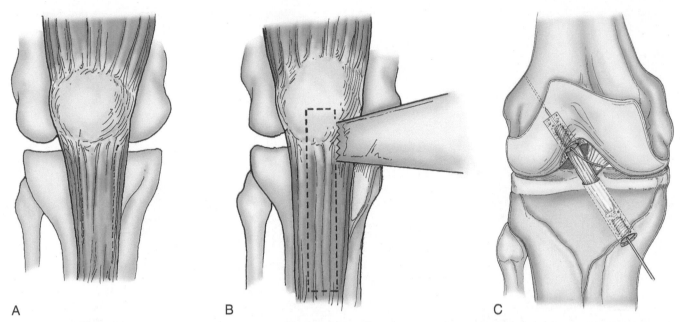

A   B   C

Fig. 47.3 **A,** Bone patellar tendon bone graft harvest. The tendon is exposed, and the paratenon is incised. An appropriately sized graft is measured, and the tendon is incised parallel to its fibers. An oscillating saw is used to remove 25-mm bone blocks from the tibia and the patella. **B,** An osteotome is used to remove the bone blocks. (Reprinted with permission from Miller MD, Howard RF, Planchar KD: Surgical Atlas of Sports Medicine. Philadelphia, Saunders, 2003, p. 46, Fig. 7-4.) **C,** Anterior cruciate ligament bone patellar bone graft fixation. (Reprinted with permission from Miller MD, Howard RF, Planchar KD: Surgical Atlas of Sports Medicine. Philadelphia, Saunders, 2003, p. 57, Fig. 7-14.)

both bundles are oriented vertically with the knee in extension, but they become horizontal when the knee is flexed 90 degrees, placing the PL insertion site anterior to the AM insertion site. When the knee is extended, the bundles are parallel; when the knee is flexed, they cross. In flexion, the AM bundle tightens as the PL bundle becomes lax, while in extension the PL bundle tightens and the AM bundle relaxes.

These observations indicate that each bundle has a unique contribution to knee kinematics at different flexion angles. Cadaver studies have shown that double-bundle reconstructions more closely restore normal knee kinematics (Tsai et al. 2009, Morimoto et al. 2009, Yagi et al. 2002), including a more normal tibiofemoral contact area (Morimoto et al. 2009), than do single-bundle reconstructions. Several prospective, randomized comparisons (level I evidence) of the two techniques have shown superior objective results with double-bundle reconstruction **but no significant differences in subjective and functional results** even in high-level athletes.

A meta-analysis of the literature (Meredick et al. 2008) found no clinically significant differences in KT-1000 or pivot shift results between double-bundle and single-bundle reconstruction. Other authors have reported significantly more rotational stability after double-bundle reconstruction than after single-bundle procedures (Tsai et al. 2009). The primary disadvantage of double-bundle reconstructions is their complexity and technical difficulty. **The creation of multiple tunnels increases the risk of tunnel misplacement and makes revision surgery extremely difficult.**

Cited advantages of single-bundle techniques include proven success, less technical difficulty, less tunnel widening, fewer complications, easier revision, lower graft cost when allograft is used, lower implant cost, and shorter surgical time (Prodromos et al. 2008).

Method of fixation. A variety of fixation devices are used for ACL reconstruction, with no consensus as to what is best.

Generally, fixation can be classified as interference screw-based, cortical, or cross-pin (Prodromos et al. 2008). Interference screw and cortical fixation can be used in both the femur and the tibia. Interference screw fixation functions by generating frictional holding power between the graft and the bone tunnel wall (Prodromos et al. 2008). Cortical fixation can be direct, compressing the graft against the cortex, or indirect, connecting the graft to the cortex with some sort of interface, often a fabric or metal loop through which the graft is passed. Cross-pinning is a relatively new fixation technique for which advocates cite the advantage of being closer to the tunnel opening than cortical fixation. This advantage, however, has not been proved. A meta-analysis showed that cortical fixation provided more stability than aperture fixation, and a prospective comparison of three fixation devices, including cross-pin fixation, found no statistically or clinically relevant differences in results at 2-year follow-up (Harilainen and Sandelin 2009). All currently used fixation techniques appear to provide adequate stability to allow early aggressive rehabilitation after ACL reconstruction (Hapa and Barber 2009).

ACL REHABILITATION RATIONALE

Protocols for rehabilitation after ACL reconstruction follow several basic guiding principles:
- Achieving full ROM and complete reduction of intra-articular inflammation and swelling before surgery to avoid arthrofibrosis
- Early weight bearing and ROM, with **early emphasis on obtaining full passive extension**
- Early initiation of quadriceps and hamstring activity
- Efforts to control swelling and pain to limit muscular inhibition and atrophy
- Appropriate use of open and closed kinetic chain exercises, avoiding early open chain exercises that may shear or tear the

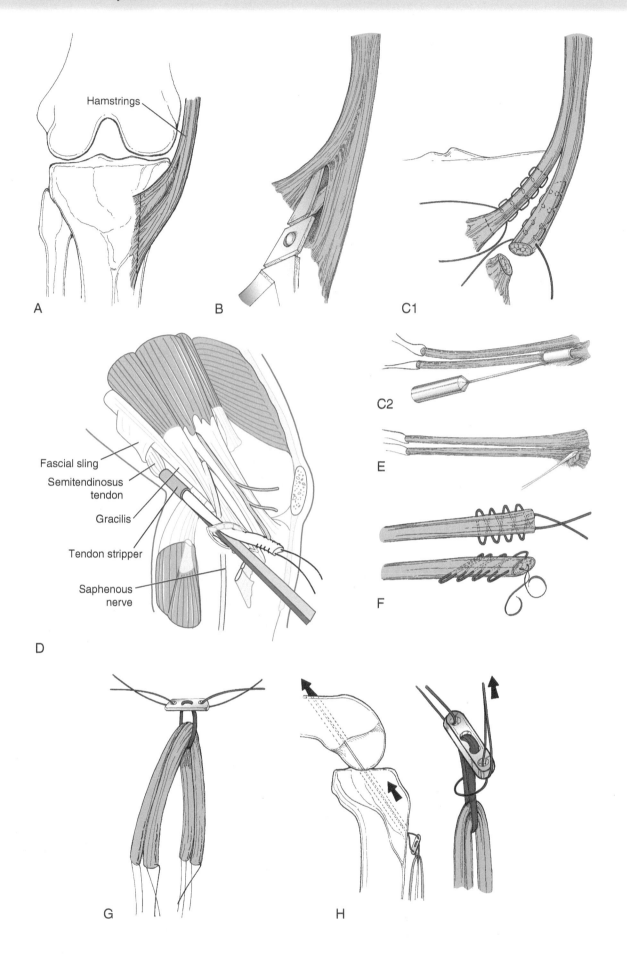

Hamstrings

A

B

C1

C2

E

F

Fascial sling

Semitendinosus tendon

Gracilis

Tendon stripper

Saphenous nerve

D

G

H

Fig. 47.4   **A** and **B,** Hamstring graft harvest. Initial dissection beneath sartorial fascia and isolation of gracilis tendon (superior) and semitendinosus tendon (inferior). **C,** Sutures placed near insertion of each tendon with a whip stitch; harvesting performed with a tendon stripper. **D,** Passage of the tendon stripper outside of the fascial sling beneath the semimembranous muscle may result in the tendon stripper's taking an aberrant path into the thigh and causing premature amputation of the semitendinosus graft. **E,** Muscle is cleared off each tendon with a curette. **F,** Sutures are placed on the free ends of the graft. **G,** A fixation device is prepared after the graft has been sized. **H,** Anterior cruciate ligament graft passage with fixation of the metal EndoButton on the lateral femoral cortex. (*A, B, C, E, F, G* Reprinted with permission from Miller MD, Howard RF, Planchar KD: Surgical Atlas of Sports Medicine. Philadelphia, Saunders, 2003, Figs. 7-5A, C, D, 7-8 A, B, C, 7-13. Part *D* adapted with permission from Brown CH, Sklar JH: Endoscopic anterior cruciate ligament reconstruction using quadrupled hamstring tendons and EndoButton femoral fixation. *Tech Orthop* 13:285, 1998.)

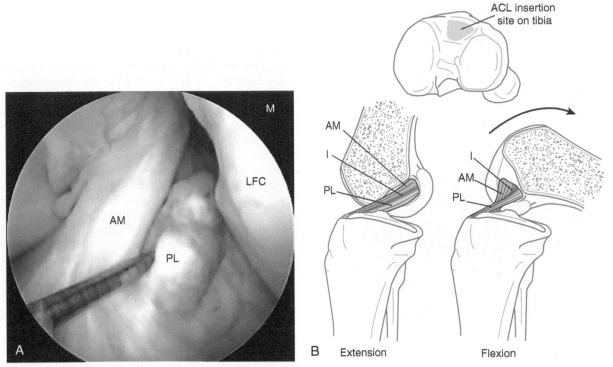

Fig. 47.5   **A,** Anterior cruciate ligament (ACL) tear of anteromedial and posterolateral bundles, each from femoral insertion. Preoperative examination demonstrated 2+ Lachman test score and 3+ pivot shift test score. (Reprinted with permission from Cole B: Surgical Techniques of the Shoulder, Elbow, and Knee in Sports Medicine. Philadelphia, Saunders, 2008, p. 664, Fig. 65-4.) **B,** The ACL is divided into three bundles based on the tibial attachment: the anteromedial (AM), the intermediate (I), and the posterolateral (PL) bundles. With knee flexion, the posterior fibers loosen and the anteromedial fibers coil around the posterolateral ones. (Redrawn with permission from Baker CL Jr: The Hughston Clinic Sports Medicine Book. Baltimore, Williams & Wilkins, 1995.)

weak immature ACL graft (see section on open and closed kinetic chain exercises)
- Comprehensive lower extremity muscle stretching and strengthening and conditioning
- Neuromuscular and proprioception retraining including perturbation training (Ch. 48)
- **Stepped progression based on achievement of therapeutic goals (i.e., criteria-based sequential progression)(Rehabilitation Protocol 47.1).**
- Functional testing and functional sport-specific training prior to return to play

Open and Closed Kinetic Chain Exercise

Considerable debate has occurred in recent years regarding the use of closed kinetic chain activity versus open kinetic chain activity after ACL reconstruction. An example of an open kinetic chain exercise is the use of a leg extension machine (Fig. 47.6). An example of closed kinetic chain exercise is the use of a leg press machine (Fig. 47.7). In theory, closed

kinetic chain exercises provide a more significant compression force across the knee with activating co-contraction of the quadriceps and hamstring muscles. It has been suggested that these two factors help decrease the anterior shear forces in the knee that would otherwise be placed on the maturing ACL graft. Because of this, closed kinetic chain exercises have been favored over open kinetic chain exercises during rehabilitation after ACL reconstruction. However, the literature supporting this theory is not definitive. Many common activities cannot be clearly classified as open or closed kinetic chain, which adds to the confusion. Walking, running, stair climbing, and jumping all involve a combination of open and closed kinetic chain components to them.

Jenkins and colleagues (1997) measured side-to-side difference in anterior displacement of the tibia in subjects with unilateral ACL-deficient knees during open kinetic chain exercise (knee extension) and closed kinetic chain exercises (leg press) at 30 and 60 degrees of knee flexion and concluded that open chain exercises at low flexion angles may produce an increase in anterior shear forces, which may cause laxity in the ACL (see Table 47.1).

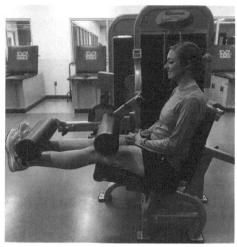

Fig. 47.6 Example of an open kinetic chain exercise (leg extension).

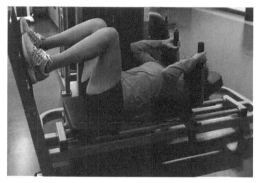

Fig. 47.7 Example of a closed kinetic chain exercise (leg press).

TABLE 47.1	Side-to-Side Difference in Anterior Displacement	
	30 degrees knee flexion (mm)	**60 degrees knee flexion (mm)**
Open kinetic chain (knee extension)	4.7	1.2
Closed kinetic chain (leg press)	1.3	2.1

(3–5 mm = abnormal; 5 mm = arthrometric failure)
(From Jenkins WL, Munns SW, Jayaraman G: A measurement of anterior tibial displacement in the closed and open kinetic chain. J Orthop Sports Phys Ther 1997; 25:49-56.)

Yack and colleagues (1993) also found increased anterior displacement during open kinetic chain exercise (knee extension) compared with closed kinetic chain exercise (parallel squat) through a flexion range of 0 to 64 degrees. Kvist and Gillquist (1999) demonstrated that displacement occurs with even low levels of muscular activity: Generation of the first 10% of the peak quadriceps torque produced 80% of the total tibial translation seen with maximal quadriceps torque. Mathematic models also have predicted that shear forces on the ACL are greater with open chain exercises. Jurist and Otis (1985), Zavetsky and coworkers (1994), and Wilk and Andrews (1993) all noted that changing the position of the resistance pad on isokinetic open kinetic chain devices could modify anterior shear force and anterior tibial displacement. Wilk and Andrews also found greater anterior tibial displacements at slower isokinetic speeds.

Beynnon and associates (1997) used implanted transducers to measure the strain in the intact ACL during various exercises and found no consistent distinction between closed kinetic chain and open kinetic chain activities. This finding contradicts the previous studies and indicates that certain closed chain activities, such as squatting, may not be as safe as the mathematic force models would predict, particularly at low flexion angles.

A protective effect of the hamstrings has been suggested based on the findings of minimal or absent strain in the ACL with isolated hamstring contraction or when the hamstrings were simultaneously contracted along with the quadriceps. Co-contraction of the quadriceps and hamstrings occurs in closed kinetic chain exercises, with a progressive decrease in hamstring activity as the flexion angle of the knee increases. Co-contraction does not occur to any significant degree during open kinetic chain exercise.

Other differences between open and closed kinetic chain exercise have been demonstrated. Closed kinetic chain exercises generate greater activity in the vasti musculature, and open kinetic chain exercises generate more rectus femoris activity. Open chain activities generate more isolated muscle activity and thus allow for more specific muscle strengthening. However, with fatigue, any stabilizing effect of these isolated muscles may be lost and can put the ACL at greater risk. Closed chain exercises, by allowing agonist muscle activity, may not provide focused muscle strengthening, but they may provide a safer environment for the ACL in the setting of fatigue.

In summary, closed chain exercises can be used safely during rehabilitation of the ACL because they appear to generate low anterior shear force and tibial displacement through most of the flexion range, although some evidence now exists that low flexion angles during certain closed kinetic chain activities may strain the graft as much as open chain activities and may not be as safe as previously thought (Table 47.2). At what level strain becomes detrimental and whether some degree of strain is beneficial during the graft healing phase are currently unknown. Until these answers are realized, current trends have been to recommend activities that minimize graft strain, so as to put the ACL at the lowest risk for developing laxity. Open chain flexion that is dominated by hamstring activity appears to pose little risk to the ACL throughout the entire flexion arc, but open chain extension places significant strain on the ACL and the patellofemoral joint and should be avoided. An assessment of randomized controlled trials found that closed kinetic chain exercises produced less pain and laxity while promoting better subjective outcome than open kinetic chain exercises (Andersson et al. 2009).

OTHER REHABILITATION CONSIDERATIONS AFTER ACL RECONSTRUCTION

Pain and Effusion

Pain and swelling are common after any surgical procedure. Because they cause reflex inhibition of muscle activity and thus postoperative muscle atrophy, it is important to control these problems quickly to facilitate early ROM and strengthening activities. Standard therapeutic modalities to reduce pain and swelling include cryotherapy, compression, and elevation.

Cryotherapy is commonly used to reduce pain, inflammation, and effusion after ACL reconstruction. Cryotherapy acts through local effects, causing vasoconstriction, which reduces fluid extravasation; inhibiting afferent nerve conduction, which decreases pain and muscle spasm; and preventing cell death, which limits the release of chemical mediators of pain, inflammation, and edema. Complications such as superficial frostbite and neuropraxia can be prevented by avoiding prolonged placement of the cold source directly on the skin. Contraindications to the use of cryotherapy include hypersensitivity to cold, such as Raynaud's phenomenon, lupus erythematosus, periarteritis nodosa, and rheumatoid arthritis.

TABLE 47.2	Criteria-Based Postoperative ACL Reconstruction		
RANK COMPARISON OF PEAK ANTERIOR CRUCIATE LIGAMENT STRAIN VALUES DURING COMMONLY PRESCRIBED REHABILITATION ACTIVITIES			
Rehabilitation Activity		**Peak Strain (0%)**	**Number of Subjects**
Isometric quads contraction at 15 degrees (30 Nm of extension torque)		4.4	8
Squatting with Sport Cord		4.0	8
Active flexion–extension of the knee with 45-N weight boot		3.8	9
Lachman test (150 N of anterior shear load)		3.7	10
Squatting		3.6	8
Active flexion–extension (no weight boot) of the knee		2.8	18
Simultaneous quads and hams contraction at 15 degrees		2.8	8
Isometric quads contraction at 30 degrees (30 Nm of extension torque)		2.7	18
Anterior drawer (150 N of anterior shear load)		1.8	10
Stationary bicycling		1.7	8
Isometric hamstring contraction at 15 degrees (to 10 Nm of flexion torque)		0.6	8
Simultaneous quadriceps and hamstring contraction at 30 degrees		0.4	8
Passive flexion–extension of the knee		0.1	10
Isometric quadriceps contraction at 60 degrees (30 Nm of extension torque)		0.0	8
Isometric quadriceps contraction at 90 degrees (30 Nm of extension torque)		0.0	18
Simultaneous quadriceps and hamstring contraction at 60 degrees		0.0	8
Simultaneous quadriceps and hamstring contraction at 90 degrees		0.0	8
Isometric hamstring contraction at 30, 60, and 90 degrees (to 10 Nm of flexion torque)		0.0	8

From Beynnon BD Fleming BC: Anterior cruciate ligament strain in-vivo: A review of previous work. J Biomech 1998; 31:519–525.

REHABILITATION PROTOCOL 47.1 ● Rehabilitation Protocol

Michael Duke, PT, CSCS, S. Brent Brotzman, MD

Phase I (Days 1–7)

Weightbearing status

- Two crutches, locked knee brace, weight bearing as tolerated after nerve block wears off

Exercises

- Heel slides/wall slides/sitting assisted knee flexion
- Ankle pumps
- Isometric quad sets in full extension with and without neuromuscular electrical stimulation (NMES) or biofeedback
- Hamstring sets (not for hamstring autograft)
- Gluteal sets
- Straight leg raise (SLR) flexion, abduction, extension with brace locked in full extension
- Prone hangs or heel propped in supine for passive knee extension
- Weight shifting in standing for weightbearing tolerance (anteroposterior and side to side)
- Continuous passive motion (CPM) 6 hours/day, increasing 5–10 degrees/day
- Gait training with crutches and brace, level ground and stairs
- Cryotherapy to reduce edema

Manual Therapy

- Patellar mobilizations
- Soft tissue mobilizations to hamstrings for spasm control

Goals

- Active range of motion (AROM) 0–90 degrees within 10 days
- Good, active quadriceps contraction
- Full weight bearing (FWB) with crutches and brace
- Edema control
- Graft protection
- Wound healing

Criteria to Progress to Phase II

- SLR with or without lag in brace
- Clean and dry wound
- Progressing range of motion (ROM)
- Able to bear weight on involved limb

Phase II (Days 8–14)

Weightbearing Status

- Weight bearing as tolerated
- Two crutches to single crutch
- Brace unlocked gradually as quad control improves (SLR without lag before unlocking brace beyond 30 degrees)

Exercises

- Stationary bike for ROM (from rocking to full revolutions)
- Isometric quad sets in full extension and at 90 degrees with and without NMES or biofeedback
- Single-leg stance in brace

Continued

REHABILITATION PROTOCOL 47.1 ■ **Rehabilitation Protocol—cont'd**

- Balance board anteroposterior in bilateral stance
- Continue ROM exercises.
- Gait training: single-leg walk (pawing) on treadmill, step-over cones forward
- Begin partial weight mini-squats (0–30 deg) on total gym/shuttle
- Heel raises
- Continue SLR, all four directions
- Terminal knee extension in standing with band
- Prone knee bridges
- Active standing hamstring curls (do not perform for postoperative hamstring autograft reconstruction)

Manual Therapy

- Continue patellar mobs as indicated.
- Continue hamstring mobs as indicated.

Goals

- AROM 0–120 degrees within 3 weeks
- SLR without quad lag
- Normal gait pattern with single crutch and unlocked brace

Criteria to Progress to Phase III

- AROM 0–90 degrees
- SLR with minimal quad lag
- Normal gait with least restrictive assistive device
- Single-leg stance on involved limb with hand-assist

Phase III (Weeks 2–4)

Weightbearing Status

- FWB, normal gait without assistive device or brace by 3 weeks

Exercises

- Stationary bike with gradual progressive resistance for endurance
- Isometric quad sets in full extension and at 90 to 60 degrees flexion with and without NMES or biofeedback until equal quad contraction bilaterally
- Closed kinetic chain squat/leg press 0 to 60 degrees, gradual progressive resistance
- Balance board bilateral in multiple planes
- Single-leg balance eyes open/closed, variable surfaces
- Sport Cord or treadmill walking forward and backward
- Standing SLRs, each LE and with resistance

Manual Therapy

- Continue patellar mobilizations as indicated.
- Initiate scar mobilizations as needed.
- Manual extension or flexion ROM as needed

Goals

- Full AROM, equal to nonsurgical knee
- Normal gait without assistive device
- Independent activities of daily living (downstairs may still be difficult)

Criteria for Progression to Phase IV

- Equal bilateral knee AROM
- Normal gait without assistive device
- Understanding of precautions regarding state of graft
- Single-leg standing without assistance

Phase IV (Weeks 4–8)

Precautions

- **State of graft at its weakest during this postoperative period.** No impact activities such as running, jumping, pivoting, or cutting, and no deep squatting (limits remain 0–60 degrees)

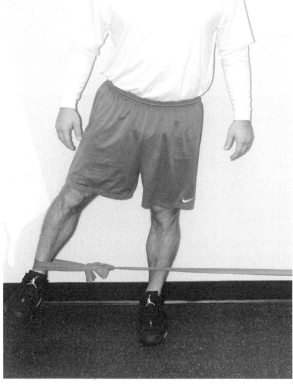

Fig. 47.8   Abduction contrakicks/steamboats.

- Pay attention to scar mobility; use manual soft tissue mobilizations as indicated

Exercises

- Stationary bike: increase resistance and some light intervals
- Squats/leg press: bilateral to unilateral (0–60 degrees) with progressive resistance
- Lunges (0–60 degrees)
- Stairs: concentric and eccentric (not to exceed 60 degrees of knee flexion)
- Calf raises: bilateral to unilateral
- Contrakicks (steamboats) (Fig. 47.8): progress from anteroposterior to side to side, then circles/random
- Rotational stability exercises: static lunge with lateral pulley repetitions
- Sport Cord resisted walking all four directions
- Treadmill walking all four directions
- Balance board: multiple planes, bilateral stance
- Ball toss to mini-tramp or wall in single-leg stance
- Single-leg deadlifts (Fig. 47.9): wait for 6–8 weeks if hamstring autograft
- Core strengthening: supine and prone bridging, standing with pulleys
- Gait activities: cone obstacle courses at walking speeds in multiple planes

Criteria for Progression to Phase V

- Bilateral squat to 60 degrees (no more) with equal weight distribution
- Quiet knee (minimal pain and effusion and no giving way)
- Quad girth within 1 to 2 cm of nonsurgical thigh at 10 cm proximal to superior patella
- Single-leg balance on involved limb >30 seconds with minimal movement

REHABILITATION PROTOCOL 47.1 ● **Rehabilitation Protocol—cont'd**

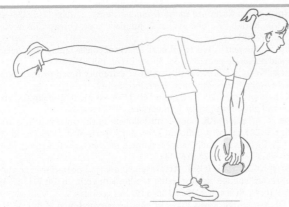

Fig. 47.9 Single-leg deadlift.

Phase V (Weeks 8–12)

Things to Watch Out for

- Patellar tendinitis

Exercises

- Squats/leg press: bilateral to unilateral (0–60 degrees) progressive resistance
- Lunges (0–60 degrees)
- Calf raises: bilateral to unilateral
- Advance hamstring strengthening
- Core strengthening
- Combine strength and balance (e.g., ball toss to trampoline on balance board, mini-squat on balance board, Sport Cord cone weaves, contrakicks)
- Advanced balance exercises (e.g., single-leg stance while reaching to cones on floor with hands or opposite foot, single-leg stance while pulling band laterally)
- Lap swimming generally fine with exception of breaststroke; caution with deep squat push-off and no use of fins yet
- Stationary bike intervals

Goals

- Equal quad girth (average gain of 1 cm per month after first month with good strength program)
- Single-leg squat to 60 degrees with good form

Criteria for Progression to Phase VI

- Nearly equal quad girth (within 1 cm)
- Single-leg squat to 60 degrees
- Single-leg balance up to 60 seconds
- Minimal, if any, edema with activity

Phase VI (Weeks 12–16)

Things to Watch Out for/Correct

- Landing during exercises at low knee flexion angles (too close to extension)
- Landing during exercises with genu varum/valgum (watch for dynamic valgus of knee and correct)
- Landing and jumping with uninvolved limb dominating effort

Exercises

- Elliptical trainer: forward and backward
- Perturbation training*: balance board, roller board, roller board with platform
- Shuttle jumping: bilateral to alternating to unilateral, emphasis on landing form
- Mini-tramp bouncing: bilateral to alternating to unilateral, emphasis on landing form
- Jogging in place with Sport Cord: pulling from variable directions
- Movement speed increases for all exercises
- Slide board exercises
- Aqua jogging

Criteria to Progress to Phase VII

- Single-leg squat, 20 repetitions to 60 degrees of knee flexion
- Single-leg stance at least 60 seconds
- Single-leg calf raise 30 repetitions
- Good landing form with bilateral vertical and horizontal jumping
- Hop testing[†]: 80% of uninvolved limb performed prior to running

Phase VII (Weeks 16–24)

Exercises

- Progressive running program[‡]
- Hop testing and training[†]
- Vertical, horizontal jumping from double to single leg
- Progressive plyometrics (e.g., box jumps, bounding, standing jumps, jumps in place, depth jumps, squat jumps, scissor jumps, jumping over barriers, skipping)
- Speed and agility drills (e.g., T-test, line drills) (make these similar in movement to specific sport of athlete)
- Cutting drills begin week 20
- Progress to sport-specific drills week 20

For Revision ACL Reconstructions

Per specific physician recommendation, follow typically similar protocol until 12 weeks, then extend weeks 12 to 16 through to 5- to 6-month timeline, when patients can then begin running and progress to functional sports activities. See Fig. 47.8 for an illustration of abduction contrakicks/steamboats (flexion, extension, and adduction contrakicks can be performed by rotating patient 90 degrees at a time).

---

*See section on perturbation training for ACL postoperative training progression.
[†]Hop testing.
[‡]Progressive running program.
Single-leg hop for distance: 80% minimum compared to nonsurgical side for running, 90% minimum for return to sport
Single-leg triple hop for distance: 80% for running, 90% for return to sport
Triple crossover hop for distance: 80% for running, 90% for return to sport
Timed 10-m single-leg hop: 80% for running, 90% for return to sport
Timed vertical hop test: 60 seconds with good form and steady rhythm considered passing
Always begin with warmup on the stationary bike or elliptical for >10 minutes prior to initiation of running.
Patient should have no knee pain following run.
Week 1: Run: walk 30 seconds: 90 seconds every other day (qod) (10–15 minutes)
Week 2: Run: walk 60:60 qod (10–20 minutes)
Week 3: Run: walk 90:30 qod (15–20 minutes)
Week 4: Run: walk 90:30 3–4 times/week (20–25 minutes)
Week 5: Run continuously 15–20 minutes 3–5 times/week

▶ Check online videos: Bridging With Side (Video 47.1), Level Ground Squats Bilateral (Video 47.2), Lunge Anterior (Video 47.3), Single Leg Balance Foam Pad (Video 47.4), Single Leg Balance Level Ground (Video 47.5) and Single Leg Balance Perturbations (Video 47.6).

REFERENCES

A complete reference list is available at https://expertconsult .inkling.com/.

FURTHER READING

Aglietti P, Insall JN, Cerulli G. Patellar pain and incongruence. I: measurements of incongruence. *Clin Orthop.* 1983;176:217–224.

Ahmed AM. The load-bearing role of the knee menisci. In: Mow VC, Arnoczky SP, Jackson DW, eds. *Knee Meniscus: Basic and Clinical Foundations.* New York: Raven Press; 1992:59–73.

Ahmed AM, Burke DL, Hyder A. Force analysis of the patellar mechanism. *J Orthop Res.* 1987;5:69–85.

Anderson DR, Weiss JA, Takai S, et al. Healing of the MCL following a triad injury: a biomechanical and histological study of the knee in rabbits. *J Orthop Res.* 1992;10:485–495.

Arms S, Boyle J, Johnson R, et al. Strain measurement in the medial collateral ligament of the human knee: an autopsy study. *J Biomech.* 1983;16:491–496.

Arnoczky SP. Meniscus. In: Fu FH, Harner CD, Vince KG, eds. *Knee Surgery.* Baltimore: Williams & Wilkins; 1994:131–140.

Arnoczky SP, Tarvin GB, Marshall JL. Anterior cruciate ligament replacement using patellar tendon: an evaluation of graft revascularization in the dog. *J Bone Joint Surg.* 1982;64A:217–224.

Arnoczky SP, Warren RF. Microvasculature of the human meniscus. *Am J Sports Med.* 1982;10:90–95.

Bach Jr BR, Levy ME, Bojchuk J, et al. Single-incision endoscopic anterior cruciate ligament reconstruction using patellar tendon autograft—minimum two year follow-up evaluation. *Am J Sports Med.* 1998;26:30–40.

Bach Jr BR, Tradonsky S, Bojchuk J, et al. Arthroscopically assisted anterior cruciate ligament reconstruction using patellar tendon autograft. *Am J Sports Med.* 1998;26:20–29.

Ballock RT, Woo SL-Y, Lyon RM, et al. Use of patellar tendon autograft for anterior cruciate ligament reconstruction in the rabbit: a long term histological and biomechanical study. *J Orthop Res.* 1989;7:474–485.

Barber FA. Accelerated rehabilitation for meniscus repairs. *Arthroscopy.* 1994;10:206–210.

Barber FA, Click SD. Meniscus repair rehabilitation with concurrent anterior cruciate reconstruction. *Arthroscopy.* 1997;13:433–437.

Barber FA, Elrod BF, McGuire DA, et al. Is an anterior cruciate ligament reconstruction outcome age dependent? *Arthroscopy.* 1996;12:720–725.

Barber-Westin SD, Noyes FR, Heckmann TP, et al. The effect of exercise and rehabilitation on anterior-posterior knee displacements after anterior cruciate ligament autograft reconstruction. *Am J Sports Med.* 1999;27:84–93.

Barrack RL, Skinner HB, Buckley SL. Proprioception in the anterior cruciate deficient knee. *Am J Sports Med.* 1989;17:1–6.

Barratta R, Solomonow M, Zhou BH, et al. Muscular coactivation: the role of the antagonist musculature in maintaining knee stability. *Am J Sports Med.* 1988;16:113–122.

Barrett DS. Proprioception and function after anterior cruciate ligament reconstruction. *J Bone Joint Surg.* 1991;73B:833–837.

Beard DJ, Kyberd PJ, Ferguson CM, et al. Proprioception enhancement for ACL deficiency: a prospective randomized trial of two physiotherapy regimens. *J Bone Joint Surg.* 1994;76B:654–659.

Bell DG, Jacobs I. Electro-mechanical response times and rate of force development in males and females. *Med Sci Sports Exerc.* 1986;18:31–36.

Bellemans J, Cauwenberghs F, Brys P, et al. Fracture of the proximal tibia after Fulkerson anteromedial tibial tubercle transfer. *Am J Sports Med.* 1998;26:300–302.

Beynnon BD, Fleming BC. Anterior cruciate ligament strain in-vivo: a review of previous work. *J Biomech.* 1998;31:519–525.

Beynnon BD, Johnson RJ. Anterior cruciate ligament injury rehabilitation in athletes: biomechanical considerations. *Sports Med.* 1996;22:54–64.

Beynnon BD, Johnson RJ, Naud S, et al. Accelerated versus nonaccelerated rehabilitation after anterior cruciate ligament reconstruction: a prospective, randomized, double-blind investigation evaluating knee joint laxity using roentgen stereophotogrammetric analysis. *Am J Sports Med.* 2011;39.12:2536–2548. Web.

Björklund K, Andersson L, Dalén N. Validity and responsiveness of the test of athletes with knee injuries: the new criterion based functional performance test instrument. *Knee Surg Sports Traumatol Arthrosc.* 2009;17(5):435–445.

Blazina ME, Kerlan RK, Jobe FW, et al. Jumper's knee. *Orthop Clin North Am.* 1973;4:665–673.

Bockrath K, Wooden C, Worrell T, et al. Effects of patella taping on patella position and perceived pain. *Med Sci Sports Exerc.* 1993;25:989–992.

Bolgla LA, Keskula DR. Reliability of lower extremity functional performance tests. *J Orthop Sports Phys Ther.* 1997;26:138–142.

Bose K, Kanagasuntheram R, Osman MBH. Vastus medialis obliquus: an anatomic and physiologic study. *Orthopedics.* 1980;3:880–883.

Boynton MD, Tietjens BR. Long-term followup of the untreated isolated posterior cruciate ligament-deficient knee. *Am J Sports Med.* 1996;24:306–310.

Brody LT, Thein JM. Nonoperative treatment for patellofemoral pain. *J Orthop Sports Phys Ther.* 1998;28:336–344.

Bush-Joseph CA, Bach Jr BR. Arthroscopic assisted posterior cruciate ligament reconstruction using patellar tendon autograft. In: Fu FH, ed. *Sports Med Arthrosc Rev.* vol. 2. 1994:106–119.

Butler DL, Grood ES, Noyes FR, et al. On the interpretation of our ACL data. *Clin Orthop.* 1985;196:26–34.

Butler DL, Guan Y, Kay MD, et al. Location-dependent variations in the material properties of the anterior cruciate ligament. *J Biomech.* 1992;25:511–518.

Butler DL, Noyes FR, Grood ES. Ligamentous restraints to anterior-posterior drawer in the human knee. *J Bone Joint Surg.* 1980;62A:259–270.

Bylski-Austrow DI, Ciarelli MJ, Kayner DC, et al. Displacements of the menisci under joint load: an in vitro study in human knees. *J Biomech.* 1994;27:421–431.

Caborn DNM, Coen M, Neef R, et al. Quadrupled semitendinosis-gracilis autograft fixation in the femoral tunnel: a comparison between a metal and a bioabsorbable interference screw. *Arthroscopy.* 1998;14:241–245.

Caborn DNM, Urban Jr WP, Johnson DL, et al. Biomechanical comparison between BioScrew and titanium alloy interference screws for bone-patellar tendon-bone graft fixation in anterior cruciate ligament reconstruction. *Arthroscopy.* 1997;13:229–232.

Caylor D, Fites R, Worrell TW. The relationship between the quadriceps angle and anterior knee pain syndrome. *J Orthop Sports Phys Ther.* 1993;17:11–16.

Cerny K. Vastus medialis oblique/vastus lateralis muscle activity ratios for selected exercises in persons with and without patello-femoral pain syndrome. *Phys Ther.* 1995;75:672–683.

Chang PCC, Lee LKH, Tay BK. Anterior knee pain in the military population. *Ann Acad Med Singapore.* 1997;26:60–63.

Clancy Jr WG, Shelbourne KD, Zoellner GB, et al. Treatment of knee joint instability secondary to rupture of the posterior cruciate ligament: report of a new procedure. *J Bone Joint Surg.* 1983;65A:310–322.

Cohn BT, Draeger RI, Jackson DW. The effects of cold therapy in the postoperative management of pain in patients undergoing anterior cruciate ligament reconstruction. *Am J Sports Med.* 1989;17:344–349.

Colby SM, Hintermeister RA, Torry MR, et al. Lower limb stability with ACL impairment. *J Orthop Sports Phys Ther.* 1999;29:444–451.

Conlan T, Garth Jr WP, Lemons JE. Evaluation of the medial soft-tissue restraints of the extensor mechanism of the knee. *J Bone Joint Surg.* 1993;75A:682–693.

Cooper DE, Xianghua HD, Burstein AL, et al. The strength of the central third patellar tendon graft. *Am J Sports Med.* 1993;21:818–824.

Corry IS, Webb JM, Clingeleffer AJ, et al. Arthroscopic reconstruction of the anterior cruciate ligament: a comparison of patellar tendon autograft and fourstrand hamstring tendon autograft. *Am J Sports Med.* 1999;27:444–454.

Cosgarea AJ, Sebastianelli WJ, DeHaven KE. Prevention of arthrofibrosis after anterior cruciate ligament reconstruction using the central third patellar tendon autograft. *Am J Sports Med.* 1995;23:87–92.

Cross MJ, Powell JF. Long-term followup of posterior cruciate ligament rupture. *Am J Sports Med.* 1984;12:292–297.

Denham RA, Bishop RED. Mechanics of the knee and problems in reconstructive surgery. *J Bone Joint Surg.* 1978;60B:345–351.

Doucette SA, Child DP. The effect of open and closed chain exercise and knee joint position on patellar tracking in lateral patellar compression syndrome. *J Orthop Sports Phys Ther.* 1996;23:104–110.

Doucette SA, Goble EM. The effect of exercise on patellar tracking in lateral patellar compression syndrome. *Am J Sports Med.* 1992;20:434–440.

Dowdy PA, Miniaci A, Arnoczky SP, et al. The effect of cast immobilization on meniscal healing: an experimental study in the dog. *Am J Sports Med.* 1995;23:721–728.

Dye SF. The knee as a biologic transmission with an envelope of function: a theory. *Clin Orthop.* 1996;325:10–18.

Eng JJ, Pierrynowski MR. Evaluation of soft foot orthotics in the treatment of patellofemoral pain syndrome. *Phys Ther.* 1993;73:62–70.

Engle CP, Noguchi M, Ohland KJ, et al. Healing of the rabbit medial collateral ligament following an O'Donoghue triad injury: the effects of anterior cruciate ligament reconstruction. *J Orthop Res.* 1994;12:357–364.

Escamilla RF, Fleisig GS, Zheng N, et al. Biomechanics of the knee during closed kinetic chain and open kinetic chain exercises. *Med Sci Sports Exerc.* 1998;30:556–569.

Falconiero RP, DiStefano VJ, Cook TM. Revascularization and ligamentization of autogenous anterior cruciate ligament grafts in humans. *Arthroscopy.* 1998;14:197–205.

Feretti A. Epidemiology of jumper's knee. *Sports Med.* 1986;3:289–295.

Fetto JF, Marshall JL. Medial collateral ligament injuries of the knee: a rationale for treatment. *Clin Orthop.* 1978;132:206–218.

Ford KR, Myer GD, Toms H, et al. Gender differences in the kinematics of unanticipated cutting in young athletes. *Med Sci Sports Exer.* 2005;37:124–129.

Frank CB, Jackson DW. The science of reconstruction of the anterior cruciate ligament. *J Bone Joint Surg.* 1997;79A:1556–1576.

Fukuda TY, Fingerhut D, Moreira VC, et al. Open kinetic chain exercises in a restricted range of motion after anterior cruciate ligament reconstruction: a randomized controlled clinical trial. *Am J Sports Med.* 2013;41.4:788–794. Web.

Fukibayashi T, Torzilli PA, Sherman MF, et al. An in vitro biomechanical evaluation of anterior-posterior motion of the knee. *J Bone Joint Surg.* 1982;64A:258–264.

Fulkerson JP, Kalenak A, Rosenberg TD, et al. Patellofemoral pain. In: Eilert RE, ed. *Instr Course Lect.* 1992;41:57–70.

Gerrard B. The patellofemoral pain syndrome in young, active patients: a prospective study. *Clin Orthop.* 1989;179:129–133.

Gilchrist J, Mandelbaum BR, Melancon H, et al. A randomized controlled trial to prevent noncontact anterior cruciate ligament injury in female collegiate soccer players. *Am J Sports Med.* 2008;36:1476–1483.

Gilleard W, McConnell J, Parsons D. The effect of patellar taping on the onset of vastus medialis obliquus and vastus lateralis muscle activity in persons with patellofemoral pain. *Phys Ther.* 1998;78:25–31.

Giove TP, Miller SJ, Kent III BE, et al. Non-operative treatment of the torn anterior cruciate ligament. *J Bone Joint Surg.* 1983;65A:184–192.

Giurea M, Zorilla P, Amis AA, et al. Comparative pull-out and cyclic-loading strength tests of anchorage of hamstring tendon grafts in anterior cruciate ligament reconstruction. *Am J Sports Med.* 1999;27:621–625.

Goldfuss AJ, Morehouse CA, LeVeau BF. Effect of muscular tension on knee stability. *Med Sci Sports Exerc.* 1973;5:267–271.

Gollehon DL, Torzilli PA, Warren RF. The role of the posterolateral and cruciate ligaments in the stability of the human knee: a biomechanical study. *J Bone Joint Surg.* 1987;69A:233–242.

Gomez MA, Woo SL-Y, Amiel D, et al. The effects of increased tension on healing medial collateral ligaments. *Am J Sports Med.* 1991;19:347–354.

Goodfellow J, Hungerford DS, Zindel M. Patello-femoral mechanics and pathology. I: functional anatomy of the patello-femoral joint. *J Bone Joint Surg.* 1976;58B:287–290.

Grabiner MD, Koh TJ, Draganich LF. Neuromechanics of the patellofemoral joint. *Med Sci Sports Exerc.* 1994;26:10–21.

Greenwald AE, Bagley AM, France EP, et al. A biomechanical and clinical evaluation of a patellofemoral knee brace. *Clin Orthop.* 1996;324:187–195.

Grelsamer RP, Klein JR. The biomechanics of the patellofemoral joint. *J Orthop Sports Phys Ther.* 1998;28:286–298.

Grood ES, Noyes FR, Butler DL, et al. Ligamentous and capsular restraints preventing straight medial and lateral laxity in intact human cadaver knees. *J Bone Joint Surg.* 1981;63A:1257–1269.

Grood ES, Stowers SF, Noyes FR. Limits of movement in the human knee: effect of sectioning the posterior cruciate ligament and posterolateral structures. *J Bone Joint Surg.* 1988;70A:88–97.

Grood ES, Suntay WJ, Noyes FR, et al. Biomechanics of the knee-extension exercise. *J Bone Joint Surg.* 1984;66A:725–734.

Habata T, Ishimura M, Ohgushi H, et al. Axial alignment of the lower limb in patients with isolated meniscal tear. *J Orthop Sci.* 1998;3:85–89.

Hakkinen K. Force production characteristics of leg extensor, trunk flexor, and extensor muscles in male and female basketball players. *J Sports Med Phys Fitness.* 1991;31:325–331.

Hardin GT, Bach Jr BR. Distal rupture of the infrapatellar tendon after use of its central third for anterior cruciate ligament reconstruction. *Am J Knee Surg.* 1992;5:140–143.

Hardin GT, Bach Jr BR, Bush-Joseph CA. Extension loss following arthroscopic ACL reconstruction. *Orthop Int.* 1993;1:405–410.

Harner CD, Hoher J. Evaluation and treatment of posterior cruciate ligament injuries. *Am J Sports Med.* 1998;26:471–482.

Harner CD, Irrgang JJ, Paul J, et al. Loss of motion after anterior cruciate ligament reconstruction. *Am J Sports Med.* 1992;20:499–506.

Harner CD, Olson E, Irrgang JJ, et al. Allograft versus autograft anterior cruciate ligament reconstruction. *Clin Orthop.* 1996;325:134–144.

Hartigan E, Axe MJ, Snyder-Mackler L. Perturbation training prior to ACL reconstruction improves gait asymmetries in non-copers. *J Orthop Res.* 2009;27:724–729.

Hashemi J, Chandrashekar N, Mansouri H, et al. The human anterior cruciate ligament: sex differences in ultrastructure and correlation with biomechanical properties. *J Orthop Res.* 2008;26:945–950.

Hewett TE, Lindenfeld TN, Riccobene JV, et al. The effect of neuromuscular training on the incidence of knee injury in female athletes. *Am J Sports Med.* 1999;27:699–706.

Hewett TE, Noyes FR, Lee MD. Diagnosis of complete and partial posterior cruciate ligament ruptures: stress radiography compared with KT-1000 Arthrometer and posterior drawer testing. *Am J Sports Med.* 1997;5:648–655.

Hewett TE, Myer GD, Ford KR. Decrease in neuromuscular control about the knee with maturation in female athletes. *J Bone Joint Surg Am.* 2004;86:1601–1608.

Holmes SW, Clancy WG. Clinical classification of patellofemoral pain and dysfunction. *J Orthop Sports Phys Ther.* 1998;28:299–306.

Howell SM, Taylor MA. Brace-free rehabilitation, with early return to activity, for knees reconstructed with a double-looped semitendinosis and gracilis graft. *J Bone Joint Surg.* 1996;78A:814–825.

Huberti HH, Hayes WC, Stone JL, et al. Force ratios in the quadriceps tendon and ligamentum patellae. *J Orthop Res.* 1984;2:49–54.

Huberti HH, Hayes WC. Contact pressures in chondromalacia patellae and the effects of capsular reconstructive procedures. *J Orthop Res.* 1988;6:499–508.

Hull ML, Berns GS, Varma H, et al. Strain in the medial collateral ligament of the human knee under single and combined loads. *J Biomech.* 1996;29:199–206.

Huston LJ, Wojtys EM. Neuromuscular performance characteristics in elite female athletes. *Am J Sports Med.* 1996;24:427–436.

Indelicato PA. Non-operative treatment of complete tears of the medial collateral ligament of the knee. *J Bone Joint Surg.* 1983;65A:323–329.

Ingersoll C, Knight K. Patellar location changes following EMG biofeedback or progressive resistive exercises. *Med Sci Sports Exerc.* 1991;23:1122–1127.

Inoue M, Yasuda K, Ohkoshi Y, et al. Factors that affect prognosis of conservatively treated patients with isolated posterior cruciate ligament injury. *Programs and Abstracts of the 64th Annual Meeting of the American Academy of Orthopaedic Surgeons.* 1997;78. San Francisco.

Inoue M, Yasuda K, Yamanaka M, et al. Compensatory muscle activity in the posterior cruciate ligament-deficient knee during isokinetic knee motion. *Am J Sports Med.* 1998;26:710–714.

Insall J, Falvo KA, Wise DW. Chondromalacia patellae. A prospective study. *J Bone Joint Surg.* 1976;58A:1–8.

Ireland ML. Anterior cruciate ligament in female athletes: epidemiology. *J Athl Train.* 1999;34:150–154.

Itoh H, Kurosaka M, Yoshiya S, et al. Evaluation of functional deficits determined by four different hop tests in patients with anterior cruciate ligament deficiency. *Knee Surg Sports Traumatol Arthrosc.* 1998;6:241–245.

Jacobs CA, Uhl TL, Mattacola CG, et al. Hip abductor function and lower extremity landing kinematics: sex differences. *J Athl Train.* 2007;42:76–83.

Juris PM, Phillips EM, Dalpe C, et al. A dynamic test of lower extremity function following anterior cruciate ligament reconstruction and rehabilitation. *J Orthop Sports Phys Ther.* 1997;26:184–191.

Karst GM, Willett GM. Onset timing of electromyographic activity in the vastus medialis oblique and vastus lateralis muscles in subjects with and without patellofemoral pain syndrome. *Phys Ther.* 1995;75:813–837.

Kartus J, Magnusson L, Stener S, et al. Complications following arthroscopic anterior cruciate ligament reconstruction. *Knee Surg Sports Traumatol Arthrosc.* 1999;7:2–8.

Keller PM, Shelbourne KD, McCarroll JR, et al. Non-operatively treated isolated posterior cruciate ligament injuries. *Am J Sports Med.* 1993;21:132–136.

King D. The healing of semilunar cartilages. *J Bone Joint Surg.* 1936;18:333–342.

Klein L, Heiple KG, Torzilli PA, et al. Prevention of ligament and meniscus atrophy by active joint motion in a non-weight-bearing model. *J Orthop Res.* 1989;7:80–85.

Kleipool AEB, Zijl JAC, Willems WJ. Arthroscopic anterior cruciate ligament reconstruction with bone-patellar tendon-bone allograft or autograft. *Knee Surg Sports Traumatol Arthrosc.* 1998;6:224–230.

Klingman RE, Liaos SM, Hardin KM. The effect of subtalar joint posting on patellar glide position in subjects with excessive rearfoot pronation. *J Orthop Sports Phys Ther.* 1997;25:185–191.

Kolowich PA, Paulos LE, Rosenberg TD, et al. Lateral release of the patella: indications and contraindications. *Am J Sports Med.* 1990;18:359–365.

Komi PV, Karlsson J. Physical performance, skeletal muscle enzyme activities, and fibre types in monozygous and dizygous twins of both sexes. *Acta Physiol Scand.* 1979;462(Suppl):1–28.

Kowall MG, Kolk G, Nuber GW, et al. Patellofemoral taping in the treatment of patellofemoral pain. *Am J Sports Med.* 1996;24:61–66.

Kwak SD, Colman WW, Ateshian GA, et al. Anatomy of the human patellofemoral joint articular cartilage: a surface curvature analysis. *J Orthop Res.* 1997;15:468–472.

Laprade J, Culham E, Brouwer B. Comparison of five isometric exercises in the recruitment of the vastus medialis oblique in persons with and without patellofemoral pain. *J Orthop Sports Phys Ther.* 1998;27:197–204.

Larsen B, Andreasen E, Urfer A, et al. Patellar taping: a radiographic examination of the medial glide technique. *Am J Sports Med.* 1995;23:465–471.

Larsen NP, Forwood MR, Parker AW. Immobilization and re-training of cruciate ligaments in the rat. *Acta Orthop Scand.* 1987;58:260–264.

Laurin CA, Levesque HP, Dussault R, et al. The abnormal lateral patellofemoral angle. A diagnostic roentgenographic sign of recurrent patellar subluxation. *J Bone Joint Surg.* 1978;60A:55–60.

Lautamies R, Harilainen A, Kettunen J, et al. Isokinetic quadriceps and hamstring muscle strength and knee function 5 years after anterior cruciate ligament reconstruction: comparison between bone-patellar tendon-bone and hamstring tendon autografts. *Knee Surg Sports Traumatol Arthrosc.* 2008;16(11):1009–1016.

Lephart SM, Kocher MS, Fu FH, et al. Proprioception following anterior cruciate ligament reconstruction. *J Sports Rehabil.* 1992;1:188–196.

Lephart SM, Pincivero DM, Rozzi SL. Proprioception of the ankle and knee. *Sports Med.* 1998;3:149–155.

Lian O, Engebretsen L, Ovrebo RV, et al. Characteristics of the leg extensors in male volleyball players with jumper's knee. *Am J Sports Med.* 1996;24:380–385.

Lieb FJ, Perry J. Quadriceps function: an anatomical and mechanical study using amputated limbs. *J Bone Joint Surg.* 1971;53A:749–758.

Lieber RL, Silva PD, Daniel DM. Equal effectiveness of electrical and volitional strength training for quadriceps femoris muscles after anterior cruciate ligament surgery. *J Orthop Res.* 1996;14:131–138.

Lipscomb Jr AB, Anderson AF, Norwig ED, et al. Isolated posterior cruciate ligament reconstruction: long-term results. *Am J Sports Med.* 1993;21:490–496.

Lundberg M, Messner K. Long-term prognosis of isolated partial medial collateral ligament ruptures. *Am J Sports Med.* 1996;24:160–163.

Lutz GE, Palmitier RA, An KN, et al. Comparison of tibiofemoral joint forces during open-kinetic-chain and closed-kinetic-chain exercises. *J Bone Joint Surg.* 1993;75A:732–739.

MacDonald P, Miniaci A, Fowler P, et al. A biomechanical analysis of joint contact forces in the posterior cruciate deficient knee. *Knee Surg Sports Traumatol Arthrosc.* 1996;3:252–255.

Magen HE, Howell SM, Hull ML. Structural properties of six tibial fixation methods for anterior cruciate ligament soft tissue grafts. *Am J Sports Med.* 1999;27:35–43.

Mangine RE, Eifert-Mangine M, Burch D, et al. Postoperative management of the patellofemoral patient. *J Orthop Sports Phys Ther.* 1998;28:323–335.

Marder RA, Raskind JR, Carroll M. Prospective evaluation of arthroscopically assisted anterior cruciate ligament reconstruction: patellar tendon versus semitendinosis and gracilis tendons. *Am J Sports Med.* 1991;19:478–484.

Mariani PP, Santori N, Adriani E, et al. Accelerated rehabilitation after arthroscopic meniscal repair: a clinical and magnetic resonance imaging evaluation. *Arthroscopy.* 1996;12:680–686.

Markolf KL, Burchfield DM, Shapiro MM, et al. Biomechanical consequences of replacement of the anterior cruciate ligament with a patellar ligament allograft. Part II: forces in the graft compared with forces in the intact ligament. *J Bone Joint Surg.* 1996;78A:1728–1734.

Markolf KL, Mensch JS, Amstutz HC. Stiffness and laxity of the knee: the contributions of the supporting structures. *J Bone Joint Surg.* 1976;58A:583–593.

Markolf KL, Slauterbeck JR, Armstrong KL, et al. A biomechanical study of replacement of the posterior cruciate ligament with a graft. Part II: forces in the graft compared with forces in the intact ligament. *J Bone Joint Surg.* 1997;79A:381–386.

McConnell J. The management of chondromalacia patellae: a long term solution. *Aust J Physiother.* 1986;32:215–223.

McDaniel WJ, Dameron TB. Untreated ruptures of the anterior cruciate ligament. *J Bone Joint Surg.* 1980;62A:696–705.

McDaniel WJ, Dameron TB. The untreated anterior cruciate ligament rupture. *Clin Orthop.* 1983;172:158–163.

McKernan DJ, Paulos LE. Graft selection. In: Fu FH, Harner CD, Vince KG, eds. *Knee Surgery.* Baltimore: Williams & Wilkins; 1994.

McLaughlin J, DeMaio M, Noyes FR, et al. Rehabilitation after meniscus repair. *Orthopedics.* 1994;17:463–471.

Merchant AC. Classification of patellofemoral disorders. *Arthroscopy.* 1988;4:235–240.

Merchant AC, Mercer RL, Jacobsen RH, et al. Roentgenographic analysis of patellofemoral congruence. *J Bone Joint Surg.* 1974;56A:1391–1396.

Mirzabeigi E, Jordan C, Gronley JK, et al. Isolation of the vastus medialis oblique muscle during exercise. *Am J Sports Med.* 1999;27:50–53.

Mok DWH, Good C. Non-operative management of acute grade III medial collateral ligament injury of the knee. *Injury.* 1989;20:277–280.

Moller BN, Krebs B. Dynamic knee brace in the treatment of patellofemoral disorders. *Arch Orthop Trauma Surg.* 1986;104:377–379.

Morgan CD, Wojtys EM, Casscells CD, et al. Arthroscopic meniscal repair evaluated by second-look arthroscopy. *Am J Sports Med.* 1991;19:632–637.

Muhle C, Brinkmann G, Skaf A, et al. Effect of a patellar realignment brace on patients with patellar subluxation and dislocation. *Am J Sports Med.* 1999;27:350–353.

Muneta T, Sekiya I, Ogiuchi T, et al. Effects of aggressive early rehabilitation on the outcome of anterior cruciate ligament reconstruction with multi-strand semitendinosis tendon. *Int Orthop.* 1998;22:352–356.

Myer GD, Ford KR, Hewett TE. Rationale and clinical techniques for anterior cruciate ligament injury prevention among female athletes. *J Athl Train.* 2004;39:352–364.

Myer GD, Paterno MV, Ford KR, et al. Rehabilitation after anterior cruciate ligament reconstruction: criteria-based progression through the return-to-sport phase. *J Orthop Sports Phys Ther.* 2006;36:385–402.

Neeb TB, Aufdemkampe G, J.H Wagener, et al. Assessing anterior cruciate ligament injuries: the association and differential value of questionnaires, clinical tests, and functional tests. *J Orthop Sports Phys Ther.* 1997;26:324–331.

Nissen CW, Cullen MC, Hewett TE, et al. Physical and arthroscopic examination techniques of the patellofemoral joint. *J Orthop Sports Phys Ther.* 1998;28:277–285.

Nogalski MP, Bach Jr BR. Acute anterior cruciate ligament injuries. In: Fu FH, Harner CD, Vince KG, eds. *Knee Surgery.* Baltimore: Williams & Wilkins; 1994.

Novak PJ, Bach Jr BR, Hager CA. Clinical and functional outcome of anterior cruciate ligament reconstruction in the recreational athlete over the age of 35. *Am J Knee Surg.* 1996;9:111–116.

Noyes FR. Functional properties of knee ligaments and alterations induced by immobilization: a correlative biomechanical and histological study in primates. *Clin Orthop.* 1977;123:210–242.

Noyes FR, Barber SD, Mangine RE. Abnormal lower limb symmetry determined by function hop tests after anterior cruciate ligament rupture. *Am J Sports Med.* 1991;19:513–518.

Noyes FR, Butler DL, Grood ES, et al. Biomechanical analysis of human ligament grafts used in knee-ligament repairs and replacements. *J Bone Joint Surg.* 1984;66A:344–352.

Noyes FR, DeMaio M, Mangine RE. Evaluation-based protocol: a new approach to rehabilitation. *J Orthop Res.* 1991;14:1383–1385.

Noyes FR, Wojyts EM, Marshall MT. The early diagnosis and treatment of developmental patella infera syndrome. *Clin Orthop.* 1991;265:241–252.

Nyland J. Rehabilitation complications following knee surgery. *Clin Sports Med.* 1999;18:905–925.

O'Connor JJ. Can muscle co-contraction protect knee ligaments after injury or repair? *J Bone Joint Surg.* 1993;75B:41–48.

O'Donoghue DH. Surgical treatment of fresh injuries to the major ligaments of the knee. *J Bone Joint Surg.* 1950;32A:721–738.

Ohno K, Pomaybo AS, Schmidt CC, et al. Healing of the MCL after a combined MCL and ACL injury and reconstruction of the ACL: comparison of repair and nonrepair of MCL tears in rabbits. *J Orthop Res.* 1995;13:442–449.

Ostenberg A, Roos E, Ekdahl C, et al. Isokinetic knee extensor strength and functional performance in healthy female soccer players. *Scand J Med Sci Sports.* 1998;8:257–264.

Osteras H, Augestad LB, Tondel S. Isokinetic muscle strength after anterior cruciate ligament reconstruction. *Scand J Med Sci Sports.* 1998;8:279–282.

Ostero AL, Hutcheson L. A comparison of the doubled semitendinosis/gracilis and central third of the patellar tendon autografts in arthroscopic anterior cruciate ligament reconstruction. *Arthroscopy.* 1993;9:143–148.

Palumbo PM. Dynamic patellar brace: a new orthosis in the management of patellofemoral pain. *Am J Sports Med.* 1981;9:45–49.

Papagelopoulos PJ, Sim FH. Patellofemoral pain syndrome: diagnosis and management. *Orthopedics.* 1997;20:148–157.

Papalia R, Vasta S, Tecame A, et al. Home-based vs supervised rehabilitation programs following knee surgery: a systematic review. *British Medical Bulletin.* 2013;108.1:55–72. Web.

Parolie JM, Bergfeld JA. Long-term results of nonoperative treatment of isolated posterior cruciate ligament injuries in the athlete. *Am J Sports Med.* 1986;14:35–38.

Paulos LE, Rosenberg TD, Drawbert J, et al. Infrapatellar contracture syndrome: an unrecognized cause of knee stiffness with patella entrapment and patella infera. *Am J Sports Med.* 1987;15:331–341.

Pincivero DM, Lephart SM, Henry TJ. The effects of kinesthetic training on balance and proprioception in anterior cruciate ligament injured knee. *J Athl Train.* 1996;31(Suppl 2):S52.

Pope MH, Johnson RJ, Brown DW, et al. The role of the musculature in injuries to the medial collateral ligament. *J Bone Joint Surg.* 1979;61A:398–402.

Popp JE, Yu JS, Kaeding CC. Recalcitrant patellar tendinitis: magnetic resonance imaging, histologic evaluation, and surgical treatment. *Am J Sports Med.* 1997;25:218–222.

Powers CM. Rehabilitation of patellofemoral joint disorders: a critical review. *J Orthop Sports Phys Ther.* 1998;28:345–354.

Powers CM, Landel R, Perry J. Timing and intensity of vastus muscle activity during functional activities in subjects with and without patellofemoral pain. *Phys Ther.* 1996;76:946–966.

Prodromos CC, Han Y, Rogowski J, et al. A meta-analysis of the incidence of anterior cruciate ligament tears as a function of gender, sport, and a knee-injury-reduction regimen. *Arthroscopy.* 2007;23:1320–1325.

Prodromos CC, Joyce BT, Shi K, et al. A meta-analysis of stability after anterior cruciate ligament reconstruction as a function of hamstring versus patellar tendon graft and fixation type. *Arthroscopy.* 2005;21:1202.

Race A, Amis AA. The mechanical properties of the two bundles of the human posterior cruciate ligament. *J Biomech.* 1994;27:13–24.

Radin EL, Rose RM. Role of subchondral bone in the initiation and progression of cartilage damage. *Clin Orthop.* 1986;213:34–40.

Reider B. Medial collateral ligament injuries in athletes. *Sports Med.* 1996;21:147–156.

Reider B, Sathy MR, Talkington J, et al. Treatment of isolated medial collateral ligament injuries in athletes with early functional rehabilitation. *Am J Sports Med.* 1993;22:470–477.

Reinold MM, Fleisig GS, Wilk KE. Research supports both OKC and CKC activities. *Biomechanics.* 1999;2(Suppl 2):27–32.

Risberg MA, Holm I, Steen H, et al. The effect of knee bracing after anterior cruciate ligament reconstruction. *Am J Sports Med.* 1999;27:76–83.

Roberts D, Friden T, Zatterstrom R, et al. Proprioception in people with anterior cruciate ligament-deficient knees: comparison of symptomatic and asymptomatic patients. *J Orthop Sports Phys Ther.* 1999;29:587–594.

Rodeo SA. Arthroscopic meniscal repair with use of the outside-in technique. *J Bone Joint Surg.* 2000;82A:127–141.

Sachs RA, Daniel DM, Stone ML, et al. Patellofemoral problems after anterior cruciate ligament reconstruction. *Am J Sports Med.* 1989;17:760–765.

Schutzer SF, Ramsby GR, Fulkerson JP. Computed tomographic classification of patellofemoral pain patients. *Orthop Clin North Am.* 1986;144:16–26.

Schutzer SF, Ramsby GR, Fulkerson JP. The evaluation of patellofemoral pain using computerized tomography: a preliminary study. *Clin Orthop.* 1986;204:286–293.

Seitz H, Schlenz I, Muller E, et al. Anterior instability of the knee despite an intensive rehabilitation program. *Clin Orthop.* 1996;328:159–164.

Sernert N, Kartus J, Kohler K, et al. Analysis of subjective, objective, and functional examination tests after anterior cruciate ligament reconstruction. *Knee Surg Sports Traumatol Arthrosc.* 1999;7:160–165.

Shelbourne KD, Davis TJ, Patel DV. The natural history of acute, isolated, non-operatively treated posterior cruciate ligament injuries. *Am J Sports Med.* 1999;27:276–283.

Shelbourne KD, Davis TJ. Evaluation of knee stability before and after participation in a functional sports agility program during rehabilitation after anterior cruciate ligament reconstruction. *Am J Sports Med.* 1999;27:156–161.

Shelbourne KD, Foulk AD. Timing of surgery in anterior cruciate ligament tears on the return of quadriceps muscle strength after reconstruction using an autogenous patellar tendon graft. *Am J Sports Med.* 1995;23:686–689.

Shelbourne KD, Nitz P. Accelerated rehabilitation after anterior cruciate ligament reconstruction. *Am J Sports Med.* 1990;18:292–299.

Shelbourne KD, Patel DV. Treatment of limited motion after anterior cruciate ligament reconstruction. *Knee Surg Sports Traumatol Arthrosc.* 1999;7:85–92.

Shelbourne KD, Patel DV, Adsit WS, et al. Rehabilitation after meniscal repair. *Clin Sports Med.* 1996;15:595–612.

Shelbourne KD, Patel DV, Martini DJ. Classification and management of arthrofibrosis of the knee after anterior cruciate ligament reconstruction. *Am J Sports Med.* 1996;24:857–862.

Shelbourne KD, Wilckens JH, Mollabaashy A, et al. Arthrofibrosis in acute anterior cruciate ligament reconstruction: the effect of timing of reconstruction and rehabilitation. *Am J Sports Med.* 1991;9:332–336.

Shellock FG, Mink JH, Deutsch AL, et al. Kinematic MR imaging of the patellofemoral joint: comparison of passive positioning and active movement techniques. *Radiology.* 1992;184:574–577.

Shelton WR, Papendick L, Dukes AD. Autograft versus allograft anterior cruciate ligament reconstruction. *Arthroscopy.* 1997;13:446–449.

Skyhar MJ, Warren RF, Oritz GJ, et al. The effects of sectioning of the posterior cruciate ligament and the posterolateral complex on the articular contact pressures within the knee. *J Bone Joint Surg.* 1993;75A:694–699.

Snyder-Mackler L, Ladin Z, Schepsis AA, et al. Electrical stimulation of thigh muscles after reconstruction of anterior cruciate ligament. *J Bone Joint Surg.* 1991;73A:1025–1036.

Steinkamp LA, Dillingham MF, Markel MD, et al. Biomechanical considerations in patellofemoral joint rehabilitation. *Am J Sports Med.* 1993;21:438–444.

Stetson WB, Friedman MJ, Fulkerson JP, et al. Fracture of the proximal tibia with immediate weightbearing after a Fulkerson osteotomy. *Am J Sports Med.* 1997;25:570–574.

Thompson WO, Thaete FL, Fu FH, et al. Tibial meniscal dynamics using three-dimensional reconstruction of magnetic resonance images. *Am J Sports Med.* 1991;19:210–216.

Torg JS, Barton TM, Pavlov H, et al. Natural history of the posterior cruciate ligament-deficient knee. *Clin Orthop.* 1989;246:208–216.

Tyler TF, McHugh MP, Gleim GW, et al. The effect of immediate weightbearing after anterior cruciate ligament reconstruction. *Clin Orthop.* 1998;357:141–148.

Uhorchak JM, Scoville CR, Williams GN, et al. Risk factors associated with noncontact injury of the anterior cruciate ligament: a prospective four-year evaluation of 859 West Point cadets. *Am J Sports Med.* 2003;31:831–842.

Vedi V, Williams A, Tennant SJ, et al. Meniscal movement: an in-vivo study using dynamic MRI. *J Bone Joint Surg.* 1999;81B:37–41.

Voloshin AS, Wosk J. Shock absorption of the meniscectomized and painful knees: a comparative in vivo study. *J Biomed Eng.* 1983;5:157–161.

Vos EJ, Harlaar J, van Ingen-Schenau GJ. Electromechanical delay during knee extensor contractions. *Med Sci Sports Exerc.* 1991;23:1187–1193.

Weiss JA, Woo SL-Y, Ohland KJ, et al. Evaluation of a new injury model to study medial collateral ligament healing: primary repair versus non-operative treatment. *J Orthop Res.* 1991;9:516–528.

Wilk KE, Davies GJ, Mangine RE, et al. Patellofemoral disorders: a classification system and clinical guideline for nonoperative rehabilitation. *J Orthop Sports Phys Ther.* 1998;28:307–322.

Williams Jr JS, Bach Jr BR. Rehabilitation of the ACL deficient and reconstructed knee. In: Grana W, ed. *Sports Med Arthrosc Rev.* vol. 3. 1996:69–82.

Woo SL-Y, Chan SS, Yamaji T. Biomechanics of knee ligament healing, repair, and reconstruction. *J Biomech.* 1997;30:431–439.

Woo SL-Y, Gomez MA, Sites TJ, et al. The biomechanical and morphological changes of the MCL following immobilization and remobilization. *J Bone Joint Surg.* 1987;69A:1200–1211.

Woo SL-Y, Hollis JM, Adams DJ, et al. Tensile properties of the human femur-anterior cruciate ligament complex. *Am J Sports Med.* 1991;19:217–225.

Woo SL-Y, Inoue M, McGurck-Burleson E, et al. Treatment of the medial collateral ligament injury II. Structure and function of canine knees in response to differing treatment regimens. *Am J Sports Med.* 1987;15:22–29.

Wright, et al. Anterior cruciate ligament reconstruction rehabilitation MOON Guidelines. *Sports Health.* Jan 2014.

Yamaji T, Levine RE, Woo SL-Y, et al. MCL healing one year after a concurrent MCL and ACL injury: an interdisciplinary study in rabbits. *J Orthop Res.* 1996;14:223–227.

Yasuda K, Erickson AR, Beynnon BD, et al. Dynamic elongation behavior in the medial collateral and anterior cruciate ligaments during lateral impact loading. *J Orthop Res.* 1993;11:190–198.

Zazulak BT, Hewett TE, Reeves N, et al. Deficits in neuromuscular control of the trunk predict knee injury risk: a prospective biomechanical-epidemiological study. *Am J Sports Med.* 2007;35:1123–1130.

Zheng N, Fleisig GS, Escamilla RF, et al. An analytical model of the knee for estimation of the internal forces during exercise. *J Biomech.* 1998;31:963–967.

Perturbation Training for Postoperative ACL Reconstruction and Patients Who Were Nonoperatively Treated and ACL Deficient

Michael Duke, PT, CSCS | S. Brent Brotzman, MD

Perturbation is defined as a small change in a physical system, most often in a system at equilibrium that is disturbed from the outside or an unconscious reaction to a sudden, unexpected outside force or movement—for example, a football running back who reacts to potential tacklers by cutting, side-stepping, stopping, and quickly starting again or a basketball player who avoids defenders by quick changes in direction and speed. **Perturbation training involves applying potentially destabilizing forces to the injured knee to enhance the neuromuscular awareness, neuromuscular response, and dynamic stability of the knee to stabilize the joint.** The goal of perturbation training is to educate the patient to elicit selective adaptive muscle reactions of the supporting knee musculature in response to force administered on the platform to gain a knee-protective neuromuscular response.

Nonoperative management of ACL rupture has had limited success in patients who wish to return to high levels of activity. Evidence supports surgical intervention for these patients if they plan to return to their high-level sport (Daniel et al. 1994, Engstrom et al. 1993). For some individuals, however, circumstances may warrant a delay in or avoidance of surgical intervention. Such individuals might include an athlete who needs to demonstrate his or her abilities for scholarship or desires to finish the competitive season, seasonal workers who want to postpone surgery until after the busy work season, or individuals for whom life circumstances or stage of life makes surgery undesirable but who want to remain active until they are able to undergo surgery.

COPERS

Among patients who opt not to have ACL reconstruction, there is a subset who are better at actively stabilizing the ACL-deficient knee through complex neuromuscular patterns (known as copers). **Copers** are distinct in their ability to return to full activity despite being ACL deficient with no instability for at least 1 year. They adopt various compensatory patterns of muscle activation that seem to be unrelated to quadriceps strength.

NONCOPERS

Noncopers are those who are not able to return to full activity and tend to demonstrate a joint-stiffening strategy or a nonadaptive generalized co-contraction of the muscles that stabilize the knee. The noncoper strategy of joint stiffening is commonly seen with early motor learning of unfamiliar activities, and as the task becomes more familiar to the individual, the individual is able to demonstrate more complex motor patterns. Those who are able to return to high functional levels demonstrate alterations in muscle activity that improve stability of the knee joint (Ciccotti et al. 1994, Gauffin and Tropp 1992, Rudolph et al. 1998). Pertubation training has also been shown to improve knee function in noncopers (Logerstedt et al. 2009) with ACL injuries.

Several theories have been proposed to explain the ability to stabilize the knee and other joints. Johansson and Sjolander suggested that an increase in sensitivity of mechanoreceptors in joint structures may result in a higher state of "readiness" of muscles to respond to challenges to joint stability (Fitzgerald et al. 2000b, Johansson and Sjolander 1993). **The implication is that if the therapist can provide progressively destabilizing challenges to the knee during rehabilitation, the neuromuscular patterns can be altered in a way that improves joint stability despite a lack of passive restraints.**

Hartigan et al. (2009) found that those who participated in a perturbation training protocol before ACL reconstruction showed no difference in knee excursion (knee flexion during gait) between the involved and uninvolved knees 6 months after ACL reconstruction. In contrast, a group who participated in only a standard strength ACL program showed significant side-to-side asymmetries. This finding indicates that some form of neuromuscular training, in particular perturbation training, is essential to restore normal movement patterns.

Given that these results show that asymmetries existed at walking speed, the problems are magnified at game speed. Similarly, a clinical trial by Risberg et al. 2007 compared a strength-based (ST) rehabilitation program and a neuromuscular control-based (NT) program. Based on their findings, Risberg advocated employing both strength- and neuromuscular control–based programs.

In reconstructing the ACL, one of the main purposes is to restore passive restraint to anterior translation of the tibia on the femur. Beard et al. (2001) studied tibial translation both preoperatively and postoperatively in patients with ACL deficiency and found that tibial translation actually transiently increased after reconstruction, which the authors attributed to reduction of the protective hypertonicity of the hamstring group, making them less able to restrain tibial movement. Given this finding and the transient loss of the stabilizing effect of the hamstrings, it becomes even more critical to retrain the neuromuscular system to prevent "giving way" episodes with resultant meniscal damage. Perturbation training has been shown to be effective at this.

TABLE 48.1	Screening Tests for Nonoperative Treatment of ACL Injury	
Test		**Passing Score**
Single, crossover, triple, and timed hop tests (Noyes et al. 1991, Reid et al. 2007)		80% or more of uninvolved limb
Reported number of giving-way episodes from the time of injury to the time of testing		No more than one episode
The Knee Outcome Survey Activities of Daily Living Scale (Irrgang et al. 1998)		80% or more
Subjective global rating of knee function (self-assessed 0%–100%)		60% or more

Several criteria have been described to select the appropriate candidate for a **successful outcome with nonoperative treatment of ACL injury** (Engstrom et al. 1993, Fitzgerald et al. 2000a):
- No evidence of joint effusion
- Full passive knee joint ROM, as compared to the uninvolved knee
- Full knee extension during a straight leg raise (SLR) on the involved limb
- A quadriceps femoris maximal voluntary contraction force on the involved limb equivalent to 75% of that on the uninvolved limb
- Tolerance for single-leg hopping on the involved limb without pain
- No concomitant ligamentous or meniscal injury

Once these criteria are met, the screening test is administered as described in Table 48.1. Patients who pass the screening test are considered good candidates for nonoperative rehabilitation.

Augmenting a standard rehabilitation protocol with perturbation training has been shown to greatly increase the likelihood of returning to the competitive season with no episodes of giving way (Fitzgerald et al. 2000c). Perturbation training generally is performed in 2 or 3 sessions a week for a total of 8 to 10 sessions, with the patient returning to sport during the last week of training.

The patient is encouraged to respond to the direction and force of the perturbations with purposeful muscle responses designed to prevent or minimize large excursions on the support surface. Gross muscular co-contraction and preparatory stiffening of the joint are discouraged and addressed with additional cues from the physical therapist.

Perturbation training consists of three techniques:
- Roller board translations
- Tilt board perturbations
- Roller board and stationary platform perturbations

Roller board translations consist of the patient standing with both feet on a rolling platform while the therapist applies translational perturbations to the platform (Fig. 48.1). Initially, safety precautions should be used, such as placing the patient in parallel bars or in a doorway, but these can be discontinued once the therapist believes there are no safety issues. The therapist instructs the patient to maintain balance on the board. Progression of the exercise can have various forms, such as the following:
- Predictable and rhythmic to random
- Weak force application to strong force
- Small translations to large translations
- Double-limb stance to single limb

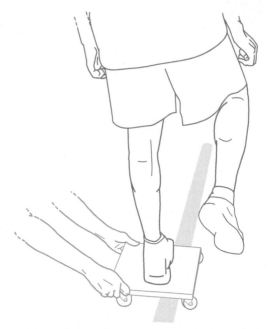

Fig. 48.1   Roller board transitional perturbation technique.

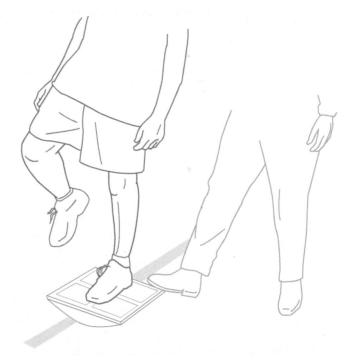

Fig. 48.2   Tilt board perturbation technique.

- Visual feedback (watching the board) to eyes closed or looking away
- Patient's focus directed on the perturbations to sports-specific distractions such as ball tossing or dribbling during perturbations

Tilt board perturbations consist of the patient standing on a tilt board while the therapist taps or steps on the edge of the board, causing the board to suddenly tip (Fig. 48.2). The patient is instructed to maintain balance and return to a neutral position after the therapist applies the perturbations. The patient can stand with the board tilting anterior and posterior, medial and lateral, or diagonally in either direction. Progression of the

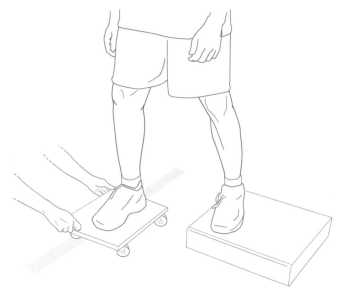

Fig. 48.3 Roller board and stationary platform perturbation technique.

exercise can include all of the aforementioned challenges, with the addition of upright posture progression to progressively deeper squat positions.

Roller board and stationary platform perturbations consist of the patient standing with one limb on the platform and one on the roller board and the therapist applying translational forces to the roller board (Fig. 48.3). The patient is instructed to "match my force" or to prevent the board from moving without co-contraction of the lower limbs. It is important for the therapist to watch for co-contractions and gauge the speed and force of response given by the patient. The patient is learning to selectively activate muscle groups in response to an external challenge. Both the response time and force should improve, indicating the need to further challenge the patient. The following progressions can be made in addition to those already mentioned:

- Side-by-side stance to front or back split stance to sports-specific stance (i.e., baseball infielder stance or quarterback throwing stance)
- Involved limb on roller board to uninvolved limb on roller board
- Wood platform to foam pad (compliant surface)
- Single direction movement to multidirectional

The therapist must be attentive to the patient's response during the training, constantly assessing response time, strength of response, ability to change directions, stability of the knee, and whether the patient demonstrates significant co-contraction. Verbal cues should be given, and appropriate responses should indicate readiness advancement to more difficult challenges.

Perturbation training also can be an effective tool in rehabilitation after ACL reconstruction. Changes in anatomic knee stability depend on the surgery; however, functional and active knee stability can be altered by rehabilitation programs. The goal of any postoperative ACL reconstruction rehabilitation program should be to enhance long-term functional outcomes, and critical to this is the patient's ability to stabilize the knee joint during high-level functional activities.

Proprioceptive recovery after ACL reconstruction is critical to joint stability. An intact ACL is known to have mechanoreceptors (Schultz et al. 1984, Schutte et al. 1987), and it has been noted by various authors that some reinnervation occurs in ACL grafts after reconstruction, although timing and extent may vary considerably (Barrack et al. 1997, Barrett 1991, Fremerey et al. 2000, Risberg et al. 2001).

Patients who have had ACL surgery demonstrate co-contraction patterns similar to those who are ACL deficient (Vairo et al. 2008). Considering the time of recovery of quadriceps strength and the need for healing of the hamstring after an autograft reconstruction, **we recommend that perturbation training begin around 12 weeks after ACL reconstruction.** Several criteria should be met before perturbation training is initiated after ACL reconstructive surgery:

- Normal gait, ROM, straight leg raise, and minimal effusion
- Single-limb balance greater than 60 seconds with minimal movement and eyes open
- Single-limb squat on the involved side to 45 degrees with no functional genu varum/valgum during the squat and good pelvic control

Once these criteria are met, a program similar to that outlined for nonoperative treatment of ACL injury can be used.

Although useful for both nonoperative and postoperative management of ACL injuries, perturbation training can be used for any condition that results in abnormal neuromuscular patterns affecting gait or sports movements. Other conditions that also may benefit from perturbation training include the following:

- Other ligament sprains of the knee
- Any joint instability of the ankle, knee, or sacroiliac joint
- Upper extremity conditions (i.e., wrist, elbow, or shoulder), with modifications
- Vestibular conditions
- Knee OA (Fitzgerald et al. 2002)

The concept of improving neuromuscular control of complicated movements through perturbation training can be successfully applied to any sport. Baseball pitchers at various phases of the throwing motion can be perturbed at the upper extremity or trunk or lower extremity. Golfers at various phases of the swing can be similarly challenged. Basketball players while in a post position or while shooting can be perturbed to improve their ability to maintain position or make a steady shot. Any running sport can benefit from single-leg balance and perturbations to improve stability and neuromuscular control to maintain position despite challenges from opponents or surface variations. Extensive study of perturbation training and ACL injury does not imply that this is its only use. Further research is necessary to determine the full extent to which perturbation can be implemented.

There is significant evidence in the literature for the use of the previously described techniques of perturbation training for knee stability. The roller board and rocker board are designed to apply destabilizing forces from the ground up, simulating various neuromuscular patterns during athletic activities where there is no contact with objects or other players. The chapter authors propose that in addition to the current perturbation protocol, athletes will benefit from a variety of perturbations from the top down.

Sports such as wrestling, basketball, football, rugby, and martial arts are all inherently contact sports, and the athletes are repeatedly exposed to external forces to knees, hips, torso, shoulders, upper extremities, head, and neck. By adding perturbing forces that begin as light and predictable and progress to functional speeds and intensity, the athlete will be better prepared for the contact that will occur during training and competition.

Standing static push perturbations consist of the patient standing, feet on floor shoulder-width apart, knees slightly bent, and eyes looking forward. The therapist can apply force to knees, hips, and shoulders in varying directions, intensity, and predictability, instructing the patient to maintain position. Add a compliant surface under the feet to increase difficulty. Add sport-specific distractions to further increase difficulty, such as dribbling a basketball, playing catch with a baseball, and the like. Given the use of hands in wrestling and other sports, incorporating upper extremities will also be valuable.

Standing stick pull perturbations consist of the patient standing in a similar position as just described, but the patient holds a stick horizontally with two hands in front, in a palm-down grip. The therapist can then apply challenges to position in all three planes of movement, again with the patient instructed to resist movement and maintain position. To provide challenges that simulate the athlete's sport, the therapist may place the athlete in positions of function to his or her sport including kneeling or half-kneeling or tandem stance or provide the training with the patient's eyes closed.

Basketball, football, rugby, and other players often encounter outside forces (other players) while in the air. Perturbation training for these athletes may include forces applied while the feet are off the ground.

Midair perturbations consist of having the patient perform vertical jumping while the therapist applies force through a Sport Cord attached around the patient's waist. With the force being applied while the patient is in midair, the landing direction has a horizontal component to it and challenges the knee stability in that way. The critical part to the exercise is the landing. The therapist should pay close attention to abnormal landing patterns that might indicate poor neuromuscular control and correct these. Jumping technique, angle of force by the therapist, amount of force, direction of jumping, and attention on task or distractions all can be modified as the athlete improves in skill.

These techniques can be applied in conjunction with perturbation training for knee rehabilitation. As with previously described perturbation training, these should be performed after an appropriate level of strength and stability has been achieved. Twelve weeks of rehabilitation should be completed for patients post-ACL surgery prior to beginning this program. The long-term benefit of these three techniques will require further research.

REFERENCES

A complete reference list is available at https://expertconsult.inkling.com/.

FURTHER READING

Bolgla LA, Malone TR, Umberger BR, et al. Hip strength and hip and knee kinematics during stair descent in females with and without patellofemoral pain syndrome. *J Orthop Sports Phys Ther.* 2008;38:12–18.

Devan MR, Pescatello LS, Faghri P, et al. A prospective study of overuse knee injuries among female athletes with muscle imbalances and structural abnormalities. *J Athl Train.* 2004;39:263–367.

Dierks TA, Manal KT, Hamill J, et al. Proximal and distal influences on hip and knee kinematics in runners with patellofemoral pain during a prolonged run. *J Orthop Sports Phys Ther.* 2008;38:448–456.

Lee TQ, Morris G, Csintalan RP. The influence of tibial and femoral rotation on patellofemoral contact area and pressure. *J Orthop Sports Phys Ther.* 2003;33:686–693.

Logerstedt D, Lynch A, Axe MJ, Snyder-Mackler L. Symmetry restoration and functional recovery before and after anterior cruciate ligament reconstruction. *Knee Surgery, Sports Traumatology, Arthroscopy Knee Surg Sports Traumatol Arthrosc.* 2012;21(4):859–868. Web.

Mascal CL, Landel R, Powers CM. Management of patellofemoral pain targeting hip, pelvis, and trunk muscle function: 2 case reports. *J Orthop Sports Phys Ther.* 2003;33:647–660.

Mizuno Y, Kumagai M, Mattessich SM, et al. Q-angle influences tibiofemoral and patellofemoral kinematics. *J Orthop Res.* 2001;19:834–840.

Powers CM. The influence of altered lower-extremity kinematics on patellofemoral joint dysfunction: a theoretical perspective. *J Orthop Sports Phys Ther.* 2003;33:639–646.

Powers CM, Ward SR, Fredericson M, et al. Patellofemoral kinematics during weight-bearing and non-weight-bearing knee extension in persons with lateral subluxation of the patella: a preliminary study. *J Orthop Sports Phys Ther.* 2003;33:677–685.

Prins MR, van der Wurff P. Females with patellofemoral pain syndrome have weak hip muscles: a systematic review. *Aust J Physiother.* 2009;55:9–15.

Shultz R, Silder A, Malone M, et al. Unstable surface improves quadriceps:hamstring co-contraction for anterior cruciate ligament injury prevention strategies. *Sports Health.* 2014;7(2):166–171. Web.

Souza RB, Powers CM. Differences in hip kinematics, muscle strength, and muscle activation between subjects with and without patellofemoral pain. *J Orthop Sports Phys Ther.* 2009;39:12–19.

Stasi SLD, Snyder-Mackler L. The effects of neuromuscular training on the gait patterns of ACL-deficient men and women. *Clinical Biomechanics.* 2012;27(4):360–365. Web.

Willson JD, Binder-Macleod S, Davis IS. Lower extremity jumping mechanics of female athletes with and without patellofemoral pain before and after exertion. *Am J Sports Med.* 2008;36:1587–1596.

Willson JD, Davis I. Lower extremity strength and mechanics during jumping in women with patellofemoral pain. *J Sport Rehabil.* 2009;18:75–89.

Willson JD, Davis I. Utility of the frontal plane projection angle in females with patellofemoral pain. *J Orthop Sports Phys Ther.* 2008;38:606–615.

Gender Issues in ACL Injury

Lori A. Bolgla, PT, PhD, MAcc, ATC

In 1972 the United States passed Title IX of the Educational Act that mandates equal treatment of females in university-level athletic programs. The passage of this act has fostered a dramatic increase in the participation of females at all levels of competition. With this change comes a significant increase in the number of injuries sustained.

ACL INJURY IN THE FEMALE ATHLETE

Overview

ACL injury represents one of the most serious knee injuries, with annual costs for management exceeding $2 billion. Although surgical reconstruction and rehabilitation significantly improve the return to recreational and occupational activities, outcomes from long-term studies suggest the eventual development of knee osteoarthritis in many ACL-injured knees. **The incidence rate of ACL tears for female athletes ranges between 2.4 and 9.7 times their male counterparts competing in similar activities.** Together, these findings have led researchers to identify risk factors and develop prevention programs aimed at reducing female ACL injuries.

More than 70% of all ACL injuries occur via a noncontact mechanism during activities such as cutting and landing. Evidence has shown that females perform these activities with the knee positioned in maladaptive femoral adduction, femoral internal rotation, and tibial external rotation (referred to as **dynamic valgus**). These combined motions apply high valgus loads onto the knee, which can lead to ACL injury (Fig. 49.1). Another contributor to ACL injury is landing from a jump with the knee in a minimally flexed position (rather than the more desired flexed knee position). This position results in greater quadriceps activation relative to the hamstrings, leading to increased anterior tibial translation on the femur.

Of note, female athletes have been shown to perform athletic maneuvers with maladaptive variation from their male counterparts on landing including decreased knee and hip flexion, increased quadriceps activation, and greater dynamic knee valgus angles and moments (Powers 2010).

Intrinsic and extrinsic factors (Box 49.1) may account for the higher incidence of ACL injury in the female athlete. **Intrinsic factors** are anatomic or physiologic in nature and are not amenable to change. **Extrinsic factors** are biomechanical or neuromuscular in nature and are potentially modifiable. Clinicians have focused much attention on these extrinsic factors for the development and implementation of ACL injury prevention and rehabilitation programs.

Intrinsic Risk Factors

ACL injury commonly occurs with the knee positioned and stressed close to **full extension,** causing an abutment of the ACL within the intercondylar notch. Although a decreased intercondylar notch size may contribute to ACL injury, data have not supported a sex difference between intercondylar notch size and ACL injury. Instead, individuals with a **smaller intercondylar notch** appear to be more susceptible to ACL injury, regardless of sex.

Recent attention has focused on **ligament stiffness.** Hashemi et al. (2008) reported that the ACL from female cadavers exhibited a decrease in length, cross-sectional area, and volume compared to males. They concluded that inherent ligament weakness, in combination with a smaller intercondylar notch size, might contribute to the ACL injury gender bias.

Physiologic laxity (e.g., general joint laxity and ligamentous laxity) represents another intrinsic factor. Because the ACL primarily limits excessive anterior tibial translation relative to the femur, injury can occur when joint movement exceeds ligamentous strength. Uhorchak et al. (2003) have reported that females with physiologic laxity have a 2.7 times higher risk for sustaining an ACL injury.

Finally, increased estrogen levels during the ovulatory and luteal phases of the menstrual cycle may increase ACL laxity, making the female athlete more prone to injury. To date, prior works have not shown a strong association between hormone fluctuations and ACL injury. The reader should note that prior works have used small sample sizes and relied on subjective histories to determine the phase of the menstrual cycle when an injury occurred. Additional investigations are needed to better understand this influence.

Extrinsic Risk Factors

Extrinsic factors include biomechanical (e.g., kinematics and kinetics) and neuromuscular (e.g., muscle strength, endurance, and activation) characteristics. Unlike intrinsic factors, clinicians can modify these factors with interventions, providing the basis for many ACL injury prevention and rehabilitation programs.

As mentioned previously, **dynamic knee valgus** applies high loads onto the ACL that can cause injury. During the past 10 years, researchers have ascertained that female athletes perform higher demanding activities in positions making them more vulnerable to ACL injury. It is important to note that structures both proximal and distal to the knee can influence ACL loading. Ireland (1999) described the **position of no return** to explain gender differences regarding trunk and lower extremity kinematics and muscle activity (Fig. 49.2). The following summarizes extrinsic factors making the female athlete more vulnerable to ACL injury during running, cutting, and landing tasks:

- Overwhelming data infer that females perform these tasks (e.g., landing) with increased dynamic knee valgus from femoral internal rotation, femoral adduction, and tibial external rotation (Fig. 49.10, *A*).

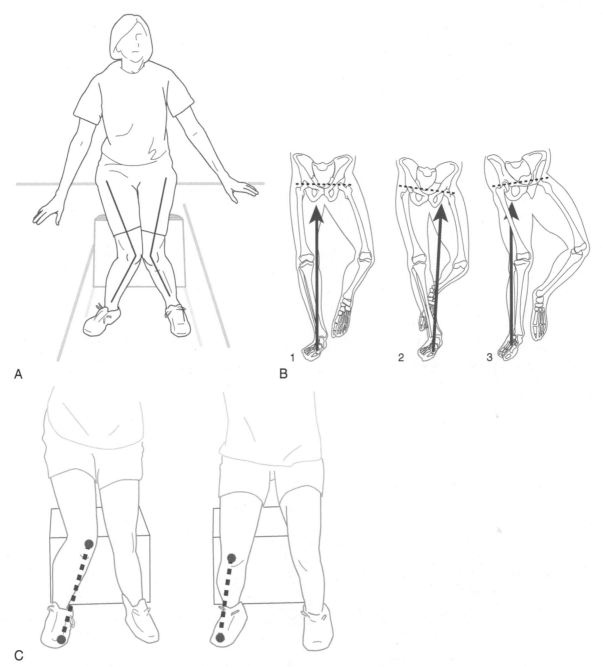

Fig. 49.1 **A,** Dynamic knee valgus resulting from excessive hip adduction and internal rotation after landing from a box jump. Because the foot is fixed to the floor, excessive frontal and transverse plane motion at the hip can cause medial motion of the knee joint, tibia abduction, and foot pronation. **B,** Frontal plane motions of the pelvis and trunk can influence the moment at the knee. This example illustrates landing from a jump on one foot. (1) With the pelvis level, the resultant ground reaction force vector passes medial to the knee joint center, thereby creating a varus moment at the knee. (2) Hip abductor weakness can cause a contralateral pelvic drop and a shift in the center of mass away from the stance limb. This increases the varus moment at the knee (i.e., the perpendicular distance from the resultant ground reaction force vector and the knee joint center increases). (3) Shifting the center of mass over the stance limb to compensate for hip abductor weakness can create knee valgus moment (i.e., the ground reaction force vector passes lateral with respect to the knee joint center). In this scenario, medial movement of the knee joint center (i.e., valgus collapse) exacerbates the problem. **C,** Low-risk and high-risk landings. The figure on the left shows a high-risk participant where the patella has moved inward and ended up medial to the first toe. The figure on the right shoes a low-risk participant where the patella has remained inward in line with the first toe.

BOX 49.1   ACL INJURY IN THE FEMALE ATHLETE

INTRINSIC FACTORS ASSOCIATED WITH FEMALE ACL INJURY

Intercondylar notch size
ACL size
Physiologic laxity (generalized joint and ligamentous)
Hormonal fluctuations

EXTRINSIC FACTORS ASSOCIATED WITH FEMALE ACL INJURY

Kinematics
Kinetics
Muscle strength
Muscle endurance
Muscle activation

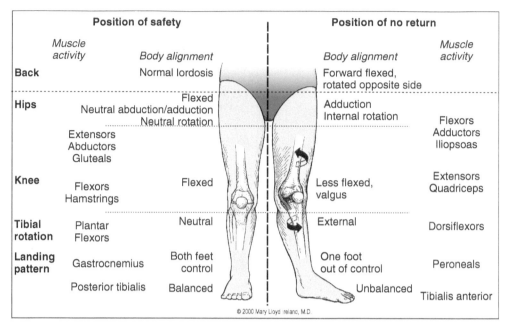

A

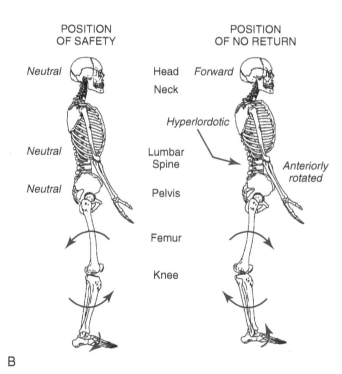

B

Fig. 49.2　**A,** Position of no return. (Copyright 2000 Mary Lloyd Ireland, MD.) **B,** In the "position of no return" (i.e., the high-risk position), the head is forward, the lumbar spine is hyperlordotic, and the pelvis is anteriorly rotated. Internal rotation at the relatively straight knee and subsequent tibial external rotation and foot pronation are also seen. The safe position shown on the left is more neutral and more flexed. (Reprinted with permission from Ireland M. The Female Athlete. Philadelphia, Saunders, 2002. Fig. 43-4.)

- Females utilize greater quadriceps activation relative to the hamstrings. This muscle imbalance can lead to excessive tibial anterior translation, especially with the knee positioned close to full extension.
- Females tend to activate the quadriceps more than other muscle groups such as the hip extensors and ankle plantar flexors. Muscle activation throughout the entire lower extremity can dampen applied ground reaction forces and reduce valgus knee loading.
- Females with evident hip musculature weakness perform demanding tasks with increased dynamic valgus. The amount of dynamic valgus exhibited during demanding tasks further increases with the onset of gluteus medius fatigue.
- Preliminary evidence infers decreased trunk neuromuscular control as a predictor of ACL injury.

ACL INJURY PREVENTION AND REHABILITATION PROGRAMS IN FEMALE ATHLETES

Identification of these extrinsic factors thought to contribute to ACL injury in the female athlete has provided the basis for the development and implementation of ACL injury prevention and rehabilitation programs. These programs typically include strengthening and neuromuscular training in combination with instruction on proper lower extremity alignment during cutting and landing tasks. Preliminary data have shown promising results for the effectiveness of these programs for preventing ACL injury in high school and collegiate-level female athletes.

ACL injury prevention programs should incorporate strengthening and neuromuscular training for the knee, hip, and trunk muscles on both stable and unstable surfaces (Figs. 49.3 through 49.6). The athlete should perform all plyometric-type exercises with the knees in a more varus, flexed position to reduce valgus loading and facilitate quadriceps/hamstring co-contraction (Fig. 49.7). Sport-specific drills that emphasize proper lower extremity alignment are another important consideration (Figs. 49.8 and 49.9). Throughout the process, the clinician should provide the athlete with continual feedback regarding proper technique when performing cutting and landing activities. The female athlete should practice proper deceleration techniques during cutting maneuvers, with a special emphasis on the avoidance of pivoting on a fixed foot. She should perform landing activities with an emphasis on keeping the knees over the toes (to minimize knee valgus) and landing as softly as possible using increased knee flexion (to dampen ground reaction forces).

An important aspect of rehabilitation prior to ACL reconstruction is the restoration of knee ROM and strength. Although quadriceps strengthening is an important component, Hartigan et al. (2009) reported on the importance of preoperative perturbation training on ACL reconstruction outcomes (see page 219). Perturbation training is a neuromuscular training program aimed at improving dynamic knee stability (Box 49.2).

Regarding postoperative ACL rehabilitation, clinicians should continue to follow protocols that emphasize symmetric knee ROM, gait normalization, and controlled weightbearing exercises. Other considerations include hip strengthening exercises (Table 49.1). The clinician also should incorporate neuromuscular retraining as indicated throughout the rehabilitation process through use of single-leg stance exercises

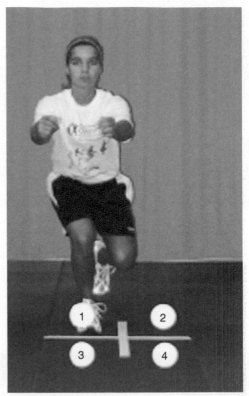

Fig. 49.3 Cross hops. The athlete faces a quadrant pattern and stands on a single limb with the support knee slightly bent. She hops diagonally, lands in the opposite quadrant, maintains forward stance, and holds the deep knee flexion landing for 3 seconds. She then hops laterally into the side quadrant and again holds the landing. Next she hops diagonally backward and holds the jump. Finally, she hops laterally into the initial quadrant and holds the landing. She repeats this pattern for the required number of sets. Encourage the athlete to maintain balance during each landing, keeping her eyes up and the visual focus away from her feet. (Reprinted with permission from Myer G, Ford K, Hewett T. Rationale and clinical techniques for anterior cruciate ligament injury prevention among female athletes. *J Athl Train* 39(4):361, 2004.)

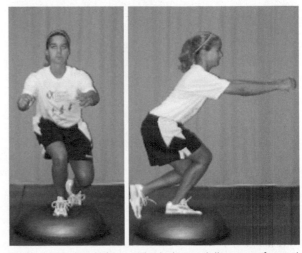

Fig. 49.4 Single-leg balance. The balance drills are performed on a balance device that provides an unstable surface. The athlete begins on the device with a two-legged stance with feet shoulder-width apart, in athletic position. As she improves, the training drills can incorporate ball catches and single-leg balance drills. Encourage the athlete to maintain deep knee flexion when performing all balance drills. (Reprinted with permission from Myer G, Ford K, Hewett T. Rationale and clinical techniques for anterior cruciate ligament injury prevention among female athletes. *J Athl Train* 39(4):361, 2004.)

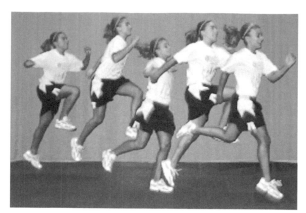

Fig. 49.5 Bounding. The athlete begins this jump by bounding in place. Once she attains proper rhythm and form, encourage her to maintain the vertical component of the bound while adding some horizontal distance to each jump. The progression of jumps advances the athlete across the training area. When coaching this jump, encourage the athlete to maintain maximum bounding height. (Reprinted with permission from Myer G, Ford K, Hewett T. Rationale and clinical techniques for anterior cruciate ligament injury prevention among female athletes. *J Athl Train* 39(4):361, 2004.)

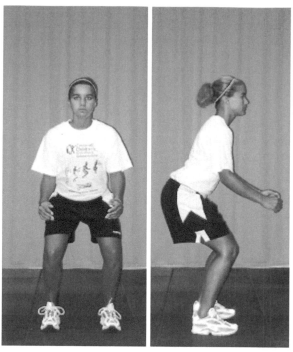

Fig. 49.7 The athletic position is a functionally stable position with the knees comfortably flexed, shoulders back, eyes up, feet approximately shoulder-width apart, and body mass balanced over the balls of the feet. The knees should be over the balls of the feet and the chest over the knees. This athlete-ready position is the starting and finishing position for most of the training exercises. During some exercises, the finishing position is exaggerated with deeper knee flexion to emphasize the correction of certain biomechanical deficiencies. (Reprinted with permission from Myer G, Ford K, Hewett T. Rationale and clinical techniques for anterior cruciate ligament injury prevention among female athletes. *J Athl Train* 39(4):361, 2004.)

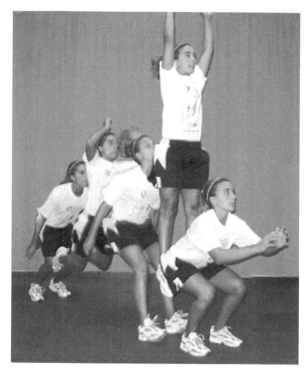

Fig. 49.6 Jump, jump, jump, vertical jump. The athlete performs three successive broad jumps and immediately progresses into a maximum-effort vertical jump. The three consecutive broad jumps should be performed as quickly as possible and attain maximal horizontal distance. The third broad jump should be used as a preparatory jump that will allow horizontal momentum to be quickly and efficiently transferred into vertical power. Encourage the athlete to provide minimal braking on the third and final broad jump to ensure that maximum energy is transferred to the vertical jump. Coach the athlete to go directly vertical on the fourth jump and not move horizontally. Use full arm extension to achieve maximum vertical height. (Reprinted with permission from Myer G, Ford K, Hewett T. Rationale and clinical techniques for anterior cruciate ligament injury prevention among female athletes. *J Athl Train* 39(4):361, 2004.)

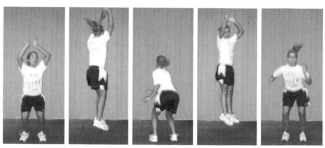

Fig. 49.8 The 180-degree jump. The starting position is standing erect with feet shoulder-width apart. The athlete initiates this two-footed jump with a direct vertical motion combined with a 180-degree rotation in midair, keeping her arms away from her sides to help maintain balance. When she lands, she immediately reverses this jump into the opposite direction. She repeats until perfect technique fails. The goal of this jump is to achieve maximal height with a full 180-degree rotation. Encourage the athlete to maintain exact foot position on the floor by jumping and landing in the same footprint. (Reprinted with permission from Myer G, Ford K, Hewett T. Rationale and clinical techniques for anterior cruciate ligament injury prevention among female athletes. *J Athl Train* 39(4):361, 2004.)

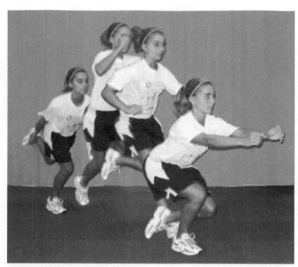

Fig. 49.9 Single-leg hop and hold. The starting position is a semi-crouched position on a single leg. The athlete's arm should be fully extended behind her at the shoulder. She initiates the jump by swinging the arms forward while simultaneously extending at the hip and knee. The jump should carry the athlete up at an angle of approximately 45 degrees and attain maximal distance for a single-leg landing. She is instructed to land on the jumping leg with deep knee flexion (to 90 degrees) and to hold the landing for at least 3 seconds. Coach this jump with care to protect the athlete from injury. Start her with a submaximal effort on the single-leg broad jump so she can experience the level of difficulty. Continue to increase the distance of the broad hop as the athlete improves her ability to "stick" and hold the final landing. Have the athlete keep her visual focus away from her feet to help prevent too much forward lean at the waist. (Reprinted with permission from Myer G, Ford K, Hewett T. Rationale and clinical techniques for anterior cruciate ligament injury prevention among female athletes. *J Athl Train* 39(4):361, 2004.)

| BOX 49.2 | ACL INJURY: PREVENTION AND REHABILITATION PROGRAMS |

COMPONENTS OF A PERTURBATION TRAINING PROGRAM

- Double-limb to single-limb stance on moveable surfaces (e.g., tilt board with progression to roller board)
- Variable direction of applied perturbations to the moving surface (e.g., anterior–posterior and medial–lateral directions)
- Variable speed of applied perturbations to the moving surface
- Variable duration of applied perturbations to the moving surface ranging from 1 to 5 seconds
- Bout of exercise ranging from 1 to 1.5 minutes each
  Progression to roller board/stationary platform exercise (Patient stands with the affected limb on a roller board and the unaffected limb on a stationary platform of equal height. The clinician applies perturbations to the roller board. The patient repeats the exercise with the unaffected limb on the moving surface and the affected limb on the stationary platform.) (Fig. 49.10)

(Adapted from Fitzgerald GK, Axe MJ, Snyder-Mackler L. The efficacy of perturbation training in nonoperative anterior cruciate ligament rehabilitation programs for physically active individuals. *Phys Ther* 80:128–140, 2000.)

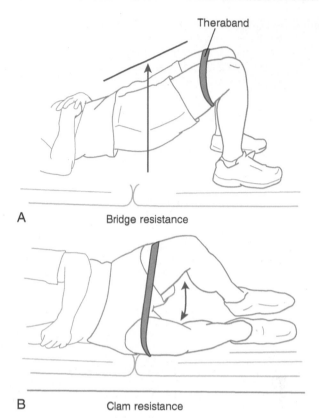

Fig. 49.10 **A,** Bridge with Theraband resistance. **B,** Hip strengthening with clam and Theraband resistance.

with a progression toward perturbation training. Later stages of rehabilitation should include plyometric-type exercises and sport-specific drills similar to those used in ACL injury prevention programs. As with ACL injury prevention programs, the clinician should provide the athlete with continuous feedback regarding proper technique when performing cutting and landing tasks.

Anterior Cruciate Ligament Reconstruction With Meniscal Repair

A lack of firm basic science and prospective outcome studies has resulted in a wide array of opinions regarding issues such as immobilization, ROM restrictions, and weightbearing status after meniscal repair combined with ACL reconstruction. An accelerated return to activities, with immediate weight bearing and no ROM limitations in the early postoperative period, has had results similar to those with more conservative rehabilitation programs. **We have found little justification for modifying the standard rehabilitation protocol after meniscal repair done with ACL reconstruction.**

TABLE 49.1	Hip-Strengthening Exercises for ACL Rehabilitation (and Patellofemoral Rehabilitation) in Female Patients: An Evidence-Based Approach for the Development and Implementation of a Progressive Gluteal Muscle Strengthening Program

Lori A. Bolgla, PT, PhD, ATC

		MUSCLE ACTIVATION*	
Exercise	Description	Gluteus Maximus (%)	Gluteus Medius (%)
Nonweightbearing standing hip abduction	Patient stands solely on the unaffected lower extremity and abducts the affected hip, keeping the pelvis in a level position.	N/A	33
Side-lying hip abduction (Fig. 49.10)	Patient positioned in side lying with the hips and knees in 0 degrees of flexion (unaffected lower extremity against the table). Patient abducts the affected hip.	39	42
Weightbearing isometric hip abduction	Patient stands solely on the affected lower extremity and abducts the unaffected hip, keeping the pelvis in a level position.	N/A	42
Bridges side-lying clam (Fig. 49.11)	Patient positioned in side lying with the hips flexed to 60 degrees and the knees flexed to 90 degrees (unaffected lower extremity against the table). Patient abducts and externally rotates the affected hip while keeping the feet together. Bridges with TheraBand resistance	39	38
Forward lunge (Fig. 49.12)	Patient stands with the lower extremities shoulder-width apart. The patient lunges forward with the affected lower extremity (to approximately 90 degrees of knee flexion) while maintaining the pelvis in a level position and the trunk in a vertical position.	44	42
Pelvic drop (Fig. 49.13)	Patient stands on the affected lower extremity on a 15-cm high step with both knees fully extended. Patient lowers the pelvis of the unaffected lower extremity toward the floor and then returns the pelvis to a level position.	N/A	57
Side hops	Patient stands with the lower extremities shoulder-width apart. The patient hops forward off the unaffected lower extremity and lands solely on the affected lower extremity.	30	57
Lateral band stepping (Fig. 49.14)	Patient stands with the lower extremities shoulder-width apart and the hips and knees in 30 degrees of flexion with an elastic band tied around the ankles. Patient steps sideways, leading with the affected lower extremity while maintaining constant elastic band tension.	27	61
Single-leg squat	Patient stands solely on the affected lower extremity with the hip and knee in 30 degrees of flexion. Patient lowers the body (keeping the knee over the toes to minimize knee valgus) until the middle finger on the opposite side touches the ground. The patient returns to the starting position.	59	64

N/A = data not available
*Expressed as a percentage of a maximum voluntary isometric contraction
Adapted from Bolgla LA, Uhl TL: Electromyographic analysis of hip rehabilitation exercises in a group of healthy subjects. J Orthop Phys Ther 35:487–494, 2005 and Distefano LJ, Blackburn JT, Marshall SW, Padua DA: Gluteal muscle activation during common therapeutic exercises. J Orthop Sports Phys Ther 39:532–540, 2009.

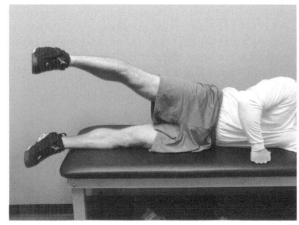

Fig. 49.11 Straight leg raise abduction.

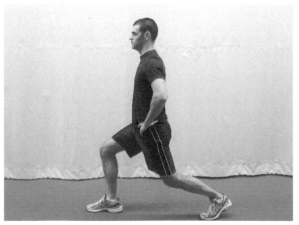

Fig. 49.12 Forward lunge.

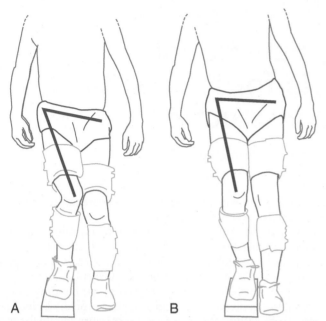

Fig. 49.13 Pelvic drop. During the exercise, the subject keeps both knees extended. The movement occurs by dropping the contralateral pelvis downward and then returning the pelvis to a level position (both lower extremities remain in an extended position). The subject uses the ipsilateral hip abductors to adduct and abduct the pelvis on the femur. Anatomically, the alignment of the subject on the right (B) shows a straight-as-an-arrow hip over knee over ankle. The subject on the left (A) demonstrates hip adduction and internal rotation with anteriorly rotated pelvis, excessive genu valgum, and external tibial rotation and subsequent pronation of the foot. (Reprinted with permission from Ireland M. The Female Athlete. Philadelphia, Saunders, 2002, p. 518, Fig. 43-2.)

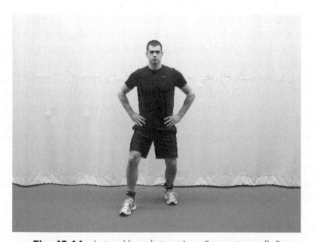

Fig. 49.14 Lateral band stepping, "monster walk."

▶ Check online video: Side-lying Clam (Video 49.1).

REFERENCES

A complete reference list is available at https://expertconsult.inkling.com/.

FURTHER READING

Aldrian S, Valentin P, Wondrasch B, et al. Gender differences following computer-navigated single- and double-bundle anterior cruciate ligament reconstruction. *Knee Surg Sports Traumatol Arthrosc.* 2013;22.9:2145–2152. Web.

Lipps DB, Oh YK, Ashton-Miller JA, et al. Morphologic characteristics help explain the gender difference in peak anterior cruciate ligament strain during a simulated pivot landing. *The American Journal of Sports Medicine.* 2011;40.1:32–40. Web.

Noonan, Benjamin, Wojtys Edward M. Gender differences in muscular protection of the knee. *ACL Injuries in the Female Athlete.* 2012:125–136. Web.

Noyes, Frank R, Barber-Westin, Sue D. ACL injuries in the female athlete: causes, impacts, and conditioning programs. N.p.: n.p., n.d. Print.

Tohyama H, Kondo E, Hayashi R, et al. Gender-based differences in outcome after anatomic double-bundle anterior cruciate ligament reconstruction with hamstring tendon autografts. *The American Journal of Sports Medicine.* 2011;39.9:1849–1857. Web.

Functional Testing, Functional Training, and Criteria for Return to Play After ACL Reconstruction

Mark V. Paterno, PhD, PT, MS, SCS, ATC | Timothy E. Hewett, PhD, FACSM

Athlete progression through the terminal phases of rehabilitation after knee injury or surgery and the criteria necessary for determination of ultimate return to sports remain a controversial topic in the sports medicine community. Current evidence lacks consensus among providers with respect to the optimal means to advance an athlete through the final steps of rehabilitation and objectively determine readiness to safely return to play. Decision to return an athlete to sport following any lower extremity injury should be based on both the athlete's physical ability to perform the desired task and whether this activity is safe for the athlete to perform.

Some authors rely on objective measures of strength to drive the decision to return to sport, whereas others rely on functional performance testing, such as hop testing. Unfortunately, no one test has proved sufficient to objectively make this clinical determination. As a result, widespread disagreement persists between practitioners regarding the safest and most optimal time to return to sports. Patients who have had ACL reconstruction are one cohort often discussed in current literature with significant controversy regarding return to sport.

RISKS WITH EARLY RETURN TO SPORT

Inherent short- and long-term risks are present once an athlete returns to sport following a lower extremity injury. The most notable short-term risk is subsequent injury. Prior epidemiologic studies investigating injury rates in high school and professional athletes demonstrate higher injury rates in athletes who experienced a previous lower extremity injury. **Rauh et al. (2007) noted that up to 25% of injured high school athletes reported multiple injuries and injured athletes were two times more likely to sustain a different injury, rather than re-injure the same location. These findings indicate prior injury may increase risk for future injury.**

A potential mechanism for this increased risk may be early return to sport prior to resolution of known impairments. This may increase risk to the involved extremity, in addition to other structures, as a result of **compensatory motor patterns** that develop in an attempt to execute an athletic task in the presence of known or unknown deficits. Neitzel et al. (2002) reported a 12-month delay following ACL reconstruction before athletes were able to equally balance forces through their involved and uninvolved extremity during a simple squatting task. Paterno et al. (2007) demonstrated that 2 years after unilateral ACL reconstruction, patients continued to place excessive loads on their uninvolved limb during dynamic functional movements, which could result in excessive stress on the previously uninjured limb. This information highlights the need to address known impairments prior to return to sport to minimize the potential risk of subsequent injury.

The most concerning long-term risk of any lower extremity injury is osteoarthritis (OA). Several authors report a high incidence in knee OA following ACL injury, regardless of nonoperative or surgical management. Injury to the meniscus or articular cartilage can increase this risk. OA of the knee has the potential to result in significant functional limitations and disability. End-stage rehabilitation after lower extremity injury should focus on addressing impaired strength and altered movement patterns to minimize abnormal stress on the joint. Current research should investigate the mechanism of the development of OA following acute knee injury and the role of rehabilitation in delaying or preventing the progression of OA.

CURRENT GUIDELINES TO RETURN TO SPORTS

Controversy regarding the optimal timing to return to sports following knee injury is ongoing. Guidelines for return to sport after ACL reconstruction serve as a template for this discussion. Current ACL rehabilitation protocols provide specific exercises and criteria to progress in the initial stages of rehabilitation; however, many fail to describe exercise prescription and detailed progressions at the end stages of rehabilitation prior to return to sport. Therefore, clinicians have less guidance to create optimal end-stage rehabilitation programs. This fact is concerning, considering recent evidence that **as many as one in four patients undergoing an ACL reconstruction suffer a second ACL injury within 10 years of their initial reconstruction.** This incidence of a second ACL injury is far greater than any population without a prior history of ACL injury, even a high-risk population of female athletes, which is typically reported to be in a range of 1 in 60 to 100 athletes.

Following ACL injury and reconstruction, these patients may continue to possess inherent neuromuscular risk factors despite extensive rehabilitation. These neuromuscular risk factors have been shown to be modifiable in an uninjured population. If the incidence of re-injury following ACL reconstruction remains high, and modifiable risk factors persist following the completion of rehabilitation, current rehabilitation programs may be failing to address these important factors in the end stages of rehabilitation. Future programs need to address these deficits.

A second deficit often present in existing ACL reconstruction protocols is a lack of appropriate objective measures to accurately determine an athlete's readiness to safely return to sport. In a systematic review of outcomes after ACL reconstruction, Kvist (2004) noted factors that influence a safe return to activity can be classified into rehabilitative, surgical, and other factors. **Rehabilitation factors** are inclusive of strength and performance, functional stability, and clinical measures to identify loss of ROM or the presence of effusion. **Surgical factors** include static knee stability and concomitant injury, whereas other factors include psychological and psychosocial variables.

Current evidence designed to quantify rehabilitative factors indicates that temporal guidelines and measures such as isokinetic strength and functional hop performance are typically utilized to determine readiness to return to sport. However, these measures, when used in isolation, have limitations. Recommendations regarding return to sport based solely on temporal guidelines are somewhat arbitrary in the medical community and neglect to consider individual patient variability in healing and progression of impairments and function. In a survey of "experts" in the sports medicine community, inclusive of orthopedic surgeons and physical therapists, Harner et al. (2001) report that some practitioners release their patients to return to strenuous sports as early as 4 months postoperative, whereas others may delay up to 18 months. The wide variability in these recommendations is unsupported by current evidence.

Evaluation of strength typically is included in current criteria to return to sport after lower extremity injury and historically has included both open and closed kinetic chain assessments. **Open kinetic chain assessments,** such as **isokinetic strength tests,** provide the clinician an opportunity to focus on a targeted muscle to determine how it functions in isolation in the absence of proximal and distal muscular contributions. Isokinetic strength deficits have shown only moderate correlations to functional performance tasks and may persist up to 24 months following reconstruction. **Closed kinetic chain assessments,** such as **functional hop tests,** have been developed with the goal to incorporate contributions from the kinetic chain to mimic functional activities and provide a more direct correlation to sports. However, Fitzgerald et al. (2001) noted that many of these tests have low sensitivity and specificity and fail to correlate to other measures of impairment or disability. Specifically, they may fail to elucidate isolated quadriceps weaknesses as a result of the development of compensatory muscle recruitment patterns. These data demonstrate that neither open nor closed kinetic chain assessment of lower extremity strength and function can be used in isolation to determine an athlete's readiness to return to sport.

Functional deficits beyond strength and success on functional hop testing often persist after lower extremity injury and are not routinely considered when determining readiness to return to sport. These variables may include biomechanics during jumping and pivoting, power, agility, balance, postural stability, and asymmetries in loading patterns. When assessed on a dynamic task, such as a drop vertical jump maneuver, subjects following ACL reconstruction demonstrated persistent at-risk deficits as long as 2 years postsurgery, despite participating in athletic tasks. More recently, Paterno et al. (2010) prospectively evaluated lower extremity biomechanics and postural stability in patients after ACL reconstruction and prior to return to sport and determined predictors of subsequent ACL injury. These factors included transverse plane hip kinetics and frontal plane knee kinematics during landing, sagittal plane knee moments at landing, and deficits in postural stability. Together, these variables predicted a second injury in this population with both high sensitivity (0.92) and specificity (0.88), yet these variables are not routinely considered when evaluating readiness to return to sport. Considering this current evidence, future research should investigate which cluster of objective assessments could potentially provide better information regarding athletes' readiness to return to sports at their previous level of function, with minimal risk of re-injury.

TARGETING END-STAGE REHABILITATION

Despite the absence of a rigorous end-stage rehabilitation protocol and a lack of a specific cluster of validated objective measures to accurately determine an athlete's readiness to safely return to sport, several authors have begun to address this topic. We attempted to specifically address these concerns related to a lack of objectivity in rehabilitation progression, optimal timing to release to activity, and absence of a criteria-based progression by creating a program designed for patients after ACL reconstruction. The goal of this program was to target specific neuromuscular imbalances believed to increase risk for ACL injury. We developed an initial model of a criteria-based progression of end-stage rehabilitation (Rehabilitation Protocol 50.1) and an algorithmic approach of progression with the ultimate criteria for determination of readiness to return to sport (Rehabilitation Protocol 50.2) (Fig. 50.6). The intent of introducing principles of ACL prevention to the end stages of rehabilitation was to target neuromuscular imbalances and potentially reduce the risk of future ACL injury in this population. This program includes specific rehabilitation phases targeting core stability, functional strength, power development, and symmetry of sports performance. Each phase was designed to specifically target a neuromuscular imbalance previously identified as a potential risk factor for ACL injury.

The ability to control the position and mobility of the center of mass during athletic maneuvers is critical for safe participation in sports. **The authors have demonstrated that deficits in trunk control and proprioception resulted in a greater incidence of knee and ACL injuries in collegiate female athletes.** In addition, the authors noted that female athletes playing high-risk sports often land with a single limb outside of their base of support. Landing with the center of mass outside the base of support often increases load on the knee and thus risk of injury. Therefore, targeted rehabilitation to control trunk motion may help athletes safely progress back to sports. The authors utilized dynamic stabilization and core stability exercises to address these impairments (Figs. 50.1 through 50.5).

Functional strength and power development also are required for successful participation in many sports. The ability to quickly absorb and generate forces during dynamic movements results in more efficient movement and improved dampening of potentially harmful forces on the lower extremity. Plyometric exercises have been shown to assist in the development of and dissipation of forces on the lower extremity. Therefore, incorporation of **plyometric exercises** in the end stages of rehabilitation following lower extremity injury may be indicated when the athletes wish to return to sports requiring dynamic and explosive movements.

Finally, a **functional reintegration phase** is critical to returning athletes to sports following lower extremity injury. The goal of this final phase is to ensure the athlete's ability to symmetrically load lower extremity forces and introduce the sports-specific movements required for the athlete to return to that sport. Prior studies have shown asymmetries in balance, strength, and loading patterns persist after lower extremity injury. If these asymmetries are unresolved when clearance to return to sport is granted, abnormal movement patterns can develop. This may ultimately result

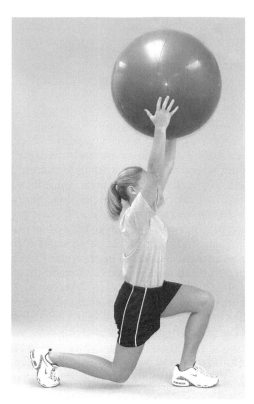

Fig. 50.1 The subject shows excellent body control position in this forward lunge, balancing the ball directly overhead. (Reprinted with permission from Ireland M. The Female Athlete. Philadelphia, Saunders 2002, p. 518, Fig. 43-5.)

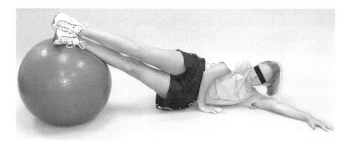

Fig. 50.2 In bridging, the left greater trochanter is lifted off the floor while maintaining balance on the ball; support is given by the upper extremity. As advanced control occurs, less hand support is required. (Reprinted with permission from Ireland M. The Female Athlete. Philadelphia, Saunders 2002, p. 518, Fig. 43-8.)

in excessive loading on the uninvolved extremity that lacks sufficient strength and motor control to absorb force when involved in a competitive, athletic situation. Resolution of these final impairments may not only lead to successful reintegration to sports but also may begin to reduce the extraordinarily high incidence of re-injury after return to sports. The program that we developed and described attempted to utilize the best current available evidence and supplemented any deficits in the literature with expert clinical opinion. The final outcome was designed as a template and may stimulate future research attempting to develop more rigorous treatment progressions designed for the end stages of rehabilitation after any lower extremity injury, in addition to designing valid, reliable, and objective means to determine the athlete's readiness to successfully and safely return to sport with minimal risk of re-injury (see Rehabilitation Protocols 50.1 and 50.2).

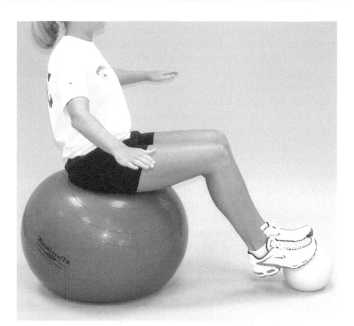

Fig. 50.3 Incorporating balance while seated on an unstable base is shown. Such advanced Swiss ball maneuvers incorporate position awareness and strength. Modifications of these exercises can be made to maintain the interest of the patient. (Reprinted with permission from Ireland M. The Female Athlete. Philadelphia, Saunders 2002, p. 518, Fig. 43-9.)

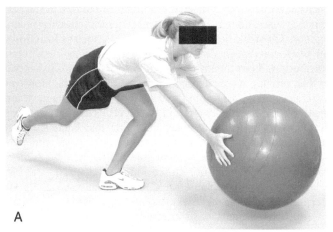

A

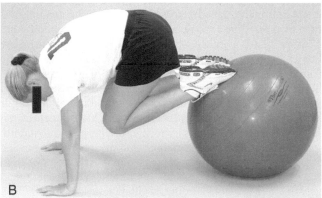

B

Fig. 50.4 A, The model is in the "around the clock" position, touching the ball to the floor and extending the right leg. B, In the prone balance position the subject maintains control; going from hip flexion and knee flexion into extension combines for core stabilization, balance, and neuromuscular control. (Reprinted with permission from Ireland M. The Female Athlete. Philadelphia, Saunders 2002, p. 518, Figs. 43-6 and 43-7.)

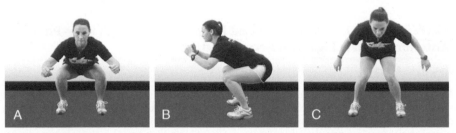

Fig. 50.5 Bilateral body weight squat (athletic position deep hold). **A,** The athlete attempts to maintain upright posture with knees in line with feet. **B,** Lateral view. Patient squats until thighs are parallel to the ground, maintaining balance while avoiding trunk flexion. **C,** Poor-quality squat with notable valgus stress of the knees and trunk flexion.

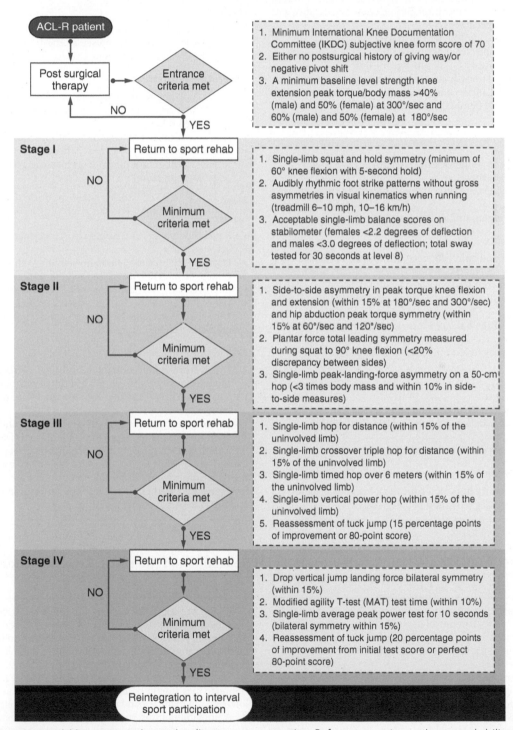

Fig. 50.6 Return-to-sports activities post anterior cruciate ligament reconstruction. Before progressing to the next rehabilitative stage in the program, the patient must meet the minimum progression criteria. *R,* reconstruction (Redrawn with permission from Myer GD, Paterno MV, Ford KR, Quatman CE, Hewett TE. Rehabilitation after anterior cruciate ligament reconstruction: criteria based progression through the return to sport phase. *J Orthop Sports Phys Ther* 36(6), 2006.)

REHABILITATION PROTOCOL 50.1 ■ **Criteria-Based Progression Through Four-Phase Return-to-Sport Rehabilitation After Anterior Cruciate Ligament Reconstruction**

G.D. Myer, M.V. Paterno, K.R. Ford

Myer et al. (2006) described a criteria-based progression through a four-stage rehabilitation program after ACL reconstruction. They suggested that return-to-sport rehabilitation progressed by quantitatively measured functional goals may improve the athlete's integration back into sport participation. Their criteria-based protocol incorporates a dynamic assessment of baseline limb strength, patient-reported outcomes, functional knee stability, bilateral limb symmetry with functional tasks, postural control, power, endurance, agility, and technique with sport-specific tasks.

Criteria for entrance into the return-to-sport phase:
- Minimum IKDC subjective knee score of 70
- No postoperative history OR negative pivot shift
- Minimum baseline strength knee extension peak torque/body mass of at least 40% (male) and 30% female at 300 degrees/s, and 60% (male) and 50% (female) at 180 degrees/s

Stage 1

Goals

- Improve single-limb weightbearing strength at increasingly greater knee flexion angles.
- Improve side-to-side symmetry in lower extremity running mechanics.
- Improve weightbearing single-limb postural balance.

Criteria for Progression

- Single-limb squat and hold symmetry (minimum 60-degree knee flexion with 5-second hold)
- Audibly rhythmic foot strike patterns without gross asymmetries in visual kinematics when running (treadmill 6 to 10 mph)
- Acceptable single-limb balance scores on stabilometer (females, less than 2.2 degrees of deflection; males, less than 3.0 degrees of deflection; total sway tested for 30 seconds at level 8)

Stage 2

Goals

- Improve lower extremity nonweightbearing strength.
- Improve force contribution symmetry during activities in bipedal stance.
- Improve single-limb landing force attenuation strategies.

Criteria for Progression

- Side-to-side symmetry in peak torque flexion and extension (within 15% at 180 degrees/s and 300 degrees/s)

- Plantar force total-loading symmetry measured during bipedal squat to 90-degree knee flexion (less than 20% discrepancy between sides)
- Single-limb peak-landing-force symmetry on a 50-cm hop (less than 3 times body mass and within 10% in side-to-side measures)

Stage 3

Goals

- Improve single-limb power production.
- Improve lower extremity muscular endurance.
- Improve lower extremity biomechanics during plyometric activities.

Criteria for Progression

- Single-limb hop for distance (within 15% of uninvolved side)
- Single-limb crossover triple hop for distance (within 15% of uninvolved side)
- Single-limb timed hop over 6 m (within 15% of uninvolved side)
- Single-limb vertical power hop (within 15% of uninvolved side)
- Reassessment of tuck jump (15 percentage point of improvement or an 80-point score)

Stage 4

Goals

- Equalization of ground reaction force attenuation strategies between limbs
- Improvement of confidence and stability with high-intensity change-of-direction activities
- Improvement and equalization of power endurance between limbs
- Use of safe biomechanics (increased knee flexion and decreased knee abduction angles) when performing high-intensity plyometric exercises

Criteria for Progression

- Drop vertical jump landing force bilateral symmetry (within 15%)
- Modified agility T-test (MAT) test time (within 10%)
- Single-limb average peak power test for 10 seconds (bilateral symmetry within 15%)
- Reassessment of tuck jump (20 percentage points of improvement from initial test score of perfect 80-point score)

Attainment of stage 4 criteria indicates that athlete can leave therapy and begin reintegration into his or her sport; however, immediate unrestricted full participation in competitive events is not recommended. Rather, the athlete should resume practice activities and begin to prepare for competitive play.

REHABILITATION PROTOCOL 50.2 ■ **Return-to-Sport Rehabilitation After ACL Reconstruction**

G.D. Myer, M.V. Paterno, K.R. Ford

Patients who are unable to develop dynamic muscular joint stabilization through neuromuscular control during walking and activities of daily living (evidenced by giving-way episodes) are excluded from progression into the aggressive return-to-sport rehabilitation program.

The first year after ACL reconstruction is a high-risk period for athletes returning to high-level sports. The algorithm of (Myer et al. 2006) aims to identify postoperative deficits and correct them through systematic progression from one stage of rehabilitation to the next, which may improve the potential for athletes to return to sport at optimal performance levels and minimize the risk of re-injury.

Use of the suggested criteria for progression of return-to-sport training was suggested to more objectively determine an athlete's readiness to return safely to sports participation and indicate that dynamic restraints are sufficient to limit both pathologic gross motion and micromotion in both the involved and uninvolved knees.

Specific exercises are not described for each phase, and rehabilitation activities should be individualized for each athlete, combining low-risk and high-demand maneuvers in a controlled environment.

A limitation of this protocol is that measurement of the progression criteria requires sophisticated equipment that may not be available in many physical therapy or sport medicine facilities.

REHABILITATION PROTOCOL 50.2 ● Return-to-Sport Rehabilitation After ACL Reconstruction—cont'd

Criteria for Beginning Return-to-Sport Rehabilitation

- Minimum IKDC Subjective Knee Form score of 70
- Either no postoperative history of giving way or negative pivot shift
- Minimum baseline strength knee extension torque/body mass of at least 40% (males) and 30% (females) at 300 degrees/second and 60% (males) and 50% (females) at 180 degrees/second

Stage I

Goals

- Improve single-limb weightbearing strength at increasingly greater knee flexion angles.
- Improve side-to-side asymmetry in lower extremity running mechanics.
- Improve weightbearing single-limb postural balance.

Activities

- Advancement of single-limb weightbearing exercises with lunge and single-limb squatting exercises
- Treadmill training with verbal and visual feedback
- Exercises stressing single-limb postural control (especially on unstable surfaces)

Criteria for Progression to Stage II

- Single-limb squat and hold symmetry (minimum 60 degrees of knee flexion with 5-second hold)
- Audibly rhythmic foot strike patterns without gross asymmetries in visual kinematics when running (treadmill 6 to 10 mph, 10 to 16 km/hour)
- Acceptable single-limb balance scores on stabilometer: females, less than 2.2 degrees of deflection; males, less than 3.0 degrees of deflection; total sway tested for 30 seconds at level 8

Stage II

Goals

- Improve lower extremity nonweightbearing strength.
- Improve force contribution symmetry during activities in bipedal stance.
- Improve single-limb land force.

Activities

- Lower extremity weightbearing strengthening
- High-intensity balance training
- Perturbation training
- Nonweightbearing lower extremity exercises
- Squatting exercises
- Single-limb landing

Criteria for Progression to Stage III

- Side-to-side asymmetry in peak torque knee flexion and extension (with 15% at 180 degrees/second and 300 degrees/second)

and hip abduction peak torque side-to-side asymmetry (within 15% at 60 degrees/second and 120 degrees/second)
- Plantar force total-loading symmetry measured during bipedal squat to 90 degrees of knee flexion (less than 20% discrepancy between sides)
- Single-limb peak-landing-force symmetry on 50-cm hop (less than three times body mass and within 10% side-to-side measures)

Stage III

Goals

- Improve single-limb power production.
- Improve lower extremity muscular endurance.
- Improve lower extremity biomechanics during plyometric activities.

Activities

- Incorporation of midlevel intensity double-limb plyometric jumps
- Introduction of low-intensity single-limb repeated hops

Criteria for Progression to Stage IV

- Single-limb hop for distance within 15% of uninvolved side
- Single-limb crossover triple hop for distance within 15% of uninvolved side
- Single-limb timed hop over 6 m within 15% of uninvolved side
- Single-limb vertical power hop within 15% of uninvolved side
- Reassessment of tuck jump (15 percentage points of improvement or 80-point score)

Stage IV

Goals

- Equalize ground reaction force attenuation strategies between limbs.
- Improve confidence and stability with high-intensity change-of-direction activities.
- Improve and equalize power endurance between limbs.
- Use safe biomechanics (increased knee flexion and decreased knee abduction angles) during high-intensity plyometric exercises.

Activities

- Power, cutting, change-of-direction exercises
- Power movements in both directions with emphasis on sufficient hip and knee flexion angles and decreased knee abduction

Criteria for Progression to Return to Sport

- Drop vertical jump landing force bilateral symmetry (within 15%)
- Modified agility T-test (MAT) test time (within 10%)
- Single-limb average peak power test for 10 seconds (bilateral symmetry within 15%)
- Reassessment of tuck jump (20 percentage points of improvement from initial score or perfect 80-point score)

 Check online video: Swiss Ball Progression Is Ys Ts (Video 50.1).

REFERENCES

A complete reference list is available at https://expertconsult.inkling.com/.

FURTHER READING

Abrams GD, Harris JD, Gupta AK, et al. Functional performance testing after anterior cruciate ligament reconstruction: a systematic review. *Orthop J Sports Med.* 2014;2.1. n. pag. Web.

Ardern CL, Webster KE, Taylor NF, et al. Return to sport following anterior cruciate ligament reconstruction surgery: a systematic review and meta-analysis of the state of play. *British Journal of Sports Medicine.* 2011;45.7:596–606. Web.

Brophy RH, Schmitz L, Wright RW. Return to play and future ACL injury risk after ACL reconstruction in soccer athletes from the Multicenter Orthopaedic Outcomes Network (MOON) Group. *The American Journal of Sports Medicine.* 2012;40.11:2517–2522. Web.

Cascio BM, Culp L, Cosgarea AJ. Return to play after anterior cruciate ligament reconstruction. *Clin Sports Med.* 2004;23(3):395–408.ix.

Ernst GP, Saliba E, Diduch DR, et al. Lower extremity compensations following anterior cruciate ligament reconstruction. *Phys Ther.* 2000;80(3):251–260.

Ford KR, Myer GD, Hewett TE. Valgus knee motion during landing in high school female and male basketball players. *Med Sci Sports Exerc.* 2003;35(10):1745–1750.

Goodstadt N, Snyder-Mackler L, et al. Functional testing to discontinue brace use for sport after ACL reconstruction. *Medicine & Science in Sports & Exercise.* 2010;42:96. Web.

Greenberger HB, Paterno MV. Relationship of knee extensor strength and hopping test performance in the assessment of lower extremity function. *J Orthop Sports Phys Ther.* 1995;22(5):202–206.

Hewett TE, Myer GD, Ford KR, et al. Biomechanical measures of neuromuscular control and valgus loading of the knee predict anterior cruciate ligament injury risk in female athletes: a prospective study. *Am J Sports Med.* 2005;33(4):492–501.

Hewett TE, Paterno MV, Myer GD. Strategies for enhancing proprioception and neuromuscular control of the knee. *Clin Orthop Relat Res.* 2002;(402):76–94.

Hewett TE, Stroupe AL, Nance TA, et al. Plyometric training in female athletes. Decreased impact forces and increased hamstring torques. *Am J Sports Med.* 1996;24(6):765–773.

Hewett TE, Torg JS, Boden BP. Video analysis of trunk and knee motion during non-contact anterior cruciate ligament injury in female athletes: lateral trunk and knee abduction motion are combined components of the injury mechanism. *Br J Sports Med.* 2009;43(6):417–422.

Hildebrandt C, Müller L, et al. Functional assessments for decision-making regarding return to sports following ACL reconstruction. Part I: development of a new test battery. *Knee Surg Sports Traumatol Arthrosc.* 2015;23.5:1273–1281. Web.

Kobayashi AHH, Terauchi M, Kobayashi F, et al. Muscle performance after anterior cruciate ligament reconstruction. *Int Orthop.* 2004;28:48–51.

Lohmander LS, Ostenberg A, Englund M, et al. High prevalence of knee osteoarthritis, pain, and functional limitations in female soccer players twelve years after anterior cruciate ligament injury. *Arthritis Rheum.* 2004;50(10):3145–3152.

Louboutin H, Debarge R, Richou J, et al. Osteoarthritis in patients with anterior cruciate ligament rupture: a review of risk factors. *Knee.* 2009;16(4):239–244.

Marshall SW, Padua D, McGrath M. Incidence of ACL injury. In: Hewett TESS, Griffin LY, eds. *Understanding and Preventing Noncontact ACL Injuries.* Champaign: Human Kinetics; 2007:5–30.

Mattacola CG, Perrin DH, Gansneder BM, et al. Strength, functional outcome, and postural stability after anterior cruciate ligament reconstruction. *J Athl Train.* 2002;37(3):262–268.

Myer GD, Ford KR, Hewett TE. Rationale and clinical techniques for anterior cruciate ligament injury prevention among female athletes. *J Athl Train.* 2004;39(4):352–364.

Myer GD, Ford KR, McLean SG, et al. The effects of plyometric versus dynamic stabilization and balance training on lower extremity biomechanics. *Am J Sports Med.* 2006;34(3):490–498.

Myer GD, Ford KR, Palumbo JP, et al. Neuromuscular training improves performance and lower-extremity biomechanics in female athletes. *J Strength Cond Res.* 2005;19(1):51–60.

Myer GD, Paterno MV, Ford KR, et al. Neuromuscular training techniques to target deficits before return to sport following anterior cruciate ligament reconstruction. *J Strength Cond Res.* 2008;22(3):987–1014.

Orchard J, Seward H, McGivern J, et al. Intrinsic and extrinsic risk factors for anterior cruciate ligament injury in Australian footballers. *Am J Sports Med.* 2001;29(2):196–200.

Paterno MV, Hewett TE, Noyes FR. The return of neuromuscular coordination after anterior cruciate ligament reconstruction. *J Orthop Sports Phys Ther.* 1998;27(1):94.

Paterno MV, Hewett TE, Noyes FR. Gender differences in neuromuscular coordination of controls, ACL-deficient knees and ACL-reconstructed knees. *J Orthop Sports Phys Ther.* 1999;29(1). Aendash45.

Pinczewski LA, Lyman J, Salmon LJ, et al. A 10-year comparison of anterior cruciate ligament reconstructions with hamstring tendon and patellar tendon autograft: a controlled, prospective trial. *Am J Sports Med.* 2007;35(4):564–574.

Shelbourne KD, Nitz P. Accelerated rehabilitation after anterior cruciate ligament reconstruction. *Am J Sports Med.* 1990;18(3):292–299.

von Porat, Roos EM, Roos H. High prevalence of osteoarthritis 14 years after an anterior cruciate ligament tear in male soccer players: a study of radiographic and patient relevant outcomes. *Ann Rheum Dis.* 2004;63(3):269–273.

Wilk KE, Arrigo C, Andrews JR, et al. Rehabilitation after anterior cruciate ligament reconstruction in the female athlete. *J Athl Train.* 1999;34(2):177–193.

Wilk KE, Reinold MM, Hooks TR. Recent advances in the rehabilitation of isolated and combined anterior cruciate ligament injuries. *Orthop Clin North Am.* 2003;34(1):107–137.

Zazulak BT, Hewett TE, Reeves NP, et al. Deficits in neuromuscular control of the trunk predict knee injury risk: a prospective biomechanical-epidemiologic study. *Am J Sports Med.* 2007;35(7):1123–1130.

Functional Performance Measures and Sports-Specific Rehabilitation for Lower Extremity Injuries: A Guide for a Safe Return to Sports

Christie C.P. Powell, PT, MSPT, STS, USSF "D"

FUNCTIONAL TRAINING

Lower extremity functional training is "purposeful" training for athletes and should include general sports skills such as running, jumping, kicking, and pivoting. According to Gambetta (2002), functional training teaches athletes how to manage and maneuver their own body weight and incorporates balance, proprioception, and kinesthesia. Boyle (2004) advises that "functional training programs need to introduce controlled amounts of instability so the athlete must react in order to regain their own stability ... and the ability to display strength in conditions of instability is actually the *highest level of strength*." Functional training prepares the athletes for their sport by using exercises and activities to train the muscles in the same manner the sport demands. Sports-specific skills can be initiated during the speed and agility phase of rehabilitation when all lower-level activities can be tolerated by the athlete with no swelling, irritation, or pain present after exercise (Fitzgerald et al. 2000a).

FUNCTIONAL PROGRESSIONS

Functional progressions are a planned sequence of progressively more difficult activities specific to the demands of the sport. This progression allows the athlete to begin adapting to the specific demands encountered in practices and games. Agility, speed, and coordination activities can be added to an athlete's rehabilitation program once general functional strength gains have been attained and tolerated.

Fitzgerald and colleagues (2000a) advise that sports-specific tasks, such as ball catching, passing, and kicking, be practiced in the context of game-playing situations. These activities should also be initiated without an opponent and then progressed to practice with an opponent (Fitzgerald et al. 2000a). There are numerous benefits of functional training and appropriate functional progressions for the athlete and the practitioner. Several areas of evaluation are needed in combination with constant clinical assessment to establish an athlete's ability to tolerate each functional progression. Core stability, good motor control, balance/proprioception, symmetric movement patterns, compensatory mechanisms, and confidence of the athlete should all be evaluated by the clinician when deciding to advance the athlete to the next level of rehabilitation.

The **Specific Adaptation to Imposed Demand Principle** (SAID principle) is often used as a guideline for functional progressions and can be used for any sport or activity. During recovery it is important to remember that the body adapts to varying degrees of stress, and it is essential to introduce the demands that an athlete will experience during sports, while keeping the appropriate healing phase in mind. The clinician will also need to consider the athlete's particular sport or sports (if multiple sports are played), the skill level and age of the athlete, and the physiologic parameters of the sport, including varying degrees of contact. An extensive criteria-based progression through the return-to-sport phase has been developed by Myer et al. (2006A, 2008) specifically for rehabilitation after anterior cruciate ligament reconstruction, but it basically can be used for all lower extremity injuries. Myer and colleagues (2006A, 2008) advise taking an athlete through four total stages of progressions with specific functional performance tests quantitatively measured in each phase to determine the athlete's readiness to move to the next level.

FUNCTIONAL PERFORMANCE MEASURES/TESTS

Functional performance measures are used by rehabilitation professionals and researchers to evaluate when an athlete can safely return to unrestricted sporting activities and are used to quantify lower limb function (Barber 1990, 1992, Noyes 1991, Juris 1997, Bolgla 1997, Itoh 1998, Fitzgerald et al. 2000a, 2001, Huston 2001, Myer 2005, 2007, 2008, Pollard 2006, Chappell 2007, Flanagan 2008, Ortiz 2008).

Barber et al. (1990, 1992) found that functional tests cannot detect specific lower extremity deficits, yet they can be clinically useful in assessing overall lower limb function. Functional performance measures incorporate numerous variables of lower extremity function that include pain, swelling, neuromuscular control and coordination, muscular and dynamic strength, and overall joint stability (Barber 1990, 1992, Fitzgerald et al. 2001).

Many functional performance tests and measures have been validated and demonstrate reliability—specifically, hop tests that include **single-leg hop** for distance (Tegner 1986, Barber 1990, 1992, Noyes 1991, Booher 1993, Hewett 1996, 1999, Bolgla 1997, Borsa 1997, Wilson 1998, Fitzgerald et al. 2000a, 2000B, 2001, Lewek 2003, Augustsson 2004, Ferris 2004, Myer 2005, 2006A, 2008, Flanagan 2008), **hop-stop tests** (Hewett 1996, 1999, Juris 1997, Fitzgerald et al. 2001, Ferris 2004, Myer 2008), and **vertical jump tests** (Barber 1990, 1992, Hewett 1996,

Fitzgerald et al. 2001, Myer 2005, 2006A, 2006B, 2006C, 2007, 2008, Rampanini 2007, Hamilton 2008).

Fitzgerald and colleagues (2001) advise hop tests should be administered during the rehabilitation process when an athlete demonstrates full knee motion, no extensor lag is noted during the straight leg raise exercise, no joint effusion is present, quadriceps strength of the injured limb is 80% of the noninjured limb, and hopping on the involved limb is pain free.

It has been suggested that to improve the sensitivity of lower extremity dynamic functional performance measures, athletes should be evaluated under conditions of fatigue (Augustsson 2004), with effective movement constraints to control for compensatory motion (Juris 1997), and using multiple single-leg hop tests (Fitzgerald et al. 2001). When attempting to determine if a functional impairment is present in an athlete prior to return to sport, it is necessary that the athlete be placed in similar conditions as found in sports that include fatigue and/or contact (Augustsson 2004). Currently, there is no functional testing paradigm that is agreed on by the medical community for the lower extremity that incorporates all the valid and reliable functional measures.

FUNCTIONAL PERFORMANCE TESTING CATEGORIES: LOWER EXTREMITIES

Performance can be measured by functional strength and dynamic joint stability, including balance and proprioception/kinesthesia; speed, agility, and coordination; plyometric features, including jumping/loading; and a running series.

Functional Strength Tests

Functional strength tests are often used to assess general strength and joint stability. **Bilateral body weight squats** (Neitzal 2002, Boyle 2004, Myer 2006B, 2006C, 2008) (Fig. 50.5), and **single-leg squats** (Zeller 2003, Ferris 2004, Myer 2006A, Myer 2008) (Fig. 51.1) are commonly used to determine general functional strength because they simulate a common athletic position and demand ankle, knee, and hip control to accomplish. In the rehabilitation setting it is critical that the athlete develop a foundation of functional strength on which to build. It has been shown that strength training alone did not alter the biomechanics of female recreational athletes during a functional performance task that includes jumping and landing (Herman 2008). As a result of the extreme forces placed on the joints during sports and other high-level activities, it is imperative the athlete's neuromuscular control and functional strength be restored while recovering from an injury, but other interventions that incorporate sports-specific activities also must be included (Herman 2008) (Table 51.1).

Dynamic Joint Stability

Balance and Proprioception/Kinesthesia. Balance is generally defined as the ability to maintain the center of mass over the base of support. In dynamic situations this requires the base of support to shift in conjunction with the center of mass. Balance can be disrupted when the mechanoreceptors found in the ankle, hip, and knee do not properly detect or correct motion to preserve the center of gravity over the base of support (Bernier

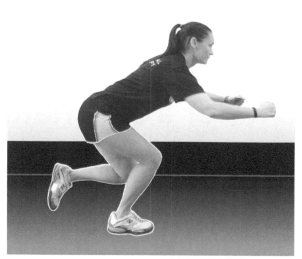

Fig. 51.1 Single-leg squat. The athlete squats on a single leg attempting to achieve 60 to 90 degrees of knee flexion with no loss of balance and good knee control. The athlete attempts to avoid internal rotation of the hip and valgus moments at the knee.

1998). These corrective and coordinated movements are critical in the execution of postural and positional corrections to avoid injury. Ergen and Ulkar (2008) describe proprioception as "a broad concept that includes balance and postural control with visual and vestibular contributions, joint kinesthesia, position sense, and muscle reaction time."

Proprioception is the ability of a joint to determine its position in space, detect precision movement and kinesthesia, and contribute to dynamic joint stability (Lephart 1997). Lephart et al. (1997) report the neuromuscular feedback system becomes interrupted following an injury and implementing a rehabilitation program that includes a proprioceptive component is highly recommended. Deficits in proprioception have been found between healthy and injured populations at the ankle and knee (MacDonald 1996, Borsa 1997, Bernier 1998, Wikstrom 2006). Information transmitted by the mechanoreceptors in the knee and ankle is responsible for detecting changes and activating dynamic restraints to avoid injury. In the knee this can be defined as the ability to maintain normal movement patterns while performing high-level activities without "unwanted" episodes of giving way (Lewek 2003, Wikstrom 2006). In general, neuromuscular control is greatly responsible for creating dynamic joint stability in the lower extremity during sports-specific activities.

Early in the rehabilitation process it is essential to implement proprioceptive and neuromuscular training to safely progress to functional and sports-specific activities following injury (Ergen 2008). Balance training to include single-leg stance activities (Bernier 1998, Sherry 2004, Myer 2008), wobble and balance/tilt boards (Bernier 1998, Fitzgerald et al. 2000b), and perturbation activities (Fitzgerald et al. 2000b, Lewek 2003) often is used in therapy (Table 51.2). Hop tests are also often used in the later stages of rehabilitation to evaluate the proprioceptive status of an injured athlete but are discussed in detail in the plyometric category (Noyes 1991, Risberg 1994).

Speed, Agility, and Coordination (Table 51.3). **Running speed** in sports is considered an important performance

TABLE 51.1	Lower Extremity Functional Strength Activities (Powell)	
Exercise	**Description**	**References**
Bilateral body weight squat/ sumo squat (athletic-position deep hold) (Fig. 50.5)	Patient places feet shoulder-width apart (or slightly wider for sumo squat) and squats until thighs are parallel to the ground while maintaining an upright posture with minimal trunk flexion.	Neitzal 2002 Boyle 2004 Myer 2006B Myer 2006C Myer 2008
Single-leg squat (60 to 90 degrees) (Fig. 51.1)	Patient stands with arms across chest and squats on a single leg, attempting to achieve 90 degrees or more of knee flexion without losing his or her balance.	Zeller 2003 Ferris 2004 Myer 2006A Myer 2006B Myer 2008
BOSU/Airex bilateral squats	Patient stands on BOSU or Airex pad and squats on both legs to 90 degrees or greater with good knee control and no loss of balance. (See full descriptions in Myer 2008 glossary of activities.)	Myer 2006B Myer 2006C Myer 2008
BOSU/Airex single-leg squats	Patient stands on BOSU or Airex pad and squats on a single leg to 60 to 90 degrees with good knee control and no loss of balance.	Myer 2006B Myer 2006C Myer 2008

TABLE 51.2	Dynamic Joint Stability: Balance and Proprioception/Kinesthesia Activities (Powell)	
Exercise	**Description**	**References**
Single-leg stance—eyes open	Patient stands on a single leg with eyes open, slightly bent knee, without moving foot, touching opposite leg or touching down for 30 seconds. Opposite leg is bent to 75 degrees behind.	Bernier 1998 Sherry 2004 Myer 2006A Myer 2008
Single-leg stance—eyes closed	Patient stands on a single leg with eyes closed, slightly bent knee, without moving foot, touching opposite leg or touching down for 30 seconds. Opposite leg is bent to 75 degrees behind.	Bernier 1998 Sherry 2004
Single-leg stance—unstable surface	Patient stands on unstable surface such as Airex pad, Dynadisc, BOSU, foam pad, half foam roll, etc., with a single leg following the same guidelines.	Myer 2008
Single-leg perturbation	Patient stands on a single leg while on a roller board and the clinician perturbates the board while the patient maintains balance.	Fitzgerald et al. 2000b Lewek 2003
Wobble board	Patient stands with various foot patterns on a wobble board and attempts to keep any board surface from touching the ground.	Bernier 1998
Balance/tilt board	Patient stands with various foot patterns on a balance/tilt board and attempts to keep any board surface from touching the ground.	Bernier 1998 Fitzgerald et al. 2000b

TABLE 51.3	Speed, Agility, and Coordination Activities (Powell)	
Exercise	**Description**	**References**
Side shuffle/side stepping	Patient instructed to move laterally right to left with change of direction as quickly as possible for various distances.	Fitzgerald et al. 2000b Sherry 2004
Carioca/grapevine stepping (Fig. 51.4)	Patient instructed to attempt forward and backward leg crossovers while moving laterally in right and left directions.	Fitzgerald et al. 2000b Sherry 2004
Shuttle run	Patient instructed to sprint forward and backward with quick starts and stops at each line. Varied distances are suggested.	Fitzgerald et al. 2000b
Multidirectional shuttle run	Patient instructed to sprint forward and use multidirectional quick starts and stops over varied distances.	Fitzgerald et al. 2000b
45-degree cutting and spinning drill	Patient instructed to sprint with change of direction at a 45-degree angle (to left and right) with spin moves intermixed.	Fitzgerald et al. 2000b
Side-step cutting	Patient instructed to run 5 meters straight then contact right foot to change direction to left (cut at 45-degree angle). Repeat to the right.	McLean 1999 Sigward 2006
Figure-of-eight run (Fig. 51.2)	Cones set 6 to 10 meters apart and patient instructed to run a figure-of-eight around the cones for two laps. Switch start position from right side of cone to the left side of the cone.	Tegner 1986 Wilson 1998 Fitzgerald et al. 2000b

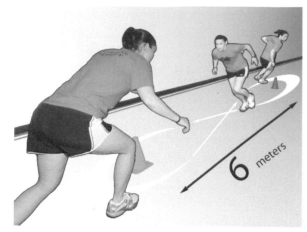

Fig. 51.2 Figure-of-eight run. Clinicians place cones 6 to 10 meters apart, and the athlete is asked to run a figure of eight around the cones without touching the cones for two total laps. The athlete starts on the right side of the cone to encourage a right turn at the far cone and then repeats from the left side of the cone.

quality of many athletes. Cissik and Barnes (2004) state sprinting requires an athlete to develop complicated movement patterns, taking place in a short period. It is critical the physical therapist or athletic trainer assess the athlete's sprinting technique during the later phases of rehabilitation because poor sprinting technique can lead to injury by placing increased stress and strain on the musculoskeletal system.

Agility activities are often used to improve lower extremity coordination, speed, and quickness, especially when changing direction. The figure-of-eight agility drill (Fig. 51.2 and Table 51.3) is commonly used by coaches, trainers, and researchers to determine an athlete's ability to coordinate sprinting, deceleration, and changing direction safely and effectively (Tegner 1986, Wilson 1998, Fitzgerald et al. 2000b). **Coordination** is a combination of optimizing intramuscular and intermuscular cooperation for skills using internal and external feedback systems (Ergen 2008). Coordination encompasses proprioception and balance abilities as the nervous system and musculoskeletal system interact to prevent injury during cutting, pivoting, and jumping activities (Ergen 2008) (Table 51.3).

Plyometric: Jumping/Loading/Landing (Table 51.4). Plyometric training refers to quick, powerful movements involving prestretching the muscle and activating the lengthen-shorten cycle to produce a subsequently stronger concentric contraction. All jumping activities are therefore considered plyometric activities and are the most commonly used to improve sports performance and establish lower extremity dynamic control. Flanagan et al. (2008) found that knee and ankle injuries are the most prevalent in athletes who participate in sports requiring cutting, pivoting, and jumping. Researchers agree jumping and landing tasks, especially those that involve a change of direction, can simulate the injury mechanism for ACL injuries (Sell 2006, Sigward 2006).

Many investigators have shown that plyometric/jump training programs significantly decrease the incidence of injury, especially with female athletes (Hewett 1999, Mandelbaum 2005), and utilize neuromuscular techniques including plyometrics to target deficits prior to returning to sport (Fitzgerald et al. 2000b, Myer 2005, 2006A, 2006B, 2006C, 2008, Chmielewski 2006). These programs often include a large variety of jumping activities that challenge an athlete in all dimensions of intensity

and difficulty. It is also appropriate to include plyometric activities when assessing an athlete's ability to return to sport because they prepare the neuromuscular system postinjury for rapid changes in movement and increased joint forces in a controlled environment (Fitzgerald et al. 2000b, Chmielewski 2006, Myer 2006A, 2006B, 2006C, 2008). Chmielewski et al. (2006) report an athlete who cannot tolerate plyometric activities in the rehabilitation setting is "unlikely to tolerate a return to sports participation."

Plyometric activities should also be included throughout the rehabilitation process to potentially provide a prophylactic effect, enhance specific performance parameters, and alter faulty biomechanics (Hewett 1996, 1999, Myklebust 2005, Mandelbaum 2005, Myer 2005, 2006A, 2006B, 2006C, 2008, Chmielewski 2006). According to a review done by Fitzgerald et al. (2001) the single-leg hop test for distance (Table 51.4 and Fig. 51.3) was the most commonly used test to assess knee function, specifically following ACL reconstruction, but it may be used for all lower extremity injuries to determine overall lower extremity function. Limb asymmetry postinjury can be exposed using plyometric functional activities as assessment tools in the rehabilitation environment (Tegner 1986, Barber 1990, Noyes 1991).

Using the **Limb Symmetry Index** (LSI) (Table 51.9), Barber et al. (1990, 1992) describe lower extremity asymmetry as less than 85% between the injured and noninjured leg, determining that an evident instability will significantly affect the distance hopped of the injured leg compared to the normal leg. During the single-leg hop, Augustsson and colleagues (2000) found the knee joint provides the major energy absorption function during the landing phase and observed 2 to 3 times greater absorbed power for the knee over the hip and 5 to 10 times greater for the knee than the ankle. Therefore, it is appropriate to use a single-leg hop test, and more difficult variations of the single-leg hop, to determine the functional performance of the lower extremity, especially the knee, because it is responsible for the majority of shock absorption upon loading and landing from a jump (Table 51.4).

Running Series. Numerous sports require running activities; therefore many clinicians may use running assessment tools to determine aerobic and anaerobic fitness. Clinicians are responsible for normalizing running mechanics in athletes returning to sports requiring running, sprinting, and cutting. Myer et al. (2006A) suggest clinicians evaluate an athlete's running kinematics on a treadmill by listening to determine arrhythmic foot strike patterns or watching to determine gross asymmetries that may limit an athlete from progressing to the next phase of the rehabilitation program.

By varying the running activities in the rehabilitation program to mimic the athletic demands of the sport, the physical therapist or athletic trainer can more accurately assess the overall function of the lower extremity (Tegner 1986, Myer 2006A, 2008). The **Repeated Sprint Ability** (RSA) test (Aziz 2008, Rampanini 2007) and **straight line running with start/stops and shuttle runs** (Fitzgerald et al. 2000b) are often used to measure the ability of an athlete to perform repeated sprints and change of direction specifically for sports such as soccer, football, lacrosse, and basketball (Table 51.5). Research is limited on running assessment tools and testing procedures to evaluate return to sport, but many of the activities can be found on individual physician protocols and used clinically, although they have not been validated in the literature. Additional research is needed to develop and implement specific running tasks that

TABLE 51.4	Plyometric: Jumping/Landing Activities (Powell)				
Exercise	**Description**	**References**	**Exercise**	**Description**	**References**
Broad jump for distance	Patient stands on line with hands behind the back, jumping off both legs as far forward as possible. Stick landing and hold for 3 to 5 seconds.	Hewett 1996 Hewett 1999 Myer 2008	Single-leg hop-hop stick	Patient stands on one leg, hops twice (or three to increase difficulty) and on second hop sticks landing for 5 seconds and repeats for a series of repetitions. Increase distance as technique improves.	Hewett 1996 Myer 2006B Myer 2006C
Squat hop/ jump vertical	Patient jumps as high as possible off both legs, raising arms overhead and landing in a squatting position touching both hands to the floor.	Hewett 1996 Hewett 1999 Myer 2006B Myer 2006C	Single-leg triple crossover hop for distance (Fig. 51.6)	Patient instructed to cross over 15.2-cm-wide (6-in) tape with each consecutive hop for a total of three on the same leg. **Total distance hopped is measured for three trials. Take average and find LSI.**	Barber 1990 Noyes 1991 Bolgla 1997 Wilson 1998 Fitzgerald et al. 2000a Fitzgerald et al. 2000b Lewek 2003 Myer 2008
Squat hop/ broad jump deep hold	Patient jumps forward as far as possible and sticks landing with knees flexed at 90 degrees (thighs parallel to ground). Holds for 3 to 5 seconds.	Hewett 1996 Hewett 1999 Myer 2008			
Single-leg hop for distance (Fig. 51.3)	Patient stands on one leg with hands placed behind the back, taking off and landing on the same foot. **Average distance measures of three trials for each leg and find limb symmetry index (LSI).**	Tegner 1986 Barber 1990 Noyes 1991 Booher 1993 Hewett 1996 Bolgla 1997 Borsa 1997 Wilson 1998 Hewett 1999 Fitzgerald et al. 2000a Fitzgerald et al. 2000b Fitzgerald et al. 2001 Lewek 2003 Augustsson 2004 Ferris 2004 Myer 2005 Myer 2006A Myer 2008 Flanagan 2008	Single-leg crossover (bound) hop-hop-hop, stick (Fig. 51.7)	Patient stands on one leg and bounds at a diagonal across a line or the body, lands on the opposite limb with the foot pointing straight ahead, and immediately redirects the jump in the opposite direction and lands on the original limb.	Myer 2005 Myer 2006C Myer 2008
			180-degree jumps	Patient jumps off two feet and rotates 180 degrees in midair, sticks landing and holds for 5 seconds, then repeats in reverse direction.	Hewett 1996 Hewett 1999 Myer 2006B Myer 2006C Myer 2008
			Triple broad jump/ vertical jump	Patient performs three broad jumps for distance and, on landing on the third jump, ends with a maximum vertical jump.	Myer 2006B Myer 2006C Myer 2008
			Bounding in place	Patient jumps from one leg to the opposite leg straight up and down, progressively increasing height and rhythm.	Hewett 1996 Hewett 1999 Myer 2006B Myer 2006C Myer 2008
Single-leg hop for time	Patient stands on one leg with hands placed behind the back, taking off and landing on the same foot. Patient jumps as quickly as possible over a distance of 6 to 20 meters. **Average time measures of three trials for each leg and find LSI.**	Barber 1990 Noyes 1991 Booher 1993 Bolgla 1997 Fitzgerald et al. 2000a Fitzgerald et al. 2000b Lewek 2003 Myer 2006A Myer 2008 Flanagan 2008	Scissor jumps/ split squats	Patient starts in stride position with one foot well in front of the other. Jump up, alternating foot positions in midair. Repeat, adding speed.	Hewett 1996 Hewett 1999 Myer 2008
			Wall jumps (ankle bounces)	Patient bounces up and down off toes with knees slightly bent and arms raised above head lightly touching the wall with each jump.	Hewett 1996 Hewett 1999 Myer 2006B Myer 2006C Myer 2008
Single-leg hop: stop forward	Patient stands on one leg, performs a single hop, and sticks it for 3 to 5 seconds and repeats for a series of repetitions.	Hewett 1999 Fitzgerald et al. 2001 Myer 2006B Myer 2008	Tuck jumps	Patient stands on two legs and jumps, bringing both knees up to the chest as high as possible. Repeat quickly for a series of repetitions.	Hewett 1996 Hewett 1999 Myer 2006A Myer 2006B Myer 2006C Myer 2008
Single-leg triple hop: stop for distance (Fig. 51.5)	Patient stands on one leg, performs three consecutive hops as far as possible, and lands on the same foot. **Total distance hopped is measured for three trials. Take average and find LSI.**	Barber 1990 Noyes 1991 Bolgla 1997 Hewett 1999 Fitzgerald et al. 2000a Fitzgerald et al. 2000b Lewek 2003 Myer 2006A Myer 2008 Hamilton 2008	Cone jumps/ barrier jumps	Patient stands on two legs and double jumps with feet together side-to-side over a cone quickly. Repeat forward and backward. To advance, patient hops on a single leg.	Hewett 1996 Hewett 1999 Myer 2006B Myer 2006C Myer 2008
			Standing vertical jump	Patient stands with hands on iliac crest, bending the knees to 90 degrees of flexion, pauses, then jumps as high as possible without knee or trunk counter-movement.	Hewett 1996 Fitzgerald et al. 2001 Myer 2005 Myer 2006B Myer 2006C Rampinini 2007 Hamilton 2008

Continued

TABLE 51.4	Plyometric: Jumping/Landing Activities (Powell)—cont'd					
Exercise	**Description**	**References**		**Exercise**	**Description**	**References**
Drop vertical jump	Patient *drops* off a box (various heights) and lands on both feet simultaneously. Immediately after landing, the patient performs a maximum vertical jump.	Pollard 2006 Myer 2006a Myer 2006B Myer 2006C Myer 2007 Myer 2008		Single-leg drop vertical jump	Patient stands on top of box (40 cm) on a single leg, then drops off box and lands on a single leg. Immediately after landing, the patient performs a maximum single-leg vertical jump.	Huston 2001 Ortiz 2008
Vertical stop-jump	Patient performs a two- to three-step approach run followed by a two-footed landing and a two-footed takeoff for maximum height.	Chappell 2007 Herman 2008		Single-leg medial drop landing	Patient balances on one leg on top of a box (13.5 cm or various heights), then *drops* off box medially from the stance limb, lands on the same leg, and sticks the landing. Hold for 2 to 3 seconds.	Myer 2006C Myer 2008
Bilateral/ single-leg hop cyclic cycles forward/ lateral	Patient stands next to a line then quickly jumps over the line in forward direction and returns to starting position as quickly as possible for multiple repetitions. Patient attempts to remain close to the line but does not land *on* the line. Repeat laterally.	Pfiefer 1999 Myer 2006B Myer 2006C Myer 2008		Single-leg stair hop	Patient hops on a single leg up and down 14 steps (20-cm height) with good control and no loss of balance.	Wilson 1998
Single-leg drop jump (Fig. 51.8)	Patient stands on top of a box (30 cm or various heights) with both feet, then *drops* off box and lands on one foot, sticking landing. Hold for 2 to 3 seconds.	Pfiefer 1999		Single-leg up–down task	Patient hops on a single leg up and down a single (20 cm) step for 10 consecutive hops.	Itoh 1998 Ortiz 2008

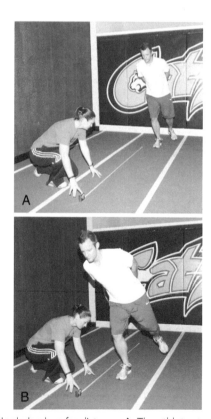

Fig. 51.3 Single-leg hop for distance. **A,** The athlete stands on one leg with hands placed behind the back (for testing only), taking off and landing on the same foot. The athlete attempts to jump as far as possible but must be able to "stick" the landing. **B,** The measurement is made from toe of stance foot and heel on landing. This activity may be used repetitively with submaximal hops for 5 to 10 repetitions to determine landing consistency. Compare distance between injured and noninjured limb. Clinicians may use the Limb Symmetry Index to determine asymmetry.

can assist in accurately assessing an athlete's ability to return to running activities safely (Table 51.5).

ADVANCED LOWER EXTREMITY SPORTS ASSESSMENT

The **Advanced Lower Extremity Sports Assessment** (ALESA) (Table 51.6) is a criteria-based tool I designed to target functional deficits in athletes with lower extremity injuries attempting to return to sports. Several investigators have determined that side-to-side imbalances noted in any of the functional performance categories including functional strength, flexibility, balance/proprioception, and coordination are helpful in predicting increased injury risk for athletes returning to sport (Tegner 1986, Barber 1990, Knapik 1991, Noyes 1991, Fitzgerald et al. 2001, Hewett 1999, McLean 1999, Myer 2005, 2006A, Paterno 2007).

ALESA has yet to be validated as a standardized assessment tool; however, most of the activities administered in the test battery have all been validated individually by numerous investigators or are currently being used clinically (Table 51.7). ALESA is currently being investigated to determine reliability as a clinical assessment tool, but it can be used currently in the clinical setting to guide functional performance testing. ALESA utilizes many of the functional performance measures previously validated in the literature that use both a qualitative and quantitative assessment of functional performance.

This assessment tool allows the clinician to observe quality of movement and quantitatively measure time, distance, or successfully completed repetitions. The scoring system is designed to assist the clinician in determining where functional deficits are present and conclude if an athlete is ready to return to sport

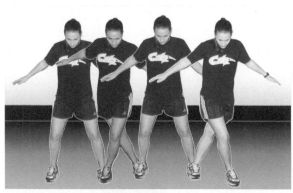

Fig. 51.4 Carioca. The athlete is instructed to attempt forward and backward crossovers while moving laterally in right and left directions. During the dynamic warmup the athlete uses the carioca foot pattern to encourage trunk rotation and increase coordination.

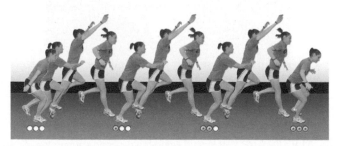

Fig. 51.5 Single-leg triple hop: stop for distance. The athlete stands on a line with hands placed behind the back (for testing only), jumping off a single leg to perform a triple hop as far as possible. The athlete must "stick" the landing. The measurement is made from toe of initial stance foot and heel on landing. This activity may be used repetitively with submaximal hops for 5 to 10 repetitions to determine landing consistency. Compare distance between injured and noninjured limb. Clinicians may use the Limb Symmetry Index to determine asymmetry.

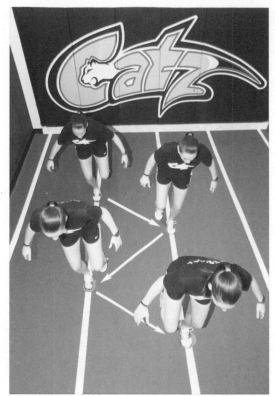

Fig. 51.7 Single-leg crossover bound (hop-hop-hop, stick). The athlete stands on one leg and bounds at a diagonal across a line or the body, lands on the *opposite* limb with the foot pointing straight ahead, and immediately redirects the jump in the opposite direction and lands on the original limb. The athlete should not take an extra hop or lose balance with each landing. This activity is useful in developing an athlete's core and knee control by demanding a change of limb and direction while decelerating through a lateral hop.

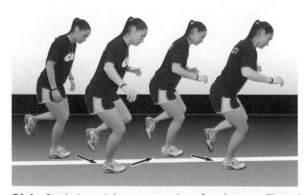

Fig. 51.6 Single-leg triple crossover hop for distance. The athlete stands on one leg with hands placed behind the back (for testing only), taking off and landing on the same foot and performing three consecutive crossover hops over a line as far as possible. The athlete must "stick" the landing. The measurement is made from toe of initial stance foot and heel on landing. This activity may be used repetitively with submaximal hops for 5 to 10 repetitions to determine landing consistency. Compare distance between injured and noninjured limb. Clinicians may use the Limb Symmetry Index to determine asymmetry.

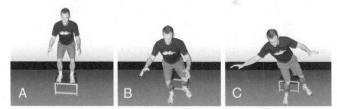

Fig. 51.8 Single-leg drop vertical jump. **A,** The athlete stands on top of a box with both feet (clinician may vary the height). **B,** The athlete then drops off the box landing on a single leg with good knee control and balance. Immediately after landing, the patient performs a maximum vertical jump. **C,** Monitor for poor landing technique with poor balance, poor core control, flexed trunk, and valgus moment noted at the knee.

by exposing potential limb asymmetries or significant imbalances noted in the lower extremity.

The battery of tests and activities for ALESA (Table 51.8) include all the functional testing categories previously listed to provide a more sensitive and reliable assessment tool. ALESA uses numerous advanced movement patterns, including several single-leg hop tests, as suggested by Fitzgerald and colleagues (2001), required for a successful return to sport. This can be used to help identify athletes with a potential risk for injury or reinjury.

Prior to using the results of ALESA to determine if an athlete is safe to return to sport, clinicians are advised to administer the same activities as part of their late-phase rehabilitation program (Myer 2006A, 2006B, 2006C, 2008). Bolgla and Keskula (1997) also emphasize adequate practice trials for athletes, prior to testing, to allow motor learning to occur.

A **simple scoring method** is used to measure the athlete's ability to establish dynamic control, static and functional

TABLE 51.5	**Running Series Activities (Powell)**	
Exercise	**Description**	**References**
Walk: jog sequence— Phase I	Patient to attempt walk:jog series—1:1 ratio 1 min. Walk:1-minute jog for total of 8–10 minutes.	Clinical
Walk: jog sequence— Phase II	Patient to attempt walk:jog series—1:1/2:1 1600-m track: 200-m walk:200-m jog for up to 1–2 miles.	Clinical
Straight-line running— build up to sprint	Patient starts with straight-line running with speeds starting at a jog and increasing speeds, then slow deceleration. Vary distances.	Clinical
Straight-line running— sprint series—start: stop ("red light/green light")	Patient starts with sprint and decelerates to a stop with verbal cuing to "stop." Clinician is to vary the distances and the verbal cues. Patient can attempt at any speed initially and progress to faster speeds as safe deceleration occurs.	Fitzgerald et al. 2000b
Hard reactive cutting/ pivoting/ twisting	Patient is to mimic sports-specific movements of cutting, pivoting, and twisting with no notable compensation or pain reported.	Clinical
Repeated-sprint ability (RSA) test	Six 40-meter (20 + 20-m) shuttle sprints separated by 20 seconds of passive recovery to assess overall fitness.	Rampinini 2007 Aziz 2008

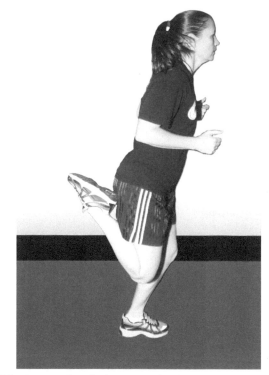

Fig. 51.9 Dynamic butt kicks. During the dynamic warmup the athlete is asked to maintain erect posture while attempting to kick heels to butt with good control and alternating with each step.

TABLE 51.6	**Advanced Lower Extremity Sports Assessment (ALESA)—Dynamic Warmup (Powell)**

Prior to Testing: 10–15 minutes: 10–20 yards
Light jog forward and backward × 2 laps
Side shuffle to the right and left × 2 laps
High knees forward and backward × 1 lap
Butt kicks forward and backwards × 1 lap (Fig. 51.9)
Skipping with high knee forward and backward × 1 lap
Carioca × 2 laps (Fig. 51.4)
Dynamic hamstring stretch forward × 1 lap (Fig. 51.10)
Dynamic hamstring stretch with rotation × 1 lap
Side lunges to the right and left × 1 lap (Fig. 51.11)
Forward lunge × 1 lap
Backward lunge with extension reach × 1 lap (Fig. 51.12)
Bilateral hopping forward and backward × 1 lap
Single-leg repeated hop right and left × 1 lap

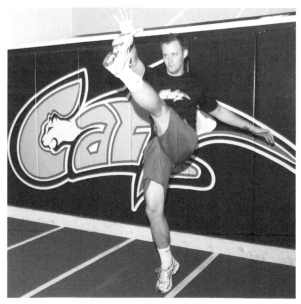

Fig. 51.10 Dynamic hamstring stretch. During the dynamic warmup the athlete mimics a kicking motion, alternating legs. For kicking sports, add rotation and full kicking motion with follow-through to mimic sports-specific movement patterns.

strength, and balance/proprioception during the simple and advanced functional performance activities (Box 51.1). This assessment tool is generally designed to test recreational to higher-level athletes involved in cutting, jumping, and pivoting sports such as soccer, basketball, football, volleyball, gymnastics, lacrosse, and the like. Each clinician can also determine which of the functional tests is appropriate for each athlete and may modify for any possible space limitations.

We advise functional performance test progression from least to most challenging preceded by a light warmup (Table 51.9)

to produce a level of fatigue that could help establish the athlete's endurance level and determine when proper technique fails, potentially leading to injury (Augustsson 2004). For all single-leg measures, start with the noninjured leg and

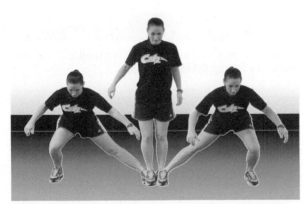

Fig. 51.11 Side lunges. During the dynamic warmup the athlete is to move through a side lunge from right to left then step through and repeat for groin/adductor stretch meant to mimic cutting and change of direction. The athlete should maintain erect posture, avoiding trunk flexion, and maintain knee in line with foot. The athlete may change foot position from forward to lateral to change target muscle group.

TABLE 51.7	ALESA Test Battery (Powell)	
ALESA Test Battery	**Authors Validating Test/ Reference**
1. Bilateral squats/sumo squats	Neitzal 2002; Boyle 2004; Myer 2006B, 2006C, 2008
2. Single-leg squat (minimum 60-degree knee flexion with 5-second hold)	Zeller 2003; Myer 2006A, 2006B, 2008
3. Broad jump for distance	Hewett 1996, 1999; Myer 2008
4. Single-leg hop for distance	Tegner 1986; Barber 1990, Noyes 1991; Hewett 1996, 1999; Bolgla 1997; Borsa 1997; Wilson 1998; Fitzgerald et al. 2000a, 2000B, 2001; Lewek 2003; Augustsson 2004; Myer 2005, 2006A, 2008; Flanagan 2008
5. Single-leg hop for time (6 m)	Barber 1990; Noyes 1991; Bolgla 1997; Fitzgerald et al. 2000a, 2000B; Lewek 2003; Myer 2006A, 2008; Flanagan 2008
6. Single-leg triple hop: stop for distance	Noyes 1991; Bolgla 1997; Hewett 1999; Fitzgerald et al. 2000a, 2000b; Lewek 2003; Myer 2006A, 2006B, 2006C, 2008; Hamilton 2008
7. Single-leg triple cross-over hop for distance	Noyes 1991; Bolgla 1997; Fitzgerald et al. 2000a, 2000b; Lewek 2003; Myer 2008; Flanagan 2008
8. Single-leg hop: stop series (×10 repetitions)	Hewett 1999; Fitzgerald et al. 2001; Myer 2006B, 2008
9. Single-leg triple hop: stop series (×5 repetitions)	Myer 2006B, 2006C, 2008
10. Single-leg balance eyes open (30 seconds)	Bernier 1998; Sherry 2004; Myer 2006A, 2008
11. Single-leg balance eyes closed (30 seconds)	Bernier 1998; Sherry 2004
12. Figure-of-eight run (6–10 m)	Tegner 1986; Wilson 1998; Fitzgerald et al. 2000b
13. Sprint series—start: stop 40 m ("red light, green light")	Clinical

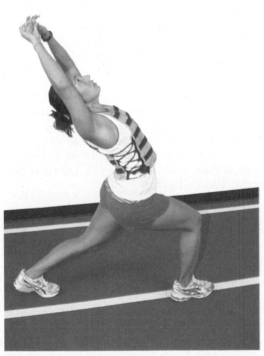

Fig. 51.12 Backward lunge with extension reach. During the dynamic warmup the athlete attempts a backward lunge with a two-handed extension reach to open abdominal area and increase trunk extension.

TABLE 51.8	ALESA Score Sheet	
Test #	**Points Earned**
#1 Bilateral squat	
#2 Single-leg squat	
#3 Broad jump for distance	
#4 Single-leg hop for distance	
#5 Single-leg hop for time (6 m)	
#6 Single-leg triple hop: stop for distance	
#7 Single-leg triple crossover hop for distance	
#8 Single-leg hop: stop series (×10 reps)	
#9 Single-leg triple hop: stop series (×5 reps)	
#10 Single-leg balance eyes open (30 inches)	
#11 Single-leg balance eyes closed (30 inches)	
#12 Figure-of-eight run (6–10 m)	
#13 Sprint series—start: stop (40 m)	
Total passing tests	/13 Total tests
ALESA score (%)	
Passing Score is 11/13 (85%)	

Created by Christie Powell, MSPT, STS, USSF D, and S. Murphy Halasz, PT, DPT, 2009.

compare with the injured lower extremity (Van der Harst 2007). Van der Harst et al. (2007) determined with healthy subjects that there are no important differences between the dominant leg and contralateral leg. The authors concluded that during functional testing (e.g., single-leg hop tests) the uninvolved leg, specifically in patients who have undergone ACL reconstruction, can be used as a "reference leg" to determine normal differences.

BOX 51.1   Advanced Lower Extremity Sports Assessment (ALESA)

Name: Date: Injury:

Dynamic Warmup: We recommend 10 to 15 minutes: 10 to 20 yards
- Light jog forward and backward
- Side shuffle to the right and left
- High knees forward and backward
- Butt kicks forward and backward
- Skipping with high knees forward and backward
- Carioca to the right and left
- Dynamic hamstring stretch, forward
- Dynamic hamstring stretch, rotation
- Side lunge to the right and left
- Forward lunge
- Backward lunge with extension reach
- Bilateral hopping forward and backward
- Single-leg repeated hop, right leg and left leg

Functional Performance Test Description: Each completed functional performance test earns 1 point or 0 points based on the distance, time, or successfully completed repetitions. Each test using repetitions requires a minimum of **80%** to earn 1 point. For PASS/FAIL tests PASS = 1 point, FAIL= 0 points. For all single-leg tests measuring distance or time, use LSI as shown in Table 51.9. **LSI 85%** or greater to PASS = 1 point.

1. Bilateral squat: The athlete is instructed to stand with feet shoulder-width apart and squat as one would sit into a chair until thighs are parallel to the ground with no loss of balance. Maintain upright posture and avoid spinal flexion. Knees must remain in line with second toe and heels must stay on the ground. *Note: Monitor for deviation off the midline and equal side-to-side limb contribution.*

   10 total repetitions. 8 complete repetitions for 80% to PASS = 1 point.

Assessment	Score	% Complete	Points
# of complete repetitions	/10		

2. Single-leg squat: The athlete is instructed to stand with arms across chest standing on a single leg and squat to 60 degrees while maintaining postural control for 5 seconds with no loss of balance. Athlete must demonstrate the ability to maintain the hip and trunk in an upright position during descent and maintain center of mass along the vertical axis. 5 total repetitions for right and left limb. **BOTH** limbs must have minimum of 80% to PASS = 1 point.

Left	Score	Right	Score
# of complete repetitions	/ 5	# of complete repetitions	/ 5
Total score % completed:		Total score % completed:	
Points:			

3. Broad jump for distance: The athlete is instructed to stand with feet at the line with hands behind back, jump as far forward as possible, and stick the landing. Knees must stay in line with second toe on takeoff and landing. Patient must jump his or her *height* to PASS. Measure distance from toe at takeoff to heel at landing for three total trials as needed to achieve height. PASS/FAIL only.

Assessment	Distance (cm)
Trial #1	
Trial #2	
Trial #3	
Patient height (cm)	
PASS or FAIL	
Points:	

4. Single-leg hop for distance: The athlete is instructed to stand on one foot at the line with hands placed behind the back and taking off and landing on the same foot. The athlete must stick the landing. Measure distance from toe at takeoff to heel at landing for three total trials. Take the average of three trials and find LSI. LSI must be 85% or greater to PASS = 1 point. Note: Monitor for valgus moment at the knees with takeoff and landing.

Left	Distance (cm)	Right	Distance (cm)
Trial #1		Trial #1	
Trial #2		Trial #2	
Trial #3		Trial #3	
Average distance		Average distance	
LSI:			
Points:			

5. Single-leg hop for time (6 m): The athlete stands on one leg with hands placed behind the back, taking off and landing on the same foot. The athlete jumps as quickly as possible over a distance of 6 meters and time is measured. Take average of three trials and find LSI. LSI must be 85% or greater to PASS = 1 point.

Left	Time (seconds)	Right	Time (seconds)
Trial #1		Trial #1	
Trial #2		Trial #2	
Trial #3		Trial #3	
Average time		Average time	
LSI:			
Points:			

6. Single-leg triple hop: stop for distance: The athlete stands on one leg with hands placed behind the back, taking off and landing on the same foot, performing three consecutive hops as far forward as possible. Distance is measured. Take average of three trials for each leg and find LSI. LSI must be 85% or greater to PASS = 1 point.

Left	Distance (cm)	Right	Distance (cm)
Trial #1		Trial #1	
Trial #2		Trial #2	
Trial #3		Trial #3	
Average distance		Average distance	
LSI:			
Points:			

7. Single-leg triple crossover hop for distance: The athlete stands on one leg with hands placed behind the back, taking off and landing on the same foot performing three consecutive *crossover* hops over a line as far as possible. Distance is measured. Take average of three trials and find LSI. LSI must be 85% or greater to PASS = 1 point.

Left	Distance (cm)	Right	Distance (cm)
Trial #1		Trial #1	
Trial #2		Trial #2	
Trial #3		Trial #3	
Average distance		Average distance	
LSI:			
Points:			

8. Single-leg hop: stop series (×10 repetitions): The athlete stands on one leg, performs a single-leg *submaximal* hop, and sticks landing for 5 seconds and repeats for a total of 10 repetitions for each leg. **BOTH** limbs must have minimum of 80% to PASS = 1 point.

Left	Score	Right	Score
# of complete repetitions	/10	# of complete repetitions	/10
Total score % completed:		Total score % completed:	
Points:			

9. Single-leg triple hop: stop series (×5 repetitions): The athlete stands on one leg, performs a single-leg *submaximal* triple hop, and sticks landing for 5 seconds and repeats for a total of five repetitions for each leg. **BOTH** limbs must have minimum of 80% to PASS = 1 point.

Left	Score	Right	Score
# of complete repetitions	/5	# of complete repetitions	/5
Total score % completed:		Total score % completed:	
Points:			

10. Single-leg balance eyes open (30 seconds): The athlete stands on a single leg with a slightly flexed knee with *eyes open* for 30 seconds on each leg. The athlete's opposite leg is bent to −75 degrees. To PASS, athlete cannot move stance foot, touch opposite leg, or touch the ground to regain balance for the *entire* 30 seconds. PASS/FAIL only. **BOTH** limbs must PASS = 1 point.

Left	Eyes Open	Right	Eyes Open
Time (s)		Time (s)	
PASS/FAIL		PASS/FAIL	
Points:			

11. Single-leg balance eyes closed (30 seconds): The athlete stands on a single leg with a slightly flexed knee with *eyes closed* for 30 seconds on each leg. The athlete's opposite leg is bent to −75 degrees. To PASS, athlete cannot move stance foot, touch opposite leg, or touch the ground to regain balance for the *entire* 30 seconds. PASS/FAIL only. **BOTH** limbs must PASS = 1 point.

Left	Eyes Closed	Right	Eyes Closed
Time (s)		Time (s)	
PASS/FAIL		PASS/FAIL	
Points:			

12. **Figure-of-eight run (6 m):** Cones set 6 meters apart and athlete is asked to run a figure-of-eight run around the cones for two laps. The athlete runs two trials for each direction (starting from right and left of cone). The athlete cannot touch a cone. Repeat trial if cone is touched. If more than three trials are necessary, athlete gets a score of 0. Take average of two trials and find LSI.

Left Start	Time (seconds)	Right Start	Time (seconds)
Trial #1		Trial #1	
Trial #2		Trial #2	
Average time		Average time	
LSI:			
Points:			

13. **Sprint series—start: stop 40 meters ("red light, green light"):** The athlete starts with sprint speed and decelerates to a stop with verbal cue to "stop." Clinician is to vary the distances for the verbal cues; attempt five total "stop" cues during 40-meter length. Athlete should come to a complete stop with no extra steps or obvious loss of balance or core control. PASS = 80% or greater. *Note: Monitor for excessive internal rotation of hips and valgus moment of knees at deceleration.*

Assessment	Score	% Complete	Points
# of successful "stops"	/5		

TABLE 51.9	Limb Symmetry Index (Powell)	
Equation for Distance Measures	**Equation for Time Measures**	
1. Find the three-trial mean distance (cm).	1. Find the three-trial mean time(s).	
2. Mean distance of INJURED limb/mean distance of NONINJURED limb	2. Mean time of NONIN-JURED limb/mean time of INJURED limb (Note this is opposite for that of distance.)	
3. Multiply by 100 to get %.	3. Multiply by 100 to get %.	
4. Find LSI score as percent-age.	4. Find LSI score as percent-age.	

Normal = greater than or equal to 85%
Asymmetry = less than 85%
Limb Symmetry Index (LSI) by Barber and Noyes 1990.

LIMB SYMMETRY INDEX

The LSI (Barber et al. 1990) (Table 51.9) will be used for all appropriate testing activities to determine asymmetry of involved versus uninvolved limbs. The author of ALESA uses the LSI to determine performance of the single-leg hop tests including single-leg hop for distance, single-leg timed hop (6 m), single-leg triple hop for distance, and single-leg crossover hop for distance (Barber et al. 1990).

To calculate the LSI for distance-measured hop tests, take the mean of the injured limb divided by the mean of the noninjured limb and multiply by 100 to get a percentage. To calculate the LSI for time-measured hop tests, take the mean of the noninjured limb divided by the mean of the injured limb, and multiply by 100 to get a percentage. For the LSI, abnormal range is considered less than 85% and normal is greater or equal to 85% when comparing injured and noninjured limbs (Barber et al. 1990) (Table 51.9).

Check online video: Single Leg Squat (Video 51.1).

REFERENCES

A complete reference list is available at https://expertconsult.inkling.com/.

FURTHER READING

Ageberg E, Friden T. Normalized motor function but impaired sensory function after normal unilateral non-reconstructed ACL injury: patients compared with uninjured controls. *Knee Surg Sports Traumatol Arthrosc.* 2008;16:449–446.

Anders J, Venbrocks R, Weinberg M. Proprioceptive skills and functional outcomes after anterior cruciate ligament reconstruction with a bone-tendon-bone graft. *Int Orthop (SICOT).* 2008;32:627–633.

Aziz A, Mukherjee S, Chia M, et al. Validity of the running repeated sprint ability test among playing positions and level of competitiveness in trained soccer players. *Int J Sports Med.* 2008;29:833–838.

Barber-Westin SD, Noyes FR. Reducing the risk of a reinjury following ACL reconstruction: what factors should be used to allow unrestricted return to sports activities? *ACL-Deficient Knee.* 2012;343–355. Web.

Barber S, Noyes F, Mangine R, et al. Quantitative assessment of functional limitations in normal and anterior cruciate ligament-deficient knees. *Clin Orthop.* 1990;255:204–214.

Barber S, Noyes F, Mangine R, et al. Rehabilitation after ACL reconstruction: functional testing. *Sports Med Rehabil Series.* 1992;15(8):969–974.

Bjordal J, Arnly F, Hannestad B, et al. Epidemiology of anterior cruciate ligament injuries in soccer. *Am J Sports Med.* 1997;25(3):341–345.

Boden B, Dean G, Feagin J, et al. Mechanisms of anterior cruciate ligament injury. *Orthopedics.* 2000;23:573–578.

Bolgla L, Keskula D. Reliability of lower extremity functional performance tests. *J Orthop Sports Phys Ther.* 1997;26(3):138–142.

Booher L, Hench K, Worrell T, et al. Reliability of three single leg hop tests. *J Sports Rehabil.* 1993;2:165–170.

Borsa P, Lephart S, Irrgang J, et al. The effects of joint position and direction of joint motion on proprioceptive sensibility in anterior cruciate ligament-deficient athletes. *Am J Sports Med.* 1997;25(3):336–340.

Button K, Van Deursen R, Price P. Measurement of functional recovery in individuals with acute anterior cruciate ligament rupture. *Br J Sports Med.* 2005;39:866–871.

Caine D, Maffulli N, Caine C. Epidemiology of injury in child and adolescent sports: injury rates, risk factors, and prevention. *Clin Sports Med.* 2008;27:19–50.

Chmielewski T, Myer G, Kauffman D, et al. Plyometric exercise in the rehabilitation of athletes: physiological responses and clinical application. *J Orthop Sports Phys Ther.* 2006;36(5):308–319.

Cissik J, Barnes M. *Sports Speed and Agility.* 1st ed. Monterey: Coaches Choice; 2004.

Ergen E, Ulkar B. Proprioception and ankle injuries in soccer. *Clin Sports Med.* 2008;27:195–217.

Ferris C, Abt J, Sell T, et al. Pelvis and hip neuromechanical characteristics predict knee biomechanics during a stop-jump task [abstract]. *J Athl Training.* 2004;39(2). Sendash34.

Fitzgerald G, Lephart S, Hwang J, et al. Hop tests as predictors of dynamic knee stability. *J Orthop Sports Phys Ther.* 2001;31(10):588–597.

Flanagan E, Galvin L, Harrison A. Force production and reactive strength capabilities after anterior cruciate ligament reconstruction. *J Athl Train.* 2008;43(3):249–257.

Gambetta V. *Gambetta Method: A Common Sense Guide to Functional Training for Athletic Performance.* 2nd ed. Sarasota: MAG Inc; 2002.

Hamilton T, Shultz S, Schmitz R, et al. Triple-hop distance as a valid predictor of lower limb strength and power. *J Athl Train.* 2008;43(2):144–151.

Herman D, Weinhold P, Guskiewicz K, et al. The effects of strength training on the lower extremity biomechanics of female recreational athletes during a stop-jump task. *Am J Sports Med.* 2008;36(4):733–740.

Hewett T, Stroupe A, Nance T, et al. Plyometric training in female athletes. *Am J Sports Med.* 1996;24(6):765–773.

Hewett T, Lindenfeld T, Riccobene J, et al. The effect of neuromuscular training on the incidence of knee injury in female athletes. *Am J Sports Med.* 1999;27(6):699–706.

Hootman J, Dick R, Agel J. Epidemiology of collegiate injuries for 15 sports: summary and recommendations for injury prevention initiatives. *J Athl Train.* 2007;42(2):311–319.

Krabak B, Kennedy D. Functional rehabilitation of lumbar spine injuries in the athlete. *Sports Med Arthrosc.* 2008;16(1):47–54.

Kvist J. Rehabilitation following anterior cruciate ligament injury. Current recommendations for sports participation. *Sports Med.* 2004;34(4):269–280.

Manske R, Reiman M. Functional performance testing for power and return to sports. *Sports Health.* 2013;5(3):244–250. Web.

Melick NE-V, Van Cingel REH, Tijssen MPW, et al. Assessment of functional performance after anterior cruciate ligament reconstruction: a systematic review of measurement procedures. *Knee Surg Sports Traumatol Arthrosc.* 2012;21(4):869–879. Web.

Orchard J, Best T, Verrall G. Return to play following muscle strains. *Clin J Sports Med.* 2005;15(6):436–441.

Pigozzi F, Giombini A, Macaluso A. Do current methods of strength testing for the return to sport after injuries really address functional performance? *Am J Physical Medicine Rehab.* 2012;91(5):458–460. Web.

Villa S, Della S, Boldrini L, et al. Clinical outcomes and return-to-sports participation of 50 soccer players after anterior cruciate ligament reconstruction through a sport-specific rehabilitation protocol. *Sports Health.* 2011;4(1):17–24. Web.

52

Treatment and Rehabilitation of Arthrofibrosis of the Knee

Scott E. Lawrance, MS, PT, ATC, CSCS | K. Donald Shelbourne, MD

INTRODUCTION

Arthrofibrosis of the knee is a common complication that can lead to loss of knee ROM, loss of strength, pain, stiffness, and inability to return to previous levels of activity. There are several definitions of arthrofibrosis in the literature; we have defined it in the past as any symptomatic loss of knee extension or flexion compared to the opposite normal knee. A patient is said to have arthrofibrosis when the limitation in knee joint ROM becomes permanent despite conservative treatments. A common cause of arthrofibrosis is improper rehabilitation or surgery for ACL reconstruction, but it can also occur after other intra-articular knee surgeries or knee injuries.

Several factors can lead to limited knee ROM after ACL surgery, including infrapatellar contracture syndrome and patella infera, inappropriate graft placement or tensioning, acute surgery on a swollen inflamed knee, "Cyclops" syndrome, concomitant medial collateral ligament (MCL) repair, and poorly supervised or designed rehabilitation programs. Prevention of arthrofibrosis is the key to successful treatment; therefore **prevention should be the focus** of every physician and rehabilitation specialist who deals with knee injuries. A good understanding of these factors and how each contributes to limitations in knee ROM is essential to developing a strategy for prevention.

Once arthrofibrosis occurs, it takes specialized medical treatment and proper rehabilitation to restore the function within a knee joint. Classification systems have been developed that can help guide treatment and provide a basis for treatment prognosis. The treatment of arthrofibrosis can be divided into preoperative rehabilitation, surgical intervention, and postoperative phases. The goals of treatment are to help restore knee ROM and increase function. **The primary focus should be on restoring full passive and active knee extension.** Once knee extension is regained and easily maintained, loss of knee flexion can be addressed. Strengthening exercises are slowly added when full ROM is restored because the focus of the procedure and rehabilitation is to address knee motion and stiffness.

PREVENTION

Preventing arthrofibrosis of the knee is based on an understanding of the potential factors that contribute to its causes and is the best way to successfully approach this complication with knee surgery. Several factors should be considered, including graft placement, associated ligamentous injuries, the timing of surgery, and postoperative rehabilitation.

ACL graft placement that is anatomically correct is important to prevent ROM problems postoperatively. If the femoral tunnel is placed too anterior, there will be a limitation in knee flexion. Tibial tunnels placed too far anteriorly will lead to graft impingement against the roof of the intercondylar notch and will not allow full knee extension.

Any ACL injury that occurs combined with either medial or lateral side knee injuries is approached by considering the ability of each structure to heal. The rationale on how to manage combined ACL/medial side knee injuries has previously been reported. To summarize, patients who sustain a combination injury to both the ACL and MCL should be treated conservatively initially because the MCL can adequately heal with good stability with proper immobilization. MCL injuries that occur proximally and avulse off the femoral condylar origin or are in the midsubstance of the ligament tend to heal with stiffness. Therefore it is important to restore full knee ROM prior to considering reconstruction of the ACL. Patients who sustain combined ACL/lateral side injuries should undergo a direct "en masse" anatomic repair of the lateral structures and reconstruction of the ACL once the knee inflammation has subsided and adequate knee ROM is obtained. Results of this technique have been previously published (see Shelbourne et al. 2007).

Timing of surgery has been previously discussed (Klootwyk 1993, Mohtadi 1991, Shelbourne and Patel 1995). **The physical condition of the knee is more important than the number of weeks from injury until reconstruction.** A knee that continues to have an active inflammatory phase or does not have full knee motion has been shown to have an increased incidence of arthrofibrosis after surgery.

Patients should not be allowed to have surgery until they have little to no swelling in the knee, full knee ROM, good leg control, and appropriate leg strength. Meeting these goals preoperatively makes postoperative rehabilitation easier and more predictable to regain full motion after the reconstruction has taken place.

An appropriate postoperative rehabilitation program that emphasizes obtaining full knee ROM and restoring good leg control can help prevent arthrofibrosis. Patients who can achieve full passive knee extension and maintain this on their own cannot develop intra-articular scarring and thus limit arthrofibrosis. Patella infera should also be avoided by stretching the patella tendon postoperatively. Flexion exercises and leg control exercises such as straight leg raise exercises stretch the patellar tendon to its full length and keep the tendon from contracting. When quadriceps muscle inhibition occurs, the tension of the hamstring muscles pulls the knee into flexion and patients are unable to stretch the patellar tendon to its maximal amount of excursion. If the quadriceps inhibition is not regained quickly, the tendon can contract, leading to patella infera. When a patient does have quadriceps inhibition, it is important to do passive full extension and passive flexion >60 degrees to prevent patellar tendon contracture and patella infera.

CLASSIFICATION

The purpose of classification schemes is to allow clinicians to better treat a condition and to make a more accurate prognosis when dealing with a condition. Shelbourne et al. (2007) reported a classification system for arthrofibrosis of the knee after ACL surgery based on ROM of the injured knee as compared to ROM in the noninjured knee (Table 52.1). The passive ROM of the knee is reported as a-b-c with "a" representing the degree of knee hyperextension, "b" representing the degree of knee extension short of 0 degrees, and "c" representing the degree of flexion present. Motion reported as 3-0-140 means that the patient's knee can hyperextend 3 degrees past zero while being able to flex to 140 degrees. In the normal population, 95% of people have some degree of hyperextension in the knee, so achieving 0 degrees of knee extension is not acceptable and the goal should be to achieve normal hyperextension equal to the noninvolved knee.

Type I arthrofibrosis is a loss of knee extension ≤10 degrees combined with normal knee flexion as compared to the opposite knee. This is usually accompanied by anterior knee pain with activity. The knee can usually passively straighten by using overpressure; however, the knee springs back into a flexed position once the pressure has been released. Tightness in the posterior capsule contributes to this inability to obtain full knee extension.

Type II arthrofibrosis is a loss of knee extension ≥10 degrees combined with normal flexion. The knee usually cannot be passively extended fully even with overpressure. This loss of extension is typically a result of the development of anterior scar as a mechanical block within the knee, mismatch of the ACL graft within the intercondylar notch, and secondary posterior capsule tightness.

Type III arthrofibrosis is a loss of knee extension >10 degrees combined with >25-degree loss of flexion. Patients with type III arthrofibrosis will be similar to the patients with type II but may also have decreased patella mobility and tight medial and lateral capsular structures. No patella infera is measured on the 60-degree lateral radiograph as compared with the opposite knee.

Type IV arthrofibrosis presents with similar ROM limitations to the patients with type III; however, patients have patella infera measured radiographically when compared to the noninvolved opposite knee.

TREATMENT

As previously described, the best treatment for arthrofibrosis is to have a comprehensive treatment plan already in place to prevent arthrofibrosis from occurring. Once a patient does have

arthrofibrosis, it is important to manage this appropriately in a goal-oriented fashion. Most surgeons prescribe physical therapy exercises, patella mobilizations, extension serial casting, continuous passive motion, and anti-inflammatory medications to help restore knee ROM before any type of surgical intervention. In our clinic, we have not seen that patella mobilizations add any benefit for patients trying to increase knee motion. Patients who can actively contract their quadriceps muscles pull the patella superiorly, and patients who can flex their knee past 90 degrees pull the patella inferiorly. Both of these movements cause greater excursion of the patella than does manual patella mobilizations performed by either a physical therapist or by the patient him or herself.

The timing of the surgical intervention is crucial and varies from case to case. Surgery during the inflammatory stage is probably contraindicated, and the importance of returning the knee to a noninflamed state prior to surgery has been described previously. Surgery should only occur when the progress from physical therapy has plateaued and the patient is mentally ready to undergo the procedure.

Preoperative Rehabilitation

The rehabilitation of arthrofibrosis is best done as a team with both the treating surgeon and physical therapist working in conjunction with one another throughout the entire process. After the diagnosis of arthrofibrosis is made, preoperative rehabilitation should begin. Physically, patients should focus on restoring knee ROM and obtaining good leg control with the primary focus on improving extension. Counseling on the significance of this condition, the difficulty in treating it, the length of rehabilitation, and prognosis for their recovery is needed.

The primary focus is restoration of knee extension until it is maximized. Exercises to increase flexion are not performed yet. Performing exercises for both knee extension and flexion is counterproductive because patients can become frustrated with the lack of any progress. Knee extension exercises include the passive towel stretch (Fig. 52.1), in which the patient stabilizes the thigh while trying to lift the heel off the ground grasping the ends of a towel that is looped around the foot. A passive knee

TABLE 52.1	Classification of Arthrofibrosis
Type I	≤10 degrees of knee extension loss with normal knee flexion
Type II	≥10 degrees of knee extension loss with normal knee flexion
Type III	>10 degrees of knee extension loss with >25 degrees of flexion loss without patella infera but with patella tightness
Type IV	>10 degrees of knee extension loss with ≥30 degrees of flexion loss accompanied by patella infera and patella tightness

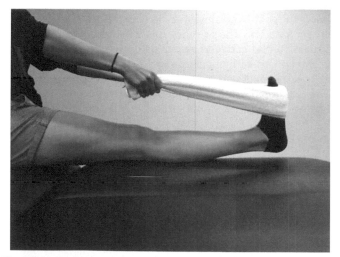

Fig. 52.1   Towel stretch for knee extension. The towel is used to lift the heel of the affected lower extremity to end-range hyperextension by pulling the end of the towel upward toward the shoulder.

extension device (Elite Seat Kneebourne Therapeutics, Noblesville, IN) is used to help restore knee extension preoperatively. The extension device (Fig. 52.2) has the advantage of allowing the patient to lie supine with relaxed hamstring muscles while controlling the amount of passive stretch applied to the knee. The patient controls the force of the passive stretch, which keeps the patient from experiencing increased amounts of pain, muscle spasm, or guarding. Patients are also instructed to stand on their involved leg (Fig. 52.3) while trying to actively contract the quadriceps muscles to lock out the knee whenever standing. Even a small amount of knee extension loss is a problem. Patients with a flexion contracture cannot comfortably stand with the knee locked into full extension. Patients will unconsciously stand with most of the weight on the noninvolved leg and will favor the involved knee by keeping it bent. The standing habit instruction is emphasized to patients because any gains patients realize from their home exercises will be lost throughout the day because of favoring the knee if not performed consistently.

Leg control is regained by performing physical therapy exercises and focusing on restoring a normal gait pattern. Exercises such as the terminal knee extension exercise (Fig. 52.4) can help encourage patients to activate the quadriceps muscles with better quality. During the gait cycle, it is important to focus on restoring heel strike to help regain leg control. Patients who have a loss of knee extension will land in a foot-flat position and not achieve heel strike. During gait, patients are instructed to slow the pace and shorten their stride to allow concentration on

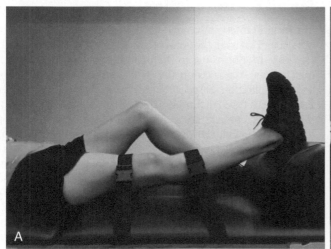
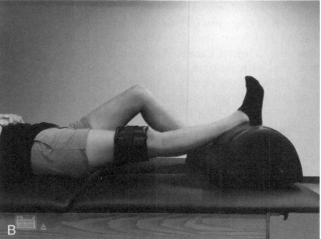

Fig. 52.2 A and B, Elite Seat device allows the patient to recline completely, which relaxes the hamstrings. The patient uses a pulley control to increase the mechanical force for knee extension. Various devices that can be used like an Elite Seat to allow relaxation of hamstrings and allow the patient to control the mechanical force for knee extension within his or her comfort limits.

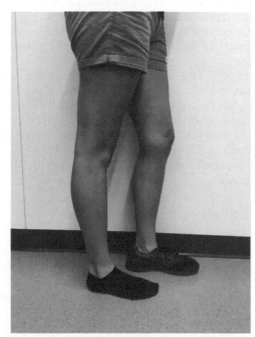
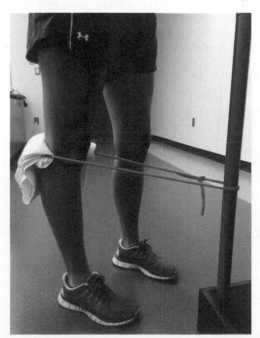

Fig. 52.3 Standing with the knee locked out into hyperextension is a habit patients should use to keep from favoring the leg and to continually work on knee extension with everyday activities.

Fig. 52.4 Terminal knee extension exercise. An elastic band is wrapped around a stable object and around the back of the patient's knee. The patient extends the knee against the resistance of the band.

using their quadriceps muscles and achieving heel strike. This keeps compensatory strategies to a minimum; as knee extension and leg control improve, the patient will be able to return to a normal gait pattern.

When a patient is able to achieve an active heel lift (Fig. 52.5), good leg control has returned and knee flexion exercises can begin. At this point, knee extension should be maximized and easily maintained through continued exercises. The heel slide exercise and/or wall slide exercise can be used to help restore flexion. However, patients should be instructed not to force knee flexion at the risk of losing knee extension. Exercises for knee flexion should be started daily once extension is maintained; however, **if the patient starts to lose knee extension, knee flexion exercises must be halted until knee extension is restored.**

Strength is not a big concern during this phase of rehabilitation and is not addressed while the patient is working on knee ROM. **It is contradictory to have patients work on both knee ROM and knee strengthening exercises at the same time because it often causes the knee to become painful and inflamed with no true gains made in knee ROM or leg strength.** However, once patients have achieved maximal knee ROM, single-leg strengthening exercises can be utilized as long as ROM is maintained. Care must be taken by both the clinician and the patient to avoid being too aggressive during this time because small losses of knee ROM will add up quickly if not checked. If losses occur, most strengthening exercises should be stopped immediately. Single-leg strengthening exercises such as the leg press are usually still tolerated well. Patients are also encouraged to exercise in a low-impact manner, such as use of the stationary bicycle, elliptical machine, or stair-stepping machine.

Patients are encouraged to improve knee ROM before surgery until it is maximized. Surgery will not be performed until improvement in ROM has plateaued. Patients who have maximized knee extension will report only anterior soreness or discomfort with stretching. If patients continue to report any posterior stretch sensations while performing knee extension exercises, they should continue rehabilitation. Patients who present with type I arthrofibrosis may be able to rehabilitate themselves to the point where surgery is not needed. Patients who regain full equal knee extension and strength that is

symmetric to the opposite noninvolved knee may elect not to have surgery and instead accept the slight limitations their knee places on them.

For patients who still have a loss of ROM despite rehabilitation, surgery becomes an option. Ongoing counseling with feedback on the goals of treatment and rehabilitation, progress made, and prognosis should be constant. Mental preparation and understanding of the treatment are as important as the actual treatment. Patients should be in good spirits and ready to tackle the challenges of surgery and the postoperative recovery. Patients still going through the grief cycle should not be operative candidates and may benefit from a referral to a licensed sports psychologist or other mental health care professional before surgical intervention.

Surgical Intervention

The surgical intervention will vary based on the preferences of the physician. However, the goals of surgery must be to restore full passive knee motion equal to the opposite, noninvolved knee. Shelbourne et al. reported on the outpatient arthroscopic technique and rehabilitation based on the type of arthrofibrosis present. Patients with **type I** arthrofibrosis are treated by excising the hypertrophied cyclops scar around the base of the ACL until the graft fits in the intercondylar notch and the patient can easily obtain full symmetric knee extension. Patients with **type II** arthrofibrosis usually require resection of the anterior scar along with resection of the extrasynovial scar tissue anterior to the proximal tibia. Notchplasty or ACL graft débridement is also performed as needed if graft impingement still occurs in full knee extension.

Patients with **type III** arthrofibrosis have scarring similar to those with type II. These patients also have extrasynovial scar present in the fibrotic fat pat between the patella tendon and the tibia. During the arthroscopy, a blunt probe is used to establish a plane between the patella tendon and the scar tissue and the scar tissue is removed distally up to the upper tibia and anteriorly to the horns of the meniscus. Once the retropatellar tendon scar tissue and anterior tibial scar tissue are resected, the fibrotic capsule is excised up to the VMO and the vastus lateralis insertion to free the patella and the patellar tendon completely.

Patients with **type IV** arthrofibrosis require a scar resection similar to those with type III; however, a more extensive resection both medial and lateral to the patella is required for these patients. In patients with type III and type IV arthrofibrosis, a knee manipulation is performed after completion of the scar resection to achieve as much flexion as possible. **A notchplasty is required for all patients with types II, III, and IV arthrofibrosis.**

Postoperative Rehabilitation

Postoperative rehabilitation begins immediately after surgery is completed. Patients are placed into antiembolic stocks and a cold/compression device (Cryo/Cuff, Aircast, A division of DJ Ortho, Vista, CA) is applied to the knee. Patients remain in the hospital for an overnight stay to prevent a knee hemarthrosis and reduce pain. After leaving the hospital, patients are restricted to bed rest with only bathroom privileges for the first 5 days. The leg is placed into a continuous passive motion machine set to move the knee from 0 to 30 degrees continuously throughout the day and night. This combination of providing

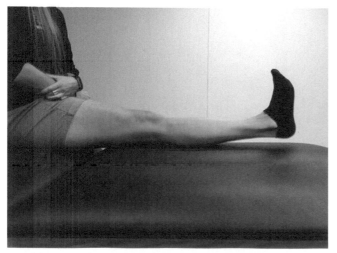

Fig. 52.5 Active heel lift exercise. The patient contracts the quadriceps muscle to fully extend the knee into full hyperextension.

cold, compression, and elevation has proved effective for preventing swelling and reducing pain.

Exercises for knee extension and leg control begin immediately and are performed four times each day. Exercises for knee extension are similar to those used preoperatively and include the towel stretch exercise with an active heel lift and use of a knee extension device. Exercises for leg control include quad sets and straight leg raises. Although both of these exercises help to increase leg control, they are also important to help prevent patellar tendon infera. By contracting the quadriceps muscles and lifting the leg, the patellar tendon is engaged and stretched to its full length, thus preventing a contracture from occurring.

Once the patient has maximized knee extension and is able to maintain active heel lift easily, gentle flexion exercises can be initiated twice a day while extension exercises are continued. Heel slide and wall slide exercises can be helpful in regaining knee flexion. Just as is the case preoperatively, patients who start to lose extension postoperatively must stop all flexion exercises and concentrate solely on regaining full knee extension. After 5 days of bed rest, patients are allowed to gradually increase their daily activities over a period of 2 to 3 days so they can return to their normal daily routine. Instructions are given to help achieve a normal gait pattern and the correct standing habits are reviewed again. Patients who were successful preoperatively with standing on the involved leg and walking with a normal gait pattern should be able to achieve these same goals postoperatively with minimal effort.

Patients are followed on a weekly basis to check for loss of knee ROM and to update the home exercise program. For type I arthrofibrosis, once knee motion is symmetric to the opposite, noninvolved knee, single-leg strengthening exercises are started along with low-impact conditioning to help restore normal leg strength. Patients with types II, III, and IV arthrofibrosis have significant losses of knee extension before surgery, and although preoperative rehabilitation improves knee extension, the mechanical block within their knee prevents them from fully stretching the posterior knee capsule preoperatively. This means that these patients will typically have to spend more time working on improving knee extension before progressing into the next phase of rehabilitation.

Once patients with type II and III arthrofibrosis have met the knee ROM goal of being symmetric to the opposite knee, they are allowed to start into a strengthening program provided full knee ROM is maintained. Patients with type IV arthrofibrosis should be able to achieve full knee extension and maintain this; however, because of the preexisting patella infera, they will not be able to regain full flexion. It is important to know how much flexion a patient is expected to recover, and communication between the physician, patient, and therapist is crucial to ensure that maximal flexion is gained.

Returning to sports activities is possible for all patients with arthrofibrosis once they have completed the rehabilitation. Patients should be able to demonstrate knee ROM symmetric to the opposite knee along with achieving strength that is within 10% of the opposite leg when tested isokinetically. Patients should carefully monitor knee ROM as they increase sports activities. Impact sports such as basketball, soccer, football, or volleyball are recommended to be performed on an every-other-day basis for the first 2 to 4 weeks to allow the knee time to recover. The cold/compression device should be used to help control inflammation and swelling within the knee after participation. Patients whose knees remain sore despite the off day or who cannot maintain full knee ROM will need further modification of their activities until they are less sore and can better maintain knee ROM. As soreness decreases and ROM is maintained, patients are allowed to increase the amount of participation accordingly. Patients are followed in the clinic until they have returned to all of their desired sports activities.

RESULTS

From January 1, 2003, until December 31, 2007, 27 patients with arthrofibrosis after ACL reconstruction were referred to our practice and treated using the surgical technique and rehabilitation program described previously. The patient sample is summarized in Table 52.2. The average ROM at initial treatment in the involved knee was 0-8-121 compared to 5-0-146 in the noninvolved knee. All patients underwent preoperative physical therapy to maximize knee ROM followed by arthroscopic scar resection and postoperative physical therapy. Postoperative ROM improved in the involved knee to 4-0-136. International Knee Documentation Committee (IKDC) subjective knee questionnaires were given to all patients and the average improved from 50 points (out of 100 points) preoperatively to 69 points postoperatively.

Preoperatively, the difference in knee extension ROM among patients was distributed evenly among the ROM categories as established by the IKDC (Fig. 52.6, A). No patient demonstrated less than 3 degrees of knee extension preoperatively. Postoperatively, all patients had an increase in their involved knee extension ROM. Twenty patients (74%) had a difference in knee extension postoperatively between 0 and 2 degrees as compared to the opposite knee, and seven patients increased their knee extension into the 3- to 5-degree category.

The difference in knee flexion preoperatively among patients can be seen in Fig. 52.6, B. Postoperatively, all patients saw an

TABLE 52.2	Change in Knee Extension and Flexion ROM With IKDC Subjective Score for Patients Preoperative to Postoperative Based on Arthrofibrosis Classification (Lawrance)						
		PREOPERATIVE DIFFERENCES		POSTOPERATIVE DIFFERENCES		IKDC	
Classification	Number of Patients (n)	Extension	Flexion	Extension	Flexion	Preoperative	Postoperative
Type I	7	7.0	4.0	1.4	1.4	57	78
Type II	5	10.6	23.0	2.0	8.6	55	68
Type III	13	16.4	40.6	1.9	16.8	47	68
Type IV	2	9.0	37.0	3.5	35.0	42	62
All patients	27	12.3	27.4	1.6	11.9	50	69

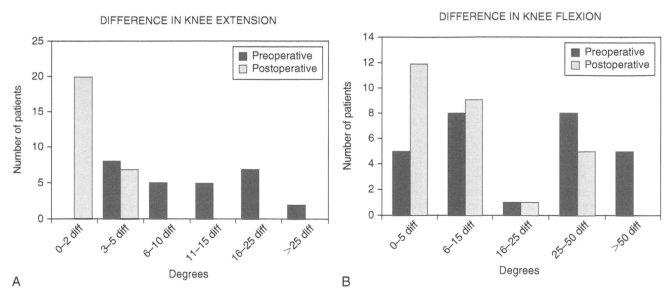

Fig. 52.6 Distribution in preoperative and postoperative knee ROM measurements for extension (*A*) and flexion (*B*).

improvement in their knee flexion. No patient lacked more than 50 degrees of flexion postoperatively.

Individuals who regained normal knee motion, according to IKDC criteria, scored higher postoperatively on their IKDC subjective questionnaires than those who did not have normal motion. Eight patients (30%) achieved normal knee motion as compared to the opposite knee, with an average postoperative IKDC score of 78. Four patients (15%) regained nearly normal extension (lacking 3 to 5 degrees), lacked greater than 16 degrees of flexion, and had an average IKDC subjective score of 43, illustrating the importance of achieving symmetric knee motion.

CONCLUSIONS

Arthrofibrosis of the knee includes a vast amount of pathology, and a good understanding of the contributing factors is vital to treat this condition successfully. The most effective method of treating this condition is taking the necessary steps initially to prevent it from occurring, because once it has occurred significant functional deficits and disability can occur. The focus of treatment should be to restore normal knee ROM with the primary focus on obtaining full knee extension first, including full hyperextension, and then obtaining full knee flexion second. Patients should be educated on the total management plan for arthrofibrosis including the prognosis for the functional status of their knee once treatment is concluded.

REFERENCES

A complete reference list is available at https://expertconsult .inkling.com/.

FURTHER READING

Chambat P, Vargas R, Desnoyer J. Arthrofibrosis after anterior cruciate ligament reconstruction. *The Knee Joint.* 2012:263–268. Web.

De Carlo MS, Sell KE. Normative data for range of motion and single-leg hop in high school athletes. *J Sport Rehab.* 1997;6:246–255.

Graf B, Uhr F. Complications of intra-articular anterior cruciate reconstruction. *Clin Sports Med.* 1988;7:835–848.

Harner CD, Irrgang JJ, Paul J, et al. Loss of motion after anterior cruciate ligament reconstruction. *Am J Sports Med.* 1992;20:499–506.

Jackson DW, Schaefer RK. Cyclops syndrome: loss of extension following intra-articular anterior cruciate ligament reconstruction. *Arthroscopy.* 1990;6:171–178.

Joseph, MF. Clinical evaluation and rehabilitation prescription for knee motion loss. *Physical Therapy in Sport.* 2012;13.2:57–66. Web.

Livbjerg, EA, Froekjaer S, et al. Pre-operative patient education is associated with decreased risk of arthrofibrosis after total knee arthroplasty. *The Journal of Arthroplasty.* 2013;28.8:1282–1285. Web.

Noyes FR, Wojtys EM, Marshall MT. The early diagnosis and treatment of developmental patella infera syndrome. *Clin Orthop Relat Res.* 1991:241–252.

Noyes FR, Mangine RE, Barber SD. The early treatment of motion complications after reconstruction of the anterior cruciate ligament. *Clin Orthop Relat Res.* 1992;277:217–228.

Nwachukwu, BU, Mcfeely ED, et al. Infrapatellar contracture syndrome. An unrecognized cause of knee stiffness with patella entrapment and patella infera. *Am J Sports Med.* 1987;15:331–341.

Rubinstein Jr RA, Shelbourne KD, VanMeter CD, et al. Effect on knee stability if full hyperextension is restored immediately after autogenous bone-patellar tendon-bone anterior cruciate ligament reconstruction. *Am J Sports Med.* 1995;23:365–368.

Salter RB, Hamilton HW, Wedge JH, et al. Clinical application of basic research on continuous passive motion for disorders and injuries of synovial joints: a preliminary report of a feasibility study. *J Orthop Res.* 1984;1:325–342.

Said S, Svend EC, Faunoe P, et al. Outcome of surgical treatment of arthrofibrosis following ligament reconstruction. *Knee Surg Sports Traumatol Arthrosc.* 2011;19.10:1704–1708. Web.

Sapega AA, Moyer RA, Schneck C, et al. Testing for isometry during reconstruction of the anterior cruciate ligament. Anatomical and biomechanical considerations. *J Bone Joint Surg Am.* 1990;72:259–267.

Shearer DW, Micheli LJ, Kocher MS. Arthrofibrosis after anterior cruciate ligament reconstruction in children and adolescents. *Journal of Pediatric Orthopaedics.* 2011;31.8:811–817. Web.

Shelbourne KD, Patel DV. Timing of surgery in anterior cruciate ligament-injured knees. *Knee Surg Sports Traumatol Arthrosc.* 1995;3:148–156.

Shelbourne KD, Patel DV, Martini DJ. Classification and management of arthrofibrosis of the knee after anterior cruciate ligament reconstruction. *Am J Sports Med.* 1996;24:857–862.

Shelbourne KD, Porter DA. Anterior cruciate ligament-medial collateral ligament injury: nonoperative management of medial collateral ligament tears with anterior cruciate ligament reconstruction. A preliminary report. *Am J Sports Med.* 1992;20:283–286.

Shelbourne KD, Wilckens JH, Mollabashy A, et al. Arthrofibrosis in acute anterior cruciate ligament reconstruction. The effect of timing of reconstruction and rehabilitation. *Am J Sports Med.* 1991;19:332–336.

Strum GM, Friedman MJ, Fox JM, et al. Acute anterior cruciate ligament reconstruction. Analysis of complications. *Clin Orthop Relat Res.* 1990;253:184–189.

Posterior Cruciate Ligament Injuries

Michael D'Amato, MD | S. Brent Brotzman, MD

Information concerning PCL injuries has expanded greatly in the past few years. Despite these advances, significant controversy still exists concerning many aspects of the evaluation and treatment of PCL injuries, especially the natural history of the PCL-injured knee. Our improved understanding of the anatomy and biomechanics of the PCL has led to a more rational and sound basis for the design of rehabilitation programs for treatment both in the nonoperative setting and after surgery.

REHABILITATION RATIONALE
Normal Posterior Cruciate Ligament

The normal PCL is a complex ligamentous structure with insertions on the posterior aspect of the proximal tibia and the lateral aspect of the medial femoral condyle. The ligament is composed of two functional bundles: a larger anterolateral bundle, which develops tension as the knee flexes, and the smaller posteromedial bundle, which develops tension in knee extension (Fig. 53.1). At its midsubstance, the anterolateral bundle is approximately twice the size of the posteromedial bundle in cross-section. The anterolateral bundle also is stiffer and has a higher ultimate load to failure. The PCL functions as the primary restraint to posterior translation of the tibia and a secondary restraint to external rotation.

Mechanism of Injury

Rupture of the PCL is usually caused by a direct blow to the proximal tibia, a fall on the knee with the foot in a plantarflexed position, or with hyperflexion of the knee. Less common causes include hyperextension or combined rotational forces. Typically, the ligament fails in its midsubstance, but avulsions of the tibial or femoral attachments have been described. The injury may be isolated to the PCL or associated with multiple ligament injuries or knee dislocation. Isolated injuries tend to occur during athletics, and combined injuries are usually the result of high-energy trauma.

EVALUATION

A number of tests are available to clinically assess the integrity of the PCL. The posterior drawer test at 90 degrees of knee flexion has been shown to be the most sensitive. Other tests include the posterior sag test, the quadriceps active test, and the reverse pivot shift test.

The rotational stability of the knee must also be evaluated to rule out any associated injury to the posterolateral ligament complex. One must also be wary when performing a Lachman test in the setting of a PCL injury. It is easy to assume that the anterior translation represents an injury to the ACL, when in fact it may be the tibia returning to a normal position from a previously abnormal posteriorly subluxated position. The collateral ligaments and menisci should also be appropriately evaluated.

Biomechanical studies have produced several key points that should be considered in the evaluation of PCL injury.
- The PCL is the primary restraint to posterior translation at all positions of knee flexion. At both 30 degrees and 90 degrees of flexion, the PCL resists 85% to 100% of posteriorly directed forces.
- PCL tear is best detected at 70 to 90 degrees of knee flexion with posterior drawer testing.
- Isolated PCL tear does not cause varus–valgus laxity or increased rotation.
- Isolated PCL tear and isolated posterolateral corner injury will produce about the same degree of posterior translation at 30 degrees of knee flexion.
- If there is varus or valgus laxity in full extension, by definition there is combined injury to the PCL and collateral complex.
- If the knee hyperextends asymmetrically, there is a combined cruciate and posterolateral corner injury.
- Posterolateral corner injury may produce mild degrees of varus laxity, but more severe degrees of varus laxity indicate PCL injury.
- A combination of PCL tear and posterolateral corner tear produces much more severe posterior translation and external rotation than either injury in isolation.
- It is difficult to have *severe* posterolateral corner instability without injury to the PCL, fibular collateral ligament, and popliteus.

Classification

Classification of PCL injuries is based on the relationship of the medial tibial plateau to the medial femoral condyle during a posterior drawer test (Fig. 53.2).
- *Grade I* injuries have 0 to 5 mm of posterior translation and maintain the position of the medial tibial plateau anterior to the medial femoral condyle.
- *Grade II* injuries have 5 to 10 mm of posterior translation and the medial tibial plateau rests flush to the medial femoral condyle.
- *Grade III* injuries have more than 10 mm of posterior translation and the medial tibial plateau falls posterior to the medial femoral condyle.

Radiographic Evaluation

Radiographs are usually negative; however, they may identify the presence of a bony avulsion that can be reattached.

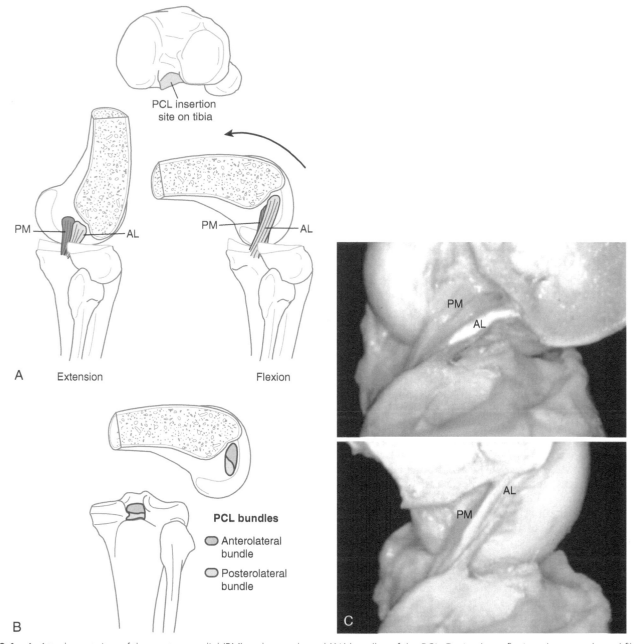

Fig. 53.1 **A,** Attachment sites of the posteromedial (PM) and anterolateral (AL) bundles of the PCL. During knee flexion, the anterolateral fibers are progressively tensed. **B,** Origin and insertion of posterior cruciate ligament anterolateral (AL) and posteromedial (PM) bands. **C,** Anatomic pictures of anterolateral (AL) and posteromedial (PM) bundles of posterior cruciate ligament. (Redrawn with permission from Harer CD, Hoher J, 1998 Evaluation and treatment of posterior cruciate ligament injuries. *Am J Sports Med* 26(3):471–482.)

Stress radiographs have been shown to compare favorably with clinical examination techniques in the diagnosis of PCL injury. Magnetic resonance imaging (MRI) is helpful to confirm the diagnosis of a PCL rupture and to evaluate the remaining structures of the knee. **Although MRI is extremely sensitive (97%) for identifying PCL tears, it is not as sensitive (67%) in differentiating partial from complete tears.** **Bone scans** can be used to demonstrate increased subchondral stress resulting from changes in knee kinematics after PCL injury. The increased stresses may predispose the knee to early degeneration, and some surgeons use the abnormal bone scan as an indication of the need for operative PCL stabilization.

BIOMECHANICS OF THE POSTERIOR CRUCIATE LIGAMENT–DEFICIENT KNEE

Injury to the PCL results in changes in the kinematics of the knee. Changes in contact pressure have been demonstrated in both the patellofemoral and the medial tibiofemoral compartments after sectioning of the PCL, with significant increases in the joint forces. In a clinical study of 14 patients with PCL-deficient knees, altered kinematics resulted in a shift of the tibiofemoral contact location and an increase in cartilage deformation in the medial compartment beyond 75 degrees of knee flexion. This alteration in the normal kinematics may explain

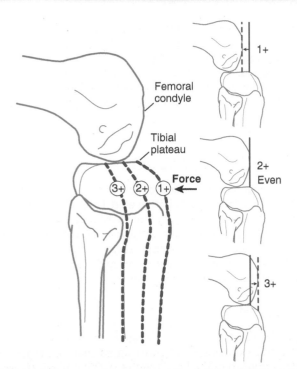

Fig. 53.2 Posterior cruciate ligament injury grading. Grading is based on the relationship of the anterior aspect of the medial tibial plateau to the anterior aspect of the medial femoral condyle. In grade I, the tibia remains anterior to the femur. In grade II, the tibia is even with the femur. In grade III, the tibia moves posterior to the femur. (From Miller MD et al. Instr Course Lect 48:199-207, ©1999 American Academy of Orthopaedic Surgeons.)

the tendency for the development of degenerative changes in these two compartments after PCL injury.

BIOMECHANICS OF EXERCISE

Markolf and colleagues (1997) demonstrated that passive ROM of the knee results in the generation of minimal force in the intact PCL throughout the entire motion arc. After reconstruction, no significant change in force production was noted except for a small increase at flexion angles greater than 60 degrees.

The **shear forces** generated in the knee during open and closed kinetic chain exercises have been closely examined. A posterior shear force occurs during closed kinetic chain exercise throughout the entire ROM of the knee, with greater forces generated as knee flexion increases. With open kinetic chain activities, there appears to be a tremendous force exerted on the PCL during flexion exercises. However, with open kinetic chain extension, minimal or no force appears to be generated in the PCL from 0 to 60 degrees, but from 60 to 90 degrees significant stress is produced in the PCL. It has been demonstrated that altering the position of the resistance pad can modify the forces generated with open kinetic chain exercises.

The magnitude of force generated in the PCL during exercise is much greater than that in the ACL, which may be a factor in the tendency for PCL grafts to stretch out after surgical reconstruction. The trend has been to avoid reconstruction of the PCL when possible, but it may be that proper rehabilitation can avoid the development of progressive laxity and improve the results of reconstruction.

O'Connor (1993) calculated that it is possible to unload the cruciate ligaments dynamically using co-contraction of the quadriceps, hamstrings, and gastrocnemius muscles. The role of the gastrocnemius in dynamically stabilizing the PCL is supported indirectly by the findings of Inoue and coworkers (1998), who demonstrated an earlier activation of the gastrocnemius before the generation of flexion torque in the knee in PCL-deficient knees compared with uninjured knees.

The goal should be to minimize the potentially deleterious generation of force during rehabilitation. It appears that passive motion can be safely performed through the entire range of flexion and extension. Active closed kinetic chain activities of any kind, in any ROM, should be used cautiously when rehabilitating the PCL, either as nonoperative therapy or after reconstruction. If these exercises are used, they should be carried out in a ROM that limits flexion of the knee to about 45 degrees or less to avoid generating higher forces in the PCL. Open kinetic chain flexion exercises generate extremely high forces in the PCL and should be avoided altogether, whereas open kinetic chain extension appears to be safe when performed at lower flexion angles (from 60 to 0 degrees). However, in this range, the patellofemoral stresses are at their greatest and the risk for development of patellofemoral symptoms is significant. Therefore, we do not routinely recommend the use of open chain exercises during rehabilitation after PCL injury or reconstruction.

NATURAL HISTORY

The natural history of isolated PCL injuries remains controversial. In a number of studies, isolated PCL injuries have been shown to do well with nonoperative treatment, whereas others have shown poor outcomes after conservative measures.

Attempts have been made to determine what variables may predict the outcome of conservatively treated PCL injuries. Increased quadriceps strength has been correlated with improved outcome in some studies, whereas others have not found a significant relationship. Shelbourne, Davis, and Patel (1999) demonstrated that subjective and objective functional outcomes were independent of knee laxity. However, all of their patients demonstrated grade II laxity or less. Shelbourne and Muthukaruppan (2005) prospectively followed 215 patients with acute, isolated grade I or II PCL injuries for an average of almost 8 years. The amount of PCL laxity did not correlate with subjective outcome scores. Of note, the subjective scores did not decrease from those at the time of injury. The authors concluded that 80% of PCL ruptures can have good or excellent results with appropriate nonoperative treatment. It is unclear what effect more severe laxity has on the results of conservative treatment.

The development of degenerative changes, particularly in the medial tibiofemoral and patellofemoral compartments, is also an area of controversy. Some studies have demonstrated increased degeneration with time after conservative treatment of PCL injuries, whereas others have not.

Unlike a torn ACL and more like a torn MCL, the PCL may regain continuity with time. Shelbourne and colleagues (1999) found that, at follow-up, 63 of 68 patients with PCL injuries had the same or less clinical laxity than at their initial evaluations. Athletes with isolated PCL injuries may be told that the amount of posterior laxity is likely to improve with time, but this does not mean a better knee subjectively.

Clearly, isolated PCL injuries may not be as benign as was once believed. The problem is not one of instability, but one of progressive disability. Most studies demonstrate reasonably good functional outcomes after conservative treatment of isolated PCL injuries, yet a significant number of patients develop pain and early degenerative change in the knee despite a good functional recovery. Unfortunately, surgical management has not been shown to consistently alter the natural history of these injuries.

REHABILITATION CONSIDERATIONS

In general, rehabilitation after PCL injury tends to be more conservative than after ACL injury. The severity of the PCL injury should also guide the aggressiveness of nonoperative therapy. Rehabilitation progression can be more rapid with grades I and II injuries, whereas rehabilitation after grade III injuries is advanced more slowly. After reconstruction, a different protocol is used, and again, a more conservative approach is used than after ACL reconstruction.

Motion

Because passive motion places negligible stress on the intact PCL and only a small stress on PCL grafts with knee flexion past 60 degrees, the use of CPM may be beneficial for grade III injuries treated nonoperatively and after reconstruction. Early active motion may expose the ligament to excessive force and lead to elongation and subsequent laxity. For grades I and II injuries treated nonoperatively, nonresisted active motion as tolerated is probably safe, but resisted motion, including weight bearing, should be limited to a 0- to 60-degree flexion arc during the early treatment phase.

Weight bearing

Weight bearing is encouraged. For mild injuries treated nonoperatively, weight bearing should be in a brace limited to 0 to 60 degrees of motion. For more severe injuries treated nonoperatively and after PCL reconstruction, weight bearing should be in a brace locked in extension during the early treatment phases and progressed gradually.

External Support

After reconstruction or during nonoperative treatment of grade III isolated PCL injuries, it is crucial to prevent posterior displacement of the tibia from the effects of gravity and the weight of the leg and from the pull of the hamstrings. Proper bracing is helpful to resist these forces, but the therapist must be aware of the potential for posterior sag to occur. If CPM devices are used, resistance straps must be included to support the proximal tibia posteriorly. Exercises also must be carried out with manual support of the tibia. Alternatively, flexion exercises can be done prone so that the posterior translational force of gravity on the tibia is eliminated.

Limited information is available concerning the efficacy of **functional bracing** after PCL injury. At this time, use of a functional brace is commonly recommended, although little scientific data supporting this recommendation can be found.

Muscle Training

Quadriceps strengthening is the foundation of rehabilitation after PCL injury. As noted earlier, the quadriceps functions to dynamically stabilize the tibia and counteract the posterior pull of the hamstrings. Open kinetic chain extension activities place the lowest strains on the PCL but result in elevated patellofemoral joint forces. We recommend the use of closed kinetic chain activities from 0 to 45 degrees as a compromise to protect both the PCL and the patellofemoral joint. Open kinetic chain flexion activities, which produce high posterior shear forces, should be avoided.

PATELLOFEMORAL JOINT

The patellofemoral joint is at particular risk for the development of symptoms during rehabilitation after PCL injury. The altered kinematics of the knee place an increased force across the joint, resulting in early degeneration of the articular surfaces. Also, open kinetic chain extension exercises at low levels of knee flexion (0 to 60 degrees) create an extremely high joint reaction force across the patellofemoral joint.

Treatment

There is still a great deal of debate regarding the treatment of PCL injuries. Currently, most agree that combined ligamentous injuries of the knee require surgical repair or reconstruction; however, there is no clear consensus as to when reconstruction is indicated for isolated PCL injuries (Figs. 53.3 and 53.4). For *acute* isolated grade I or II PCL injuries, the common recommendation is nonoperative rehabilitation (Rehabilitation Protocol 53.1). For acute isolated grade III injuries, the clear indication for surgery is an avulsion or "pull-off" injury of the ligament at the bony insertion site. Less clear are the indications for surgical treatment of midsubstance rupture of the ligament. Some advocate nonoperative treatment for all acute isolated grade III PCL injuries, whereas others recommend reconstruction in younger, high-demand patients.

For *chronic* injuries, grade I and most grades II and III injuries are treated with rehabilitation and activity modification. Surgery is indicated for symptomatic chronic grades II and III injuries. The symptoms are typically pain or instability. A positive bone scan, indicating kinematic changes leading to early joint degeneration, may prompt surgical reconstruction in an attempt to forestall the progression of joint arthrosis.

Nonoperative Treatment

For grades I and II injuries, progression can proceed rapidly, with minimal immobilization, early strengthening, proprioception and neuromuscular training, and a return to full activity relatively quickly. Outcomes after grade III injuries are less predictable, and the likelihood of an undetected posterolateral corner injury is significant. Therefore, with grade III injuries, a more conservative approach is recommended. These injuries are generally treated with a short course of immobilization, with passive rather than active motion in the early healing phase, and a less aggressive strengthening program. A long-term follow-up study (6 to 12 years) found that patients who had surgery within 1 year of injury had significantly better functional results than those who had surgery later; the authors recommended that the nonoperative period not be extended longer than 1 year from injury.

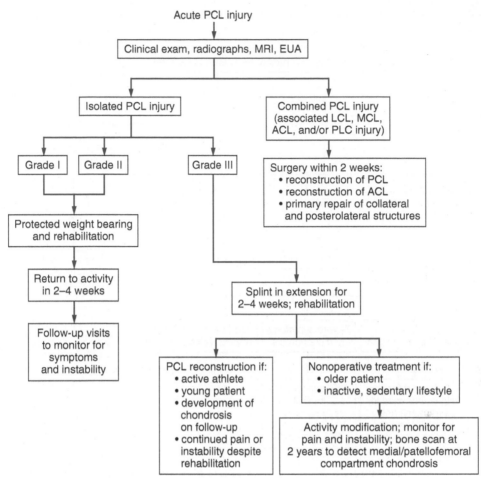

Fig. 53.3 Treatment algorithm from acute posterior cruciate ligament (PCL) injury. (Reprinted with permission from Miller MD, Cole BJ: Textbook of Arthroscopy. Philadelphia, WB Saunders, 2004.)

Operative Treatment

Historically, the surgical approach to PCL reconstruction has involved transtibial fixation, in which the graft is passed proximally and posterior through the tibia, making a 90-degree turn around the superior edge of the posterior opening of the tibial tunnel before entering the knee joint ("killer curve") (Fig. 53.5). Because friction at this point can cause graft elongation and failure, a tibial inlay technique was developed to avoid placement of the graft in this position. The tibial inlay technique involves arthroscopic placement of the femoral tunnel or tunnels and open creation of a trough in the posterior tibial bone, securing the graft to the anatomic tibial attachment footprint. A comparison of the tibial inlay and transtibial techniques in 20 patients found no significant differences in functional outcomes at a minimum 2-year follow-up; 90% of patients were satisfied with their results, regardless of the technique used. Arthroscopic tibial-inlay techniques (single and double bundle) have been reported to obtain results similar to those with open techniques.

As with the ACL, recent focus has been on reconstructing both bundles of the PCL in an attempt to restore more normal knee anatomy and function. Biomechanical testing of double-bundle PCL reconstruction has produced conflicting data, and clinical studies have not shown the double-bundle technique to produce superior functional results. A systematic review of the literature concluded that **the superiority of single-bundle or double-bundle PCL reconstruction remains uncertain**. Chhabra et al. (2006) suggested guidelines for selecting the appropriate PCL reconstruction technique based on the injury pattern: single-bundle reconstruction for acute (<3 weeks from injury), isolated, or combined PCL injuries (PCL/posterolateral corner, PCL/MCL, knee dislocation) and acute or chronic PCL injuries in which the posteromedial bundle and meniscofemoral ligaments remain intact and double-bundle reconstruction when all three components of the PCL complex are ruptured (anterolateral and posteromedial bands and meniscofemoral ligaments).

Because drilling two tunnels in the femoral condyle may interfere with condylar blood supply and increase the risk of fracture, Wiley et al. (2007) recommended a period of protected weight bearing in the early postoperative period to reduce the risk of fracture in patients who have a double-bundle reconstruction. No clinical study, however, has specifically evaluated the effect of postoperative rehabilitation on clinical outcomes of double-bundle reconstruction.

Regardless of the technique used, Fanelli et al. (2007) listed keys to successful PCL reconstruction: identify and treat all pathology, use strong graft material, accurately place tunnels in anatomic insertion sites, minimize graft bending, use

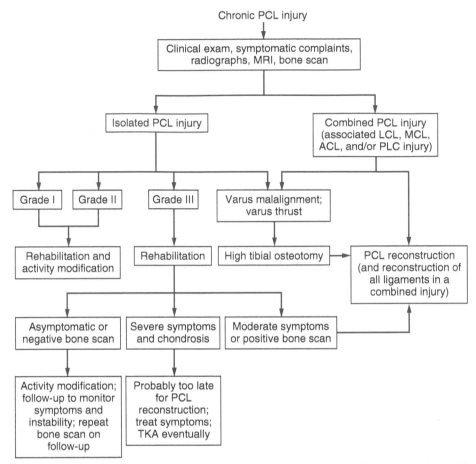

Chronic PCL injury

Clinical exam, symptomatic complaints, radiographs, MRI, bone scan

Isolated PCL injury

Combined PCL injury (associated LCL, MCL, ACL, and/or PLC injury)

Grade I · Grade II · Grade III · Varus malalignment; varus thrust

Rehabilitation and activity modification

Rehabilitation

High tibial osteotomy

PCL reconstruction (and reconstruction of all ligaments in a combined injury)

Asymptomatic or negative bone scan

Severe symptoms and chondrosis

Moderate symptoms or positive bone scan

Activity modification; follow-up to monitor symptoms and instability; repeat bone scan on follow-up

Probably too late for PCL reconstruction; treat symptoms; TKA eventually

Fig. 53.4 Treatment algorithm from chronic posterior cruciate ligament (PCL) injury. (Reprinted with permission from Miller MD, Cole BJ: Textbook of Arthroscopy. Philadelphia, WB Saunders, 2004.)

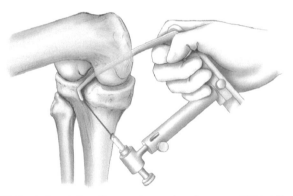

Fig. 53.5 Arthotek Fanelli posterior cruciate ligament (PCL) drill guide positioned to place guide wire in preparation for drilling of the transtibial PCL tibial tunnel. (Redrawn with permission of Arthotek, Inc., Warsaw, IN.)

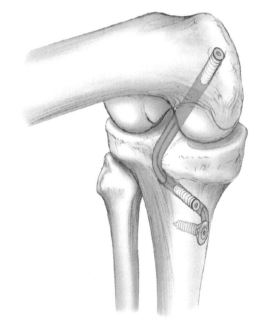

Fig. 53.6 Final graft with primary backup fixation. (Redrawn with permission of Arthotek, Inc., Warsaw, IN.)

a mechanical graft-tensioning device, use primary and backup graft fixation, and use the appropriate postoperative rehabilitation program (Fig. 53.6).

The rehabilitation protocol after reconstruction of the PCL is conservative when compared with that after ACL reconstruction, primarily because of the greater posterior shear forces generated during activity and motion of the knee. Prevention of posterior sag and hamstring activity is paramount in avoiding residual laxity. Despite this conservative approach, motion problems are rare after PCL reconstruction. As the biology of graft healing becomes better understood and

surgical techniques improve, accelerated rehabilitation protocols may be shown to be safe, but at present, the information regarding aggressive rehabilitation is limited and protection of the graft from potentially deleterious forces must be enforced (Rehabilitation Protocol 53.2).

REHABILITATION PROTOCOL 53.1 ● Nonoperative Treatment of Posterior Cruciate Ligament Injuries

Michael D'Amato, MD, Bernard R. Bach, MD

Phase 1

Days 1–7

- Range of motion (ROM) 0–60 degrees
- Weight bearing with two crutches
- Electrical muscle stimulation to quadriceps
- Exercises
  - Quadriceps sets
  - Straight leg raise (SLR)
  - Hip adduction and abduction
  - Mini-squats/leg press (0–45 degrees)

Weeks 2–3

- ROM 0–60 degrees
- Weight bearing without crutches
- Progress exercises using weights
- Bike (week 3) for ROM
- Pool program
- Leg press (0–60 degrees)

Phase 2

Week 3

- ROM to tolerance
- Discontinue brace
- Bike, Stairmaster, rowing

- Progress exercises with weights
- Mini-squat (0–60 degrees)
- Leg press (0–60 degrees)
- Step-ups
- Hip abduction and adduction
- Toe-calf raises

Weeks 5–6

- Continue all exercises.
- Fit functional brace.
- Pool running

Phase 3

Weeks 8–12

- Begin running program.
- Continue all strengthening exercises.
- Gradual return to sports activities
- Criteria to return to sports:
  - No change in laxity
  - No pain, tenderness, or swelling
  - Satisfactory clinical examination
  - Functional testing 85% of contralateral knee
  - Quadriceps strength 85% of contralateral knee

REHABILITATION PROTOCOL 53.2 ● Criteria-Based Rehabilitation After Surgical Reconstruction of the Posterior Cruciate Ligament

Michael D'Amato, MD, Bernard R. Bach, MD

General Guidelines

- No open chain exercises
- Caution against posterior tibial translation (by gravity, muscle action)
- No continuous passive motion
- Resistance for hip progressive resistance exercises (PREs) is placed above the knee for hip abduction and adduction; resistance may be distal for hip flexion.

Phase 1: Weeks 0–4

Goals

- Protect healing bony and soft tissue structures.
- Minimize the effects of immobilization.
- Early protected ROM (protection against posterior tibial sagging)
- PREs for quadriceps, hip, and calf, with emphasis on limiting patellofemoral joint compression and posterior tibial translation
- Patient education for a clear understanding of limitations and expectations of the rehabilitation process and need for supporting proximal tibia and avoiding sag

Bracing

- Brace locked at 0 degrees for 1 week
- At 1 week after surgery, brace is unlocked for passive ROM done by physical therapist or athletic trainer.

- Patient is instructed in self-administered passive ROM with the brace on, with emphasis on supporting the proximal tibia.

Weight bearing

- As tolerated with crutches, brace locked in extension

Special Considerations

- Pillow under proximal posterior tibia at rest to prevent posterior sag

Therapeutic Exercises

- Patellar mobilization
- Prone passive flexion and extension
- Quadriceps sets
- Straight leg raise (SLR)
- Hip abduction and adduction
- Ankle pumps
- Hamstring and calf stretching
- Calf exercise with Theraband, progressing to standing calf raise with full knee extension
- Standing hip extension from neutral
- Functional electrical stimulation (may be used for trace to poor quadriceps contraction)

Phase 2: Weeks 4–12

Criteria for Progression to Phase 2

- Good quadriceps control (good quadriceps set, no sag with SLR)
- Approximately 60 degrees of knee flexion
- Full knee extension
- No signs of active inflammation

Goals

- Increase ROM (flexion).
- Restore normal gait.
- Continue quadriceps strengthening and hamstring flexibility.

Continued

REHABILITATION PROTOCOL 53.2 ● **Criteria-Based Rehabilitation After Surgical Reconstruction of the Posterior Cruciate Ligament—cont'd**

Bracing

- 4–6 weeks: brace is unlocked for controlled gait training only (patient may walk with brace unlocked while attending physical therapy or when at home).
- 6–8 weeks: brace is unlocked for all activities.
- 8 weeks: brace is discontinued (as allowed by physician).

Weight bearing

- 4–8 weeks: weight bearing as tolerated with crutches
- 8 weeks: may discontinue crutches if patient exhibits no quadriceps lag with SLR
- Full knee extension
- Knee flexion 90–100 degrees
- Normal gait pattern (patient can use one crutch or cane until normal gait is achieved)

Therapeutic Exercises

Weeks 4–8
- Wall slides (0–45 degrees)
- Mini-squats (0–45 degrees)
- Leg press (0–60 degrees)
- Four-way hip exercises for flexion, abduction, adduction, extension from neutral with knee fully extended
- Ambulation in pool (work on restoration of normal heel-toe gait pattern in chest-deep water)

Weeks 8–12
- Stationary bike (foot placed forward on pedal without use of toe clips to minimize hamstring activity, seat set slightly higher than normal)
- Stairmaster, elliptical stepper, NordicTrack
- Balance and proprioception activities
- Seated calf raises
- Leg press (0–90 degrees)

Phase 3: Months 3–6

Criteria for Progression to Phase 3

- Full, pain-free ROM (*Note*: It is not unusual for flexion to be lacking 10–15 degrees for up to 5 months after surgery.)
- Normal gait
- Good to normal quadriceps strength
- No patellofemoral complaints
- Clearance by physician to begin more concentrated closed kinetic chain progression

Goals

- Restore any residual loss of motion that may prevent functional progression.
- Progress functionally and prevent patellofemoral irritation.
- Improve functional strength and proprioception using closed kinetic chain exercises.
- Continue to maintain quadriceps strength and hamstring flexibility.

Therapeutic Exercises

- Continue closed kinetic chain exercise progression.
- Treadmill walking
- Jogging in pool with wet vest or belt
- Swimming (no frog kick)

Phase 4: Month 6–Full Activity

Criteria for Progression to Phase 4

- No significant patellofemoral or soft tissue irritation
- Presence of necessary joint ROM, muscle strength, endurance, and proprioception to safely return to athletic participation

Goals

- Safe and gradual return to athletic participation
- Maintenance of strength, endurance, and function

Therapeutic Exercises

- Continue closed kinetic chain exercise progression.
- Sport-specific functional progression, which may include but is not limited to
  - Slide board
  - Jog/run progression
  - Figure-of-eight, carioca, backward running, cutting
  - Jumping (plyometrics)

Criteria for Return to Sports

- Full, pain-free ROM
- Satisfactory clinical examination
- Quadriceps strength 85% of contralateral leg
- Functional testing 85% of contralateral leg
- No change in laxity testing

REFERENCES

A complete reference list is available at https://expertconsult.inkling.com/.

FURTHER READING

Årøen A, Verdonk P. Posterior cruciate ligament, exploring the unknown. *Knee Surg Sports Traumatol Arthrosc.* 2013;21(5):996 997. Web.

Cavanaugh JT, Saldivar A, Marx RG. Postoperative rehabilitation after posterior cruciate ligament reconstruction and combined posterior cruciate ligament reconstruction-posterior lateral corner surgery. *Operative Techniques Sports Med.* 2015. n. pag. Web.

Montgomery SR, Johnson JS, Mcallister DR, et al. Surgical management of PCL injuries: indications, techniques, and outcomes. *Curr Rev Musculoskelet Med.* 2013;6(2):115–123. Web.

Pierce CM, O'Brien L, Griffin LW, et al. Posterior cruciate ligament tears: functional and postoperative rehabilitation. *Knee Surg Sports Traumatol Arthrosc.* 2012;21(5):1071–1084. Web.

Sakai T, Koyanagi M, Nakae N, et al. Evaluation of a new quadriceps strengthening exercise for the prevention of secondary cartilage injury in patients with PCL insufficiency: comparison of tibial movement in prone and sitting positions during the exercise. *Brit J Sports Med.* 2014;48(7):656. Web.

54

Medial Collateral Ligament Injuries

Michael Angeline, MD | Bruce Reider, MD

CLINICAL BACKGROUND

An understanding of both the anatomic and biomechanical properties of the MCL is important in formulating a treatment strategy for MCL and associated injuries. As popularized by Warren and Marshall, the three-layer concept describes the anatomic structures of the medial side of the knee. The first layer is composed of the fascia investing the sartorius muscle. The second layer contains the superficial MCL, the medial patellofemoral ligament, and the ligaments of the posteromedial corner of the knee.

Known as the primary static medial stabilizer of the knee, the superficial MCL is composed of parallel and oblique fibers. These parallel fibers blend posteriorly with the oblique fibers of the third layer to form the posteromedial capsule (PMC). Within this condensation of fibers, Hughston identified the posterior oblique ligament (POL), which acts to assist the dynamic function of the semimembranosus tendon. The third layer is formed from the true capsule of the knee joint and the deep MCL, which is composed of the meniscofemoral and meniscotibial ligaments (Fig. 54.1).

The superficial MCL is the primary restraint to tibial valgus stress across the arc of knee flexion and plays a secondary role of resistance to external rotation and anterior–posterior translation. The PMC controls posterior translation of the tibia when the knee is extended, and the deep MCL functions as a secondary stabilizer against tibial valgus stress. Biomechanical testing has shown that the sequential failure of the medial layers of the knee goes from the deep to superficial layers, and **it also has been noted clinically that the deep MCL is ruptured more frequently than the superficial MCL.**

MECHANISM OF INJURY

Most isolated MCL injuries result from a direct blow to the outer aspect of the upper leg or lower thigh creating a valgus force (Fig. 54.2). Noncontact external rotation mechanisms also can cause MCL injuries, but these indirect mechanisms typically also result in associated injuries, usually involving the cruciate ligaments. A careful history should include the mechanism of injury, the location of pain, the ability to ambulate after the injury, and the onset of swelling. The patient may report a popping or tearing sensation on the medial aspect of the knee. An absence of an effusion may indicate a severe tear, which allows fluid to extravasate outside the joint and into the surrounding tissues (Box 54.1).

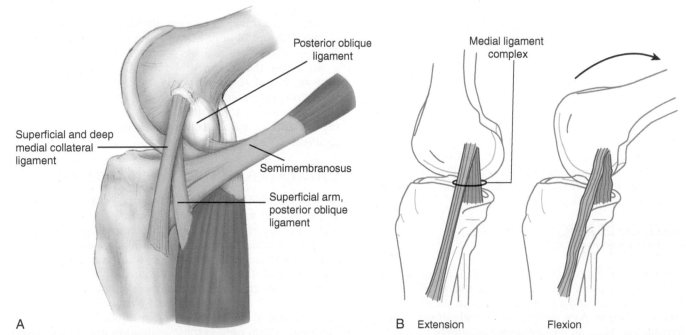

Fig. 54.1 **A,** Normal anatomy of the medial side of the knee. The superficial and deep portions of the medial collateral ligament and the posterior oblique ligament are seen. (Reprinted with permission from Cole B. Surgical Techniques of the Shoulder, Elbow, and Knee in Sports Medicine. Philadelphia, Saunders, 2008. Fig. 70-1.) **B,** In extension, the posterior fibers of the medial ligament complex are relatively tight. In flexion, the tension in the fibers decreases.

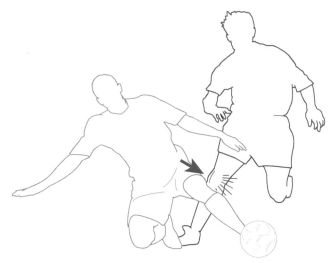

Fig. 54.2 Medial collateral ligament (MCL) injury mechanism. A direct blow to the lateral aspect of the knee creates a valgus stress, disrupting the MCL.

BOX 54.1 CLASSIFICATION OF MEDIAL COLLATERAL LIGAMENT SPRAIN

Grade	Damage to Ligament	Clinical Examination	Laxity on Examination (mm)
1	Microtrauma with no elongation	Tender ligament Normal valgus laxity	0–5
2	Elongated but intact	Increased valgus laxity with firm endpoint on valgus stress at 20 degrees of knee flexion	5–10
3	Complete disruption	Increased valgus laxity with soft endpoint on valgus stress at 30 degrees of knee flexion	>10

Most MCL injuries occur at the femoral origin or in the midsubstance over the joint line, although tibial avulsions do occur. MCL sprains may be isolated or combined with other knee injuries. To diagnose associated injuries, the clinician should look for clues that appear in the history and examination or while monitoring the patient's clinical progress.

DIAGNOSIS AND PHYSICAL EXAMINATION

The differential diagnosis of an isolated MCL injury includes a medial knee contusion, a medial meniscal tear, patellar dislocation or subluxation, and a physeal fracture in patients who are skeletally immature. A careful physical examination will help to differentiate an MCL injury from other pathology.

A large effusion is suggestive of an intra-articular injury, such as a cruciate ligament injury, a meniscal tear, or a fracture.

The Lachman, posterior drawer, and varus stress tests can help rule out concomitant ACL, PCL, and lateral cruciate ligament (LCL) complex injuries.

Because the MCL is an extra-articular structure, isolated injuries rarely result in extensive intra-articular swelling; however, there may be localized edema over the course of the MCL and moderate effusions may occur. Injuries to the femoral origin of the MCL may be characterized by an increase in the normal prominence of the medial epicondyle.

Once visual inspection of the knee has been completed, the knee should be palpated along the entire course of the MCL to locate the area or areas of maximal tenderness. An injury at the origin of the MCL may be associated with tenderness near the adductor tubercle or the medial retinaculum adjacent to the patella, but this can also be related to a patellar dislocation or subluxation with a concomitant VMO avulsion or medial retinacular tear. To help distinguish an MCL injury from an episode of patellar instability, a patellar apprehension test can be used. Additionally, medial joint line tenderness may indicate an MCL injury or a medial meniscal tear or chondral injury.

The valgus stress test with the knee in 30 degrees of flexion is the crucial test for evaluating an injury to the MCL. With the injured leg over the side of the examination table, the examiner places one hand under the heel to support the leg and with the other hand applies a valgus force. Rotation of the thigh should be prevented during this maneuver, and the examination should be compared with the contralateral knee as a control for the amount of joint line opening.

Injuries to the MCL are graded based on the amount of laxity to valgus stress testing:
- Grade I injury: no increase in medial joint line opening compared to the opposite knee at 30 degrees of knee flexion and tenderness along the ligament
- Grade II injury: more generalized tenderness with 5 to 10 mm of joint line opening on examination but a moderately firm endpoint
- Grade III injury: complete disruption of the ligament and >10 mm of joint line opening with only a vague endpoint, if any

To assess the integrity of the MCL and posteromedial capsule, valgus stress testing is done with the knee in full extension. Increased laxity with the knee in full extension suggests a severe injury of the MCL and the posteromedial capsule and a possible injury to one or both of the cruciate ligaments.

RADIOGRAPHIC EXAMINATION

For evaluation of an acute MCL injury, routine plain radiographs of the knee including anteroposterior, lateral, and Merchant views are obtained. Stress radiographs may be helpful to exclude physeal injuries in adolescents. In both a cadaver biomechanical study and an in vivo study in adults, Laprade et al. found that more than 3 to 4 mm of medial compartment gapping compared to the opposite knee (with the knee in 20 degrees of flexion) was indicative of a grade III MCL injury. In patients with chronic MCL injuries at the proximal origin, radiographic evaluation may reveal heterotopic calcification near the medial epicondyle (Pellegrini-Stieda lesion).

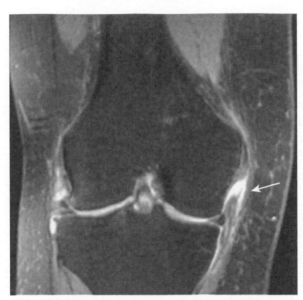

Fig. 54.3 Coronal magnetic resonance imaging sequence showing full-thickness injury to the medial collateral ligament at its femoral attachment site. (Reprinted with permission from Cole B. Surgical Techniques of the Shoulder, Elbow, and Knee in Sports Medicine. Philadelphia, Saunders, 2008. Fig. 70-3.)

Magnetic resonance imaging evaluation usually is not indicated for an isolated MCL injury unless the examination is equivocal, but it may be useful to rule out a concomitant cruciate ligament injury if suspected based on clinical findings. A T2-weighted coronal imaging sequence is the most valuable (Fig. 54.3); low signal intensity is observed in intact fibers, whereas disruption in the continuity of the fibers or an increased signal is indicative of an MCL injury.

TREATMENT OF ISOLATED AND COMBINED MEDIAL COLLATERAL LIGAMENT INJURIES

For all grades of isolated MCL injuries, a nonoperative early functional rehabilitation (EFR) treatment protocol with a rapid return to sports participation is advocated. EFR has been shown in several studies to have an acceptable re-injury rate and to enable a more rapid recovery, with results equivalent or superior to those with surgery or prolonged immobilization.

A lightweight hinged knee brace is used during the rehabilitation process to allow early motion while protecting the knee from valgus stress. Full weightbearing with quadriceps and hamstring strengthening is encouraged once the pain has subsided. As a result of this goal-oriented rehabilitation program, secondary muscle atrophy is minimized and the attainment of functional goals rather than an arbitrary period of time are the main factors limiting the patient's return to sport. Additionally, studies exploring the effects of motion on healing of MCL injuries in rabbit and rat models suggest that it may lead to improvements in ligament strength and stiffness.

Although most MCL injuries are treated nonoperatively, it is important to be aware of special situations involving a complete ligament disruption, which may require operative intervention. **Indications for operative treatment of MCL injury** include the following:

- A large bony avulsion
- A concomitant tibial plateau fracture
- Associated cruciate ligament injury
- Intra-articular entrapment of the end of the ligament

Surgical fixation of the MCL usually is done within 7 to 10 days after the injury and can be through a primary repair or reconstruction with autograft or allograft augmentation. No prospective randomized (level 1) studies have compared repair and reconstruction. A recent evidence-based systematic review found satisfactory results with both repair and reconstruction; the authors were unable to make any evidence-based recommendations for either technique (Kovachevich et al. 2009).

In combined ACL and MCL injuries, treatment of the cruciate injury is important to not only restore the overall stability of the knee, but also to optimize the environment for MCL healing. For this reason, most authors advocate reconstruction of the ACL with nonoperative functional rehabilitation of the MCL injury. A prospective randomized trial (level 1 evidence) of 47 patients with combined ACL and MCL injuries compared outcomes in those with and without surgical treatment of the MCL. At a mean follow-up of 27 months, there were no differences between the groups with regard to knee function, stability, ROM, strength, and return to activity. A hinged knee brace and EFR protocol are used for combined ACL/MCL injuries.

Occasionally, there is persistent laxity to valgus stress of the knee in full extension (>4 mm compared to the contralateral side) after the ACL has been reconstructed. In such cases, the MCL injury also is treated surgically, by primary repair or reconstruction according to the quality of tissue available. Repair or reconstruction of the MCL also is done in combined ACL/PCL/MCL injuries after the ACL and PCL have been reconstructed.

REHABILITATION AFTER MCL INJURY

The EFR program for MCL injuries is divided into three distinct phases, with a focus on early return to sports participation. Each functional goal must be attained before the athlete can progress to the next phase.

For full return to competitive play, the athlete must fulfill four criteria:

- Minimal or no pain
- Full ROM
- Quadriceps and hamstring strength equal to 90% of the contralateral limb
- Completion of one session of the EFR running program

Overall, the average time of return to competitive play varies with both the sport and grade of MCL injury. Patients with grade I injuries require about 10 days to complete the functional training program, whereas patients with grade II or III injuries require about 3 to 6 weeks (Rehabilitation Protocols 54.1 and 54.2).

REHABILITATION PROTOCOL 54.1 ■ Isolated Medial Collateral Ligament Injury

Michael Angeline, MD, Bruce Reider, MD

Phase 1

Goals

- Normal gait
- Minimal selling
- Full range of motion (ROM)
- Baseline quadriceps control

Cryotherapy

- Therapeutic cold via ice packs or other means is applied to the medial aspect of the knee for 20 minutes every 3 to 4 hours for the first 48 hours.
- Early cryotherapy provides anesthesia and local vasoconstriction to minimize initial hemorrhage and reduce secondary edema. Leg elevation also helps limit swelling.

Weight bearing

- Weight bearing is allowed as tolerated.
- Crutches are used until the patient ambulates without a limp, which takes approximately 1 week.
- For grades 2 and 3 sprains, a lightweight hinged brace is worn. The brace should protect against valgus stresses of daily living but should not restrict motion or inhibit muscle function. The brace is worn at all times except for bathing during the initial 3 to 4 weeks.
- Use of knee immobilizers and full-leg braces is discouraged because they tend to inhibit motion and prolong the period of disability.

Exercises

- ROM exercises are begun immediately. A cold whirlpool bath may make these exercises easier.
- Exercises such as towel extension exercises and prone hangs are used to obtain extension or hyperextension equal to the contralateral side. A heavy shoe or light ankle weight can be used with prone hangs to aid extension.
- To promote flexion, the patient sits at the end of a table, allowing gravity to aid in flexion. The uninjured limb assists by gently pushing the injured leg into further flexion.
- A similar technique of the uninjured limb assisting can be used during supine wall slides.
- To achieve greater than 90 degrees of flexion, heel slides are done with the patient sitting and grabbing the ankle to flex the knee farther.
- A stationary bicycle also aids in the restoration of motion. The bicycle seat is initially set as high as possible and gradually lowered to increase flexion.
- Isometric quadriceps sets and straight leg raises are begun immediately to minimize muscle atrophy.

- Electrical stimulation may be helpful by limiting reflex muscle inhibition.

Phase 2

Goal

- Restoration of the strength of the injured leg to approximately 80% to 90% of the uninjured leg

Bracing

- Continued use of the lightweight hinged brace

Exercises

- Strengthening exercise begins with 4-inch step-ups and 30-degree squats without weights.
- Light resistance exercises of knee extensions, leg presses, and curls on a standard isotonic weight bench or dedicated resistance machine. Sets with lighter weights but a higher number of repetitions are usually used.
- Recurrent pain and swelling are signs of too rapid progression. If they occur, the strengthening program should be slowed.
- Upper body, aerobic, and further lower extremity conditioning are achieved with swimming, stationary cycling, and/or a stair climber.

Phase 3

Goals

- Completion of a running program
- Completion of a series of sport-specific activities

Bracing

- Continued use of the brace is recommended during this phase and for the rest of the athletic season. This may protect against further injury and at least provides psychological support.

Exercises

- A progressive running program commences with fast-speed walking and advances to light jogging, straight-line running, and then sprinting. Next, agility is achieved with cutting and pivoting activities such as figure-of-eight drills and cariocas.
- If pain or swelling occurs, the program is amended appropriately.
- Continued input from a trainer or physical therapist will be helpful in providing progress reports and guidance in appropriate performance of the activities.

Return to Sport

- Permitted when the athlete can complete a functional testing program including a long run, progressively more rapid sprints, cutting and pivoting drills, and appropriate sport-specific tests.

REHABILITATION PROTOCOL 54.2 ■ Progression of Rehabilitation After Medial Collateral Ligament Injury

Michael Angeline, MD, Bruce Reider, MD

	Phase 1	Phase 2	Phase 3		Phase 1	Phase 2	Phase 3
Bracing				Squats		X	X
Lightweight brace	X	X	X	Knee extensions		X	X
Weight Bearing				Leg presses		X	X
Full	X	X	X	Leg curls		X	X
Crutches until normal gait	X			**Conditioning**			
Range of Motion				Stationary bike	X	X	X
Cold whirlpool	X			Swimming		X	X
Extension exercises	X			Elliptical trainer		X	X
Towel extensions	X			**Agility/Sport-Specific Training**			
Prone hangs	X			Running program			
Flexion exercises				Fast-speed walking			X
Sitting off table	X			Light jogging			X
Wall slides	X			Straight-line running			X
Heel slides	X			Sprinting			X
Strengthening				Figure-of-eight drills			X
Isometric quadriceps sets	X	X		Cariocas			X
Straight leg raise	X	X		Sport-specific drills			X
Step-ups		X	X				

REFERENCES

A complete reference list is available at https://expertconsult.inkling.com/.

FURTHER READING

Andia, I, Maffulli N. Use of platelet-rich plasma for patellar tendon and medial collateral ligament injuries: best current clinical practice. *J Knee Surg.* 2014;28.01:011–018. Web.

Laprade, RF, Wijdicks CA. The management of injuries to the medial side of the knee. *J Orthop Sports Phys Ther.* 2012;42.3:221–233. Web.

Lundblad M, Walden M, Magnusson H, et al. The UEFA injury study: 11-year data concerning 346 MCL injuries in professional football. In: *Br J Sports Med.* 2014;48.7:629. Web.

55

Meniscal Injuries

Michael D'Amato, MD | S. Brent Brotzman, MD | Theresa M. Kidd, BA

CLINICAL BACKGROUND

The importance of the menisci in preserving the health and function of the knee has been well established. Most of the functions performed by the menisci relate to protecting the underlying articular cartilage (Fig. 55.1, *A* and *B*).

- By increasing the effective contact area between the femur and the tibia, the menisci lower the load-per-unit area borne by the articular surfaces. Total meniscectomy results in a 50% reduction in contact area.
- The menisci transmit central compressive loads out toward the periphery, further decreasing the contact pressures on the articular cartilage.
- Half of the compressive load in the knee passes through the menisci with the knee in full extension, and 85% of the load passes through the knee with the knee in 90 degrees of flexion.
- **Meniscectomy has been shown to reduce the shock absorption capacity of the knee by 20%.**
- **Partial meniscectomy has reduced morbidity compared to total meniscectomy. Shelbourne and Dickens (2007) found 88% of patients who underwent partial medial meniscectomy had joint space narrowing of 2 mm or less at a mean follow-up of 12 years. Of patients, 88% to 95% subjectively reported good to excellent results.**
- Repeat surgery after partial meniscectomy is uncommon; Chatain et al. (2003) reported only 2.2% of patients required a second surgery in the same compartment as the previous partial medial meniscectomy.
- Although degenerative changes are known to follow total medial meniscectomy, degenerative change after partial medial meniscectomy is infrequently reported (Shelbourne and Dickens 2007).

MENISCAL MOVEMENT

The lateral meniscus has been shown to be more mobile than the medial meniscus. In each meniscus, the anterior horn has greater mobility than the posterior horn. The reduced mobility of the posterior medial meniscus may result in greater stresses in this area, leading to increased vulnerability to injury. This would explain the higher rate of meniscal tears that occur in the posterior medial meniscus.

Weight bearing has been shown to effect few changes in the movement of the menisci, although it has been suggested that meniscal loading may lead to distraction of radial tears. ROM of the knee, especially increasing rotation and flexion of the knee past 60 degrees, results in significant changes in the anteroposterior position of the menisci. Clinically, second-look arthroscopy has shown that extension of the knee maintains a posterior horn meniscal tear in a reduced position, and knee flexion results in displacement of the tear.

Meniscal Healing

King, in 1936, first noted that communication with the peripheral blood supply was critical for meniscal healing. Arnoczky and Warren, in 1982, described the microvasculature of the menisci. In children, the peripheral blood vessels permeate the full thickness of the meniscus. With age, the penetration of the blood vessels decreases. In adults, the blood supply is limited to only the outer 6 mm or about a third of the width of the meniscus (Fig. 55.2). It is in this vascular region that the healing potential of a meniscal tear is greatest. This potential drops off dramatically as the tear progresses away from the periphery.

Meniscal healing is also influenced by the pattern of the tear (Fig. 55.3). Longitudinal tears have a more favorable healing potential compared with radial tears. Simple tear patterns are more likely to heal than complex tears. Traumatic tears have higher healing rates than degenerative tears, and acute tears heal better than chronic tears. Fig. 55.4 demonstrates a bucket handle meniscal tear that often results in locking of the knee (inability to fully straighten) when the bucket handle displaces toward the midline.

REHABILITATION CONSIDERATIONS

Weight Bearing and Motion

Although weight bearing has little effect on displacement patterns of the meniscus and may be beneficial in approximating longitudinal tears, it may place a displacing force across radial tears. Several studies have confirmed the benefits of early motion by demonstrating meniscal atrophy and decreased collagen content in menisci after immobilization. ROM of the knee before 60 degrees of flexion has little effect on meniscal displacement, **but flexion angles greater than 60 degrees translate the menisci posteriorly. This increased translation may place detrimental stresses across a healing meniscus.** As knee flexion increases, compressive loads across the meniscus also increase. The combination of weight bearing and increasing knee flexion must be carefully balanced in the development of a rehabilitation protocol.

Axial Limb Alignment

Varus malalignment tends to overload the medial compartment of the knee, with increased stress placed on the meniscus, and **valgus malalignment** has the same effect on the lateral compartment and lateral meniscus. These increased stresses may interfere or disrupt meniscal healing after repair. Patients with limb malalignment tend to have more degenerative meniscal tears, which have been suggested to have an inherently poorer healing capacity. The use of an "unloader" brace

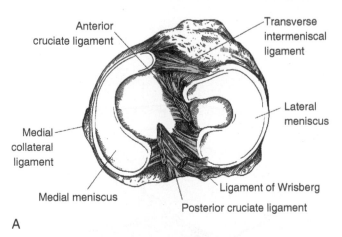

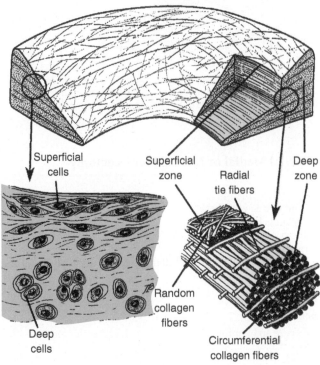

Fig. 55.1 **A,** Anatomy of the menisci viewed from above. Note the differences in position and shape of the medial and lateral menisci. (Adapted with permission from Pagnani MJ, Warren RF, Arnoczky SP, Wickiewics TL. Anatomy of the knee. In Nicholas JA, Hershman EB, eds. The Lower Extremity and Spine in Sports Medicine, ed 2. St. Louis, Mosby, 1995, pp. 581–614.) **B,** Collagen ultrastructure and cell types in the meniscus. The illustration demonstrates the collagen fiber orientation in the surface and deep zones. The radial tie fibers are also shown. Superficial meniscal cells tend to be fibroblastic, whereas the deep cells have a rounded morphology. (Reprinted with permission from Kawamura S, Lotito K, Rodeo SA. Biomechanics and healing response of the meniscus. In Drez D, DeLee JC, eds. Operative Techniques in Sports Medicine. Philadelphia, WB Saunders, 2003, pp. 68–76.)

has been recommended to help protect the healing meniscus, although no scientific data exist to support this approach.

Rehabilitation After Partial Meniscectomy

Because there is no anatomic structure that must be protected during a healing phase, rehabilitation may progress aggressively (Rehabilitation Protocol 55.1). The goals are early control of

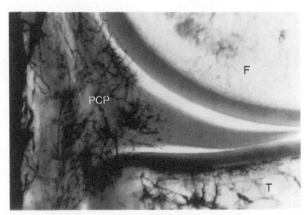

Fig. 55.2 Scan of 5-mm thick frontal section of the medial compartment of the knee (Spalteholz 3×). Branching radial vessels from the peromeniscal capillary plexus (PCP) can be seen penetrating the peripheral border of the medial meniscus in very young patients. The PCP recedes to the very periphery with age. *F,* femur; *T,* tibia. (Reprinted with permission from Arnoczky SP, Warren RF. Microvasculature of the human meniscus. *Am J Sports Med* 1982;10(2):90–95.)

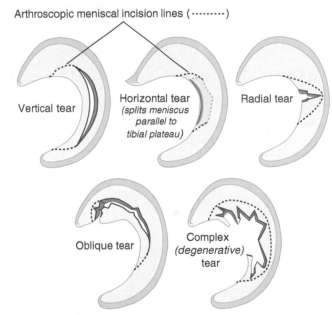

Fig. 55.3 Various meniscus tears.

pain and swelling, immediate weight bearing, obtaining and maintaining a full ROM, and regaining quadriceps strength.

Rehabilitation After Meniscal Repair

Current studies support the use of unmodified accelerated ACL rehabilitation protocols after combined ACL reconstruction and meniscal repair (Rehabilitation Protocol 55.2). In tears with decreased healing potential (such as white–white tears, radial tears, or complex pattern tears), limiting weight bearing and limiting flexion to 60 degrees for the first 4 weeks have been suggested to better protect the repair and increase the healing potential of these difficult tears. However, we are unaware of any published studies that support these measures.

Rehabilitation after isolated meniscal repair remains controversial. The healing environment clearly is inferior to that with concomitant ACL reconstruction, but good results have been

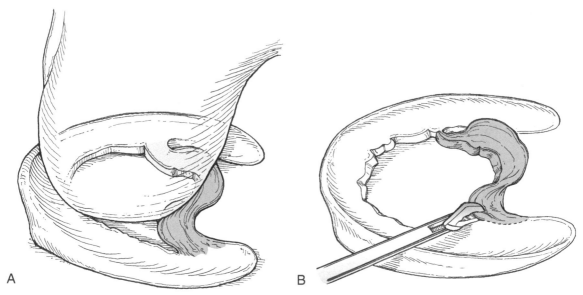

Fig. 55.4   **A,** Arthroscopic partial meniscectomy of a bucket handle tear of the meniscus. Tear displaced into the notch. This often results in a locked knee, which manifests as the inability to extend (straighten) the knee the last 5 to 15 degrees. **B,** Arthroscopic partial resection of meniscus torn in the avascular zone with no potential for healing. (Reprinted with permission from Miller M. Surgical Atlas of Sports Medicine. Philadelphia, Saunders, 2003. Fig. 2-8.)

REHABILITATION PROTOCOL 55.1   After Arthroscopic Partial Medial or Lateral Meniscectomy

Phase 1: Acute Phase

Goals

- Diminish inflammation and swelling.
- Restore range of motion (ROM).
- Re-establish quadriceps muscle activity.

Days 1–3

- Cryotherapy
- Quadriceps sets
- Straight leg raise (SLR)
- Electrical muscle stimulation to quadriceps
- Hip adduction and abduction
- Knee extension
- 30-degree mini-squats
- Active-assisted ROM stretching, emphasizing full knee extension (flexion to tolerance)
- Weight bearing as tolerated (two crutches)
- Light compression wrap

Days 4–7

- Cryotherapy
- Electrical muscle stimulation to quadriceps
- Quadriceps sets
- Knee extension 90 to 40 degrees
- SLR
- Hip adduction and abduction
- 30-degree mini-squats
- Balance/proprioceptive drills
- Active-assisted and passive ROM exercises
- ROM 0 to 115 degrees (minimal)
- Stretching (hamstrings, gastrosoleus, quadriceps)
- Weight bearing as tolerated (one crutch)
- Continued use of compression wrap or brace
- High-voltage galvanic stimulation/cryotherapy

Days 7–10

- Continue all exercises.
- Leg press (light weight)
- Toe raises
- Hamstring curls
- Bicycle (when ROM is 0 to 100 degrees with no swelling and able to make a full revolution)

Phase 2

Goals

- Restore and improve muscular strength and endurance.
- Re-establish full nonpainful ROM.
- Gradual return to functional activities

Days 10–17

- Bicycle for motion and endurance
- Lateral lunges
- Front lunges
- Half squats
- Leg press
- Lateral step-ups
- Knee extension 90 to 40 degrees
- Hamstring curls
- Hip abduction and adduction
- Hip flexion and extension
- Toe raises
- Proprioceptive and balance training
- Stretching exercises
- Active-assisted and passive ROM knee flexion (if necessary)
- Elliptical trainer

Day 17–Week 4

- Continue all exercises.
- Pool program (deep-water running and leg exercises)
- Compression brace may be used during activities.

REHABILITATION PROTOCOL 55.1 ■ After Arthroscopic Partial Medial or Lateral Meniscectomy—cont'd

Phase 3: Advanced Activity Phase: Weeks 4–7*

Criteria for Progression to Phase 3

- Full, nonpainful ROM
- No pain or tenderness
- Satisfactory isokinetic test
- Satisfactory clinical examination (minimal effusion)

Goals

- Enhance muscular strength and endurance.
- Maintain full ROM.
- Return to sport/functional activities.

Exercises

- Continue to emphasize closed kinetic chain exercises.
- May begin plyometrics
- Begin running program and agility drills.

*Patients can begin phase 3 when criteria are met, which may be earlier than week 4.

REHABILITATION PROTOCOL 55.2 ■ Accelerated Rehabilitation After Meniscal Repair

Bernard R. Bach, MD, Michael D'Amato, MD

Phase 1: Weeks 0–2

Goals

- Full motion
- No effusion
- Full weight bearing

Weight Bearing

- As tolerated

Treatment

- ROM as tolerated (0–90 degrees)
- Cryotherapy
- Electrical stimulation as needed
- Isometric quadriceps sets
- Straight leg raise (SLR)

Phase 2: Weeks 2–4

Criteria for Progression to Phase 2

- Full motion
- No effusion
- Full weight bearing

Goals

- Improved quadriceps strength
- Normal gait

Therapeutic Exercises

- Closed kinetic chain resistance exercises 0 to 90 degrees
- Bike and swim as tolerated
- Early-phase functional training

Phase 3: Weeks 4–8

Criteria for Progression to Phase 3

- Normal gait
- Sufficient strength and proprioception for advanced functional training

Goals

- Strength and functional testing at least 85% of contralateral side
- Discharge from physical therapy to full activity

Therapeutic Exercises

- Strength work as needed
- Sport-specific functional progression
- Advanced-phase functional training

obtained with accelerated rehabilitation protocols after isolated meniscal repairs.

REFERENCES

A complete reference list is available at https://expertconsult.inkling.com/.

FURTHER READING

Anderson AF, Anderson CN. Correlation of Meniscal and Articular Cartilage Injuries in Children and Adolescents With Timing of Anterior Cruciate Ligament Reconstruction. *Am J Sports Med.* 2014;43.2:275–281. Web.

Bhatia S, Laprade CM, Ellman MB, et al. Meniscal Root Tears: Significance, Diagnosis, and Treatment. *Am J Sports Med.* 2014;42.12:3016–3030. Web.

Herrlin, Sylvia V, Peter O, et al. Is Arthroscopic Surgery Beneficial in Treating Non-traumatic, Degenerative Medial Meniscal Tears? A Five Year Follow-up. *Knee Surg Sports Traumatol Arthrosc.* 2012;21.2:358–364. Web.

Noyes, Frank R, Barber-Westin Sue D. Treatment of Meniscus Tears During Anterior Cruciate Ligament Reconstruction. *Arthrosc J Arthroscopic Relat Surg.* 2012;28.1:123–130. Web.

Katz JN, Brophy RH, Chaisson CE et al. Surgery versus Physical Therapy for a Meniscal Tear and Osteoarthritis. *N Engl J Med.* 2013;369(7):683. Web.

Patellofemoral Disorders

S. Brent Brotzman, MD

CLINICAL BACKGROUND

Patellofemoral pain syndrome (PFPS), or anterior knee pain, is one of the most common lower extremity conditions reported in physically active populations, affecting one in four people. PFPS remains the most common orthopedic injury among active young women (Wilson et al. 2008). The patellofemoral joint is a complex articulation that depends on both dynamic and static restraints for stability (Fig. 56.1). Anterior knee pain encompasses numerous underlying disorders and cannot be treated by a single treatment algorithm.

The key to successful treatment of patellofemoral pain is obtaining an accurate diagnosis by a thorough history and physical examination. For example, the treatment of reflex sympathetic dystrophy syndrome (RSDS) is different from that for excessive lateral pressure syndrome (ELPS), and the correct diagnosis must be made to allow appropriate treatment (Box 56.1).

Chondromalacia has been incorrectly used as an all-inclusive diagnosis for anterior knee pain. Chondromalacia actually is a pathologic diagnosis that describes articular cartilage changes seen on direct observation (Fig. 56.2). This term should not be used as a synonym for patellofemoral or anterior knee pain. Often, the articular cartilage of the patella and femoral trochlea is normal, and the pain originates from the densely innervated peripatellar retinaculum or synovium. All peripatellar structures should be palpated and inspected. Other nociceptive input is possible from the subchondral bone, paratenon, tendon, and subcutaneous nerves in the patellofemoral joint.

Dye (1996) introduced the concept of loss of normal tissue homeostasis after overload of the extensor mechanism. The presence of excessive biomechanical load overwhelms the body's capacity to absorb energy and leads to microtrauma, tissue injury, and pain. Dye described the knee as a biological transmission system that functions to accept, transfer, and dissipate loads. During normal ambulation, the muscles about the knee actually absorb more energy than they produce for propulsive forces.

Dye also described an "envelope of function" that considers both the applied loads at the knee and the frequency of loading. This model is useful in conceptualizing both direct trauma and overuse repetitive trauma as a cause of patellofemoral pathology. Either an excessive single loading event or multiple submaximal loading variables over time could exceed the limits of physiologic function and disrupt tissue homeostasis. For healing and homeostasis to occur, the patient must keep activities and rehabilitation efforts within the available envelope of function. Therefore, submaximal, pain-free exercise and avoidance of "flaring" activities (increased patellofemoral joint reactive forces [PFJRFs]) are important parts of rehabilitation of patellofemoral injuries.

CLINICAL PEARLS FOR PATELLOFEMORAL PAIN

- Factors that potentially alter the orientation of the quadriceps reaction force historically have been felt to contribute to development of PFPS. This alteration of the quadriceps reaction force changes the load across the retropatellar surface, thereby increasing retropatellar articular cartilage stress and subsequent injury.
- Previous literature has suggested that the causes of PFPS are multifactorial. Imbalance of the vastus medialis and vastus lateralis, abnormally large quadriceps angle (Q-angle), tibiofemoral abduction angular impulse, or a high pelvis width to femoral length ratio have been suspected contributors in the literature. Each of these factors alters the orientation of the quadriceps reaction force.
- Utting et al. 2005 suggested that patients with PFPS are likely to develop patellofemoral osteoarthritis later in life. **These**

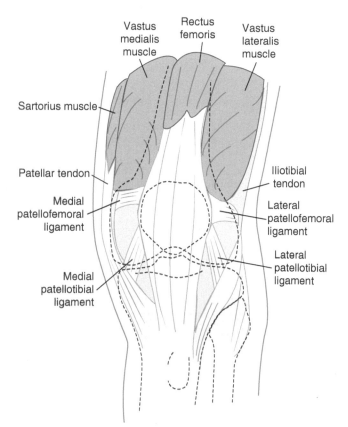

Fig. 56.1 Stabilizing anatomy of the anterior aspect of the knee. (Redrawn with permission from Baker CL Jr.: The Hughston Clinic Sports Medicine Book. Baltimore, Williams & Wilkins, 1995.)

BOX 56.1   POSSIBLE ETIOLOGIES OF PATELLOFEMORAL PAIN

Acute patellar dislocation
Patellar subluxation (chronic)
Recurrent patellar dislocation
Jumper's knee (patellar tendinitis)
Osgood-Schlatter disease
Sinding-Larsen-Johansson syndrome (inferior pole of patella)
Excessive lateral patellar compression syndrome (ELPS)
Global patellar pressure syndrome (GPPS)
Iliotibial band friction syndrome (lateral knee at Gerdy's tubercle)
Hoffa's disease (inflamed fat pad)
Bursitis
Medial patellofemoral ligament pain or tear
Trauma
Patellofemoral arthritis
Sickle cell disease
Anterior blow to patella
Osteochondritis dissecans (OCD)
Reflex sympathetic dystrophy syndrome (RSDS)
Hypertrophic plica (runner)
Turf knee, wrestler's knee
Patellar fracture
Quadriceps rupture
Contusion
Tibial tubercle fracture
Prepatellar bursitis (housemaid's knee)
Patella baja
Patella alta
Medial retinaculitis
Referred hip pain
Gout
Pseudogout (chondrocalcinosis)

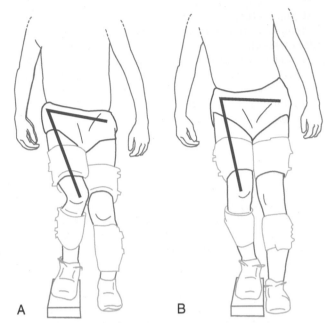

Fig. 56.3 Patient performing step-down maneuver pretreatment (*A*) and post-treatment (*B*). Both show the same knee flexion angle (as assessed by motion analysis). Pretreatment, the patient demonstrates a greater amount of hip internal rotation and adduction and contralateral hip drop.

Outerbridge Classification

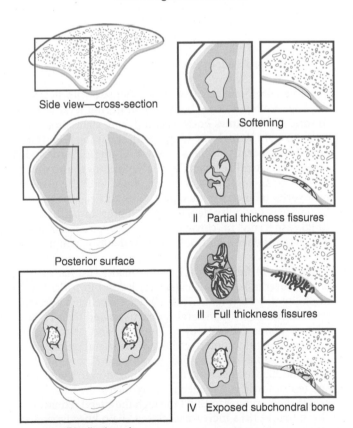

Side view—cross-section

I   Softening

II   Partial thickness fissures

Posterior surface

III   Full thickness fissures

IV   Exposed subchondral bone

Distribution of chondromalacia changes

Fig. 56.2   Outerbridge classification of chondromalacia.

authors found 22% of the 118 patients with patellofemoral arthritis had retropatellar knee pain as an adolescent.

- Recent studies suggest several additional factors may contribute to PFPS. **Boling et al. (2009) found risk factors for the development of PFPS include decreased knee flexion angle during jump-landing task and increased hip internal rotation angle and decreased vertical ground reaction force during the same task.**
- **Women with PFPS often have been found to possess ipsilateral decreased hip strength compared with healthy control groups in several, though not all, studies (Willson et al. 2008). In our own patients with PFPS we always test hip strength and implement hip strengthening exercises as part of the rehab regimen.**
- Females with PFPS produced 13% to 24% less hip and trunk force during strength testing than the control group. With exertion females with PFPS showed increased contralateral **pelvic drop** (a clinical sign of hip abductor insufficiency). This appears to contribute to greater **hip adduction** (Fig. 56.3) noted on the involved side. Increased hip adduction appears to contribute to the origin of PFPS through two primary mechanisms. First, increased hip adduction can increase the Q-angle, which increases retropatellar stress (Huberti et al. 1984). Second, hip adduction tensions the iliotibial (IT) band; the latter reinforces the lateral patellar retinaculum. This tension on the IT band leads to greater lateral force on the patella through the lateral patellar retinaculum.
- Hip and trunk muscle weakness may also increase retropatellar stress and promote PFPS symptoms. Decreased strength of hip abductors, hip external rotators, and trunk lateral flexors increases the likelihood of hip adduction and internal rotation during weight bearing. This internal rotation increases retropatellar stress. Trunk strengthening and control should also be addressed in PFPS rehabilitation.

- **Fatigued athletes participating in strenuous athletics have been noted to have an increased tendency for abnormal lower extremity mechanics.** Biomechanical studies of jumping reveal an increase in the relative contribution of the hip joint musculature as the jumping athlete becomes progressively more fatigued. Note that many women with PFPS have less hip strength compared to controls. Therefore these fatigued patients, already prone to abnormal hip mechanics and now further fatigued, have an even greater reliance on relatively weaker hip musculature. There is a resultant increase in PFPS symptoms (Willson and Davis 2009).
- Excessive hip adduction and internal rotation can cause the knee joint center to move medially relative to the foot. Because the foot is fixed to the ground, this inward movement of the knee joint causes the tibia to abduct and the foot to pronate, the end result being dynamic knee valgus (Powers 2010).
- Dynamic knee valgus (see Fig. 49.1) is a contributor to ACL injury and in this case patellofemoral joint dysfunction. It has been reported that hip adduction is the primary contributor to excessive dynamic knee valgus.
- Pollard et al. (2009) suggest that higher knee valgus angles and moments observed in female athletes represent a movement strategy in which there is insufficient utilization of the hip extensors during deceleration of the body center of mass.
- Powers (2003) found that the altered patellofemoral joint kinematics in females with PFPS was the result of excessive internal rotation of the femur (twice the control group). This suggests control of femur rotation is important in therapeutic attempts to restore normal patellofemoral joint kinematics.
- Pollard et al. (2009) suggest that improving use and strength of the gluteus maximus in the sagittal plane may serve to unload the knee by decreasing the need for compensatory quadriceps action to absorb impact forces.
- To supplement static or isometric strength testing, it is useful to perform **functional strength testing** for the entire lower extremity to determine abnormal movement patterns. The **step-down test** (Fig. 56.4) (patient stands with involved limb on edge of step and is asked to slowly lower opposite foot to floor and then return to starting position) will often point out hip abduction weakness with resultant uninvolved limb pelvic drop or drift of the weightbearing limb into dynamic genu valgum at low flexion angles, thus indicating weak quads and hip musculature.

Other Important Patellofemoral Pearls

- Arthroscopic lateral release is only effective in patients with a positive lateral tilt (i.e., a tight lateral retinaculum) who have failed exhaustive conservative measures (Fig. 56.5, A and B) (Rehabilitation Protocol 56.1). However, a lateral release should never be used to treat patellar instability or the patient with generalized ligamentous laxity and its associated patellar hypermobility. A common complication of this procedure incorrectly used for the patient with patellar instability rather than a tight lateral retinaculum is iatrogenic medial patellar subluxation or worsened instability.

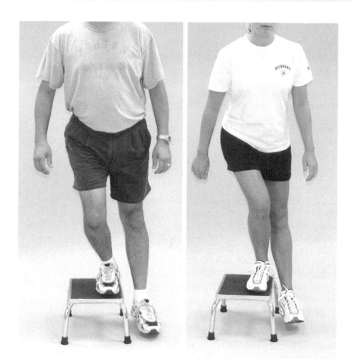

Fig. 56.4   These individuals were instructed to perform a step-down maneuver. Anatomically, the alignment of the male, on the left, shows a straight-as-an-arrow hip over knee over ankle. The female, on the right, demonstrates hip adduction and internal rotation with anteriorly rotated pelvis, excessive genu valgum, and external tibial rotation and subsequent pronation of the foot. (Reprinted from Ireland M: The Female Athlete. Philadelphia, Saunders, 2002, Fig. 43.2.)

- Osteochondral fractures of the lateral femoral condyle or the medial facet of the patella have been documented by arthroscopy in 40% and 50% of patellar dislocations.
- Success rates of patellar operative procedures are directly related to the procedure selected and the number of previous surgeries.
- Patellofemoral joint reactive forces increase with flexion of the knee from 0.5 times body weight during level walking, to three to four times body weight during stair climbing, to seven to eight times body weight with squatting (Fig. 56.6).
- **Females generally have a greater Q-angle than males. However, critical review of available studies found no evidence that Q-angle measures correlated with the presence or severity of anterior knee pain.**
- Quadriceps flexibility deficits are common in patients with PFPS, especially in chronic cases. Quadriceps stretching exercises produce significant improvement in symptoms in these patients.
- Restoration of **flexibility** (IT band, quadriceps, hamstrings) is often overlooked but is extremely helpful in patients with flexibility deficits (Fig. 56.7, A–C). Excessive lateral pressure syndrome with a tight lateral retinaculum and tight IT band often responds dramatically to iliotibial band stretching and low-load, long-duration stretching of the lateral retinaculum.
- In addition to a flexibility program for the IT band, quadriceps, and hamstrings, soft tissue mobilization to the IT band and tensor fascia lata is effective at reducing the lateral tightness that contributes to ELPS through the lateral retinaculum.
- Given that PFJRFs increase as closed chain knee flexion angles increase, shallow squats and/or leg press exercises with good form are effective at quadriceps strengthening without increasing symptoms.

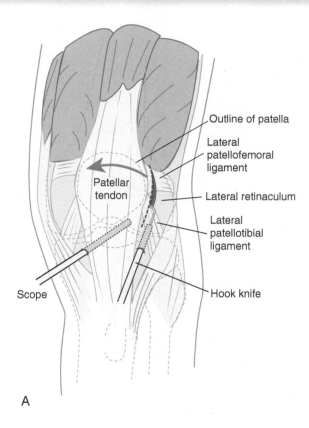

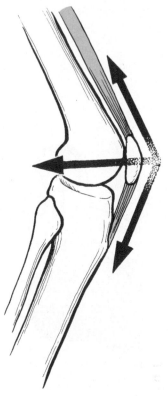

Fig. 56.6 Patellofemoral resultant force increases with knee flexion because of position and muscle actions. (Reprinted with permission from DeLee J: Delee & Dreez's Orthopaedic Sports Medicine, ed 2. Philadelphia, Saunders, 2002, p. 1817, Fig. 28E7.6.)

- Patellar tendinitis (jumper's knee)
- Quadriceps tendinitis
- Osgood-Schlatter disease (tibial tubercle)
- Sinding-Larsen-Johansson syndrome (inferior aspect of the patella)
- **Patellar compression syndrome**
- Excessive lateral pressure syndrome
- Global patellar pressure syndrome (GPPS)
- **Soft tissue lesions**
- Iliotibial band friction syndrome (lateral knee)
- Symptomatic plica syndrome
- Inflamed hypertrophic fat pad (Hoffa's disease)
- Bursitis
- Medial patellofemoral ligament pain
- **Biomechanical linkage problems**
- Foot hyperpronation
- Limb-length discrepancy
- Loss of lower limb flexibility
- **Direct trauma**
- Articular cartilage lesion (isolated)
- **Fracture**
- Fracture dislocation
- Osteochondritis dissecans
- **RSDS**

EVALUATION OF THE PATELLOFEMORAL JOINT

Signs and Symptoms

- *Instability.* Often, patients complain of the patella "giving way" during straight-ahead activities or stair climbing (versus insta-

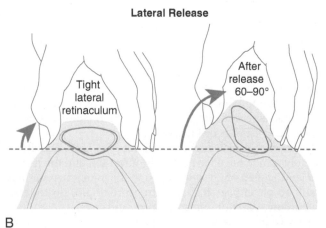

Lateral Release

Fig. 56.5 **A,** Arthroscopic lateral release of tight lateral retinaculum. **B,** After lateral release of the tight lateral retinaculum, the patella should be able to be tilted 60 to 90 degrees on patellar tilt testing. (Part *B* redrawn with permission from Banas MP, Ferkel RD, Friedman MJ: Arthroscopic lateral retinacular release of the patellofemoral joint. *Op Tech Sports Med* 1994;2:291–296.)

CLASSIFICATION

Confusion over classification of patellofemoral disorders exists in the literature. Wilk and associates (1999) noted that a comprehensive patellofemoral classification scheme should (1) clearly define diagnostic categories, (2) aid in the selection of appropriate treatment, and (3) allow the comparison of treatment approaches for a specific diagnosis.

- **Patellar instability**
- Acute patellar dislocation
- Chronic patellar subluxation
- Recurrent patellar dislocation
- **Overuse syndromes**

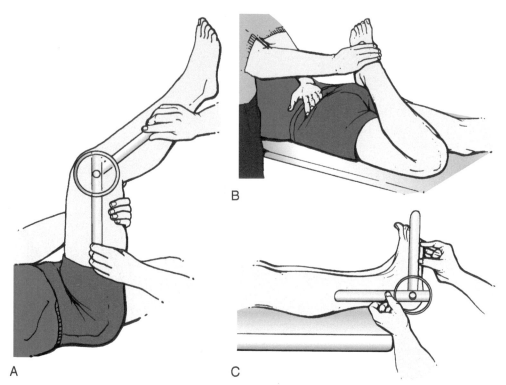

Fig. 56.7 **A,** Measurement of hamstring tightness. With the hip flexed 90 degrees, if the knee will not extend completely, the residual knee flexion angle is measured and recorded as hamstrings tightness. **B,** Measurement of quadriceps flexibility. With the patient prone, the knee is flexed as far as possible. The anterior pelvis rising off the examination table, a sensation of tightness along the anterior thigh, or lack of knee flexion compared with the opposite side may all indicate quadriceps tightness. **C,** Measurement for heel cord tightness. With the knee fully extended and the foot slightly inverted, the ankle is dorsiflexed as far as possible. The normally flexible gastrocnemius–soleus complex should allow 15 degrees of dorsiflexion beyond neutral. (Reprinted with permission from DeLee J: Delee & Dreez's Orthopaedic Sports Medicine, ed 2. Philadelphia, Saunders, 2002, p. 1817, Figs. 28E2.26, 28E2-29, and 28E2-27.)

bility owing to ACL or PCL injury, which typically is associated with giving way during pivoting or changing directions). **Patellar subluxation** typically lacks a history of trauma found with ACL-related instability. With frank episodes of patellar dislocation, the patella may spontaneously reduce or reduction may require pushing the patella medially and/or extending the knee. Dislocations typically are followed by a large bloody effusion (versus recurrent patellar subluxation).

- *Overuse or training errors.* Training errors or overuse should be suspected in athletes, patients who are obese, patients who climb stairs or squat all day, and the like.
- *Localization of pain.* Pain may be diffuse or discretely localized to the patellar tendon (patellar tendinitis), medial or lateral retinaculum, quadriceps tendon, or inferior patella (Sinding-Larsen-Johansson syndrome).
- *Crepitance.* Crepitance is often a result of underlying articular cartilage damage in the patellofemoral joint, but it may result from soft tissue impingement. Many patients describe asymptomatic crepitance with stair climbing.
- *Aggravating activities.* Painful popping with hill running may indicate only plica or iliotibial band syndrome. Aggravation of symptoms by stair climbing, squatting, kneeling, or rising from sitting to standing (movie theater sign) suggests a patellofemoral articular cartilage or retinacular source (often GPPS or ELPS).
- *Swelling.* Perceived knee swelling with patellofemoral pain is infrequently a result of an actual effusion, but it is more commonly a result of synovitis and fat pad inflammation. Large effusions are seen after patellar dislocations, but otherwise an effusion should imply other intra-articular pathology.

- *Weakness.* Weakness may represent quadriceps inhibition secondary to pain or may be indicative of extensive extensor mechanism damage (patellar tendon rupture, fractured patella, or patellar dislocation).
- *Night pain.* Pain at night or without relation to activity may imply tumor, advanced arthritis, infection, and the like. Unrelenting pain out of proportion to the injury, hyperesthesia, and so on implies RSDS, neurogenic origin, postoperative neuroma, symptom magnification, and so on.
- Associated hip abductor weakness

Physical Examination

Both lower extremities should be examined with the patient in shorts only and without shoes. The patient should be examined and observed standing, walking, sitting, and lying supine. The ipsilateral knee, hip, foot, and ankle should be examined and compared with the opposite limb for symmetry, comparison of thigh muscular girths, Q-angles, and other factors.

Physical examination also should include evaluation of the following:

- Generalized ligamentous laxity (positive thumb to wrist test, elbow or finger hyperextension, positive sulcus sign of shoulder), which raises a red flag for possible patellar subluxation
- Strength testing of hip abductors (gluteus medius and minimus) and hip musculature
- Functional strength testing (step-down test; see Fig. 56.4)
- Gait pattern
- Extensor mechanism alignment

- Q-angle (standing and sitting) and/or frontal plane projection angle (FPPA)
- Genu valgum, varum, recurvatum (see Fig. 47.2)
- Tibial torsion
- Femoral anteversion
- Patellar malposition (baja, alta, squinting)
- Pes planus or foot pronation
- Hypoplastic lateral femoral condyle
- Patellar glide test: lateral glide, medial glide, apprehension (Fairbank sign)
- Patellofemoral tracking
- J-sign (if present): a sharp jump of the patella into the trochlear groove during patellar tracking indicating late centering of the patella
- Patellofemoral crepitance
- VMO atrophy, hypertrophy
- Effusion (large, small, intra-articular, extra-articular)
- Peripatellar soft tissue point tenderness
- Medial retinaculum
- Lateral retinaculum
- Bursae (prepatellar, pes anserinus, iliotibial)
- Quadriceps tendon
- Patellar tendon
- Palpable plica
- Iliotibial band/bursa
- Enlarged fat pad
- Atrophy of thigh, VMO, calf
- Flexibility of lower extremity
- Hamstrings
- Quadriceps
- Iliotibial band (Ober test)
- Leg-length discrepancy
- Lateral pull test
- Areas of possible referred pain (back, hip)
- RSDS signs (temperature or color change, hypersensitivity)
- Hip ROM limitation or pain, flexion contracture of hip

CLINICAL TESTS FOR PATELLOFEMORAL DISORDERS

Q-angle

The Q-angle is the angle formed by the intersection of lines drawn from the anterior superior iliac spine to the center of the patella and from the center of the patella to the tibial tubercle (Fig. 56.8). In essence, these lines represent the lines of action of the quadriceps musculature and patellar tendons, respectively, on the patella. It should be measured with the knee slightly flexed, to center the patella in the trochlear groove. Foot pronation (pes planus or flat feet) and limb internal rotation both increase the Q-angle. The range of normal for the Q-angle varies in the literature, and there is controversy whether the wider pelvic anatomy in women contributes to a greater Q-angle. The reported values of normal Q-angles are 10 degrees for men and 15 degrees for women. It is well accepted that patellar alignment is somewhat affected by the degree of valgus at the knee; however, the degree of valgus present at the knee is not a dependable pathologic marker for severity of symptoms.

Soft Tissue Stabilizers of the Patella

In addition to the bony stabilizers, there are medial and lateral soft tissue restraints to the patella. The medial restraints

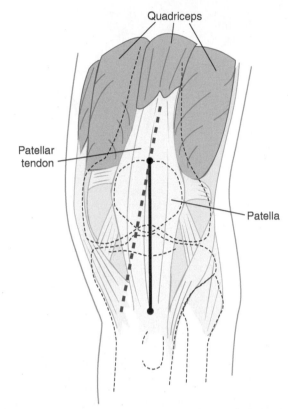

Fig. 56.8 The quadriceps angle (Q-angle) is the angle formed among the quadriceps, the patella, and the patellar tendon in extension. (Reprinted with permission from Micheli L: The Pediatric and Adolescent Knee. Philadelphia, Saunders, 2006, Fig. 2.7.)

consist of the medial retinaculum, the medial patellofemoral ligament, and the VMO. The VMO is the most important dynamic stabilizer of the patella to resist lateral displacement. Its fibers are oriented at about a 50- to 55-degree angle to the long axis of the femur (Fig. 56.9). It inserts normally into the superomedial aspect of the patella along about one-third to one-half its length. However, in some cases of instability, the muscle may be absent or hypoplastic or may insert proximal to the patella.

The lateral restraints consist of the lateral retinaculum, the vastus lateralis, and the iliotibial band. Contracture or tightness in any of these structures may exert a tethering effect on the patella (e.g., ELPS), and they must be appropriately assessed during evaluation of the patellofemoral region.

Standing Alignment of the Extensor Mechanism

Inspection of the entire lower extremity should be performed not only to assess the alignment of the extensor mechanism but also to look for pes planus, tibial torsion, genu varum or valgum, genu recurvatum, femoral anteversion, or limb-length discrepancy, all of which can contribute to patellofemoral dysfunction. It is important to evaluate the patient in a standing position. The weightbearing position may unmask otherwise-hidden deformities such as excessive forefoot pronation (which increases the relative standing Q-angle) or limb-length discrepancies. Observation of the gait pattern may reveal abnormalities in mechanics, such as foot hyperpronation, or avoidance patterns during stair descent. Muscular atrophy can be visualized qualitatively or measured quantitatively (circumferentially from

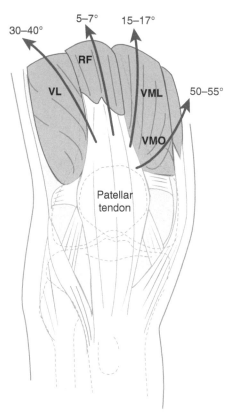

Fig. 56.9   Fiber orientation of quadriceps muscle groups. *RF*, rectus femoris; *VL*, vastus lateralis; *VML*, vastus medialis longus; *VMO*, vastus medialis oblique.

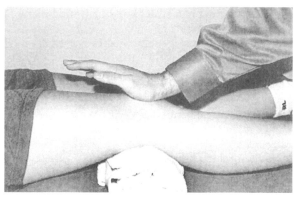

Fig. 56.10   Patellar grind or compression test. The examiner evaluates articular pain and crepitus by compressing the patella into the trochlea at various angles of knee flexion. Avoid compressing the peripatellar soft tissues by pressing the patella with the thenar eminence of the hand. The flexion angles that elicit pain during compression will indicate the likely location of the lesions.

a fixed point) with a tape measure. The presence of erythema or ecchymosis in a particular area may offer an additional clue to the underlying pathology.

Local Palpation

Palpation also reveals any tenderness that may be present in the soft tissues around the knee. Tenderness along the medial retinacular structures may be the result of injury occurring with patellar dislocation. As the patella dislocates laterally, the medial retinaculum has to tear to allow the lateral displacement of the patella.

Lateral pain may be secondary to inflammation in lateral restraints, including the iliotibial band. Joint-line tenderness typically indicates an underlying meniscal tear. Tenderness resulting from tendinitis or apophysitis in the quadriceps or patellar tendon will typically present with distinctly localized point tenderness at the area of involvement. Snapping or painful plicae may be felt, typically along the medial patellar border.

Range of Motion (Hip, Knee, and Ankle)

ROM testing should include not only the knee but also the hip, ankle, and subtalar joints. Pathology in the hip may present as referred knee pain, and abnormal mechanics in the foot and ankle can lead to increased stresses in the soft tissue structures of the knee that may present as pain. While ranging the knee, the presence of crepitation and patellar tracking should be assessed. Palpable crepitus may or may not be painful and may

or may not indicate significant underlying pathology, although it should raise the suspicion of articular cartilage injury or soft tissue impingement. The patellar grind or compression test (Fig. 56.10) will help to elucidate the etiology. To perform this test, one applies a compressive force to the patella as the knee is brought through a ROM. The reproduction of pain with or without accompanying crepitus is indicative of articular cartilage damage. More experienced examiners may be able to further localize the pain to specific regions of the patella or trochlea with subtle changes in the site of compression.

Flexibility of the Lower Extremity

Flexibility of the lower extremity must be evaluated. Quadriceps, hamstring, or IT band tightness may all contribute to patellofemoral symptoms. Quadriceps flexibility may be tested with the patient in a prone or lateral position. The hip is extended and the knee progressively flexed. Limitation of knee flexion or compensatory hip flexion is indicative of quadriceps tightness. Hamstring flexibility should also be tested.

The Ober test (Fig. 56.11) is used to assess iliotibial band flexibility. The test is done with the patient in a side-lying position with the leg being measured up above the other. The lower hip is flexed to flatten lumbar lordosis and stabilize the pelvis. The examiner, positioned behind the patient, gently grasps the leg proximally just below the knee, flexes the knee to apply a mild stretch on the quadriceps, and flexes the hip to 90 degrees to flatten the lumbar lordosis. The hip is then extended to neutral, and any flexion contracture is noted. With the opposite hand at the iliac crest to stabilize the pelvis and prevent the patient from rolling backward, the examiner maximally abducts and extends the hip. The abducted and extended hip is then allowed to adduct by gravity while the knee is kept flexed, the pelvis stabilized, and the femur in neutral rotation. Generally, the thigh should adduct to a position at least parallel to the examining table. Palpation proximal to the lateral femoral condyle with the IT band on stretch is frequently painful to patients with IT band and lateral retinacular tightness. When this is found, IT band stretches become a valuable part of the treatment plan. Again, bilateral comparison is important. Ober's position is useful in the treatment (stretching) and diagnosis of iliotibial band tightness.

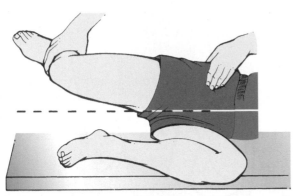

Fig. 56.11 Ober test assesses iliotibial band tightness. The unaffected hip and the knee are flexed. The involved knee is flexed 90 degrees, and the ipsilateral hip is abducted and hyperextended. A tight iliotibial band will prevent the extremity from dropping below the horizontal. (Reprinted with permission from DeLee J: Delee & Dreez's Orthopaedic Sports Medicine, ed 2. Philadelphia, Saunders, 2002, Fig. 28E10.4.)

J-Sign

The J-sign refers to the inverted J path the patella takes in early knee flexion (or terminal knee extension) as the patella begins its path from a laterally subluxated starting position and then suddenly shifts medially as it engages the bony femoral trochlear groove (or the reverse in terminal extension). It is indicative of possible patellar maltracking and/or patellar instability (Fig. 56.12).

Examination for knee instability should include a full evaluation of the cruciate and collateral ligaments to assess for any rotatory component and to examine the patellar restraints. Patients with posterolateral corner knee instability may develop secondary patellar instability owing to a dynamic increase in the Q-angle. Similarly, patients with chronic MCL laxity may also develop secondary patellar instability. Apprehension on medial or lateral displacement testing of the patella should raise the suspicion of underlying instability in the patellar restraints. Superior and inferior patellar mobility should also be assessed; they may be decreased in situations of global contracture.

Patellar Glide Test

The patellar glide test is useful to assess the medial and lateral patellar restraints. In full extension, the patella lies above the trochlear groove and should be freely mobile both medially and laterally. As the knee is flexed to 20 degrees, the patella should center in the trochlear groove, providing both bony and soft tissue stability.

Lateral Glide Test

The lateral glide test evaluates the integrity of the medial restraints. Lateral translation is measured as a percentage of patellar width (Fig. 56.13). Translations of 25% of patellar width are considered normal; translations greater than 50% indicate laxity within the medial restraints. The medial patellofemoral ligament (MPFL) has been noted to provide 53% of the stabilizing force to resist lateral subluxation and normally presents with a solid endpoint when the lateral glide test is performed. Reproduction of the patient's symptoms with passive lateral translation of the patella pulling on the medial structures is referred to as a positive lateral apprehension sign. This signals lateral patellar instability.

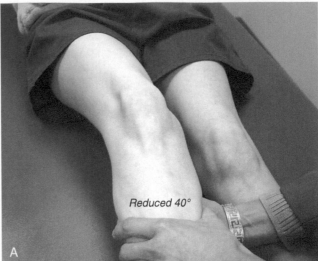

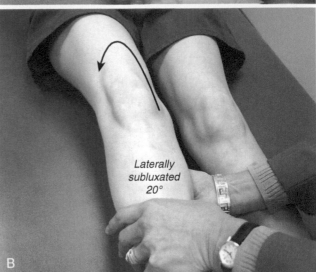

Fig. 56.12 A and B, A positive "J" sign is demonstrated as the patient's patella is at 40 degrees of flexion and subluxes laterally at 20 degrees of flexion. Asking the patient to straighten the leg against examiner's resistance can demonstrate this sign of lateral patellar instability. (Copyright 2002, ML Ireland.)

Lateral Patellar Glide Test

Lateral

25 50 75 100
%

Femoral condyles

Patient in supine position with knee flexed 30°

Fig. 56.13 Lateral patellar glide test.

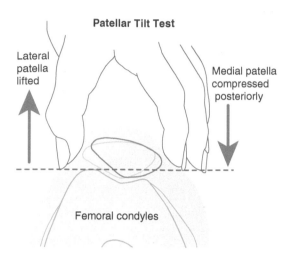

Patient in supine position with leg straight

Fig. 56.14 Patellar tilt test.

Medial Glide Test

The medial glide test is performed with the knee in full extension. The patella is centered on the trochlear groove, and medial translation from this "zero" point is measured in millimeters. Greater than 10 mm of translation is abnormal. The lateral retinacular laxity may result from a hypermobile patella or, less commonly, medial instability. Medial patellar instability is rare and usually presents as an iatrogenic complication following patellar realignment surgery, typically from an overaggressive lateral release. Six to 10 mm of translation is considered normal. Translation less than 6 mm medially indicates a tight lateral restraint and may be associated with ELPS. See Rehabilitation Protocol 56.2 for procedures following distal and/or proximal patellar realignment procedures.

Patellar Tilt

A tight lateral restraint may contribute to patellar tilt. Patellar tilt is evaluated as the knee is brought to full extension and an attempt is made by the examiner to elevate the lateral border of the patella (Fig. 56.14). Normally, the lateral border should be able to be elevated 0 to 20 degrees above the medial border. Less than 0 degrees indicates tethering by a tight lateral retinaculum, vastus lateralis, or IT band. Presence of clinical and radiographic lateral patellar tilt is indicative of tight lateral structures. This may be responsible for ELPS. If extensive rehabilitation fails, the presence of a lateral patellar tilt correlates with a successful outcome after lateral release.

Patellar tilt is evaluated by the patellofemoral angle. This angle is formed by the lines drawn along the articular surfaces of the lateral patella facet and the lateral wall of the trochlear groove. The lines should be roughly parallel. Divergence is measured as a positive angle and is considered normal, whereas convergence of the lines is measured as a negative angle and indicates the presence of abnormal patellar tilt.

Bassett Sign

Tenderness over the medial epicondyle of the femur may represent an injury to the medial patellofemoral ligament in the patient with an acute or recurrent patellar dislocation.

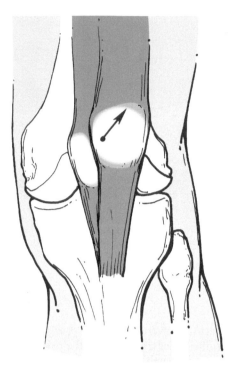

Fig. 56.15 Lateral pull sign. In this left knee, when the quadriceps is contracted, the patella moves in an exaggerated lateral and proximal direction. This also indicates predominance of lateral forces. (Reprinted with permission from DeLee J: Delee & Dreez's Orthopaedic Sports Medicine, ed 2. Philadelphia, Saunders, 2002, Fig. 28E2.21.)

Lateral Pull Test/Sign

The lateral pull test is performed by contraction of the quadriceps with the knee in full extension. Test results are positive (abnormal) if lateral displacement of the patella is observed. This test demonstrates excessive dynamic lateral forces (Fig. 56.15).

Radiographic Evaluation

Three views of the patella—an AP, a lateral in 30 degrees of knee flexion, and an axial image—should be obtained. The AP view can assess for the presence of any fractures, which should be distinguished from a bipartate patella, a normal variant. The overall size, shape, and gross alignment of the patella can also be ascertained. The lateral view is used to evaluate the patellofemoral joint space and to look for patella alta or baja. In addition, the presence of fragmentation of the tibial tubercle or inferior patellar pole can be seen. Both the AP and the lateral views can also be used to confirm the presence and location of any loose bodies or osteochondral defects that may exist. An axial image, typically a Merchant (knee flexed 45 degrees and x-ray beam angled 30 degrees to axis of the femur) or skyline view, may be the most important. It is used to assess patellar tilt and patellar subluxation. The anatomy of the trochlear groove is also well visualized, and the depth and presence of any condylar dysplasia can be determined. One important point deserves mention. The radiographs visualize only the subchondral bone of the patella and trochlea and do not show the articular cartilage. The articular surfaces are not necessarily of uniform thickness in these regions. Therefore, any measurements made from plain radiographs are only an indirect indication of the actual anatomic structure.

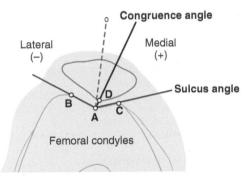

Fig. 56.16 Sulcus angle and congruence angle. The sulcus angle is formed by lines BA and AC. The congruence angle is formed by a line bisecting the sulcus angle and a line drawn through the lowest point on the patella articulate surface (represented by D in this diagram). A sulcus angle of greater than 150 degrees indicates a shallow trochlear groove, predisposing to patellar instability. Patellofemoral subluxation is evaluated by the congruence angle.

Assessment begins with the measurement of the **sulcus angle** (Fig. 56.16). A line is drawn along the medial and lateral walls of the trochlea. The angle formed between them is the sulcus angle. Greater than 150 degrees is abnormal and indicates a shallow or dysplastic groove that may have a predisposition for patellar instability.

Patellofemoral subluxation is evaluated by measurement of the **congruence angle** (Fig. 56.16). The angle is formed by a line drawn from the apex of the trochlear groove bisecting the sulcus angle and a line drawn from the apex of the groove to the apex of the patella. A lateral position of the patella apex relative to the apex of the trochlea is considered positive. A normal congruence angle has been described as −6 degrees ±6 degrees.

IMPORTANT POINTS IN REHABILITATION OF PATELLOFEMORAL DISORDERS
Patellar Instability

- Patellar instability refers to symptoms secondary to episodic lateral (rarely medial) subluxation or dislocation of the patella. Lateral patellar subluxation is common (Rehabilitation Protocol 56.3).
- Medial subluxation is typically rare, iatrogenic, and a result of excessive or ill-advised lateral release.
- Predisposing risk factors contributing to patellar instability include the following:
  - Previous patellar dislocation
  - Generalized ligamentous laxity
  - Genu valgum/increased Q-angle
  - Structural malalignment (e.g., deficient femoral trochlea and patella alta)
  - Quadriceps tightness or generalized quad weakness
  - Pes planus
  - Iatrogenic over-release of lateral retinaculum (medial instability rather than typical lateral instability)
  - Atrophy or delayed VMO activation
  - Femoral anteversion

Patellar subluxation generally describes the transient lateral movement of the patella during early knee flexion. Often, this subluxation is reported as "something jumps or comes out of place" or is "hung up."
- Palpation often elicits medial retinacular tenderness.

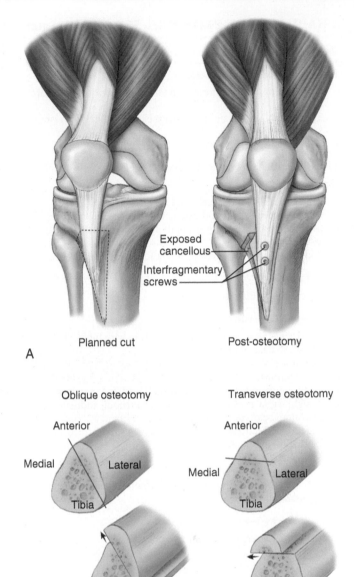

Planned cut   Post-osteotomy

A

Oblique osteotomy   Transverse osteotomy

Anterior   Anterior

Medial   Lateral   Medial   Lateral

Tibia   Tibia

B

Fig. 56.17 **A,** Overview of anteromedialization. **B,** Orientation of the oblique AMZ osteotomy (*left*) and of the flat osteotomy of TTM (*right*). (Reprinted with permission from Cole B: Surgical Techniques of the Shoulder, Elbow, and Knee in Sports Medicine. Philadelphia, Saunders, 2008, Fig. 74.3.)

- Patient apprehension (positive Fairbank sign) is common on examiner displacing the patella laterally.
- Patellar mobility should be evaluated by displacing the patella medially and laterally with the knee flexed 20 to 30 degrees. If more than 50% of the total patellar width can be displaced laterally over the edge of the lateral femoral condyle, patellar instability should be suspected.
- Inspection of patellar tracking should be done with particular attention to the entrance and exit of the patella into the trochlea between 10 and 25 degrees of knee flexion. An abrupt lateral movement of the patella on terminal knee extension (extension subluxation) indicates patellar instability or subluxation.
- Conlan and coworkers (1993) in a biomechanical study of medial soft tissue restraints that prevent lateral patellar subluxation found that the medial patellofemoral ligament provides 53% of the total restraining force.

REHABILITATION PROTOCOL 56.1 ▪ After Lateral Retinacular Release

Michael D'Amato, MD, Bernard R.Bach, MD

Indications for Lateral Release

- Recalcitrant patellofemoral pain with a positive lateral tilt of the patella.
- Tight lateral retinaculum—positive excessive lateral pressure syndrome.
- Lateral retinacular pain with positive lateral tilt.

Phase 1: Immediately After Surgery–2 Weeks

Goals

- Protect healing soft tissue structures.
- Improve knee flexion and extension.
- Increase lower extremity strength, including quadriceps muscle re-education.
- Education of patient regarding limitations and rehabilitation process.

Weight bearing

- As tolerated with two crutches.

Therapeutic Exercises

- Quadriceps sets and isometric adduction with biofeedback for vastus medialis obliquus.
- Heel slides.
- Ankle pumps.
- Nonweightbearing gastrosoleus and hamstring exercises.
- Straight leg raise (SLR) in flexion with turnout, adduction, and extension; begin hip abduction at approximately 3 weeks.
- Functional electrical stimulation can be used for trace to poor quadriceps contraction.
- Begin aquatic therapy at 2 weeks (when wound is healed) with emphasis on normalization of gait.
- Stationary bike for range of motion when sufficient knee flexion is present.

Phase 2: Weeks 2–4

Criteria for Progression to Phase 2

- Good quadriceps set.
- Approximately 90 degrees of active knee flexion.
- Full active knee extension.
- No signs of active inflammation.

Goals

- Increase flexion.
- Increase lower extremity strength and flexibility.
- Restore normal gait.
- Improve balance and proprioception.

Weight bearing

- Ambulation as tolerated without crutches if following criteria are met:
  - No extension lag with SLR.
  - Full active knee extension.
  - Knee flexion of 90 to 100 degrees.
  - Nonantalgic gait pattern.
  - May use one crutch or cane to normalize gait before walking without assistive device.

Therapeutic Exercises

- Wall slides from 0 to 45 degrees of knee flexion, progressing to mini-squats.

- Four-way hip exercises for flexion, extension, and adduction.
- Calf raises.
- Balance and proprioception activities (including single-leg stance, kinesthetic awareness trainer (KAT), biomechanical ankle proprioception system (BAPS) board.
- Treadmill walking with emphasis on normalization of gait pattern.
- Iliotibial band and hip flexor stretching.

Phase 3: Weeks 4–8

Criteria for Progression to Phase 3

- Normal gait.
- Good to normal quadriceps strength.
- Good dynamic control with no evidence of patellar lateral tracking or instability.
- Clearance by physician to begin more concentrated closed kinetic chain progression.

Goals

- Restore any residual loss of ROM.
- Continue improvement of quadriceps strength.
- Improve functional strength and proprioception.

Therapeutic Exercises

- Quadriceps stretching when full knee flexion has been achieved.
- Hamstring curl.
- Leg press from 0 to 45 degrees knee flexion.
- Closed kinetic chain progression.
- Abduction on four-way hip exercises.
- Stairmaster or elliptical trainer.
- NordicTrack.
- Jogging in pool with wet vest or belt.

Phase 4: Return to Full Activity–Week 8

Criteria for Progression to Phase 4

- Release by physician to resume full or partial activity.
- No patellofemoral or soft tissue complaints.
- No evidence of patellar instability.
- Necessary joint ROM, muscle strength and endurance, and proprioception to safely return to athletic participation.

Goals

- Continue improvements in quadriceps strength.
- Improve functional strength and proprioception.
- Return to appropriate activity level.

Therapeutic Exercises

- Functional progression, which may include but is not limited to the following
  - Slide board.
  - Walk/jog progression.
  - Forward and backward running, cutting, figure-of-eight, and carioca.
  - Plyometrics.
  - Sport-specific drills.

REHABILITATION PROTOCOL 56.2 ● After Distal and/or Proximal Patellar Realignment Procedures (Fig. 56.17)

Michael D'Amato, MD, Bernard R. Bach, MD

General Guidelines
- No closed kinetic chain exercises for 6 weeks.
- Same rehabilitation protocol is followed for proximal and distal realignments, except for weightbearing limitations as noted.
- After a combined proximal and distal realignment, the protocol for distal realignment is used.

Phase 1: Immediately Postoperative—Weeks 1–6
Goals
- Protect fixation and surrounding soft tissues.
- Control inflammatory process.
- Regain active quadriceps and vastus medialis obliquus (VMO) control.
- Minimize adverse effects of immobilization through continuous passive motion (CPM) and heel slides in the allowed range of motion (ROM).
- Obtain full knee extension.
- Patient education regarding the rehabilitation process.

Range of Motion General Guidelines
- 0–2 weeks: 0–30 degrees of flexion.
- 2–4 weeks: 0–60 degrees of flexion.
- 4–6 weeks: 0–90 degrees of flexion.

Brace
- 0–4 weeks: locked in full extension for all activities except therapeutic exercises and CPM use; locked in full extension for sleeping.
- 4–6 weeks: unlocked for sleeping, locked in full extension for ambulation.

Weight bearing
- As tolerated with two crutches for proximal realignment procedure; 50% with two crutches for distal realignment procedure (Fig. 56.17).

Therapeutic Exercises
- Quadriceps sets and isometric adduction with biofeedback and electrical stimulation for VMO (no electrical stimulation for 6 weeks with proximal realignment).
- Heel slides from 0 to 60 degrees of flexion for proximal realignment and 0 to 90 degrees for distal realignment.
- CPM for 2 hours, twice daily, from 0 to 60 degrees of flexion for proximal realignment and 0 to 90 degrees of flexion for distal realignment.
- Nonweightbearing gastrocnemius soleus, hamstring stretches.
- Straight leg raise (SLR) in four planes with brace locked in full extension (can be done standing).
- Resisted ankle ROM with Theraband.
- Patellar mobilization (begin when tolerated).
- Begin aquatic therapy at 3 to 4 weeks with emphasis on gait.

Phase 2: Weeks 6–8
Criteria for Progression to Phase 2
- Good quadriceps set.
- Approximately 90 degrees of flexion.
- No signs of active inflammation.

Goals
- Increase range of flexion.
- Avoid overstressing fixation.
- Increase quadriceps and VMO control for restoration of proper patellar tracking.

Brace
- Discontinue use for sleeping, unlock for ambulation as allowed by physician.

Weight bearing
- As tolerated with two crutches.

Therapeutic Exercises
- Continue exercises, with progression toward full flexion with heel slides.
- Progress to weightbearing gastrocnemius soleus stretching.
- Discontinue CPM if knee flexion is at least 90 degrees.
- Continue aquatic therapy.
- Balance exercises (single-leg standing, kinesthetic awareness trainer (KAT), biomechanical ankle proprioception system (BAPS) board).
- Stationary bike, low resistance, high seat.
- Wall slides progressing to mini-squats, 0 to 45 degrees of flexion.

Phase 3: 8 Weeks–4 Months
Criteria for Progression to Phase 3
- Good quadriceps tone and no extension lag with SLR.
- Nonantalgic gait pattern.
- Good dynamic patellar control with no evidence of lateral tracking or instability.

Weight bearing
- May discontinue use of crutches when following criteria are met:
  - No extension lag with SLR.
  - Full extension.
  - Nonantalgic gait pattern (may use one crutch or cane until gait is normalized).

Therapeutic Exercises
- Step-ups, begin at 2 inches and progress toward 8 inches.
- Stationary bike, add moderate resistance.
- Four-way hip for flexion, adduction, abduction, extension.
- Leg press for 0 to 45 degrees of flexion.
- Swimming, elliptical trainer for endurance.
- Toe raises.
- Hamstring curls.
- Treadmill walking with emphasis on normalization of gait.
- Continue proprioception exercises.
- Continue flexibility exercises for gastrocnemius soleus and hamstrings; add iliotibial band and quadriceps as indicated.

Phase 4: 4–6 Months
Criteria for Progression to Phase 4
- Good to normal quadriceps strength.
- No evidence of patellar instability.
- No soft tissue complaints.
- Clearance from physician to begin more concentrated closed kinetic chain exercises and resume full or partial activity.

Goals
- Continue improvements in quadriceps strength.
- Improve functional strength and proprioception.
- Return to appropriate activity level.

Therapeutic Exercises
- Progression of closed kinetic chain activities.
- Jogging/running in pool with wet vest or belt.
- Functional progression, sport-specific activities.

REHABILITATION PROTOCOL 56.3 ■ General Guidelines for Nonoperative Treatment of Recurrent (Not Acute) Patellar Instability (Lateral)

Goals

- Decrease symptoms and instability.
- Increase quadriceps strength and endurance (vastus medialis obliquus [VMO] > lateral structures).
- Use of passive restraints (Palumbo-type bracing, McConnell taping) to augment stability during transition.
- Enhance patellar stability by dynamic stabilization or passive mechanisms.

Exercises

- Modify or avoid activities that aggravate or induce symptoms (running, squatting, stair climbing, jumping, high-impact activities).
- Rest, ice, limb elevation.
- Use of cane or crutches if needed.
- NSAIDs (if not contraindicated) for anti-inflammatory effect; no steroid injection.
- Modalities to modify pain, reduce effusion and edema.
- Electrical stimulation.
- Biofeedback for VMO strengthening.
- External Palumbo-type lateral buttress bracing or McConnell taping based on patient preference and skin tolerance to taping.
- Orthotics posted in subtalar neutral to control foot pronation, decrease Q-angle, or correct leg-length discrepancy.
- General conditioning and cross-training.
- Aqua exercises, deep pool running.
- Swimming.
- Avoid bicycling in the early phases.
- Pain-free quadriceps strengthening exercises with VMO efficiency enhancement.
- Medial patellar mobilizations for lateral retinacular stretching.
- Hip abduction strengthening both in open chain and closed chain.
- No exercises isolate the VMO but several produce high electromyographic activity of the VMO.
- Leg press.
- Lateral step-ups.
- Isometric quadriceps setting.
- Hip adduction exercises.
- Gradual restoration of flexibility (stretching) for noted deficits.
- Iliotibial band.
- Quadriceps.
- Hamstrings.
- Gastrocnemius soleus.
- Avoid mobilization of the medial retinaculum.
- Re-establish knee proprioception skills.

 Check online videos: Squatting (Video 56.1) and Squatting With Therapist Tapping (Video 56.2).

REFERENCES

A complete reference list is available at https://expertconsult.inkling.com/.

57

Medial Patellofemoral Ligament Reconstruction

Charles E. Giangarra, MD | Jace R. Smith, MD

There are many factors that may be associated with patella instability, ranging from developmental conditions such as malalignment or a dysplastic femoral groove to physiologic conditions such as a weak VMO or hyperlaxity. Over the past 20 years, the importance of the medial patella femoral ligament has been identified (Conlant 1993, Sanders 2001, Ahmad 2000, Desio 1998). It has been shown that in most patella dislocations there is some injury to the MPFL (Nomura 2002, Sallay 1996) (Fig. 57.1).

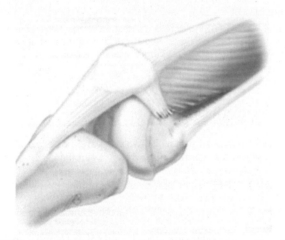

Fig. 57.1 Anatomy of medial patella femoral ligament tear. From Handy (Operative Techniques Sports Medicine, Vol 9, #3, pg. 166 Fig. 1 "B").

ANATOMY

The MPFL is found in layer two of the medial aspect of the knee between the medial retinaculum and joint capsule (Warren 1979). It is extracapsular. It is a fanlike ligament that measures approximately 6 cm in length, is wider at its patella attachment, and narrows as it approaches the femoral attachment. It attaches on the superior two-thirds of the patella and inserts approximately 4 mm distal and 2 mm anterior to the adductor tubercle (Baldwin 2009, Laprade 2007, Nomura 2005) (Fig. 57.2).

PATHOGENESIS

The usual mechanism of injury is a twisting injury with the knee slightly flexed and foot planted. Occasionally a direct blow is connected with the injury. Often the patients will spontaneously reduce the patella when they extend the knee (Fig. 57.3). A large hematoma is often associated with the acute injury and occasionally there may be associated osteochondral injuries with loose body formation (Fig. 57.4).

TREATMENT

Treatment for first-time dislocation should be nonoperative unless there is a loose body formation or another associated injury that would require surgical intervention. Initial

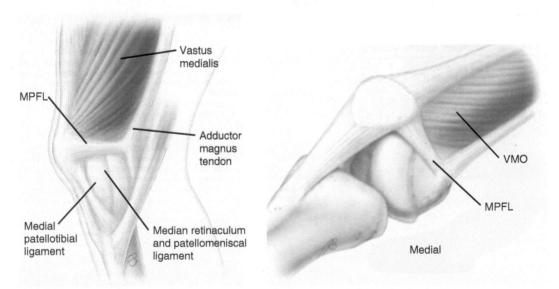

Fig. 57.2 Anatomy of intact MPFL. From Elliott (Operative Techniques Sports Medicine, Vol 9, #3, pg 114 Fig. 3).

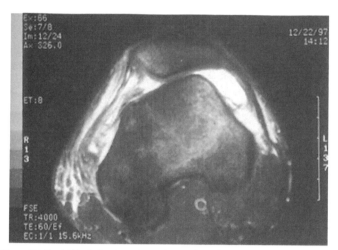

Fig. 57.3 MRI following lateral patella dislocation with tear of MPFL. From Handy (Operative Techniques Sports Medicine, Vol 9, #3, pg 167 Fig. 3).

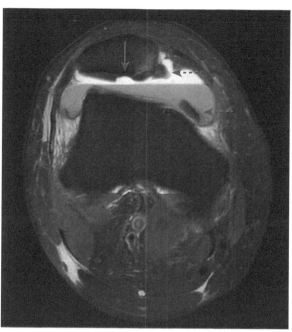

Fig. 57.4 MRI following patella dislocation with patella cartilage injury (arrow), lipohemarthrosis, and two loose bodies (dotted arrows). From Schulz (Operative Techniques Sports Medicine, Vol 18, #2, 2010 pg 76 Fig. 17).

treatment for first-time dislocation would include a period of immobilization in extension followed by standard quad strengthening and patella stabilization program as this has been shown to be effective (Sillanpaa 2008, Fithian 2004, Christiansen 2008).

When nonoperative treatment fails, surgery needs to be considered. As the MPFL has been shown to be injured in most cases of recurrent patella instability, a number of procedures have been described (Gomes 2004, Ahmad 2009, Christiansen 2008, Drez 2001, Fithian 2010).

The majority of surgeons will use a hamstring autograft to recreate the sling and check rain to prevent lateral subluxation of the patella. All associated pathology must be taken into consideration at the time of the reconstruction (Reagan 2014). The key to a successful procedure is the accurate placement of the graft (Fig. 57.5).

The indication for MPFL reconstruction is recurrent lateral patella dislocation in spite of trial of appropriate, supervised nonoperative treatment. Contraindications include patella femoral pain syndrome, patella femoral arthritis, and severe malalignment syndrome.

Postoperative Rehab

Postoperatively, most protocols involve a period of immobilization with progression to return to full activity in approximately 4 months (Boselli 2010, Reagan 2014). A typical protocol is summarized below.

Week 0–2: Full weight bearing in knee immobilizer without activation of quads

Week 2: Start formalized PT with passive and active-assisted ROM.

Week 6: More aggressive strengthening of quads and hamstrings as well as hip and core muscles (stationary bike with minimal resistance, closed chain double leg exercises)

Week 12: Agility and running permitted (start single leg closed chain exercises)

Week 16: Return to full activity.

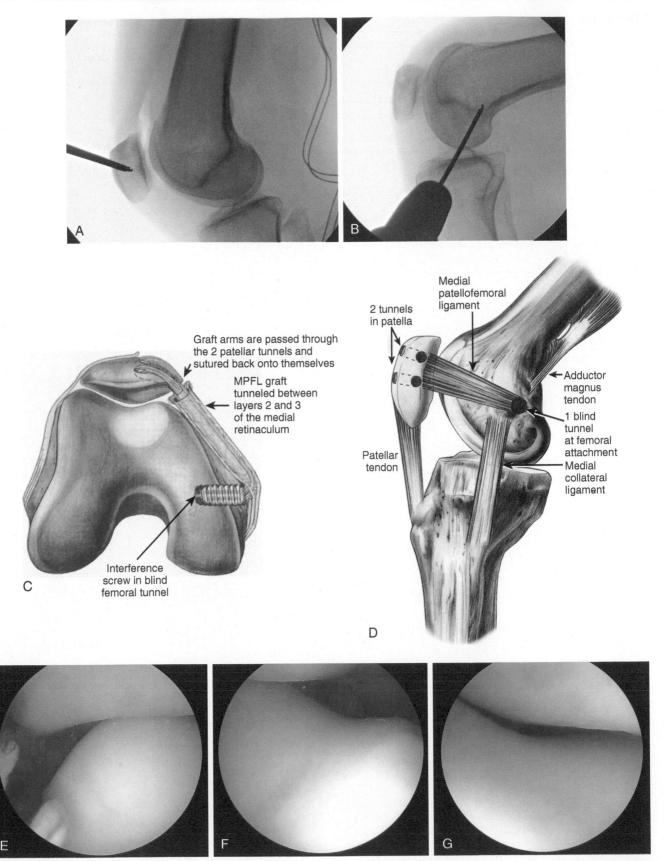

Fig. 57.5 **A,** X-ray confirmation for placement of patella tunnels during MPFL Reconstruction. From Reagan (Clinics Sports Medicine, 7/14 pg 506 Fig. 4). **B,** X-ray confirmation for placement of femoral attachment. From Reagan (Clinics Sports Medicine, 7/14 pg 507 Fig. 6). **C and D,** Schematic representation of completion of a reconstruction technique. From Lithian (Operative Techniques in Sports Medicine, Vol 18 #2, 2010 pg 95 Fig. I). **E–G,** Personal arthroscopic photographs.

REFERENCES

A complete reference list is available at https://expertconsult.inkling.com/.

FURTHER READING

Baldwin JL. The anatomy of the medial patellofemoral ligament. *AMJSM.* 2009;37:2355–2362.

Boselli K, Bowers A, Shubin Stein B, et al. Medial patellofemoral ligament reconstruction: docking technique. *Open Techniques Sports Med.* 2010;18(2):98–106.

Desio SM, Burks RT, Bachn KN. Soft tissue restraints to lateral patella translation in the human knee. *AJSM.* 1998;26:59–65.

Meininger A, Miller M, eds. Understanding the patellofemoral joint from instability to arthroplasty. *Clin Sports Med.* 2014;33(3).

Reagan J, Kullar R, Burke R. Medial patellofemoral ligament reconstruction: technique and results. *Clin Sports Med.* 2014;33(3):501–516.

58

Hip Strength and Kinematics in Patellofemoral Syndrome

Lori A. Bolgla, PT, PhD, ATC

Much research has focused on the presence of hip weakness and faulty lower extremity kinematics (especially of the hip) predominantly in females with patellofemoral pain syndrome. Findings from most studies have shown that females with PFPS demonstrate weakness of hip abductor and external rotator musculature. Using handheld dynamometry to measure muscle force, researchers have reported that females with PFPS generally generate hip abductor force equal to or less than 25% of body weight and hip external rotator force equal to or less than 15% of body weight. Clinicians may use these values as a threshold for identifying females with PFPS and hip weakness.

Conflicting data exist regarding an absolute association between hip weakness and faulty lower extremity kinematics. Bolgla et al. (2008) reported that females with PFPS and hip weakness completed a stair descent task with similar hip and knee kinematics as matched controls. However, other researchers have found lower extremity kinematic differences when assessing females with PFPS during more demanding activities such as running, repetitive single-leg jumping, and bilateral drop landings. Kinematic discrepancies between more and less demanding activities suggest that females with PFPS may use compensatory patterns.

Clinicians may use the **frontal plane projection angle** during a single-leg squat to determine excessive knee valgus that a female may exhibit during dynamic tasks (Fig. 58.1). The clinician can calculate the FPPA by taking a digital photograph while the female performs a single-leg squat at 45 degrees of knee flexion. The clinician then imports the photograph into a digital software program to draw the FPPA. The FPPA is similar to the Q-angle with the following exceptions. The line on the femur is drawn from the ASIS to the middle of the tibiofemoral joint (not the midpoint of the patella). The line on the tibia is drawn from the middle of the tibiofemoral joint (not the midpoint of the patella) to the middle of the ankle mortise (not the tibial tubercle). Like the Q-angle, an increased FPPA infers greater knee valgus.

Willson and Davis (2008) have reported a moderate association between an increased FPPA and the amount of hip adduction and tibial external rotation during running and single-leg jumping for females with PFPS. Therefore, a female's inability to perform a single-leg squat with an increased FPPA may infer decreased hip and knee control during dynamic activities.

ADDITIONAL PATELLOFEMORAL PAIN SYNDROME REHABILITATION CONSIDERATIONS

Mascal et al. (2003) first reported on the effectiveness of using a rehabilitation program that focused on trunk, pelvis, and hip strengthening to treat two females with PFPS who initially demonstrated altered lower extremity movement patterns (as evidenced by increased hip adduction and hip internal rotation during a step-down maneuver). Since this time, findings from subsequent studies have supported the use of **hip strengthening** for the treatment of this patient population. Although designed to target the hip muscles, exercises included in these investigations likely also affected the knee extensors because subjects performed most exercises in weightbearing positions. This limitation makes it difficult to ascertain the absolute effect that hip strengthening had on symptom reduction. Future studies should compare the separate effects of isolated hip strengthening and isolated knee strengthening for the treatment of PFPS.

At this time, overwhelming evidence continues to support quadriceps exercise for the treatment of PFPS. However, a specific cohort of patients with PFPS and hip weakness may benefit from additional hip strengthening exercises. The gluteus medius and gluteus maximus control hip adduction and internal rotation, and clinicians routinely prescribe nonweightbearing and weightbearing exercises to strengthen these muscles. Researchers have assessed muscle activity using electromyography (EMG) during various hip strengthening exercises to make inferences about the strength gains a patient may receive from various exercises. They believe that exercises that require greater EMG activity will result in greater strength gains. Clinicians can use these data to develop and implement a progressive hip strengthening program (Table 58.1).

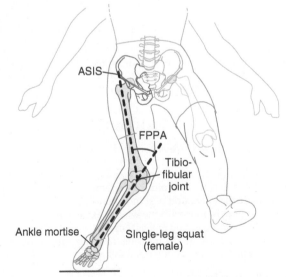

Fig. 58.1 The frontal plane projection angle (FPPA) is similar to the Q-angle with the following exceptions. The line on the femur is drawn from the ASIS to the middle of the tibiofemoral joint rather than the midpoint of the patella. The line on the tibia is drawn from the middle of the tibiofemoral joint rather than the midpoint of the patella to the middle of the ankle mortise (not the tibial tubercle). Like the Q-angle, an increased FPPA infers greater knee valgus.

PATELLAR EXCESS PRESSURE SYNDROMES (GPPS VERSUS ELPS)

The most important clinical finding differentiating global patellar pressure syndrome (GPPS) from excessive lateral pressure syndrome (ELPS) is patella mobility (Rehabilitation Protocols 58.1, 58.2, and 58.3). In GPPS mobility is restricted in both the medial and the lateral directions. Often, superior mobility is also restricted. With ELPS tightness is present **only** in the lateral retinacular structures.

The rehabilitation program for ELPS focuses on stretching the tight lateral retinacular structures and includes medial mobilization with medial glides and tilts, McConnell taping to "medialize" or normalize the patella (correct the tilt), and low-load long-duration stretching of the tight lateral structures. Musculotendinous stretching should include the hamstrings, quadriceps, and IT band. Improving quadriceps strength, especially the VMO, is emphasized. Open-chain knee extension and bicycling are not used in early rehabilitation. NSAIDs can be used for synovitis and inflammation and modalities such as high-voltage galvanic stimulation and cryotherapy. Daily home

exercises are done, and the patient is educated about which activities to avoid (stairs, squatting, kneeling, jumping, running) and counseled about changing sports.

GPPS is treated in a similar manner, with a few important changes. Patellar mobility in all planes must be re-established or improved before initiation of any aggressive rehabilitation to decrease inflammation and cartilage degeneration. Modalities such as a warm whirlpool bath and ultrasound can be used before mobilization of the patella. The glide is held for at least 1 to 2 minutes, 10 to 12 minutes if possible, during mobilization. Mobilization of the quadriceps insertion is used. The patient performs unrestricted knee motion several times a day to maintain soft tissue mobility. Restoration of full passive knee extension is vital to preserve the integrity of patellofemoral articular cartilage. Initially, multiangle quadriceps isometric contraction, straight leg raises, and 40-degree mini-squats are used until patellar mobilization improves. Then leg press, lunge, and wall squat can be added. Bicycling, deep knee bends, deep squats, and resisted knee extension should be avoided until patellar mobility is restored. Bracing or taping is **not** used in patients with GPPS because it restricts and compresses the patella.

TABLE 58.1	Hip Strengthening Exercises for ACL Rehabilitation (and Patellofemoral Rehabilitation) in Female Patients: An Evidence-Based Approach for the Development and Implementation of a Progressive Gluteal Muscle Strengthening Program		

Lori A. Bolgla, PT, PhD, ATC

Exercise	Description Gluteus Maximus (%)	Gluteus Medius (%)
Nonweightbearing standing; Patient stands solely on the unaffected lower extremity and hip abduction abducts the affected hip, keeping the pelvis in a level position.	NA	33
Side-lying hip abduction: Patient positioned in side lying with the hips and knees in 0 degrees (Fig. 49.10) of flexion (unaffected lower extremity against the table). Patient abducts the affected hip.	39	42
Weightbearing isometric: Patient stands solely on the affected lower extremity and abducts the unaffected hip, keeping the pelvis in a level position.	NA	42
Bridges side-lying clam: Patient positioned in side lying with the hips flexed to 60 degrees (Fig. 49.11) and the knees flexed to 90 degrees (unaffected lower extremity against the table). Patient abducts and externally rotates the affected hip while keeping the feet together.	39	38
Bridges with Theraband resistance		
Forward lunge (Fig. 49.12): Patient stands with the lower extremities shoulder-width apart. The patient lunges forward with the affected lower extremity (to approximately 90 degrees of knee flexion) while maintaining the pelvis in a level position and the trunk in a vertical position.	44	42
Pelvic drop (Fig. 49.13): Patient stands on the affected lower extremity on a 15-cm high step with both knees fully extended. Patient lowers the pelvis of the unaffected lower extremity towards the floor and then returns pelvis to a level position.	NA	57

REHABILITATION PROTOCOL 58.1 ■ McConnell Patellar Taping Techniques

Michael D'Amato, MD, Bernard R. Bach, MD

- The knee is cleaned, shaved, and prepared with an adhesive spray. If possible, try to avoid shaving immediately before taping to decrease the likelihood of skin irritation.
- Patellar taping is done with the knee in extension.
- Leukotape P is the taping material used.
- Correction is based on the individual malalignment, with each component corrected as described following.

Correcting Lateral Glide

- The tape is started at the midlateral border.
- It is brought across the face of the patella and secured to the medial border of the medial hamstring tendons while the patella is pulled in a medial direction.
- The medial soft tissues are brought over the medial femoral condyle toward the patella to obtain a more secure fixation.

Correcting Lateral Tilt

- The tape is started in the middle of the patella.
- It is brought across the face of the patella and secured to the medial border of the medial hamstring tendons, lifting the lateral border of the patella.
- The medial soft tissues are brought over the medial femoral condyle toward the patella to obtain a more secure fixation.

Correcting External Rotation

- The tape is applied to the middle of the inferior border of the patella.
- The inferior pole of the patella is manually rotated internally.
- The tape is secured to the medial soft tissues in a superior and medial direction while the manual correction is maintained.

REHABILITATION PROTOCOL 58.1 ● McConnell Patellar Taping Techniques—cont'd

Alternatively, if there is also a component of **inferior tilt,** the tape can be started on the middle of the superior pole. After manual correction of the rotational deformity, the tape is secured in a superior and lateral direction. This not only corrects patellar rotation but also lifts the inferior pole away from the fat pad. Care must be taken not to create a lateral patellar glide when using this alternative method.

Correcting Inferior Patellar Tilt

- Correction of inferior tilt is always combined with correction of lateral tilt or glide component.
- To correct the inferior tilt component, the starting position of the tape is shifted from the midportion of the patella to the superior portion of the patella. Correction is then carried out as explained earlier for each individual component of glide or tilt. The superior starting position of the tape lifts the inferior pole of the patella away from the fat pad.

Technical Taping Considerations

- The tape is never left on for more than 24 hours at a time and should not be worn during nighttime sleep.
- The average duration of continuous taping treatment is 2 weeks, followed by a weaning period during which the tape is worn only during strenuous activities. Taping may be continued as long as 6 weeks, if tolerated.
- The tape must be removed slowly and carefully to prevent skin irritation, which will limit further taping. Commercial solvents are available to aid in tape removal.
- The application of rubbing alcohol to the skin after tape removal helps toughen the skin and prevent skin breakdown.
- Application of a skin moisturizer overnight will nourish the skin; the moisturizer is removed before tape is applied the next day.
- Allergic reaction to the tape may occur in a few first-time patients. The knee will develop an itchy rash, usually at 7 to 10 days after the start of taping. Topical cortisone creams may limit the rash. Only hypoallergenic tape should be used in patients who develop an allergic reaction.

REHABILITATION PROTOCOL 58.2 ● Principles of McConnell Taping

- Taping is used as an adjunct to exercise and muscular balancing.
- The vastus medialis obliquus–to–vastus lateralis ratio has been shown to improve during taping.
- The ability to truly change patellar position is debated.
- To tape correctly, the position of the patella relative to the femoral condyle must be evaluated.
- Four positional relationships are evaluated statically (sitting with the legs extended and quadriceps relaxed) then dynamically by doing a quadriceps set.

Glide component is the relationship of the medial and lateral poles of the patella to the femoral condyles. Statically, the patella should be centered in the condyles; dynamically, this relationship should be maintained. With a quadriceps set, the patella should move superiorly without noticeable lateral movement. Most athletes require correction of the glide component for static or dynamic malalignment.

Tilt component is evaluated by comparing the anterior and posterior relationships of the medial and lateral borders of the patella. With the patient supine and the knee extended, the borders should be horizontal, both statically and dynamically. Frequently, the lateral border will be pulled posteriorly by the lateral retinaculum into the lateral condyle. This may also occur after the glide is corrected by taping.

Rotational component is the relationship between the long axis of the patella and the long axis of the femur. The ideal position is for the axes to be parallel. Frequently, the inferior pole of the patella is lateral to the axis of the femur, which would be described as lateral rotation.

Anteroposterior tilt is the anterior and posterior relationship of the superior and inferior poles of the patella. When the inferior pole of the patella is posterior, fat pad irritation is common.

After the patellar position is evaluated, an activity is identified that consistently provokes the patient's symptoms. Stepping off from an 8-inch step is often effective. After taping, the test should be done again to ensure the effectiveness of taping in eliminating pain.

Taping Procedure

- Corrections are typically done in the order of evaluation, but the most significant alteration in position should be corrected first.
- Leukosport tape (Beiersdorf, Inc., Wilton, CT) is commonly used.
- Tape that is strong and tacky enough to be effective requires a protective cover next to the skin, such as "Cover Roll Stretch."
- To correct the glide component, the tape is anchored on the lateral pole of the patella and the patella is manually glided medially and taped in this position.
- The tilt component is corrected by starting the tape in the middle of the patella and pulling the medial pole of the patella posteriorly and anchoring over the tape used for the glide correction.
- A rotational fault is corrected by anchoring on the lateral aspect of the inferior pole of the patella and pulling toward the medial joint line.
- If an anteroposterior tilt is present, it is corrected by taping the glide or tilt on the superior aspect of the patella to pull the inferior aspect of the patella out of the fat pad.
- Not all components have to be corrected if the pain is eliminated with one or two corrections.
- A provocation test should be done after each stage of taping to check its effectiveness.
- Taping is worn during activities that produce pain (just with athletics or with all activities of daily living).
- Once muscular control of the patella is improved, the patient is weaned from the tape; it is not intended for long-term use.

(Protocol adapted from Bockrath K, Wooden C, Worrell T, et al. Effects of patella taping on patella position and perceived pain. Med Sci Sports Exerc 1993;25:989–992.)

REHABILITATION PROTOCOL 58.3 ▪ Patellofemoral Compression Syndromes: Excessive Lateral Pressure Syndrome (ELPS) And Global Patellar Pressure Syndrome (GPPS)

Michael D'Amato, MD, Bernard R. Bach, MD

Phase 1

Goals

- Reduce pain and inflammation.
- Increase patellar mobility, mobilize contracted peripatellar structures.
- Regain quadriceps control.
- Improve patellofemoral movements.

Taping/Bracing

- ELPS: McConnell taping to correct tilt
- GPPS: no bracing or taping

Therapeutic Exercises

- Ice, electrical stimulation, and NSAIDs to decrease inflammation and pain
- Quadriceps sets and straight leg raises (SLR), multiangle quadriceps isometrics
- Hip strengthening adduction and abduction, flexion and extension exercises
- Begin patellar mobilization techniques.
- ELPS: mobilize tight lateral patellar tissues.
- GPPS: mobilize medial, lateral, superior peripatellar tissue.

Phase 2

Criteria for Progression to Phase 2

- Minimal pain
- Minimal inflammation

Goals

- Good quadriceps set with no extension lag
- Improve range of motion.
- Increase patellar mobility (*Note:* Avoid aggressive strengthening with GPPS until patellar mobility is significantly improved.)

Therapeutic Exercises

- Continue patellar mobilization.
- Fit patella stabilizing brace or use McConnell taping (ELPS) to correct patellar tilt.
- Continue ice and electrical stimulation (especially after exercise) and NSAIDs.
- SLR, quadriceps sets
- Flexibility exercises for quadriceps, hamstrings, iliotibial band, gastrocnemius, soleus
- Closed chain exercises: mini-lunges, wall slides, lateral step-ups, mini-squats
- Avoid bicycling, deep knee bends, deep squats, resisted knee extension.

- Pool exercises, swimming
- Advance exercises for hip flexors and extensors, abductors and adductors, and muscles of the lower leg and foot, increasing weight as tolerated, doing 3 to 10 sets and increasing weight by 2 pounds.

Phase 3

Criteria for Progression to Phase 3

- No increase in pain or inflammation
- Good quadriceps strength

Goals

- Full knee range of motion (ROM)
- Improved strength and flexibility

Bracing

- Continue using brace or taping if helpful.

Therapeutic Exercises

- Advance hamstring strengthening exercises.
- Bicycling, swimming, stair-stepping, or walking for cardiovascular and muscle endurance; increase duration, then speed
- Continue flexibility exercises.
- Progress closed chain activities

Phase 4

Criteria for Progression to Phase 4

- Full knee ROM
- Quadriceps strength 80% of normal

Goal

- Return to full activity.

Brace

- Brace or tape is worn for sports participation if desired. Tape up to 6 weeks, then discontinue. Continue brace as needed.

Therapeutic Exercises

- Add slow return to running if desired; increase distance, then speed.
- Warm up well.
- Use ice after workout.
- Continue aerobic cross-training.
- Start jumping, cutting, and other sport-specific exercises.

Return to Full Activity

- Full pain-free ROM
- Strength and functional tests 85% of normal

REFERENCES

A complete reference list is available at https://expertconsult.inkling.com/.

FURTHER READING

Ferber Reed, Bolgla Lori, Jennifer E, et al. Strengthening of the hip and core versus knee muscles for the treatment of patellofemoral pain: a multicenter randomized controlled trial. *J Athl Train.* 2015;50.4:366–377. Web.

Fukuda, Yukio Thiago, Melo William Pagotti, Zaffalon Bruno Marcos, et al. Hip posterolateral musculature strengthening in sedentary women with patellofemoral pain syndrome: a randomized controlled clinical trial with 1 year follow-up. *J Orthop Sports Phys Ther.* 2012;42.10:823–830. Web.

Khayambashi Khalil, Fallah Alireza, Movahedi Ahmadreza, et al. Posterolateral hip muscle strengthening versus quadriceps strengthening for patellofemoral pain: a comparative control trial. *Arch Phys Med Rehabil.* 2014;95.5:900–907. Web.

Khayambashi Khalil, Mohammadkhani Zeynab, Ghaznavi Kourosh, et al. The effects of isolated hip abductor and external rotator muscle strengthening on pain, health status, and hip strength in females with patellofemoral pain: a randomized rcontrolled trial. *J Orthop Sports Phys Ther.* 2012;42.1:22–29. Web.

Overuse Syndromes of the Knee

S. Brent Brotzman, MD

Overuse syndromes involving the extensor mechanism are commonly grouped together under the term "jumper's knee." **Patellar tendinitis** or tendinopathy is the most common, typically presenting with pain near the insertion of the tendon at the inferior pole of the patella (see Fig. 59.1). Less commonly, the symptoms may be localized to the distal tendon insertion at the tibial tubercle or the quadriceps tendon insertion at the proximal pole of the patella. In adolescents, it typically presents as a form of apophysitis, occurring at the tibial tubercle (Osgood-Schlatter) or distal patellar pole (Sinding-Larsen-Johansson) (Fig. 59.2).

HISTORY OF PATELLAR TENDINITIS (JUMPER'S KNEE)

The typical history of patellar tendinitis is that of an insidious onset of anterior knee pain, localized to the site of involvement, that develops during or soon after repetitive running or jumping activities. Jumper's knee is an insertional tendinopathy that most commonly affects the patellar tendon origin on the inferior pole of the patella (Fig. 59.2). It is not an inflammatory condition (Bahr et al. 2006).

- Histologically, there is hypercellularity, neovascularization, lack of inflammatory cells, and loss of the tightly bundled collagen appearance. This has been termed a "failed healing response". It occurs most often in basketball, volleyball, and track and field athletes. One theory is that it results from the accumulation of damage after recurrent episodes of microtrauma to the tendon. It has

been shown that, compared with asymptomatic athletes, athletes with jumper's knee have an ability to generate greater force during jumping activities, indicating an overload phenomenon as a possible cause. The type of playing surface may also play a role, with activities on hard surfaces (concrete floors) leading to an increased incidence of tendon symptoms.

- **An epidemiologic study by Lian et al. (2005) showed the average duration of substantial pain and reduced knee function is almost 3 years.**
- The prevalence of jumper's knee has been estimated to range between 40% and 50% among high-level volleyball players and between 35% and 40% among elite basketball players.
- **Decreased ankle dorsiflexion is implicated in patellar tendon tendinopathy,** increasing the rate and amount of loading on the tendon. This finding if present should be addressed in rehabilitation.
- Age appears to contribute not by degeneration but by a reduction in proteoglycans and an increase in cross-links as the tendon ages, making the tendon stiffer and less capable of tolerating load.
- Eccentric single-leg squat exercises involving active lengthening of the muscle tendon unit are effective in treating patellar tendinopathy, and the results are enhanced using a decline board (Fig. 59.3) to perform these eccentric exercises (Purdam et al. 2004, Young et al. 2005).
- Eccentric single-leg squats on a 25-degree decline board are performed twice daily consisting of three sets of 15

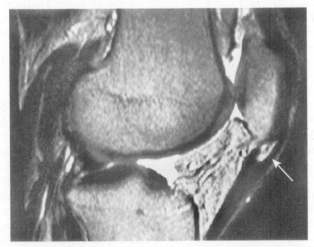

Fig. 59.1 Magnetic resonance imaging scan of a patient with jumper's knee (patellar tendinopathy), demonstrating the classic location of the lesion (*arrow*) associated with this condition. (Reprinted with permission from Lavignino M, Arnoczky SP, Elvin N, Dodds J: Patellar tendon strain is increased at the site of jumper's knee lesion during knee flexion and tendon loading. *Am J Sports Med* 36(11):2110–2114, 2008.)

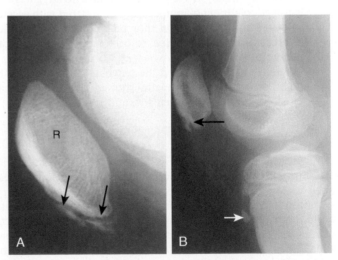

Fig. 59.2 **A,** Sinding-Larsen-Johansson changes (*arrows*) in a symptomatic 11-year-old basketball player. **B,** Concomitant Sinding-Larsen-Johansson (*long arrow*) and Osgood-Schlatter (*short arrow*) changes. The 12-year-old patient had symptoms at the patellar inferior pole. He was asymptomatic at the tibial tubercle. (Reprinted with permission from DeLee J: Delee & Dreez's Orthopaedic Sports Medicine, ed 2. Philadelphia, Saunders, 2002, Figs. 28E7-38, 28E7-40.)

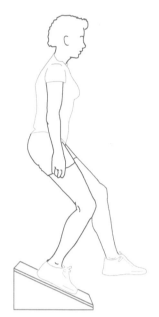

Fig. 59.3 Eccentric decline squat.

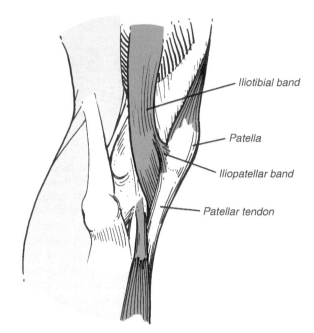

- Iliotibial band
- Patella
- Iliopatellar band
- Patellar tendon

Fig. 59.4 Lateral structures of the knee: the superficial aspect. (Reprinted with permission from DeLee J: Delee & Dreez's Orthopaedic Sports Medicine, ed 2. Philadelphia, Saunders, 2002, Figs. 28E7-38, 28E2-6.)

repetitions performed consistently for 12 weeks. The patients are instructed to perform the exercise by slowly flexing the knee to 90 degrees of flexion, perform eccentric loading of the quad only, and return to the starting position using the noninjured leg. The downward (eccentric) component was performed with the affected leg; the upward (concentric component) was performed with the unaffected leg. The authors felt the decline board reduced calf muscle tension, allowing better isolation of the knee extensor mechanism and accounting for better results in this group than the standard squat group.

- Young et al. (2005) recommended implementation of the 12-week protocol in the off-season if possible because of some of the patellar tendon pain associated with the eccentric-based program.
- Bahr et al. (2006) in a level 1 study found no advantage to surgical treatment of jumper's knee compared with eccentric strength training and thus recommended 12 weeks of eccentric training tried prior to any open surgical tenotomy.
- A review of 23 studies on the outcome of surgical treatment of patellar tendinopathy showed favorable surgical outcomes ranging between 46% and 100%.

ILIOTIBIAL BAND FRICTION SYNDROME

Repetitive activity can also lead to irritation of the soft tissues, such as the iliotibial band friction syndrome, which is very common in runners. The iliotibial band is a thick fibrous tissue band that runs along the lateral aspect of the thigh and inserts at the Gerdy tubercle on the anterolateral aspect of the proximal tibia. It has small attachments to the lateral patellar retinaculum and to the biceps femoris. As a result of the femoral and tibial attachments of the iliotibial band, it is possible that atypical hip, knee, and foot mechanics can play a role in the development of iliotibial band syndrome (ITBS).

The primary functions of the IT band are to serve as a lateral hip and knee stabilizer and to resist hip adduction and knee internal rotation. As the knee moves from full extension to flexion, the IT band shifts from a position anterior to the lateral femoral epicondyle to a position posterior to the epicondyle (Fig. 59.4). Orchard et al. (1996) suggested that frictional forces between the IT band and the lateral femoral condyle are greatest at 20 to 30 degrees of knee flexion, which occur during the first half of the stance phase of running. The repetitive flexion and extension of the knee in running can lead to irritation of the IT band as it passes back and forth over the lateral femoral epicondyle. Subsequently, the surrounding tissues and bursa become inflamed and painful.

Abnormal hip mechanics (weak hip abductor–gluteus medius) may potentially lead to an increase in hip adduction angle, increasing the strain on the IT band. Fredrickson et al. (2000) reported that runners with ITBS had significantly reduced hip abductor muscle strength in the affected limb compared to the unaffected limb and as compared to healthy controls. These authors reported that following a 6-week hip abductor strengthening program, 22 of 24 runners became pain free with running (Powers 2010).

Niemeth et al. (2005) also found significantly reduced hip abductor muscle strength in the involved ITBS limb. Thus hip abductor weakness and knee internal rotation often lead to increased hip adduction during the stance phase of running, and these factors may be related to the development of ITBS.

Miller et al. (2007) reported that runners at the end of an exhaustive run demonstrated a greater rearfoot inversion angle (rearfoot invertor moments) at heel strike compared to controls. They hypothesized this contributed to a greater peak knee (tibial) internal rotation velocity and thus torsional strain to the IT band.

In a prospective study by Noehren et al. (2007) the authors concluded that runners who developed ITBS exhibited increased hip adduction and knee internal rotation angles compared to uninjured runners. As a result, in our own running lab

REHABILITATION PROTOCOL 59.1 ● Iliotibial Band Friction Syndrome Rehab

S. Brent Brotzman, MD, Michael Duke, PT, CSCS

- Rest from running until asymptomatic
- Dynamic stretching prior to initiation of exercise
- Ice area after exercise
- Oral NSAIDs may be of some temporary initial benefit.
- Relative rest from running and high flexion–extension activities of the knee (cycling, running, stair descent, skiing)
- Avoid downhill running.
- Avoid running on surfaces with a pitched drainage grade to the road.
- Use of soft, new running shoes rather than hard shoes
- Use of iontophoresis if helpful
- Steroid injection into bursa if required

Hip and thigh musculature strengthening
- Stretching exercises
- Two-man Ober stretch
- Self-Ober stretch
- Lateral fascial stretch
- Posterior fascial stretch plus gluteus maximus and piriformis self-stretch
- Standing wall lean for lateral fascial stretch
- Rectus femoris self-stretch
- Iliopsoas with rectus femoris self-stretch
- Seated external stretching (passive) of knee at 90 degrees of flexion and near full extension

---

(Athletic Performance Lab) we focus in part on hip abductor strengthening and passive external stretching of the knee to address possible internal rotation contracture at the knee.

HISTORY AND EXAMINATION

Patients typically complain of a gradual onset of pain, tightness, or burning at the lateral aspect of the knee that develops during the course of a run. Symptoms usually resolve with rest. Examination reveals tenderness and possibly localized swelling at the lateral femoral epicondyle or at Gerdy's tubercle, and when the knee is put through ROM, pain, snapping, popping, or crepitation may be felt as the IT band crosses the epicondyle. Iliotibial band contracture is associated with the presence of symptoms and this can be evaluated by the Ober test (see Fig. 56.11).

PREDISPOSING FACTORS

Factors that may also predispose runners to IT band friction syndrome include inexperience, a recent increase in distance, and running on a track. Other potential etiologies include leg-length discrepancies, a lack of lower extremity flexibility, hyperpronation of the foot, hip muscular weakness, and running repetitively in one direction on a pitched surface.

TREATMENT OF ILIOTIBIAL BAND FRICTION SYNDROME

The basic progression of treatment is early reduction of the acute inflammation, followed by stretching of the IT band and strengthening of the hip abductors to alleviate soft tissue contracture, and then education in proper running techniques and institution of an appropriate running/training program to prevent recurrence (Rehabilitation Protocol 59.1).

REFERENCES

A complete reference list is available at https://expertconsult .inkling.com/.

FURTHER READING

Alfredson H, Pietila T, Jonsson P, et al. Heavy-load eccentric calf muscle training for the treatment of chronic achilles tendinosis. *Am J Sports Med.* 1998;26:360–366.

Hartigan EH, Axe MJ, Snyder-Mackler L. Time line for noncopers to pass return-to-sports criteria after anterior cruciate ligament reconstruction. *J Orthop Sports Phys Ther.* 2010;40(3):141–154.

Neumann DA. Kinesiology of the hip: a focus on muscular actions. *Orthop Sports Phys Ther.* 2010;40(2):82–94.

Purdam CR, Jonsson P, Alfredson H, et al. A pilot study of the eccentric decline squat in the management of painful chronic patellar tendinopathy. *Br J Sports Med.* 2004;38:395–397.

Rahnama L, Salavati M, Akhbari B, et al. Attentional demands and postural control in athletes with and without functional ankle instability. *J Orthop Sports Phys Ther.* 2010;40(3):180–187.

Strauss EJ, et al. Iliotibial band syndrome: evaluation and management. *J Am Acad Orthop Surg.* Dec. 2011;19(12).

Tenforde Adam S, Sayres Lauren C, Mccurdy Mary L, et al. Overuse injuries in high school runners: lifetime prevalence and prevention strategies. *PM R.* 2011;3(2):125–131. Web.

Tonley JC, Yun SM, Kochevar RJ, et al. Treatment of an individual with piriformis syndrome focusing on hip muscle strengthening and movement reeducation: a case report. *J Orthop Sports Phys Ther.* 2010;40(2):103–111.

Tonoli C. Incidence, risk factors and prevention of running related injuries in long distance running: a systematic review. *ARSPA Annals of Research in Sport and Physical Activity.* 2011;2:134–135. Web.

Warden SJ. Extreme skeletal adaptation to mechanical loading. *J Orthop Sports Phys Ther.* 2010;40(3):188.

Young MA, Cook JL, Purdam CR, et al. Eccentric decline squat protocol offers superior results at 12 months compared with traditional eccentric protocol for patellar tendinopathy in volleyball players. *Br J Sports Med.* 2005;39:102–105. Erratum in: *Br J Sports Med.* 39:246, 2005.

Patellar Tendon Ruptures

Matthew J. Matava, MD | Ryan T. Pitts, MD | Suzanne Zadra Schroeder, PT, ATC

BACKGROUND

Rupture of the patellar tendon is an uncommon but potentially disabling injury, with a reported incidence of less than 1 per 100,000 patients. Most of these injuries are unilateral and occur in athletic patients younger than age 40. When bilateral injuries occur, a systemic illness or collagen disorder should be suspected. In the strictest sense, the term "patellar tendon" is incorrect because this structure connects two bones—the patella and tibia—and therefore should be defined as a ligament. However, because the patella is a sesamoid bone, the term "patellar tendon" has been the more widely recognized term.

ANATOMY AND BIOMECHANICS

The thickened anterior fibers of the rectus femoris tendon, along with contributions from the medial and lateral retinaculi, form the extensor mechanism. The patellar tendon is the main component of this structure and inserts into the proximal tibia at the tibial tubercle. Patellar tendon ruptures usually involve the retinacular tissues also. Consequently, these other structures should also be treated during the surgical repair of the tendon.

Active knee flexion with the joint at approximately 60 degrees of flexion generates the greatest amount of tensile strain within the tendon. Previous studies have shown that maximal strain occurs at the bony insertion sites of the tendon. This finding, along with decreased collagen fiber stiffness in these areas, likely explains why ruptures most commonly occur at or near the proximal insertion site.

ETIOLOGY

Two main mechanisms cause failure of the patellar tendon, and both involve an eccentric quadriceps contraction. A sudden load against an actively firing quadriceps or a strong contraction against a fixed structure both may produce sufficient force to cause failure of the tendon. Most acute patellar tendon ruptures occur after longstanding tendon degeneration. Related mucoid, hypoxic, calcific, and lipomatosis degeneration and tendinopathy commonly contribute to a weakened tendon structure that leads to subsequent rupture. Chronic diseases such as autoimmune conditions, diabetes mellitus, and chronic kidney failure may contribute to tendon degeneration and failure even during nonstrenuous activity. As noted earlier, these metabolic conditions predispose the tendons to a weakened state that may also lead to bilateral injuries.

Injection of corticosteroids in or around the patellar tendon also has been associated with patellar tendon rupture. This practice should be avoided because the resulting collagen necrosis and disorganization lead to a weakened tendon prone to rupture. Surgical procedures also may disturb the normal structure of the patellar tendon, such as the exposure for a total knee arthroplasty or harvest of a bone–patellar tendon–bone graft for ACL reconstruction. The subsequent surgical treatment and altered rehabilitation protocols necessitated by tendon repair or reconstruction may compromise the long-term outcome of the index procedure, and meticulous technique during these procedures should be used at all times.

CLINICAL EVALUATION
Physical Examination

Common findings after acute patellar tendon rupture include pain, the inability to bear weight, loss of active knee extension, and a large hemarthrosis. Palpation of the extensor mechanism will reveal a defect in the tendon. The patella also will be noted to reside in a proximal position compared to the contralateral knee as a result of unopposed tensile pull of the quadriceps musculature. A thorough knee examination to rule out any associated injuries is also mandatory in the setting of a traumatic mechanism of injury.

Radiographic Evaluation

Although the diagnosis of a patellar tendon rupture can often be made clinically, plain radiographs (most importantly a lateral view at 30 degrees of flexion) can be used to confirm the clinical suspicion. The most common finding is patella alta on the lateral view; the patella–tibial tubercle distance is more than twice the length of the patella (the Insall ratio) (Fig. 60.1). It is important to note the presence of a patellar fracture or any avulsed fragments of bone that may be attached to the tendon.

Magnetic resonance imaging often is used to confirm the diagnosis of a patellar tendon rupture (Fig. 60.2). Although MRI is an excellent tool to evaluate the extensor mechanism, it is expensive and often unnecessary. On MRI tendon rupture is diagnosed by discontinuity of the tendon proper and hemorrhage between the two tendon ends with retraction of the patella. MRI also can confirm the exact location of the rupture (proximal, distal, or midsubstance). A more practical use for MRI is to rule out any concomitant injuries, which may be difficult to evaluate through a thorough physical examination in a patient with an acute injury. McKinney et al. 2008 found that 10 of 33 patients with patellar ruptures had associated injuries, most often ACL and medial meniscal injuries; six of eight with a high-energy, direct-impact mechanism of injury had associated injuries.

Ultrasound also can be used to confirm both acute and chronic patellar tendon ruptures. On high-resolution sagittal images obtained with a linear array transducer, complete rupture is indicated by an area of hypoechogenicity (Fig. 60.3). With a chronic patellar tendon rupture, thickening and disruption of the tendon's normal echo pattern are typically seen.

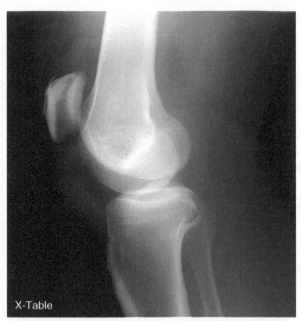

Fig. 60.1 The patella–tibial tubercle distance is more than twice the length of the patella.

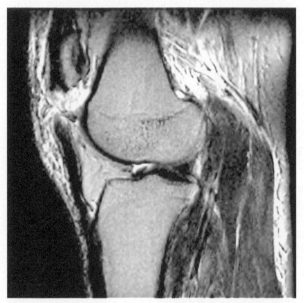

Fig. 60.2 Magnetic resonance imaging (MRI) often is used to confirm the diagnosis of a patellar tendon rupture.

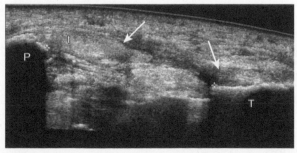

Fig. 60.3 High-resolution sagittal images obtained with a linear array transducer. Complete rupture is indicated by an area of hypoechogenicity. Arrows define area of rupture of patella tendon.

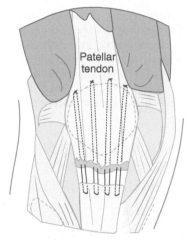

Fig. 60.4 Repair of patellar tendon rupture.

The main disadvantage of ultrasound is its dependence on the skill and experience of the technician and radiologist evaluating the images. As a result, despite its relatively low cost and ease of performance, the accuracy of ultrasound varies among institutions.

Classification

There currently is no universally accepted system to classify patellar tendon ruptures. Various systems have focused on the location, configuration, and chronicity of the injury, with the most widely used classification focusing on the time between injury and repair. Siwek and Rao (1981) grouped patellar tendon ruptures into two categories: those repaired *immediately* (less than 2 weeks from injury) and those repaired in a *delayed* fashion (more than 2 weeks from injury). This classification system has shown a correlation between the chronicity of rupture and both the method of treatment and final outcome, allowing surgeons to determine if repair or reconstruction should be done. With respect to differences in rehabilitation protocols, rehabilitation should be tailored more to the method of treatment than the type of rupture.

Treatment

Unless medical comorbidities preclude general anesthesia, all complete patellar tendon ruptures should be repaired surgically (Fig. 60.4). Repair should be undertaken as soon after injury as possible to optimize outcome and avoid the need for complex reconstructive techniques. Multiple methods for surgical repair have been described. When possible, simple end-to-end repair, with a permanent, braided suture woven in a locking fashion (with or without a cerclage suture) has been the method of choice. For more proximal ruptures without sufficient tendon for an end-to-end repair, sutures placed through patellar bone tunnels have been the preferred method, although newer techniques using suture anchors have also shown acceptable results. Distal avulsion injuries can be repaired with woven sutures placed through drill holes in the tibial tuberosity.

For patellar tendon injuries older than 6 weeks, contraction and scarring of the extensor mechanism may make direct repair impossible. In these situations, passive ROM or preoperative distal traction on the patella may allow the tendon ends to be approximated for repair. If tendon apposition is possible but the tendon ends are too damaged to allow a strong repair, augmentation can be done with various allograft tissues (i.e., Achilles or patellar tendon), autograft tissue (i.e., semitendinosus or fascia lata), or synthetic materials. If no native tendon tissue remains, reconstruction of the extensor mechanism with either an Achilles or bone–patellar tendon–bone allograft can be attempted, but patients must be warned of the inferior results associated with these salvage reconstructions.

REHABILITATION FOLLOWING SURGICAL TREATMENT OF PATELLAR TENDON RUPTURE
General Principles

To optimize function after patellar tendon repair, the rehabilitation protocol must balance soft tissue healing and the biomechanical principles of effective muscle strengthening and conditioning (Rehabilitation Protocols 60.1 and 60.2). Early joint mobilization and gradual application of force across the repair site progress to normalization of movement and quadriceps strengthening. Ideally, this is accomplished with a multiphase approach that incorporates functional rehabilitation activities aimed at allowing full daily activities and return to sports participation. Any rehabilitation program should be tailored to the individual patient, taking into consideration any comorbidities or behaviors (i.e., smoking, noncompliance) that negatively affect normal tissue healing. A "cookbook" approach to postoperative rehabilitation is discouraged because the timing of various rehabilitation milestones must be tempered by the ease with which the patient is able to progress from one phase to the next.

Termination of Rehabilitation

Rehabilitation can be discontinued when full ROM and strength of 85% to 90% of that of the contralateral side is obtained on isokinetic testing. Resumption of strenuous sporting activities is not allowed until a minimum of 4 to 6 months postoperatively. A full functional assessment, including the one-legged hop test and sports-specific functional activities, should be done before return to sports is allowed.

REHABILITATION PROTOCOL 60.1 ■ **Outline After Repair of Acute Unilateral Patellar Tendon Tear**

Matthew J. Matava, MD, Ryan T. Pitts, MD

Weeks 0–2
- Hinged knee immobilizer locked at 15 degrees flexion, braced in extension
- Touch-down weight bearing
- Quadriceps isometric exercises
- Upper body ergometer

Weeks 3–6
- Hinged knee immobilizer locked at 0 degrees of flexion
- Weight bearing as tolerated
- 0 to 45 degrees active flexion with passive extension (in brace)
- Active flexion range of motion (ROM) increased by 15 degrees each week
- Full ROM achieved by 6 weeks
- Quadriceps isometrics
- Upper body ergometer
- Stationary bike, no resistance

Weeks 7–8
- Hinged knee immobilizer discontinued
- Full weight bearing
- Quadriceps isometrics
- Open chain exercises
- Short arc quadriceps
- Straight leg raise

- Closed chain exercises
- Double-leg mini-squats
- Leg press
- Stationary bike, progressive resistance

Weeks 9–12
- Open chain exercises
- Closed chain exercises
- Isokinetics
- Stationary bike, progressive resistance
- Treadmill walking

Months 4–6
- Open chain exercises
- Closed chain exercises
- Isokinetics
- Stationary bike, progressive resistance
- Treadmill walking
- Jogging/running
- Sport-specific conditioning
- Plyometrics
- Slide board
- Running, sprinting, figures-of-eight
- Advanced isokinetics

REHABILITATION PROTOCOL 60.2 ■ **Repair of Acute Unilateral Patellar Rupture**

Matthew J. Matava, MD, Ryan T. Pitts, MD, Suzanne Zadra Schroeder, PT, ATC

Phase 1: Immobilization and Protection
Weeks 0–2
Bracing
- Hinged knee brace locked in full extension
- All activities, including exercises, are done in the brace. The brace can be removed for bathing and showering once surgical incision has healed.

Weight bearing
- Toe-touch weight bearing with axillary crutches and knee braced
- Placement of a heel lift in opposite shoe will facilitate swing phase of the involved leg during gait.
Modalities
- Ice, elevation, compression, and electrical stimulation for edema control

REHABILITATION PROTOCOL 60.2 ● **Repair of Acute Unilateral Patellar Rupture—cont'd**

Range of Motion
- 0 to 15 degrees of flexion

Therapeutic Exercise
- Gentle patellar mobilizations inferior to superior and medial to lateral
- Quadriceps isometrics emphasizing the vastus medialis obliquus; electrical stimulation may be used to facilitate a contraction
- Ankle pumps and gluteal isometrics
- Isometrics: Three sets of 10 repetitions, two times daily. Hold each repetition for 10 seconds. The focus of strengthening in this phase is for muscle re-education.
- Gentle hamstring and gastrocnemius–soleus stretching
- Upper body ergometry for aerobic fitness

Phase 2: Range of Motion and Light Strength

Weeks 3–6
Bracing
- Hinged knee brace open from 0 to 45 degrees of flexion
- Open brace starting at 0 to 60 degrees until the end of week 4; progress to 0 to 90 degrees by week 5 to 6

Weight bearing
- Progress to weight bearing as tolerated with brace locked in full extension.
- Progression to full weight bearing should be achieved by 6 weeks.
- May progress to one crutch on opposite side of involved leg as progressing toward full weight bearing
- Normalize gait pattern as full weight bearing is achieved.

Modalities
- Continue with modalities for edema control.
- Continue with electrical stimulation if needed for quad and vastus medialis obliquus re-education.

Range of Motion
- 0 to 45 degrees of active knee flexion in hinged knee brace with passive extension in brace. Full range of motion (ROM) should be achieved by 6 weeks with knee flexion increasing 15 degrees each week.
- ROM performed two to three times a day for 5 minutes
- Stationary bike with NO PEDAL RESISTANCE

Therapeutic Exercise
- Continue quadriceps and gluteal isometrics and patellar mobilizations.
- Ankle resistive exercises
- Open kinetic chain gluteus medius, gluteus maximus, and adductor strengthening
- Strength focus should be on longer contractions for endurance training.
- Gentle hamstring and gastrocnemius–soleus stretching
- Start closed kinetic chain strengthening at the end of 6 weeks.
- Upper body ergometry for aerobic conditioning
- Initiate balance and proprioceptive exercises in brace.

Phase 3: Progressive Strengthening

Weeks 7–12
Bracing
- Discontinue brace once good quadriceps control is obtained, the patient is able to perform a straight leg raise without an extension lag, and full ROM and a normal gait are achieved.

Weight bearing
- Full weight bearing should be achieved.

Modalities
- Continue with modalities as needed for edema control.

Range of Motion
- Joint ROM should be full; incorporate stretching of the hamstrings, hip flexors, quadriceps, hip rotators, iliotibial band, gastrocnemius and soleus, and prone hangs for knee extension.

Therapeutic Exercise
- Open kinetic chain straight leg raise with no extension lag and good vastus medialis obliquus contraction, gluteal strength, short-arc quadriceps, and hamstring curls from 0 to 90 degrees of flexion
- Closed kinetic chain wall squats not to go beyond 70 degrees of knee flexion; heel raises, leg press, terminal knee extension in standing, forward step-ups, and lateral step-ups
- Combine long holds and short holds for varied muscle fibers.

Phase 4: Advanced Strengthening and Functional Exercises

Weeks 12–16
Modalities
- Continue with ice if needed for pain and edema.

Range of Motion
- Continue stretching for any muscle imbalances. Make sure to check nonsurgical side and upper body for return to sport and activities of daily living.

Therapeutic Exercise
- Focus should be on balancing muscle strength for control of neutral alignment and beginning sports-specific and functional activity.
- Continue with open kinetic strengthening 2 days a week for correct muscle firing pattern and continue with core and upper body strengthening.
- Closed kinetic chain exercises should progress to squats away from the wall and proceed to single-leg squats with good control.
- Exercises incorporating the sports cord in forward and lateral directions and retro-walking
- Side-stepping (Fig. 60.5) and "monster walk" with Theraband around the ankles to increase the strength of hips
- Continue with leg press bilateral and unilateral, hamstring curls, and start leg extensions 0 to 30 degrees at 16 weeks.
- Proprioception and balance training with progression to a single leg
- Light agility drills
- Aquatic therapy if pool available
- Start pool running and transition to land running at the end of the phase. Running should be introduced gradually no more than three times per week. Allow 1 day for recovery. Start on a level surface and at a comfortable speed. Do not change more than one variable (i.e., speed, mileage, and surface) per week with running.
- Continue elliptical trainer and Stairmaster for endurance training.
- Isokinetic strengthening

Phase 5: Sports-Specific Drills and Plyometrics

Weeks 16–24
Modalities
- Ice as needed

Range of Motion
- Continue stretching as needed.

Therapeutic Exercise
- Focus on neutral alignment to decrease stress on knee.
- Basic open kinetic chain exercises for vastus medialis obliquus, straight leg raises, gluteus medius, and gluteus maximus for muscle memory; hamstring curls and leg extensions avoiding terminal knee extension
- Continue closed kinetic chain exercises: squats, leg press, Sport Cord and lunges not going beyond 70 degrees of knee flexion.
- Unilateral closed kinetic chain single-leg squats and balance progressing to an unstable surface (i.e., Bosu board, foam, or proprioceptive device)
- Triplanar strength with lunges and single-leg activity

Continued

REHABILITATION PROTOCOL 60.2 ■ Repair of Acute Unilateral Patellar Rupture—cont'd

- Advance agility drills.
- Advance running drills.
- Begin sprinting and progress to start cutting, quick changes of directions, start and stop activity, and figure-of-eights.
- Plyometrics: start with bilateral exercises and progress to unilateral strengthening. *Do not allow valgus stress on the knee.*

- Tailor exercise to meet demands of the sport(s).
- Sports-specific upper body and core strengthening
- Advanced multispeed isokinetics
- Transition to return to sport and emphasize the need to continue with a home exercise program to avoid re-injury.

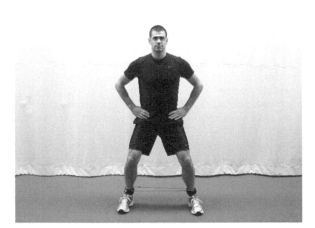

Fig. 60.5   Side-stepping.

REFERENCES

A complete reference list is available at https://expertconsult .inkling.com/.

FURTHER READING

Antich T, Brewster C. Modification of quadriceps femoris muscle exercises during knee rehabilitation. *Phys Ther.* 1986;66:1246–1251.

Aoki M, Ogiwara N, Ohata T, et al. Early active motion and weightbearing after cross-stitch Achilles tendon repair. *Am J Sports Med.* 1998;26:794–800.

Bonomo JJ, Krinick RM, Sporn AA. Rupture of the patellar ligament after use of its central third for anterior cruciate reconstruction: a report of two cases. *J Bone Joint Surg.* 1985;196A:253–255.

Burks RT, Delson RH. Allograft reconstruction of the patellar ligament: a case report. *J Bone Joint Surg.* 1994;76A:1077–1079.

Carroll TJ, Abernethy PJ, Logan PA, et al. Resistance training frequency: strength and myosin heavy chain responses to two and three bouts per week. *Eur J Appl Physiol.* 1998;78:270–275.

Cervellin M, De Girolamo L, Bait C, et al. Autologous platelet-rich plasma gel to reduce donor-site morbidity after patellar tendon graft harvesting for anterior cruciate ligament reconstruction: a randomized, controlled clinical study. *Knee Surg Sports Traumatol Arthrosc.* 2011;20.1: 114–120. Web.

Davies SG, Baudouin CJ, King JD, et al. Ultrasound, computed tomography and magnetic resonance imaging in patellar tendinitis. *Clin Radiol.* 1991;43:52–56.

Dervin GF, Taylor DE, Keene G. Effects of cold and compression dressings on early postoperative outcomes for the arthroscopic anterior cruciate ligament reconstruction patient. *J Orthop Sports Phys Ther.* 1998;27:403–406.

Diaz-Ledezma Claudio, Orozco Fabio R, Delasotta Lawrence A, et al. Extensor mechanism reconstruction with Achilles tendon allograft in TKA: results of an abbreviate rehabilitation protocol. *J Arthroplasty.* 2014;29.6:1211–1215. Web.

Ecker ML, Lotke PA, Glazer RM. Late reconstruction of the patellar tendon. *J Bone Joint Surg.* 1979;61A:884–886.

Emerson Jr RH, Head WC, Malinin TI. Reconstruction of patellar tendon rupture after total knee arthroplasty with an extensor mechanism allograft. *Clin Orthop.* 1990;260:154–161.

Evans PD, Pritchard GA, Jenkins DHR. Carbon fibre used in the late reconstruction of rupture of the extensor mechanism of the knee. *Injury.* 1987;18:57–60.

Gould III JA, Davies GJ, eds. *Orthop Sports Phys Ther.* St. Louis: Mosby; 1985.

Greenberger HB, Paterno MV. Relationship of knee extensor strength and hopping test performance in the assessment of lower extremity function. *J Orthop Sports Phys Ther.* 1995;22:202–206.

Hsu KY, Wang KC, Ho WP, et al. Traumatic patellar tendon ruptures: a follow-up study of primary repair and a neutralization wire. *J Trauma.* 1994;36:658–660.

Ismail AM, Balakrishnan R, Rajakumar MK. Rupture of patellar ligament after steroid infiltration: report of a case. *J Bone Joint Surg.* 1969;51B:503–505.

Jones D, Rutherford O. Human muscle strength training: the effects of three different regimes and the nature of the resultant changes. *J Physiol.* 1987;391:1–11.

Kannus P, Jozsa L. Histopathological changes preceding spontaneous rupture of a tendon: a controlled study of 891 patients. *J Bone Joint Surg.* 1991;73A:1507–1525.

Kennedy JC, Willis RB. The effects of local steroid injections on tendons: a biomechanical and microscopic correlative study. *Am J Sports Med.* 1976;4:11–21.

Magnussen RA, Demey G, Archbold P, Neyret P. Patellar tendon rupture. In: Bentley G, ed. *Eur Surg Orthop Traumatol.* Berlin, Germany: Springer; 2014:3019–3030.

McNair PJ, Marshall RN, Maguire K. Swelling of the knee joint: effects of exercise on quadriceps muscle strength. *Arch Phys Med Rehabil.* 1996;77: 896–899.

Mortensen NH, Skov O, Jensen PE. Early motion of the ankle after operative treatment of a rupture of the Achilles tendon. *J Bone Joint Surg.* 1999;81A:983–990.

Palmitier R, An K-N, Scott S, et al. Kinetic chain exercise in knee rehabilitation. *Sports Med.* 1991;11:402–413.

Rutherford O. Muscular coordination and strength training: implications for injury rehabilitation. *Sports Med.* 1998;5:196–202.

Siwek CW, Rao JP. Ruptures of the extensor mechanism of the knee joint. *J Bone Joint Surg.* 1981;63A:932–937.

Takai S, Woo S, Horibe S, et al. The effects of frequency and duration of controlled passive mobilization on tendon healing. *J Orthop Res.* 1991;9:705–713.

Tejwani NC, Lekic N, Bechtel C, et al. Outcomes after knee joint extensor mechanism disruptions. *J Orthop Trauma.* 2012;26.11:648–651. Web.

Tepperman PS, Mazliah J, Naumann S, et al. Effect of ankle position on isometric quadriceps strengthening. *Am J Phys Med.* 1986;65:69–74.

Vadalà A, Iorio R, Bonifazi AM, et al. Re-revision of a patellar tendon rupture in a young professional martial arts athlete. *J Orthopaed Traumatol.* 2011;13.3:167–170. Web.

Vergso J, Genuario S, Torg J. Maintenance of hamstring strength following knee surgery. *Med Sci Sports Exerc.* 1985;17:376–379.

Webb LX, Toby EB. Bilateral rupture of the patella tendon in an otherwise healthy male patient following minor trauma. *J Trauma.* 1986;26:1045–1048.

Wigerstad-Lossing, Grimby G, Jonsson T, et al. Effects of electrical stimulation combined with voluntary contractions after knee ligament surgery. *Med Sci Sports Exerc.* 1988;20:93–98.

Woo S, Maynard J, Butler D, et al. Ligament, tendon, and joint capsule insertions to bone. In: Woo SL-Y, Buckwalter JA, eds. *Injury and Repair of the Musculoskeletal Soft Tissues.* Park Ridge, Ill: American Academy of Orthopaedic Surgeons; 1988:133–166.

Yu JS, Petersilge C, Sartoris DJ, et al. MR imaging of injuries of the extensor mechanism of the knee. *Radiographics.* 1994;14:541–551.

61

Articular Cartilage Procedures of the Knee

G. Kelley Fitzgerald, PhD, PT | James J. Irrgang, PhD, PT, ATC

CLINICAL BACKGROUND

Designing successful rehabilitation programs after articular cartilage surgical procedures requires careful consideration of the healing process and a thorough understanding of the potential stresses applied to articular surfaces during therapeutic exercise. Although it is important to begin early rehabilitation to promote tissue healing and to restore joint motion, muscular strength, and functional capacity, rehabilitation procedures must be applied in a manner that does not interfere with or disrupt the healing articular lesion.

Cole et al. (2009) have developed a treatment algorithm for the treatment of focal articular lesions in the knee (Fig. 61.1).

TYPES OF MOTION

Evidence from animal studies suggests that early active and passive motion exercises after articular cartilage lesions can enhance the quality of tissue healing, limit the adverse effects of joint immobilization on the remaining healthy articular cartilage, and reduce the risk of adhesions. Complete immobilization is not recommended after surgical procedures that involve the articular cartilage.

However, the application of shear stress while the healing articular lesion is under compression may have adverse effects on the healing process. ROM exercises should be done in a controlled manner to avoid excessive shear loads while the joint is under compression. This can be accomplished by emphasizing passive, active-assisted, and unloaded-active ROM exercises in the early postoperative period (0 to 6 weeks).

MUSCLE STRENGTHENING

Muscle performance training is an essential component of postoperative rehabilitation after articular cartilage surgical procedures. Muscles need to be strong enough to assist in absorbing shock and dissipating loads across the joint. The resistance exercise program should be tailored to minimize shear loading across the lesion during the healing period. In general, exercises that have the potential for producing high shear stress coupled with compression, such as closed chain exercises, should be avoided in the early phases of rehabilitation.

We believe isometric exercises are the safest option for restoring muscle strength during early rehabilitation. Isometric quadriceps exercises in full knee extension may be effective in preventing or resolving a knee extensor lag, and most articular lesions will not be engaged with the knee in full extension. Isometric exercise at 90 degrees of flexion may also be a safe option

because it is unlikely to result in excessive compression or shear loads across most articular cartilage lesions. In addition, it has been shown that isometric quadriceps training at 90 degrees of flexion can result in increased muscle force production at other joint angles. Isometric exercises at angles between 20 and 75 degrees should be used with caution because most articular lesions would be engaged in this arc of motion. If open chain leg extension exercises are to be used, it is essential that the arc of motion is limited to ranges that do not engage the lesion. This requires effective communication between the surgeon and the therapist regarding ROM limitations for resistive exercises.

WEIGHT BEARING PROGRESSION

Progression of weight bearing and functional activities is a gradual process that begins in the intermediate phase of postoperative rehabilitation. The weightbearing status after surgery is dependent on the size, nature, and location of the lesion and the surgical procedure that has been used to treat it. Progression of weight bearing is also dependent on the resolution of joint motion and muscular strength impairments in the early rehabilitation period.

After arthroscopic débridement, patients are usually permitted to bear weight as tolerated with crutches. Weight bearing can be progressed as long as increased loading does not result in increased pain or effusion. Crutches can be discontinued when the patient has full passive knee extension and at least 100 degrees of knee flexion, can perform an SLR without an extensor lag, and can walk without pain or limp.

When patients have undergone abrasion arthroplasty, microfracture procedure (Fig. 61.2), fixation of an articular cartilage defect, or osteochondral graft (Fig. 61.3), weight bearing is usually delayed for 6 weeks to allow adequate initial healing of the lesion. Nonweight bearing or touch-down weight bearing with crutches is allowed in the immediate postoperative period. In some cases, depending on the location of the lesion or stability of fixation, partial weight bearing or weight bearing as tolerated with crutches may be permitted in conjunction with use of a rehabilitation brace locked in full knee extension. Progressive weight bearing is usually begun 6 weeks after surgery. At this time, fibrocartilage should have begun to fill in the articular defect, and an osteochondral graft or articular cartilage fragment should have united with adjacent subchondral bone. Crutches can be discontinued when the patient has full passive knee extension and at least 100 degrees of knee flexion, can perform an SLR without an extensor lag, can walk without an extensor lag, and can walk without pain or limp. Therapists should monitor patients for increases in pain or effusion during

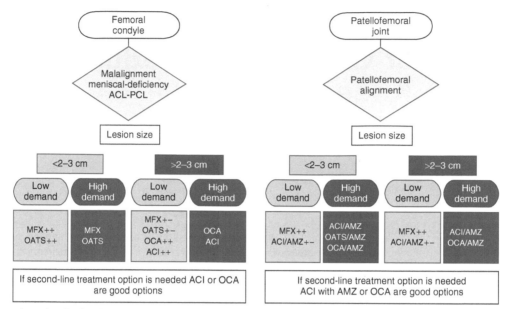

Fig. 61.1 Treatment algorithm for focal chondral lesions. Before treatment, it is important to assess the presence of correctable lesions. Surgical treatment should be considered for trochlear and patellar lesions only after use of rehabilitation programs has failed. The treatment decision is guided by the size and location of the defect, the patient's demands, and whether it is first- or second-line treatment. *ACL,* anterior cruciate ligament; *PCL,* posterior cruciate ligament; *MFX,* microfracture; *OATS,* osteochondral autograft transplantation; *ACI,* autologous chondrocyte implantation; *OCA,* osteochondral allograft; *AMZ,* anteromedialization; *++,* best treatment option; *+–,* possible option depending on patient's characteristics. (From Cole BJ, Pascual-Garrido C, Grumet RC. Surgical management of articular defects in the knee. *JBJS Am* 91:1778–1790, 2009, Fig. 1.)

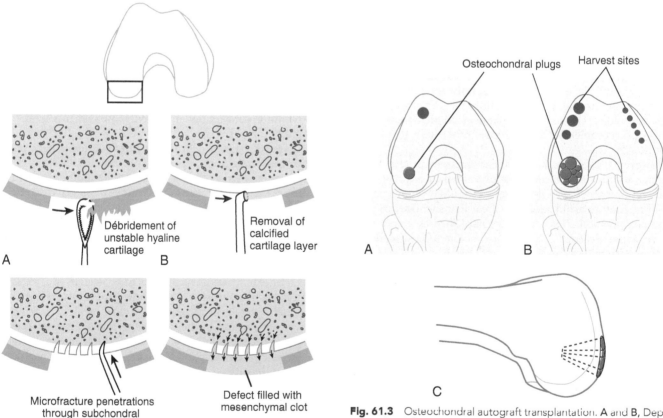

Fig. 61.2 Cartilage repair with the microfracture technique involves several steps, including débridement to a stable cartilage margin (*A*), careful removal of the calcified cartilage layer (*B*), and homogenous placement of microfracture penetrations within the cartilage defect (*C*), with resultant complete defect fill by well-anchored mesenchymal clot (*D*). (Redrawn with permission from Mithoefer K. Clinical efficacy of the microfracture technique for articular cartilage repair in the knee. *Am J Sports Med* 37(10):2053, 2009, Fig. 1.)

Fig. 61.3 Osteochondral autograft transplantation. **A** and **B**, Depending on the defect size, one or more multiple osteochondral plugs can be used to fill the defect. The plugs are often harvested from the intercondylar notch or from the margins of the lateral or medial condyles above the sulcus terminalis. **C**, This sagittal section shows how the osteochondral graft should be placed to fill the defect. (Redrawn from Mithoefer K. *Am J Sports Med* 37(10):2053 Fig 1, ©2009 Sage Publications.)

progressive weight bearing and reduce the progression if these iatrogenic effects arise.

The progression from protected weight bearing to full weight bearing can be facilitated by using techniques that gradually increase the load on the knee. Deweighting devices can be used for treadmill ambulation and running. Unloading of body weight by the deweighting device is increased to the point that allows performance of the activity without pain or gait abnormalities. The unloading is then gradually reduced over time until the patient can perform the activity in full weight bearing without pain. A pool can also be used to unload body weight for ambulation and running activities. These activities can be initiated in shoulder-deep water and then gradually progressed by decreasing the depth of the water.

Once the patient has progressed to pain-free full weight bearing, a variety of low-impact aerobic activities, such as walking, cycling, and use of step or cross-country ski machines, can be employed to improve local muscular and cardiovascular endurance. Returning to sports activities may not be possible for some patients, depending on the severity of joint damage. These patients should be counseled with respect to appropriate activity modifications. For patients who wish to return to recreational or sports activities, a functional retraining program involving agility training and sport-specific skill training should be incorporated into the program. These activities should be delayed until the patient can perform low-impact aerobic activities without recurrent pain or effusion. Agility and sport-specific skill training should be progressed gradually from 50% effort to full effort. The therapist should continue to monitor the patient for changes in pain and effusion as these activities are progressed.

IMPORTANT REHABILITATION CONSIDERATIONS

- The surgeon should include on the physical therapy referral form the type of surgical procedure, the location of the lesion, and restrictions in ROM during exercise. A diagram of the lesion site is also helpful. Therapists must adhere to the surgeon's ROM limitations so that the lesion is not engaged during exercise.
- Unloaded passive or active-assisted ROM exercises should begin as soon as possible after surgery. Closed chain exercises should be avoided in the first 6 weeks after surgery.
- Isometric exercises with the knee in full extension or 90 degrees of flexion should be emphasized for early strength training. Open chain exercises can be used in arcs of motion that do not engage the lesion.
- Protected weight bearing with the use of crutches, and in some cases a rehabilitation brace, should be incorporated in the first 6 weeks after surgery. Assistive devices can be discontinued when the patient has full knee extension and 100 degrees of knee flexion, can perform an SLR without an extensor lag, and can walk without pain or limp.
- Progression of weightbearing activities can be made easier by gradually increasing the load on the knee. This can be accomplished with the use of deweighting devices or doing pool activities. A gradual progression of agility and sport-specific skill training should be completed before the patient is allowed to return to full sports activity.

REHABILITATION PROTOCOL

Our articular cartilage rehabilitation protocol (Rehabilitation Protocol 61.1) is divided into three phases: early postoperative phase (0 to 6 weeks), intermediate phase (6 to 12 weeks), and return to activity phase (12 weeks and beyond). The time frames for these phases are only estimated guidelines. Progression to each phase depends on meeting criteria based on the type of surgical procedure, estimated periods of healing, restoration of joint mobility and strength, and potential recurrence of pain and joint effusion. Individual patients are able to progress at different intervals, and the surgeon and therapist are required to use their clinical judgments in determining when progression should be delayed or can be accelerated.

TROUBLESHOOTING TECHNIQUES AFTER ARTICULAR CARTILAGE PROCEDURES
Pain and Effusion With Exercise or Activity Progression

Monitoring of pain and effusion in response to exercise or activity progression is important to maintain a safe and effective rehabilitation process. Pain and effusion in response to exercise may indicate that the articular lesion is being harmed or the intensity of exercise is too rigorous. Therapists should reconsider the ROM restrictions that are being used and perhaps modify them to re-establish pain-free ranges. The frequency and duration of joint mobility exercise or the magnitude of loading during resistance exercises may also have to be reduced.

Recurrent pain and effusion that occur during progression of weight bearing or functional retraining activities indicate that the joint is not ready to progress to higher levels of activity. Progression of activity may need to be delayed in these circumstances.

Footwear and activity surface types should also be considered. Patients may need to obtain footwear that provides better cushioning or biomechanical foot orthotics to compensate for faulty foot mechanics. Activities may need to be begun on softer surfaces to acclimate to more rigorous ground reaction forces as higher activity levels are introduced.

Persistent effusion in the early postoperative period may result in quadriceps inhibition (reduced ability to voluntarily activate the quadriceps muscles). This can significantly retard progress with the rehabilitation program. Use of cold treatments, compression bandaging, limb elevation, and intermittent isometric contractions of the thigh and leg muscles may help resolve problems with effusion. If significant effusion persists more than 1 or 2 weeks after surgery, the therapist should notify the surgeon.

Quadriceps Inhibition or Persistent Knee Extensor Lag

Some patients may have difficulty with voluntary activation of the quadriceps muscles after surgery. This problem may be indicated by the inability to perform a full, sustained, isometric quadriceps contraction or the presence of a knee extensor lag on SLR. If patients exhibit this problem, they may not respond well to voluntary exercises alone. In addition, prolonged inability to actively achieve full knee extension may result in a knee flexion contracture that could, in turn, result in gait abnormalities and excessive loading of the knee during weightbearing activities. Other treatment adjuncts to enhance quadriceps muscle activation such as neuromuscular electrical stimulation or EMG biofeedback may need to be incorporated into the program. If these treatment adjuncts are administered, the intensity of the treatment stimulus should be great enough to produce a full, sustained contraction of the quadriceps as evidenced by superior glide of the patella during the quadriceps contraction. Superior glide of the patella is important to prevent patellar entrapment in the intercondylar groove, which may sometimes be a causative factor in knee extensor lags (Table 61.1).

TABLE 61.1	
Typical Findings in Common Knee Conditions Chapter Overview	

Acute Patellar Dislocation
Patient often reports "the knee shifted"
Tender over medial retinaculum (torn)
Usually a tense effusion (hemarthrosis)
Positive patellar apprehension test and increased lateral excursion on lateral glide test
May have an osteochondral fracture of patella or subluxed position of patella on sunrise view

Anterior Cruciate Ligament Tear
Acute injury
Rapid effusion (<2 hours)
Inability to continue play
Subjective instability
Positive Lachman test, pivot shift test
Positive anterior drawer sign (usual)

Baker's Cyst
Posterior mass in back of knee
May transilluminate
High incidence of associated intra-articular pathology (e.g., meniscal tear)

Iliotibial Band Syndrome
Lateral knee pain and tenderness over the iliotibial band
Runner
Training errors such as hill climbing, rapid progression (variable)
Pain on hill climbing, Stairmaster, or deep flexion exercises

Jumper's Knee
Pain at the patellar tendon
Tender on the palpation of the patellar tendon
History of repetitive jumping, running, or overuse syndrome

Medial Collateral Ligament Injury
Forced valgus mechanism (acute)
Medial pain and tenderness over medial collateral ligament
Minimal localized effusion (variable) over MCL
Pain or opening on valgus stress testing at 30 degrees of knee flexion with type 2 or 3 MCL injury

Meniscal Tears
True locking is almost pathognomic (locking also seen with a loose body)
Medial or lateral joint line pain and tenderness
Pain with twisting or deep knee flexion at joint line
Positive McMurray test
Locked knee or lack of extension if a large (bucket handle) tear
Apley compression test positive (variable)

Osgood-Schlatter Disease

Active, skeletally immature athlete
Tender tibial tubercle
Prominent tibial tubercle

Osteoarthritis
Insidious or gradual onset
Angular deformity (variable)
Effusion (variable)
Joint line narrowing on standing AP films
Tenderness and pain over affected joint lines
Osteophytes (variable)

Osteochondritis Dissecans
Vague, insidious onset of clicking, popping, locking, mild swelling
Radiographs (tunnel view) often reveal an OCD lesion
MRI useful to some degree for diagnosis and staging

Patellofemoral Syndrome (Anterior Knee Pain)
Anterior knee pain
Often bilateral
Exacerbated by activities that increase patellofemoral joint reaction forces (squatting, jumping, running, stair climbing)
Often underlying biomechanical changes (see patellofemoral section) such as increased Q-angle, patellar tilt, pes planus, patella alta
No mechanical symptoms or findings
Tender on patellar facet palpation, may have crepitance

Posterior Cruciate Ligament Tear
Abnormal posterior drawer test
Posterior cruciate ligament mechanism of injury (see section)
Effusion (variable)
Drop-back sign

Posterolateral Capsuloligamentous Injury
Dropback sign
Posterior Drawer sign positive
External rotation (Loomer) test positive
Often other ligament injuries associated

Prepatellar Bursitis (Housemaid's Knee)
Swollen, large bursa noted over anterior aspect of knee
Often a history of repetitive shearing force to anterior aspect of knee (repetitive kneeling on knee [e.g., carpet layer], etc.)
Aspiration of knee joint is negative—NO intra-articular effusion

Sinding-Larsen-Johansson Syndrome
Tender at inferior pole of patella
Radiographic changes noted at inferior pole of patella (traction apophysitis)
May have bump palpable at inferior pole of patella

REHABILITATION PROTOCOL 61.1 ■ After Articular Cartilage Procedures

G. Kelley Fitzgerald, PhD, PT, James J. Irrgang, PhD, PT, ATC

Early Postoperative Phase (0–6 Weeks)

	Joint Mobility	**Muscle Performance**	**Weight bearing**
Arthroscopic débridement	Passive and active-assisted ROM with no restrictions on ROM. Full knee extension should be obtained in 1 week and full flexion in 3 weeks.	Initiate training with isometric exercises. May progress to open chain resisted exercises* when tolerated. Closed chain resisted exercises† initiated when patient meets criteria for full weight bearing.	Weight bearing as tolerated with crutches until patient has full extension, 100 degrees of flexion, no knee extensor lag, and ambulates without pain or effusion. Initiate low-impact aerobic activities (walking program, stationary cycling, swimming) at 3 to 6 weeks, when patient meets full weightbearing status.
Abrasion arthroplasty, subchondral drilling, microfracture procedures	Passive and active-assisted ROM in pain-free range for 6 weeks. Full extension should be achieved in 1 week and full flexion in 3 weeks.	Isometric exercises in ROM that does not engage the lesion site. Open chain exercises with light resistance may be initiated at 4 to 6 weeks in ROM that does not engage lesion site. Avoid closed chain exercises.	Nonweight bearing or toe-touch weight bearing with crutches
Osteochondral grafts	Passive and active-assisted ROM in range restrictions that do not engage lesion site. Full knee extension should be obtained in 1 week and full flexion in 6 weeks.	Isometric exercises in ROM that does not engage the lesion site. Open chain exercises with light resistance may be initiated at 4 to 6 weeks in ROM that does not engage lesion site. Avoid closed chain exercises.	Nonweight bearing or toe-touch weight bearing with crutches
Osteotomy	Passive and active ROM exercises in pain-free ROM. Full knee extension should be achieved in 1 week and full flexion in 8 weeks.	Isometric exercises for 4 to 6 weeks. No open or closed chain resisted exercises for 4 to 6 weeks to avoid loading across the osteotomy site	Touch-down weight bearing for first 2 weeks, partial weight bearing 2 to 4 weeks, weight bearing as tolerated with crutches 4 to 8 weeks. Rehabilitation brace locked in full extension.

Intermediate Phase (6–12 weeks)

Arthroscopic débridement	Full motion should be achieved at this time. Continue with maintenance active ROM. Progress open and closed chain resistance exercises‡,§ as tolerated.	Agility‖ and sport-specific skill training initiated at 50% effort and progressed to full effort as tolerated. Initiate return to full activity when these activities do not induce recurrent pain or effusion.
Abrasion arthroplasty, subchondral drilling, microfracture procedures	Progress to full-range active ROM. Progress loading of resistive exercises. May initiate closed chain exercise when full weight bearing is achieved. Restrict to ranges that do not engage lesion site.	Discontinue use of crutches at 6 to 8 weeks when patient has achieved full knee extension, 100 degrees of flexion, and no extensor lag and can ambulate without pain or effusion. May use deweighting device¶ or pool activities in making transition to full weight bearing.
Osteochondral grafts	Progress to full-range active ROM. Progress loading of resistive exercises. May initiate closed chain exercise when full weight bearing is achieved. Restrict to ranges that do not engage lesion site.	Discontinue use of crutches at 6 to 8 weeks when patient has achieved full knee extension, 100 degrees of flexion, and no extensor lag and can ambulate without pain or effusion. May use deweighting device or pool activities in making transition to full weight bearing. Low-impact aerobic activities may be initiated when patient achieves full weightbearing status.
Osteotomy	Progress to full-range active ROM. Progress loading of resistive exercises. May initiate closed chain exercise when full weight bearing is achieved. Restrict to ranges that do not engage lesion site.	Discontinue rehabilitation brace. Progress to full weight bearing without crutches when patient has achieved full knee extension, 100 degrees of flexion, and no extensor lag and can ambulate without pain or effusion. May use deweighting device or pool activities in making transition to full weight bearing. Low-impact aerobic activities may be initiated when patient achieves full weightbearing status.

Continued

REHABILITATION PROTOCOL 61.1 ■ After Articular Cartilage Procedures—cont'd

Return to Activity Phase (12 Weeks and Beyond)

	Joint Mobility and Muscle Performance	Functional Retraining and Return to Activity
Arthroscopic débridement		Patients should have returned to full activity by this time period.
Abrasion arthroplasty, subchondral drilling, microfracture procedures	Continue with maintenance full active ROM exercise. Continue with progression of resistance for open and closed chain exercises as tolerated in ranges that do not engage lesion site.	Initiate agility and sport-specific skill training when tolerating low-impact aerobic activities without recurrent pain or effusion. Agility and sport-specific skill training should be initiated at 50% effort and progressed to full effort as tolerated. Running should be delayed until 6 months postsurgery. May initiate return to activity when tolerating running and agility and sport-specific skill training without recurrent pain or effusion.
Osteochondral grafts	Continue with maintenance full active ROM exercise. Continue with progression of resistance for open and closed chain exercises as tolerated in ranges that do not engage lesion site.	Initiate agility and sport-specific skill training when tolerating low-impact aerobic activities without recurrent pain or effusion. Agility and sport-specific skill training should be initiated at 50% effort and progressed to full effort as tolerated. Running should be delayed until 6 months postsurgery. May initiate return to activity when tolerating running and agility and sport-specific skill training without recurrent pain or effusion.
Osteotomy	Continue with maintenance full active ROM exercise. Continue with progression of resistance for open and closed chain exercises as tolerated in ranges that do not engage lesion site.	Initiate agility and sport-specific skill training when tolerating low-impact aerobic activities without recurrent pain or effusion. Agility and sport-specific skill training should be initiated at 50% effort and progressed to full effort as tolerated. Running should be delayed until 6 months postsurgery. May initiate return to activity when tolerating running and agility and sport-specific skill training without recurrent pain or effusion.

*Resisted open chain exercises refers to nonweightbearing leg extensions for quadriceps strengthening and leg curls for hamstring strengthening.
†Resisted closed chain exercises include leg press, partial range squats, wall slides, and step-ups.
‡Resisted open chain exercises refer to nonweightbearing leg extensions for quadriceps strengthening and leg curls for hamstring strengthening.
§Resisted closed chain exercises include leg press, partial range squats, wall slides, and step-ups.
‖Agility training includes activities such as side slides, cariocas, shuttle runs, cutting and pivoting drills, and figure-of-eight running.
¶A deweighting device is a pelvic harness that is suspended above the treadmill from a frame. Cables attached to the harness are connected to an electric motor that can be programmed to apply an upward-lifting load on the pelvis through the harness, which, in turn, will reduce the loading effect of the patient's body weight on the lower extremities while the patient is ambulating on the treadmill. The upward-lifting load is set high enough to allow performance of walking on the treadmill without reproducing the patient's pain. Treatment is progressed over several sessions by gradually reducing the upward-lifting load as tolerated by the patient, until the patient is able to ambulate in full weight bearing on the treadmill without pain.

REFERENCES

A complete reference list is available at https://expertconsult.inkling.com/.

FURTHER READING

Bandy WD, Hanten WP. Changes in torque and electromyographic activity of the quadriceps femoris muscles following isometric training. *Phys Ther.* 1993;73:455–465.

Bostrom. Fracture of the patella. A study of 422 patella fractures. *Acta Orthop Scand Suppl.* 1972;143:1–80.

Buckwalter J. Effects of early motion on healing musculoskeletal tissues. *Hand Clin.* 1996;12:13–24.

Filardo G, Kon E, Andriolo L, et al. Does patient sex influence cartilage surgery outcome? Analysis of results at 5-year follow-up in a large cohort of patients treated with matrix-assisted autologous chondrocyte transplantation. *The Am J Sports Med.* 2013;41.8:1827–1834. Web.

Houghton GR, Ackroyd CE. Sleeve fractures of the patella in children: a report of three cases. *J Bone Joint Surg Br.* 1979;61B(2):165–168.

Mithoefer K, Hambly K, Logerstedt D, et al. Current concepts for rehabilitation and return to sport after knee articular cartilage repair in the athlete. *J Orthop Sports Phys Ther.* 2012;42.3:254–273. Web.

Montgomery SR, Foster BD, Ngo SS, et al. Trends in the surgical treatment of articular cartilage defects of the knee in the United States. *Knee Surg Sports Traumatol Arthrosc.* 2014;22.9:2070–2075. Web.

Murray IR, Benke MT, Mandelbaum BR. Management of knee articular cartilage injuries in athletes: chondroprotection, chondrofacilitation, and resurfacing. *Knee Surg Sports Traumatol Arthrosc.* 2016;24(5):1617–1626.

Rosenberg TD, Paulos LE, Parker RD, et al. The forty-five-degree posteroanterior flexion weight bearing radiograph of the knee. *J Bone Joint Surg.* 1988;70A:1479–1483.

Salter RB, Minster R, Bell R, et al. Continuous passive motion and the repair of full-thickness articular cartilage defects: a 1-year follow-up [abstract]. *Trans Orthop Res Soc.* 1982;7:167.

Salter RB, Simmonds DF, Malcolm BW, et al. The biological effect of continuous passive motion on healing of full-thickness defects in articular cartilage: an experimental study in the rabbit. *J Bone Joint Surg.* 1980;62A:1232–1251.

Solheim E, Hegna J, Øyen J, et al. Osteochondral autografting (mosaicplasty) in articular cartilage defects in the knee: results at 5 to 9 years. *The Knee.* 2010;17.1:84–87. Web.

Suh J, Aroen A, Muzzonigro T, et al. Injury and repair of articular cartilage: related scientific issues. *Oper Tech Orthop.* 1997;7:270–278.

62

The Arthritic Knee

David A. James, PT, DPT, OCS, CSCS | Cullen M. Nigrini, MSPT, MEd, PT, ATC, LAT | Robert C. Manske, PT, DPT, MEd, SCS, ATC, CSCS | Alexander T. Caughran, MD

Osteoarthritis of the knee is a widespread health problem that affects more than 46 million people in the United States (Centers for Disease Control, 2006). As the population continues to age, this number will continue to rise to an estimated 67 million by 2030. The causes of OA of the knee are multiple and include aging (wear and tear), obesity, and previous knee trauma or surgery. Most often (80%) OA affects the medial compartment of the knee, and as the bone wears away medially a varus or "bow-legged" appearance develops. Much less frequently patients develop lateral compartment OA that results in a valgus or "knock-kneed" deformity. A small percentage of patients have rotatory deformities of the tibia that cause significant patellar maltracking or subluxation.

The most frequently cited cause of OA of the knee is older age, with the accumulation of years of wear-and-tear trauma on the joint, but other risk factors have been identified (see Box 62.1).

The diagnostic criteria for OA are not clearly defined, in part because of discordance between symptoms and radiologic evidence of OA. What appears on radiographs to be substantial OA may not create severe symptoms, whereas relatively mild OA on radiographs may produce disabling pain and stiffness (Bland and Cooper 1984, Dieppe et al. 1997, Felson. 2004, Hannan et al. 2000, Kellgren and Lawrence 1952, Lawrence et al. 1966, Lethbridge-Cejku et al. 1995, Scott et al. 1995, Szebenyi et al. 2006). The American College of Rheumatology lists six clinical criteria, three of which must be met, in addition to pain in the knee, for the diagnosis of OA of the knee:

- Age 50 years or older
- Morning stiffness lasting less than 30 minutes
- Crepitus with active motion
- Bony tenderness
- Bony enlargement
- No warmth to touch

When four laboratory criteria are added, five of the nine criteria must be met for the diagnosis to be made: ESR <40 mm/hour, rheumatoid factor (RF) <1:40, and synovial fluid signs of OA.

Other conditions in the knee can occur concomitantly with OA, including synovial irritation that causes synovial profusion and swelling; intra-articular subchondral bone sclerosis; and marginal osteophytes that lead to hypertrophic changes in the ends of the long bones, capsule, ligaments, tendons, and muscles. These secondary pathologies can be potent pain generators leading to disuse and progressive decline of physical function.

CLASSIFICATION

Arthritic deformities of the knee are classified as varus or valgus, with or without patellar involvement. Patellofemoral arthritis is common in an arthritic knee but seldom is the major source of symptoms. Articular surface damage is commonly classified according to severity: **minimal**, no radiologic narrowing is seen; **mild**, loss of one third of the joint space; **moderate,** two thirds of the joint space is narrowed; and **severe**, evidence of bone-on-bone contact.

DIAGNOSIS

Examination of the knee for arthritis can be done by moving the joint under a load (e.g., to examine medial compartment, a varus strain is applied to the knee and for the lateral compartment a valgus load is applied as the knee is moved through a ROM). Crepitus can be felt under the hand applying the varus or valgus strain and pain will be reproduced. Both collateral and cruciate ligaments should be examined. A slight increase in varus/valgus motion may be produced in a patient with a significant amount of joint space narrowing as the buttress effect of the meniscus and articular cartilage may be lost. The presence of any fixed flexion deformity (e.g., lack of passive extension of the knee) should be noted. The patellar position (central or subluxed) is important, as is the presence of a rotator deformity of the tibia. When the patient stands, any genu varum or valgum should be noted.

A thorough history and examination of the arthritic knee should obtain the following information:

1. Symptom location
   - Isolated (medial, lateral, or patellofemoral)
   - Diffuse
2. Type of symptoms
   - Swelling
   - Giving way, instability (ligament tear or weak quadriceps)
   - Diminished ROM
   - Mechanical (crepitance, locking, catching, pseudolocking)
3. Timing of onset
   - Acute
   - Insidious
4. Duration
5. Exacerbating factors
6. Prior intervention (e.g., NSAIDs, physical therapy, injections, or surgery) and the patient's response

RADIOGRAPHIC EVALUATION

For the standard patient with osteoarthritis of the knee, radiographic evaluation consists of four x-rays: an AP (anterior–posterior) weightbearing view, a PA (posterior–anterior) weightbearing view (taken with the knee in 30 degrees of flexion), a lateral view of the knee, as well as a merchant (or skyline) view of the knee to evaluate the patellofemoral joint. This helps to get an overall sense of the severity and location of the arthritis within the three compartments of the knee. In patients whose arthritis is located primarily in the lateral compartment

Bosomworth NJ. Exercise and knee osteoarthritis: benefit or hazard? *Can Fam Phys* 55:871–878, 2009.

BOX 62.1   CONTRIBUTION OF SPECIFIC RISK FACTORS TO THE DEVELOPMENT OF OSTEOARTHRITIS IN THE KNEE

Risk Factor	Contribution
Older age	Incidence increases with age
Female sex	Greater prevalence of OA in women
Obesity	Higher incidence of OA in patients who are obese
Osteoporosis	Associated with higher incidence and slower progression of OA
Occupation	Higher incidence of OA with repetitive squatting, kneeling, bending
Sports activities	Increased risk of OA with high-impact contact, torsional loads, and overuse
Previous trauma	Increase in OA in athletes postinjury
Muscle weakness/dysfunction	Increases in OA with inactivity, poor training, and injury
Proprioceptive deficit	Increases in OA with age, comorbid illness, and anterior cruciate ligament injury
Genetic factors	Neither preventable or modifiable—variable expression

of the knee, the so-called valgus knee, where the wear pattern is primarily on the posterior femur or tibia as opposed to the central wear seen in the varus knee, the AP view can underestimate the severity of the arthritis. The standing PA view is the best radiographic view to evaluate this wear pattern. Furthermore, if surgery is contemplated, a hip-to-ankle view can also be obtained to determine the overall mechanical alignment of the lower extremity and can also be useful in detecting any deformities or pathology of the joints above and below the knee (e.g., a valgus or varus deformity of the ankle, prior surgeries, or arthritic changes of the ankle/hip).

TREATMENT OPTIONS

Physical Therapy

Both manual therapy and exercise have been shown to be beneficial for those with knee OA. Studies by Deyle et al. (2000, 2005) have demonstrated a significant effect on pain and physical function with use of manual therapy in treatment of those with knee OA. Because knee OA may be partially caused by restrictions of periarticular mobility as a result of adhesions from repetitive bouts of inflammatory reagents, biomechanical forces at the joint level may be responsible for some of the pain and disease progression. Manual therapy may decrease restricted mobility, allowing increased excursion of these tissues and allowing reduced pain and stiffness. This reduction in pain may allow patients to participate more fully in therapeutic exercise programs such as those described here.

Currier et al. (2007) developed a clinical prediction rule that when followed appears to provide short-term relief in patients with knee pain and clinical evidence of knee OA. Patients with symptomatic knee OA may benefit from hip mobilizations if they have two or more of the following criteria: (1) hip or groin

pain or paresthesia, (2) anterior thigh pain, (3) passive knee flexion less than 122 degrees, (4) passive hip medial (internal) rotation less than 17 degrees, and (5) pain with hip distraction.

Furthermore, exercise has been shown to be effective in multiple studies in patients with OA (Baker et al. 2001; Fitzgerald and Oatis 2004; Deyle et al. 2005; Fransen et al. 2001, 2002; Petrella and Bartha 2001; Peloquin et al. 2002). Therapeutic exercises that have been proved to be beneficial include the following:

- Quadriceps sets
- Standing terminal knee extensions
- Seated leg presses
- Partial squats (not deep)
- Step-ups
- Flexibility and ROM exercises
- Calf, hamstring, and quadriceps stretching
- Knee flexion to extension
- Stationary biking

Systematic reviews and randomized clinical trials on the immediate effect of exercise on knee OA have demonstrated increased function and decreased pain (Baar et al. 1999, Rogind et al. 1998, O'Reilly et al. 1999), but at longer-term follow-up there appears to be a decline in effects over time (Baar et al. 2001). Therefore, a continued program or at minimum follow-up exercise sessions must be stressed to maintain positive results.

Quadriceps strengthening has been a mainstay of conservative treatment for knee OA because muscle weakness can lead to functional disability (Anderson and Felson 1988, Baker et al. 2004, Brandt et al. 1998, Fisher and Pendergast 1997, Slemenda et al. 1998, Wessel 1996). Very strong quadriceps can considerably delay the necessity for surgery. If the patella is painful, extension exercises should be carried out only over the last 20 degrees of extension. Activities such as deep squatting, kneeling, and stair climbing that increase the patellofemoral joint reaction forces (PFJRFs) increase pain. Those activities should be avoided.

Bosomworth (2009) found in a literature review that the best evidence suggests that exercise, at least at moderate levels, does not accelerate knee OA and running seems to be particularly safe. There might be an increased risk of OA with competitive sports participation, particularly when started early in life, although the presence of OA following this does not typically lead to an increased level of disability. Other problems may increase risk such as obesity, trauma, occupational stress, and lower extremity alignment problems.

Aerobic exercise may be beneficial because it not only increases cardiovascular endurance but also helps with weight control and reduction. Aerobic programs can also reduce pain and stiffness, improve and maintain balance, and increase walking speed and agility (Minor et al. 1989, Rogind et al. 1998). Both land-based and aquatic-based programs have been shown to be beneficial for those with knee OA (Wyatt et al. 2001). A randomized controlled trial (Hinman et al. 2007) found that patients who participated in aquatic physical therapy had less pain and joint stiffness and greater physical function, quality of life, and hip muscle strength than those who did not. The authors suggested several benefits over land-based physical therapy: buoyancy reduces loading across joints affected by pain and allows performance of closed-chain exercises that may be too difficult on land; water turbulence can be used as a method of increasing resistance; the percentage of body weight borne by the affected extremity can be increased or decreased by varying the depth of immersion; and the warmth and pressure of the water may further assist with pain relief, swelling reduction, and ease of movement.

Lin et al. (2009) compared nonweightbearing proprioceptive training and strength training in more than 100 patients with knee OA and found that both types significantly improved function: Proprioceptive training led to greater improvement in walking speed on spongy surfaces, while strength training resulted in a greater improvement in walking speed on stairs. They suggested that nonweightbearing exercise may be an option in individuals who are unable to exercise in a weightbearing position because of pain or other reasons.

Unloading Braces

Counterforce bracing can be used to "unload" the medial or lateral joint. Typically, these braces are custom made/fit to the patient to allow an intrinsic valgus or varus correction of several degrees that will allow small individual alterations to be made depending on symptoms. The brace, by applying an appropriate stress to the knee, may allow a partial restoration of the more "normal neutral" knee position that has been reduced by loss of articular cartilage and allow for the mechanical weightbearing axis to be transferred to the healthy compartment. Biomechanical studies have shown that pain, joint position sense, strength, and function can be altered by an unloading brace (Finger and Paulos 2002, Lindenfeld et al. 1997, Pollo et al. 2002, Self et al. 2000). More recently, Ramsey et al. (2007) determined that a brace in neutral alignment performs as well as or better than one that has a valgus alignment for those with medial compartment arthritis. They suggested that the symptom relief and improved function may actually be the result of diminished muscle co-contractions rather than from actual medial compartment unloading.

Insoles

Keating et al. (1993) found that of 85 patients with medial compartment arthritis in the knee, more than 75% had significant improvement in Hospital for Special Surgery pain scores at 12 months follow-up while using a lateral-wedge insole. By placing the calcaneus in a valgus position, a medial unloading may take place more proximal up the kinematic chain at the knee. Sasaki and Yasuda in two articles (Sasaki and Yasuda 1987, Yasuda and Sasaki 1987) both demonstrated reduced medial joint surface loading with the use of a lateral-wedge insole. For most, the cost effectiveness of a lateral-wedge insole is its greatest benefit.

Weight Loss

Weight loss may be an important adjunct to other therapies. Although the mechanism is not clearly understod yet, it seems empirically that people who are overweight or obese may have an increased risk for developing knee OA. Reduced body weight may help by reducing loads on weightbearing joints (Felson 1996, Felson et al. 1997, Messier et al. 2000, Toda et al. 1998) and improving overall physical function (Christensen et al. 2005). Recent evidence has shown that, although obesity may be a risk factor for incident knee OA, no overall relationship between obesity and the progression of knee OA coul d be found in a study of 5159 knees of patients who were overweight (Niu et al. 2009). Niu et al. (2009) found obesity not to be associated with OA progression in knees with varus alignment; however, it did increase the risk of progression in knees with neutral or valgus alignment. Therefore, location of OA may predicate effectiveness of weight loss in preventing progression of structural damage in OA knees. Weight loss alone may not be effective in those with varus alignment placing increased stress on the medial knee compartment.

Oral Therapy

Acetaminophen can be useful in the treatment of knee osteoarthritis. It provides an inflammatory effect and acts as an inhibitor of COX-1 and COX-2 in the central nervous system and has been shown to be significantly superior to placebo for pain relief (Towheed et al. 2006). It is among the safest of the oral analgesics but does carry a small risk for hepatic toxicity, although this is rare at doses of 4 g/day or less.

Oral NSAIDs are primarily effective in limiting pain by their capacity to reduce inflammation and nociceptor pain through COX-2 inhibition. Because of the risks of gastric and cardiovascular complications, these agents should be used at the lowest dose possible and for as short a time as possible.

Topical Agents

To avoid some of the side effects of oral therapy, topical agents have been recommended to apply analgesia to specific joints. Topical agents that have been used for OA of the knee include salicylates, capsaicin, and NSAID preparations. Salicylates have not been shown to be effective for pain relief in patients with OA. Capsaicin provides an analgesic effect by irritating the nerve endings, causing depletion of nociceptor pain transmitters. The primary side effect of capsaicin, which is derived from chili peppers, is a burning sensation for several days when first used. Studies of the use of capsaicin for relief of pain in OA have had mixed results, with some showing no benefit and others showing significant improvement in pain scores.

Diclofenac sodium gel (DSG), an NSAID topical agent, has been in use in Europe for many years but has only received U.S. Food and Drug Administration approval in the past 5 years. Some studies have reported effective pain relief for 2 to 3 months. Although benefits of topical agents have not been firmly established, given their limited systemic effects, they may be an attractive option for patients in whom oral NSAIDs are contraindicated, such as elderly patients and those with an increased risk of gastrointestinal irritability.

Intra-Articular Corticosteroid Injection

The primary action of intra-articular corticosteroid injection is anti-inflammatory. This treatment generally is recommended for moderate to severe pain when other methods, such as oral NSAIDs, have failed. A Cochrane review of corticosteroid injections for OA of the knee found benefit and limited side effects with short-term use. Because of the risk of a variety of side effects, corticosteroid injections should not be done more than four times a year.

Viscosupplementation

Viscosupplementation is a highly used palliative treatment for knee OA because of ease of application and theoretical ability to relieve symptoms by restoring and replenishing hyaluronate component into the knee joint. Multiple studies have demonstrated that these forms of treatment are clinically safe and suggest that this treatment may be effective for short-term symptom relief in patients with OA and may delay the need for total knee arthroplasty (Bellamy et al. 2006, Dagenais 2006, Divine et al. 2007, Conrozier and Chevalier 2008, Chevalier 2010); however, these positive findings may be a result of a robust placebo effect (Brockmeier and Shaffer 2006). Even if hyaluronate supplementation does partially restore intra-articular lubricating properties, it is not a form of treatment that is effective for those with severely damaged articular cartilage (Chen et al. 2005). In common practice, the viscosupplementation is reserved for those with mild to moderate arthritis.

The American Academy of Orthopaedic Surgeons (AAOS) released in 2013 a summation of the AAOS clinical practice guidelines, "Treatment of Osteoarthritis of the Knee, 2nd edition." In this body of work is contained all the current evidence-based treatment recommendations for nonoperative management of the arthritic knee. This can be found on their website: www.aaos.org/guidelines.

Operative Treatment

Arthroscopic débridement is of temporary if any value in arthritic knees, simply cleaning out the tags and meniscal tears and flushing from the joint fluid that contains pain-producing peptides. Cole and Harners' (1999) article on the evaluation and management of knee arthritis provides an excellent overview on arthroscopy in patients with knee arthritis.

Livesley et al. (1991) compared the results in 37 painful arthritic knees treated with arthroscopic lavage by one surgeon against those in 24 knees treated with physical therapy alone by a second surgeon. The results suggested that there was better pain relief in the lavage group at 1 year. Edelson et al. (1995) reported that lavage alone had good or excellent results in 86% of their patients at 1 year and in 81% at 2 years using the Hospital for Special Surgery scale.

Jackson and Rouse (1982) reported on the results of arthroscopic lavage alone versus lavage combined with débridement, with 3-year follow-up. Of the 65 patients treated with lavage alone, 80% had initial improvement, but only 45% maintained improvement at follow-up. Of the 137 patients treated with lavage plus débridement, 88% showed initial improvement and 68% maintained improvement at follow-up. Gibson et al. (1992) demonstrated no statistically significant improvement with either method, even in the short term.

Patients who present with flexion deformities associated with pain or discomfort and osteophyte formation around the tibial spines may benefit from osteophyte removal and notchplasty, as demonstrated by Puddu et al. (1994).

The true efficacy of lavage with or without débridement is controversial. More recent randomized controlled studies performed by Kirkley et al. (2008) and Moseley et al. (2002) found no benefit to arthroscopic lavage in patients with moderate to severe arthritis of the knee.

GENERAL CONSIDERATIONS

Operative treatment frequently is required for disabling knee pain, particularly in patients with post-traumatic knee OA. Reconstruction options include osteotomy, arthrodesis, and arthroplasty. In general, corrective osteotomy is done in younger patients with single-compartment degenerative change and angular malalignment. Osteotomy that corrects the angular malalignment also unloads the arthritic compartment and can delay disease progression and the need for total knee arthroplasty. Relative contraindications to osteotomy include tricompartmental arthritis, symptomatic patellofemoral degenerative changes, inflammatory arthritis, and age older than 60 years (Bedi and Haidukewych 2009). A downside to osteotomy is that changing the joint-line orientation with the osteotomy increases the technical difficulty of ensuing total knee arthroplasty.

For large, isolated traumatic lesions in young patients, fresh osteochondral allografting has been done in conjunction with the unloading osteotomy, with about 85% graft survival at 10 years (Ghazavi et al. 1997, Gross et al. 2005). Arthrodesis can be effective in relieving pain, but the functional limitations are substantial and ipsilateral back and hip pain may develop because of increased stress on these joints. Conversion of knee arthrodesis to total knee arthroplasty is difficult, has a high complication rate, and produces less than excellent outcomes.

Osteotomy of the Knee

Osteotomy of the knee is a mechanical load-shifting procedure. The mechanical axis of the knee is "shifted" from the worn compartment (usually medial) to the good compartment. **Closing wedge osteotomies** have an inherent disadvantage in that the tibiofibular joint must be disrupted with some degree of shortening and joint-line alteration. Because the joint line must remain "horizontal," in OA with a valgus deformity the osteotomy is done through the supracondylar region of the femur; for varus deformity it is done through the proximal tibia. Contraindications to tibial osteotomy include tricompartmental arthritis, severe patellofemoral disease, severely restricted ROM (loss of more than 15 to 20 degrees of extension or flexion less than 90 degrees), and inflammatory arthritis. There are very few contraindications to a varus osteotomy other than damage to the medial compartment. Outcome after a valgus osteotomy depends on the varus thrust force. This force, however, can be detected only by the use of a very sophisticated force plate analysis, of which there are very few available worldwide, and other indications must be used. Strength-to-weight ratio is extremely important, meaning that the older the patient and the heavier he or she is, the less the indication. A straight tibial diaphysis will result in an oblique joint line. A pagoda-shaped or sloping surface of the tibial plateaus usually produces a poor result. Lateral subluxation of the tibia on the femur and flexion contracture of more than 7 degrees also tends to produce a poor result.

No osteotomy will last indefinitely. Supracondylar femoral osteotomies do not interfere with subsequent total knee replacement because the osteotomy is done above the level of the collateral ligaments. Tibial osteotomy will produce an inferior result with a total knee replacement because the osteotomy is done inside the collateral ligaments and patellar tendons and may produce a patella baja deformity. Eventually, a total knee replacement will be required in these patients. For this reason, osteotomies are seldom done in the United States, although they remain moderately popular in many places in the world. New **"opening wedge"** techniques with Puddu plate type fixation are currently being evaluated. Their purported value is that the open wedge does not adversely affect the joint line in subsequent total knee replacement.

Total Knee Arthroplasty Rationale

When discussing primary total knee replacements in the United States, the major distinguishing feature from one operation to another is determined by whether the implant is cemented or not (cemented versus cementless) and whether the PCL is transected (posterior stabilized or PS knee, also known as cruciate substituting or CS knee) or retained (cruciate retaining or CR knee) (Fig. 62.1). Regardless of implant choice, the rehabilitation program is essentially the same. For cementless total knees, the rationale is that the initial fixation of noncemented femoral and tibial components is in general so good that loosening is uncommon. The tibia is largely loaded in compression. The stability achieved with pegs, screws, and stems on modern implants is now adequate to allow full weight bearing. However, if the bone is exquisitely soft, weight bearing may sometimes be delayed. The progression to weight bearing, therefore, must be based solely on the surgeon's discretion and intraoperative observations.

The guidelines for rehabilitation given here are general guidelines and should be tailored to individual patients. Concomitant osteotomies, intraoperative fracture, or significant structural bone grafting are indications for limited weight bearing until healing has been achieved. Similarly, if the bone is extremely osteoporotic, full weight bearing may be delayed until the peri-implant bone plate develops. Exposure problems requiring a tibial tubercle osteotomy or a quadriceps tendon division may require that straight leg raises be avoided until adequate healing has occurred, which typically takes 6 to 8 weeks.

Component design, fixation methods, bone quality, and operative techniques all affect perioperative rehabilitation. The implant choice no longer determines rehabilitation methods. It does not or should not make much difference whether the implant is unconstrained, semi-constrained, or fully constrained.

Postoperative return of 90 degrees of knee flexion is generally considered the minimal requirement for activities of daily living with an involvement of one knee. However, if both knees are replaced, it is essential that one knee reach more than 105 degrees of knee bend to allow the patient to rise from a normal low toilet seat. Furthermore, to descend stairs reciprocally, without hip or trunk substitution, requires 115 to 117 degrees of knee flexion.

Continuous passive motion (CPM) may be used after surgery, but there is a certain increase in wound problems with it. Furthermore, if the patient is left on it for long periods, a fixed flexion contracture of the knee tends to develop. If CPM is to be used, therefore, the patient must come off the machine for part of the day and work at achieving full extension. We limit aggressive or prolonged CPM use in patients with the potential for wound problems (such as those with diabetes or those who are obese).

Immediately after surgery, patients frequently have a flexion contracture because of hemarthrosis and irritation of the joint. These flexion contractures generally resolve with time and appropriate rehabilitation. However, patients who have been left with a fixed flexion contracture at the time of the surgery frequently are unable to achieve full extension. It is important, therefore, that full extension be achieved in the operating room.

Manipulation under anesthesia occasionally may be required. This is an individual decision on the part of the surgeon. Generally, it is preferable to carry out a full manipulation under anesthesia using muscle relaxant if the patient has not achieved greater than 70 degrees of flexion by 1 week. The usual area at which adhesions develop is the suprapatellar pouch. Many surgeons rarely perform any manipulations under anesthesia and believe that the patient will be able to work through the motion loss. Late manipulation under anesthesia (after 4 weeks) requires great force and can be associated with complications such as ligamentous rupture or periprosthetic fracture. Alternatively, arthroscopic lysis of adhesions in the suprapatellar pouch can be done with an arthroscopy obturator or a small periosteal elevator.

Reflex sympathetic dystrophy syndrome (RSDS) of the knee is uncommon after total knee replacement and is usually diagnosed late. The hallmarks are chronic pain that is present 24 hours a day and allodynia or skin tenderness. Such patients usually fail to achieve a reasonable ROM and usually also develop a flexion contracture. If this is suspected, a lumbar sympathetic block may be of not only diagnostic but also therapeutic value and should be carried out as soon as possible.

GOALS OF REHABILITATION AFTER TOTAL KNEE ARTHROPLASTY

- Prevent hazards of bed rest (e.g., DVT, PE, pressure ulcers).
- Assist with adequate and functional ROM:
  - Strengthen thigh musculature.
  - Assist patient in achieving functional independent activities of daily living.
- Achieve independent ambulation with an assistive device.

Perioperative Rehabilitation Considerations

Component design, fixation method, bone quality, and operative technique (osteotomy, extensor mechanism technique) will all affect perioperative rehabilitation. Implants can be posterior cruciate ligament (PCL)-sacrificing, PCL-sacrificing with substitution, or PCL-retaining. See the box for advantages and disadvantages of these component designs.

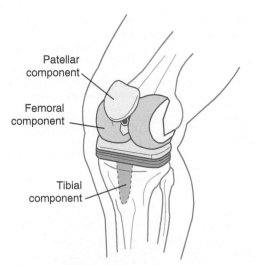

Patellar component

Femoral component

Tibial component

Fig. 62.1 Total knee arthroplasty.

Continuous Passive Motion

Data are conflicting regarding the long-term effects of CPM on ROM, DVT, PE, and pain relief. Several studies have shown a shorter period of hospitalization with the use of CPM by shortening the length of time required to achieve 90 degrees of flexion. However, an increased incidence of wound complications has also been reported. Reports vary on whether there is any long-term (1 year) improvement of postoperative flexion in patients using CPM versus those who do not. A 2003 Cochrane review (Milne et al.) of 14 trials found CPM combined with PT resulted in increased active knee flexion and decreased length of stay. CPM also related to a decreased need for postoperative manipulation, although CPM usage did not improve passive knee flexion and extension or active extension. They also note that, although CPMs are commonly included in the postoperative plan of care, protocols vary considerably. If specific physician instructions are not given, use the CPM for 4 to 6 hours per day with a limit of 40 degrees for the first 4 days postoperatively and progression of 10 degrees per day thereafter.

Transcutaneous oxygen tension of the skin near the incision for total knee replacement has been shown to decrease significantly after the knee is flexed more than 40 degrees. Therefore, a CPM rate of one cycle per minute and a maximal flexion limited to 40 degrees for the first 3 days is recommended.

If a CPM unit is used, the leg seldom comes out into full extension. Such a device must be removed several times a day so that the patient can work to prevent the development of a fixed flexion deformity.

Deep Vein Thrombosis Prophylaxis

The incidence of DVT after total knee arthroplasty is much higher than originally suspected. Based on clinical detection, the DVT rate after total knee arthroplasty ranges from 1% to 10%. However, more sensitive techniques (radioactive fibrinogen scans) have revealed a much higher incidence (50% to 70%). Prophylactic treatment is indicated.

Management of Rehabilitation Problems After Total Knee Arthroplasty

Recalcitrant Flexion Contracture (Difficulty Obtaining Full Knee Extension)

- Initiate backward walking.
- Perform passive extension with the patient lying prone with the knee off the table, with and without weight placed across the ankle. This should be avoided if contraindicated by the PCL status of the arthroplasty.

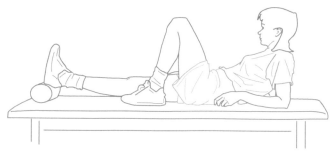

Fig. 62.2   Passive range of motion exercises for knee extension. The patient places a towel under the foot. Use a slow, sustained push with the hands downward on the quadriceps.

- Perform eccentric extension. The therapist passively extends the leg and then holds the leg as the patient attempts to lower it slowly.
- With the patient standing, flex and extend the involved knee. Sports cord or rubber bands can be used for resistance.
- Use electric stimulation and VMO biofeedback for muscle re-education if problem is active extension.
- Passive extension is also performed with a towel roll placed under the ankle and the patient pushing downward on the femur (or with weight on top of the femur) (Fig. 62.2).

Delayed Knee Flexion

- Passive stretching into flexion by therapist
- Wall slides for gravity assistance
- Stationary bicycle. If patient lacks enough motion to bicycle with saddle high, then begin cycling backward, then forward, until able to make a revolution. Typically, this can be done first in a backward fashion.

REFERENCES

A complete reference list is available at https://expertconsult.inkling.com/.

FURTHER READING

Brennan G, et al. Outpatient rehabilitation care process factors and clinical outcomes among patients discharged home following unilateral total knee arthroplasty. *J of Arthroplasty.* 2015;30:885–890.

Husain A, Gwo-Chin L. Establishing Realistic Patient expectations following Total Knee arthroplasty. *J Am Acad Ortho Surg.* 2015;23(12):707–713.

Jogi P, et al. Effectiveness of balance exercises in the acute post-operative phase following total hip and knee arthroplasty: a randomized clinical trial. *SAGE Open Medicine.* 2015:1–9.

Larsen K. Cost-effectiveness of Accelerated Periopererative Care and Rehabilitation After Total Hip and Knee Arthroplasty. *J Bone Joint Surg Am.* 2009;91:761–772.

Mahomed N, et al. Inpatient Compared with Home-based Rehabilitation Following Primary Unilateral Total Hip or Knee Replacement: a randomized controlled trial. *J Bone Joint Surg Am.* 2008;90:1673–1680.

Ong K, et al. Prevalence and Costs of Rehabilitation and Physical Therapy after Primary Total Joint Arthroplasty. *J of Arthroplasty.* 2015;30:1121–1126.

Total Knee Replacement Protocol

David A. James, PT, DPT, OCS, CSCS | Cullen M. Nigrini, MSPT, MEd, PT, ATC, LAT

Recent evidence indicates extensive variation in outcome measures used in clinical trials of knee and hip arthroplasty published since 2000. Riddle et al. (2009) found this heterogeneity led to confusion in attempts at conducting systematic reviews and applying evidence to clinical practice. More confusion is created when the available literature reports little difference in long-term outcomes between therapy, home exercise, and CPM groups. Minns-Lowe et al. (2007) in a meta-analysis found physiotherapy to result in short-term benefit following total knee arthroplasty, although differences were minimal after 1 year.

Because of the lack of a guiding consensus behind rehabilitation protocols, clinicians must continue to utilize their skills and apply their knowledge. Each patient must be given individual tasks based on individual goals. Valtonen et al. (2009) concluded that the major goals for musculoskeletal rehabilitation are to restore a person's mobility and functional capacity while preventing mobility disability. These authors felt that muscle power needed to be a focus of rehabilitation, finding significant power deficits in the postoperative limb in bilateral comparison 10 months after joint replacement. Strength should remain a focal point of rehabilitative activity, and the majority of patients benefit from strength training. Balance, mobility, coordination of movement, and gait should all be addressed also. Functional movement cannot be overlooked, and total body progression must take place for a patient to truly benefit from rehabilitation. Compensatory patterns developed while with pain and dysfunction can be identified and addressed after the pain of the arthritic knee has been treated. All of these factors must be adjusted for each patient depending on their progress, goals, and desired outcomes (Rehabilitation Protocol 63.1).

If patients are staying active longer, returning to activities will more often include return to sport. DeAndrade (1993) recommended return to sport by evaluating the demands of each sport. He concluded that high-impact sports such as jogging, racquetball, and tennis and jumping sports including basketball and volleyball should be avoided. More recently, the International Federation of Sports Medicine (www.FIMS.org) released a position statement on return to sport following joint replacement. They pointed out that joint implants have dramatically risen in popularity over the past 20 years and indications for the procedure have also expanded. Younger patients are undergoing total joint replacement and may have higher levels of desired activity following rehabilitation.

The group agreed with the general trend that lower-impact sports with cyclic performance and low-impact force are recommended. Evidence suggests that low-impact exercise can improve clinical outcomes. This position statement argues against automatic dismissal of return to high-impact sport. The group felt this should be evaluated on a case-by-case basis. They do note avoidance of forces that might result in luxation relative to the surgical technique and sports with increased injury rates. Seyler et al. (2006) agree there is conflicting advice for high-impact sport return and careful selection is needed, as are randomized controlled trials within this topic. Several considerations were identified by the FIMS to help determine the risks and rewards of return to a particular sport.

A patient's prior experience in his or her sport should play a major role in the decision. They also feel 6 months should have passed prior to resuming heavy activity and the patient should be systemically cleared for activity. Interaction with or evaluation by the patient's general physician, cardiologist, or internist can offer support in these areas. Radiologic evidence of proper axial alignment with no signs of loosening should also be confirmed. As far as contraindications, instability of the joint, loosening of the implant, and infection were listed. Relative contraindications were listed as prior revision of the endoprosthesis, muscular insufficiency, and obesity (body mass index >30). Table 63.1 lists the recommendations for return to sport as per the FIMS. Because of limited data on sport return, Healy et al. (2001) suggest physicians should provide information for the patient to evaluate the risk and then recommend appropriate athletic activities.

The literature does contain some sport-specific return-to-play data. Wylde et al. (2008) evaluated 2085 patients 1 to 3 years after total hip or total knee arthroplasty and found 61.4% returned to their sports including swimming, walking, and golf, whereas only 26% were unable to return as a result of the joint replacement. Jackson et al. (2009) reported on 151 golfers, finding 57% of patients who received total knee arthroplasty returned to golf 6 months postoperatively. Of these golfers, 81% noted less pain and were golfing as often as or more frequently than they were prior to the operative procedure. Of these golfers, 86% reported utilizing a golf cart, raising the question of desire versus ability to walk long distance.

Although objective discharge criteria following surgery exist and are listed in Rehabilitation Protocol 63.1, objective data should also be obtained. The Knee injury and Osteoarthritis Outcome Score (KOOS) has been validated in the literature as reliable, valid, and responsive (Roos and Toksvig-Larsen 2003). The KOOS was developed as an extension of the Western Ontario and McMasters Universities Osteoarthritis Index (WOMAC) and can be downloaded at http://www.koos.nu. The WOMAC is also a viable option, as are the Knee Society Score, Global Knee Scale, and standard forms such as the SF-36.

TABLE 63.1	Recommended, Recommended With Limitations, and Less Recommended Types of Sport After Total Joint Replacement of Hip, Knee, and Shoulder Joints		
Joints	**Recommended**	**Recommended With Limitations**	**Less Recommended**
Hip joint	Aerobics (without jumps)	Aerobics (without jumps)	Basketball
	Aqua jogging	Alpine skiing	Figure skating
	Ergometer training	Golf	Speed skating
	Individual gymnastics	Bowling	Soccer
	Bowling	Weight training	Gymnastics
	Cycling (saddle height)	Running/jogging	Handball
	Horse riding	Horse riding	Hockey
	Rowing	Cross-country skiing	Inline skating
	Darts	Tennis	Martial arts/combat sport
	Swimming	Table tennis	Rock climbing
	Dancing		Athletics (jumps)
	Walking/Nordic walking		Mountain biking
	Hiking		Squash
			Volleyball
Knee joint	Aerobics (without jumps)	Alpine skiing	Basketball
	Individual gymnastics	Weight training	Figure skating
	Bowling	Running/jogging	Speed skating
	Horse riding	Horse riding	Soccer
	Darts	Rowing	Handball
	Swimming	Cross-country skiing	Hockey
	Dancing	Tennis	Rock climbing
	Walking/Nordic walking	Golf	Squash
	Hiking		Volleyball
Shoulder	Aqua jogging	Alpine skiing	Basketball
	Individual gymnastics	Golf	Figure skating
	Running/jogging	Weight training	Speed skating
	Cycling	Running/jogging	Soccer
	Horse riding	Horse riding	Handball
	Walking/Nordic walking	Rowing	Hockey
	Hiking	Swimming	Martial arts/combat sports
			Rock climbing
			Mountain biking
			Squash
			Volleyball

From *Int Sport Med J* 9(1):39–43, 2008, http://www.ismj.com.

REHABILITATION PROTOCOL 63.1A ● Total Knee Replacement Exercise

Overall patient health, age, prior level of function, and patient progress may change.

Preoperative (>3 Weeks Prior to Surgery)

- Patient education on the surgical procedure/process and expected outcome.
- Introduction to the acute postoperative exercise program.
- Assessment of the patient's living situation and addressing possible needs.
  - Direct visit(s) are favorable, but pamphlets/literature can be created in lieu of or in addition.

Postoperative Acute (Days 1–5 or Discharge to Rehabilitation Unit/Home)

Acute/Inpatient Rehabilitation Care and Home Exercise Preparation

- Numeric pain rating scale pretreatment and post-treatment (0–10).
- Rest.
- Ice ± Cryotherapy device.
- Compression.

- Elevation ± continuous passive motion (CPM) with daily flexion increases to 40 degrees until day 4, then as tolerated.
- Review of weightbearing status (based on physician-specific guidelines).
- Monitor for changing/worsening symptoms affecting but not limited to circulation, sensation, and cardinal signs of infection.
- Visual inspection of wound and review of wound precautions.
- Bedside exercises (to be initiated 2–4 hours postoperatively).
  - Ankle pumps.
  - Quadriceps sets, progression to straight leg raise if extension lag absent.
  - Gluteal max sets (isometric hip extensions) unilateral and bilateral.
  - Heel slides (PROM → active-assisted ROM → active ROM as tolerated).
  - Adjust level of assist as tolerated by patient pain and able cognition.
  - Terminal knee extensions with pillow or small bolster.
  - CPM as directed on discharge from facility or after day 4: 4–6 hours per day and 10-degree increase daily if no specific instruction.

REHABILITATION PROTOCOL 63.1A ■ **Total Knee Replacement Exercise—cont'd**

- Goal of independence with home exercise program with handout provided.

Range of Motion Guidelines

- A minimum of 60 to 90 degrees of flexion should be established.
  - Goal of 0 to 90 degrees active-assisted ROM for discharge.

Gait Restoration and Training

- Gait training with appropriate assistive device.
  - Goal of ambulation ×150 feet with a rolling walker.

Transfer and Mobility Training to Ensure Patient Safety

- Bed mobility.
  - Assistance with involved lower extremity from person, gait belt, etc.
- Gait and transfer training with utilization of assistive devices.
  - Sit ↔ stand.
  - Toilet transfers.
  - Rolling walker instructions.
  - Goal of independence with transfers alone or with caregiver and minimally assisted to modified independence with stairs as needed for home environment using assisted device and/or caregiver.

Postoperative Weeks 1–4

- Focus on full-extension restoration, gait normalization, and flexion increases.
- Progress from 90 to 120 degrees of flexion.
- Progress to independent function with activities of daily living.
- Eliminate need for assisted devices and restore gait pattern to safety and tolerance.
- Functional transfer training (such as sit to/from stand, toilet transfers, bed mobility).
- Stretching hamstrings, gastroc–soleus, iliotibial band/tensor fascia lata, and general lower extremity.
- Improve balance.
- Progress ambulation tolerance and distance.
- RICE as needed.
- Ready patient for outpatient rehabilitation.
- Focus on full-extension restoration, gait normalization, and flexion increases.
  - Restore quadriceps and gluteal max neuromuscular control.
  - Quad sets/straight leg raises.
  - Gluteal sets.
  - Progress supine hook-lying gluteus max from isometric to bridging.
  - Range of motion, circulation active-assisted ROM—active ROM exercises in seated or supine.
  - Recumbent bike.
  - Portable lower-body ergometer (LBE).
  - Heel slides with assistance and/or friction reduction.
  - Continued bedside exercises for HEP.
- Low-load long duration extension restoration.
- Standing terminal knee extension with Theraband exercises for active ROM, active-assistive ROM, and terminal knee extension.

- Hip AROM standing or supine abduction/adduction.
- Gluteal medius/external rotator progression (i.e., clam shells [see Fig. 49.10]).
- Isometrics.
- Strengthening exercises (e.g., ankle pumps, heel slides, straight leg raises, and isometric hip adduction).

Postoperative Weeks 4–12

- Gait restoration.
  - Unilateral treadmill with uninvolved leg and bilateral upper extremity support.
  - Closed kinetic chain gait NMR involved leg heel strike ↔ Toe-off UE support as needed.
  - Parallel bars.
- Progression of ROM and strengthening exercises to the patient's tolerance.
  - Bridging with progression to unilateral or unstable surface (physioball).
  - Quad sets/straight leg raises with neuromuscular electrical stimulation ± biofeedback for NMR.
  - Short-arc quadriceps.
  - Terminal knee extension (both directions).
  - Isometric open kinetic chain extension at 90 degrees with submaximal contraction and no pain.
  - Progress hip abduction/adduction strengthening exercises.
  - Proprioceptive neuromuscular facilitation patterns of the hip with Theraband or manual resistance.
- Progression of ambulation on level surfaces and stairs (if applicable) with the least restrictive device or independent.
- Progression of activities of daily living (ADLs) training.
- Progress balance training.
  - Adding external factors as performance improves.
  - Perturbation, vector pull with sport cord, unstable surfaces, upper extremity involvement, etc.
- Progress lateral movement.
  - Again utilizing external factors to progress rather than adding weight.
- Progress to functional activities if return to sport is desired and with MD clearance.
  - Work with components of sport.
  - Upper extremity movement with club/racket with lower extremity on unstable surface, etc.
  - Work with low-velocity and short arc/isometric movements, progress.

Weeks 12 and Beyond

- Determine exercise progression and discharge plan based on patient status.
  - Age, desired level of activity, ROM and strength, MD clearance.
  - Patient may be readied for discharge to home exercises program or fitness/wellness program.
  - Patient may be in need of sport-specific training to ensure gradual return.

REHABILITATION PROTOCOL 63.1B ■ Total Knee Arthroplasty

Mintken et al.

Inpatient Rehabilitation Exercise Program

Postoperative Day 1

- Bedside exercise: ankle pumps, quadriceps sets, gluteal sets, hip abduction (supine), short-arc quads, straight leg raise (if able).
- Knee range of motion (ROM): heel slides.
- Bed mobility and transfer training (bed to/from chair).

Postoperative Day 2

- Exercise for active ROM, active-assisted ROM, and terminal knee extension.
- Strengthening exercises (e.g., ankle pumps, quadriceps sets, gluteal sets, heel slides, short-arc quads, straight leg raise, supine hip abduction), 1 to 3 sets of 10 repetitions for all strengthening exercises, twice per day.
- Gait training with assistive device on level surfaces and functional transfer training (e.g., sit to/from stand, toilet transfers, bed mobility).

Postoperative Days 3–5 (or on discharge to rehabilitation unit)

- Progression of ROM with active-assisted exercises and manual stretching, as necessary.
- Progression of strengthening exercises to the patient's tolerance, 1 to 3 sets of 10 repetitions for all strengthening exercises, twice per day.
- Progression of ambulation distance and stair training (if applicable) with the least restrictive assistive device.
- Progression of activities-of-daily-living training for discharge to home.

Outpatient Rehabilitation Exercise Program

Range of Motion

- Exercise bike (10–15 min), to be started with forward and backward pedaling with no resistance until enough ROM for full revolution.
  - Progression: lower seat height to produce a stretch with each revolution.
- Active-assisted ROM for knee flexion, sitting or supine, using other lower extremity to assist.
- Knee extension stretch with manual pressure (in clinic) or weights (at home).
- Patellar mobilization as needed.

Strength

- Quad sets, straight leg raises (without knee extension lag), hip abduction (side-lying), hamstring curls (standing), sitting knee extension, terminal knee extensions from 45 degrees to 0 degrees, step-ups (5- to 15-cm block), wall slides to 45-degree knee flexion, 1–3 sets of 10 repetitions for all strengthening exercises.
- Criteria for progression: exercises are to be progressed (e.g., weights, step height, etc.) only when the patient can complete the exercise and maintain control through 3 sets of 10 repetitions.

Pain Swelling

- Ice and compression as needed.

Incision Mobility

- Soft tissue mobilization until incision moves freely over subcutaneous tissue.

Functional Activities

- Ambulation training with assistive device, as appropriate, with emphasis on heel strike, push-off at toe-off, and normal knee joint excursions.
- Emphasis on heel strike, push-off and toe-off, and normal knee joint excursions when able to walk without assistive device.
- Stair ascending and descending step over step when patient has sufficient concentric/eccentric strength.

Cardiovascular Exercise

- 5 min of upper body ergometer until able to pedal full revolutions on exercise bicycle, then exercise bicycle.
  - Progression: duration of exercise progressed up to 10–15 min as patient improves endurance; increase resistance as tolerated.

Monitoring Vital Signs

- Blood pressure and heart rate monitored at initial evaluation and as appropriate.

Mintken PE, Carpenter KJ, Eckhoff D, Kohrt WM, Stevens JE. Early Neuromuscular Electrical Stimulation to Optimize Quadriceps Function After TKA: A Case Report, *J Orthop Sports Phys Ther* 37:364-371, 2007.

REFERENCES

A complete reference list is available at https://expertconsult.inkling.com/.

FURTHER READING

Brennan G, et al. 2015 Outpatient rehabilitation care process factors and clinical outcomes among patients discharged home following unilateral total knee arthroplasty. *J of Arthroplasty.* 2015;30:885–890.

Husain A, Gwo-Chin L. Establishing realistic patient expectations following total knee arthroplasty. *J Am Acad Ortho Surg.* 2015;23(12):707–713.

Jogi P, et al. Effectiveness of balance exercises in the acute post-operative phase following total hip and knee arthroplasty: a randomized clinical trial. *SAGE Open Med.* 2015;1:1–9.

Larsen K. Cost-effectiveness of accelerated periopererative care and rehabilitation after total hip and knee arthroplasty. *J Bone Joint Surg Am.* 2009;91:761–772.

Mahomed N, et al. Inpatient compared with home-based rehabilitation following primary unilateral total hip or knee replacement: a randomized controlled trial. *J Bone Joint Surg Am.* 2008;90:1673–1680.

Ong K, et al. Prevalence and costs of rehabilitation and physical therapy after primary total joint arthroplasty. *J Arthroplasty.* 2015;30:1121–1126.

Hip Injuries

64

Hip Injuries

Erik P. Meira, PT, SCS, CSCS | Mark Wagner, MD | Jason Brumitt, PT, PhD, ATC, CSCS

Effective rehabilitation of the hip joint begins with proper diagnosis. Advances in magnetic resonance imaging technology and hip arthroscopy have greatly improved and refined the diagnosis of hip pathology in recent years. The use of these diagnostic tools has increased the understanding of the hip joint and provided insight into the underlying pathology of many types of hip joint dysfunction.

Pathology around the hip can be classified into three groups: **intra-articular, extra-articular, and hip mimickers** (Table 64.1). Intra-articular pathology includes injuries to the hip joint itself. These include more global diagnoses such as osteoarthritis, avascular necrosis, and femoroacetabular impingement (FAI) and more focal diagnoses such as acetabular labral tears, chondral defects, and ligamentum teres tears. Extra-articular pathology includes injuries to structures around the hip such as internal and external coxa saltans, gluteus medius tears, and muscle strains. Hip mimickers include injuries to more remote regions that refer pain into the region of the hip such as athletic pubalgia, osteitis pubis, or lumbar radiculopathy.

TREATMENT OF INTRA-ARTICULAR HIP PATHOLOGY

Treatment of intra-articular pathology often requires surgical management. As with most synovial joints, blood supply to many structures inside the hip is limited, which limits the success of conservative management. Surgical procedures to the hip can be performed open or, more recently, arthroscopically. Postoperative rehabilitation is guided by the specific healing considerations of the structures involved, motivation of the patient, and ultimate goals for final level of function.

Nonsurgical management of intra-articular pathology begins with an attempt to protect the damaged structures and reduce the acute symptoms. As with other acute orthopedic injuries, the use of rest, ice, compression, and elevation is indicated. As symptoms become controlled, gentle exercises are begun to attempt to restore strength and ROM to the area. The patient is then progressed as tolerated through exercises and activities increasing in intensity similar to the postoperative protocol. After initial control of the symptoms has been achieved, many patients with minor pathology are content to limit their higher intensity activities, thereby minimizing their symptoms. Patients with frequent continued exacerbations of symptoms from more severe pathology or higher intensity activities of daily living (such as patients involved in athletics) often require surgical correction to achieve acceptable outcomes.

HIP ARTHROSCOPY

Although first introduced in 1931, hip arthroscopy was not embraced as much as similar procedures in the knee and shoulder in North America until recently. Anatomically the femoral head is deeply recessed into the acetabulum. The thick fibrocapsular tissue surrounding the hip joint limits the amount of distension allowed for arthroscopy, making the available working space restricted. Many diagnoses being treated with arthroscopy today were not originally treated with open procedures in the past. Surgical arthrotomy of the hip was reserved more for advanced disease states, whereas minor pathology was often undiagnosed and untreated.

Currently hip arthroscopy is a useful option for treating many of these previously untreated pathologies such as acetabular labral tears, ligamentum teres tears, FAI, and focal chondral pathology. Because many recent studies have shown that the presence of osteoarthritis in the hip joint is inversely related to successful outcome, this should be taken into consideration when evaluating for surgical intervention.

There are five main categories of arthroscopic procedures in the hip: repair, débridement, osteoplasty, capsular modification, and microfracture (Table 64.2). Repair procedures most often involve the anchoring of a detached acetabular labrum. Débridement of loose tissue that cannot be repaired such as fraying of the acetabular labrum, tears of the ligamentum teres, or chondral defects is often sufficient for symptom relief. In cases of FAI, osteoplasty of the femoral head (cam deformity) and/or the acetabular rim (pincer deformity) must be performed to correct the impingement and subsequent labral damage caused by the deformity. Patients with reported instability often undergo capsular modification to provide increased stability to the joint. Microfracture is often done to minimize the future progression of a chondral defect into more advanced osteoarthritis.

TABLE 64.1	Potential Causes of Groin/Hip Pain in Athletes	
Intra-Articular	**Extra-Articular**	**Hip Mimickers**
Acetabular labral tears	Internal coxa saltans	Athletic pubalgia (sports hernia)
Ligamentum teres tears	External coxa saltans	Osteitis pubis
Femoroacetabular impingement	Gluteal tears	Genitourinary disorders
Chondral defects	Muscle strains	Intra-abdominal disorders
Osteoarthritis	Piriformis syndrome	Lumbar radiculopathy
Osteonecrosis	Slipped capital femoral epiphysis	
Dysplasia	Fractures	

POSTOPERATIVE REHABILITATION FOLLOWING HIP ARTHROSCOPY

Although there are many different procedures performed arthroscopically in the hip, the postoperative rehabilitation for each is similar. There is little description of postoperative rehabilitation following hip arthroscopy, but most accepted protocols include a **protective phase, strengthening phase, and return to functional baseline phase** (Table 64.3). In cases of multiple procedures, precautions of the most restrictive procedure performed should be followed.

TABLE 64.2	Hip Arthroscopy Procedures and Specific Guidelines
Procedure	**Specific Guidelines**
Labral repair	Tolerable range of motion only for first 2 weeks
	Limit hip flexor activity for first 4 weeks
	Weight bearing as tolerated
	No impact (running) for at least 12 weeks
Débridement	Tolerable range of motion only for first 2 weeks
	Weight bearing as tolerated
	Progress all activity as tolerated (no specific time restrictions)
Osteoplasty	Tolerable range of motion only for first 2 weeks
	Limit hip flexor activity for first 4 weeks
	20 pounds partial weight bearing progressing to weight bearing as tolerated at 4 to 6 weeks
	Progress activity as tolerated after 6 weeks
Capsular modification	Tolerable range of motion only for first 2 weeks
	Limit extension and external rotation range of motion for first 4 weeks
	Weight bearing as tolerated
	No impact (running) for at least 12 weeks
Microfracture	Tolerable range of motion only for first 2 weeks
	Limit hip flexor activity for first 4 weeks
	20 pounds partial weight bearing progressing to weight bearing as tolerated at 4 to 6 weeks
	No impact (running) for at least 12 to 16 weeks

Protective Phase

In each case, the initial phase involves significant protection of the joint during the first 2 weeks after surgery. During this phase, ROM is progressed only as tolerated to avoid exacerbating the joint. After capsular modification, forced extension and external rotation are avoided for the first 4 weeks to protect the capsule. Activation of the hip flexors is discouraged during this phase as this causes increased pressure to the hip joint and may also exacerbate any postoperative irritation.

Weight bearing precautions vary depending on the specific procedure performed. After simple débridement or labral repair, weight bearing is as tolerated. Because the acetabular labrum is not a weight bearing structure, the use of crutches is discontinued when the patient is able to ambulate pain free without any significant gait deviation. When femoral osteoplasty is performed to correct for FAI, patients begin with partial weight bearing of 20 pounds, progressing to weight bearing as tolerated at 4 to 6 weeks. This is to protect the modified femoral neck from possible fracture while still providing enough load to optimize bone formation during healing. This is also true for microfracture procedures in the hip. Because of the better distribution of loads across the spherical femoral head compared to the flatter load-bearing surfaces of the knee, microfracture procedures of the hip tend to progress faster than those performed at the knee.

Isometric strengthening exercises in all directions except flexion can be performed immediately after surgery. These include isometrics such as gluteal squeezes, adduction isometrics against a ball (Fig. 64.1), and prone heel squeezes (Fig. 64.2). Gentle ROM exercise can be begun on a stationary bicycle as tolerated after surgery. To avoid excessive hip flexion the bike should be an upright model instead of semi- or full recumbent and the seat should be higher than normal for the first 2 weeks after surgery. After 2 weeks, the seat can be lowered into a normal position and the patient can begin progressing the duration of the workout as tolerated, usually in 5-minute increments. Active ROM exercises may also begin at 2 weeks (Fig. 64.3).

Strengthening Phase

Typically between 4 and 6 weeks after surgery the patient has achieved full ROM and is now permitted to apply full body weight to the involved lower extremity. Patients should be

TABLE 64.3	Postoperative Phases of Hip Arthroscopy: Suggested Intervention and Goals	
Phase	**Intervention**	**Goals to Progress to Next Phase**
Protective	Gentle passive range of motion (first 2 weeks)	Minimize postsurgical inflammation
	Isometrics (first 2 weeks)	Full range of motion
	Active range of motion (after 2 weeks)	Ambulating without assistive device
	Stationary bicycle (elevated seat height for first 2 weeks)	
	Manual therapy and modalities as indicated	
	Assistive device as indicated	
Strengthening	Stretching as indicated	No increased symptoms with current activities
	Progress to elliptical and pool activities	
	Closed kinetic chain exercises progressing from double leg to single leg; increasing intensity	Balance within normal limits
		Lower extremity strength within 80% uninvolved side
Return to functional baseline	Continue strengthening activities	Single-leg hop distance within 80% of uninvolved side
	Progress to running as tolerated	
	Cutting and other sport-specific activities	Return to baseline activities without increased symptoms
	Progress from double-leg jump to single-leg hop as tolerated	

progressed from activities such as the exercise bicycle to more weight bearing training. Elliptical training is useful in this phase because it adds a weight bearing component while still minimizing impact forces. Patients may also progress through higher intensity swimming workouts as tolerated. After procedures involving tissue repairs, impact activities should be avoided for at least 12 weeks to avoid excessive load to the still-healing structures.

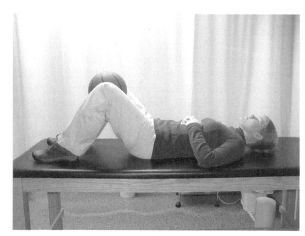

Fig. 64.1   Isometric adduction against a ball.

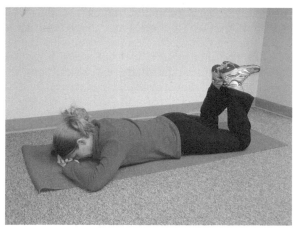

Fig. 64.2   Prone heel squeezes.

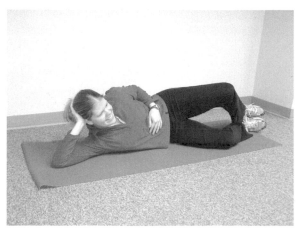

Fig. 64.3   Side-lying abduction/external rotation with hip flexed to 45 degrees.

The gluteus medius has been identified as a major stabilizer of the hip joint and should demand a large amount of attention during this phase of the rehabilitation. Patients should be progressed through exercises that increasingly challenge the hip abductors as tolerated (Table 64.4). As patients achieve greater strength and coordination in this muscle group, they should begin incorporating more functional total lower extremity exercises and greater intensity (Fig. 64.4). Patient tolerance should guide the progression through this phase.

Toward the end of this phase, patients should be participating in higher intensity closed kinetic chain exercises that involve minimal impact to prepare the patient for the return to functional baseline phase. They should progress through squats, lunges in multiple directions (Fig. 64.5), and core stability exercises such as planks. As with all postoperative rehabilitation, single-leg activities should be integrated into the program to ensure that the involved joint is able to tolerate the stresses necessary to increase strength (Fig. 64.6). Progress through this phase should be based on incrementally challenging criteria and limited by patient tolerance.

Return to Functional Baseline Phase

After repair, capsular modification, or microfracture patients should not enter the return to functional baseline phase until at least 12 to 16 weeks after surgery. This allows the involved structures to become strong enough to tolerate impact forces

TABLE 64.4	Sample Hip Abductor Strengthening Progression

- Gluteal squeezes (isometric)
- Prone heel squeezes (isometric)
- Side-lying abduction/external rotation with hip flexed to 45 degrees
- Standing hip abduction bearing weight on uninvolved lower extremity
- Bridging
- Bridging with marching
- Side-lying abduction in neutral hip position
- Standing hip abduction bearing weight on involved lower extremity
- Single-leg mini-squats with external rotation
- Shoulder-width lunges
- Shoulder-width lunges with trunk rotation

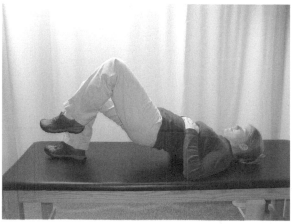

Fig. 64.4   Bridging with marching.

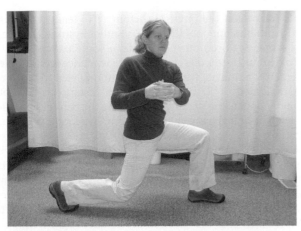

Fig. 64.5 Shoulder-width lunges with trunk rotation.

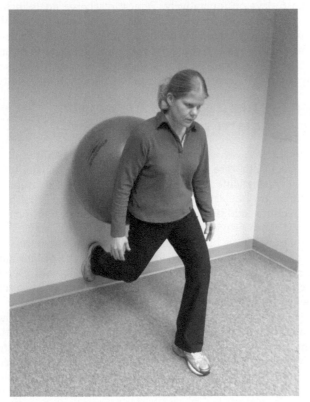

Fig. 64.6 Single-leg mini-squats with external rotation. Note that body weight is shifted toward the outside of the foot to maintain external rotation at the hip.

involved in many activities such as running, cutting, and jumping. Patients with procedures such as osteoplasty or simple débridement may enter this phase any time that the goals of the strengthening phase have been met. As with the strengthening phase, progress through this phase should be based on incrementally challenging criteria and limited by patient tolerance.

Many of the more advanced exercises from the strengthening phase are continued into this final phase. Patients begin incorporating light running into their cardiovascular routine, usually starting with 5 minutes and increasing by 5-minute increments as tolerated until they reach their personal running goal. Cutting progression usually begins with side shuffles followed by cutting away from the involved side ending with cutting toward

the involved side (cross-over cuts). Single-leg hops are useful during this phase to compare involved versus uninvolved power and to assess the patient's confidence in the joint. Dysfunction that can be hidden in double-leg activities becomes much more apparent during single-leg activities.

As the patient returns to normal baseline activities, he or she should follow up with the rehabilitation professional to assure an acceptable return to preinjury function. This is especially true with athletes who often do not perceive their limitations until after they have been released to return to practice. As with all orthopedic surgeries, continuous communication between the patient, rehabilitation professional, and the surgeon will help assure an optimal outcome.

OPEN PROCEDURES OF THE HIP

When arthroscopic procedures are not practical for diagnosis or treatment, open procedures must be explored. Diagnoses that often require open correction include intra-articular pathologies such as osteonecrosis (ON) and severe osteoarthritis and extra-articular pathologies such as slipped capital femoral epiphysis (SCFE) and femoral neck fractures. In cases of ON, core decompression is often performed to increase blood flow to the femoral head. An attempt to pin the femoral head in its "slipped" position is performed for SCFE. Attempting to reposition the slipped femoral head into its original position can often lead to ON. When possible, femoral neck fractures are openly reduced and internally fixed as with other fractures. In all of these diagnoses, severe involvement usually leads to total hip arthroplasty.

TOTAL HIP ARTHROPLASTY

A total hip arthroplasty (THA) is indicated for individuals who experience pain and/or functional loss as a result of pathology at the hip. The primary diagnosis associated with a THA is osteoarthritis at the hip. A hip replacement may also be indicated for those suffering from pain or functional loss as a result of a hip fracture, rheumatoid arthritis, bone tumors, or ON.

Physical therapists are among the many health care providers who will provide treatment to the patient both before and after the total hip replacement surgery. Advances in surgical procedures have allowed for accelerated rehabilitation programs and improved patient outcomes. Despite improvements in surgical procedures, physical therapists in acute care, home health, skill nursing, and outpatient orthopedics will likely provide rehabilitation services for this patient population.

PREOPERATIVE PATIENT EDUCATION

Physical therapists routinely conduct hospital-based education seminars for patients prior to their respective total hip replacement surgery. These classes educate the patient as to the surgical procedure and the rehabilitation course the patient should expect. In addition, these courses may help to reduce preoperative fears or concerns, help the patient to identify medical equipment that may be needed at home (e.g., elevated toilet seat), and prepare family members as to the level of support needed to facilitate recovery. Participation in the course may also help to reduce the postoperative pain experienced by the patient and reduce the risk of experiencing a postoperative dislocation.

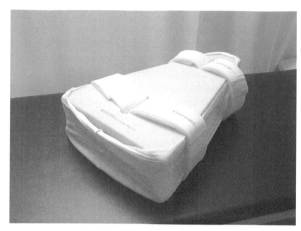

Fig. 64.7   Abduction splint.

Research supports the use of preoperative joint replacement educational courses. Vukomanović et al. (2008) report that patients who both performed the postoperative exercises and received preoperative education demonstrated the ability to perform functional activities significantly earlier than those who were randomly assigned to the control group. These functional activities included being able to walk up and down stairs earlier, use the toilet and chair sooner, transfer independently, and ambulate independently.

POSTOPERATIVE PHYSICAL THERAPY

The hospital-based physical therapy staff is responsible for supporting and continuing the immediate postoperative management initiated by the nursing staff. Surgical room nurses are responsible for the initial monitoring of lower extremity circulation and fitting the patient with his or her abductor splint. The acute care nursing staff continues initial management, monitoring vital signs and administering medication. Ice is routinely applied by the nursing staff to the patient's surgical site to help modulate pain. An **abductor splint** (also known as a **hip abduction pillow**) (Fig. 64.7) is a triangular-shaped piece of foam that *helps to limit the patient's lower extremity movement including hip adduction and internal rotation.*

Physical therapy services are initiated the day after surgery. The goals for the first physical therapy session are to assess the patient's mobility status and to initiate therapeutic activities. With the patient lying supine in the bed, the physical therapist should observe the patient's positioning, assess for signs of a deep vein thrombosis (DVT), note the state of the dressing, and record the range of motion and strength of the uninvolved leg. If signs of a DVT are present or if there is excessive drainage noted on the dressing, the nursing staff should be immediately informed prior to continuing the treatment session.

Prior to assessing the patient's mobility status, the physical therapist must identify which surgical approach was performed and review the physician's mobility orders. The hip joint is purposefully dislocated during the surgery to allow the physician the ability to gain access to the joint. The trauma associated with the surgical procedure weakens the inherent stability of the joint. As a result, there is an increased risk of hip dislocation postoperatively associated with specific movement patterns. These precautions are kept in place for 6 to 12 weeks.

It is the role of the physical therapy (PT) team to establish the patient's baseline mobility status and determine the degree of assistance required during transfers. Some patients may be able to demonstrate a high level of independence and be able to immediately ambulate with an ambulation device weight bearing as tolerated (WBAT) for significant distances. PT should frequently update the nursing staff during the patient's inpatient stay when he or she has a change in his or her mobility or transfer status.

Therapeutic exercises should also be initiated during the initial visit. Day 1 exercises could consist of lower extremity isometrics (quadriceps, hamstrings, gluteal sets) and ankle pumps. Initially, a patient may only be able to tolerate passive ROM; however, he or she should be able to demonstrate increased active ROM tolerance over the course of the inpatient stay. Therapeutic exercises are frequently added daily to the patient's routine.

Patients are discharged from the acute care hospital between 4 and 6 days postoperatively. Typical discharge goals include independence with transfers, demonstrating mobility for functional distances with or without an ambulation device, good recall of one's home exercise program, and good recall of one's precautions. Individuals who are unable to meet these goals may need additional rehabilitation at a skilled nursing facility.

SKILLED NURSING AND HOME HEALTH INTERVENTIONS

Physical therapists who work at skilled nursing facilities or for a home health care organization may provide rehabilitation services to patients recovering from a total hip arthroplasty. A patient may be referred to a skilled nursing facility if he or she requires additional nursing and rehabilitation services beyond those provided during the acute hospital stay. Often, a patient will have one or more comorbidities that necessitate the additional care. The physical therapist in the skilled nursing setting should continue the previously established exercise program with the goal of advancing the patient to maximum independence.

Patients may also receive physical therapy services in their home. For some, these services are provided as a transition from the acute care setting to the outpatient orthopedic clinic. However, some patients are now completing their postoperative rehabilitation exclusively at home. In these cases, the home health physical therapist is responsible for maximizing the home exercise program.

OUTPATIENT ORTHOPEDIC PHYSICAL THERAPY

Patients are routinely referred to outpatient physical therapy centers to maximize their postoperative function. The outpatient orthopedic physical therapist will first need to evaluate the patient's ambulation ability, muscle strength (manual muscle test and functionally), and ROM. This information combined with the patient's goals will allow the PT to develop a comprehensive rehabilitation program. Typically, a patient should be either able to demonstrate or be working toward the following **clinical goals:**

- Achieving full, allowed active ROM at the hip by the end of the sixth postoperative week (e.g., hip flexion 90 degrees, hip abduction 40 degrees for the patient who has had a posterior approach surgery)

- Additional ROM may be restored through stretching exercises once the physician's postoperative precautions have been lifted
- Progress to functional strengthening, including closed kinetic chain and balance exercises
- Independent ambulation by week 12 (and without the use of an assistive device for those who did not require their utilization preoperatively)
- Patient able to drive by the end of the sixth postoperative week
- Patient able to assume side-lying position on operative hip by the end of the sixth postoperative week
- Return to most recreational/sports pursuits by the end of the twelfth week postoperative (see later discussion)

Isometrics (Figs. 64.8 through 64.10), open kinetic chain exercises (Figs. 64.11 through 64.13), closed kinetic chain exercises (Figs. 64.14 and 64.15), and balance exercises (Fig. 64.16) may be prescribed to address weakness. Progressive overload to the muscles may be performed manually by the physical therapist, with the application of ankle weights or with the use of elastic resistance bands. Initial exercise prescription should consist of one to three sets of 15 to 20 repetitions. This volume of training will help to improve muscular endurance while minimizing the risk of excessive postexercise muscular soreness or pain. As endurance capacity increases, strength training volumes of two to four sets of 6 to 10 repetitions may be performed.

RETURN TO SPORT

Physical activity levels may affect the lifespan of the total hip replacement. Wear and tear on the replaced joint or a traumatic event may necessitate a revision surgery at a later date. However, having a hip replaced does not require an end to the patient's recreational or sport pursuits. Exercise and activity are necessary for maintaining overall health. Instead of restricting activity, physicians have developed recommendations and guidelines for those who wish to return to activities that are more strenuous than walking.

SPORT-SPECIFIC EXERCISES FOR THE GOLFER WITH A TOTAL HIP REPLACEMENT

It is generally agreed that golfing is an acceptable sport to return to and that it places a low degree of stress on the hip implant

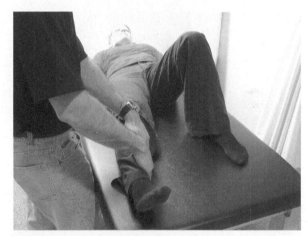

Fig. 64.10 Manually applied hip adduction isometric exercise (hip is maintained at neutral to slightly abducted).

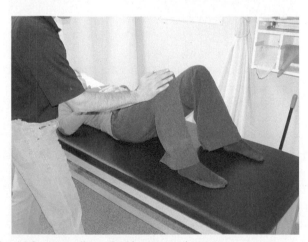

Fig. 64.8 Manually applied hip external rotation isometric exercise.

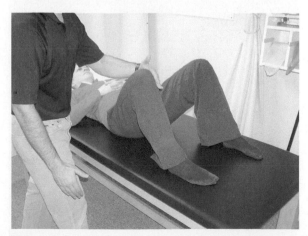

Fig. 64.9 Manually applied hip internal rotation isometric exercise (hip is maintained at neutral to slightly externally rotated).

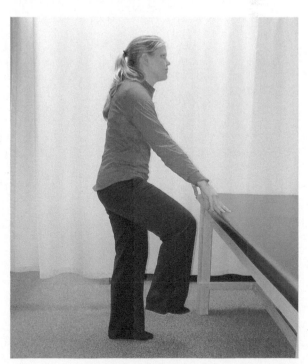

Fig. 64.11 Standing hip flexion.

(Fig. 64.17). Because of the multiplanar nature of the golf swing and the unique forces placed on the body (specifically the core), the rehabilitation and strength training program for the golfer who has had a total hip replacement should include sport-specific exercises.

Sport-specific training will likely not occur until the patient's physician has lifted precautions. However, the initial therapeutic exercises prescribed will establish a functional strength base from which additional exercise prescription can proceed.

Many sport-specific exercises should address core stability and multiplanar movement patterns. Core endurance capacity should be addressed with exercises such as a front plank with hip extension (Fig. 64.18), the bird dog, and the side plank. With improved core endurance, the golfer should be prescribed

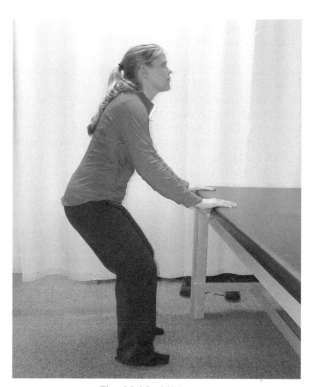

Fig. 64.14 Mini-squat.

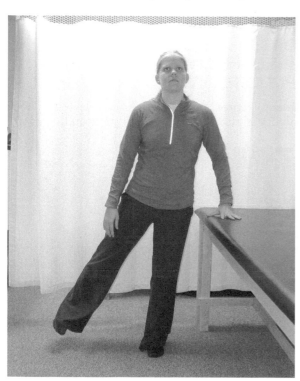

Fig. 64.12 Standing hip abduction.

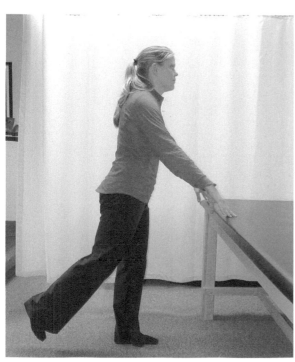

Fig. 64.13 Standing hip extension.

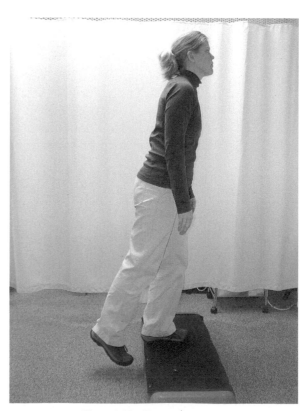

Fig. 64.15 Forward step-up.

multiplanar exercises such as the lunge with trunk rotation (see Fig. 7.50), kettle bell squats (Fig. 64.19), plyometric ball tosses (Fig. 64.20), and proprioceptive neuromuscular facilitation chop and lift patterns performed against resistance.

TREATMENT OF EXTRA-ARTICULAR HIP PATHOLOGY

Extra-articular pathology of the hip includes injuries of the soft tissues and extrinsic support structures of the femoroacetabular joint. These injuries may involve one or more of the following types of tissues: tendons, muscles, bursae, fascia, and nerves. Accurately diagnosing pathology associated with these hip structures may be clinically challenging; many of the conditions

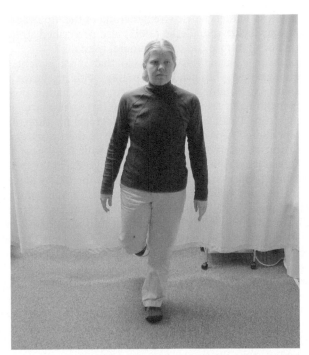

Fig. 64.16   Single-leg balance.

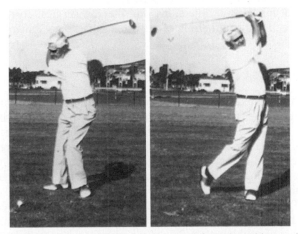

Fig. 64.17   Professional senior golfer with bilateral total hip replacements. (From Clifford PE, Mallon WJ. Sports after total joint replacement. *Clin Sports Med* 2005;24(1):178. Fig. 5.)

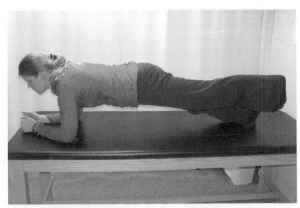

Fig. 64.18   Front plank with hip extension.

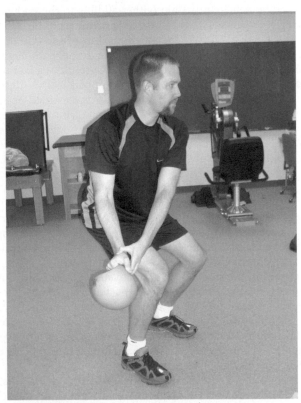

Fig. 64.19   Kettle bell squat with rotation.

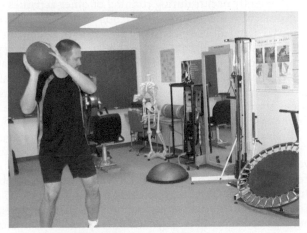

Fig. 64.20   Plyometric ball tosses with rebounder.

lack sensitive or specific special tests. Imaging studies or arthroscopy may be necessary to establish a final diagnosis.

Prior to conducting the physical evaluation of the patient with an injured hip, the physical therapist must take a careful and complete history. The information obtained from the history may be as (or more) important to the information collected during the physical examination. Many of the signs and symptoms of extra-articular hip pathology are similar. The mechanism of injury, the location of pain, the associated mechanical symptoms such as a reported "catching" and/or "snapping," and identification of exacerbating and relieving factors will help the clinician when establishing the initial diagnosis.

COXA SALTANS

Coxa saltans (also known as "snapping hip") is a condition marked by a snap at the hip (either audible to the patient and therapist or palpable to the therapist) and hip pain during activity (White et al. 2004). The **snapping hip syndrome** may be the result of intra-articular, internal, or external pathology. The **intra-articular snapping hip** is often the result of a labral tear, chondral damage, loose bodies, or other pathology within the hip joint. The **extra-articular snapping** is classified as either internal or external. The internal snapping hip is caused by movement of the iliopsoas tendon over a bony prominence, whereas the external snapping hip occurs when movement of the iliotibial band "rubs" over the greater trochanter.

Internal Coxa Saltans

The **internal snapping hip** occurs when the iliopsoas tendon moves over the iliopectineal eminence, the femoral head, or the lesser trochanter. Athletes whose sport requires frequent hip movements into high flexion angles combined with additional external and internal hip rotation are susceptible to this injury. Athletes who participate in dance, martial arts, soccer, gymnastics, and football have an increased risk of experiencing an internal snapping hip. The clinician is challenged when attempted to distinguish between the internal and the intra-articular snapping hip. The patients' pain and symptom complaints for both are frequently similar in nature.

Diagnosis is frequently established from the patient's history. The chief complaint is of a painful, repetitive clicking and sometimes "clunking" in the anterior hip. These symptoms may even be able to be reproduced voluntarily by the patient. The snapping frequently occurs during running or other activities (ballet, gymnastics) that require contraction of the iliopsoas while the hip is extended. The patient will present with a deep catch or "clunk" sensation in the anterior hip and groin when being passively moved from a position of hip flexion and external rotation to extension with internal rotation. The examiner can confirm the diagnosis by applying pressure to the iliopsoas tendon as the patient attempts to reproduce the snapping. The pressure will inhibit the snapping sensation, helping to confirm the diagnosis.

Physical therapy interventions should address asymmetries in muscular flexibility and deficits in core strength. Conservative treatment of internal snapping hip should consist of rest, stretching exercises, and general hip strengthening. Jacobson and Allen (1990) suggested stretching the hip flexors for 6 to 8 weeks should help to resolve symptoms associated with snapping hip syndrome. Gruen et al. (2002) reported a 63% success rate with a 3-month training program that included iliopsoas stretching, concentric strengthening of the external and internal

hip rotators, and eccentric strengthening of the hip flexors and extensors. Taylor and Clarke (1995) also prescribed stretching and included ultrasound to the femoral triangle.

Johnston et al. (1998) suggested that most patients with internal snapping hip syndrome present with hip flexor tightness and hip rotator weakness. Their rehabilitation program begins with daily external and internal hip rotator strengthening in sitting (with hip flexed to 90 degrees) for three sets of 20 repetitions. After 2 weeks, a patient is then progressed to side-lying abduction/external rotation with the knees flexed to 90 degrees and the hip flexed to 45 degrees. In this position the subject abducts and externally rotates the hip by spreading the knees apart against a resistance band while maintaining the feet in contact with each other. This exercise is also performed daily for three sets of 20 repetitions. After an additional 2 weeks, the final prescribed exercise was external and internal rotation strengthening, performed in standing, with the hip in neutral flexion/extension. The individual stands against a wall for support while performing a single-leg mini-squat on the affected side. During the mini-squat, the knee must remain over the lateral foot to keep the hip in external rotation. This exercise was performed two to three times a week for a total of three sets of 20 repetitions. Subjects are also instructed to perform daily stretching of the iliopsoas.

If a conservative treatment fails, an injection of lidocaine and corticosteroids into the iliopsoas bursa under fluoroscopy may be helpful. When the patient fails to improve with the use of medication, injections, and therapy, surgical correction by fractional lengthening of the psoas muscle has shown to be successful.

External Coxa Saltans

External coxa saltans is the most common cause of snapping in the hip. Symptoms occur when the iliotibial band (IT band) rubs over the greater trochanter of the femur. The repetitive rubbing causes the bursae around the greater trochanter to become inflamed. The pain associated with the friction produced is often referred to as iliotibial band syndrome.

Patients frequently complain of pain over the lateral aspect of the hip and occasionally report experiencing a sensation similar to that of a subluxation. Pain is experienced when an individual is lying on the affected side and during sit-to-stand transitions. Other provocative activities include running, stair climbing, incline walking, and other higher-impact activities. During the physical examination the patient often has pain with palpation over the greater trochanter and may report an increase in symptoms with external rotation of the hip in 90 degrees of flexion. The physical therapist should palpate the greater trochanter with the patient lying on the unaffected side. Positioning the patient in this manner allows for better exposure of the greater trochanter. The Ober test may provide important information regarding IT band flexibility. The clinician performs this test by placing the patient on the unaffected side with the symptomatic hip abducted and extended and the knee bent to 90 degrees. The symptomatic extremity is then adducted while maintaining extension looking for flexibility restriction. The snapping may be reproduced during the Ober test or during external and internal rotation in the same side-lying position with the hip abducted and externally rotated.

Conservative treatment for external coxa saltans consists of rest, NSAIDs, gentle stretching, strengthening exercises

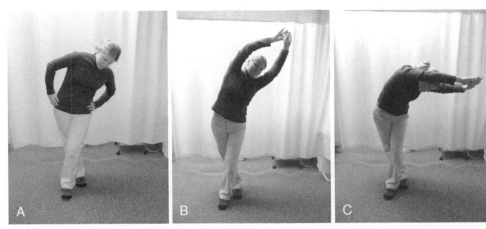

Fig. 64.21 Different positions for iliotibial band stretch. Positions **A**, **B**, and **C**. Position "B" has been shown to be most effective.

(especially hip abduction and hip external rotation), ice, and other modalities for inflammation control. When conservative measures fail to alleviate symptoms, a corticosteroid injection into the bursa is indicated. Once the initial inflammation has subsided, increasing the intensity of stretching to the IT band may commence. Fredericson (2002) compared the effectiveness of three different IT band stretches (Fig. 64.21, A–C). In the first stretching position (Fig. 64.21, A), the subject in standing position extends and adducts the affected leg, placing it behind the unaffected side. Next the subject side bends the trunk away from the symptomatic side until a stretch is experienced. The second stretch (Fig. 64.21, B) is similar to the first position except the hands are clasped over the head with the arms extended. The third stretch (Fig. 64.21, C) is similar to the second position except that the arms are stretched diagonally downward away from the affected hip. The authors report that all stretches were effective; however, the second stretch produced the greatest results followed by the third stretch.

GLUTEAL TEARS

The gluteal tendons at the greater trochanter have been called the rotator cuff of the hip. Tendinopathy and subsequent tearing may be a degenerative process similar to that in the shoulder. Studies have shown the presence of gluteal tears in nearly 20% of patients with femoral neck fracture and in those who are electing to have total hip arthroplasty. The exact cause of pathology is unknown but is thought to be from direct mechanical trauma or through progressive degeneration. Researchers have hypothesized that progressive degeneration initially begins as a tendonitis. Tendonitis can then lead to tendon thickening and progress to partial and then complete tearing of both the gluteus medius and minimus. Excessive tensioning of the iliotibial band over the greater trochanter may further contribute to these ruptures. This condition has been reported to occur most frequently during the fourth through sixth decades of life and has been described as being four times more common in women than in men, possibly because of the wider female pelvis.

Patients often complain of a dull ache with tenderness to palpation over the greater trochanter. They may also complain of a "grinding" sensation along with pain when lying on the affected side and with single-leg stance activities such as climbing stairs. On evaluation they often demonstrate hip abductor weakness. Patients may demonstrate this weakness by presenting with a Trendelenburg gait, leaning over the involved lower

extremity during the stance phase and causing passive abduction of the hip to decrease load to the gluteals. Patients may also have pain during passive and resisted external rotation with the hip flexed to 90 degrees and with single-leg stance for more than 30 seconds. Patients diagnosed with trochanteric bursitis that does not respond to conservative care should be further evaluated for gluteal tendon pathology because clinical presentation may initially appear to be trochanteric bursitis. Plain radiographs are usually negative but may sometimes show calcification at the tendon insertion. MRI is useful to determine the severity of damage to the tendon along with fatty deposition of the gluteal muscles and calcification of the tendon insertion.

As with rotator cuff pathology of the shoulder, management of gluteal tendinopathy depends on severity. Initial intervention is similar to that of trochanteric bursitis and should include the use of NSAIDs, rest, ice, and other modalities for inflammation control such as ultrasound. As patients become less symptomatic, they can begin progressive strengthening of the hip abductors (Table 64.4). Strengthening programs should include all motions of the hip along with exercises to strengthen the abdominals, lower back, and other trunk musculature. If conservative management fails, endoscopic repair of the tendon may be beneficial.

Check online videos: Hip Abduction Side-lying (Video 64.1), Hip Extension (Video 64.2), Isometric Hip Abduction Wall (Video 64.3), Single Leg Balance Hip Rotation (Video 64.4) and Standing Hip Abduction (Video 64.5).

REFERENCES

A complete reference list is available at https://expertconsult .inkling.com/.

FURTHER READING

Engebretsen AH, Myklebust G, Holme I, et al. Intrinsic risk factors for groin injuries among male soccer players: a prospective cohort study. *Am J Sports Med.* 2010;38:2051–2057.

Hammoud S, Bedi A, Voos JE, et al. The recognition and evaluation of patterns of compensatory injury in patients with mechanical hip pain. *Sports Health: A Multidisciplinary Approach 6.2.* 2014:108–118.

Quinn A. Hip and groin pain: physiotherapy and rehabilitation Issues. *Open Sports Med J.* 2010;4:93–107.

Ryan J, Deburca N, Mc Creesh K. Risk factors for groin/hip injuries in field-based sports: a systematic review. *J Sports Med.* 2014;48(14):1089–1096.

65

The Arthritic Hip

Alexander T. Caughran, MD | Charles E. Giangarra, MD

Osteoarthritis (OA) is the most prevalent joint disease in the United States, afflicting an estimated 43 million people. A report by the Centers for Disease Control and Prevention indicated that patients with arthritis have substantially worse health-related quality of life than those without it.

Pathology around the hip can be classified into three groups: intra-articular, extra-articular, and hip mimickers (Table 65.1).
- Intra-articular pathology includes injuries to the hip joint itself. These include more global diagnoses such as osteoarthritis, osteonecrosis (AVN), femoroacetabular impingement (FAI), and more focal diagnoses such as acetabular labral tears, chondral defects, and ligamentum teres tears.
- Extra-articular pathology includes injuries to structures around the hip such as internal and external "snapping hip" (coxa saltans), gluteus medius tears, and muscle strains.
- Hip mimickers include injuries to more remote regions that refer pain into the region of the hip such as athletic pubalgia, osteitis pubis, or lumbar radiculopathy. Hip mimickers and non-arthritic etiology are discussed in the Special Topics chapter.

CLINICAL BACKGROUND

Arthritis of the hip can result from many causes, such as childhood sepsis, slipped capital epiphysis (SCFE), FAI, osteoarthritis, and rheumatoid arthritis. About 30% of all patients with hip arthritis have a mild form of acetabular dysplasia (a shallow socket), and 30% have a retroverted socket. Both of these conditions reduce the contact area of the femoral head in the acetabulum, which increases the pressure and makes wear more likely. Approximately 30% of patients have no obvious risk factors.

Arthritis of the hip is marked by progressive loss of articular cartilage with joint space narrowing and pain. The loss of articular cartilage encourages osteophyte formation (bone spurs) as the joint tries to distribute the joint reactive forces over a broader surface area. The abnormal morphology of the ball and socket joint (a "square peg in a round hole") as well as these osteophytes, which put tension on the surrounding soft tissues, creates a stiff hip that makes it difficult for the patient to even put on socks and shoes. Eventually, this wear pattern leads to a general picture of shortening, adduction deformity, and external rotation of the hip, often with a fixed flexion contracture. Bone loss usually occurs slowly, but in some instances (e.g. with osteonecrosis) this can occur rather precipitously.

GENERAL FEATURES OF OSTEOARTHRITIS

According to Dieppe (1984), the following are general features of osteoarthritis:
- A heterogeneous group of conditions that share common pathologic and radiographic features

- Focal loss of articular cartilage in part of a synovial joint is accompanied by hypertrophic reaction in the subchondral bone and joint margin.
- Radiographic changes of joint space narrowing, subchondral sclerosis, cyst formation, and marginal osteophytes
- Common and age related, with identified patterns of involvement targeting the hands, hips, knees, and apophyseal joints of the spine
- Clinical findings often include joint pain with use, stiffness of joints after a period of inactivity, and lost range of motion (ROM).

PRIMARY SYMPTOMS AND SIGNS OF OSTEOARTHRITIS

Symptoms

- Pain during activity
- Stiffness after inactivity (stiffness usually lasts less than 30 minutes)
- Loss of movement (difficulty with certain tasks)
- Feelings of insecurity or instability
- Functional limitations and handicap

Signs

- Tender spots around joint margin
- Firm swellings of the joint margin
- Coarse crepitus (creaking or locking)
- Mild inflammation (cool effusions)
- Restricted, painful movements
- Joint "tightness"
- Instability (obvious bone or joint destruction)

CLASSIFICATION OF HIP ARTHRITIS

The radiographic appearance of OA can be classified as (1) **concentric,** in which there is uniform loss of articular cartilage, (2) **downward and medial migration** of the femoral head, or (3) **upward migration** and **superolateral migration** of the femoral head. This is important if a corrective osteotomy is considered but is otherwise of no significance.

DIAGNOSIS OF HIP ARTHRITIS

The source of hip pain can be wide varying from true intra-articular pathology (most often groin pain symptoms), to lateral-sided hip pain (most often from trochanteric bursitis), or to referred pain (from the lumbar spine from herniated disc, spinal stenosis, or even vascular causes such as stenosis of the internal iliac artery). Therefore a proper physical exam should rule out

TABLE 65.1	Potential Causes of Groin Pain in Athletes	
Intra-Articular	**Extra-Articular**	**Hip Mimickers**
Acetabular labral tears	Internal coxa saltans	Athletic pubalgia (sports hernia)
Ligamentum teres tears	External coxa saltans	Osteitis pubis
Femoroacetabular impingement	Gluteal tears	Genitourinary disorders
Chondral defects	Muscle strains	Intra-abdominal disorders
Osteoarthritis	Piriformis syndrome	Lumbar radiculopathy
Avascular necrosis	Slipped capital femoral epiphysis	
Dysplasia	Fractures	

these extraarticular sources of pain. The classic clinical test for hip arthritis is internal rotation of the hip in flexion. With hip arthritis, this internal rotation is limited and painful. Patients with trochanteric bursitis are focally tender along the greater trochanter and may have limitations with hip adduction (Ober test). Those with spinal pathology often have a history suggestive of radicular or neurologic symptoms, as well as positive physical exam findings (straight leg raise or reverse straight leg raise).

Differential diagnoses include hip dislocation, hip fracture, pelvic fracture or disruption, entrapment of the lateral femoral cutaneous nerve, FAI or labral pathology, tendinitis of the piriformis or gluteus maximus or minimus tendons, trochanteric bursitis, L3–4 sciatica, spinal referred pain, internal iliac artery stenosis, and strain or contusion of the quadriceps or hamstring muscles.

Radiographic examination includes an anteroposterior (AP) view of the pelvis and AP and cross-table lateral views of the hip. The cross-table lateral view is helpful in looking at the posterior aspect of the hip joint, as 10% of patients with intra-articular pathology can present with buttock pain as opposed to the typical groin pain. Serologic investigations are seldom required. The only indication for further imaging studies such as bone scanning and magnetic resonance (MRI) is suspected osteonecrosis in the absence of radiographic findings.

The American College of Rheumatology lists several criteria for the diagnosis of OA of the hip.

- Pain in the hip AND internal hip rotation <15 degrees AND erythrocyte sedimentation rate (ESR) ≤45/hour or hip flexion ≤115 degrees if ESR unavailable
- Pain in the hip AND internal hip rotation ≤15 degrees, pain with internal hip rotation, morning hip stiffness lasting 60 minutes or less, and age older than 50 years
- Adding radiographic criteria, OA is diagnosed if two of three criteria are met in addition to pain in the hip: ESR <20 mm/hour, radiographic evidence of femoral and/or acetabular osteophytes, radiographic evidence of joint space narrowing.

TREATMENT OF HIP ARTHRITIS
Nonoperative Treatment

Nonoperative treatment is initially indicated for nearly all patients with hip osteoarthritis. This may include activity modifications, assistive devices, and medications. Although some high-impact activities such as running and jumping should be avoided, it is important to maintain as much activity and joint motion as possible. Swimming, cycling, and leisurely walking are all low-impact activities that can help maintain range of motion, strength, and function. Staying active also can help with weight loss, which is an important part of the management of hip arthritis. For patients who are overweight, losing

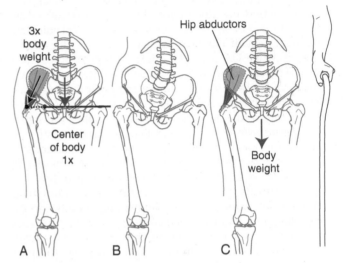

Fig. 65.1 Use of a cane redirects the force across the hip. Without the cane, the resultant force across the hip is about three times body weight because the force of the abductors acts on the greater trochanter to offset body weight and levels the pelvis in single stance. A, Without cane normal force across hip joint 3x body weight; B, Abductors work to level pelvis in single stance phase; C, Properly fitted cane will level pelvis and unload hip by decreasing forces by abductors. (Redrawn from Kyle RF. Fractures of the hip. In Gustilo RB, Kyle RF, Templeton D (eds.). Fractures and Dislocations. St. Louis: Mosby, 1993.)

20 pounds or more may decrease pain and delay the need for surgery by decreasing the joint reactive forces around the hip.

A cane in the opposite hand helps to unload the hip significantly (Fig. 65.1). A properly fitted cane should reach the top of the greater trochanter of the patient's hip while wearing shoes. Doing stretching and strengthening exercises or joining a yoga class can be of surprising value in terms of regaining ROM because it is not uncommon that stiffness of periarticular structures (e.g., the inability to put on shoes and socks) rather than pain makes surgery necessary.

Medical Treatment

Anti-inflammatories and analgesics are of some value (albeit limited). In general, nonsteroidal anti-inflammatory drugs (NSAIDs) act by reversibly inhibiting the cyclo-oxygenase or lipo-oxygenase side of arachidonic acid metabolism. This effectively blocks the production of proinflammation agents such as prostaglandins and leukotrienes. Also inhibited are the beneficial effects of prostaglandins, including protective effects on the gastric mucosal lining, renal blood flow, and sodium balance. Unlike aspirin, which has an irreversible antiplatelet effect persisting for the life of the platelet (10 to 12 days), NSAID bleeding times usually correct within 24 hours of their discontinuation. Dyspepsia (gastrointestinal upset) is the most common side effect of NSAIDs. Other potential side effects include gastrointestinal ulceration, renal toxicity, hepatotoxicity, and cardiac failure. Contraindications to the use of NSAIDs include history of gastrointestinal disease, renal disease, hepatic disease, or simultaneous anticoagulation therapy. The American College of Rheumatology recommends annual complete blood count, liver function, and creatinine testing in patients on a course of prolonged NSAID use. Hemograms and fecal occult blood testing are recommended both before initiating NSAIDs and regularly thereafter.

Acetaminophen is the most commonly used oral medication for OA. In addition to its anti-inflammatory effect, acetaminophen acts as an inhibitor of cyclo-oxygenase (COX)-1 and COX-2 in the central nervous system. Several clinical guidelines for the treatment of OA recommend its use for the relief of mild to moderate OA pain (American College of Rheumatology [www.rheumatology.org], Osteoarthritis Research Society International [www.oarsi.org], European League Against Rheumatism [www.eular.org]). A 2006 Cochrane review (Towheed et al.), however, found that although acetaminophen was significantly superior to placebo for pain relief, the clinical significance of the improvement was dubious. Although acetaminophen is among the safest oral analgesics, it does carry some risk for hepatic toxicity, although rarely at doses of 4 g/day or less.

Neutraceuticals such as glucosamine and chondroitin sulfate are popular but unproven. Glucosamine and chondroitin sulfate are synergistic endogenous molecules in articular cartilage. Glucosamine is thought to stimulate chondrocyte and synoviocyte metabolism, and chondroitin sulfate is believed to inhibit degradative enzymes and prevent formation of fibrin thrombi in periarticular tissues (Ghosh et al. 1992). A minimum of 1 g of glucosamine and 1200 mg of chondroitin sulfate per day are the standard recommended doses. The average cost of this oral therapy is $50 per month. In our practice, we will recommend that patients try these medications daily for 4 weeks and then continue or discontinue its use depending on whether it is effective.

Injections of steroids can provide temporary relief but are not of lasting benefit and should not be done more than every 3 months because of the risk of side effects such as weakening of the soft tissues around the hip joint and possibly the bone itself. Furthermore, data have shown that intra-articular injections performed within 3 months prior to a hip replacement place the patient at increased risk for prosthetic joint infection. More recently, hyaluronate injections have been reported to be effective in some patients (Migliore et al. 2009), whereas others have reported no benefit (Richette et al. 2009). This treatment currently is investigational for hip arthritis and is considered an "off-label" use.

Operative Options for Hip Arthritis

Osteotomies, such as pelvic and intertrochanteric osteotomies, were popular in the past, and they still may have a limited role in selected situations. **Arthrodesis (fusion)** still does have a role in select cases (e.g., a laborer with severe arthritis who is too young for a hip replacement); however, the mainstay of surgical treatment is total hip replacement (Fig. 65.2). In most modern hip replacements, the femoral and acetabular components are "press fit" into place, such that over time bony ingrowth into the implants can occur to promote long-term fixation. In rare cases, such as severely osteoporotic bone, the implants are cemented in place because the cement is better able to interdigitate and provide the long-term fixation. In revisions with poor-quality bone, the surgeon makes fixation choices based on intraoperative findings.

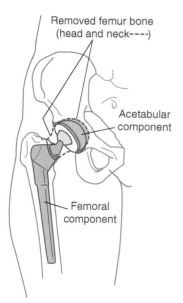

Fig. 65.2   Total hip replacement.

Weightbearing restrictions are largely the same after arthroplasty whether cemented and cementless hip implants were used, unless intraoperative findings suggest otherwise. Cement is as strong as it will ever be 15 minutes after insertion. Some surgeons believe that some weightbearing protection should be provided until the bone at the interface with the cement (which has been damaged by mechanical and thermal trauma) has reconstituted with the development of a peri-implant bone plate. This phenomenon takes 6 weeks. Most surgeons, however, believe that the initial stability achieved with cement fixation is adequate to allow immediate full weight bearing with a cane or walker. For patients who have cementless fixation, the stem is "press fit" such that a three-point mold is held that provides the temporary fixation until the bony ingrowth occurs.

This stability is usually adequate by 6 weeks; however, maximal stability is probably not achieved until approximately 6 months. Regardless, the majority of surgeons believe that the initial stability achieved is adequate to allow weight bearing as tolerated immediately after surgery.

Straight leg raises (SLR) can produce very large out-of-plane loads on the hip and should be avoided in the postoperative period after total hip arthroplasty. Side-leg-lifting in the lying position also produces large loads on the hip. Even vigorous isometric contractions of the hip abductors should be practiced with caution, especially if a trochanteric osteotomy has been done.

Initial rotational resistance of a noncemented hip may be low, and it may be preferable to protect the hip from large rotational forces for 6 weeks or more. The most common rotational load comes when arising from a sitting position, so pushing with hands from a chair is strongly recommended.

After full weight bearing is established, it is essential that the patient continue to use a cane in the contralateral hand until the limp stops. This helps prevent the development of a **Trendelenburg gait,** which may be difficult to eradicate at a later date. In some difficult revisions in which implant or bone stability has been difficult to establish, a patient may be advised to continue to use a cane indefinitely. In general, when a patient gets up and walks away, forgetting about the cane, this is an indicator that the cane may be safely discarded.

REFERENCES

A complete reference list is available at https://expertconsult.inkling.com/.

FURTHER READING

Barrett, et al. Prospective Randomized Study of Direct Anterior v Postero-lateral Approach for Total Hip arthroplasty. *J of Arthroplasty.* 2013;28:1634–1638.

Jogi P, et al. Effectiveness of balance exercises in the acute post-operative phase following total hip and knee arthroplasty: a randomized clinical trial. *SAGE Open Medicine.* 2015:1–9.

Larsen K. Cost-effectiveness of Accelerated Perioperative Care and Rehabilitation After Total Hip and Knee Arthroplasty. *J Bone Joint Surg Am.* 2009;91:761–772.

Mahomed N, et al. Inpatient Compared with Home-based Rehabilitation Following Primary Unilateral Total Hip or Knee Replacement: a randomized controlled trial. *J Bone Joint Surg Am.* 2008;90:1673–1680.

Snow R, et al. Associations Between Preoperative Physical Therapy and Post-Acute Care Utilization Patterns and cost in Total Joint Replacement. *J Bone Joint Surgery.* 2014;96:e165(1–8).

Taunton M, et al. Direct Anterior Total Hip Arthroplasty Yields more Rapid Voluntary Cessation of All walking Aids: a prospective, randomized clinical trial. *J of Arthroplasty.* 2014;29:169–172.

66

Total Hip Replacement Rehabilitation: Progression and Restrictions

Morteza Meftah, MD | Amar S. Ranawat, MD | Anil S. Ranawat, MD | Alexander T. Caughran, MD

The success of total hip replacement (THR) is a result of predictable pain relief, improvements in quality of life, and restoration of normal function (Brown et al. 2009). Postoperative rehabilitation is one of the factors that can affect outcomes after THR. The main goal of postoperative rehabilitation protocols is achieving maximal functional performance by focusing on reducing pain, increasing ROM, and strengthening the hip muscles (Brander et al. 1994).

Because the majority of functional performance is gained within the first 6 months postoperatively (Gogia et al. 1994), a proper rehabilitation program that addresses the aforementioned goal is of paramount importance. Several factors influence the results of these programs, such as preoperative management, surgical approach, multimodal pain control modalities, hip precautions, postoperative protocols, weight-bearing status, and the level of rehabilitative care.

PREOPERATIVE MANAGEMENT

Patient education regarding postoperative pain management, restrictions, independent walking, and proper rehabilitation is an important first step in achieving satisfactory results after THR. Preoperative classes can facilitate patients' understanding of reasonable expectations of recovery, increase their motivation, and help expedite the rehabilitation learning process (Giraduet-Le Quintrec et al. 2003). Vukomanovic (Vukomanovi et al. 2008) reported that patients who both performed the "postoperative" exercises and received preoperative education demonstrated the ability to perform functional activities significantly earlier than those who were randomly assigned to the control group. These functional activities included being able to walk up and down stairs earlier, use the toilet and chair sooner, transfer independently, and ambulate independently.

Patient education also has been shown to be directly related to faster postoperative ambulation, reductions in hospital length of stay, and less use of narcotic pain medications (Spaulding 1995). A major part of preoperative educational classes should be dedicated to prevention of postoperative dislocation by appropriate explanation of hip precautions, if they are needed.

For patients planning to undergo total hip replacement, many surgeons will require a course of preoperative physical therapy prior to proceeding with the replacement. The benefit of this therapy, however, is unclear in the literature. Some studies have shown that preoperative strengthening exercises have a significant correlation with longer postoperative walking distance and may improve early return to ambulatory function after THR (Gilbey et al. 2003; Wang et al. 2002; Whitney and Parkman 2002); others have shown that these exercises have no significant impact on the outcomes (Gocen et al. 2004; Rooks et al. 2006). More recently, preoperative physical therapy has been linked to decreased health costs in the postoperative time period as it can cut down on costs associated with skilled nursing, home health, or even inpatient rehab (Snow et al. 2014).

SURGICAL APPROACH

One of the factors influencing postoperative recovery and rehabilitation is the surgical approach. The patient's gait may be compromised with approaches in which the hip abductors are altered (i.e., lateral or anterolateral approaches). Inadequate repair or weakness of the abductor muscles after these approaches may result in prolonged limping. The posterolateral approach spares the hip abductors but is associated with a slightly higher dislocation rate. This dislocation rate can be reduced with the use of larger femoral heads and proper repair of the posterior soft tissues (Pellicci et al. 1998; Woo and Morrey, 1982). The direct anterior approach is a "muscle sparing" approach that has a slightly faster initial time to recovery, allowing patients to cease use of a walking aid on average 6 days sooner than those performed through a posterior approach (Taunton et al. 2014). The downside to the direct anterior approach is that it has a steep learning curve and may require specialized equipment such as fracture table or intraoperative fluoroscopy (Peak et al. 2005). Minimally invasive THR has been widely marketed, but the claims of significantly reduced pain, less morbidity, better function, and improved patient satisfaction appear to be unfounded (Khan et al. 2009). Based on recent reports, minimally invasive THR does not appear to affect the short-term or intermediate-term outcomes after the THR (Howell et al. 2004; Inaba et al. 2005; Lawlor 2005). Complications of minimally invasive THR include wound-healing problems, component malposition, and increased risk of femoral fractures (Howell et al. 2004; Lawlor 2005).

The anterior approach to the hip (also referred to as the "Smith-Petersen" approach) is the one truly internervous approach to the hip, meaning that the approach is made between muscles that have separate innervations. The interval is found superficially between the sartorius (innervated by the femoral nerve) and the tensor fascia lata (innervated by the superior gluteal nerve). This dissection is carried down deeper between the rectus femoris and the gluteus medius, innervated by femoral and superior gluteal nerve, respectively, prior to entering the hip capsule. The posterior approach, however, is an intramuscular plane. A lateral incision to the hip is made and dissection is carried down through the gluteus maximus superiorly and the tensor fascia lata. The piriformis muscle along with the short

TABLE 66.1	Precautions Associated With Total Hip Arthroplasty Surgical Approaches
Surgical Approach	**Precautions**
Anterior	Do not extend hip beyond neutral. No lying in prone Do not externally rotate and extend the hip. Do not perform the bridging exercise.
Posterior	Do not flex the hip greater than 90 degrees. Do not internally rotate the hip beyond neutral. Do not adduct the leg beyond neutral.

external rotators is then detached from the posterior aspect of the greater trochanter and the hip joint is entered posteriorly. It is because these muscles are violated that these patients must obey hip precautions during the postoperative phase.

MULTIMODAL PAIN MANAGEMENT

Severe pain after THR is one of the greatest fears patients have before surgery and is the leading cause of delayed discharge. Pain remains a poorly understood, complex phenomenon that plays a significant role in limiting patients' functional recovery and participation in postoperative physical therapy (Ranawat and Ranawat 2007). Optimal pain control promotes earlier ambulation and faster return to normal gait (Singelyn et al. 1998). Decreased postoperative range of motion due to pain commonly contributes to arthrofibrosis and inferior results (Ryu et al. 1993). A multimodal pain regimen is a relatively new concept that has shown excellent results in terms of improving postoperative pain, reducing the need for narcotic medications, and increasing patients' motivation and participation in postoperative physical therapy (Brown et al. 2009, Busch et al. 2006, Hebl et al. 2005, Maheshwari et al. 2006, Peters et al. 2006). The key to multimodal pain control is the use of various pain medications with different mechanisms of action that results in superior pain control while minimizing their adverse side effects. Several postoperative pain control protocols exist, including patient-controlled anesthesia pumps (PCA), femoral nerve blocks (FNBs), continuous or one-time psoas compartment block (cPCB), and continuous lumbar plexus block (cLPB) (Becchi et al. 2008; Siddiqui et al. 2007). The use of local infiltration through an intra-articular catheter after THR has been shown to reduce the hospital stay and reduce the opioid-related side effects, such as nausea and vomiting, compared to continuous epidural infusion (Andersen et al. 2007). Local periarticular injections have also been used in a multimodal pain regimen that has been shown to reduce postoperative pain and improve patient satisfaction and functional recovery (Pagnano et al. 2006; Parvataneni et al. 2007).

HIP PRECAUTIONS

Postoperative hip restrictions are used to protect the soft tissue repair after a posterior approach and thereby avoid hip dislocation (Masonis and Bourne 2002). Table 66.1 presents the common precautions associated with each surgical approach; however, variations may exist regionally. These precautions can be difficult to adhere to and may interfere with the postoperative rehabilitation process (Peak et al. 2005). Dislocation after THA through the posterior approach commonly occurs when

the hip is adducted past midline, internally rotated, and flexed more than 90 degrees. To prevent this, an **abduction pillow** (Fig. 64.7) is placed between the patient's knees while in bed or a small cushion can be situated between the thighs while sitting (Rao and Bronstein 1991). In some cases, especially in revisions or in patients who are noncompliant, it may be necessary to use knee immobilizers or hip abduction orthoses for 6 to 12 weeks postoperatively to restrict hip adduction and flexion (Venditolli et al. 2006).

After an anterior or anterolateral approach, patients should avoid extreme external rotation, adduction, and extension because this could increase the chance for dislocation. However, newer reports have shown that removal of hip precautions after the anterior or anterolateral approach poses no increased risk on short-term dislocation rates (Peak et al. 2015, Talbot et al. 2002).

POSTOPERATIVE TOTAL HIP ARTHROPLASTY REHABILITATION PROGRAMS

Although a wide variety of exercise programs exist based on surgeon preference and geographic location, most protocols include quadriceps sets, gluteal sets, ankle pumps, and active hip flexion (heel slides) exercises (Enloe et al. 1996). Progressive hip abductor strengthening is also advocated because the abductors maintain the pelvis level during the stance phase and prevent tilting of the contralateral hip during the swing phase (Enloe et al. 1996, Soderberg 1986). Most exercise programs address this issue initially by concentric hip abduction in a supine position and later through isometric hip abduction against resistance (Munin et al. 1995). **The straight-leg raising exercise has been shown to apply a force of 1.5 to 1.8 times body weight and should be allowed only when partial or full weight bearing is permitted** (Davy et al. 1988). If pain occurs, hip flexion and knee extension exercises can be done separately with placement of a bolster under the knee to minimize hip stress (Davy et al. 1988, Trudelle-Jackson et al. 2002). Several reports have shown persistent quadriceps atrophy or weak thigh flexors of the operated hip compared to the contralateral hip (Bertocci et al. 2004, Reardon et al. 2001, Shih et al. 1994).

Functional tasks of daily living targeted in the rehabilitation program include weight transfer to the nonoperated hip, gait training on both level and uneven surfaces, stair climbing, and lower extremity dressing. Transferring of weight to the uninvolved side is initiated by leading with the nonoperated limb both into and out of bed and then is progressed to both sides of the bed. This method is also used with stair climbing: Patients are instructed to lead with the uninvolved hip while ascending and lead with the operated hip while descending the stairs to optimize control of body weight through the uninvolved leg (Strickland et al. 1992).

WEIGHT BEARING

Weightbearing restrictions after hip replacement, such as toe-touch weight bearing (TTWB) or partial weight bearing (PWB), directly affect the level of functional independence after surgery. PWB refers to 30% to 50% of the body weight, but studies have shown that patients have difficulty estimating and maintaining this percentage and commonly violate the restricted weight bearing (Davy et al. 1988). In TTWB, no more than 10% of body weight should be applied. TTWB is preferred over non-weight bearing (NWB) because the latter may actually create greater pressures over the hip joint as a result of muscle forces maintaining the correct pelvic positioning (Davy et al. 1988). Full weight bearing (FWB) has been shown to promote faster recovery and shorter hospital stays (Kishida et al. 2001). This is a result of reduced reliance on the upper extremities for weight bearing, resulting in earlier strengthening of the operative hip abductors and improved functional outcomes.

Assistive devices such as walkers, crutches, and canes are used to unload the operated joint and provide support and balance (Holder et al. 1993, Strickland et al. 1992). Progression from one to another is dependent on several factors such as age, comorbidities, and weightbearing restrictions. Walkers are usually the first choice after THR and provide the greatest stability by increasing the patient's base of support and unloading the affected leg (Davy et al. 1988). Because walkers require the use of both hands, carrying objects and performing self-care activities are challenging. In addition, walkers occasionally do not fit through doorways and are not recommended for use on stairs. Rolling walkers have higher self-selected walking speeds than standard walkers (Palmer and Toms 1992). Most patients advance easily from gait training with a walker to crutches or a cane. Axillary and forearm crutches are more appropriate for younger, more agile patients because they allow faster gait and yield better energy efficiency in NWB healthy subjects (Holder et al. 1993), but they have the least stability and require more control of the lower extremity and overall balance (Palmer et al. 1992). A potential complication of axillary crutches is axillary nerve compression injuries from incorrect use (O'Sullivan and Schmitz 1988). Canes are usually used on the contralateral side of the hip replacement and can transfer 10% to 20% of body weight by decreasing vertical hip contact forces (Brander et al. 1994, Deathe et al. 1993, Stineman et al. 1996). The basic function of a cane is to extend the base of support and to provide stability. Canes should be used only for patients who are fully weight bearing. Canes are inexpensive, allow a reciprocal walking pattern, can be used on stairs, and can be sized according to the patients' height. The crook of the handle should be even with the radial styloid process when the elbow is flexed at 15 to 30 degrees (O'Sullivan and Schmitz 1988).

LEVELS OF REHABILITATIVE CARE

Different rehabilitation settings include acute hospital care, inpatient rehabilitation, skilled nursing facilities, and home or outpatient rehabilitation centers. Selecting the appropriate postoperative rehabilitation that best serves the patient is often confusing to both the patient and health care professionals. In acute hospital care, postoperative physical therapy is usually started on the same day of surgery or the next morning. The goals for the first physical therapy session are to assess the patient's mobility status and to initiate therapeutic activities. With the patient lying supine in the bed, the physical therapist should observe the patient's positioning, assess for signs of a deep vein thrombosis (DVT) (Table 66.2), note the state of the dressing, and record the ROM and strength of the uninvolved leg. If signs of a DVT are present or if there is excessive drainage noted on the dressing, the nursing staff should be immediately informed prior to continuing the treatment session.

TABLE 66.2	Signs Associated With a Deep Vein Thrombosis

Lower leg swelling
Patient reporting pain in the calf and/or thigh
Redness in the calf
Pain reported by the patient when the calf and/or thigh are palpated

TABLE 66.3	Sample Week 1 Total Hip Replacement Postoperative Exercise Program*

Postoperative Day	Prescribed Exercises
Day 1	Isometrics (quadriceps sets, hamstring sets, gluteal sets)
	Ankle pumps
Day 2	Continue previous exercises.
	Supine hip range of motion within allowed ranges (passive to active as tolerated)
	Hip abduction active assisted to active range of motion
	Heel slides (heel toward buttocks)
	Bridging
Days 3–4	Continue previous exercises.
	Sitting heel raises
	Large-arc quads
Days 5–7	Continue previous exercises.
	Mini-squats
	Standing hip flexion to 90 degrees (surgical leg)
	Standing hip extension (surgical leg)
	Standing hip abduction (surgical leg)
	Forward step-up

*This sample program is based on a posterior surgical approach.

Initial training includes strength assessments, sit-to-stand transfers, and gait and balance teaching. Transfers from bed to chair are usually done twice a day for half an hour at a time. Patient education further involves lower extremity dressing, bathing, and toilet transfers using appropriate equipment to maintain hip precautions. Transfers and gait training exercises are advanced depending on the patients' weightbearing status, preoperative level of ambulation, age, and amount of improvement, progressing from simple walking to attempting curbs and ramps based on the patient's needs. Medical management includes aggressive multimodal pain control, bowel regimens, DVT prophylaxis, and management of any comorbidities.

Therapeutic exercises initiated during the initial visit may consist of lower extremity isometrics (quadriceps, hamstring, gluteal sets) and ankle pumps. Initially, a patient may be able to tolerate only passive ROM; however, he or she should be able to demonstrate increased active ROM tolerance over the course of the inpatient stay. Therapeutic exercises frequently are added daily to the patient's routine. Table 66.3 presents a sample therapeutic exercise progression during the first postoperative week.

Comprehensive inpatient rehabilitation is different from acute hospital care because it is more focused on physical therapy and interdisciplinary treatment in combination with intensive family training. Inpatient rehabilitation is reserved for patients who require more than a few days of continuous skilled care, are able to physically tolerate at least 3 hours of therapy per day, and have a good chance of returning home within a reasonable time frame (Stineman et al. 1996). Medical management is similar to the acute hospital care setting. Reports have shown that older patients without family support and patients with comorbid medical conditions usually need inpatient rehabilitation after THR (Munin et al. 1995, Weingarten et al. 1994). The subacute nursing facility (SNF) was developed as a complement to inpatient rehabilitation and has grown as an alternative to it. The SNF is reserved for patients who cannot tolerate the 3 hours of therapy per day required in an inpatient rehabilitation program and are not at risk for medical instability (Haffey and Welsh 1995).

Because of recent increasing pressure to discharge patients more quickly after surgery, it is important to assess if a patient can be safely discharged home. With improved surgical and pain management techniques, some patients may go home as early as the first postoperative day, whereas others with more comorbidities require longer lengths of hospital stay.

General criteria for home discharge include the following:
- Independent ambulation farther than 150 feet on level indoor surfaces
- Adherence to hip precautions
- Achieving basic functional activities of daily living using adaptive equipment (Brander et al. 1994, Erickson and Perkins 1994, Hughes et al. 1993, Möller et al. 1992, Munin 1995).

POSTOPERATIVE PROTOCOL AFTER PRIMARY TOTAL HIP REPLACEMENT

Our routine protocol after primary THR includes progression of quad sets and calf raises, each twice a day, up to 20 lifts each time. We recommend walking as far as possible every day with the physical therapist and with an assistive device (walker), stationary bicycling with no resistance for 15 to 20 minutes each day, and eventually swimming as tolerated. After THA through a posterolateral approach, hip precautions usually are continued for 6 weeks after surgery.

Management of Common Problems after Total Hip Replacement

1. Trendelenburg gait (weak hip abductors)
   - Concentrate on hip abduction exercises to strengthen abductors.
   - Evaluate leg-length discrepancy.
   - Have patient stand on involved leg while flexing opposite (uninvolved) knee 30 degrees. If opposite hip drops, have patient try to lift and hold in an effort to re-educate and work gluteus medius muscle (hip abductor).
   - Walk stance weight shifts: In a walk stance position patient should shift weight forward over the involved hip until unable to control hip/pelvic drop and then shift back, progressing to full weight shift and weight bearing on involved limb over time as the hip abductor strength improves.
   - Manual or pulley resistance at the pelvis with lateral walking.
2. Flexion contracture of the hip
   - **AVOID** placing pillows under the knee after surgery.
   - Walking backward helps stretch flexion contracture. Perform a Thomas stretch of 30 stretches a day (five stretches six times per day). Pull the uninvolved knee to the chest

while supine. Push the involved (postoperative) leg into extension against the bed. This stretches the anterior capsule and hip flexors of the involved leg.

Gait Faults

Gait faults should be watched for and corrected. Chandler et al. (1982) pointed out that most gait faults either are caused by or contribute to flexion deformities at the hip. These faults generally are attributable to the patient's attempts to avoid extension of the involved hip because such extension causes an uncomfortable stretching sensation in the groin.

The most common gait fault occurs when the patient takes a large step with the involved leg and a short step with the uninvolved leg. The patient should be taught to concentrate on taking longer strides with the uninvolved extremity.

A second common gait fault occurs when the patient breaks the knee in late stance phase. This is associated with flexion of the knee and early and excessive heel rise at late stance phase. The patient should be instructed to keep the heel on the ground in late stance phase.

A third common gait fault occurs when the patient flexes forward at the waist in mid and late stance. To correct this, teach the patient to thrust the pelvis forward and the shoulders backward during mid and late stance phase of gait.

One additional fault, a limp, occasionally arises simply as a habit that can be difficult to break. A full-length mirror is a useful adjunct in gait training because it allows patients to observe themselves while walking toward it.

Outpatient Total Hip Arthroplasty Physical Therapy Protocol

Typically, a patient should be either able to demonstrate or be working toward the following clinical goals:
- Achieving full, allowed active ROM at the hip by the end of the sixth postoperative week.
  - For example: hip flexion 90 degrees, hip abduction 40 degrees for the patient who has had a posterior approach surgery
- Additional ROM may be restored through stretching exercises once the physician's postoperative precautions have been lifted.
- Progress functional strengthening; including closed kinetic chain and balance exercises.
- Independent ambulation by week 12 (and without the use of an assistive device for those who did not require their utilization preoperatively).
- Patient able to drive by the end of the sixth postoperative week.
- Patient able to assume side-lying on operative hip by the end of the sixth postoperative week.
- Return to most recreational/sports pursuits by the end of the twelfth week postoperative (see later discussion).
  Exercises to increase muscle strength include the following:
- Isometrics (see Figs. 64.8 through 64.10)
- Open kinetic chain exercises (see Figs. 64.11 through 64.14)
- Closed kinetic chain exercises (see Figs. 64.14 and 64.15)
- Balance exercises (see Fig. 64.16)
  - Recent reports have suggested that adding balance exercises to the typical post THA protocol can significantly improve the patients' overall balance and functional

mobility quicker in such tests as the Timed Up and Go and the Berg balance scale (Jogi et al. 2015). This could have implications on how quickly patients discontinue assistive aids and also prevent postoperative falls.

Progressive overload to the muscles can be applied manually by the application of ankle weights or with the use of elastic resistance bands. The initial exercise prescription should consist of one to three sets of 15 to 20 repetitions. This volume of training will help to improve muscular endurance while minimizing the risk of excessive postexercise muscular soreness or pain. As endurance capacity increases, strength training can be increased to volumes of two to four sets of 6 to 10 repetitions. Table 66.4 presents frequently prescribed therapeutic exercises that address muscular weakness. The exercises are grouped by the muscles trained and in the order of difficulty.

RETURN TO SPORT AFTER TOTAL HIP REPLACEMENT

Physical activity levels may have an impact on the lifespan of the total hip replacement. Wear and tear on the replaced joint or a traumatic event may necessitate a revision surgery at a later date; however, having a hip replaced does not mean that one must end his or her recreational or sport pursuits. Exercise and activity are necessary for maintaining overall health. Instead of restricting activity, physicians have developed recommendations and guidelines for those who wish to return to activities that are more strenuous than walking. Table 66.5 presents examples of activities and sports, their associated levels of impact on the hip replacement, and recommendations as to the safety of performing and participating in a particular sport.

Table 66.6 provides a list of sports that are considered acceptable for participation, those that are possibly acceptable for participation, and those that are not recommended. Sports are designated "possibly acceptable" or "not recommended" based on the risk of falling or traumatic contact. Falling or experiencing traumatic forces may contribute to hip dislocation, hip fracture, or failure of the hip replacement.

SPORT-SPECIFIC EXERCISES FOR THE GOLFER WITH A TOTAL HIP REPLACEMENT

It is generally agreed that golfing is an acceptable sport to return to and that it places a low degree of stress on the hip implant (see Fig. 64.17). Because of the multiplanar nature of the golf swing and the unique forces placed on the body (specifically the core), the rehabilitation and strength training program for the golfer who has had a total hip replacement should include sport-specific exercises once the patient's physician has lifted hip precautions. Most sport-specific exercises should address core stability and multiplanar movement patterns.

Exercises to increase core endurance capacity include front plank with hip extension (see Fig. 64.18), the bird dog, and the side plank. With improved core endurance, the golfer should be prescribed multiplanar exercises such as the lunge with trunk rotation (see Fig. 64.19), kettle bell squats (Fig. 66.1), plyometric ball tosses (see Fig. 64.20), and proprioceptive neuromuscular facilitation chop and lift patterns performed against resistance (Fig. 66.2).

TABLE 66.4	Therapeutic Exercises Frequently Prescribed in the Outpatient Orthopedic Physical Therapy Setting	
Muscle Group	**Exercises***
Hip flexors	Isometric hip flexion
	Sitting hip flexion (no greater than 90 degrees initially)
	Manually resisted active hip flexion (patient supine, no greater than 90 degrees initially)
	Straight leg raise
	Standing hip flexion (no greater than 90 degrees initially)
	Standing hip flexion—full ROM when precautions are lifted
	Multihip machine flexion
Hip extensors	Gluteal sets
	Bridging
	Manually resisted hip extension (patient supine with leg starting in a position of hip flexion)
	Standing hip extension
	Bridging with lower extremity extension
	Prone hip extension
	Multihip machine extension
	Forward step-up
	Mini-squats
	Lateral step-down
Hip abductors	Lateral heel slides (hip abduction supine)
	Manually resisted hip abduction (patient supine)
	Standing hip abduction
	Multihip machine abduction
	Side-lying hip abduction (when precautions are lifted)
	Lateral step-downs
Hip adductors	Hip adductor isometrics (with the patient supine and the hip in neutral or slightly abducted)
	Manually resisted hip adduction to neutral from a hip-abducted position
	Standing hip adduction (when precautions are lifted)
	Side-lying hip adduction (when precautions are lifted)
Hip external rotators	Manually applied hip external rotation isometric (patient supine in hook-lying)
	Manually applied hip external rotation with active hip external rotation from neutral (patient supine in hook-lying)
Hip internal rotators	Manually applied hip internal rotation isometric (patient supine in hook-lying with hip positioned in neutral or slightly externally rotated)
	Manually applied hip internal rotation with active hip internal rotation from a starting position of external rotation to neutral (patient positioned in supine)
Knee extensors	Quadriceps set
	Short-arc quad
	Straight leg raise
	Large-arc quad
	Forward step-up
	Mini-squat
	Lateral step-down
	Leg press
Knee curl	Hamstring sets
	Heel slides toward buttock
	Standing hamstring curls
	Leg curl machine (sitting): double-legged and single-legged curls
Gastrocnemius and soleus	Sitting heel raise
	Standing heel raise

*Exercises are presented by their relative degree of difficulty.

TABLE 66.5	Sport Participation Recommendations and Associated Levels of Impact on the Total Joint Replacement	
Level of Impact	**Examples**	**Recommendations**
Low	Stationary cycling Calisthenics Golf Stationary skiing Swimming Walking Ballroom dancing Water aerobics	Can improve general health Desirable for most patients, but may increase rate of wear Orthotics and activity modifications can reduce impact loads. Concentration on conditioning and flexibility rather than strengthening
Potentially low	Bowling Fencing Rowing Isokinetic weight lifting Sailing Speed walking Cross-country skiing Table tennis Jazz dancing and ballet Bicycling	Desirable for most patients, but may increase rate of wear Requires preactivity evaluation, monitoring, and development of guidelines by surgeon Balance and proprioception must be intact. Orthotics and activity modifications can reduce impact loads. Emphasize high number of repetitions with minimal resistance.
Intermediate	Free-weight lifting Hiking Horseback riding Ice skating Rock climbing Low-impact aerobics Tennis In-line skating Downhill skiing	Appropriate only for selected patients Require preactivity evaluation, monitoring, and development of guidelines for participation by surgeon Excellent physical condition is necessary. Orthotics, impact-absorbing shoes, and activity modification frequently necessary.
High	Baseball/softball Basketball/volleyball Football Handball/racquetball Jogging/running Lacrosse Soccer Water skiing Karate	Should be avoided Significant probability of injury and need for revision

From Clifford PE, Mallon WJ: Sports participation for patients with joint replacements based upon level of impact loading. Clin Sports Med 2005 2005; 24(1):182, Table 1.

TABLE 66.6	Sports Participation Recommendations for Patients With a Total Hip Replacement		
Acceptable	**Possible**	**Not Recommended**
Ballroom dancing	Ballet dancing	Baseball/softball
Bicycling	Calisthenics	Basketball
Bowling	Downhill skiing	Football
Cross-country skiing	Fencing	Handball/racquetball
Golf	Hiking	Karate
Horseback riding	Jazz dancing	Lacrosse
Ice skating	Jogging/running	Soccer
In-line skating	Rock climbing	Volleyball
Low-impact aerobics	Table tennis	
Rowing	Tennis	
Sailing	Water skiing	
Speed walking		
Stationary cycling		
Stationary skiing		
Swimming		
Walking		
Water aerobics		

Adapted from Clifford PE, Mallon WJ: Sports participation for patients with joint replacements based upon level of impact loading. Clin Sports Med 2005; 24(1):183, Table 2.

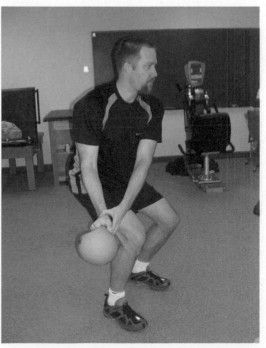

Fig. 66.1 Kettle bell squat with rotation.

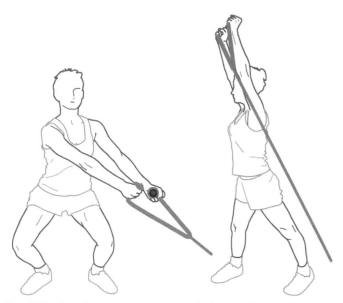

Fig. 66.2 Proprioceptive neuromuscular facilitation chop and lift patterns with pulleys.

REFERENCES

A complete reference list is available at https://expertconsult .inkling.com/.

FURTHER READING

Barrett, et al. Prospective randomized study of direct anterior v postero-lateral approach for total hip arthroplasty. *J Arthroplasty.* 2013;28:1634–1638.

Larsen K. Cost-effectiveness of accelerated periopererative care and rehabilitation after total hip and knee arthroplasty. *J Bone Joint Surg Am.* 2009;91:761–772.

Lima D, Magnus R, Paprosky WG. Team management of hip revision patients using a post-op hip orthosis. *J Prosthet Orthop.* 1994;6:20–24.

Mahomed N, et al. Inpatient compared with home-based rehabilitation following primary unilateral total hip or knee replacement: a randomized controlled trial. *J Bone Joint Surg Am.* 2008;90:1673–1680.

Talbot NJ, Brown JH, Treble NJ. Early dislocation after total hip arthroplasty: are postoperative restrictions necessary? *J Arthroplasty.* 2002;17:1006–1008.

Groin Pain

Michael P. Reiman, PT, DPT, OCS, SCS, ATC, FAAOMPT, CSCS | S. Brent Brotzman, MD

BACKGROUND

Groin pain is a broad, general term that means different things to different people. Patients may describe "I pulled my groin" (groin strain), or "I got kicked in the groin" (testicle), or "I have a lump in my groin" (lower abdominal wall). It is estimated that 5% to 18% of athletes experience activity-restricting groin pain. This groin pain is common in sports involving repetitive kicking, twisting, or turning at high speeds. The complex anatomy and multitude of differential diagnoses make the identification of a specific cause difficult, as do the often diffuse, insidious, and nonspecific symptoms. Adding to the diagnostic dilemma is the fact that two or more injuries may coexist. The keys to this diagnostically challenging problem are thorough history taking and examination.

Initially it is important to establish accurately whether this is an acute injury (usually musculoskeletal) or a chronic symptom (often nonmusculoskeletal in origin). Second, the correct anatomic area being described should be identified (e.g., hip adductors [medial], hip, testicle, lower abdominal wall). The commonly accepted definition of a groin strain focuses on injury to the hip adductors and includes the iliopsoas, rectus femoris, and sartorius musculotendinous units (Fig. 67.1). An accurate area of anatomic pain must be delineated by the examiner (e.g., adductor origin or testicular pain with radiation).

In a study of 207 athletes with groin pain (Hölmich 2007), adductor-related dysfunction was the primary clinical entity (58%), followed by iliopsoas-related dysfunction (36%) and rectus abdominus–related dysfunction (6%). Multiple clinical entities were found in 33%.

HISTORY

Careful history taking is required to avoid missing a potentially catastrophic problem (e.g., stress fracture of the femoral neck).

Acute (Traumatic) Injuries

- Mechanism of injury (e.g., change of direction, pivoting)
- Hear or feel a pop?
- Swelling or bruising noted? If so, location?
- Previous groin injury?
- Recent change in training regimen?
- Pain with walking? If so, location?

Chronic Injuries or Those With No Clearcut Traumatic, Musculoskeletal Mechanism

- Pain at rest or at night (neoplasm possible)
- Does the pain radiate (e.g., to the back, thigh, hip, scrotum, or perineum)?
- What alleviates pain (e.g., physical therapy, rest, NSAIDs)?

- Associated numbness (look for a dermatomal pattern emanating from the back)
- Pain on coughing or sneezing, which increases intra-abdominal pressure (hernia or low back disc)
- Can patient reproduce pain with exertion or certain movements?
- Does patient complain of popping, catching, or clicking deep in hip? (possible intra-articular hip pathology; i.e., labral tear, snapping hip, etc.)
- Fever or chills (possible infection or neoplasm)
- Activities that cause the pain
- Recent weight loss (neoplasm)
- Urinary symptoms such as dysuria, urgency, frequency, hematuria (possible sexually transmitted disease, urinary tract infection, stones)
- Bowel symptoms such as blood in stool, mucus, diarrhea (Crohn's disease, ulcerative colitis)

EXAMINATION

Examination should include the groin, hip area, back, genitourinary, and lower abdominal wall (Tables 67.1 and 67.2). If the patient's complaint is anatomically hip pain rather than groin

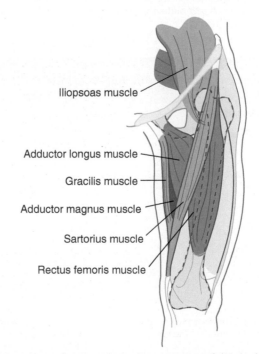

Fig. 67.1 Among the musculotendinous injuries of the thigh that can cause groin pain, adductor longus muscle injuries are the most common. Any injury to the iliopsoas, rectus femoris, sartorius, or gracilis muscle can also produce groin pain. (Redrawn from DeLee JC, Drez D Jr, Orthopaedic Sports Medicine: Principles and Practice. Philadelphia, WB Saunders, 1994.)

TABLE 67.1	Physical Examination of the Groin	
Patient's Position	**Procedure**	**Details**
Standing	Observe posture, gait, limb alignment, muscle wasting, ability to sit and stand up, swelling.	Have the patient point to the area of pain and the pattern of radiation.
		Have the patient reproduce painful movements.
	Examine the low back: active ROM.	Forward flexion, side bending, extension.
	Examine the hip: active ROM.	Trendelenburg's sign (hip adductor strength), ability to squat and duck walk.
	Examine the hernia.	Palpate the inguinal region (have the patient cough or strain down).
Supine	Examine the abdomen.	Palpate for abdominal aortic aneurysm, pain, rebound, guarding, hernia, pulses, nodes.
		Test for costovertebral angle tenderness (renal area).
		When appropriate, perform a rectal examination to palpate the prostate and rule out occult blood.
	Examine male genitalia.	Palpate for a testicular mass, varicocele, or tender epididymis.
	Pelvic examination in women, if appropriate.	Look for purulent vaginal discharge of pelvic inflammatory disease and bluish cervix of pregnancy (ectopic).
		Palpate for tender cervix or adnexa, ovarian mass.
	Examine low back, sciatic nerve roots.	Perform SLR, test for Lasègue sign and Bragard sign (dorsiflexion of ankle).
	Examine hip motion.	Evaluate flexion, external rotation, internal rotation, abduction, adduction, joint play, quadrant tests, any groin pain with internal rotation.
		Perform passive SLR, Thomas, and rectus femoris stretch tests.
	Palpate pelvic structures.	Palpate symphysis, pubic rami, iliac crests, adductor insertions, ASIS, PSIS, ischial tuberosities.
	Examine sacroiliac joints.	Perform Patrick (flexion, abduction, external rotation, extension [FABERE]).
	Look for leg-length discrepancy.	Verify grossly and determine true length by measuring from ASIS to lateral malleoli.
Prone	Examine hip motion.	Evaluate extension and internal and external rotation.
		Perform Ely and femoral nerve stretch tests.
Side lying	Examine iliotibial band.	Perform Ober test.
Sitting	Evaluate muscle strength.	Test hip flexion (L2, L3), hip extension (L5, S1, S2), abduction (L4, L5, S1), adduction (L3, L4).
	Test reflexes.	Assess patellar tendon (L4).
	Test sensation.	Assess lower abdomen (T12), groin (L1), medial thigh (L2), anterior quadriceps (L3).

ASIS, anterior superior iliac spine; *PSIS*, posterior superior iliac spine; *ROM*, range of motion; *SLR*, straight leg raises.
From Lacroix VJ. A complete approach to groin pain. Phys Sportsmed 2000;28(1):66.

TABLE 67.2	Potential Causes of Groin Pain: Key Features and Treatments	
Causes	**Key Features**	**Treatment Options**
MUSCULOSKELETAL		
Abdominal muscle tear	Localized tenderness to palpation; pain with activation of rectus abdominis	Relative rest, analgesics
Adductor tendinitis	Tenderness over involved tendon, pain with resisted adduction of lower extremity	NSAIDs, rest, physical therapy
Avascular necrosis of the femoral head	Radiation of pain into the groin with internal rotation of hip; decreased hip ROM	Recommend MRI
		Mild: conservative measures, possible core decompression; *Severe:* total hip replacement, needs orthopedic hip specialty consult
Avulsion fracture	Pain on palpation of injury site; pain with stretch of involved muscle, x-ray positive, felt a pop when "turning on speed"	Relative rest; ice; NSAIDs; possibly crutches; evaluate for ORIF of fragment if >1 cm displacement
Bursitis	Pain over site of bursa	Injection of cortisone, anesthetic, or both; avoid injections around nerves (e.g., sciatic)
Conjoined tendon dehiscence	Pain with Valsalva maneuver	Surgical referral (general surgeon)
Herniated nucleus pulposus	Positive dural or sciatic tension signs	Physical therapy or appropriate referral (spine specialist)
Legg-Calvé-Perthes disease	Irritable hip with pain on rotation, positive x-rays, pediatric (usually ages 5–8 yr)	Pediatric orthopedic surgeon referral
Muscle strain	Acute pain over proximal muscles of medial thigh region; swelling; occasional bruising	Rest; avoidance of aggravating activities; initial ice, with heat after 48 hr; hip spica wrap; NSAIDs for 7–10 days; see section on treatment

TABLE 67.2	Potential Causes of Groin Pain: Key Features and Treatments—cont'd	
Causes	**Key Features**	**Treatment Options**
Myositis ossificans	Pain and decreased ROM in involved muscle; palpable mass within substance of muscle, x-ray shows calcification, often history of blow (helmet) to area	Moderately aggressive active or passive ROM exercises; wrap thigh with knee in maximum flexion for first 24 hr; NSAIDs used sparingly for 2 days after trauma
Nerve entrapment	Burning or shooting pain in distribution of nerve; altered light-touch sensation in medial groin; pain exacerbated by hyperextension at hip joint, possibly radiating; tenderness near superior iliac spine	Possible infiltration of site with local anesthetic; topical cream (e.g., capsaicin)
Osteitis pubis	Pain around abdomen, groin, hip, or thigh, increased by resisted adduction of thigh; tender on palpation of pubis symphysis; x-ray positive for sclerosis irregularity; osteolysis at the pubis symphysis; bone scan positive	Relative rest; initial ice and NSAIDs; possibly crutches; later, stretching exercises
Osteoarthritis	Groin pain with hip motion, especially internal rotation	Non-narcotic analgesics or NSAIDs; hip replacement for intractable pain; see Section 6
Pubic instability	Excess motion at pubic symphysis; pain in pubis, groin, or lower abdomen	Physical therapy, NSAIDs; compression shorts
Referred pain from knee or spine	Hip ROM and palpation response normal	Identify true source of referred pain
Seronegative spondyloarthropathy	Signs of systemic illness, other joint involvement	Refer to rheumatologist
Slipped capita femoral epiphysis*	Inguinal pain with hip movement; insidious development in ages 8–15 yr; walking with limp, holding leg in external rotation	Discontinue athletic activity; refer to orthopedic surgeon for probable pinning, crutches; TDWB
STRESS FRACTURE		
Pubic ramus	Chronic ache or pain in groin, buttock, and thighs	Relative rest; avoid aggravating activities, crutches PWB
Femoral neck*	Chronic ache or pain in groin, buttock, and thighs or pain with decreased hip ROM (internal rotation in flexion)	Refer to orthopedist if radiographs or bone scan shows lesion; TDWB crutches and cessation of all weightbearing activities until orthopedic consult
NONMUSCULOSKELETAL		
Genital swelling or inflammation		
Epididymitis	Tenderness over superior aspect of testes	Antibiotics if appropriate or refer to urologist
Hydrocele	Pain in lower spermatic cord region	Refer to urologist
Varicocele	Rubbery, elongated mass around spermatic cord	Refer to urologist
Hernia	Recurrent episodes of pain; palpable mass made more prominent with coughing or straining; discomfort elicited by abdominal wall tension	Refer for surgical evaluation and treatment (general surgeon)
Lymphadenopathy	Palpable lymph nodes just below inguinal ligaments; fever, chills, discharge	Antibiotics, work-up, also rule out underlying sexually transmitted disease
Ovarian cyst	Groin or perineal pain	Refer to gynecologist
PID	Fever, chills, purulent discharge + chandelier sign, "PID shuffle"	Refer to gynecologist
Postpartum symphysis separation	Recent vaginal delivery with no prior history of groin pain	Physical therapy, relative rest, analgesics
Prostatitis	Dysuria, purulent discharge	Antibiotics, NSAIDs
Renal lithiasis	Intense pain that radiates to scrotum	Pain control, increased fluids until stone passes; hospitalization sometimes necessary
Testicular neoplasm	Hard mass palpated on the testicle; may not be tender	Refer to urologist
Testicular torsion or rupture†	Severe pain in the scrotum; nausea, vomiting; testes hard on palpation or not palpable	Refer immediately to urologist
Urinary tract infection	Burning with urination; itching; frequent urination	Short course of antibiotics

*Nonweightbearing until orthopedic evaluation to avoid fracture.
†Emergent immediate referral.
MRI, magnetic resonance imaging; *NSAIDS,* = nonsteroidal anti-inflammatory drugs; *ORIF,* = open reduction and internal fixation; *PID,* = pelvic inflammatory disease; *PWD,* = partial weight bearing; *ROM,* = range of motion; *TDWB,* touch-down weight bearing.
Modified from Ruane JJ, Rossi TA. When groin pain is more than just a strain. Phys Sportsmed 26(4):78.

TABLE 67.3	Differential Diagnosis of Hip Pain in Athletes

- Hip dislocation
- Hip subluxation with or without acetabulum or labrum injury
- Osteochondritis dissecans
- Acetabulum or pelvis fracture or stress fracture
- Femoral neck fracture or stress fracture
- Anterior superior iliac spine avulsions (sartorius or rectus femoris origin)
- Iliac spine contusion (hip pointer)
- Adductor muscle strain
- Osteitis pubis
- Inguinal hernia
- Lateral femoral cutaneous nerve entrapment or injury (meralgia paresthesia)
- Femoral artery or nerve injury
- Idiopathic avascular necrosis of the femoral head
- Idiopathic chondrolysis
- Slipped capital femoral epiphysis
- Legg-Calvé-Perthes disease
- Metabolic disorders
- Sickle cell disease
- Inflammatory disease
- Lumbar disc disease
- Neoplastic abnormalities of the pelvis acetabulum or femur
- Piriformis syndrome

From Lacroix VJ. A complete approach to groin pain. *Phys Sportsmed* 2000;28(1):66–86.

pain, differential diagnosis can include a number of possible causes of hip pain in athletes (Table 67.3).

Although the diagnosis usually is made clinically, radiographs can be useful for excluding fractures or avulsions, and MRI can confirm muscle strain or tears and partial and complete tendon tears. Ultrasound also can be used to identify muscle and tendon tears.

TREATMENT

The location of a tear of adductor musculature has important therapeutic and prognostic implications. With acute tears at the musculotendinous junction, a relatively aggressive rehabilitation program can be used, whereas a partial tear at the tendinous insertion of the adductors on the pubis usually requires a period of rest before pain-free physical therapy is possible. Generally initial treatment includes physical therapy modalities, such as rest, ice, compression, and elevation, that help prevent further injury, followed by restoration of ROM and prevention of atrophy. Then the patient focuses on regaining strength, flexibility, and endurance. *Restoration of at least 70% of strength and a pain-free full ROM are criteria for return to sport; this may require 4 to 6 weeks for an acute strain and up to 6 months for a chronic injury.*

A systematic review of the available literature concerning exercise therapy for groin pain (Machotka et al. 2009) found that exercise, particularly strengthening of the hip and abdominal musculature, can be an effective treatment for athletes with groin pain. The evidence suggested that strengthening exercises may need to be progressed, from static contractions to functional positions, and performed through a ROM. Duration of therapy of 4 to 16 weeks was generally recommended. In a group of 19 National Football League (NFL) players (Schlegel et al. 2009), 14 who were treated nonoperatively returned to play at an average of 6 weeks, whereas 5 treated operatively returned to play at an average of 12 weeks.

Although some have suggested that an exercise program may help prevent groin injuries, a study of 977 soccer players randomized to an exercise program targeting groin injury prevention (strengthening [concentric and eccentric], coordination, and core stability exercises for the muscles related to the pelvis) or their usual training regimen found that the risk of a groin injury was reduced by 31%, but this reduction was not significant. A univariate analysis showed that **having had a previous groin injury almost doubles the risk of developing a new groin injury and playing at a higher level almost triples the risk of developing a groin injury** (Hölmich et al. 2010).

Schilders et al. (2007) reported that a single injection of a local anesthetic and corticosteroid into the adductor enthesis was effective in 28 recreational athletes and 24 competitive athletes. Five minutes after the injection all patients reported resolution of their groin pain, but pain relief was lasting only in those with normal findings on MRI; 16 of 17 competitive athletes with enthesopathy on MRI had recurrence within an average of 5 weeks, whereas none of 7 with normal MRI findings had recurrence. Most recreational athletes (75%) had pain relief at 1 year regardless of MRI findings.

For chronic adductor-related groin pain, adductor release has been reported to be successful in about 70% of patients (Atkinson et al. 2009). If a sports hernia is identified, operative treatment usually is required (Garvey et al. 2010), with return to preinjury level of activity at approximately 3 months postoperatively.

REFERENCES

A complete reference list is available at https://expertconsult.inkling.com/.

FURTHER READING

Almeida, Matheus O, Brenda Ng Silva, et al. Conservative interventions for treating exercise-related musculotendinous, ligamentous and osseous groin pain. *Cochrane Database Syst Rev*. 1996. n. pag. Web.

Anderson K, Strickland SM, Warren R. Hip and groin injuries in athletes. *The Am J Sports Med*. 2001;29(4):521–530.

Farber AJ, Wilckens JH. Sports hernia: diagnosis and therapeutic approach. *The Am Acad Orthop Surg*. 2007;15:507–514.

Lacroix VJ. A complete approach to groin pain. *Physician Sports Med*. 2000;28(1):32–37.

Leibold MR, Huijbregts PA, Jensen R. Concurrent criterion-related validity of physical examination tests for hip labral lesions: a systematic review. *J Man Manipul Ther*. 2008;16(2):E24–E41.

Maffey L, Emery C. What are the risk factors for groin strain injury in sport? *Sport Med*. 2007;37(10):881–894.

Michalski Max, Larsn Engebretse. Bone and joint problems related to groin pain. *Sports Injuries*. 2015:705–721. Web.

Serner A, Van Eijck CH, Beumer BR, et al. Study quality on groin injury management remains low: a systematic review on treatment of groin pain in athletes. *Br J Sports Med*. 2015;49.12:813. Web.

Suarez JC, Ely EE, Mutnal AB, et al. Comprehensive approach to the evaluation of groin pain. *J Am Acad Orthop Surg*. 2013;21(9):558–570. Web.

Swain R, Snodgrass S. Managing groin pain, even when the cause is not obvious. *Physician Sports Med*. 1995;23.1:54–62.

Swan Jr KG, Wolcott M. The athletic hernia: a systematic review. *Clin Orthop Relat Res*. 2007;455:78–87.

Weir A, Jansen JACG, Van De Port IGL, et al. Manual or exercise therapy for long-standing adductor-related groin pain: a randomised controlled clinical trial. *Man Ther*. 2011;16.2:148–154. Web.

Hamstring Muscle Injuries in Athletes

J. Allen Hardin, PT, MS, SCS, ATC, LAT, CSCS | Clayton F. Holmes, PT, EdD, MS, ATC

Hamstring muscle injuries are a significant cause of lost playing time and disability in high school, college, and professional sports. One study found that hamstring strain injuries were second in frequency only to knee sprains in a group of professional football players over a 10-year period (Woods et al. 2004). Another study of the NFL found that hamstring injuries comprised 12% of all injuries over a two-season period (Levine et al. 2000).

Hamstring injuries are most frequent in sports that require sprinting, such as football, rugby, soccer, basketball, and track, but hamstring injuries also occur in sports that do not require significant running and sprinting. For example, dancers have susceptibility to hamstring injuries but most often sustain the injury during slow stretching (Askling et al. 2006, 2007). Wrestling, which may require a high forceful shortening against resistance of the hamstring, can also lead to hamstring injuries.

The average hamstring injury can cause an athlete to miss up to 3 weeks of activity. Torn hamstrings can be much more serious and lead to prolonged loss of time from sport or surgery. A troubling aspect of hamstring injuries is the high re-injury rate, ranging from 12% to 30% in the literature (Orchard and Best 2002). **Two major factors implicated by Schneider-Kolsky et al. (2006) in re-injury of the hamstrings are an inadequate rehabilitation program and a premature return to sport.**

CONSIDERATIONS OF APPLIED ANATOMY AND BIOMECHANICS

The most common type of hamstring injury is a hamstring strain. The most common type of hamstring strain occurs at the musculotendinous junction of the biceps femoris muscle. Because of diminished blood supply of the tendon unit, injuries to musculotendinous junctions and tendons themselves can be particularly challenging to rehabilitate.

Because the typical presentation of acute hamstring strains includes very specific anatomic identification, it is important to understand the anatomy of the hamstrings. The hamstrings are a group of muscles that compose the posterior thigh and cross both the hip and knee joints. Concentrically, when activated prone against resistance, the hamstrings flex the knee and/or extend the hip. More important, during function, the most intense type of contraction occurs during the second half of the swing phase of walking or running. In other words, the hamstring functions to slow the leg during the swing phase of running. This is essentially an eccentric contraction.

The hamstring is comprised of three muscles: the semimembranosus, the semitendinosus, and the biceps femoris (Fig. 68.1). It is important to note that all three muscles, with the exception of the short head of the biceps femoris (the biceps femoris includes both a long and short head), cross both the hip and the knee posteriorly with the tendon of the biceps attaching distally to the head of the fibula and the tendinosus and

membranosus attaching to the tibia medially (Fig. 68.2). These muscles, like all musculotendinous units, consist of the muscle and the surrounding tendons attaching to the bone. This is important because the clinical examination includes application of the principles of selective tissue tension testing, which distinguishes between contractile and noncontractile tissue.

CLASSIFICATION OF HAMSTRING INJURY

In 1985, Agre categorized musculotendinous injuries, based on their etiology, as a result of either indirect or direct trauma. The primary etiology of injuries in the hamstring is indirect trauma. These injuries are often referred to as hamstring strains and have been classified as grades 1 through 3 based on severity of the injury, increasing with the grade. A grade 1 is considered a mild strain, grade 2 a moderate strain, and grade 3 a severe strain. More specifically, the classification system is based on clinical presentation and the assumed underlying soft tissue damage (Table 68.1).

It should be noted that, although grading the injury is important relative to prognosis, specific clinical and functional findings are better indicators of prognosis and treatment.

ETIOLOGIC CONCERNS

The most common hamstring injury is a hamstring strain sustained in a running sport, and the most common presentation is symptoms along the musculotendinous junction of the biceps femoris and the semitendinosus muscles. The mechanism of injury and the tissue injured have an important prognostic value in estimating rehabilitation time needed to return to preinjury level of performance. Injuries to an intramuscular tendon or aponeurosis and adjacent muscle fibers (biceps femoris during high-speed running) require shorter rehabilitation time than injuries involving a proximal, free tendon (semimembranosus during dance or kicking).

In 1992, Worrell and Perrin described the primary predisposing factors for hamstring strains: strength (including strength imbalances in either unilateral extensors or flexors), flexibility, and fatigue. The two most common factors in hamstring injury are lack of adequate flexibility and strength imbalances in the hamstrings (flexor-to-extensor and right-to-left imbalance).

The clinical history of a running athlete often includes a description of being unable to finish his or her activity and "pulling up." The athlete may also report feeling or hearing a "pop" in the posterior thigh. If this injury occurs early during an athletic activity (i.e., early in practice), the primary factor may be assumed to be a lack of flexibility, whereas injuries occurring later during the athletic event (practice or competition) may be believed to be associated with fatigue. In reality, multiple factors may be involved, including intrinsic factors such as muscle

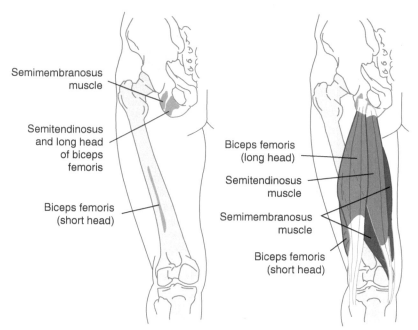

Fig. 68.1 Origins of the hamstring tendons *(left)* and muscles of the hamstring group *(right)*. (From Clanton TO, Coupe KJ. Hamstring strains in athletes: Diagnosis and treatment. © 1998 American Academy of Orthopaedic Surgeons. Reprinted from the *Journal of the American Academy of Orthopaedic Surgeons*, Volume 6 (4), pp. 237–248, with permission.)

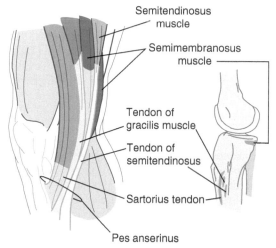

Fig. 68.2 *Left,* Attachment of the semitendinosus with the pes anserinus at the proximal medial aspect of the tibia. *Right,* Insertions of the gracilis (G), sartorius (S), semimembranosus (SM), and semitendinosus (ST). (From Clanton TO, Coupe KJ. Hamstring strains in athletes: diagnosis and treatment. © 1998 American Academy of Orthopaedic Surgeons. Reprinted from the *Journal of the American Academy of Orthopaedic Surgeons*, Volume 6 (4), pp. 237–248, with permission.)

TABLE 68.1	Classification of Muscle Strains	
Type	**Severity**	**Clinical Signs**
1	Mild, damage to a few muscle fibers	Sensation of muscle "cramping" and tightness
		Slight pain with muscle stretch and contraction
		Signs may not be present until after activity
2	Moderate, more extensive damage to muscle fibers, partially torn but still intact	Immediate pain
		More severe pain with stretch and contraction
		Soreness over hamstring muscle
		Slight bruising 2 to 3 days after injury
3	Severe, complete rupture of the muscle	Immediate burning or stabbing pain
		Inability to walk
		Palpable mass of muscle tissue at tear
		Severe bruising 2 to 3 days after injury

weakness, strength and balance, fatigue, inadequate flexibility, abnormal biomechanics, disturbed posture, poor running technique, and psychosocial factors. Extrinsic factors include warmup and training procedures, fatigue related to excessive activities, poor playing surfaces, unsuitable training, and sports-specific activities. No single risk factor has been found to have a significant association with hamstring injury.

PHYSICAL EXAMINATION

If the athlete presents with a primary acute hamstring strain, the examination begins with having the athlete point with one finger to the pain or to the "epicenter" of pain. Very often this will direct the physical examination and lead to a diagnosis.

Inspection may or may not reveal ecchymosis and swelling depending on the severity and acuity of the injury. When these signs are present, they are not necessarily reflective of the site of injury because of the width of the hamstring and the blood supply available to the hamstring muscle group. However, in general, ecchymosis and swelling in the posterior thigh are indicative of a hamstring injury.

Palpation of a grade 1 strain may reveal tenderness at the associated site (correlated with the athlete's report of the site of pain) and increased tension at the site (possibly muscle spasm). An indentation in the soft tissue is indicative of a partial or complete rupture as with a grade 3 strain. The latter findings are more evident the earlier the examination occurs relative to the injury.

Inspection and palpation should be done with the athlete prone and the knee in three positions:
1. Relaxed (relative extension)
2. Slightly flexed (15 degrees)
3. Flexed (90 degrees)

Light resistance should be applied to the heel posteriorly, with the knee moving into flexion. All three of these positions should be used because of the relative length of the hamstring muscle group in each of these positions. It is common for abnormal palpation findings to be present with the knee in the 90-degree position with light manual resistance.

In patients with acute injuries, strength and ROM are generally not tested because of pain. With subacute injuries, pain and swelling often decrease the validity of these findings; ecchymosis and swelling often are present.

Several special tests have been described that may strongly correlate with prognosis:

- **Passive straight leg raise.** This is performed in the same way as the typical supine straight leg raise test for back pain, but the athlete is asked to report the first stretch or discomfort/stiffness. The degree of hip flexion is measured by an inclinometer or goniometer.
- **Measurement of active knee extension.** The supine athlete is asked to maintain the hip at 90 degrees of flexion against a wooden frame with the noninjured leg measured first. The athlete is asked to extend the knee with light contact against the horizontal part of the frame. A temporary myoclonus of alternating contraction and relaxation of the quadriceps and hamstring muscle groups tends to occur at the maximal angle of active knee extension. The athlete is instructed not to push the knee extension beyond this "shaking." The angle of knee flexion indicates the point of hamstring resistance. This measure is then correlated with the dorsiflexion passive straight leg raise (DPSLR) test and the initial complaint of pain.
- **Manual muscle testing** of hamstring muscles. This is not a classic manual muscle test in the sense of grading strength; rather, this test is used to elicit pain. A positive test is one in which pain is elicited, and a negative test is one in which resistance is applied and no pain is reproduced.
- **Slump test.** This neural tension testing is aimed at distinguishing between soft tissue (e.g., hamstring) and neurologic tissue involvement. The knee of the limb to be assessed is manually extended. If it reaches full extension, the ankle is then dorsiflexed. If this maneuver reproduces the patient's symptoms, he or she is asked to extend the cervical spine. If the nervous system/neural tension is implicated in producing the symptoms, the symptoms will reduce. Alternatively, the patient may be instructed to plantar flex and dorsiflex the ankle. Again, symptoms associated with spinal cord and sciatic/tibial nerve should lessen in plantarflexion. False positives are common.

DIAGNOSTIC IMAGING

Although there have been many advancements in diagnostic imaging, thorough clinical examination remains the gold standard of evaluation. The use of ultrasonography and MRI in the evaluation of hamstring injuries has not demonstrated increased sensitivity relative to the clinical examination. Thorough clinical examination has demonstrated accuracy at least equivalent to MRI in determining ultimate prognosis.

HAMSTRING INJURIES OTHER THAN STRAINS

Specific consideration during examination and evaluation should be given to the avulsions of the ischial tuberosity and severe injuries to the distal tendons of the hamstrings.

Avulsions

Differentiating between proximal hamstring avulsions and proximal muscle strains is critically important to the long-term prognosis. One study indicated that as many as 12% of hamstring injuries may include hamstring avulsions (Koulouris 2003). Proximal hamstring injuries should be evaluated with imaging techniques, which are not necessary for typical hamstring strains, to rule out an avulsion. It is also important to note that examination findings in proximal hamstring injuries, regardless of osseous involvement, typically include dramatic ecchymosis and swelling with associated morbidity and a less positive prognosis. If a hamstring avulsion is complete, a palpable gap is present at the hamstring attachment. Again, as with all clinical findings, palpation findings become less valid as swelling and ecchymosis become present.

Tendinous avulsions are most accurately diagnosed with MRI. A classification system has been described that is based on the anatomic location of the injury, the degree of avulsion (complete or incomplete), the degree of muscle retraction (if avulsion is complete), and the presence or absence of sciatic nerve tethering (Wood et al. 2008). Classification facilitates preoperative planning to determine the type of surgery required.

Distal tears of hamstring tendons cause symptoms similar to those of typical hamstring strains at the musculotendinous junction of the biceps femoris. Reported symptoms include weakness and pain during knee flexion and a sense of instability of the knee joint. Other findings include tenderness at the site of the injury and localized swelling and ecchymosis. As with other hamstring strains, a proximally retracted muscle belly and palpable defect may also be present.

Other sources of pain and disability that may present as chronic hamstring muscle pain include a tendon or musculotendinous junction tear or an avulsion of the biceps femoris tendon from the head of the fibula. Differential diagnosis of an apparent unresolved hamstring muscle strain should consider such pathologies.

Rehabilitation of Hamstring Injuries

The primary objective of a rehabilitation program is to return the athlete to sport at the highest level of function with minimal risk of re-injury. Returning the athlete with a hamstring muscle injury to sport may require the use of multiple rehabilitation strategies, consisting of both direct and indirect techniques. The high recurrence rate and chronicity associated with hamstring injuries have placed significant emphasis not only on appropriate treatment of these injuries after they occur but also on developing and implementing strategies to prevent hamstring injuries.

Several factors may contribute to the high recurrence rate of hamstring injuries: (1) persistent hamstring muscle weakness, (2) scar tissue formation that results in reduced extensibility of the musculotendon unit, and (3) biomechanical and neuromuscular adaptations as a result of the injury. Therefore, therapeutic interventions that address these factors must be identified and incorporated.

The recurrence rate for hamstring injuries is as high as 12% to 31%, and estimates indicate that approximately one in three athletes re-injure their involved hamstring within 1 year of returning to sport. These data suggest that these injuries can be difficult to rehabilitate effectively, particularly because symptoms can be persistent and healing can be slow, and that inappropriate criteria are used to determine suitability for return to sport or traditional rehabilitation methods are insufficient for reducing the risk of recurrence.

Rehabilitation of Acute Hamstring Injuries

Rehabilitation programs are typically based on the tissue's theoretical healing response. Worrell (1994) suggested a four-phase program, which proposed that progressive stretching and strengthening of the injured tissue would lead to tissue remodeling and collagen fiber alignment in the developing scar tissue:
1. The acute phase (2 to 4 days), focusing on controlling inflammation and regaining early motion
2. The subacute phase, incorporating isolated hamstring strengthening and pain-free stretching
3. The remodeling phase, with continued hamstring strengthening and the addition of eccentric muscle strengthening
4. The functional period, during which jogging, running, sprinting, functional training, and sport-specific drills are added

These rehabilitation phases are loosely guided by and take into consideration the time since injury; however, specific interventions and progression should be dictated by the athlete's status. The interventions described in the following paragraphs should be implemented into the rehabilitation program using the phased structure as a guide. The methods, techniques, and interventions described here are not all-inclusive, and the treatment chronology must be adapted according to the severity of the injury and the individual features and symptoms of the injury.

Acute hamstring injuries result in pain and disability, manifested in decreased ROM, decreased strength, and decreased functional abilities. The initial focus of rehabilitation of hamstring injuries should be on minimizing the acute effects of the injury and promoting tissue healing. Management of acute hamstring injuries begins with an emphasis on indirect interventions to decrease the inflammation and pain associated while promoting tissue healing and protecting the scar formation. Interventions include low-intensity therapeutic exercise, modalities, medications, and protection.

Protection

The injured extremity is protected with modified ambulation. Full weight bearing ambulation, using shorter strides to protect the injured tissue from excessive stretching, is allowed if tolerated. If symptoms are more disabling and weight bearing needs to be limited, crutches can be used for ambulation.

NSAIDS

Nonsteroidal anti-inflammatory medications are often used during the initial days following an acute hamstring injury to control pain and inflammation. Controversy exists regarding this widely accepted approach, however, because of the demonstrated lack of benefit and a potentially negative effect on healing muscle tissue. The most controversial aspect of NSAID use is regarding the timing of administration. Although short-term use starting immediately after injury is the most common recommendation, it may be beneficial to delay treatment several days to avoid interfering with chemotaxis of cells necessary for repair and remodeling of regenerating muscle. Analgesics are an alternative to NSAIDs with fewer associated risks.

ICE

Application of ice, or cryotherapy, is used for decreasing pain and inflammation. It can be used acutely. Ice should be applied to the injured area several times a day. The duration of the treatment depends on the method(s) used (ice pack, ice massage, etc.), but generally ice should be applied for 10 to 20 minutes to be effective.

Intramuscular Corticosteroid Injection

The use of corticosteroid injections for the treatment of hamstring muscle injuries is highly controversial, primarily because of the temporal relationship with tendon or fascial rupture. However, in one retrospective study no adverse effects were found when intramuscular corticosteroid injections were used to decrease the inflammatory response and limit the loss of playing time in athletes with severe, discrete intramuscular or myotendinous hamstring injuries (Levine et al. 2000). This suggests that intramuscular corticosteroid injections may speed an athlete's return to sport without increasing the risk of recurrence.

Therapeutic Exercise

Rehabilitation protocols for acute muscle strains have traditionally emphasized isolated muscle stretching and strengthening. Sherry and Best (2004), however, reported a **significant reduction in the rate of recurrence in individuals with hamstring injuries when a progressive agility and trunk stabilization program was used.** The program emphasized early movement and coordination of the pelvis and trunk muscles, suggesting that improved neuromuscular control of the lumbopelvic region allows the hamstrings to function at safe lengths and loads during athletic movement, thereby reducing the risk of re-injury. Although this evidence is encouraging, a program that incorporates various aspects of isolated muscle stretching and strengthening *and* progressive agility and trunk stabilization may be most appropriate.

Exercises and movements designed to promote neuromuscular control should be implemented within a protected ROM to minimize the risk of damage to healing tissue. Submaximal, *pain-free* isometric exercises of the hamstring muscles should be initiated early in the rehabilitation program to prevent atrophy and promote healing. If the athlete experiences pain, the intensity should be decreased until pain-free contraction can be accomplished. Additionally, low-intensity stepping exercises,

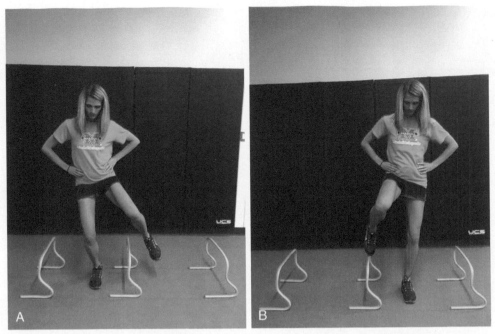

Fig. 68.3 Side-stepping.

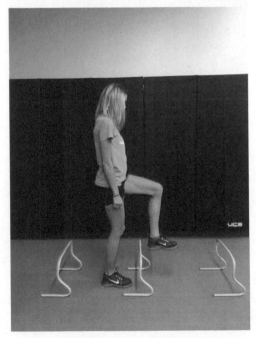

Fig. 68.4 Forward stepping.

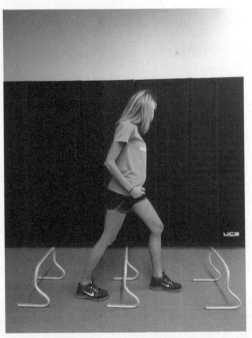

Fig. 68.5 Backward stepping.

including side, forward, and backward stepping, single-leg stance exercises, and lumbopelvic isometric exercises such as prone bridging, supine bent knee bridging, and side bridging, should be performed. See Figs. 68.3 through 68.10.

As the athlete's functional abilities improve and tolerance for increased exercise intensity builds, in conjunction with progression into the subacute and remodeling phases of rehabilitation, direct interventions aimed at increasing flexibility, strength, neuromuscular control, and function may be appropriate to incorporate into the program. Eccentric hamstring strengthening should be incorporated when sufficient tissue regeneration has occurred to allow the muscle to withstand the greater forces induced by such a contraction. Additionally, emphasis should be placed on hamstring muscle stretching to regain normal flexibility of the healing tissue. Athletes with injured hamstrings who undergo a more intensive stretching regimen regain motion faster and have a shorter rehabilitation period. Other therapeutic exercises that aim to improve functional abilities may include side-shuffling, grapevine jogging, boxer shuffling, rotating body bridges, supine bent knee body bridges with walkouts, single-leg stance windmill touches without weight, lunge walk with trunk rotation, single-leg stance with trunk forward lean, and opposite hip extension. See Figs. 68.11 through 68.18.

Finally, as the athlete nears symptom-free function and strength and neuromuscular control has substantially improved, therapeutic exercises that integrate postural control and high-demand

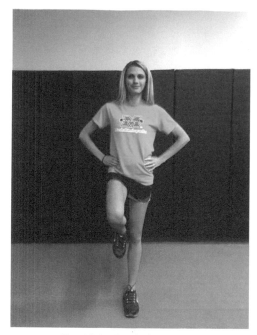

Fig. 68.6   Single-leg stance.

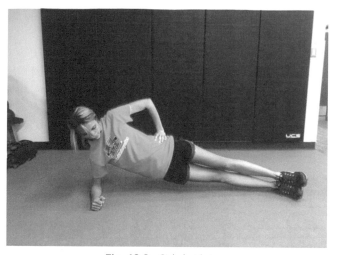

Fig. 68.9   Side bridging.

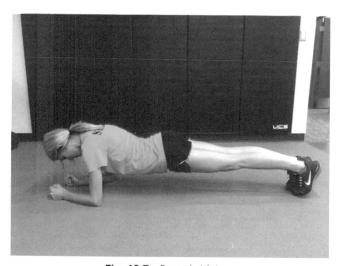

Fig. 68.7   Prone bridging.

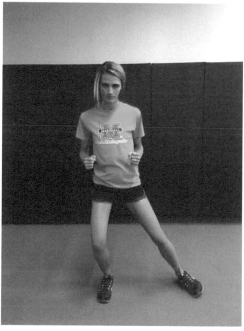

Fig. 68.10   Side-shuffling.

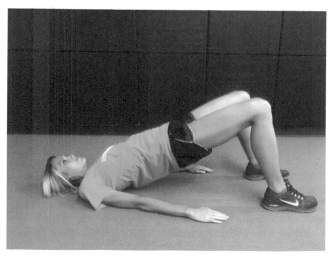

Fig. 68.8   Supine bent-knee bridging.

sport-specific activities can be implemented. Suggested therapeutic exercises include more aggressive static and dynamic flexibility training with incorporation of anterior pelvic tilt, eccentric muscle strengthening with the muscle in elongated position, skipping exercises, forward and backward accelerations, rotating body bridges with dumbbells, supine single-limb chair bridge, lunge walk with trunk rotation, and sport-specific drills that replicate sport-specific movements near maximal speed while incorporating postural control. See Figs. 68.19 through 68.23.

Soft Tissue Mobilization Techniques

Loss of muscle flexibility, in part from connective tissue scar formation, is a characteristic of hamstring injuries. Although evidence remains mostly anecdotal, the use of manual soft tissue mobilization techniques aimed at altering the mechanical environment of the injured muscle is common. The theoretic benefit of techniques such as various forms of massage and

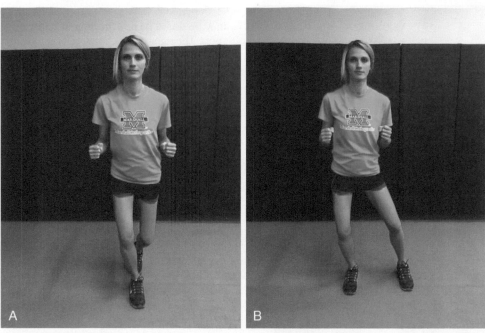

Fig. 68.11 Grapevine jogging.

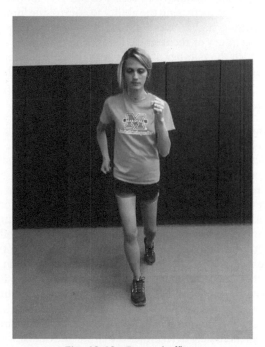

Fig. 68.12 Boxer shuffling.

augmented soft tissue mobilization is limitation of the residual effects of scar tissue formed early in the remodeling process, resulting in increased soft tissue extensibility. Scar tissue formation may result in changes in musculotendinous properties that can alter the mechanical environment, affect muscle fiber stretch, and therefore contribute to risk of recurrence.

The use of specific augmented soft tissue mobilization techniques does not appear to improve muscle strength. However, although largely unsubstantiated in the literature, these techniques may be of benefit in reducing the residual effects present in a previously injured muscle—namely, the restrictions in muscle fibers created by the formation of scar tissue that is stiffer

than the contractile tissue it replaces. Furthermore, because tendon nodularity secondary to scar formation may result in recurrent strain injury, soft tissue mobilization may be used to prevent exuberant scar tissue formation. These techniques may be beneficial in hastening recovery and should be considered by clinicians appropriately trained in their administration.

FUNCTIONAL PROGRESSION AND RETURN-TO-PLAY GUIDELINES

Pain-free participation in sports-specific activities is perhaps the best indicator of readiness to return to sport. Additionally, the healing process after a hamstring injury may be much slower than the clinical findings would indicate, resulting in athletes and clinicians alike underestimating the recovery time necessary to return to sport. Evidence suggests that often the injury has not fully resolved at the time of return to sport. Because return to competition prior to pain-free participation may result in recurrent or more severe injury, using an appropriate functional progression and adhering to return-to-play guidelines are critical to optimal recovery.

Functional progression toward return to play involves a goal-oriented approach to rehabilitation. While the progression should be criteria based and not time based, it must nonetheless respect the time constraints associated with the theoretic healing response. The rehabilitation program must be designed in a sequential progression, with each phase demanding slightly more ability (or strength, flexibility, or neuromuscular control) or requiring slightly more skilled movements or movement patterns that replicate sport.

Hamstring injuries are often associated with sports that involve stretch-shortening cycle activities, such as high-speed sprinting, high-intensity running, stopping, starting, quick changes of direction, and kicking. Although uncertainty remains regarding the phase in the gait cycle in which the muscle is most susceptible to injury, it may be the late swing phase when the hip is flexed and the knee is extended. Evidence indicates that potential conditions

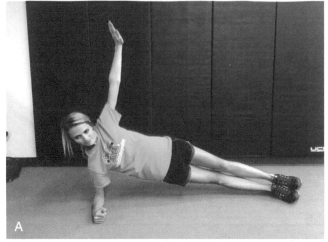

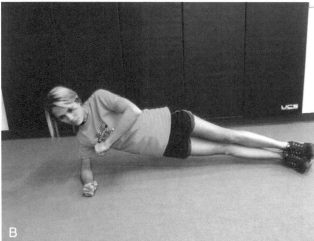

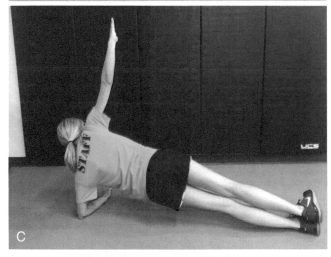

Fig. 68.13 Rotating body bridging.

for muscle strain injury occur at this point, prior to foot contact, in which peak hamstring stretch occurs while the hamstrings are active, thus undergoing an active lengthening contraction. It has been suggested that it is during this time in which there is a rapid change from eccentric to concentric function that the muscle is most vulnerable. Therefore, a program that simulates this condition should be implemented and mastery of this task should be a prerequisite for return to sport, particularly in sports that require higher-speed skilled movements such as sprinting. See Rehabilitation Protocol 68.1 for acute hamstring strain.

Functional tests that mimic skills or sport-specific activities may be useful in determining an athlete's suitability for return to sport. The rigor of functional tests can be increased by adding tasks beyond what is normally expected of athletes in their respective sports; however, these additional tests should be used as risk assessors rather than absolute requirements for return to play.

PREVENTION
Risk Factors

Prevention, rather than treatment, of hamstring injuries is the goal when managing the care of athletes. Understanding the individual risk factors for injury is an important basis for developing preventative measures. Although evidence-based information on risk factors for hamstring injuries is somewhat limited, it appears that these injuries invariably result from the interaction of several risk factors, both modifiable and nonmodifiable. **Nonmodifiable risk factors** include age and previous hamstring injuries; **modifiable risk factors** may include muscle fatigue, lower extremity strength imbalances (low hamstring-to-quadriceps ratio), greater training volume, insufficient warmup, poor muscle flexibility, cross-pelvic posture (anterior pelvic tilt with increased lumbar lordosis), and poor lumbopelvic strength and stability. The ability to mitigate modifiable risk factors, such as increasing the ability to control the lumbopelvic region during higher-speed skilled movements, may prevent hamstring injury or recurrence. Further, there may be a threshold at which the number of risk factors produces an injury, and some factors may be more predictive of injury than others.

Stretching

Although there is limited evidence supporting the role of passive and active warmup and muscle stretching before activity in reducing the incidence of hamstring injuries, these strategies have been suggested as effective in injury prevention. Because of the retrospective nature of the evidence, it remains unclear, however, if decreased hamstring flexibility is a cause or a consequence of hamstring injury. Many studies examining hamstring injury risk have failed to show decreased flexibility as a risk factor for injury, yet others demonstrate evidence supporting the role of stretching, suggesting that athletes who sustain a hamstring muscle injury have significantly less flexibility in the hamstring muscles before their injury than uninjured athletes and that stretching is of great importance and improves the effectiveness of the rehabilitation program. Stretching of the muscle theoretically determines the stress lines along which collagen will be oriented after injury. Failure of this to occur may result in decreased tensile strength, limited function, and pain that may predispose to recurrence.

The type, duration, and frequency of stretching are factors that may influence the effectiveness of the stretching program. Injured muscles with altered viscoelasticity may require longer stretches or more repetitions to obtain maximal benefit. Static stretching techniques in which the pelvis remains in an anterior tilt may be performed for 30 seconds four or more times per day or, more arbitrarily, based on clinician or athlete preference. Potential benefits of stretch-induced alterations in hamstring muscle tissue include a short-term increase in ROM and long-term increased tissue strength and stretch tolerance.

Finally, evidence suggests that the **contralateral hip flexor muscles** may have as large an influence on hamstring stretch

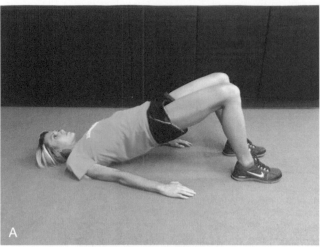
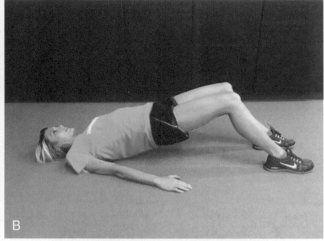

Fig. 68.14 Supine bent-knee body bridging with walk-out.

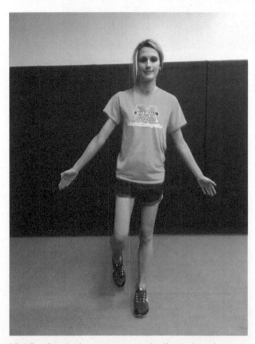

Fig. 68.15 Single-leg stance windmill touch without weight.

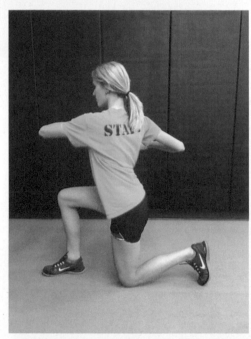

Fig. 68.17 Lunge walking with trunk rotation.

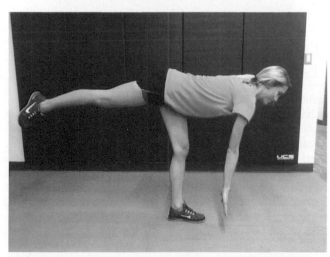

Fig. 68.16 Single-leg stance windmill touch without weight.

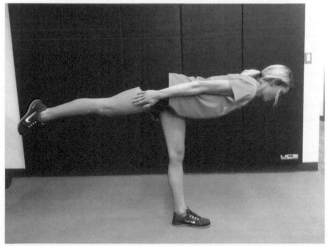

Fig. 68.18 Single-leg stance with trunk forward lean and opposite hip extension.

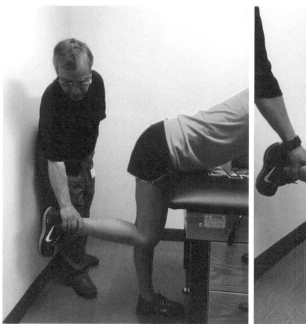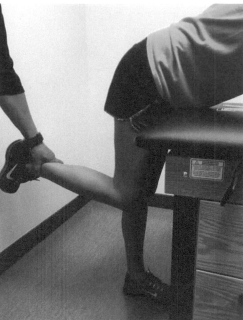

Fig. 68.19 Manual resist eccentric strength with hamstring muscle elongated (hip flexed).

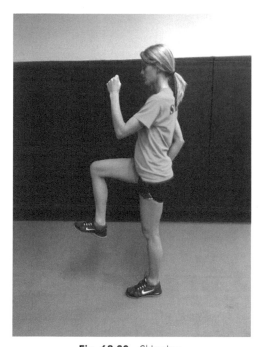

Fig. 68.20 Skipping.

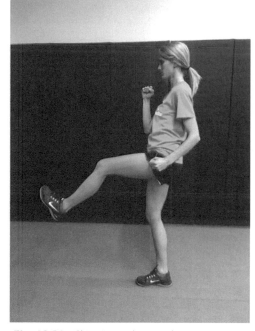

Fig. 68.21 Skipping with active knee extension.

as the hamstring muscles themselves because the iliopsoas can directly induce an increase in anterior pelvic tilt, which in turn necessitates greater hamstring stretch.

Hamstring Stretching Regimen

Single-Leg Hamstring Stretch. For the single-leg hamstring stretch, the athlete should lie supine with both legs flat on the table, loop a towel around the foot and hold the ends of the towel with both hands, with the knee straight and the foot in dorsiflexion (pointing toward the ceiling). The leg is pulled up toward the ceiling until a stretch is felt in the back of the leg; the stretch is sustained for 30 seconds. Then the leg is relaxed and the stretch is repeated (Fig. 68.24).

Straddle Groin and Hamstring Stretch. For the saddle groin and hamstring stretch, the athlete sits on the floor with both legs straddled (Fig. 68.25). The knees are kept straight with the kneecap facing the ceiling and the feet in dorsiflexion (pointing toward the ceiling). The back is kept straight and the athlete bends forward at the hips. First, the athlete reaches straight forward until a stretch is felt in the hamstring and sustains the stretch for 30 seconds. Then he or she relaxes and reaches to the right until a stretch is felt and holds this stretch for 30 seconds. The stretch is relaxed and the athlete then reaches to the left.

Side-Straddle Groin and Hamstring Stretch. For the side straddle, the athlete sits on the floor with the injured leg straight,

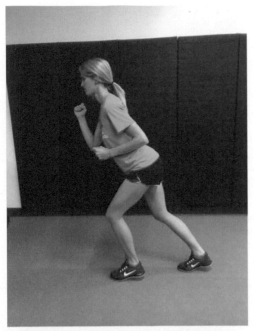

Fig. 68.22   Forward/backward accelerations.

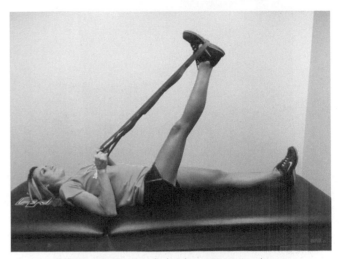

Fig. 68.24   Single-leg hamstring stretch.

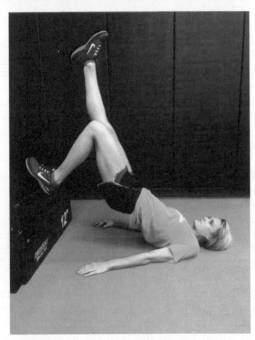

Fig. 68.23   Supine single-limb chair bridging.

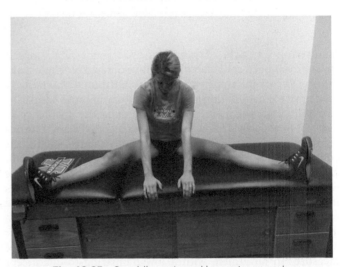

Fig. 68.25   Straddle groin and hamstring stretch.

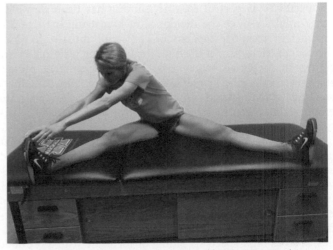

Fig. 68.26   Side-straddle groin and hamstring stretch.

keeping the kneecap facing the ceiling and the foot pointing toward the ceiling. The uninvolved leg is relaxed with the knee bent, and the athlete bends forward at the hips, keeping the back straight, reaching for the injured leg's ankle until a hamstring stretch is felt. This stretch is sustained for 30 seconds (Fig. 68.26), then relaxed and repeated.

Pelvic-Tilt Hamstring Stretch. For the pelvic-tilt, the athlete sits on the edge of the chair with the injured leg resting straight. The uninjured leg is bent at 90 degrees (Fig. 68.27). With the back straight, the athlete bends forward at the hips with both hands resting on the thighs for support. The athlete leans forward until a stretch is felt, holds for 30 seconds then relaxes and repeats the stretch.

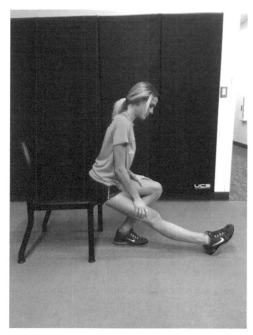

Fig. 68.27 Hamstring stretch with anterior pelvic tilt.

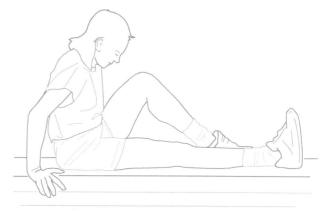

Fig. 68.28 Isometric hamstring exercise. The patient pushes down against the bed with the left (involved) leg.

Hamstring Muscle Strengthening. Hamstring muscle strength has been considered predictive of recurrent hamstring injury. Recurrent injuries are often attributed, in part, to inadequate rehabilitation after initial injury because hamstring strengthening has been shown to reduce the incidence of hamstring muscle strains. Nevertheless, controversy remains regarding whether strength imbalances are solely the consequence of the initial injury, a current causative factor for re-injury, or both. **Evidence demonstrates that athletes with untreated strength imbalances were four to five times more likely to sustain a hamstring injury when compared to athletes with no such problems.** Recognizing strength imbalances as a potential modifiable risk factor represents justification for incorporating strengthening as a preventive measure. In an athlete with a low hamstring-to-quadriceps ratio, efforts to restore a normal balance between agonist and antagonist muscle groups are warranted to decrease the risk of injury.

The incorporation of eccentric hamstring strengthening exercises as part of routine training has been shown to substantially reduce the incidence of hamstring injuries. An insufficient eccentric capacity of hamstring muscles to offset the concentric action of the quadriceps during terminal swing results in increased injury risk. Because persistent muscle strength abnormalities may lead to recurrent hamstring injuries, an individualized preventative/rehabilitation program emphasizing eccentric strength training based on specific deficits is suggested.

Because muscle strength disorders cannot provide an explanation for all the recurrent hamstring muscle problems and etiologic factors are rarely independent of one another, a preventative program that incorporates activities aimed at improving hamstring muscle flexibility and strength, and lumbopelvic neuromuscular control, should be prescribed for athletes participating in sports that involve stretch-shortening cycle activities, such as high-speed sprinting, or for those with a previous history of hamstring muscle injury.

Hamstring Strengthening Regimen for Injury Prevention

Hamstring strengthening exercises are also used to improve the quadriceps-to-hamstring ratio and any asymmetry between the hamstrings of the right and left legs. Strong, symmetric hamstrings should be less prone to injury.

Isometric Hamstring Curls. For isometric hamstring curls, the athlete sits on the floor with the uninjured leg straight. The involved leg is bent with the heel on the floor, and the heel is pushed into the floor and then pulled toward the buttocks to tighten the hamstring muscle (Fig. 68.28). The contraction is held for 5 seconds, then relaxed. The athlete begins with one set of 12 to 15 repetitions and progresses to perform two to three sets of 12 to 15 repetitions.

Prone Hamstring Curls. For prone hamstring curls, an ankle weight is placed on the involved leg. The athlete lies prone, with a pillow under the involved knee if needed. With the foot in position, as shown in Fig. 68.29, the heel is brought toward the buttocks in a slow, controlled manner. The athlete begins with one set of 12 to 15 repetitions and progresses to two to three sets of 12 to 15 repetitions.

Standing Hamstring Curls. For standing hamstring curls, an ankle weight is placed on the involved leg. The athlete stands with the feet shoulder-width apart. Holding on to a support, the heel is curled toward the buttocks in a slow, controlled manner, taking care to maintain proper knee alignment with the uninvolved leg. The athlete begins with one set of 12 to 15 repetitions and progresses to two to three sets of 12 to 15 repetitions (Fig. 68.30).

Hamstring Curl Machine. The exercise can be performed on a prone or a standing hamstring machine. The weight will be at the ankle. The leg is curled against resistance by bringing the heel toward the buttocks. The athlete begins with one set of 12 to 15 repetitions and progresses to two to three sets of 12 to 15 repetitions.

Seated Walking. While sitting on a rolling stool with wheels, the athlete begins walking forward while sitting on the stool (Fig. 68.31).

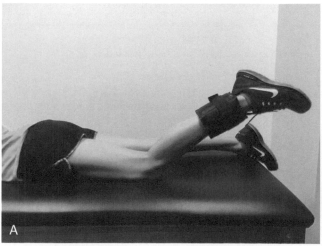

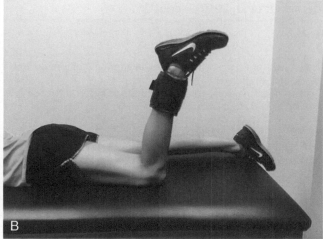

Fig. 68.29 A and B, Prone hamstring curls with weight.

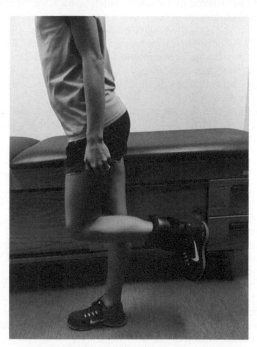

Fig. 68.30 Standing hamstring curls.

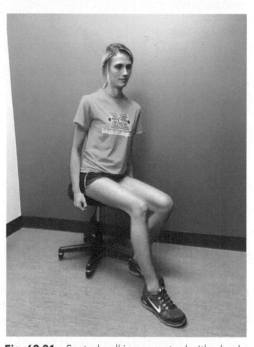

Fig. 68.31 Seated walking on a stool with wheels.

REHABILITATION PROTOCOL 68.1 ● Rehabilitation Protocol for Acute Hamstring Strain (Heiderscheit et al. 2010)

Phase 1

Goals

- Protect scar development.
- Minimize atrophy.

Protection

- Avoid excessive active or passive lengthening of the hamstrings.

Ice

- Two to three times a day

Therapeutic Exercise (daily)

- Stationary bike × 10 min
- Side-step × 10 min, 3 × 1 min, low to moderate intensity, pain-free speed and stride
- Grapevine × 10 min, 3 × 1 min, low to moderate intensity, pain-free speed and stride
- Fast feet stepping in place, 2 × 1 min
- Prone body bridge, 5 × 10 sec
- Supine body bridge, 5 × 10 sec
- Single-limb balance progressing from eyes open to closed, 4 × 20 sec

Criteria for Progression to Next Phase

- Normal walking stride without pain
- Very-low-speed jog without pain
- Pain-free isometric contraction against submaximal (50%–70%) resistance during prone knee flexion (90-degree) manual strength test

Continued

REHABILITATION PROTOCOL 68.1 ◼ **Rehabilitation Protocol for Acute Hamstring Strain (Heiderscheit et al. 2010)—cont'd**

Phase 2

Goals

- Regain pain-free hamstring strength, beginning in midrange and progressing to a longer hamstring length.
- Develop neuromuscular control of trunk and pelvis with progressive increase in movement speed.

Protection

- Avoid end-range lengthening of hamstrings while hamstring weakness is present.

Ice

- Postexercise, 10 to 15 min

Therapeutic Exercise (5–7 days/week)

- Stationary bike × 10 min
- Side-step × 10 min, 3 × 1 min, moderate to high intensity, pain-free speed and stride
- Grapevine × 10 min, 3 × 1 min, moderate to high intensity, pain-free speed and stride
- Boxer shuffle × 10 m, 2 × 1 min, low to moderate intensity, pain-free speed and stride
- Rotating body bridge, 5-sec hold each side, 2 × 10 reps
- Supine bent knee bridge with walk-outs, 3 × 10 reps
- Single-limb balance windmill touches without weight, 4 × 8 reps per arm each limb
- Lunge walk with trunk rotation, opposite hand-toe touch and T-lift, 2 × 10 steps per limb
- Single-limb balance with forward trunk lean and opposite hip extension, 5 × 10 sec per limb

Criteria for Progression to Next Phase

- Full strength (5/5) without pain during prone knee flexion (90 degrees) manual strength test
- Pain-free forward and backward jog, moderate intensity

Phase 3

Goals

- Symptom-free (no pain or tightness) during all activities
- Normal concentric and eccentric hamstring strength through full range of motion and speeds
- Improve neuromuscular control of trunk and pelvis.
- Integrate postural control into sport-specific movements.

Protection

- Avoid full intensity if pain, tightness, or stiffness is present.

Ice

- Postexercise, 5 to 10 minutes as needed

Therapeutic Exercise (4–5 days/week)

- Stationary bike × 10 min
- Side-shuffle × 30 m, 3 × 1 min, moderate to high intensity, pain-free speed and stride
- Grapevine jog × 30 m, 3 × 1 min, moderate to high intensity, pain-free speed and stride
- Boxer shuffle × 10 m, 2 × 1 min, moderate to high intensity, pain-free speed and stride
- A and B skips, starting at low knee height and progressively increasing, pain free
- A skip: hop-step forward movement that alternates from leg to leg and couples with arm opposition (similar to running). During the hop, the opposite knee is lifted in a flexed position and then the knee and hip extend together to make the next step.
- B skip: progression of the A skip, but opposite knee extends before the hip extends, recreating the terminal swing phase of running. The leg is then pulled backward in a pawing-type action. The other components remain the same as in the A skip.
- Forward-backward accelerations, 3 × 1 min, start at 5 m, progress to 10 m, then 20 m
- Rotating body bridge with dumbbells, 5-sec hold each side, 2 × 10 reps
- Supine single-limb chair bridge, 3 × 15 reps, slow to fast speed
- Single-limb balance windmill touches with dumbbells, 4 × 8 reps per arm each leg
- Lunge walk with trunk rotation, opposite hand dumbbell toe touch and T-lift, 2 × 10 steps per limb
- Sport-specific drills that incorporate postural control and progressive speed

Criteria for Return to Sport

- Full strength without pain
- Four consecutive repetitions of maximal effort manual strength test in each prone knee flexion position (90 degrees and 15 degrees)
- Less than 5% bilateral deficit in eccentric hamstrings (30 degrees/sec); concentric quadriceps (240 degrees/sec) ratio during isokinetic testing
- Bilateral symmetry in knee flexion angle of peak isokinetic concentric knee flexion torque at 60 degree/sec
- Full range of motion without pain
- Replication of sport-specific movements near maximal speed without pain (incremental sprint test for running athletes)

▶ Check online videos: Prone Eccentric Hamstrings Manual Resistance (Video 68.1) and Supine Hamstring Curl (Video 68.2).

REFERENCES

A complete reference list is available at https://expertconsult .inkling.com/.

FURTHER READING

Arnason A, Andersen TE, Holme I, et al. Prevention of hamstring strains in elite soccer: an intervention study. *Scand J Med Sci Sports*. 2008;18:40–48.

Arnason A, Sigurdsson SB, Gudmundsson A, et al. Risk factors for injuries in football. *Am J Sports Med*. 2004;32:5S–16S.

Askling C, Tengvar M, Saartok T, et al. Sports related hamstring strains— two cases with different etiologies and injury sites. *Scand J Med Sci Sports*. 2000;10:304–307.

Askling CM, Heiderscheit BC. Acute hamstring muscle injury: types, rehabilitation, and return to sports. *Sports Injuries*. 2013:1–13. Web.

Bahr RHI. Risk factors for sports injuries—a methodological approach. *Br J Sports Med*. 2003;37:384–392.

Brooks JH, Fuller CW, Kemp SP, et al. Incidence, risk, and prevention of hamstring muscle injuries in professional rugby union. *Am J Sports Med*. 2006;34:1297–1306.

Clanton T, Coupe K. Hamstring strains in athletes: diagnosis and treatment. *J Am Acad Orthop Surg*. 1998;6:237–247.

Croisier J. Factors associated with recurrent hamstring injuries. *Sports Med*. 2004;34:681–695.

Croisier J, Forthomme B, Namurois M, et al. Strength imbalances and prevention of hamstring injury in professional soccer players. A prospective study. *Am J Sports Med*. 2008;36:1469–1475.

Croisier J, Forthomme B, Namurois M, et al. Hamstring muscle strain recurrence and strength performance disorders. *Am J Sports Med*. 2002;30:199– 203.

Cyriax J. *Textbook of Orthopaedic Medicine: Vol. 1: Diagnosis of Soft Tissue Lesions*. London: Bailliere Tindall; 1982.

Delos D, Maak TG, Rodeo SA. Muscle injuries in athletes: enhancing recovery through scientific understanding and novel therapies. *Sports Health*. 2013;5.4:346–352. Web.

Devlin L. Recurrent posterior thigh symptoms detrimental to performance in rugby union: predisposing factors. *Sports Med*. 2000;29:273–287.

Drezner JA. Practical management: hamstring muscle injuries. *Clin J Sport Med*. 2003;13:48–52.

Feeley BT, Kennelly S, Barnes RP. Epidemiology of National Football League training camp injuries from 1998 to 2007. *Am J Sports Med*. 2008;36:1597–1603.

Goldman EF, Jones DE. Interventions for preventing hamstring injuries (review). *Cochrane Database Syst Rev*. 2010.

Hawkins RD, Hulse MA, Wilkinson C, et al. The association football medical research programme: an audit of injuries in professional football. *Br J Sports Med*. 2001;35:43–47.

Heiser TM, Weber J, Sullivan G, et al. Prophylaxis and management of hamstring muscle injuries in intercollegiate football players. *Am J Sports Med*. 1984;12:368–370.

Hoppenfeld S. *Physical Examination of the Spine and Extremities*. 1st ed. East Norwalk: Appleton-Century-Crofts; 1976.

Kellett J. Acute soft tissue injuries-a review of the literature. *Med Sci Spor Ex*. 1986;18:489–500.

Kerkhoffs GM, van Es N, Wieldraaijer T, et al. Diagnosis and prognosis of acute hamstring injuries in athletes. *Knee Surg Sports Traumatol Arthrosc*. 2012;21.2:500–509. Web.

Koulouris GCD. Imaging of hamstring injuries: therapeutic implications. *Eur Radiol*. 2006;16:1478–1487.

Lempainen L, Sarimo J, Mattila K, et al. Distal tears of the hamstring muscles: review of the literature and our results of surgical treatment. *Br J Sports Med*. 2007;41:80–83.

Magee DJ, Zachazewski JE, Quillen WS. *Pathology and Intervention in Musculoskeletal Rehabilitation*. 1st ed. St. Louis: Saunders Elsevier; 2009.

Malliaropoulos N, Papalexandris S, Papalada A, et al. The role of stretching in rehabilitation of hamstring injuries: 80 athletes follow-up. *Med Sci Spor Ex*. 2004;36:756–759.

Mason Dl, Dickens V, Vail A. Rehabilitation for hamstring injuries. *Protocols The Cochrane Database of Systematic Reviews*. 1996. n. pag. Web.

Mendiguchia Jurdan, Brughelli Matt. A return-to-sport algorithm for acute hamstring injuries. *Physical Therapy in Sport*. 2011;12.1:2–14. Web.

Mishra DK, Friden J, Schmitz MC, et al. Anti-inflammatory medication after muscle injury. A treatment resulting in short-term improvement but subsequent loss of muscle function. *J Bone Joint Surg Am*. 1995;77:1510–1519.

Neumann DA. *Kinesiology of the Musculoskeletal System*. 2nd ed. Mosby: St. Louis: Elsevier; 2010.

Orchard J, Best TM, Verrall GM. Return to play following muscle strains. *Clin J Sport Med*. 2005;15:436–441.

Petersen J, Holmich P. Evidence based prevention of hamstring injuries in sport. *Br J Sports Med*. 2005;39:319–323.

Rahusen FT, Weinhold PS, Almekinders LC. Nonsteroidal anti-inflammatory drugs and acetaminophen in the treatment of an acute muscle injury. *Am J Sports Med*. 2004;32:1856–1859.

Reiman MP, Manske RC, Smith BS. Immediate effects of soft tissue mobilization and joint manipulation interventions on lower trapezius strength. AAOMPT conference abstract. *J Man Manip Ther*. 2008;16:166.

Reynolds JF, Noakes TD, Schwellnus MP, et al. Non-steroidal anti-inflammatory drugs fail to enhance healing of acute hamstring injuries treated with physiotherapy, *S Afr Med J* 85:517–522.

Thelen DG, Chumanov ES, Sherry MA, et al. Neuromusculoskeletal models provide insights into the mechanisms and rehabilitation of hamstring strains. *Exerc Sport Sci Rev*. 2006;34:135–141.

Verrall GM, Kalairajah Y, Slavotinek JP, et al. Assessment of player performance following return to sport after hamstring muscle strain injury. *J Sci Med Sport*. 2006;9:87–90.

Verrall GM, Slavotinek JP, Barnes PG. The effect of sports specific training on reducing the incidence of hamstring injuries in professional Australian rules football players. *Br J Sports Med*. 2005;39:363–368.

Witvrouw E, Danneels L, Asselman P, et al. Muscle flexibility as a risk factor for developing muscle injuries in male professional soccer players. A prospective study. *Am J Sports Med*. 2003;31:41–46.

Athletic Pubalgia

Charles Andrew Gilliland, BS, MD

INTRODUCTION

Athletic pubalgia (a.k.a., chronic/acute groin pain, sports hernia, sportsman hernia, Gilmore's groin, hockey hernia, pubic inguinal pain syndrome, inguinal disruption) is not only an ailment without a clear identity, it is also widely regarded as one of the most difficult to diagnose and treat maladies encountered in musculoskeletal medicine. This is felt largely due to the intricate overlapping musculoskeletal anatomy involved and the proximity of multiple organ systems in a relatively compact region. This has lead to varied opinions regarding its true cause (Gilmore 1992, Taylor et al. 1991).

All of these variables add layers of complexity not often seen with other musculoskeletal conditions and create challenges for the musculoskeletal practitioner.

The purpose of this section is to outline the presentation, diagnosis, management, and rehabilitation of athletic pubalgia. Consideration will also be given to the athletic population, as well as closely related pathology often encountered. Further discussion will elaborate on considerations for return to sport. Attention will also be paid to outlining diagnostic testing and the role of imaging in diagnosing this condition.

EPIDEMIOLOGY/SPECIAL POPULATION (ATHLETIC)

Athletic pubalgia is not exclusively seen in the athletic population but it is in this realm that much of the literature is focused. It is generally seen in athletes who engage in agility-focused activities with rapid changes in velocity (Minnich 2011). It is very commonly seen in sports such as American/Australian rules football, ice hockey, and soccer but there are reports throughout nearly all realms of sport involving change in direction or violent adduction. It is believed that groin injuries can be attributed to up to 5% of athletic injury (Moeller 2007).

It is more often seen in males but can be seen in females as well (Garvey 2010, Meyers et al. 2008). This gender difference is felt primarily to be due to the differentiations of the inguinal canal and genitourinary anatomy. It has been reported that up to 50% of chronic groin pain in athletes can be attributed to some iteration of inguinal disruption (Lovell 1995).

Athletic pubalgia typically results in significant time lost and has a high recurrence rate.

CLINICAL PRESENTATION

Athletic pubalgia typically presents as a complaint of vague lower abdominal pain that worsens with extension-based activity (Litwin et al. 2011). It may be unilateral or bilateral and resolves with rest only to resume upon initiation of activity. It is not uncommon for the athlete to be unable to recall an inciting injury, lending credence to the theory that athletic pubalgia is an overuse injury resulting in breakdown of the posterior abdominal wall/inguinal musculature. It is important to note, however, that

some athletes are able to recall an inciting event. The pain can radiate into the thigh, scrotum, or perineal region and is often exacerbated by activities that increase intra-abdominal pressures (Hackney 1993, Meyers et al. 2000, Larson and Lohnes 2002).

The athlete with pubalgia often presents after months of vague complaints with no clear causative agent. Its diagnosis is entirely dependent on the practitioner evaluating the athlete. Conservative management has often been attempted but failed (Morelli and Smith 2001).

RISK FACTORS

Important attention should be paid to athletes "at risk" for this condition. It is well established that poor muscular control of core musculature as well as deficiencies in range of motion of the hips are primary risk factors for athletic pubalgia (Whittaker et al. 2015). Other risk factors of note include previous history of groin injury and limb-length discrepancy (Ryan et al. 2014).

These athletes may be identified as at risk during their annual participation physical if required. If identified as at risk, special attention during strength and conditioning activities in the pre-/off-season should be given with additional core and pubic strengthening being a focus.

DIFFERENTIAL DIAGNOSIS

Given the complexity of anatomy within the region, it is important for the evaluating musculoskeletal practitioner to have a deep understanding of other conditions that may mimic athletic pubalgia. Box 69.1 presents a broad overview of consideration, but two ailments of specific interest should be highlighted. It is not uncommon for osteitis pubis or signs of femoroacetabular impingement to be present along with athletic pubalgia (Economopolous et al. 2014, Beatty 2012, Macintyre et al. 2006).

This is likely due to the pelvic pivot joint theory. In this theory, forces transferred through a pathologic lower abdominal wall/pubic ring aponeurosis result in more stress being taken on by neighboring joints. The pubic symphysis and hip joint are most commonly affected and can create a difficult mixture of presenting complaints with separate underlying pathologies. It may be necessary for the evaluating practitioner to include treatments for these other interrelated maladies to successfully fully rehabilitate the athlete.

ANATOMY

The anatomy involved in the lower abdominal/groin region is quite complex. It is important to note that the evaluation and management of athletic pubalgia can be biased by the type of specialist evaluating (e.g., urologists may focus on genitourinary considerations whereas a surgeon may focus on the intraabdominal or abdominal wall musculature). It is essential for evaluation to be multidisciplinary if there is doubt regarding the primary anatomic cause. The abdominal-adductor aponeurosis consists of the lower abdominal wall musculature (external oblique, internal oblique, transversus abdominis, trasversalis), rectus abdominis, and conjoint tendon. These comprise the cephalad component of the muscular insertions onto the pubic bone whereas in the caudad aspect we take into consideration the hip adductors and gracilis (Larson, 2014).

BOX 69.1 DIFFERENTIAL DIAGNOSES

- True abdominal hernia
- Synovitis
- Lumbosacral pain
- AVN of femur/Legg-Calvé-Perthes
- Slipped capital femoral epiphysis
- Arthritis (inflammatory, osteo, rheumatoid, infectious)
- SIJ dysfunction
- PID
- Pubic stress
- Femoral neck stress fracture
- Muscular rupture/avulsion/physeal injury
- Snapping hip
- Inflammatory bowel/GI
- GU causes (PID, PCOS, ectopic, prostatitis, STD)
- Intra-abdominal mass
- Nerve entrapment
- Pubic symphysitis

Figs. 69.1 and 69.2 outline the muscular and genitourinary anatomy, as well as the vector forces that are transferred through the pelvic bone (Caudill et al. 2008, Meyers, 2007).

The interplay between these muscles and structures results in the pelvic joint acting as a dynamic fulcrum.

PHYSICAL EXAMINATION

Physical examination should consist of a complete evaluation of the lower abdominal viscera, musculature, and genitourinary structures including pelvic examination if felt needed. Visual inspection should reveal no clear alternative pathology. Palpation of the lower abdominal/pelvic musculature at their sites of origin and insertion should be undertaken. The examiner should also engage in provocative testing such as resisted sit-up, Valsalva maneuver, and direct palpation of the inguinal ring (Farber and Wilckens 2007).

Evaluation should also include evaluation of the hip and pubic symphysis to assess for possible comorbidity from femoroacetabular impingement or osteitis pubis. Generally, pain along the superior aspect of the pubic tubercle is appreciated while there is no other clear causative pathology including hernia findings. It is not uncommon to find tenderness along the hip adductor. Finally, depending upon specialty and comfort level, the examiner should examine along the inguinal ring and possibly the testicle.

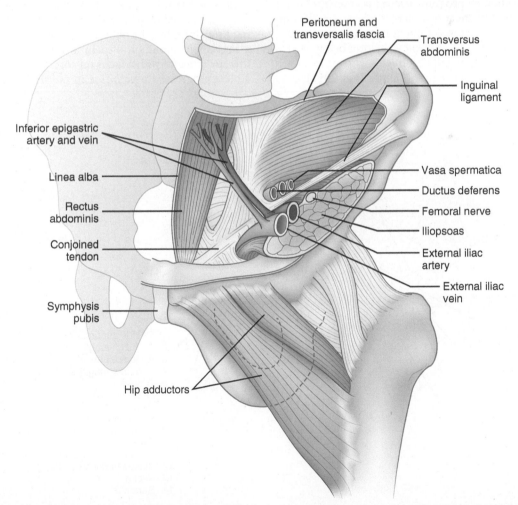

Fig. 69.1 The anatomic considerations of the inguinoabdominal region. (From Caudill P, Nyland J, Smith C, et al.: Sports hernias: a systematic literature review. Br J Sports Med 42(12):954-964, 2008.)

DIAGNOSIS

Definitive diagnosis is generally only considered in the postoperative state with complete resolution of the symptomatology. Athletic pubalgia is a diagnosis of exclusion and requires vigilant testing by the treating practitioner to rule out all other causes. It is often expected for the treating team to be multidisciplinary to assess for all possibilities. X-ray imaging may be useful to rule out bony abnormalities such as CAM deformities on hip x-ray (Lischuk et al. 2010).

Although the accepted imaging modality is MRI, it is often common to see no irregularity. As a general rule there are two patterns seen on MRI if findings are present. These patterns are segmented by age with the younger population demonstrating a more diffuse picture of edema whereas the older population will have more focal findings (Albers et al. 2001).

Ultrasound can be useful in the skilled hand because it may be able to demonstrate a functional defect in the posterior abdominal wall. Herniography can be considered in some instances but has fallen out of fashion.

MANAGEMENT

Management of athletic pubalgia should be focused on pain control and limiting time lost (Sheen et al. 2014). Conservative management should consist of relative rest, followed by an intensive physiotherapy program (Hegedus et al. 2013). It is important to note that medications such as NSAIDs or prednisone can be used to assist. It is not uncommon to see ilioinguinal nerve blocks or even radiofrequency ablation being used as an adjunctive treatment, especially in athletes who are in season and choose to continue to participate (Comin et al. 2013).

There is not a great amount of evidence suggesting a superior rehabilitation method. The focus of most rehab programs centers around the athlete being initially pain free at rest followed by progression of ROM. This is followed by focused region-specific exercises specific to the affected athlete. Upon completion of this, a global "whole-body" approach is undertaken including agility-based/total body exercises (LeBlanc and LeBlanc 2003). This is an effort to return the athlete to his or her sport-specific activities. If the athlete fails to progress through the rehabilitation program, other treatments including surgery should be considered (Lynch and Renstrom 1999).

If surgical management is deemed necessary the surgery is generally an attempt to reinforce the posterior abdominal wall and to alleviate pathologic tension. Surgical approach can either be laparoscopic or open with either mesh repair or suture repair commonly used. There is no clear evidence to suggest a superior surgical approach at this time and experience/comfort should decide operative technique. Laparoscopic approaches may offer a more rapid return when compared to their open counterpart (Harmon 2007). There is good success in the postoperative athlete independent of approach and thus it should be strongly considered in athletes who fail conservative treatment.

OUR APPROACH

Whenever an athlete presents to our medical team with groin pain, whether it be insidious in onset or acute in nature, relative rest coupled with high-dose NSAIDs is the first step. Imaging modalities may be obtained and typically include MRI and x-ray. Upon resolution of pain at rest using the VAS, physiotherapy is begun with a focus on core/pelvic musculature. If the athlete progresses to pain free in physiotherapy, an attempt to

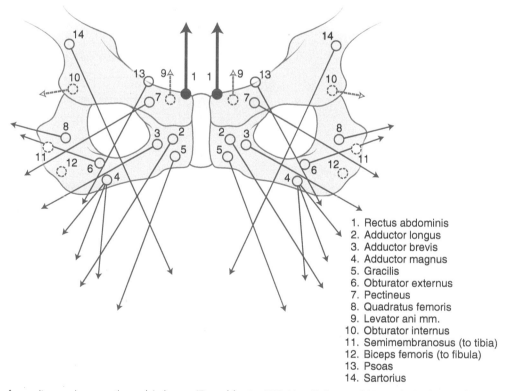

1. Rectus abdominis
2. Adductor longus
3. Adductor brevis
4. Adductor magnus
5. Gracilis
6. Obturator externus
7. Pectineus
8. Quadratus femoris
9. Levator ani mm.
10. Obturator internus
11. Semimembranosus (to tibia)
12. Biceps femoris (to fibula)
13. Psoas
14. Sartorius

Fig. 69.2 Muscular force dispersal across the pelvic bone. (From Meyers WC, Yoo E, Devon ON, et al.: Understanding "sports hernia" (athletic pubalgia): the anatomic and pathophysiologic basis for abdominal and groin pain in athletes. Oper Tech Sports Med 15(4):165-177, 2007. [Figure 3])

return to sport specific exercise is then considered. If the athlete remains pain free, he/she may return to the respective sport as tolerated. As a general rule, failure to progress within 2 months is considered failure of conservative management and thus requires surgical consideration. Return is then based on resolution of symptomatology.

CONCLUSION

Athletic pubalgia is a very difficult to manage condition requiring skilled practitioners of musculoskeletal medicine. It usually presents as vague lower abdominal/groin pain and may be insidious in nature or accompanied by an inciting event. It is typically seen in athletes who participate in agility-based activity. Limiting time lost from sport and pain resolution should be the focus of treatment. Awareness of comorbidity is key to expediting return to play. Careful history and physical examination are the core tenets to a successful outcome.

Athletic pubalgia is a diagnosis of exclusion and, given the complexity of the region, a multidisciplinary team should be utilized. This team should include surgeons, physiotherapists, and specialists in abdominal and genitourinary pathology. Groin MRI is the accepted standard for imaging modality. Conservative management may be successful but often surgical treatment is required for complete resolution.

REFERENCES

A complete reference list is available at https://expertconsult .inkling.com/.

70

Femoro-acetabular Impingement: Labral Repair and Reconstruction

Tigran Garabekyan, MD | Damien Southard, MPT | Jeff Ashton, PT

INTRODUCTION

Femoro-acetabular impingement (FAI) is a diagnosis describing painful abutment of the upper femur against the rim of the acetabulum occurring with certain provoking activities (Beck 2005). The impingement typically affects the front of the hip joint and is precipitated by deep flexion and rotation as in squatting, kicking, or pivoting. Over time, repetitive impingement may result in tearing of the interposed labrum or articular cartilage, giving rise to mechanical symptoms including clicking, catching, and locking. Left untreated, symptomatic FAI can result in progressive and irreversible joint damage leading to early onset arthritis (Beck 2005, Ganz 2008, Ganz 2003).

RELEVANT ANATOMY

The bony hip joint is composed of the acetabulum or hip socket and the deeply seated femoral head. There is a ring of cartilage attached to the acetabular rim called the labrum that forms a suction seal around the femoral head. The labrum functions to lubricate the articular cartilage and stabilize the joint (Seldes 2001, Stafford 2009). With progressive impingement, the labrum becomes torn and detached from the rim, leaving the adjacent articular cartilage vulnerable to injury (Fig. 70.1) (Beck 2005, Ganz 2008, Ganz 2003, Seldes 2001, Stafford 2009, Masjedi 2013).

Cam impingement is one common variant of FAI and results from excessive bone about the upper femur (Cobb 2010). This abnormal bone is thought to develop during peak adolescent growth, maturing as the growth plate closes (Ganz 2008). It functions to limit the clearance anteriorly with flexion, reducing motion and causing pain (Fig. 70.2). Over time, repetitive impingement causes progressive articular cartilage injury leading to delamination from the underlying bone and painful mechanical symptoms (Fig. 70.3) (Beck 2005, Ganz 2008).

CONSERVATIVE MANAGEMENT AND PREOPERATIVE REHABILITATION

All patients with FAI undergo initial nonoperative management consisting of activity modification, use of nonsteroidal anti-inflammatories, and in most cases an intra-articular corticosteroid injection. Specific modalities aim to restore core and paraspinal muscle strength, as well as hip abductor strength. Tight hip flexors and adductors are addressed with tissue mobilization and stretching techniques to improve joint range of motion and function.

Patients who fail to improve with conservative management are evaluated preoperatively to establish a baseline functional status with which periodic comparisons can be made to establish whether expected measurable progress is occurring. In our clinic, whenever possible, this evaluation occurs immediately preoperatively, as this is the condition from which we seek to generate improvement. In addition to traditional gait assessment, two outcome measures are used: the modified Harris Hip Score, originally published in 1969 as an assessment of

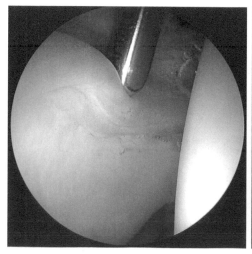 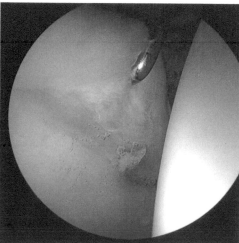

Fig. 70.1   Tearing of the anterior labrum and detachment from the acetabular rim.

the results of hip surgery, and the short form International Hip Outcome Tool (IHOT), developed by Mohtadi et al. (2012) as a means of assessing a patient's ability to return to an active lifestyle by obtaining subjective measures of symptoms, as well as determining emotional and social health status (Griffin 2012, Mohtadi 2012). The IHOT was developed for younger and more active patients with hip pathology. In addition to these initial measures, the patient is counseled on anticipated postoperative range of motion and weightbearing restrictions.

SURGICAL TREATMENT

Patients with persistent painful impingement despite conservative measures are candidates for arthroscopic surgery. The operation is carried out under general anesthesia utilizing

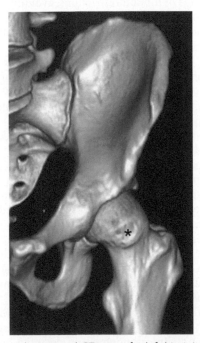

Fig. 70.2 Three-dimensional CT scan of a left hip joint. The red star denotes the cam lesion, or area of abnormal bone on the upper femur, which causes a painful limitation in flexion.

distraction to create space in the hip joint for access and instrumentation (Fig. 70.4). Two to three small incisions allow access to the hip joint to address the intra-articular pathology typically encountered in FAI including labral tears, articular cartilage lesions, and cam lesions (Fig. 70.5).

POSTOPERATIVE REHABILITATION GUIDELINES

The stages and exercise progressions described in this chapter are based on a protocol by Dr. Marc Philippon (Fig. 70.6) (Philippon 2009). The time frames are *guidelines,* and advancement (or regression) is based on how each individual is feeling and performing. The clinician should use his or her judgment when deciding to add or remove exercises. Modalities such as cryotherapy and electrical stimulation may be helpful in controlling or minimizing pain and inflammation. Although numerous publications have outlined various ways to rehabilitate the hip, there is currently no consensus on the optimal approach (Cheatham 2015, Enseki 2014, Malloy 2013, Stalzer 2006, Voight 2010, Wahoff 2011).

Postoperative rehabilitation begins with re-instruction in range of motion precautions and training in proper crutch use. The crutches must first be adjusted properly to enable the patient to approximate normal gait pattern and to protect the nerves and vascular structures passing through the axillary region. The length should be adjusted so that two fingers will easily fit between the top of the crutch and the axilla. Hand grips are adjusted so that they line up with the crease of the wrist with the patient standing upright, arms hanging to the outsides of the crutches. Weight bearing is limited initially to 25% or less and the time frame for weaning varies depending on the arthroscopic procedure(s) performed—usually ranging from 10 days to 6 weeks postoperatively. When advancing weight bearing, the patient's level of pain and degree of muscular control should be taken into account. The progression should not produce pain and the gait pattern should not degenerate. Avoid teaching "toe-touch" weight bearing, as this technique results in the patient holding the operative hip and knee in flexion, continuously activating the hip flexor mechanism. Both the psoas major and the iliacus travel directly over the area of surgical repair, and contraction of these muscles should

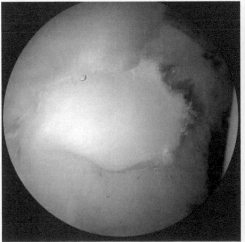
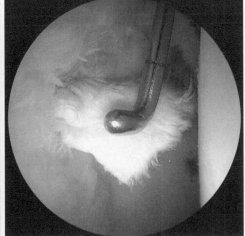

Fig. 70.3 Large full-thickness articular cartilage delamination of the acetabulum due to long-standing FAI.

be minimized during the initial postoperative period to protect the healing tissue and prevent hip flexor tendinitis, a common complication.

Range of motion limitations are necessary for up to 6 weeks postoperatively to protect the healing tissues. Flexion is limited to no more than 90 degrees to avoid stress on the anterior labral repair. Abduction and external rotation are discouraged to preserve the mending joint capsule; however, this restriction may be lifted if a capsular closure has been performed. The patient should limit sitting to less than 30 minutes at a time during the first week and maintain relative hip extension. When traveling in a car, we suggest a slightly reclined seat to open the angle of the hip joint.

IMMEDIATE POSTOPERATIVE REHABILITATION

On the evening of surgery, or on postoperative day 1, the patient initiates upright stationary bicycle exercises with resistance at its lowest setting. Seat height is adjusted to allow the patient to easily reach the bottom of the pedal stroke while limiting hip flexion to 90 degrees at the top of the cycle (Fig. 70.7). Daily cycling for 15 to 20 minutes is essential to reduce the incidence of postoperative adhesions, a complication that may necessitate revision surgery.

A typical complaint in the first 2 weeks following surgery is paresthesia/numbness in the foot or lower leg on the operative side. These symptoms are most likely caused by compression of peripheral nerve branches by the boot while applying traction during surgery. Meticulous attention to detail while padding the foot will reduce the incidence of paresthesias and the patient may be reassured that the vast majority of such symptoms resolve within 6 weeks. If a post is used for counter-traction, paresthesias/numbness may also be reported in the perineum and follow a similarly benign course. By limiting traction time to 2 hours and avoiding excessive force, the surgeon may reduce the incidence of these transient complications. In our practice,

we have transitioned away from using a post for counter-traction and instead place the operative table in 5 to 15 degrees of Trendelenburg (depending on the patient's weight).

OUTPATIENT REHABILITATION

Outpatient therapy begins following discharge from the hospital and is divided into four phases: initial exercises, intermediate exercises, advanced exercises, and sport-specific training.

Phase 1: Initial Exercises (Initiated Postoperative Week 1)

Goals during the initial phase of rehabilitation following hip arthroscopy are as follows:
- Protection of the operative hip (adherence to weightbearing and range of motion restrictions, avoiding prolonged hip flexion, patient education)
- Mobilization of the operative hip to prevent adhesions
- Restoration of muscular control/activation

Initial visits (first week after surgery) are focused primarily on reinforcing principles of safe mobilization and muscle activation:
- Stationary bicycle for 15 to 20 minutes daily with appropriate precautions
- Isometric muscle contractions including abdominals, gluteals, quadriceps, hamstrings
- Ankle pumps
- Passive range of motion

Passive range of motion should be kept within pain-free limits in all planes, progressing to recommended restrictions. The patient may need frequent verbal cueing to relax. Guarding is common, especially when there is postsurgical discomfort and when the patient is nervous or tense. In addition to passive movement in the cardinal planes (sagittal, coronal), log rolling allows for pain-free internal rotation, and circumduction provides combined movements (Fig. 70.8).

Week 2 exercise progression is listed below. All exercises do not have to be added at once and again therapists should use observation and clinical judgment in deciding how much and when to progress. Scar tissue mobilization (portal sites) and muscular mobilization are useful in preventing adhesions and restoring mobility between muscle and soft tissue layers.
- Quadruped rocking
- Standing hip internal rotation
- Isometric hip abduction
- Prone hip internal and external rotation with Theraband resistance
- Uninvolved knee to chest stretch

With quadruped rocking (Fig. 70.9, *A–B*), initially the forward-rocking movement should be emphasized, returning to a neutral position with the hips at 90 degrees of flexion. In the later stages of Phase 1, the patient may begin to rock backward beyond 90 degrees of hip flexion as long as doing so does not elicit pain. The muscle contraction produced by the weight bearing in this position (closed chain) stabilizes the femoral head position with respect to the acetabulum and labrum. Prone hip rotation with Theraband resistance should be done carefully, particularly with external rotation, avoiding rotation beyond 30 degrees (Fig. 70.9, *D–E*). Isometric hip abduction can be done with a stabilizing strap or gait belt (Fig. 70.9, *F*). The uninvolved knee-to-chest stretch is done with the operative leg relaxed

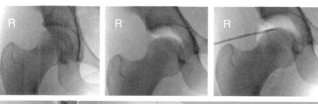

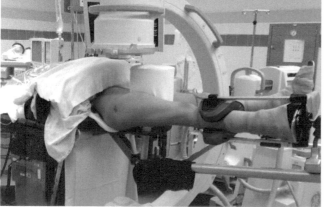

Fig. 70.4   *Above:* Fluoroscopic images demonstrating distraction of hip joint for safe instrumentation. *Below:* Intra-operative picture showing patient positioning.

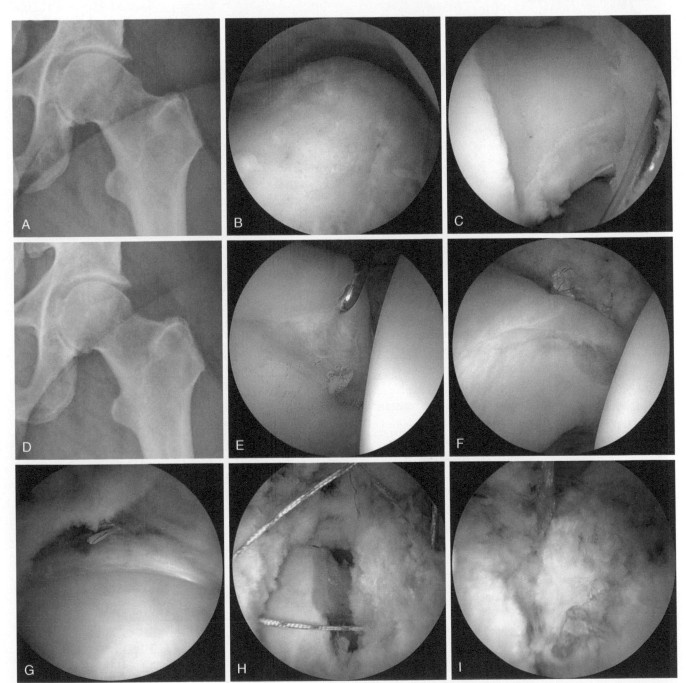

Fig. 70.5 Typical intra-articular pathology encountered in FAI surgery. Images *A–D* demonstrate decompression of a cam lesion. Images *E–G* illustrate labral repair with subsequent restoration of suction seal against femoral head. Images *H–I* show capsular closure at the conclusion of the procedure to restore anatomy and stability to the hip.

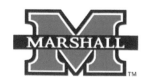

Hip Arthroscopy Protocol

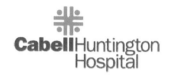

Phase 1: Initial Exercises

ROM limits (6 wks):
Flexion < 90
Abduction < 25
Avoid active hip flexion
Avoid abduction + ER

Weight-bearing:
[ ] 25% WB x 10 days

[ ] 25% WB x 3 wks
   50% starting wk 4
   100% starting wk 5

[ ] Toe-touch for 6 wks

Stationary Cycling:
[ ] 15 – 20 min daily
   Low resistance

Weeks

Exercise	1	2	3	4	5	6	7	9	13	17	19	21	25
Phase 1: Initial Exercises													
Ankle pumps	X	X	X										
Gluteal, quad, HS, T-ab isometrics	X	X	X										
Stationary biking with minimal resistance	X	X	X	X									
Passive ROM (IR and circumduction)	X	X	X	X	X								
Passive supine hip roll IR	X	X	X	X	X								
Quadruped rocking		X	X	X	X	X							
Standing hip IR		X	X	X	X								
Hip abductor isometrics		X	X	X	X								
Uninvolved knee to chest		X	X	X	X								
Prone IR/ER (band resistance)		X	X	X	X	X							
2 way leg raises (abduction, extension)			X	X	X	X							
Clam			X	X	X	X							
Double leg bridges with band			X	X	X	X							
Kneeling hip flexor stretch			X	X	X	X							
Leg press (limited weight)			X	X	X	X							
Phase 2: Intermediate Exercises													
Double 1/3 knee bends				X	X	X	X						
Side supports				X	X	X	X						
Stationary biking with resistance/outdoor				X	X	X							
Swimming				X	X	X							
Manual long axis distraction					X	X	X						
Manual A/P mobilizations					X	X	X						
Dyna-disc single leg stance					X	X	X						
Advanced bridging (single leg, Swiss ball)					X	X	X						
Standing IR/ER (band resistance)						X	X	X					
Pilates skaters						X	X	X					
Side stepping						X	X	X					
Single knee bends (lateral step downs)						X	X	X					
Elliptical / stair-climber						X	X	X					
Phase 3: Advanced Exercises													
Lunges							X	X	X				
Water bounding / plyometrics							X	X	X				
Side to side lateral agility							X	X	X				
Forward / Backward running with cord							X	X	X				
Running progression							X	X	X				
Phase 4: Sport-Specific Training													
Z-cuts / W-cuts								X	X	X	X	X	X
Cariocas								X	X	X	X	X	X
Sports specific drills								X	X	X	X	X	X

Fig. 70.6 Early passive range of motion to facilitate joint mobilization.

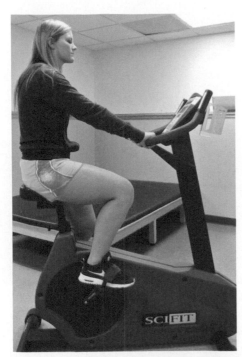

Fig. 70.7 Stationary bicycle exercises initiated on postoperative day 1.

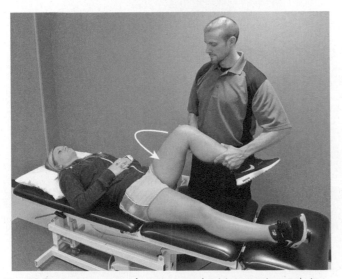

Fig. 70.8 Passive range of motion, emphasizing rotation and circumduction within restrictions.

and extended, indirectly producing a gentle, passive extension stretch (Fig. 70.9, *G*).

During week 3, controlled open and closed chain exercises are introduced. These activities should not produce pain and range of motion limitations should continue to be observed.

- Two-way leg raises (abduction and extension)
- Water jogging
- Clam
- Double-leg bridges with tubing
- Leg press (light weight)
- Kneeling hip flexor stretch

Two-way leg raises are performed on both hips, adhering to postoperative motion restrictions for the operative hip (Fig. 70.10, *A–B*). Light Theraband resistance may be utilized for the

clam exercises, performed in the side-lying or supine position (Fig. 70.10, *C*). Double-leg bridges may be performed statically, maintaining the bridge with slight stretch of the band, or dynamically with active bridges and knee flares (Fig. 70.10, *D*). Leg press is pictured with a wedge behind the patient's back to allow for a more recumbent position providing greater movement without violating the 90-degree hip flexion constraint (Fig. 70.10, *E*). The kneeling hip flexor stretch should be monitored closely to ensure that the patient is not too aggressive (Fig. 70.10, *F*). In hypermobile individuals, if normal range of motion is achieved quickly, it may be counterproductive to continue this exercise.

Phase 2: Intermediate Exercises (Initiated Postoperative Week 4)

Phase 2 is begun when phase 1 exercises are pain free. The transition time frame is dependent on the surgical procedure and how the patient is progressing. Goals for this stage are the following:

- Regain muscular strength
- Establish trunk stability and pelvic control
- Progress weight bearing if appropriate
- Restore normal gait pattern
- Achieve stable single-leg stance on the operative leg
Week 4 exercise additions include:
- Double 1/3 knee bends
- Side supports
- Stationary bicycle with progressive resistance
- Swimming (no breaststroke)

Double 1/3 knee bends, or partial squats, should be done with weight toward the heels and the lower legs as vertical as possible (Fig. 70.11, *A*). Using the extended upper extremities as a counterweight is helpful in maintaining balance. Side supports are modified side planks with the knees bent (Fig. 70.11, *B*). These may be advanced to traditional side planks as the patient progresses. Bicycle resistance is increased to the point that there is moderate muscle fatigue, ensuring that no groin pain occurs.

In week 5, careful hip joint mobilizations are introduced along with 2 exercises:

- Dyna-Disc single-leg stance
- Advanced bridging—single leg or Swiss ball
- Manual long axis distraction
- Manual A/P mobilizations

The Dyna-Disc single-leg stance consists of the patient standing with the operative leg on a Dyna-Disc while using one hand on a support surface for balance (Fig. 70.12, *A*). Initially, the goal is to achieve control. Over the weeks, mini single-leg squats may be added. Advanced bridging with a Swiss ball incorporates core and hip stabilization. Single-leg bridging should be supervised carefully—inadequate hip strength and/or improper form may cause this activity to be counterproductive (Fig. 70.12, *B–C*). Manual long axis distraction and A/P mobilizations should not be aggressive at this point and must be pain free.

Week 6 activities grow more functional and include the following:

- Standing resisted IR/ER
- Pilates skaters
- Side-stepping
- Single-leg knee bends/lateral step-downs
- Elliptical machine/stair climber

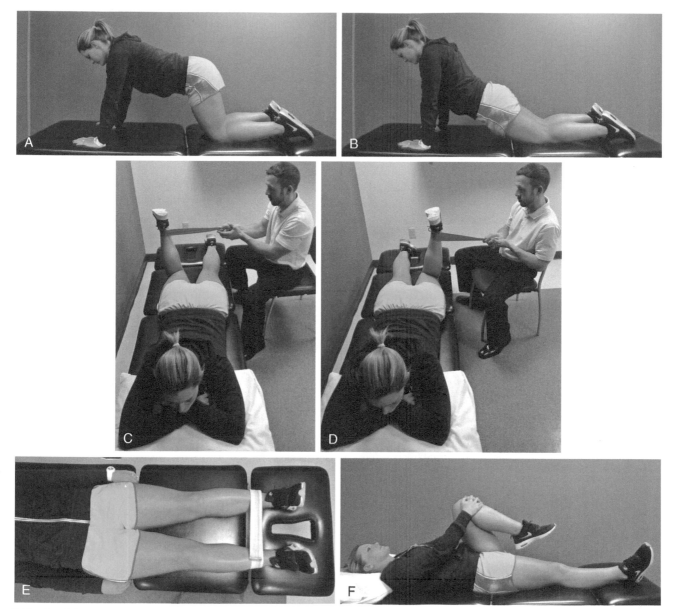

Fig. 70.9 Week 2 exercises. Images *A–B* illustrate proper form during quadruped rocking. Images *C–D* show prone resisted hip internal and external rotation, respectively. Image *E* illustrates supine isometric hip abduction. Image *F* depicts the uninvolved knee to chest stretch, bringing the nonoperative leg to the chest and generating gentle extension stretch of the operative hip.

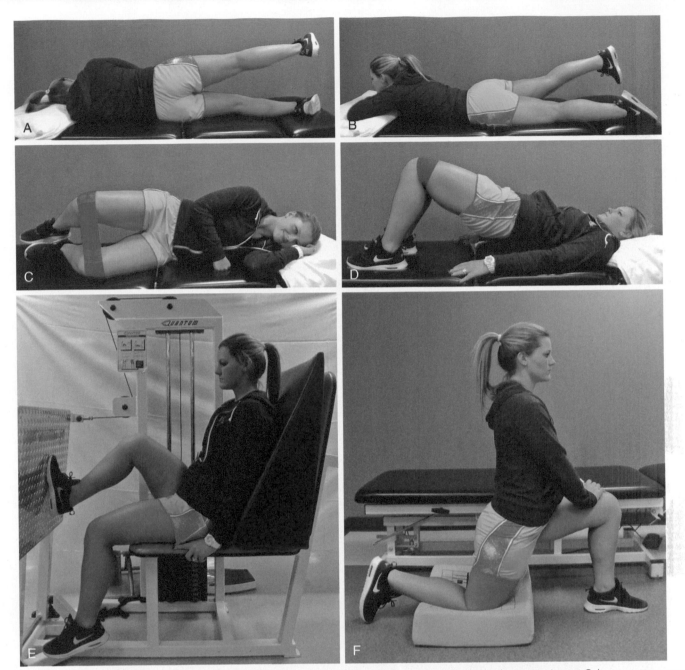

Fig. 70.10 Week 3 exercises. Image *A*, lateral leg raise and image *B*, prone leg raise comprise the two-way leg raises. Image *C* demonstrates proper technique for the clam exercise. Image *D* illustrates the double-leg bridge. Image *E* illustrates proper technique for single-leg press while maintaining hip flexion <90 degrees by utilizing a wedge. Image *F* depicts the kneeling hip flexor stretch.

Similar to prone hip rotation with band resistance, standing resisted rotation requires more core stability (Fig. 70.13, *A*). Pilates skaters incorporate both concentric and eccentric work for the lateral hip musculature. Side-stepping can be performed with or without resistance bands and may be combined with partial squats (Fig. 70.13, *B*). Single-leg knee bends can be done on the floor from a single-leg stance, stepping down from a solid surface (box or step), or from an unstable surface such as a Dyna-Disc to integrate proprioception and stabilization (Fig. 70.13, *C*). Proper pelvic control should be emphasized. When using a stair climber, be wary of hip flexor irritation, which could potentially result from repetitive hip flexion.

Phase 3: Advanced Exercises (Initiated Postoperative Week 7)

Phase 3 is begun when phase 2 exercises are pain free. The transition time frame is dependent on the surgical procedure and how the patient is progressing. Goals for this stage are the following:

- Running progression
- Lateral mobility
- Plyometrics and conditioning

Weeks 7 to 9 include early sport-specific activities when appropriate, along with the following advanced exercises:

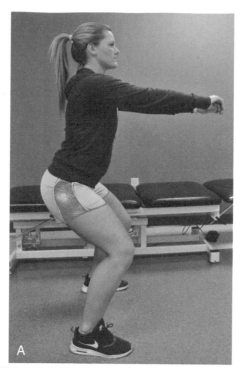

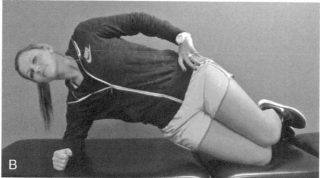

Fig. 70.11   Week 4 exercises. Image *A* shows double-third knee bends. Image *B* depicts side supports.

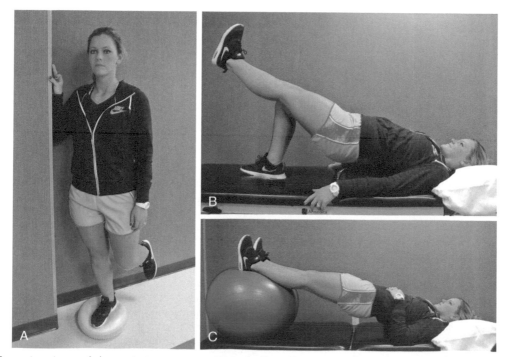

Fig. 70.12   Week 5 exercises. Image *A* demonstrates proper stance on the Dyna-Disc. Images *B–C* demonstrate advanced bridging techniques with single leg and use of a Swiss ball, respectively.

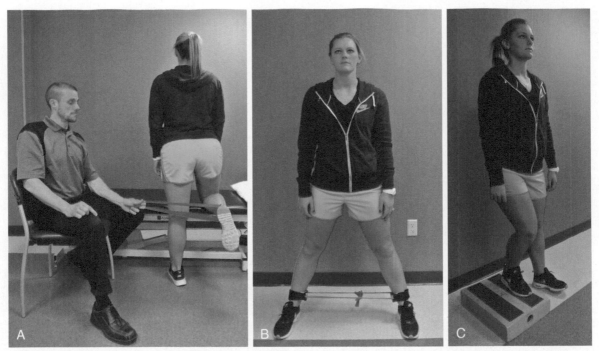

Fig. 70.13 Week 6 exercises. Image *A* demonstrates standing resisted hip internal rotation with Theraband. Image *B* illustrates resisted side-stepping. Image *C* demonstrates lateral step-down.

- Lunges
- Water bounding/plyometrics (if available)
- Side-to-side lateral agility
- Forward/backward running with cord
- Running progression

During lunges observe the anterior leg and note stability. The ability to maintain normal alignment during lunges is a necessary prerequisite to initiating running and sport-specific activities (Fig. 70.14, *A–B*). Valgus knee collapse may result from inadequate strength in the lateral hip musculature. Lateral agility (Fig. 70.14, *C–D*) and running with cord resistance (Fig. 70.14, *E–F*) should begin with light resistance and gradually increase displacement as the patient progresses. Running progression should be a gradual pain-free walk/jog progression with careful attention to form abnormalities, which may result in regression.

Phase 4: Sport-Specific Training (Initiated Postoperative Week 9)

Phase 4 is begun when phase 3 exercises are pain free. The transition time frame is dependent on the surgical procedure and how the patient is progressing. Goals for this stage are the following:

- Back pedaling
- Side shuffles
- Z cuts
- W cuts
- Cariocas
- Ghiardellis
- Sport-specific drills

Week 9 marks the beginning of agility drills and sport-specific activities. Exercises included should relate to skills necessary for the sport to which the patient intends to return, such as running, cutting, jumping, twisting, or throwing. Cariocas should be carried out while maintaining contraction of the core musculature (Fig. 70.15, *A–C*). Ghiardellis require balance while maintaining the upper body over the weightbearing joints (Fig. 70.15, *D–F*). Ghiardellis should be introduced on the non-operative leg first and progressively performed on the operative extremity, as long as the terminal part of the exercise does not incite groin pain.

There are a number of tests available for determining when an athlete is ready to return to sport, and it is important to select a sport-appropriate assessment tool. Agility tests such as the hop/jump test, T-test, and the lower extremity functional test (LEFT) have been used to determine safe return to play after lower extremity rehabilitation but have not been validated for patients with hip pathology. Further study is needed to establish reliable functional performance tests for athletes who have undergone hip preservation surgery.

More important than meeting established testing norms is that the patient performs the evaluations, as well as the specific activities to which he or she intends to return, without pain, apprehension, or compensation due to weakness. Subtle signs of compensation may include:

- Pelvic asymmetry (Trendelenburg sign)
- Valgus collapse (knee collapsing into medial rotation and adduction)
- Knee locking in extension during gait (quadriceps weakness)
- Patella extending past the toe during squats (core weakness)
- General form degradation

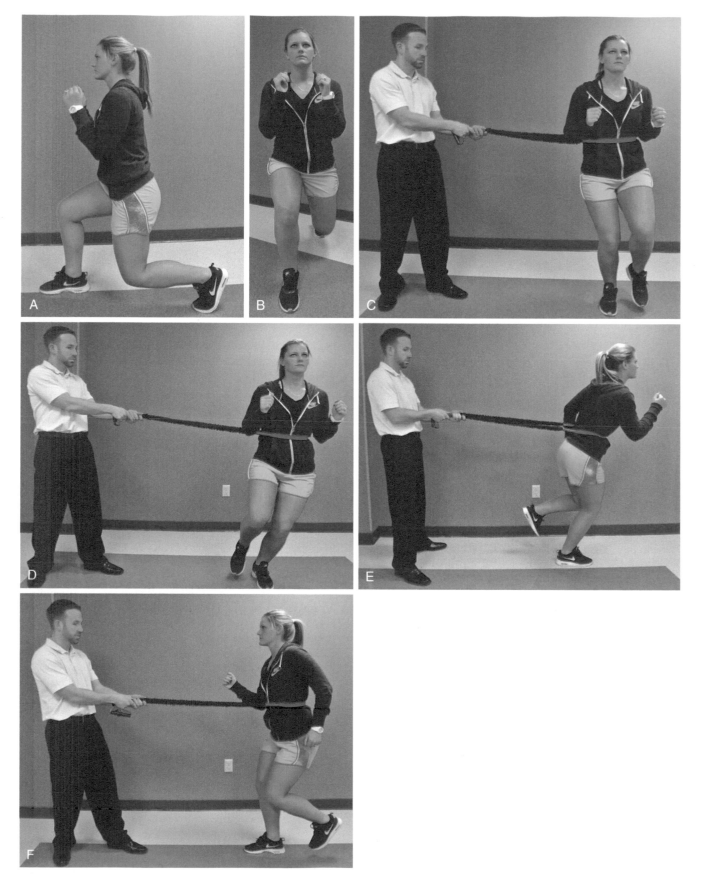

Fig. 70.14 Week 7 exercises. Images *A–B* demonstrate proper form during lunges. Images *C–D* demonstrate starting and ending positions, respectively, for side-to-side agility drills. Images *E–F* demonstrate resisted forward and backward running drills, respectively.

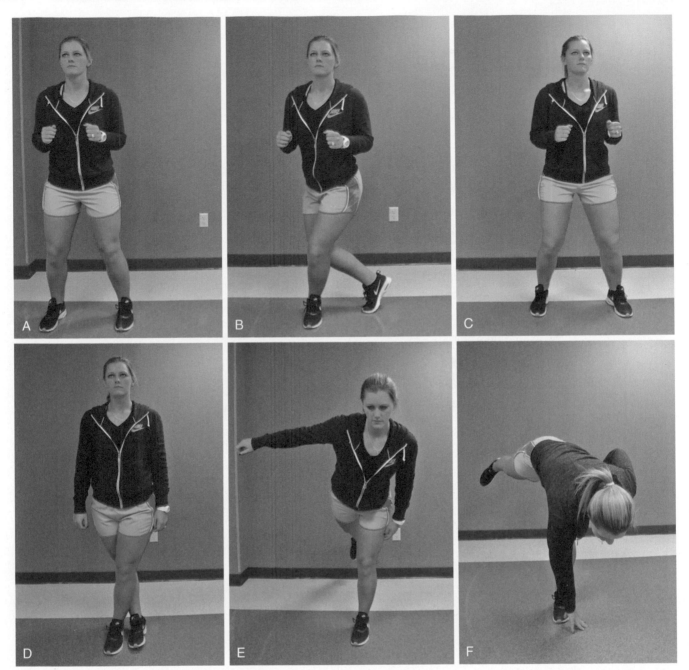

Fig. 70.15 Week 9 exercises: Images *A–C* demonstrate proper form during Cariocas. Images *D–F* demonstrate proper form while performing Ghiardellis.

REFERENCES

A complete reference list is available at https://expertconsult .inkling.com/.

FURTHER READING

Beck M, Kalhor M, Leunig M, et al. Hip morphology influences the pattern of damage to the acetabular cartilage: femoroacetabular impingement as a cause of early osteoarthritis of the hip. *J Bone Joint Surg Br.* 2005;87(7):1012–1018.

Ganz R, Leunig M, Leunig-Ganz K, et al. The etiology of osteoarthritis of the hip: an integrated mechanical concept. *Clin Orthop Relat Res.* 2008; 466(2):264–272.

Malloy P, Malloy M, Draovitch P. Guidelines and pitfalls for the rehabilitation following hip arthroscopy. *Curr Rev Musculoskelet Med.* 2013;6(3): 235–241.

Philippon MJ, Christensen JC, Wahoff MS. Rehabilitation after arthroscopic repair of intra-articular disorders of the hip in a professional football athlete. *J Sport Rehabil.* 2009;18(1):118–134.

Stalzer S, Wahoff M, Scanlan M. Rehabilitation following hip arthroscopy. *Clin Sports Med.* 2006;25(2):337–357. x.

SECTION 7

Spinal Disorders

ACKNOWLEDGMENT

We would like to acknowledge the review work done by Dr. BJ Lehecka, DPT Assistant Professor, Wichita State University, for the Spinal Disorders section that has greatly enhanced the quality of the section.

Whiplash Injury: Treatment and Rehabilitation

Adriaan Louw, PT, MAppSc (Physio), CSMT

THE WHIPLASH EPIDEMIC

In 1928 Harold Crowe introduced the term "whiplash" to describe an injury mechanism of sudden hyperextension followed by hyperflexion of the neck. Although several other terms (e.g., necklash, hyperextension injury, and acceleration injury) have been suggested, the term "whiplash" has stood the test of time. Unfortunately, the term "whiplash," which was used originally to graphically describe the manner in which the head was suddenly moved, has become a commonly used diagnostic label (Bogduk 2003). The biggest criticism associated with the labeling is the lack of information regarding the diagnosis, injury, prognosis, or treatment. Whiplash can best be described as a sudden acceleration and deceleration of the head in space (Fig. 71.1) (Bogduk 2003, Spitzer et al. 1995). This describes the process of the sudden movement and slowing down of the head in space that can occur during a motor vehicle collision (MVC), sport, or activity of daily living (ADL) (Spitzer et al. 1995). Patients presenting for the treatment of signs and symptoms associated with whiplash injury are said to have a whiplash-associated disorder (WAD) (Spitzer et al. 1995).

Whiplash injuries have been called the "disease of the century" with ever-increasing numbers of people diagnosed with WAD and seeking treatment (Bogduk 2003). Motor vehicle collisions are the leading cause of death among Americans 1 to 34 years old, and according to the U.S. Department of Transportation, the total societal cost of crashes exceeds $230 billion (U.S. Department of Transportation 2014) annually. With the increasing number of patients with WAD, little information available regarding the epidemiology, and nothing written on diagnosis, prognosis, and various interpretations of the treatments, therapists often describe whiplash as being challenging and frustrating to treat (Holm et al. 2007, Spitzer et al. 1995). Several studies have shown that WAD leads to high rates of chronic pain and disability (Holm et al. 2007, Sterling et al. 2006). It is now accepted that approximately one in four or even as many as one in three patients may develop pain lasting more than 2 years after an MVC (Bogduk 2003, Spitzer et al. 1995). No management approach treating acute whiplash has substantially reduced the incidence of transition to chronicity of this disorder (Spitzer et al. 1995).

DIAGNOSIS

Before any attempt is made to treat WAD, consideration must be given to proper diagnosis. Several studies have shown the high incidence of missed injuries, including fractures on standard imaging studies such as x-ray, magnetic resonance imaging (MRI), and computerized tomography (CT) (Bogduk 2003,

Spitzer et al. 1995). Because of the poor ability of these studies to truly identify tissue pathology, current emergency department (ED) guidelines do not routinely prescribe the use of imaging techniques. This creates a problem: A patient has significant pain and dysfunction, yet imaging tests are unable to "find a cause" of the pain. This has, unfortunately, also caused patients with WAD to be viewed as malingerers, dishonest, or even neurotic (Spitzer et al. 1995, Sterling et al. 2006). Several studies have shown that a valid way to determine disability following whiplash is via a thorough history and evaluation of the patient's disability (Carroll et al. 2009, Spitzer et al.1995). In fact, the neck disability index (NDI), which was originally designed for mechanical neck pain, was validated for use in patients with WAD. A high NDI indicates significant disability as a result of WAD, regardless of imaging test results. A thorough history and questions regarding function and/or the use of the NDI are currently the preferred tests to evaluate the effect of the WAD on the patient.

A second common fault in dealing with whiplash injuries is that patients with mechanical neck pain and traumatic neck pain (whiplash) often are grouped together (Jull et al. 2007). It is clear from the research that this is not only wrong but also poses significant problems for patients and health care providers. Whiplash is not a homogeneous entity, with evidence indicating that WAD presents as a heterogeneous complaint in terms of the levels of pain and disability and changes in the sensory, motor, and psychological systems (Jull et al. 2007); however, such classification does little to direct physical therapy management. It is recommended that therapists utilize two models: idiopathic neck pain and neck pain following trauma. Moreover, whiplash can be subclassified using the following grades: Grade 0 includes no complaint about the neck or physical signs; Grade I includes complaint of neck pain, stiffness, or tenderness only, and no other physical signs; Grade II includes neck complaints and musculoskeletal signs of impairment including decreased range of motion (ROM) and point tenderness; Grade III is similar to Grade II with the exception of the inclusion of neurologic signs such as decreased or absent tendon reflexes, myotomal weakness, and sensory deficits; and Grade IV is the classification used to describe neck complaint and fracture or dislocation (South Australian Centre for Trauma and Injury Recovery 2008) (Fig. 71.2).

TREATMENT: REVIEW OF THE LITERATURE

For treatment of whiplash Crowe suggested, "the less the treatment, the better it is." Gay and Abott (1698) advised bed rest during the first 24 to 72 hours and sedation as part of the

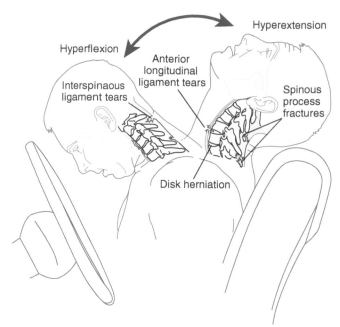

Fig. 71.1 Whiplash is the sudden acceleration–deceleration of the head in space.

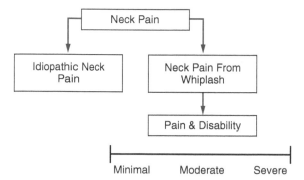

Fig. 71.2 Subclassification of neck pain and whiplash-associated disorders.

medical approach and concluded that "constant use of a cervical collar resulted in atrophy and worsening of symptoms." The first studies on exercise emerged in the 1960s, in which authors such as Knott and Barufaldi (1961) recommended traction and isometric exercises, followed by relaxation exercises. The first major study was published by Janes and Hooshmand (1965), who investigated 10,000 patients with whiplash between 1956 and 1963. The following was determined:

- 80% of their patients improved in the first year
- Immobilization in a Peterson brace (hard brace) was recommended for 6 weeks
- Muscle relaxers and moist heat
- Steroid injections in the trigger points
- Patients immobilized for 6 weeks had significantly less pain after removal of the collar

In the mid-1970s the controversies surrounding mobilization started when authors began describing the benefits and precautions of applying mobilization and/or manipulation. When reviewing the literature on the use of cervical spine soft collars, it is interesting to note a variance between minimum

periods of 2 weeks up to 1 year after MVC. Numerous early studies recommended the immediate start of therapeutic traction, with or without the application of heat. Clinical trials soon followed in 1989. Mealy et al. (1986) compared soft collars to Maitland mobilization techniques and showed greater improvement in the mobilized group in terms of ROM and pain ratings. McKinney et al. (1989) compared rest, active physiotherapy, and self-care, showing no significant difference, and Pennie and Agambar (1990) compared cervical traction, self-care, and neck and shoulder exercises, showing no significant difference.

In 1995 a landmark study on whiplash was published—The Quebec Task Force Study (Spitzer et al. 1995)—in which 10,382 articles published on whiplash over a 10-year period were reviewed and 62 studies were found relevant and meritorious. The Task Force summarized the results of the most commonly used treatments for whiplash (Table 71.1). This review, although dated, is still seen by many as the gold standard and is used as a template for treatment. The Task Force concluded that:

> *Anti-inflammatories and analgesics, short term manipulations and mobilization by trained persons, and active exercises are useful in the treatment of whiplash injuries, but prolonged use of soft collars, rest, or inactivity probably prolongs the disability of whiplash. The key message to the whiplash patient is that the pain is not harmful, is usually short-lived and controllable.*

Since the Task Force's recommendation and the emergence of evidence-based practice, several high-quality randomized controlled trials (RCTs) and systematic reviews of RCTs have been conducted on whiplash, providing evidence for the following:

- Manual therapy, exercise, and educational interventions
- Postural exercises and neck stabilization exercises (Drescher et al. 2008)
- The need for more research (Verhagen et al. 2007)
- "Rest makes rusty," whereas active interventions have a tendency to be more effective in patients with whiplash injury
- Early education via means of video (Oliveira et al. 2006)
- Exercise and advice
- Supervised training is more favorable than home training (Bunketorp et al. 2006)

When considering the development of physical therapy treatments for patients with whiplash, it is helpful to group the injury into three phases: acute, subacute, and chronic.

TREATMENT OF ACUTE WHIPLASH (0 TO 3 WEEKS)

The first 3 weeks are chosen as the acute phase based on tissue healing time, clinical observation regarding referral to physical therapy, and important research related to timelines associated with whiplash (Sterling et al. 2003a). This phase includes the immediate post-whiplash examination and treatment in the ED. After the ED visit, patients typically are referred to their primary care physician for follow-up. Based on clinical observation, it is typical that injury, ED visit, physician follow-up, and subsequent referral to physical therapy occur around the third week. Based on the current best evidence into WAD treatment, some therapists may view this as inadequate and believe that therapy should start sooner. From a pain science perspective, it may be worthwhile to have a patient "rest" for a few days and psychologically "cope with the injury." However, significant

TABLE 71.1	Summary of the Quebec Task Force Findings on the Treatment of Whiplash-Associated Disorders (WAD)
Treatment	**Summary and Recommendation by the Task Force**
Collars	Commonly prescribed; may delay recovery, causing increased pain, and decrease range of motion (ROM). Soft collars do not adequately immobilize the spine.
Rest	Commonly prescribed for the first few days. Should be limited to less than 4 days. Detrimental to recovery from WAD.
Cervical pillows	No studies
Manipulation	Single manipulation reduced asymmetry but showed the results lasted less than 48 hours. Comparing mobilization to manipulation, no clear benefit of one over the other in decreasing pain and increasing ROM. Long-term manipulation is not justified in the treatment of WAD.
Mobilization	Several studies. Maitland and McKenzie mobilization versus rest showed significantly greater improvement in pain and ROM for the mobilization groups. One study showed that patients given active exercises and advice recovered just as well as the mobilized group. Another study showed that mobilization was more effective than a combination of analgesics and education in the decrease of pain and increase of ROM. Mobilization appears to be beneficial in the short term, but the long-term benefits need to be established. Physical therapy should emphasize early return to usual activity and promote mobility.
Exercise	No independent effect of exercise has been evaluated. The evidence suggests exercise as part of a multimodal intervention may be beneficial (short- and long-term).
Traction	No independent effects of traction were found. One study tested different types of traction (static, intermittent, manual), but no significant differences were found on the different traction types.
Posture	No studies
Spray and stretch	No studies
Transcutaneous electrical stimulation (TENS)	No accepted studies
Electrical stimulation	No studies
Ultrasound	No studies
Laser, diathermy, heat, ice, massage	No independent studies. The modalities were part of the combination of passive modalities in different studies.
Surgery	No studies on surgery or nerve blocks
Injections Epidural Intrathecal Intra-articular	No studies. Not justified in the management of WAD patients.
Pharmacology Analgesics Anti-inflammatories	Shown to be effective with the use of physical modalities.
Muscle relaxants	No studies
Psychosocial	No studies
Acupuncture	No studies

evidence suggests that early education and encouragement to move soon after the injury are of great value. This is different from aggressive early mobilization/manipulation. Several authors have questioned this approach because of the significant injuries associated with whiplash and the high incidence of missed fractures (Bogduk, 2003). Two recent RCTs showed that patients who received educational videos in the ED regarding the pathology, self-help ideas, prognosis, plan of care, and goals performed much better than patients receiving "usual care"—ED waiting room, tests, medicine, and referral to their primary care physicians (Oliveira et al. 2006). Therefore, in the acute phase (0–3 weeks) therapists may consider the following:

- Arrange patient visits as soon as possible to give quality advice and education. Therapists may consider viewing the patient with acute WAD similar to a "crutch trainer." Therapists may even consider developing a program where therapists attend to the patient with WAD in the ED. The educational session should address four key issues: what is wrong with them (diagnosis), how long it will take (prognosis), what they should do for it at home (self-help), and what therapy can do for them (plan of care). All of the information should be delivered in a nonthreatening, calming manner, avoiding phrases or words that induce fear, such as "torn," "ripped," or "fracture."
- Inform the patient regarding the pathology and healing process. For example, "Damage has been done and you have had

a nasty injury, but the healing process has already begun." "You have had a big injury, but it will not be like this forever. There is work you can do that will help recovery given time." "Research shows the more you move—provided it's gentle, little, and often—the better the results."

- Encourage self-management. Teach the patient strategies to deal with the pain at home, including cardiovascular exercise, moving other joints, breathing, trying relaxation methods, and heat/cold as needed. If pain wakes the patient at night, he or she should engage in these treatment strategies to ease pain and reduce fear.
- Reduce pain as soon as possible. This may include the use of medication and modalities. Engage in frequent short rest periods only for a limited time. Perform relaxed, gentle, oscillating movements little and often.
- If possible, encourage the patient to return to work as soon as possible, even if it is light or restricted duty. People who work follow certain habits or routines, and once they get out of them it is more challenging to return to them. It is also a powerful coping strategy.
- Use modalities for a limited time as a means of reducing pain.
- Consider bracing. The majority of the research follows the sports medicine model of movement; however, there is some evidence and concern by several authors that aggressive, early movement may not be the best. It is recommended that

clinicians carefully examine patients, and patients who are on the more severe end of the scale of the injury or disability use a collar for a short time. This may be a few days to a week. Wean the patient off the brace as soon as possible (Kongsted et al. 2007, Spitzer et al. 1995). Brace wearing should either be time or function dependent rather than pain dependent. This way the patient is less focused on the pain and uses the brace only during a certain functional task and/or for a certain amount of time. Therapists may even consider using a brace in therapy (e.g., having a patient with acute WAD get the benefit of aerobic exercise on a treadmill while the braced spine is relaxed and protected).

- Therapists who choose to engage patients with acute WAD in exercises should perform exercises with the patient supine. With the increased understanding of pain inhibition on the stabilizing muscles of the cervical spine, therapists should aim to increase movement without producing pain.
- Move other joints. Therapists should encourage movement of the extremities and trunk to prevent further dysfunction in the body.

TREATMENT OF SUBACUTE WHIPLASH (3 WEEKS TO 3 MONTHS)

Most patients seen in physical therapy for WAD are seen in the subacute phase. These patients follow the traditional model of injury: ED visit, referral to their primary care physician, and then referral to physical therapy approximately 3 weeks after the injury. These patients usually present with neck pain, scapular pain, headaches, decreased ROM, decreased function, and possible neurologic deficit (Bogduk 2003, Spitzer et al. 1995). Treatment of the patient with subacute whiplash includes all of the acute whiplash principles and current best-evidence strategies.

In general, patients in the subacute phase should be able to engage in some movement and have some decrease in pain. Patients most likely are finding improvement in some functions and ROM, although they are still limited in others. After a thorough examination, therapists should focus on alleviating the specific physical dysfunctions and may consider the following:

Exercise

Exercises for patients with whiplash can be divided into active ROM (AROM) exercises, postural exercises, spinal stabilization exercises, balance/proprioception exercises, and cardiovascular exercises.

AROM Exercises

After the initial supine exercises aimed at encouraging movement, therapists should progress AROM exercises in a weight-bearing (upright) position and during functional tasks. AROM exercises should aim to engage all planes of movement and be performed into slight resistance or discomfort. A stretch, ache, or pain does not signal damage but rather the sensitivity of the tissue. By slowly "nudging" the exercises into slight discomfort, AROM will improve. Exercises that stop short of pain will over time cause patients to decrease their movement, whereas the "no pain, no gain" mantra leads to "boom-bust" cycles in which

patients ignore pain and pay for it in the days to follow. Over time this model will also cause patients to move less.

Postural Exercises

It is common for patients with whiplash to present with a forward head, rounded shoulder posture after a whiplash injury. Pain inhibition, protective mechanisms, and fear cause the patient to adopt a posture of comfort or safety. This is normal. Anterior cervico-thoracic muscles develop adaptive shortening, whereas posterior thoracic muscles tend to lengthen and become weak, leading to postural changes (Drescher et al. 2008). Therapists should develop exercises aimed at stretching shortened overactive muscles, while working on strengthening weak muscles. Therapists should also encourage patients to routinely check posture throughout the day with cues such as a cell phone ringing or signing on to check e-mail.

Spinal Stabilization Exercises (Sterling et al. 2003b)

There is a large body of research regarding segmental spinal stabilization in the lumbar spine. Similar research is now emerging about the cervical spine (Jull et al. 2007, Sterling et al. 2003b). The cervical spine helps support and orient the head in relation to the thoracic spine and provides two key elements: stability and mobility. Similar to the lumbar spine, the deeper muscles closer to the spine contribute to stability, whereas the larger, superficial muscles that span multiple joints contribute more to movement. The deeper muscles have control strategies and proper morphology to stabilize the neck. In healthy individuals, the deep neck flexors provide a low-level, tonic contraction prior to movement of the extremities to protect the cervical spine. However, following injury, several changes occur to the deep cervical flexors:

- Reduced activation of the deep neck flexors
- Augmented superficial muscle activity
- Change in feedforward activity
- Prolonged muscle activation after voluntary contraction
- Reduced relative rest periods
- Change in muscle fiber type from type I (slow twitch) to type II (fast twitch)
- Increased fatigue
- Muscle atrophy
- Fatty tissue infiltration
- Changes in fiber/capillary ratios

All of these changes indicate that patients with neck pain (i.e., WAD) will demonstrate limited endurance, greater fatigability, less strength, altered proprioception, and reorganized motor control. The cranio-cervical flexion test (CCFT) is used to evaluate the ability of the deep cervical flexors to produce low-load tonic submaximal contractions (Fig. 71.3) (Jull et al. 2008). Therapists should concentrate part of the rehabilitation of the patient with whiplash to retraining the deep neck flexors of the cervical spine. These exercises should aim to provide protection to the cervical spine during ADLs. Once local stabilizers have been activated and retrained, therapists should have patients perform various exercises incorporating weights and resistive bands while engaging the deep neck flexors. Stabilization exercises should focus on low-load, tonic contractions, which should be progressed by increasing the time the

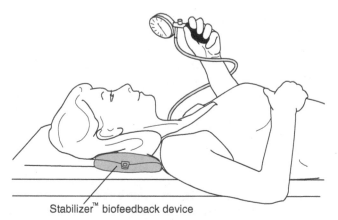

Stabilizer™ biofeedback device

Fig. 71.3 Cranio-cervical flexion test (CCFT). Assessing the deep neck flexor activity with the Stabilizer biofeedback device.

patient contracts the deep neck flexors (their endurance, in other words).

Proprioception/Balance Exercises

The previous section on spinal stabilization describes the function of the cervical spine muscles as a means to help orient the head in space. Studies have shown that patients with WAD and patients with mechanical neck pain have difficulty repositioning their head in space. Because the cervical spine muscles not only contribute to segmental control but also head positioning, therapists should evaluate and treat joint positioning errors. Therapists should develop exercises that help retrain balance and proprioception by increasingly challenging the postural system (i.e., altering foot position and visual input).

Cardiovascular Exercises

Therapists should help patients develop a home exercise program that includes aerobic exercise. The neurophysiologic mechanisms behind aerobic exercise include increasing blood flow and oxygenation of muscles and neural tissue, regulating stress chemicals such as adrenaline and cortisol, boosting the immune system, improving memory, decreasing sleep disturbance, and providing distraction.

Manual Therapy (Spitzer et al. 1995)

The Quebec Task Force study and subsequent systematic reviews and RCTs have shown that manual therapy techniques such as spinal mobilization and manipulation may benefit patients with subacute whiplash. Following a thorough examination, therapists are encouraged to carefully progress through the grades of movement/resistance to alleviate pain and dysfunction associated with specific physical dysfunction of specific joints/spinal levels. Manual therapy can be applied to both the cervical spine and thoracic spine. Evidence suggests that patients with neck pain respond favorably to manipulative therapy applied to the thoracic spine. Considering the concerns about missed fractures and significant tissue injury with whiplash, it is recommended that therapists perform skilled evaluations, continually reassess the patient, and adhere to a principle taught by manual therapy pioneer Geoffrey Maitland (2005) of "using the least amount

of force to gain the desired outcome." Qualitative studies have shown that patients want to receive hands-on treatment, and studies that compared hands-on to exercise-only interventions have found that hands-on treatment leads to better outcomes in the short term (Miao 2011, Koes et al. 1993).

Neural Tissue Mobilization

To date, no studies have investigated the effect of neural tissue mobilization on patients with WAD; however, studies have shown that patients with WAD demonstrate decreased slump tests and upper limb neurodynamic tests (Koes 1993, Yeung et al. 1997). There is growing evidence that active and passive neural tissue mobilization may facilitate a faster return to work and recreational activities, increase the ROM associated with the neurodynamic test, decrease the need for surgery, and decrease pain. It is recommended that therapists incorporate active and passive neural tissue mobilization techniques into the treatment regimen for whiplash. This includes neural mobilization techniques of the lower extremities, upper extremities, and trunk.

Based on the current best-available evidence regarding the treatment of subacute whiplash, a multimodal approach combining exercise, modalities, manual therapy, and education should be part of the treatment plan (Jull et al. 2007). All of the movement-based treatments should be complemented with continuous education focused on reducing fear, explaining treatments, setting goals, offering encouragement, and providing a safe healing environment.

Consideration also should be given to strategies aimed at reducing the chance of a patient with subacute whiplash developing chronic WAD. Therapists who treat patients in the acute and subacute phases have a unique opportunity to help a patient progress through these phases and not move on to the chronic phase. Several factors have been identified in the development of chronicity, including factors associated with the accident (head position, signs and symptoms, the accident site, male/female, stationary car, etc.) and patient attributes (poor coping skills, extended rest, etc.) (Bogduk 2003, Jull et al. 2008, Spitzer et al. 1995). Some factors can be positively affected by a therapist in the acute and subacute phases.

Education

Therapists should aim to educate their patients suffering whiplash and thus reduce fear. Fear of pain, injury, or re-injury may be the most potent factor in the development of chronic spinal pain. This has led to the development of questionnaires to examine the level of fear a patient may have. The most commonly used "fear questionnaire" is the fear-avoidance belief questionnaire (FABQ). The FABQ is a 16-item questionnaire that was designed to quantify fear and avoidance beliefs in individuals with low back pain. The FABQ has two subscales: a seven-item scale to measure fear-avoidance beliefs about work and a four-item scale to measure fear-avoidance beliefs about physical activity. Higher scores represent an increase in fear-avoidance beliefs. The FABQ is a valid and reliable measure of fear-avoidance beliefs (Askary-Ashanti et al. 2014).

Low levels of physical activity: Incorporating exercise and movement is an active strategy in dealing with pain and disability, compared to a passive approach. Therapists should encourage movement and exercise.

Visiting many health care providers: Indirectly, therapists guide patients' treatment choices. By providing high-quality care, therapists may decrease the need for patients to seek additional help.

Overuse of medication: Although therapists do not prescribe or address issues related to medication, therapists can utilize and teach patients strategies, such as the use of modalities, rest, education, and exercise to manage pain and reduce dependency on medication.

Passive coping strategies: Numerous studies encourage an active approach. Therapists should use hands-on, passive approaches and not make the patient "dependent" on passive strategies for managing spinal pain.

Belief that activity causes pain or injury: Education, encouragement, and realistic goals associated with exercise and movement should aim to change patient beliefs.

TREATING CHRONIC WHIPLASH (3 MONTHS AND MORE)

Although patients with subacute whiplash may be the group most frequently presenting to physical therapy, patients with chronic whiplash are the most challenging. Three months is chosen specifically for the chronic phase because several studies have shown that patients who do not have significant decrease in their symptoms by 3 months postinjury have a very high likelihood of developing chronic pain associated with the whiplash injury (Spitzer et al. 1995, Sterling et al. 2003, Sterling et al. 2006). This population also includes patients with whiplash who show up months or even years after injury seeking help for the pain and disability.

It is important to realize that the patient with chronic whiplash described here is the patient who has experienced an upregulated central nervous system (CNS). With all the issues associated with the accident (stress, anxiety, fear, failed treatment, different explanations of the injury), the CNS heightened its sensitivity as a means of survival, a process referred to as central sensitivity or secondary hyperalgesia. Now input from tissues such as muscles or joints from exercises, examinations, and treatments may be registered as pain. (For more information, refer to the section on chronic pain.) Common clinical signs and symptoms include:

- Ongoing pain. Reasoning based on tissue models (anatomy, pathoanatomy, etc.) has the therapist thinking, "The tissues should have healed by now."
- Summation and latency. After an activity, there is pain that not only lasts but increases. For example, working 30 minutes at the computer leads to 3 days of severe pain.
- Unpredictability. The patient's symptoms do not respond in a typical stimulus response predictability. Therapists often find themselves "chasing the pain" through the body.
- Pain description. "Everything hurts and the pain is everywhere."
- Highly unstable nature. All movements hurt, including the cervical spine and adjacent joints.
- Pain out of dermatomal fields. The original pains have spread.
- Mirror pains. Pain that is felt on the left side of the body is also found on the right side of the body.
- Sudden stabs of pain. Pain with a mind of its own. "Pain comes when it wants to."
- Poor or inconsistent responses to treatment. The same treatment may on one day provide significant relief, whereas if the same treatment is repeated on another day, the pain is increased.
- Association with anxiety and depression.
- Variable diagnoses such as late whiplash syndrome, myofascial syndrome, or fibromyalgia.

A detailed description of the latest evidence in treating chronic spinal pain is given in the section on managing chronic pain. The key points are highlighted here with an emphasis on whiplash:

1. Identify patients with "red flags." Even in the chronic phase, therapists should always be on the lookout for red flags (i.e., symptoms of vertebral basilar insufficiency) by continually assessing the patient. Patients with a red flag should be referred for additional testing and medical management.
2. Educate the patient about the nature of the problem. Education has been discussed in detail. Recent research has evaluated the use of neuroscience education in decreasing pain and disability among patients with chronic pain. It is recommended that therapists educate patients more regarding their pain as opposed to only using anatomy models. Additionally, neuroscience education has been shown to decrease fear and change a patient's pain perception (Oliveira et al. 2006).
3. Provide prognostication. Focus on function rather than pain. Set attainable goals related to exercise, function, and social interaction.
4. Promote self-care. A powerful management strategy for patients with chronic pain is to teach them strategies to help themselves. This fosters greater independence and helps with the development of coping strategies—teaching patients that they are able to manage their own pain. This also creates less dependence on the health care provider.
5. Get patients moving and active as early as possible and appropriately after injury. Movement is essential. There are many reasons to get patients to move soon after injury, including (from a biological perspective) blood flow, removal of irritant substances, and (from a psychological aspect) coping strategies, empowerment, and more.
6. Decrease unnecessary fear related to movement, leisure, and work activities. Several factors are associated with the development and maintenance of a pain state. As mentioned earlier, several authors believe that fear of pain, injury, or re-injury may be the most potent factor in the development of chronic spinal pain. Use the FABQ to examine the patient's fear levels and address fear issues related to activity, exercise, and movement.
7. Help the patient experience success. Encouragement is important. Patients with chronic pain have numerous psychological comorbidities such as depression, poor body image, and lack of self-confidence.
8. Perform a skilled physical examination, and communicate results to the patient. Study has shown that patients want to be physically examined (Connan, 2009). It is recommended that clinicians consider a skilled "low-tech" examination. This implies the evaluation is thorough, yet more geared toward a global view of the physical test findings. Patients with chronic pain exhibit increased widespread sensitivity (hyperalgesia), which decreases the relevance of specific physical dysfunction. Carefully analyze the findings of the physical tests. Once the evaluation is complete, communicate findings to the patient in a nonthreatening manner.

9. Make any treatment strategy as closely linked to evidence of the biological nature of the problem rather than syndrome or geography. Clinicians are encouraged to get away from syndromes and areas of pain. Neck pain or scapular pain only refers to the fact that the area of pain is in or around the neck. The geography (where the pain is) does not tell the patient anything about the underlying pathology or explain why treatments may be of benefit. Neither do syndromes. Late whiplash syndrome only informs the patient he or she has persistent pain after whiplash. There is growing evidence that the more patients understand the biology behind their pain, the better understanding of the pathology they have and the better their understanding of the proposed treatment plan. This is another cornerstone of neuroscience education— "biologizing" a patient's pain. The clinician should explain to the patient what happens on a biological level that causes the pain and what can be done.

10. Use any measures possible to reduce pain. With all the knowledge now available on the development of central sensitization, it seems imperative to decrease the constant barrage of danger messages to the CNS as soon as possible. With persistent input from the periphery, the CNS will upregulate, which may lead to long-lasting changes. Clinicians should use any and all means to decrease pain. This includes the skillful application of medication, modalities, education, hands-on treatment, and more.

11. Minimize number of treatments and contacts with medical personnel. The ideal scenario is for a patient with chronic pain to develop a greater understanding of his or her pain and develop a treatment plan focused on developing independence and an ability to self-manage the condition. Therapists should aim to develop this independence through encouragement, home exercise programs, and education.

12. Consider multidisciplinary management. The sad reality of chronic pain is that these patients have many comorbidities, long-lasting physical and emotional changes, and medication needs. This implies that patients may benefit from several health care providers including a physical therapist, psychologist, pain management physician, art therapist, dietician, and more. This does not mean all patients need it. Clinicians should, based on their experience and evaluation, decide if a patient may need additional help. This needs to be discussed with the patient and his or her physician.

13. Manage identified and relevant physical dysfunctions. Patients present in physical therapy with various physical dysfunctions (e.g., stiff joints, muscles not recruiting). The important aspect is to determine if these are relevant. This may be more apparent in an acute tissue-based pain state but less obvious in the patient with chronic pain. Relevance relates to function. Correcting a dysfunction should help a patient function better. Therapists should manage these dysfunctions but always be aware of the larger picture of the patient's pain state.

14. Assess and assist recovery of general physical fitness. A vast body of evidence supports the use of aerobic exercise in the management of patients with chronic pain. Therapists should help patients develop a home exercise program that includes a large focus on aerobic exercise.

15. Assess the effects on the patient's creative outlets. Therapists should embrace a holistic approach to management— embracing each patient's individualism, goals, strengths, and weaknesses—and design a treatment approach that will help the patient achieve his or her goals.

Probably the most important aspect in treating chronic whiplash is to properly identify the patient as in a centralized pain state. These patients should be educated regarding their pain and managed through the development of an active, self-help program of exercises and coping strategies, focused on function rather than pain.

The treatments outlined here are suggestions aimed at the patient with WAD in the first 3 weeks after the injury. There are many variables to consider, such as the extent of the injury, patient goals and coping skills, referring physician's preferences, and more. Sound clinical reasoning cannot be stressed enough. A patient may present to physical therapy 1 week after the injury and have little disability and may be treated with more advanced approaches (such as in the subacute phase), whereas another patient may show up at the end of week 3 but may not be ready for advanced treatments because of pain, fear, increased disability, and more. It is highly recommended that therapists use the NDI to determine the patient's level of disability and conduct a thorough, skilled subjective and objective examination. Good-quality education and encouragement as soon as possible after the injury cannot be stressed enough. Researchers are now showing that a subgroup of patients with whiplash may develop an instant upregulation (sensitivity) of the nervous system as soon as 3 weeks after the injury. Every possible attempt should be made to calm the nervous system as soon as possible after the injury.

REFERENCES

A complete reference list is available at https://expertconsult.inkling.com/.

FURTHER READING

Bogduk N. Epidemiology of whiplash. *Ann Rheum Dis*. 2000;59:394–395. author reply 5–6.

Bogduk N. Regional musculoskeletal pain. The neck. *Baillieres Best Pract Res Clin Rheumatol*. 1999;13:261–285.

Bogduk N. Whiplash can have lesions. *Pain Res Manag*. 2006;11:155.

Brison RJ, Hartling L, Dostaler S, et al. A randomized controlled trial of an educational intervention to prevent the chronic pain of whiplash associated disorders following rear-end motor vehicle collisions. *Spine*. 2005;30:1799–1807.

Busch AJ, Barber KA, Overend TJ, et al. Exercise for treating fibromyalgia syndrome. *Cochrane Database Syst Rev*. 2007:CD003786.

Butler D. *The Sensitive Nervous System*. Adelaide: Noigroup Publications; 2000.

Cleland JA, Childs JD, Fritz JM, et al. Development of a clinical prediction rule for guiding treatment of a subgroup of patients with neck pain: use of thoracic spine manipulation, exercise, and patient education. *Phys Ther*. 2007;87:9–23.

Cleland JA, Fritz JM, Childs JD. Psychometric properties of the fear-avoidance beliefs questionnaire and Tampa Scale of Kinesiophobia in patients with neck pain. *Am J Phys Med Rehabil*. 2008;87:109–117.

Coppieters M, Alshami A. Longitudinal excursion and strain in the median nerve during novel nerve gliding exercises for carpal tunnel syndrome. *J Orthop Res*. 2007;25:972–980.

Coppieters MW, Bartholomeeusen KE, Stappaerts KH. Incorporating nerve-gliding techniques in the conservative treatment of cubital tunnel syndrome. *J Manipulative Physiol Ther*. 2004;27:560–568.

Coppieters MW, Stappaerts KH, Wouters LL, et al. The immediate effects of a cervical lateral glide treatment technique in patients with neurogenic cervicobrachial pain. *J Orthop Sports Phys Ther*. 2003;33:369–378.

Drechsler WI, Knarr JF, Snyder-Mackler L. A comparison of two treatment regimens for lateral epicondylitis: a randomized trial of clinical interventions. *Journal of Sport Rehabilitation* 1997;6(3):226–234 (*13 ref*);6:226–34.

Falla DL, Jull G, Edwards S, et al. Neuromuscular efficiency of the sternocleidomastoid and anterior scalene muscles in patients with chronic neck pain. *Disabil Rehabil*. 2004;26:712–717.

Falla DL, Jull G, Hodges PW. Feedforward activity of the cervical flexor muscles during voluntary arm movements is delayed in chronic neck pain. *Exp Brain Res.* 2004;157:43–48.

Falla DL, Jull G, Rainoldi A, et al. Neck flexor muscle fatigue is side specific in patients with unilateral neck pain. *Eur J Pain.* 2004;8:71–77.

Falla DL, Campbell CD, Fagan AE, et al. Relationship between cranio-cervical flexion range of motion and pressure change during the cranio-cervical flexion test. *Man Ther.* 2003;8:92–96.

Falla DL, Jull GA, Hodges PW. Patients with neck pain demonstrate reduced electromyographic activity of the deep cervical flexor muscles during performance of the craniocervical flexion test. *Spine.* 2004;29:2108–2114.

Fernandez-de-las-Penas C, Cleland JA. Management of whiplash-associated disorder addressing thoracic and cervical spine impairments: a case report. *J Orthop Sports Phys Ther.* 2005;35:180–181.

Gifford LS. Pain mechanisms in whiplash. In: Gifford LS, ed. *Physiotherapy Pain Association Yearbook.* Falmouth: NOI Press; 1997.

Grotle M, Vollestad NK, Brox JI. Clinical course and impact of fear-avoidance beliefs in low back pain: prospective cohort study of acute and chronic low back pain: II. *Spine.* 2006;31:1038–1046.

Guramoorthy D, Twomey L. The Quebec Task Force on Whiplash-Associated Disorders. *Spine.* 1996;21:897.

Hurwitz EL, Carragee EJ, van der Velde G, et al. Treatment of neck pain: noninvasive interventions: results of the Bone and Joint Decade 2000-2010 Task Force on Neck Pain and Its Associated Disorders. *Spine.* 2008;33:S123–S152.

Jull G, Kristjansson E, Dall'Alba P. Impairment in the cervical flexors: a comparison of whiplash and insidious onset neck pain patients. *Man Ther.* 2004;9:89–94.

Jull G, Sterling M, Kenardy J, et al. Does the presence of sensory hypersensitivity influence outcomes of physical rehabilitation for chronic whiplash?–A preliminary RCT. *Pain.* 2007 May;129(1-2):28–34. Epub 2007 Jan 10.

Knott M, Barufaldi D. Treatment of whiplash injuries. *Phys Ther Rev.* 1961;41:573–577.

Koes BW, Bouter LM, van Mameren H, et al. A randomized clinical trial of manual therapy and physiotherapy for persistent back and neck complaints: subgroup analysis and relationship between outcome measures. *J Manipulative Physiol Ther.* 1993 May;16(4):211–219.

Kornberg C, Lew P. The effect of stretching neural structures on grade one hamstring injuries. *J Orthop Sports Phys Ther.* 1989;10:481–487.

Kornberg C, McCarthy T. The effect of neural stretching technique on sympathetic outflow to the lower limbs. *J Orthop Sports Phys Ther.* 1992;16:269–274.

Loudon JK, Ruhl M, Field E. Ability to reproduce head position after whiplash injury. *Spine.* 1997;22:865–868.

Mealy K, Brennan H, Fenelon GC. Early mobilization of acute whiplash injuries. *Br Med J (Clin Res Ed).* 1986;292:656–657.

Moseley GL. Evidence for a direct relationship between cognitive and physical change during an education intervention in people with chronic low back pain. *Eur J Pain.* 2004;8:39–45.

Moseley GL. Joining forces—combining cognition-targeted motor control training with group or individual pain physiology education: a successful treatment for chronic low back pain. *J Man Manip Therap.* 2003;11(2):88–94.

Moseley GL. Widespread brain activity during an abdominal task markedly reduced after pain physiology education: fMRI evaluation of a single patient with chronic low back pain. *Aust J Physiother.* 2005;51:49–52.

Moseley GL, Hodges PW, Nicholas MK. A randomized controlled trial of intensive neurophysiology education in chronic low back pain. *Clin J Pain.* 2004;20:324–330.

O'Leary S, Falla D, Hodges PW, et al. Specific therapeutic exercise of the neck induces immediate local hypoalgesia. *J Pain.* 2007;8:832–839.

Peeters GG, Verhagen AP, de Bie RA, et al. The efficacy of conservative treatment in patients with whiplash injury: a systematic review of clinical trials. *Spine.* 2001;26:E64–E73.

Pennie B, Agambar L. Patterns of injury and recovery in whiplash. *Injury.* 1991;22:57–59.

Poiraudeau S, Rannou F, Baron G, et al. Fear-avoidance beliefs about back pain in patients with subacute low back pain. *Pain.* 2006;124:305–311.

Rozmaryn LM, Dovelle S, Rothman ER, et al. Nerve and tendon gliding exercises and the conservative management of carpal tunnel syndrome. *J Hand Ther.* 1998;11:171–179.

Stewart MJ, Maher CG, Refshauge KM, et al. Randomized controlled trial of exercise for chronic whiplash-associated disorders. *Pain.* 2007;128:59–68.

Sweeney J, Harms A. Persistent mechanical allodynia following injury of the hand. Treatment through mobilization of the nervous system. *J Hand Ther.* 1996;9:328–338.

Treleaven J, Jull G, Low Choy N. The relationship of cervical joint position error to balance and eye movement disturbances in persistent whiplash. *Man Ther.* 2006;11:99–106.

U.S. Department of Transportation. *Safety Facts and Statistics. U.S. Department of Transportation;* October 15, 2014. http://safety.fhwa.dot.gov/facts_stats/. Accessed 8/8/15.

Vicenzino B, Collins D, Wright A. The initial effects of a cervical spine manipulative physiotherapy treatment on the pain and dysfunction of lateral epicondylalgia. *Pain.* 1996;68:69–74.

Waddell G, Newton M, Henderson I, et al. A fear-avoidance beliefs questionnaire (FABQ) and the role of fear avoidance beliefs in chronic low back pain and disability. *Pain.* 1993;52:157–168.

Wallin MK, Raak RI. Quality of life in subgroups of individuals with whiplash associated disorders. *Eur J Pain.* 2008.

Weirich SD, Gelberman RH, Best SA, et al. Rehabilitation after subcutaneous transposition of the ulnar nerve: immediate versus delayed mobilization. *J Shoulder Elbow Surg.* 1998;7:244–249.

Yeung E, Jones M, Hall B. The response to the slump test in a group of female whiplash patients. *Aust J Physiother.* 1997;43(4):245–252.

Therapeutic Exercise for the Cervical Spine

Christopher J. Durall, PT, DPT, MS, SCS, LAT, CSCS

Neck pain affects most adults at some point in their lives, and nearly 20% of the population suffers from persistent or recurrent symptoms (Croft et al. 2001, Binder 2006). Individuals with neck pain may have deficits in coordination (Falla et al. 2004a, Chui et al. 2005), strength, endurance (O'Leary et al. 2007b), repositioning acuity (Kristjansson et al. 2003, Sjolander et al. 2008), postural stability (Michaelson et al. 2003), or oculomotor control (Treleaven et al. 2005a). Patients with neck pain may also have mobility deficits in the cervical and/or upper thoracic regions (Childs et al. 2008). Therapeutic exercise has shown considerable promise as an intervention for individuals with neck pain (Kay et al. 2005, Gross et al. 2007), despite a lack of consensus among clinicians and researchers on optimal exercises or guidelines. In this section, exercises intended to correct deficits are discussed, with the objectives of reducing symptoms, improving function, and preventing recurrence.

EXERCISES TO IMPROVE MUSCULAR COORDINATION, ENDURANCE, OR STRENGTH

Deficits in cervical muscle performance may occur rapidly following the onset of neck pain and may persist despite symptom reduction or resolution (Sterling et al. 2003). Research has shown that exercises to improve coordination, endurance, or strength can aid neck symptom resolution (Sarig-Bahat 2003). This is logical given that the neck musculature provides nearly 80% of the mechanical stability of the cervical spine (Panjabi et al. 1998).

The deep cervical flexor (DCF) muscles (longus capitus and colli, rectus capitus anterior and lateralis, hyoid muscles) and deep cervical extensor (DCE) muscles (semispinalis cervicis, multifidus, rectus capitus posterior major and minor), in particular, appear prone to impairment in patients with neck pain (Sterling et al. 2003). These muscles have a high density of type I fibers and muscle spindles and are vulnerable to pain inhibition (Boyd-Clark et al. 2002). Reduced control and capacity of the deeper neck muscles can result in unwanted segmental motion or buckling during contraction of the multisegmental superficial muscles (Winters & Peles 1990). Thus the initial rehabilitation emphasis should be toward improving performance or coordination of the deeper cervical muscles.

EXERCISES TO IMPROVE MUSCULAR COORDINATION

Patients with neck pain tend to have impaired DCF activity and elevated superficial cervical flexor (SCF; sternocleidomastoid [SCM], anterior scalene) activity during craniocervical flexion (Falla et al. 2004a, Chui et al. 2005). One exercise reported to help reverse this aberrant neck flexor synergy uses a pressure device positioned inferior to the occiput to provide feedback (Fig. 72.1). For this exercise the patient attempts to flatten the cervical lordosis, which requires DCF contraction (Mayoux-Benhamou et al. 1994), while minimizing SCF activation. The contractile effort with this exercise should be low and the patient should focus on precise control of the movement. Low-load exercises (20% maximal voluntary contraction) have been shown to facilitate more selective activation of the deeper cervical flexor and extensor muscles, while minimizing activity in their more superficial synergists (O'Leary et al. 2007a). Gentle, low-load exercise has also been shown to produce a superior, immediate hypoalgesic effect relative to higher-load exercise and is more appropriate when pain is a primary concern. Exercising above the pain threshold can impair neuromuscular control (Falla et al. 2007).

The pressure device–assisted craniocervical flexion exercise is as effective at increasing cervical flexion strength as an endurance exercise program in patients with chronic neck pain (Falla et al. 2006). Moreover, the perception that the exercise program was beneficial was roughly 10% greater in the group that performed craniocervical flexion with a pressure device. Of interest, this exercise was shown to improve repositioning acuity in people with neck pain to nearly the same extent as a proprioceptive training regimen (Jull et al. 2007).

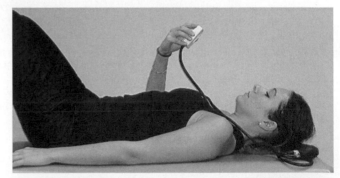

Fig. 72.1 With the patient hook-lying and in neutral craniocervical spine alignment, a pneumatic pressure device is inflated to 20 mm Hg and placed between the upper cervical spine (below occiput) and table. The patient is instructed to slowly and subtly nod his or her head as though saying "yes" while trying to keep the superficial cervical flexor (SCF) relaxed. The nodding movement will flatten the cervical lordosis and increase device pressure. The clinician should monitor for unwanted SCF activation, which is usually most apparent in the sternocleidomastoid (SCM). The patient can place the tongue on the roof of the mouth, with lips together but teeth slightly apart, to decrease platysma and/or hyoid activation. Initially, the patient can practice controlling and varying pressure in the device. As tolerated, the patient should practice holding increased levels of pressure until he or she can sustain 30 mm Hg for 10 seconds with minimal SCF activation.

Controlled craniocervical flexion can also be done without a pressure device (Fig. 72.2). This exercise can be done sitting or standing initially to minimize gravity resistance and then reclined as tolerated to increase gravity resistance. Once the patient can nod while supine with minimal SCF activation, he or she can practice flexing the lower cervical spine while sustaining upper cervical flexion (Fig. 72.3). The SCMs are required to flex the lower cervical segments, so the patient does not need to palpate the SCMs during the combined movement. Inability to sustain upper cervical flexion during this exercise results in head protrusion (Fig. 72.4), which indicates that the exercise is too challenging and should be regressed. Krout and Anderson (1966) reported that 12 of 15 patients with nonspecific neck pain who performed controlled head/neck flexion while supine experienced good to complete recovery. This exercise and the craniocervical flexion exercise described previously involving the pressure device were shown to produce equivalent neck flexor strength gains following 6 weeks of twice-weekly training in a group of women with mild neck pain and disability (O'Leary et al. 2007a). Exercises for the DCFs can be particularly

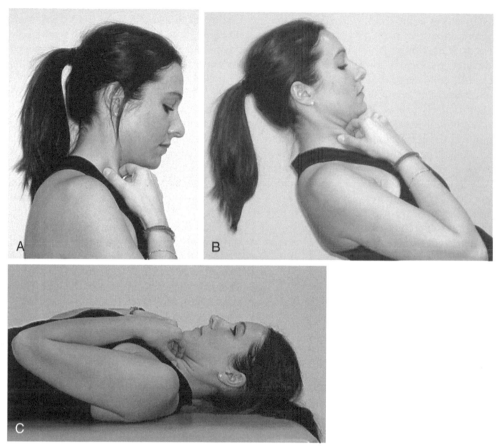

Fig. 72.2 In sitting or standing, patient slowly and subtly nods head as though saying "yes" while palpating sternocleidomastoids (SCMs) to ensure minimal activation (*A*). The starting position is sequentially reclined to increase gravity resistance (*B, C*).

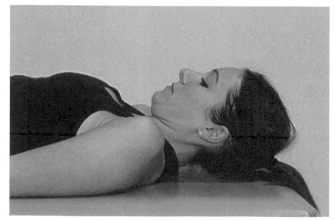

Fig. 72.3 In supine, the patient nods the head as though saying "yes" and sustains this while flexing the lower cervical spine.

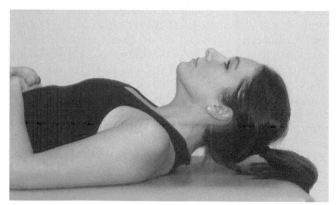

Fig. 72.4 Head protrusion (i.e., upper cervical spine extension) from inadequate deep cervical flexor (DCF) activation.

important for patients with cervicogenic headaches, who are prone to have poor DCF strength and endurance (Watson & Trott 1993, Jull et al. 1999) and weak cervical extensors (Placzek et al. 1999).

Compared to the DCF, evidence-based recommendations for facilitating selective activation of the DCE muscles are lacking. O'Leary and colleagues (2009) proposed that flexing and extending the lower cervical spine while maintaining a neutral craniocervical spine challenges the deep lower cervical extensors while minimizing activity of the more superficial extensors (Fig. 72.5). One method for training the cervical extensors is shown in Fig. 72.6. This exercise provides patient-controlled, progressive resistance to the cervical extensors. Whether this exercise selectively activates the DCE is unknown. Low-intensity isometric exercises for the cervical rotators also have been suggested to facilitate co-contraction of the neck flexors and extensors (Jull et al. 2007).

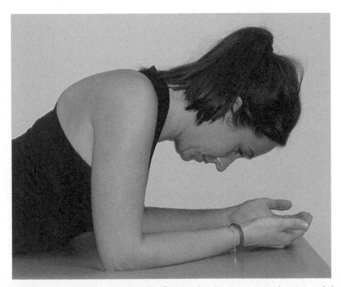

Fig. 72.5 Patient eccentrically flexes the lower cervical spine while maintaining a neutral craniocervical spine (i.e., head and upper cervical spine do not flex or extend), then slowly returns to the starting position. This exercise can be performed in four-point kneeling, prone on elbows, or sitting.

EXERCISES TO IMPROVE MUSCULAR ENDURANCE OR STRENGTH

When an acceptable foundation of muscular coordination has been established, endurance and strength conditioning may be introduced. Previous studies have shown that endurance training and/or strength training can reduce pain and disability in patients with cervical strain, degenerative or herniated discs, and chronic or recurrent neck disorders. An endurance training approach utilizing low loads should be considered initially to avoid symptom aggravation. Of note, several investigators have found endurance training and strength training to be equally efficacious in reducing chronic neck pain, at least in women (Waling et al. 2000, Ylinen et al. 2006). Exercises to increase fatigue resistance of cervical and upper thoracic muscles may be particularly useful for patients with neck pain associated with sustained postures. Patients with neck pain have been found to adopt a more forward-head posture and have difficulty maintaining an upright posture when seated (Szeto et al. 2002). Corrected posture in sitting significantly reduces cervical, upper thoracic, shoulder, and facial muscle activity compared to forward-head posture (McLean 2005).

Individuals with neck pain may also have impaired performance of the axioscapular muscles (levator scapulae, trapezius) (Falla et al. 2004b). This phenomenon may be explained by the dual influence of the axioscapular muscles on the cervical spine and the shoulder girdle (Behrsin & Maguire 1986). Weakness of the trapezius muscles in particular has been reported to coincide with neck disorders (Andersen et al. 2008). Exercises known to elicit high levels of activation in the trapezius muscles are listed in Table 72.1 (Moseley et al. 1992, Ballantyne et al. 1993, Cools et al. 2007). Performing shoulder abduction while standing with the back against a wall (Fig. 72.7) may help correct deficits in trapezius performance and structural alignment simultaneously (Sahrmann 2002). Additional exercises for the axioscapular muscles have been used in various neck rehabilitation protocols (e.g., shoulder abduction, flexion, extension, scapular retraction, wall or floor push-ups, latissimus pull-downs, arm cycling), and associated pain reduction benefits have been reported (Randløv et al. 1998, Waling et al. 2000).

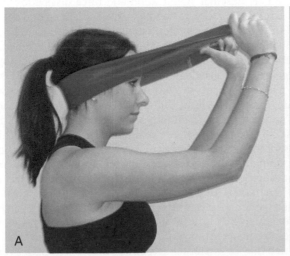
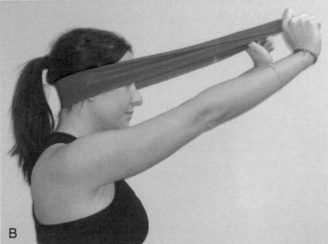

Fig. 72.6 While maintaining neutral craniocervical spine alignment in sitting or standing, the patient passes an elastic band around the cervical spine (*A*), then slowly extends the elbows to provide progressive isometric challenge to the cervical extensors (*B*).

TABLE 72.1	Exercises With High Levels of Trapezius Electromyographic Activity

EXERCISES WITH HIGH LEVELS OF UPPER TRAPEZIUS EMG ACTIVITY
Prone rowing
Military press
"T" with neutral rotation or w/ER
Shoulder shrugs
Lateral raises
Upright rows

EXERCISES WITH HIGH LEVELS OF MIDDLE TRAPEZIUS EMG ACTIVITY
Prone extension
Prone rowing
Side-lying ER
Side-lying forward flexion
"T" with neutral rotation or w/ER

EXERCISES WITH HIGH LEVELS OF LOWER TRAPEZIUS EMG ACTIVITY
Abduction
Bilateral ER at 0 degrees of abduction
Empty-can in standing
Flexion in standing/sitting or side lying
Prone ER at 90 degrees of abduction
Prone rowing
Side-lying ER
"T" with ER
"Y"

EMG, electromyography; "T", prone horizontal abduction, starting at 90 degrees of abduction; ER, external rotation; empty-can, scaption w/ glenohumeral internal rotation; "Y", prone horizontal abduction, starting ≈120 degrees of abduction.

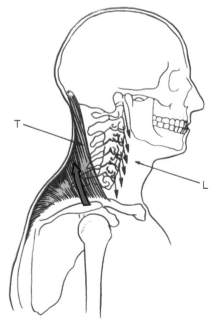

Fig. 72.8 Sagittal view of the cervical spine showing the synergistic relation between the trapezius and longus capitus and colli. The longus capitus must prevent the occiput from extending for the trapezius to use this fixed origin from which to elevate the shoulder girdle. *L*, force vectors for the longus colli and capitus muscles; *T*, trapezius. (From Porterfield JA, DeRosa C: Mechanical Neck Pain: Perspectives in Functional Anatomy. Philadelphia, WB Saunders Co., 1995. **Fig. 3-6, p. 54.)

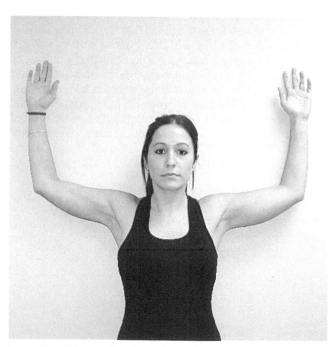

Fig. 72.7 With scapulae, buttocks, and occiput contacting the wall, the patient abducts both arms along the wall as far as possible while maintaining contact with the wall.

It is worth noting that the cervical spine and head must be fixed during upper trapezius or levator scapulae activation for meaningful force transmission to the scapulae. During arm elevation, for instance, the head and cervical spine attachments of the upper trapezius must be fixed to enable the muscle to upwardly rotate the scapula. Inadequate fixation will result in craniocervical extension. Thus, in this example, the DCF muscles must be activated to stabilize the head and cervical spine by neutralizing the extension moment of the upper trapezius (Fig. 72.8) (Porterfield & DeRosa 1995). This reinforces the importance of creating a foundation of motor control/coordination in the deeper cervical muscles before higher-resistance training exercises are introduced.

Higher-resistance training of the cervical musculature may be necessary to significantly reduce pain and disability in individuals with chronic or recurrent neck disorders or to provide adequate muscular stabilization and force dissipation in select patients (e.g., wrestlers, football players). Ylinen and colleagues (2006) reported the greatest strength gains and symptom reduction in women with chronic neck pain occurred during the first 2 months with strength training or endurance training. This suggests a concerted effort may be required for at least 8 weeks to reap the benefits of endurance or strength training on neck pain. In another study, Ylinen et al. (2007a) reported the gains in neck strength and motion achieved during a 12-month exercise program were largely maintained 3 years later. This suggests patients should be encouraged to continue endurance and/or strength training, presumably with an independent "maintenance" program, for up to 1 year to prevent symptom recurrence.

Endurance and/or strength training can be particularly effective for women (Ylinen et al. 2003, 2006, 2007a, 2007b). Women have a greater incidence of neck pain and higher prevalence of chronic neck pain than men (Hagen et al. 2000), which may be attributable to lower muscle strength (Vasavada et al. 2008). Maximal moments of the neck muscles are roughly 1.5 to 2.5 times lower in women than men, even when adjusted for body size (Jordan et al. 1999). Consequently the neck flexors and extensors are roughly 30% and 20% weaker, respectively, in healthy females than in males (Vasavada et al. 2008). This suggests that, in women, the mechanical demands on the neck muscles may be closer to their maximal moment-generating capacity. As a result, neck muscles may fatigue sooner in women, diminishing the muscles' capacity to stabilize the cervical spine.

The intensity, volume (repetitions and sets), and frequency of endurance and strengthening exercises should be "titrated" to stimulate the desired adaptive changes without undesirable side effects such as symptom aggravation or poor adherence (Haskell 1994). Patients with high irritability may tolerate only brief bouts of very-low-intensity exercise through a limited arc, whereas patients with moderate or low irritability may be tolerant of longer and more intense exercise sessions.

Evidence suggests that the majority of strength gains occur in response to the first exercise set stimulus (Pollock et al. 1993, Durall et al. 2006). Accordingly, the American College of Sports Medicine (2002) recommends one set per exercise, with each set performed to volitional exhaustion. Pollock and colleagues (1993) reported that strength gains in the cervical extensors were not statistically different between healthy subjects who performed one set of 8 to 12 repetitions or two sets of 8 to 12 repetitions twice each week for 12 weeks. Randløv et al. (1998) found no difference in pain, ADLs, strength, or endurance outcomes between groups of patients who performed one set or five sets of cervical and shoulder exercises over 3 months.

EXERCISES TO IMPROVE REPOSITIONING ACUITY, OCULOMOTOR CONTROL, OR POSTURAL STABILITY

Research has shown that people with chronic or recurrent neck disorders or neck pain secondary to cervical spine trauma are prone to deficits in head/neck repositioning acuity (Kristjansson et al. 2003, Sjolander et al. 2008), postural stability (Michaelson et al. 2003, Treleaven et al. 2005b), and oculomotor control (Treleaven et al. 2005b)—apparently as a result of impaired afferentiation from cervical mechanoreceptors (Dejong et al. 1977). A growing body of evidence supports the use of exercises to ameliorate these deficits (Sarig-Bahat 2003).

Repositioning acuity can be fostered by using a light source (e.g., focused-beam headlamp or laser pointer affixed to a headband) and a target (e.g., dart board, archery target) (Fig. 72.9). Relocation exercises, like the one demonstrated in Fig. 72.9, are commonly performed sitting but also can be done standing. Labile surfaces (e.g., ball, dome, wobble board) can be used to increase the challenge.

Oculomotor exercises, designed to improve eye/head coupling and gaze stability, can be progressed from eye movements with the head stationary to trunk and/or head movements with visual fixation on a target. These exercises can be made more challenging by increasing the speed and range of eye, head, or trunk movements or by altering backgrounds and visual targets. Exercises to improve oculomotor control (Table 72.2) have been shown to reduce dizziness and pain and to improve postural control, cervical ROM, and function (Revel et al. 1994, Taimela et al. 2000).

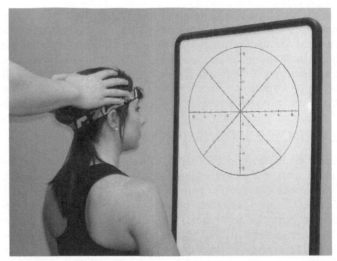

Fig. 72.9 Starting with eyes open, the patient's head/neck is moved passively until the light is aimed at a designated focal point on the target (e.g., bulls-eye). Next, with eyes closed or covered, the patient's head is passively moved in multiple directions to disorient him or her (as for "Pin the Tail on the Donkey"). Following this, the patient actively repositions the head/neck in an effort to aim the light source at the designated focal point again. While holding this position, the patient opens or uncovers his or her eyes to assess repositioning accuracy.

TABLE 72.2	Exercises to Improve Oculomotor Control

"Skywriting" or tracing patterns on wall with eyes with head stationary
Rotate eyes and head to same side, in both left and right directions.
Move eyes to target followed by head with eyes remaining focused on the target.
Move eyes then head to look between two targets positioned horizontally or vertically.
Maintain fixed gaze on target while weight shifting or rotating torso (passively or actively).
Maintain fixed gaze on target while head is passively or actively rotated.
Quickly move head and/or eyes, then focus on designated location on target.
Move eyes and head in opposite directions.

TABLE 72.3	Exercises to Improve Postural Stability

Seated weight shifting on different surfaces (stool, dome, wobble board, ball)
Balancing on floor or labile surface (pillow, foam, dome, trampoline, wobble board) with different stances (preferred, narrow, tandem, single leg)
Standing weight shifting on various surfaces
Moving upper extremities in different patterns while balancing
Playing "catch" while balancing
Walking while rotating or flexing/extending head
Walking while balancing foam pad or pillow on vertex of head
Performing oculomotor or repositioning exercises while balancing

Activities intended to improve postural stability are listed in Table 72.3. Postural stability exercises are often progressed from stable to labile surfaces and from bilateral to unilateral stances. These exercises are not unique to cervical spine treatment, and other techniques for challenging postural stability can be incorporated. Taimela et al. (2000) reported that patients with chronic neck pain who received eye fixation exercises, seated wobble board training, exercises to improve cervical muscle endurance and coordination, along with relaxation training and behavioral support had greater reductions in neck symptoms, improvements in general health, and improvements in their ability to work than patients who were educated on neck care or instructed in a traditional cervical spine home exercise program.

EXERCISES TO IMPROVE MOBILITY

Some evidence supports the use of self-stretching exercises to relieve pain, at least in the short term, in patients with neck pain. Ylinen et al. (2007b) compared the effectiveness of twice-weekly manual therapy (deep muscle massage, stretching, and joint-specific mobilization techniques) with a stretching regimen (lateral flexion, ipsilateral flexion plus rotation, flexion—each held 30 seconds and repeated three times plus neck retraction performed five times for 3 to 5 seconds) performed five times a week in patients with nonspecific chronic neck pain. Stretching and manual therapy were found to be equally effective in abolishing pain at the 4- and 12-week follow-ups. Manual therapy was slightly more effective in decreasing disability and neck stiffness compared with stretching, but the clinical difference was minimal.

Childs and colleagues (2008) suggested that flexibility exercises should be considered for the anterior/medial/posterior scalenes, upper trapezius, levator scapulae, pectoralis minor, and pectoralis major. Stretching of the SCF muscles may be a necessary emphasis, especially the anterior scalene and SCM (Fig. 72.10), which promote a forward-head posture when shortened. Addressing length impairments in other muscles may be beneficial for certain patients. For instance, patients with neck pain associated with an increased thoracic kyphosis may benefit from pectoralis minor stretching and/or thoracic extension self-mobilization using a chair back or foam roller to create a fulcrum (Fig. 72.11).

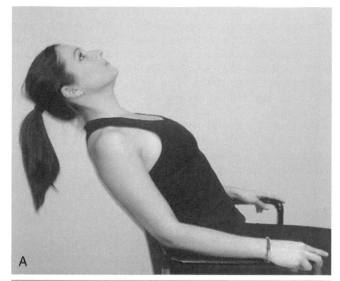

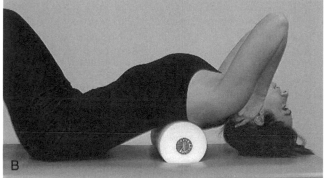

Fig. 72.11 Thoracic spine extension self-mobilization using a chair back (A) or a foam roller (B) to create a movement fulcrum.

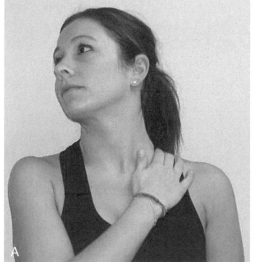
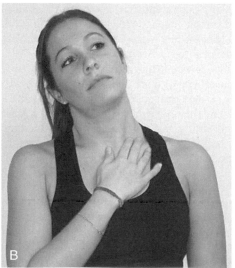

Fig. 72.10 To stretch the anterior and middle scalene, the ipsilateral first rib is firmly stabilized, then the head/neck is extended and laterally flexed (A). To stretch the sternocleidomastoid (SCM), the clavicle is stabilized, then the head/neck is extended, laterally flexed, and contralaterally rotated, and the upper cervical spine is flexed (as if nodding "yes") (B).

Patients lacking cervical rotation may benefit from active or active-assisted rotation on a partially inflated beach ball (Fig. 72.12). To facilitate rotation, a nylon or cotton strap can be used to impart an anteriorly directed force on the contralateral articular process of the hypomobile cervical segment as the patient actively rotates. This facilitated rotation exercise (performed sitting without a beach ball) was reported to be effective in reducing cervicogenic headache symptoms by 50% within 4 weeks in patients who had a loss of rotation in full flexion of 10 degrees or more (Hall et al. 2007).

A strap, pillow case, or towel can also be used to create a fulcrum for extension below a hypomobile cervical segment (Fig. 72.13, A). Alternatively, patients can be educated to use their index and/or middle fingers to create a dynamic, accommodating fulcrum, thereby "biasing" the extension movement to the restricted motion segment (Fig. 72.13, B).

Nerve mobilization techniques may be beneficial for patients with neck and arm pain to facilitate improved nervous tissue gliding (Murphy et al. 2006). Coppieters et al. (2009) reported that nerve excursion was greater with a gliding technique (alternate ends of nerve are concurrently tensed and slacked) than with a tensioning technique. Readers are encouraged to consult additional sources for nerve mobilization techniques.

Patients with radicular or referred symptoms may also benefit from directionally specific exercises. McKenzie (2009) advocated performing repeated movements (with concurrent manual procedures as needed) in directions that promote distal-to-proximal symptom migration ("centralization"). At the time of this writing there were no published clinical trials using specific exercise movements to promote symptom centralization exclusively in patients with cervical radiculopathy, so the efficacy of centralization procedures for this particular subgroup of patients is unknown. However, it is evident that patients with cervical radiculopathy benefit from a multimodal treatment approach (Costello 2008). Kjellman and Oberg (2002) reported that the McKenzie method was no more effective than general exercise or low-intensity ultrasound in combination with education in reducing disability in patients with nonspecific neck pain.

A popular exercise in the McKenzie approach, cervical retraction (Fig. 72.14), can be used to increase flexion ROM in the upper cervical segments (Ordway et al. 1999), reduce anterior shearing of the lower cervical segments, and train the DCFs and cervical extensors in synchrony (Mayoux-Benhamou et al. 1994). This may be particularly important for patients with a more forward-head posture. As previously described, a strap or the index and middle fingers can be used to focalize the lower cervical extension that occurs during retraction.

The heterogeneous, multifactorial nature of neck pain makes it difficult to develop "one-size-fits-all" exercise programs. Clinicians should select exercises according to identified deficits, functional limitations, and the patient's irritability level. Comprehensive exercise programs for patients with neck pain should include exercises to improve aerobic conditioning and performance of the trunk/torso muscles (See Rehabilitation Protocol 72.1).

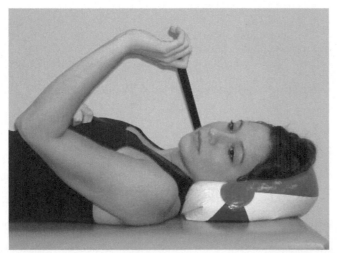

Fig. 72.12 Facilitated head/neck rotation using a partially inflated beach ball and/or a strap.

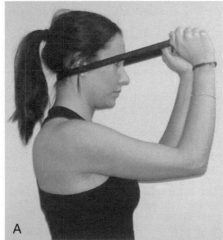 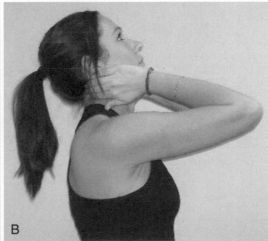

Fig. 72.13 Cervical extension self-mobilization using a strap (A) or the index and/or middle fingers (B) to create a dynamic, accommodating movement fulcrum.

REHABILITATION PROTOCOL 72.1 ● Sample Therapeutic Exercise Program for Patient With Nonspecific Neck Pain

Phase 1

- **Status:** High irritability; nearly constant pain that limits activities of daily living (ADLs)
- Emphasis: Slow, controlled, minimally painful exercises to improve muscle coordination and proprioception
- Chin nods in sitting (phase 1 of deep cervical flexor progression) or using pressure device
- Light targeting (or other target practice)
- Walking while balancing foam pad on head
- Weight shifting or rotating torso on stool or therapy ball with fixed gaze
- Side-lying shoulder external rotation and/or prone shoulder extension
- Repeated movement(s) in direction of symptom centralization (if indicated)
- Daily walking for 10 to 20 minutes

Phase 2

- **Status:** Low to moderate irritability; pain with increased activity
- **Emphasis:** Muscular endurance
- Four-way neck isometrics with low-resistance elastic band/tubing
- Isometric retraction with low-resistance elastic band/tubing (see Fig. 72.8)
- Prone horizontal shoulder abduction starting at 90 degrees of abduction ("T"), with shoulder external rotation

- Bilateral shoulder external rotation at 0 degrees abduction with low to moderate resistance elastic band/tubing
- Shoulder abduction standing with back against wall (aka wall slide)
- Side-lying shoulder flexion
- Progress proprioceptive exercises
- Sternocleidomastoid, anterior scalene, pec minor stretching
- Thoracic spine extension self-mobilization using foam roller
- Low to moderate intensity aerobic exercise for 20+ minutes

Phase 3

- **Status:** Very low or no irritability; very little or no pain with activity
- **Emphasis:** Muscle strengthening
- Shoulder flexion with contralateral leg extension in quadruped (aka Bird dog or Pointer exercise)
- Four-way isometrics with moderate to heavy resistance elastic band/tubing
- Isometric retraction with moderate to heavy resistance elastic band/tubing (see Fig. 72.8)
- I, Y, Ts with dumbbells
- Chest press, rows, shoulder raises
- Progress proprioceptive exercises as needed (PRN)
- Continue stretching and thoracic spine extension self-mobilization PRN
- Moderate to high intensity aerobic exercise for 20+ minutes

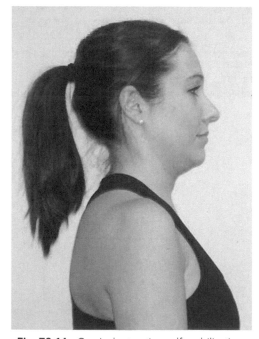

Fig. 72.14 Cervical retraction self mobilization.

REFERENCES

A complete reference list is available at https://expertconsult .inkling.com/.

FURTHER READING

Berg HE, Berggren G, Tesch PA. Dynamic neck strength training effect on pain and function. *Arch Phys Med Rehabil.* 1994;75:661–665.

Bexander CS, Mellor R, Hodges PW. Effect of gaze direction on neck muscle activity during cervical rotation. *Exp Brain Res.* 2005;167:422–432.

Bovim G, Schrader H, Sand T. Neck pain in the general population. *Spine.* 1994;19(12):1307–1309.

Clare H, Adams R, Maher CG. A systematic review of the efficacy of McKenzie therapy for spinal pain. *Aust J Physiother.* 2004;50:209–216.

Cote P, Cassidy J, Carroll L. The Saskatchewan health and back pain survey. The prevalence of neck pain and related disability in Saskatchewan adults. *Spine.* 1998;23:1689–1698.

Ekstrom RA, Donatelli RA, Soderberg GL. Surface electromyographic analysis of exercises for the trapezius and serratus anterior muscles. *J Orthop Sports Phys Ther.* 2003;33:247–258.

Galea V, Teo A, MacDermid JC. Performance of patients with mechanical neck disorders on a reach and grasp task: neural strategies. *Orthopaedic Division Review.* 2006;35.

Highland TR, Dreisinger TE, Vie LL, et al. Changes in isometric strength and range of motion of the isolated cervical spine after eight weeks of clinical rehabilitation. *Spine.* 1992;17:S77–S82.

Jull G. Deep cervical flexor muscle dysfunction in whiplash. *J Musculoskel Pain.* 2000;8:143–154.

Jull G, Trott P, Potter H, et al. A randomized controlled trial of exercise and manipulative therapy for cervicogenic headache. *Spine.* 2002;27(17):1835–1843.

Jull G, Amiri M, Bullock-Saxton J, et al. Cervical musculoskeletal impairment in frequent intermittent headache. Part 1: subjects with single headaches. *Cephalalgia.* 2007;27:793–802.

Levoska S, Keinanen-Kiukaanniemi S. Active or passive physiotherapy for occupational cervicobrachial disorders? A comparison of two treatment methods with a 1-year follow-up. *Arch Phys Med Rehabil.* 1993;74:425–430.

Makela M, Heliovaara M, Sievers K, et al. Prevalence, determinants, and consequences of chronic neck pain in Finland. *Am J Epidemiol.* 1991;134:1356–1367.

Mayoux-Benhamou MA, Revel M, Vallee C. Selective electromyography of dorsal neck muscles in humans. *Exp Brain Res.* 1997;113:353–360.

McCabe RA. Surface electromyographic analysis of the lower trapezius muscle during exercises performed below ninety degrees of shoulder elevation in healthy subjects. *N Am J Sports Phys Ther.* 2007;2:34–43.

McDonnell MK, Sahrmann SA, Van Dillen L. A specific exercise program and modification of postural alignment for treatment of cervicogenic headache: a case report. *J Orthop Sports Phys Ther.* 2005;35(1):3–15.

Nederhand MJ, IJzerman MJ, Hermens HJ, et al. Cervical muscle dysfunction in the chronic whiplash associated disorder grade II (WAD-II). *Spine.* 2000;25:1938–1943.

Picavet HSJ, Schouten JSAG. Musculoskeletal pain in the Netherlands: prevalences, consequences and risk groups, the DMC3-study. *Pain.* 2003;102:167–178.

Staudte HW, Duhr N. Age- and sex-dependent force related function of the cervical spine. *Eur Spine J.* 1994;3:155–161.

Teo A, Galea V, MacDermid JC, et al. Performance of patients with mechanical neck disorders on a reach and grasp task: coordination dynamics. *Ortho Div Rev.* 2006;35.

Tjell C, Rosenthall U. Smooth pursuit neck torsion test: a specific test for cervical dizziness. *Am J Otol.* 1998;19:76–81.

Treleaven J, Jull G, LowChoy N. The relationship of cervical joint position error to balance and eye movement disturbances in persistent whiplash. *Man Ther.* 2006;11:99–106.

Vasavada AN, Li S, Delp SL. Three-dimensional isometric strength of neck muscles in humans. *Spine.* 2001;26:1904–1909.

Ylinen J, Ruuska J. Clinical use of neck isometric strength measurement in rehabilitation. *Arch Phys Med Rehabil.* 1994;75:465–469.

Treatment-Based Classification of Low Back Pain

Michael P. Reiman, PT, DPT, OCS, SCS, ATC, FAAOMPT, CSCS

Low back pain (LBP) is the most prevalent of all musculoskeletal conditions and one of the primary reasons an individual visits a primary care physician (Woolf and Pfleger 2003). LBP affects nearly everyone some time in his or her lifetime and about 4% to 33% of the population at any given point (Woolf and Pfleger 2003).

BACKGROUND

Despite extensive research into the assessment and treatment of LBP, it remains a twentieth-century health care enigma (Waddell 1996). In the 1990s much of the evidence for efficacious treatment remained elusive (van Tulder et al. 1997). The reason for some treatments failing to demonstrate efficacy in randomized, controlled trials may be a false assumption that sufferers of LBP are a homogeneous group (Delitto et al. 1995). The importance of identifying homogeneous subgroups in randomized, controlled trials has been emphasized to avoid problems with sample heterogeneity (Binkley et al. 1993, Spratt et al. 1993, Delitto et al. 1995, Fritz and George 2000, Bendebba et al. 2000). The process of developing criteria for the identification of homogeneous subgroups within the LBP population is classification. Different potential types of classification schemes might include the following:

- Signs and symptoms: LBP classified according to patient presentation of specific signs and symptoms
- Pathoanatomic: LBP classified according to lumbar structure pathology
- Psychological: LBP classified according to psychological criteria
- Social: LBP classified according to social criteria

Although there are potentially other types of classification schemes, and each of those listed has relevance, the literature currently supports the classification scheme based on signs and symptoms. Signs and symptom classification and the appropriate subsequent treatment have been termed treatment-based classification (TBC).

HISTORY

TBC is based on the premise that subgroups of patients with LBP can be identified from key history and clinical examination findings (Delitto et al. 1995). Delitto et al. (1995) also hypothesized that each subgroup would respond favorably to a specific intervention but only when applied to a matched subgroup's clinical presentation. Seven intervention classification groups were originally described in TBC; however, recent investigations have collapsed the seven groups to four: manipulation, specific exercise (flexion, extension, and lateral shift patterns), stabilization, and traction (Table 73.1).

The clusters of examination findings and matched interventions used in the TBC approach were principally derived from expert opinion, with little evidence. Proper classification of patients into the appropriate category has proved reliable (Fritz and George 2000, Heiss et al. 2004, Fritz et al. 2006). However, it is also recognized that refinement is needed, given only moderate inter-rater reliability for multiple categories and also because significant numbers of patients met criteria for either multiple or no (Henry 2012, Stanton 2011) categories. The manipulation clinical prediction rule (see Table 73.1) has the best supportive evidence because it has been validated (Childs et al. 2004). Perhaps most important to consider regarding TBC is whether overall outcomes are improved when it is used in comparison to an alternative approach. Fritz et al. (2003) and Brennan et al. (2006) both provided support for the use of a TBC approach and matched intervention for patients with LBP.

TABLE 73.1	Treatment-Based Classification and Matched Treatment in Patients With Acute Low Back Pain	
Classification	**Key History and Clinical Findings**	**Matched Intervention**
Manipulation	Clinical prediction rule variables (Flynn et al. 2002) Variables: 1. Duration of symptoms <16 days 2. FABQ work subscale <19 3. At least one hip with a >35 degrees of internal rotation range of motion 4. Hypomobility of at least one segment in the lumbar spine 5. No symptoms distal to knee	Manipulation of the lumbopelvic region with the technique utilized by Flynn et al. 2002 or Cleland et al. 2006 (see Figs. 73.1 and 73.2)

TABLE 73.1	Treatment-Based Classification and Matched Treatment in Patients With Acute Low Back Pain—cont'd	
Classification	**Key History and Clinical Findings**	**Matched Intervention**
Specific Exercise 1. Extension 2. Flexion 3. Lateral Shift	1. Symptoms centralize with extension and peripheralize with flexion of lumbar spine Symptoms often distal to buttock Postural and directional preference for extension 2. Symptoms improve with flexion and worsen with extension of lumbar spine Postural and directional preference for flexion Typically older in age (>50 years) Imaging evidence of lumbar spinal stenosis 3. Visible frontal plane deformity, shoulders relative to pelvis Directional preference for lateral translation movements of pelvis	1. Mobilization and exercise to promote extension; avoidance of flexion of lumbar spine 2. Mobilization or manipulation of the lumbar spine to promote flexion; avoidance of extension of lumbar spine Body-weight–supported treadmill ambulation 3. Exercises (either by clinician or patient him or herself) to correct lateral shift Mechanical or autotraction
Stabilization	Clinical prediction rule variables (Hicks et al. 2005) Variables (in order of importance): 1. Age <40 years 2. Average straight-leg raise >91 degrees 3. Positive prone instability test (see Figs. 74.1 and 74.2) 4. Aberrant movement present Postpartum patients: 1. Positive posterior pelvic pain provocation test (see Fig. 74.3) 2. Positive active straight-leg raise test Positive modified Trendelenburg test	Trunk stabilization training Promotion of local stabilizing muscle groups (transverse abdominis, multifidus, etc.) Strength training of larger, global muscle groups (erector spinae, oblique abdominals, etc.) Progression of local and global muscle group training in functional positions
Traction	1. No movement (specifically neither flexion, extension, or lateral shift correction) centralizes symptoms 2. Signs and symptoms suggestive of nerve root compression	Mechanical or autotraction

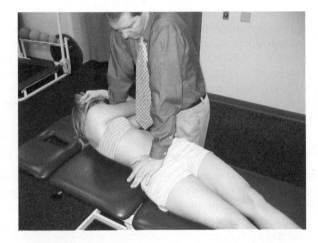

Fig. 73.1 Supine SI regional manipulation. Clinician side bends patient to the involved side (right in this case) and then rotates patient's spine in contralateral direction (left in this case) until slack is taken up. Thrust to the right side is performed in direction as shown.

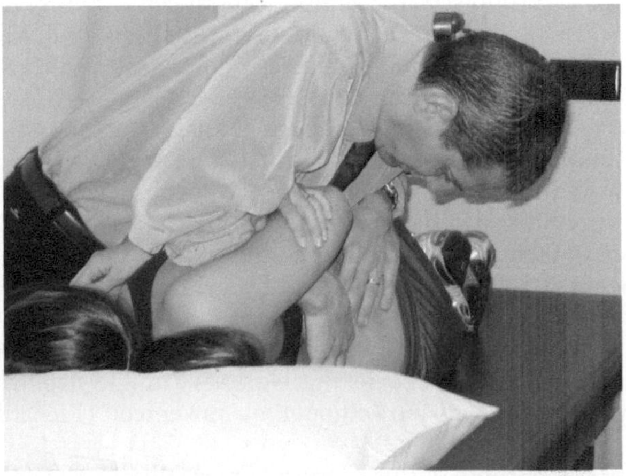

Fig. 73.2 Side-lying lumbar spine gapping manipulation. Clinician locks the segment via hip flexion and upper trunk rotation to the involved segment as shown. Clinician maintains this setup and then log rolls the patient to him as a unit. Clinician's cranial hand blocks the cranial spinous process of the segment. Using the left forearm in this case the clinician provides a thrust in an anterior direction, gapping the right facet joint of the involved segment.

REFERENCES

A complete reference list is available at https://expertconsult.inkling.com/.

FURTHER READING

George SZ, Delitto A. Clinical examination variables discriminate among treatment-based classification groups: a study of construct validity in patients with acute low back pain. *Phys Ther*. 2005;85(4):306–314.

Hestbaek L, Leboeuf-Yde C, Manniche C. Low back pain: what is the long-term course? A review of studies of general patient populations. *Eur J Spine*. 2003;12(2):149–165.

Pengel LH, Herbert RD, Maher CG, et al. Acute low back pain: systematic review of its prognosis. *BMJ*. 2003;327(7410):323–327.

Core Stabilization Training

Barbara J. Hoogenboom, EdD, PT, SCS, ATC | Kyle Kiesel, PT, PhD, ATC, CSCS

The common prerequisite for participation and success in dynamic function is a strong and stable body core. Control of the spinal segments during upright posture is required not only for activities of daily living but also for balance, stability, and coordination during occupational tasks and complex or high-level sports activities (Ebenbichler et al. 2001). This stability enables an individual to transmit forces from the earth through the body's kinetic chain, resist externally applied loads and forces, and ultimately propel the body or an object using the limbs. The concept of core stabilization of the trunk and pelvis as a prerequisite for movements of the extremities was described biomechanically in 1991 (Bouisset 1991). Subsequently, core training for stabilization has become a major trend in treatment of spinal injuries and pathologies, after spinal surgery, and in training regimens for enhancement of athletic/work performance and injury prevention.

Many descriptive terms and rehabilitation programs are associated with the concept of core stability, including: abdominal bracing, lumbar stabilization, dynamic stabilization, motor control (neuromuscular) training, neutral spine control, muscular fusion, and trunk stabilization (Akuthota and Nadler 2004). The core has been conceptually described as either a box or a cylinder (Richardson et al. 1999) because of its anatomic and structural composition. The abdominals create the anterior and lateral walls, the paraspinals and gluteals form the posterior wall, and the diaphragm and pelvic floor create the top and bottom of the cylinder, respectively (Fig. 74.1). Additionally, muscles of the hip girdle reinforce and support the bottom and sides of the cylinder. Envisioning this cylindrical system helps to understand core function as that of a dynamic muscular support system, described by some authors as the powerhouse, engine, or a "muscular corset that works as a unit to stabilize the body and spine, with and without limb movement" (Richardson et al. 1999).

For the purpose of this chapter, core stabilization is defined as the muscular balance and control required about the pelvis, hips, and trunk (lumbar, thoracic, and cervical spines) to maintain functional stability of the entire human body. Static stabilization of the core is a prerequisite, but it is merely a starting point and not sufficient for all demands introduced during functional activity. Core stability must be further understood as the ability to control movement of the core that occurs during *dynamic* trunk and extremity movement tasks.

Proximal stability as a requisite for distal mobility is a commonly understood principle of human movement originally described by Knott and Voss (1968) and applied in the concepts of proprioceptive neuromuscular facilitation. Without proximal core control, athletes could not effectively use the lower extremities to propel the body during running and jumping or eccentrically control the pelvis and limbs during the loading phases of running and landing. Furthermore, during activities that require use of the upper extremities to properly support

or propel the body (e.g., gymnastics and swimming), manipulate an object (e.g., tennis racquet or golf club), or throw objects (e.g., shot put or pitching), sufficient proximal core control is essential. Simply put, the core, as a result of its position in the middle of the human kinetic chain, serves as a link that allows for energy transfer between the upper and lower extremities. According to Kibler et al. (1998):

> *Injuries or adaptations in some areas of the kinetic chain can cause problems not only locally but distally, as other distal links have to compensate for the lack of force or energy delivered through the more proximal links. This phenomenon, called* catch-up, *is both inefficient in the kinetic chain and dangerous to the distal link because it may create more load of stress than the link can safely handle.*

When the core is functioning optimally, muscles throughout the kinetic chain can also function optimally, allowing the individual to produce strong, functional movements of the extremities (Kibler et al. 1998, Andrews et al. 2004) (Table 74.1).

Even small alterations within the kinetic chain have serious repercussions on other portions of the kinetic chain and thus on skills that require efficient, coordinated utilization of segments (Kibler et al. 1998). Without proper stabilization and dynamic concentric and eccentric control of the trunk during functional tasks, the extremities or "transition zones" between the core and extremities (e.g., hip and shoulder joints) can be overstressed, resulting in injury or tissue damage.

ANATOMY

Stability of the core requires both passive (bony and ligamentous structures) and dynamic (coordinated muscular contractions) stiffness. A spine without the contributions of the muscular system is unable to bear essential compressive loads associated with normal upright activities and remain stable (McGill 2002). Anatomists have known for decades that a compressive load of as little as 2 kilograms causes buckling of the lumbar spine in the absence of muscular contractions (Morris et al. 1961). Additionally, significant microtrauma of structures within the lumbar spine can occur with as little as two degrees of segmental rotation, demonstrating the vital stabilizing function of the trunk core muscles (Gracovetsky et al. 1985, Gardner-Morse and Stokes 1998). Core stabilization is important not only for protection of the lumbar spine but also to transmit the wide variety of forces that are placed on the spine and core muscles by moving limbs.

Many authors have described classifications of local and global (Richardson et al. 1999, Punjabi et al. 1989, McGill 2002) or superficial and deep muscles, which together contribute to stability of the core. The local or intersegmental muscles are hypothesized to function primarily as stabilizers, and the global or multisegmental muscles are hypothesized to function primarily as producers of movement (Kavcic et al. 2004) (Table 74.2). Panjabi et al. (1989) suggested that global muscles may play an important role in stabilization because of their ability to efficiently produce stiffness in the entire spinal column, as compared with local muscles acting on only a few levels. The global muscle system, although important

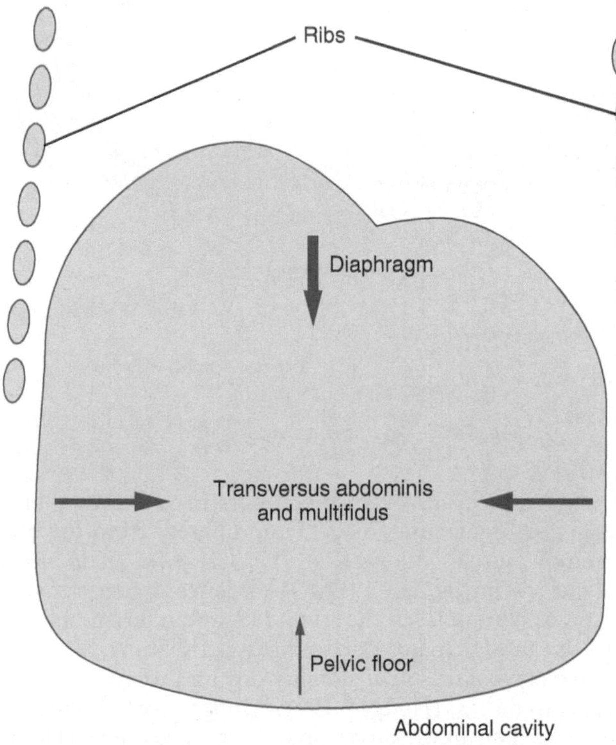

Fig. 74.1 Muscular support of the abdominal cavity.

for movement and total spinal stability, contributes primarily compressive forces to stability and is limited in its ability to control segmental shear forces (Richardson et al. 1999). Even if the global muscle system is performing adequately, the local system working insufficiently to control segmental motion may cause local instability. In fact, excessive use of global muscles in co-contraction during light functional tasks may indicate inappropriate trunk muscle control in patients with low back pain (O'Sullivan et al. 1997). Global muscles that link the trunk to the extremities (e.g., the iliacus in the lower extremity and the latissimus dorsi in the upper extremity) may actually challenge or adversely affect segmental stabilization. Segmental spinal stability must be maintained in the presence of contractions of powerful global muscles during functional activities (Richardson et al. 1999). Local and global muscles both contribute to postural segmental control and general multisegmental stabilization during static and dynamic tasks (Akuthota and Nadler 2004, Richardson et al. 1999, McGill 2002); however, debate continues over which muscles are important stabilizers. Debate also continues about how to better train the neuromuscular control system to prepare it to provide sufficient stability of the core to withstand the three-dimensional torque demands imposed upon it. Cholewicki et al. (1996, 2002) reported on the basis of biomechanical analyses that no single local or global muscle owns a dominant responsibility for lumbar spine stability. Stability and movement likely depend on appropriate length and excursion, facilitated co-contractions, and coordinated muscular activity (both concentric and eccentric) in *all* core muscles. The emergent view by many prominent authors is that continual, low-level, local muscle contractions, in addition to neuromuscular coordination and motor control, are requisite for all functional activities (Richardson et al. 1999, McGill 2002). Additionally, the timing of activation and ability to demonstrate volitional control of local muscles are important precursors to higher

TABLE 74.1	Core Demands, Kinetic Chain Relationships, and Outcomes of Example Tasks		
Functional Activity	**Core Demands**	**Kinetic Chain Relationships**	**Outcome**
Baseball or softball pitch	Rotational and flexion/extension stability. Acceleration and deceleration of trunk	Transmission of forces from ground to LEs through trunk to UE to ball	Velocity, location, rotation of pitched ball Delivery of various types of pitches (fastball, sinker/drop, rise, breaking ball, etc.)
Gymnastics: Vault event	Rotational and flexion/extension stability. Power with punch from horse	Transmission of forces from horse to UEs through trunk to propel body in airborne positions	Conversion of horizontal energy to vertical; speed, position, and trajectory of body through space
Tennis serve	Rotational and flexion/extension stability. Acceleration and deceleration of trunk	Transmission of forces from ground to LEs through trunk to UE through racquet to ball	Velocity, location, spin of served ball (80–120 mph). Delivery of various types of serves
Swimming: Butterfly stroke	Flexion/extension stability	Transmission of forces from UEs to trunk to LEs to team with butterfly kick	Efficient propulsion of body through water. Avoid excess trunk flexion and extension
Golf swing (drive), but could be applied to all swinging strokes	Extreme rotation and extension range of motion at spine and hips. Acceleration and deceleration of trunk	Transmission of forces from ground to LEs, through trunk to UEs to club to ball	Club head acceleration, speed, accuracy at impact, and velocity, distance the ball travels
Lifting a heavy object	Rotational and flexion/extension stability. Stability of core for UEs and LEs to provide power for lift	Transmission of forces from ground to LEs through trunk to UE to object Stability of core while directing and placing object	Successful lift of object with protection of the trunk from excessive sagittal plane motion (flexion), shear and rotational forces

LE, lower extremity; UE, upper extremity.

TABLE 74.2	Local and Global Muscles of the Core	
Local Muscles (Postural, Tonic, Segmental/Joint Stabilizers)	**Global Muscles (Dynamic, Phasic, Torque Producing)**	
Intertransversarii and interspinales (function primarily as proprioceptive organs)	Rectus abdominis	
Multifidi	External oblique	
Transversus abdominis	Internal oblique (anterior fibers)	
Quadratus lumborum (medial portion)	Longissimus (thoracic portion)	
Diaphragm	Iliocostalis (thoracic portion)	
Internal oblique (posterior fibers)	Quadratus lumborum (lateral portion)	
Iliocostalis and longissimus (lumbar portions)	Latissimus dorsi	
Psoas major (posterior portion, when working on the spine, not as a hip flexor)	Iliacus	
	Psoas major (anterior portion, when working as a hip flexor)	
Hip rotators*	Hip adductors	
Hip abductors*	Hip extensors	
	Quadriceps	
	Hamstrings	
	Hip rotators*	
	Hip abductors*	

*Disagreement exists about whether these are local or global.
(Adapted from Richardson, Panjabi, McGill.)

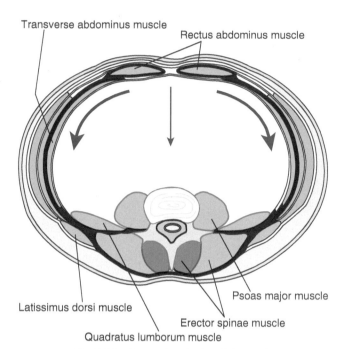

Fig. 74.2   Anatomic cylinder of the trunk.

level core strengthening. (Hodges 2003, Macedo et al. 2009, Tsao and Hodges 2008).

Although as a society we are fixated on the rectus abdominis and its classic "six-pack" appearance, the importance of the local muscles diminishes the functional importance of this global muscle. The rectus abdominis is a trunk flexor with a large movement capacity of the trunk that often substitutes for contractions of the important local muscles. Overuse of the rectus abdominis provides a substantial flexion moment, and associated flexion of the spine, rather than stabilization. Many fitness programs incorrectly overemphasize the training of the rectus abdominis (Akuthota and Nadler 2004) and inappropriately induce shear forces by the flexion moments produced by its contraction. The shear forces induced by the contraction of the rectus abdominis are counterproductive to the goal of segmental and total core control, which is the primary goal of core strengthening or neuromuscular training. Furthermore, there are associated concerns of repeated segmental flexion of the lumbar spine and the potential for increased posterior-directed disc pressure.

Contemporary research has illuminated the roles of two important local muscle groups: the transversus abdominis (TA) (Cresswell et al. 1994, Hodges 1999) and the multifidus (Wilke et al. 1995, Hides et al. 1994). The TA, the deepest of the abdominal muscles, uses its horizontal fiber alignment and attachment to the thoracolumbar fascia to increase intraabdominal pressure (IAP), thereby making the core cylinder more stable. Although increased IAP had been associated with the control of spinal flexion forces and a decrease in load on the extensor muscles (Thomson 1988), it is probable that the TA is most important in its ability to assist in intersegmental control (Richardson et al. 1999). The TA offers "hooplike" cylindrical stresses to enhance segmental stiffness to limit both translational and rotational movement of the spine (Ebenbichler 2001, McGill and Brown 1987). Bilateral contraction of the TA performs the movement of "drawing in of the abdominal wall" (Richardson et al. 1999) and does not produce spinal movement. The TA is active throughout the movements of

both trunk flexion and extension, suggesting a unique stabilizing role during dynamic movement, different from the other abdominal muscles (Cresswell 1993, Cresswell et al. 1994). Finally, electromyographic (EMG) evidence suggests that the more internal muscles of the trunk (TA and internal obliques) behave in an anticipatory or feedforward manner to provide proactive control of spinal stability during movements of the upper extremities (Hodges 1997, Hodges and Richardson 1997), regardless of the direction of limb movements (Hodges and Richardson 1997). The results of Allison et al. (2008) suggest that the feedforward mechanism that affects the TA originally described by Hodges and Richardson may exhibit asymmetry and directional selectivity based on task performance. As methods to examine the function of the core muscles improve, the functional specificity of training will likely become more differentiated.

Among the posterior spinal muscles, the multifidus is important for its contribution to control of the neutral or stable position of the spine (Punjabi et al. 1989, Wilke et al. 1995). As a result of its unique anatomic structure and segmental innervation, the multifidus is important for providing segmental stiffness, proprioceptive input to the central nervous system, and motion control. The tonically active multifidus is reported to offer two-thirds of the increase in segmental stiffness at the L4–L5 segment when contracted (Wilke et al. 1995). Dysfunction of the multifidus that occurs after injury to the spine (Hides et al. 1994) makes this muscle group an important focus for rehabilitation (Macdonald et al. 2006). Clinical and preliminary experimental evidence suggests that a biomechanically beneficial co-contraction of the TA and multifidi occurs during specific exercises (Richardson et al. 1999) (Fig. 74.2). This specific and specialized relationship provides increased stiffness within spinal structures, offering critical tonic cylindric stabilization for the core, and is the basis for rehabilitation.

The importance of the top and bottom of the core, the diaphragm, and the pelvic floor, respectively, must not be underestimated. The diaphragm, like the TA, functions in anticipatory

TABLE 74.3	Muscle Group Categories
Specific Muscle Group	**Primary Responsibility**
Transversus abdominis	Maintaining neutral lumbopelvic position by abdominal drawing/cylindrical stabilization
Ipsilateral internal and external obliques	Trunk side flexion
Contralateral internal and external obliques	Trunk rotation
Multifidus	Segmental lumbar stability
Erector spinae	Trunk extensor
Gluteus maximus	Hip extensor
Gluteus medius	Hip abductor/lateral rotator and eccentric control of pelvic alignment
Hip lateral rotators	Eccentric control of internal rotation of limb
Diaphragm	Proximal "cylinder" stabilization and intra-abdominal pressure
Pelvic floor	Distal "cylinder" stabilization and intra-abdominal pressure

postural control by firing prior to extremity musculature during the movement of shoulder flexion (Hodges et al. 1997). Also, contraction of the diaphragm occurs concurrently with activation of the TA but independent of the phase of respiration (Hodges et al. 1997). Although beyond the scope of this chapter discussion, restoring diaphragmatic breathing may be an important component of core training to consider prior to the initiation of core strengthening (Akuthota and Nadler 2004). The pelvic floor has been shown to be active during lifting tasks and to be instrumental in increased activation of the TA when voluntarily contracted (Richardson et al. 1999). Conversely, EMG activity of the pubococcygeus increased during activation of the abdominal muscles. Thus, the bottom of the cylinder, the pelvic floor, cannot be ignored during core strengthening (Table 74.3).

Reviewing and considering the anatomy of the core allows medical and allied health professionals to best understand principles of injury and rehabilitation. This sets the stage for attempting to persuade patients, athletes, coaches, and other professionals to decrease the preoccupation with the training of the rectus abdominis and other "high-profile" global muscles of the core, which may detract focus from effective functional performance and rehabilitation.

MECHANISMS OF INJURY TO THE CORE

The early portion of this chapter describes many mechanisms of injury and possible sources of pain and progressive dysfunction. Spinal injuries occur in both deconditioned and well-conditioned individuals. Injury to the trunk, abdomen, and low back is not gender specific, and males and females are injured in similar mechanisms. Cholewicki et al. (2000) suggested that a common factor for injury to athletes may be the inability to generate sufficient core stability to resist external forces imposed on the body during high-speed events. Other authors suggest deficient endurance of the trunk stabilizing musculature predisposes individuals to the negative effects of repetitive forces over time (Richardson et al. 1999), motor control deficits, and imbalances of the local (TA and multifidus) and global

musculature (rectus abdominis and erector spinae). A weak or inefficient core may result in altered functional movements, altered postures, and an increased potential for both macrotraumatic and microtraumatic injury in workers and athletes (Andrews et al. 2004).

Like the extremities, the core may be injured in macrotraumatic mechanisms such as contusions, muscle strains, and tears and during injuries such as fractures or dislocations. Subsequent to macrotraumatic injuries, development of laxity in spinal joints and ligaments may occur and contribute to segmental instability. The core can also be injured over time by repetitive microtrauma as a result of poor posture, repetitive excessive movements (e.g., hyperextension and rotation in activities such as lifting, gymnastics, and golf), improper muscle activation patterns during functional tasks, and strength imbalances. Segmental instability of the lumbar spine has been implicated as a possible cause of functional limitations, positional dysfunctions, strains, and pain. Increased or excessive motion of segments results in the loss of sensory motor contributions to stability and the ability to maintain a neutral or supported position during function.

Two examples of microtraumatic injuries that can occur in workers and athletes are spondylolysis and spondylolisthesis. The athletic population is more prone to these conditions and is more likely to be symptomatic from these injuries than nonathletes because of the extreme extension/flexion reversals in trunk posture demanded by many sports. Spondylolytic microfracture of the pars is believed to occur as a result of shear forces that occur during repetitive flexion and extension (Swedan 2001). Athletes with high rates of this type of microtraumatic injury include gymnasts (Hall and Thein Brody 1999), divers, figure skaters, swimmers who perform the butterfly stroke (Swedan 2001), and volleyball players (Hall and Thein Brody 1999). In fact, gymnasts younger than age 24 have a four times greater incidence of spondylolysis than the general female population (Swedan 2001). Spondylolytic microfractures can lead to a subsequent spondylolisthesis condition.

Microtraumatic injuries may also occur as a result of muscular imbalances, from uncontrolled shear forces acting on the spine (Swedan 2001, Hall and Thein Brody 1999), or because of a lack of synchronized muscular control and stabilization by the core musculature. Sports such as golf, diving, and softball provide potential mechanisms for microtraumatic injury to the core induced in a similar manner. Rather than being a result of straight plane flexion and extension, these injuries are related to extreme rotation, often in combination with extension. Careful assessment of motor strategies and subsequent corrective movement training by the therapists may be a key to preventing many microtraumatic injuries in a wide variety of athletes and workers.

Findings from diagnostic ultrasound measurements taken on patients with acute LBP indicate that rapid multifidus atrophy, as measured by cross-sectional area, occurs on the same side as the low back pain, even as quickly as within 24 hours after injury (Hides et al. 1994). This effect is likely a result of muscular inhibition. After a first episode of acute low back pain, recovery of multifidus function and cross-sectional area does not occur without specific, targeted intervention (Hides et al. 1996). In a study of male high-performance rowing athletes, multifidus muscle dysfunction was present *despite* their rigorous training (Roy et al. 1990). In this same study, the fatigue rates of the multifidus were used to successfully discriminate

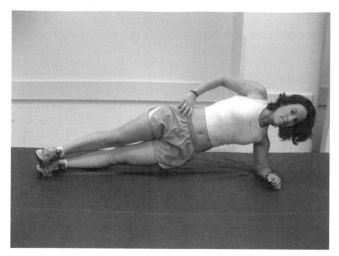

Fig. 74.3 Side bridge/plank.

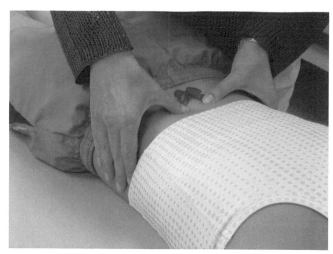

Fig. 74.4 Palpation test for multifidus muscular activation. Palpation position as shown. An inability to properly activate the segmental multifidus is indicated by palpating little or no muscle tension developing under the fingers after the verbal command. A rapid and superficial (nonsustained) development of tension is also unsatisfactory.

between controls and subjects with low back pain. Fortunately, regular training with specific, localized muscular contractions of the core can facilitate recovery of the multifidus muscle (Roy et al. 1990). Understanding the support function of the local muscles is relevant to treatment of a wide variety of conditions including generalized low back pain, disc derangement, facet joint irritation and dysfunctions, sacroiliac dysfunction, incontinence, and respiratory disorders (Richardson et al. 1999).

REHABILITATION: ASSESSMENT AND INTERVENTION

Examination

The functions of the deep, local muscles of the core are best objectively examined using fine-wire EMG (Gardner-Morse and Stokes 1998, Stokes et al. 2003) or real-time ultrasound (Hodges 2003, Kiesel 2007a, Koppenhaver et al. 2009, Teyhen 2006) and magnetic resonance imaging (MRI) (Kiesel 2007a). The use of real-time ultrasound by the rehabilitation professional has been designated as rehabilitative ultrasound imaging (RUSI) (Teyhen 2006).

RUSI can be used for various aspects of spinal rehabilitation including assessment of muscle activation by the measurement of thickness change from rest to activation and muscle girth. Thickness-change deficits have been identified in both the TA and lumbar multifidus muscles in patients with LBP. Additionally, research has been conducted on the use of RUSI for biofeedback during motor control training (Kiesel 2007a, Henry and Westervelt 2005, Teyhen et al. 2005, Frantz Pressler et al. 2006).

Although RUSI is not widely used in the clinical setting, its use has been growing steadily and perhaps clinical practice of the future will allow for increased use of this tool for both examination and intervention (Teyhen 2007, Teyhen et al. 2007).

Simple, reliable, and objective clinical tests for dynamic motor control of the core are not readily available. Clinically, therapists can use manual muscle tests that examine isometric holding of muscles (e.g., Kendall tests for upper and lower abdominals or Sahrmann tests for lower abdominals), positional holding tests (plank or side plank) (Fig. 74.3) for endurance in isometric positions, and pressure biofeedback to assess the ability of a patient to hold the core stable during

dynamic tasks. Sahrmann (2002) subscribes to the premise of activating the lower abdominal group (TA and external obliques) to provide proper lumbopelvic control while adding dynamic LE movements of progressive levels of difficulty. She originally described a functional grading system on a 0 to 5 scale, which was later expanded to include several descriptors of lower-level function (e.g., levels 0.3 to 0.5). This system provides a construct to assist the therapist in determining the appropriate starting point for the lower abdominal exercise progression. The patient is given the command to "pull the belly button toward the spine," which recruits the TA (Goldman 1987). The assessment grades indicate that the patient is able to successfully maintain appropriate lumbopelvic control with the specific LE perturbation. Sahrmann's lower abdominal scale is shown in Table 74.3 (Sahrmann 2002), and it should be noted that it does not correlate with the Kendall and McCreary (1983) grading system of 1 to 5 as used in manual muscle testing.

A subjective clinical test for the multifidus involves the activation of the multifidus at various segments under the palpating fingers of a therapist (Richardson et al. 1999). The **multifidus activation test** is performed with the patient prone using the command, "Gently swell out your muscles under my fingers without using your spine or pelvis. Hold the contraction while breathing normally" (Richardson et al. 1999). This test includes both side-to-side and multiple-level comparisons to assess for segmental activation or inhibition of the lumbar multifidi (Fig. 74.4).

Richardson et al. (1999) described the **abdominal drawing in** test for function of the deep abdominal muscles and subsequently developed the air-filled pressure biofeedback unit in an attempt to quantify this task. This clinical test of deep muscle cocontraction is performed in prone, by performing the drawing in task while concurrently using the pressure biofeedback device (Richardson et al. 1999). Intra- and inter-rater reliability for the use of pressure biofeedback for assessing lumbopelvic stability have been shown to be good to excellent (ICC = 0.6–0.95) and fair to excellent (ICC = 0.4–0.86), respectively (Fig. 74.5).

In addition to the basic performance of this task, the physical therapist must also monitor the patient for the ability to

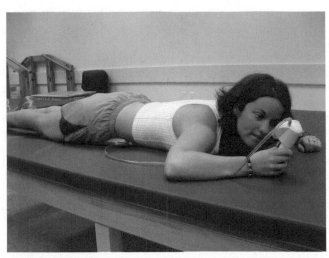

Fig. 74.5 Prone abdominal drawing in test using air-filled pressure biofeedback (The Stabilizer Pressure Biofeedback, manufactured by Chattanooga Pacific, Queensland, Australia). Device is centered with distal edge of the pad in line with the ASISs, inflated to 70 mm Hg. Motor contraction test should attempt to draw the abdomen off the pad and hold for 10 seconds. Note the pressure change. A successful test reduces the pressure by 6 to 10 mm Hg. A drop of less than 2 mm Hg, no change in pressure, or an increase in pressure is considered a poor result.

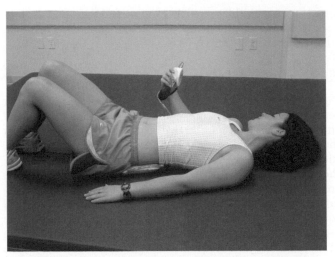

Fig. 74.6 Hook-lying abdominal drawing in test with air-filled pressure biofeedback; supine biofeedback with varied levels of leg loading. Test is performed by inflating the cuff to approximately 40 mm Hg and positioning the patient in hook-lying position. Begin with low-load tests of short lever leg (bent knee) loading and progress difficulty, using larger load tests (unsupported and extended legs).

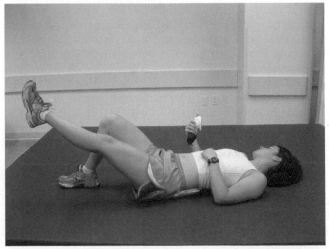

Fig. 74.7 Hook-lying abdominal drawing in test with extremity movement using air-filled pressure biofeedback. The patient is asked to pre-contract the transversus abdominis with the drawing in maneuver, then hold the pressure reading steady during various maneuvers including the single-leg slide with contralateral support, single-leg slide without contralateral support, and unsupported leg slide with contralateral support.

hold a tonic, smooth contraction of the TA without resorting to the use of the global muscles. The prone position is useful because it minimizes the ability of the patient to use the rectus abdominis for the contraction. In a single-blind study of subjects with and without back pain, it was determined that only 10% of patients with a history of LBP could perform the TA test using The Stabilizer (Chatanooga Rehabilitation Products, Chatanooga, TN) as compared to 82% of the patients without back pain (Richardson et al. 1999, 2004).

Testing of control of lumbopelvic posture as a measure of core stability against a load is accomplished clinically by performing various leg-loading activities in supine using the pressure biofeedback device (Figs. 74.6 and 74.7). The test examines the ability of the core to hold the lumbopelvic region steady during various progressive leg-loading activities (Sahrmann 2002). The pressure biofeedback device provides information to the patient about loss of support or neutral position during functional tasks. Posterior pelvic tilt motion of the pelvis results in an increase in baseline pressure, whereas anterior pelvic tilt results in a decrease in pressure from baseline. Other tasks in prone and supine positions, such as movement of the extremities and loading activities, can be assessed. Effective contraction of the TA solicits a co-contraction of the multifidus and vice versa (Richardson et al. 1999).

Unfortunately, the use of the pressure biofeedback device is limited to activities that involve a surface to offer counterforce to read the pressure exerted onto the device. It is not yet clinically possible to evaluate dynamic core stability and measure activity of deep stabilizing musculature in the upright position, and clinicians must rely on motor performance taught in other positions to "carry over" to more demanding positions. Richardson et al. (1999) advocated frequent repeat prone formal testing using the biofeedback device to check efficiency of the local core stabilizers because "assessment in functional tasks by means of observation and palpation only does not give a reliable indication of the improvement in deep muscle capacity."

Henry and Westervelt (2005) explored the use of RUSI for teaching the abdominal "drawing in" or abdominal hollowing maneuver to healthy subjects. This feedback tool decreased the number of trials needed to consistently perform this maneuver. The authors stated that RUSI is a beneficial teaching tool for facilitating consistency of performance of the abdominal hollowing maneuver compared to verbal and cutaneous feedback, which are the teaching methods used presently by most clinicians. Teyhen et al. (2005) demonstrated that RUSI can be used reliably to measure the thickness of the TA in both contracted and relaxed states. Studies to assess the value of using RUSI for feedback when learning to volitionally activate the multifidus have also shown favorable results. Van et al. (2006) also demonstrated that visual feedback improved the ability of subjects to perform the multifidus swelling exercise and that variable feedback was superior to constant feedback on long-term retention trials (Herbert et al. 2008).

Exercises/Training Techniques

Contemporary thinkers refer to the concept of **neuromuscular retraining** of the core (contributing to segmental stability and stiffness) rather than pure strengthening of muscles supporting the core (Ebenbichler et al. 2001, Akuthota and Nadler 2004, Richardson et al. 1999). To effectively provide core stabilization, the patient must use the neuromuscular system to coordinate contractions of many local and global muscles that are able to influence the position of the pelvis, hips, and spine. In vitro studies demonstrated that local muscles can effectively provide segmental stabilization of the lumbar spine (Wilke et al. 1995). Thus, recruitment and tonic activity of local musculature are the hallmark of contemporary rehabilitation and training activities, as compared with older programs that focused on contractions of the global musculature. Motor control programs for functional performance of skills used by patients (both healthy and injured) are widely varied, are complex, and may involve alterations in both feedback and feedforward mechanisms (Richardson et al. 1999). Multifidus muscle dysfunction, which may be present in highly skilled athletes despite their excellently trained condition, supports the use of an alternative (training of local stabilizers) exercise approach rather than the traditional exercise regimen often used for core strengthening with a focus on global musculature (Roy et al. 1990). Jemmet (2003) described such an alternative approach as a shift away from treating multifidus dysfunction using a strengthening model to a model based on motor re-education.

According to Richardson, Jull, Hodges, and Hides (1999), rehabilitation has three distinct phases: (1) formal motor skill training, (2) gradual incorporation into light functional tasks, and (3) progression to heavy-load functional tasks. The last phase of rehabilitation must be tailored to include high-level work and sport-specific demands performed by the patient in a wide variety of body positions, whether during a prevention or rehabilitation program. Therapeutic exercise in more advanced activities must have two different goals in mind:

1. Ensure that the deep local muscles remain functional stabilizers of the lumbopelvic region when higher load exercises are added and when movement or control of movement is necessary.
2. Assess and treat any dysfunction that is identified in the function of global musculature during task performance (Richardson et al. 1999, McGill 2002).

Current evidence supports the concept that training efforts should not focus on any single muscle; rather, they should have components of local and global muscle training (Cholewicki and McGill 1996, Cholewicki and Van Vliet 2002, McGill 2002).

WHERE TO BEGIN: FORMAL MOTOR SKILL TRAINING

The key to training the local stabilizers is teaching the abdominal drawing-in or hollowing exercise, an action specific to the TA. Drawing in of the abdominal wall was originally described by Kendall and McCreary (1983) and later further described by DeTroyer et al (1990) as "drawing the belly in." The patient

must be cued to "narrow your waist" or "pull your belly button away from your waistband" without using the other abdominal muscles or holding his or her breath.

Sahrmann (2002) described using lower-level exercises initially to develop control versus higher-level exercises focused on more strength development. Her lower abdominal exercise progression, directed toward proper recruitment of both the obliques and TA, is initiated in a supine position with hips and knee flexed. The patient is instructed to "pull your belly button toward the spine" for all exercise levels described in Table 74.3. Based on the results of the evaluation described earlier in this section, the patient must maintain lumbopelvic control while adding the specific LE perturbations. The exercise progression is essentially the same as the assessment, only done in repetition and to the tolerance of the patient. **It is important that if the patient is no longer able to maintain proper lumbopelvic control, then the exercise is stopped.** The therapist needs to use good clinical judgment to determine if the patient is at the appropriate level or if the exercise needs to be regressed or progressed based on periodic reassessment.

Another important feature of teaching the skill of abdominal bracing is that the patient understands the corset-like circular function of the TA so he or she can envision it working to draw in the waist or hollow the abdomen. The difficulty of core exercises must be tailored to the level of achievement of the abdominal drawing-in exercise (Andrews et al. 2004) and progressed from there. The patient must also understand that this action occurs without producing any movement of the spine and requires only low-level activation of the TA, <10% of the maximal voluntary isometric contraction (McGill 2002, Richardson et al. 1999). Movement of the spine or pelvis indicates global muscles are being used to attempt the task, rather than effectively recruiting and using the local TA. The quadruped position can be used initially to teach this task and then other positional instruction can be added (e.g., supine, prone, sitting, standing, and half kneeling) (Fig. 74.8).

Exercises should be progressed in difficulty only when the patient can maintain spinal stability and contraction of the TA

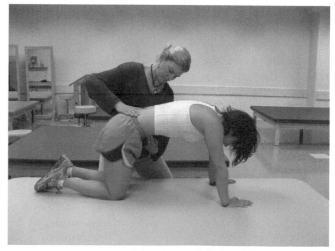

Fig. 74.8 Quadrupled abdominal drawing in with tactile cueing by the therapist. Note: This is an excellent teaching position, but the patient must progress to more functional positions such as standing and half kneeling (most difficult because it removes the lower extremity contribution to stabilization).

while breathing normally (Andrews et al. 2004). The drawing-in maneuver should then be taught in the plank exercise, which helps to develop endurance of the TA and multifidus in a semifunctional position.

Maintaining the drawing-in maneuver during the ideal lumbopelvic position is critical because the patient often has a tendency to be too flexed or too extended in the trunk. Use the cue "keep your back flat like a table top" while performing the plank exercise for a timed bout (Fig. 74.9). Patients often have difficulty assuming and holding the plank position because of poor abdominal performance or concurrent UE weightbearing difficulty. Athletes with excellent core control and endurance have been known to hold this position for more than 3 minutes. The average athlete begins with 30 to 60 seconds and works up in time duration. For patients who have trouble maintaining the position for 30 seconds, an alternative position with the knees flexed and supporting the trunk can be used, which decreases core demands by shortening the control lever arm. Many patients are challenged by 15 seconds or less.

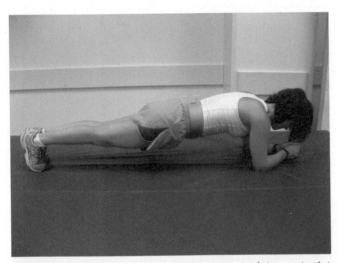

Fig. 74.9 Full plank position. (Note the position of the trunk. If the patient cannot maintain this position, the exercise can be done in a modified half-plank position, bearing weight on the knees, much like a modified push-up).

Finally, appropriate recruitment of the multifidi for segmental stability is critical in managing low back pain in patients/athletes. After the patient learns how to recruit the multifidi in the prone position (see earlier prone multifidus test of Richardson, Hodges, and Hides), then he or she progresses to the quadruped position for training multifidus activation and neuromuscular training. In a multifidus neuromuscular control exercise, the patient in quadruped is cued to lift the knee straight toward the ceiling approximately 1 inch without lifting the toes off the ground or laterally shifting the hips or trunk. If the patient has difficulty performing this exercise properly, it may be necessary to stabilize the contralateral side against a stable surface (e.g., wall or couch). The progression for this exercise is placement of a towel roll under the contralateral knee to increase the range of segmental lumbar motion (Fig. 74.10).

INCORPORATION INTO LIGHT FUNCTIONAL TASKS

Once the patient is able to properly demonstrate recruitment and control of the local core exercises (e.g., drawing in for TA, plank, multifidus), the program must be advanced to include light dynamic functional tasks. The next stage is to progress to more general functional exercises that target the key muscle groups in isolation but move closer toward the specific movement and loading patterns necessary for the patient's activities. The key muscle groups are listed in Table 74.4 with their primary responsibility as they relate to the neuromusculoskeletal system.

Functional progression of core stabilization activities is the most important part of the program when used either for prevention or rehabilitation. Functional progressions require therapist knowledge of work- or sport-specific demands along with a good sense of creativity. Without progression through relevant functional tasks, appropriate motor learning cannot be achieved because carryover from lower functional or developmental level tasks cannot be assumed. The most basic functional task requiring tonic deep muscular support is the transition from sitting to standing. Maintenance of neutral core while rising to standing from a sitting posture is functional for almost every patient (Fig. 74.11). Instruction

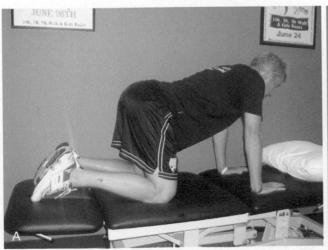
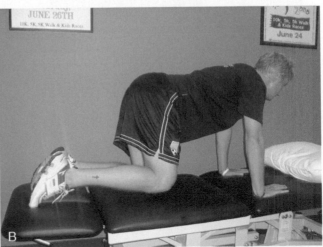

Fig. 74.10 Four-point multifidus exercise. A, Start position. B, End position.

in monitoring of the core and repetition of this simple task is a low-level start. After sit to stand is mastered, the next functionally relevant task is walking. An early dynamic exercise is to teach the patient to activate the TA and multifidus while walking and breathing normally (Richardson et al. 1999).

TABLE 74.4	**Sahrmann's Lower Abdominal Grading**

Test position: In supine, all tests begin in hook-lying position. Instruct the patient to maintain a flat, silent, stable lumbar spine while performing the following movement.

LEVELS OF DIFFICULTY

Level 0.3	Single bent knee lift less than 2 inches off the table, while other foot remains on the table. Keep pelvis silent.
Level 0.4	Using hands, *passively* hold one knee firmly to the chest (hip >90 degrees), then perform single bent knee lift as in 0.3.
Level 0.5	Using hands, *passively* hold one knee lightly toward chest (hip at 90 degrees), then perform single bent knee lift as in 0.3.
Level 1A	Single bent knee lift (as 0.3), with opposite hip held *actively* at greater than 90 degrees of flexion
Level 1B	Single bent knee lift (as 0.3), opposite hip held *actively* at 90 degrees of flexion
Level 2	Bring both hips to 90 degrees of flexion, *actively* hold one there while sliding the other heel on table until knee is fully extended, and return.
Level 3	Bring both hips to 90 degrees of flexion, *actively* hold one there while gliding the other heel to (glide = unsupported by table) until full knee extension, and return.
Level 4	Double-leg knee extension (heels supported by table)
Level 5	Double-leg knee extension (heels unsupported by table)

Note: Each movement is performed unilaterally, to assess for rotational function, until grades 4 and 5, which are performed bilaterally.
(Adapted from Sahrmann SA: Diagnosis and treatment of movement system impairments, St. Louis, 2002, Mosby Inc.)

Difficulty can be added to exercises by changing body positions, using less stable positions (e.g., therapeutic balls, foam rollers, Dyna-Discs, or other unstable surfaces), adding equipment for perturbations (e.g., band, tubing, or cable pulleys), or increasing load during tasks. The plank can be made more difficult and somewhat dynamic in the side plank position by adding UE and LE challenges (Fig. 74.12). Examples of additional developmental postures to use during dynamic exercises include tall kneeling and half kneeling, shown in Figs. 74.13 and 74.14.

We use many types of equipment such as medicine balls, elastic resistance bands, the Body Blade, and the Sport Cord (Medco Sports Medicine, Tonawanda, NY) to add resistance to typical functional movements and maneuvers in a wide variety of developmental postures, thereby challenging the patient's core stability during movement.

With a logical functional progression and relatively inexpensive equipment, the rehabilitation professional is limited only by his or her own creativity in designing intermediate and advanced functional, core stabilization exercises.

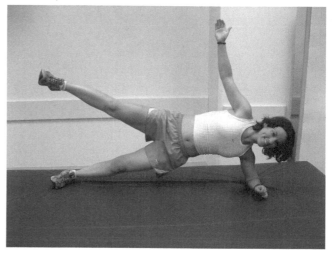

Fig. 74.12 Side plank with upper extremity (UE) and lower extremity (LE) challenge. The LE and UE can move or oscillate between a rest position and an elevated position as shown.

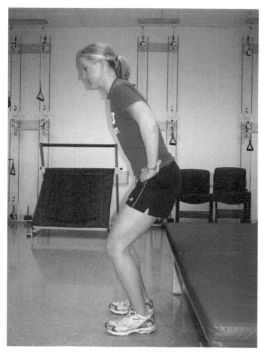

Fig. 74.11 Sit to and from stand, low-level training.

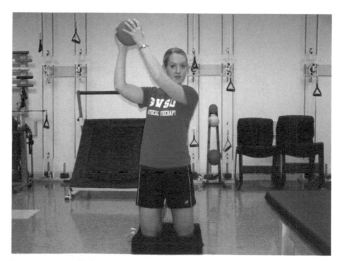

Fig. 74.13 Tall kneeling lift, using weighted ball for stabilization challenge.

Finally, the practice of isolated training of a specific group of muscles to reduce compressive loads on the spine must be examined (Kavcic et al. 2004). Strength training of the lumbar extensors has traditionally been a part of low back rehabilitation. The lumbar extensors are considered global muscles. They serve as prime movers into trunk extension and may need to be included in strengthening exercise programs for athletes after injury to the low back. Many exercises directed at strengthening the lumbar extensors as a group, however, fail to place the pelvis in a stable, neutral position and prevent substitution of the gluteals. In fact, many commercially available "low back strengthening" exercise machines do not attempt to stabilize the pelvis and place the spine in a lordotic or hyperextended position. Graves et al. (1994) studied the effect of pelvic stabilization on retraining of the lumbar extensors and found that strengthening should be performed with the pelvis stabilized. It should be noted, however, that in their research they used a machine that provided passive external stabilization to the lumbar spine (because of machine design), but a successfully maintained active pelvic stabilization may be more appropriate. Techniques of core stabilization using local musculature can be applied during various strengthening tasks involving global muscles of the trunk and extremities. Kavcic et al. (2004) concluded that it is "justifiable to train motor patterns that involve the contribution of many of the potentially important lumbar spine stabilizers" during rehabilitation and that focus on a single muscle or group appears to be misdirected if the goal is the development of a stable spine.

Table 74.5 gives several examples of exercise progression for core stabilization.

GENERAL FUNCTIONAL EXERCISES

The important role of the deep local stabilizers has been well documented. Specifically, the TA and the multifidus have vital roles in core stabilization and the successful management of LBP, both chronic and acute. Once the patient/athlete has demonstrated appropriate recruitment patterns and control with the exercises described, it is imperative that the rehabilitation professional progress the exercise program to a more functionally based routine to achieve optimal results. Several intermediate-level functional exercises are described in the following paragraphs.

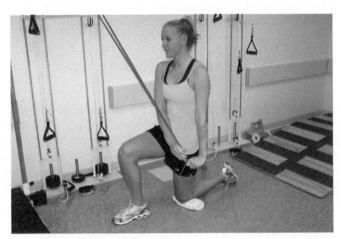

Fig. 74.14 Half-kneeling chop with Theraband, start and end positions.

TABLE 74.5	Progression of Core Stabilization Exercises	
Beginning Exercises	**Intermediate Exercises**	**Advanced Exercises**
Isometric holding exercises: 1. The abdominal hollowing exercise 2. Pelvic floor contractions, best started in supine, hook-lying 3. Lumbar multifidus contractions (Fig. 74.4) 4. Diaphragmatic breathing Abdominal hollowing in alternate static positions: 1. Prone, knees straight with Stabilizer (Fig. 74.5) 2. Supine, knees bent (Fig. 74.6) 3. Quadruped with therapist cues (Fig. 74.8) Abdominal hollowing with challenges: 1. Supine bridging 2. Movement of UEs with Stabilizer, aka "dead bug" 3. Movement of LEs into leg-loading tasks with Stabilizer (Fig. 74.7) 4. Four point with UE or LE movements	Functional positions: 1. Sitting to/from standing (Fig. 74.11) 2. Pelvic floor contractions with bridge on ball (Fig. 74.18) 3. Quadruped multifidus exercise (Fig. 74.10) Planks: 1. Half side planks (knees flexed) 2. Side planks, LEs extended (Fig. 74.3) 3. Half front planks (knees flexed, modified push-up position) 4. Full front planks (Fig. 74.9) Dynamic activities during side planks: 1. LE movements 2. Side plank on BOSU (Fig. 74.16) 3. UE/LE movements (Fig. 74.12) 4. Use of tubing, weights, ab roller with various plank positions	Progress to advanced positions: 1. Tall kneeling lift with core ball (Fig. 74.13) 2. Half-kneeling chop with Theraband (Fig. 74.14) 3. Standing with UE perturbations (Fig. 74.15)*Consider the Body Blade Other training postures: 1. Standing on unstable surfaces with trunk or UE movements with or without resistance (Figs. 74.17, 74.23, 74.25, and 74.28) 2. Squat with overhead lift (Fig. 74.20); lunge to BOSU with core ball (Fig. 74.19) Dynamic sport/work positions: 1. Overhead medicine ball toss (Fig. 74.22) 2. Half-kneeling medicine ball rotation toss (Fig. 74.24) 3. Core ball punch on unstable surface (Fig. 74.27) 4. Single-limb dead lift (Fig. 74.28)

UE, upper extremity; LE, lower extremity.

Notes: It is important to provide the patient with clear explanations and use a variety of teaching "tools" such as verbal analogies/descriptors, visual aids, clinician demonstration, and tactile cues. The patient must be educated to the type of skill and motor retraining that needs to occur. This includes a discussion about precision and intensity of contractions (mild to moderate contractions of the involved musculature, rather than maximal contractions, are indicated). The patient must understand from the outset the subtlety and precise natures of the contractions involved and then apply to all activities. Be certain to monitor for signs of unwanted global muscle activity during activities. These signs include pelvic or spine movement, rib cage depression, no change in diameter of the abdominal wall (should draw in laterally and anteriorly), aberrant breathing patterns, inability to perform normal breathing during tasks, and coactivation of thoracic portions of erector spinae. Methods of observation include visual observation, palpation, and electromyographic assessment. Be creative in designing and progressing activities of core stabilization; your only limitation is your own imagination.

Transversus Abdominis With Ue Perturbations

Exercise: Drawing-in technique with bilateral tubing pulls standing on Airex pad (Fig. 74.15).

Description: The patient is instructed to perform a proper drawing-in technique in a partial squat position while performing repeated bilateral UE pull-downs with tubing or band with the goal of maintaining an isometric hold of the trunk.

Ipsilateral IO/EO—Side Flexion

Exercise: Side plank with elbow resting on a BOSU (BOSU, Shanghai PYC Industrial, Shanghai, China) ball (Fig. 74.16).

Description: The patient is instructed to maintain a side-plank position with elbow resting on a more unstable surface using the BOSU ball. The goal is to maintain the proper trunk alignment in both the frontal and sagittal planes. Perturbations can be added by moving the arm not bearing weight.

Contralateral IO/EO—Rotation

Exercise: Isometric oblique punches with tubing standing on a foam mat (Fig. 74.17).

Description: The tubing or band is placed in the door at elbow level. The patient is instructed to stand on the foam mat and punch straight forward while holding onto the band or tubing. The goal is to maintain an isometric hold and not allow any trunk rotation to occur.

Diaphragm and Pelvic Floor

Exercise: Supine bridge with feet on exercise ball with cued breathing (Fig. 74.18).

Description: Lying supine with both feet on a small exercise ball, the patient is instructed to lift the hips off the table to a position where the thighs are in line with the trunk. The key to this exercise is to have the athlete *exhale on exertion*. This coordinated breathing pattern will facilitate the co-contraction of the diaphragm and pelvic floor.

DYNAMIC, PROGRESSIVE FUNCTIONAL CHALLENGES

The stresses placed on the tissues during sporting events and work tasks tend to be repetitive and may need to be sustained for several hours. Thus, the focus of the prescribed exercises may need to be more endurance than strength. The following examples provide dynamic, progressively more difficult exercises, which could be dosed for strength or endurance.

Lunge Onto Unstable Surface Using Exercise Ball

Description: Standing on one leg, the athlete lunges forward with the other leg and places foot onto the BOSU ball (Fig. 74.19). The athlete is instructed to perform the lunge while maintaining a stable core and concurrently reaching with the core ball. Note: External perturbation may be provided by the therapist using a dowel to push on the patient's pelvis during the lunge.

Squat With Overhead Sustained Lift

Description: With feet shoulder-width apart, knees slightly bent, spine in neutral, the athlete starts by lifting a piece of dowel overhead and maintaining while performing a form squat (Fig. 74.20). The emphasis is on having the patient maintain a neutral spine position throughout the entire squatting motion. This exercise is progressed by adding weights (e.g.,

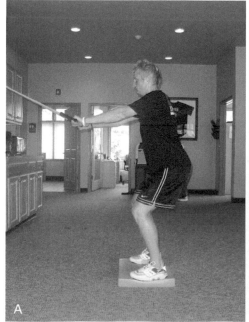 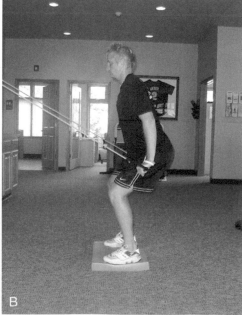

Fig. 74.15 Transversus abdominis stabilization in standing with upper extremity perturbations. **A,** Starting position. **B,** Finish position.

dumbbells, barbell, or barbell with weights) in the overhead position.

Four-Way Tubing Pulls on Unstable Surface

Description: With tubing anchored low, the athlete places one end around one ankle while standing on an unstable surface (e.g., Airex pad, foam roller, or Dyna-Disc [Dynadisk R. Exertools, Petaluma, CA]) (Fig. 74.21). With the stance leg in slight knee flexion, the athlete is instructed to pull against the tubing away from the anchor point. The exercise is repeated with changes in direction for hip extension, abduction, flexion, and adduction. The emphasis is on having the athlete maintain proper lumbopelvic alignment, especially in the frontal and sagittal planes.

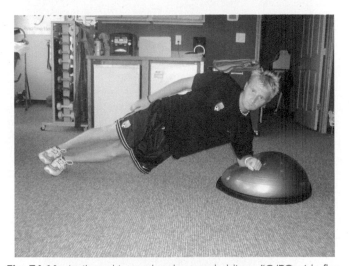

Fig. 74.16 Ipsilateral internal and external oblique (IO/EO; side flexion) on BOSU ball.

Overhead Medicine Ball Toss Kneeling on Bosu Ball

Description: The patient kneels on a BOSU ball and performs an overhead toss and catch with a medicine ball either with another person or against a Plyoback Rebounder (Plyoback Elite Rebounder®, Exertools, Petaluma, CA) (Fig. 74.22). The emphasis is on having the patient maintain good trunk alignment, avoiding flexion or extension of the lumbar spine. This can be made more difficult by having the patient not allow the feet to touch the ground.

Single-Limb Stance on Bosu Ball With Repeated Rowing

Description: With the tubing anchored at chest height the patient assumes a single-limb stance in a partial-squat position on the BOSU and performs repeated rowing motions with the tubing (Fig. 74.23). The emphasis is on having the patient maintain neutral lumbopelvic alignment, especially in the frontal and sagittal planes.

The movement patterns encountered during sport and work often generate a great deal of rotational joint and tissue stress at the spine. It is important to challenge the core stabilizers in a rotational manner with the primary goal of maintaining the ideal transverse plane spine position specific to the individual sport or industrial demand.

Half-Kneeling Medicine Ball Side Toss

Description: While in a half-kneeling position (near leg up) and sideways to the Plyoback Rebounder, the patient performs a rotational toss and catch, allowing trunk rotation to occur in a controlled midrange of motion (Fig. 74.24). The emphasis is on having the obliques not only generate the rotational movement during the toss phase but also control the eccentric movement during the catching phase. The exercise is performed from both sides.

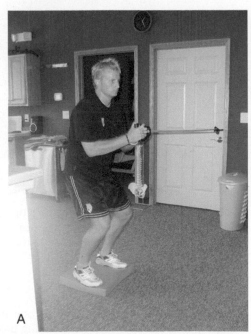
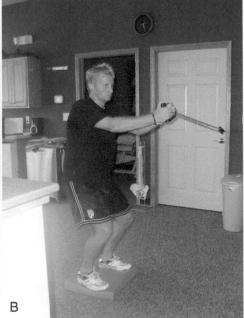

A   B

Fig. 74.17 Contralateral internal and external oblique (IO/EO; rotation) on foam support. **A,** Starting position. **B,** Finish position.

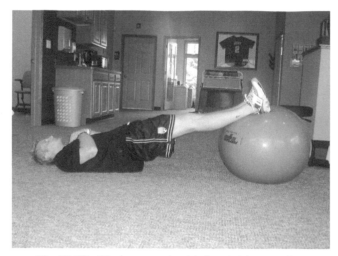

Fig. 74.18   Diaphragm and pelvic floor bridge exercise.

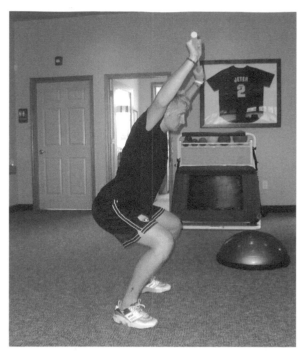

Fig. 74.20   Squat with overhead sustained lift.

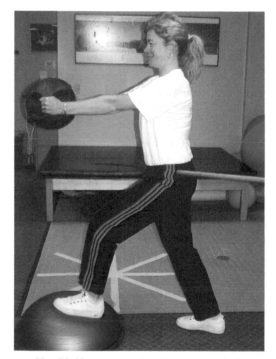

Fig. 74.19   Lunge to BOSU using core ball.

Diagonal Tubing Pulls on Unstable Surfaces

Description: Diagonal tubing pulls can be done in both D_1 and D_2 patterns either with single (Fig. 74.25) or double arm pulls (Fig. 74.26). By placing the athlete on unstable surfaces (e.g., Airex pad, foam rollers, Dyna-Disc, or BOSU) and in different stance positions (e.g., double limb, single limb, tandem stance, lunge position, squat position, or sport-specific stance), the exercise can be tailored to meet the needs of any athlete.

Core Ball Punch on Unstable Surface

Description: While in a double-limb stance on an unstable surface (e.g., Dyna-Discs, foam rollers, or BOSU) and holding a core ball against the chest, the athlete performs a forward punching motion (arms parallel to the ground), then

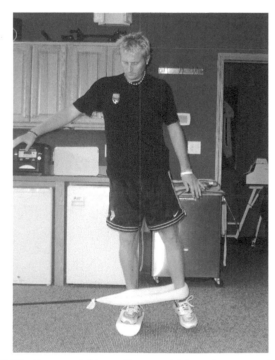

Fig. 74.21   Four-way tubing pulls on unstable surface, example of abduction.

returns to the chest (Fig. 74.27). The emphasis is on maintaining the ideal spine position during all phases of the exercise. This exercise can be modified by moving the ball diagonally or rotationally.

Single-Limb Dead Lift

Description: The patient stands on one limb with the knee slightly flexed (Fig. 74.28). Maintaining proper spine and pelvis and upright trunk, the patient lowers one or both hands

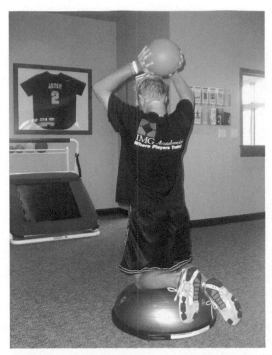

Fig. 74.22 Overhead medicine ball toss kneeling on BOSU.

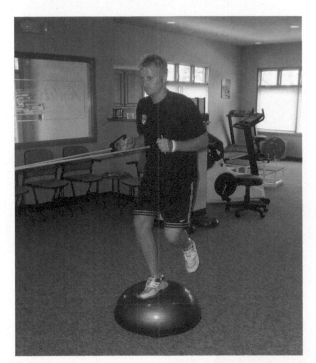

Fig. 74.23 Single-limb stance on BOSU with repeated rowing.

toward the floor while flexing at the hip and then returns to the upright starting position. It is imperative that the slight lordosis (neutral spine) is not lost during the motion. The movement is accomplished by the gluteus maximus and, to a lesser extent, the hamstrings on the stance leg. This motion is also known as a flat back or golfer's lift and may be functional for lifting light loads.

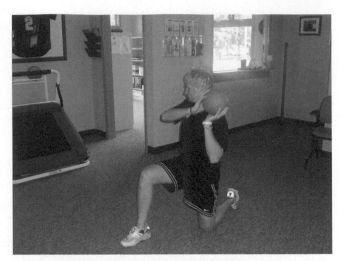

Fig. 74.24 Half kneeling medicine ball side toss.

CONCLUSION

Core stability training is increasing in popularity as clinicians have become aware of the relationship that a poorly functioning core has to performance and injury. Experts agree that retraining of the deep local muscles of the core must be incorporated into rehabilitation of patients with injury to the low back to effectively accomplish functional rehabilitation (Richardson et al. 1999). Core training routines can be creatively designed and progressed by the rehabilitation professional to facilitate complete return to occupation or sport. It must be acknowledged that the concept of core stabilization is not intended to replace many other systems and philosophies of treatment; rather it is but one part of the big picture of spinal rehabilitation. Motor re-education of the deep core stabilizers may need to precede more general exercise and be incorporated into subsequent exercises to successfully educate or re-educate deep local muscles in their essential stabilizing function. Local muscular exercises must be carefully assessed, taught, and mastered using available clinical tools and techniques before training the global muscles of the core. Successful use of local muscles during exercises and function may prevent or correct motor control problems that contribute to recurrent injury and incorrect use of the muscles of the core. As more evidence emerges regarding the use of RUSI, and it becomes more available to clinicians, it likely will gain popularity as a tool for clinical muscular assessment and biofeedback during rehabilitation. No matter the exercise approach or applied theory, the clinical outcomes of core stability programs have not been well researched. The specific exercises and theories described in this chapter need further investigation both for rehabilitation of injuries of the low back, pelvis, and associated core muscles and for use in strength training and performance-enhancement programs. Incorporation of core stabilization techniques into rehabilitative, fitness, preventive, and wellness programs will continue to be important in the ever-evolving practice of spinal rehabilitation.

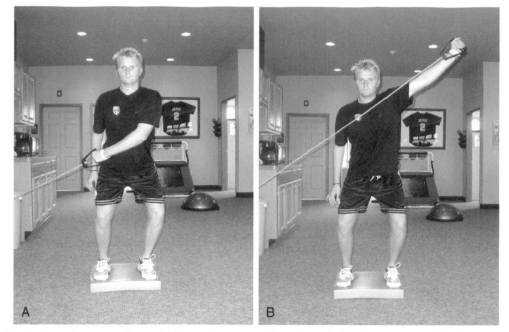

Fig. 74.25 Single-arm diagonal tubing pulls on unstable surfaces. **A,** Starting position. **B,** Finish position.

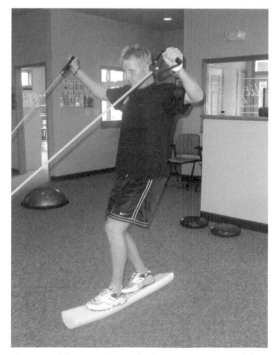

Fig. 74.26 Double-arm diagonal tubing pulls on unstable surfaces.

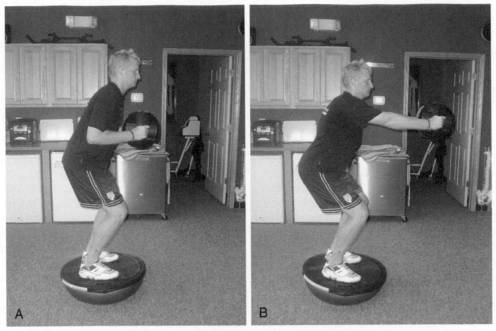

Fig. 74.27   Core ball punch on unstable surface. **A,** Starting position. **B,** Finish position.

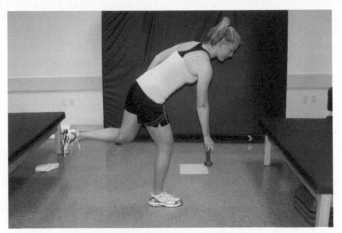

Fig. 74.28   Single-limb dead lift.

REFERENCES

A complete reference list is available at https://expertconsult .inkling.com/.

FURTHER READING

Cresswell AG, Thorstensson A. Change in intra-abdominal pressure, trunk muscle activation and force during isokinetic lifting and lowering. *Eur J Appl Physiol*. 1994;68:315–321.

Hides J, Gilmore C, Stanton W, et al. Multifidus size and symmetry among chronic LBP and healthy asymptomatic subjects. *Man Ther*. 2008;13(1):43–90. Epub 2006 Oct 27.

Hodges PW, Richardson CA. Delayed postural contraction of transverse abdominis in low back pain associated with movement of the lower limb. *J Spinal Disord*. 1998;1:46–56.

Hodges PW, Pengel LH, Herbert RD, et al. Measurement of muscle contraction with ultrasound imaging. *Muscle Nerve*. 2003;27(6):682–692.

Hodges PW, Moseley GL. Pain and motor control of the lumbopelvic region: effect and possible mechanisms. *J Electromyogr Kinesiol*. 2003;13(4):361–370.

Kiesel KB, Uhl TL, Underwood FB, et al. Measurement of lumbar multifidus muscle contraction with rehabilitative ultrasound imaging. *Man Ther*. 2007;12(2):161–166.

Kiesel K, Underwood F, Matacolla C, et al. A comparison of select trunk muscle thickness change between subjects with low back pain classified in the treatment-based classification system and asymptomatic controls. *J Orthop Sports Phys Ther*. 2007;37(10).

McKenzie Approach to Low Back Pain

Barbara J. Hoogenboom, EdD, PT, SCS, ATC | Jolene Bennett, PT, MA, OCS, ATC, Cert MDT

The rehabilitation professional caring for patients with low back pain must use an evidence-based, efficient, and effective treatment approach. In this light, it must be recognized that evidence for the effectiveness of a McKenzie approach to low back pain is limited (Machado et al. 2006). Evidence suggests patients show slightly greater improvement in low back pain if they are treated by physical therapists with McKenzie training rather than nontrained therapists (Deutscher et al. 2014). However, other research suggests the McKenzie method has limited effect on patients' pain and disability (Machado et al. 2010). The objectives of this section are to present an introduction to the McKenzie classification system, describe evaluation techniques, and present treatment interventions common to the McKenzie system for the lumbar spine. A case study describing lumbar pain/pathology in a baseball player is used to illustrate the importance of a thorough evaluation process to determine the correct treatment approach. This section of the chapter is to be considered only as an introduction to the McKenzie system and is not to be used as a substitute for attendance at the courses offered by the McKenzie Institute or thorough reading of the textbooks related to the lumbar spine written by Robin McKenzie and Stephen May (McKenzie and May 2004).

TYPES OF PAIN

As noted in chapter 77, any anatomic structure that has a nerve supply is capable of causing pain or nociceptive impulses. In the lumbar spine these structures may include the capsules of the facet and sacroiliac joints, the outer part of the intervertebral discs, the interspinous and longitudinal ligaments, the vertebral bodies, the dura mater, nerve root sleeve, connective tissue of nerves, blood vessels of the spinal canal, or local muscles (Bogduk 1997, Butler 1991). The large number of nociceptors within the lumbar region makes it impossible, even for the most experienced clinician, to determine the exact tissue that is the source of the pain. Kuslich et al. (1991) determined that compressed nerve roots are the source of significant leg pain, and the outer wall of the annulus fibrosus is the source of significant back pain. Other authors determined that most pain in the lumbar spine and leg is attributable to the intervertebral disc, whereas the facet and sacroiliac joints play a lesser role (Bogduk 1993 and 1994).

There are four possible types of pain; however, somatic and neurogenic/radicular pains are the two most common types encountered in the rehabilitation environment. Somatic pain is pain generated by musculoskeletal tissue, and neurogenic pain is initiated by the nerve root, dorsal root ganglion, and dura. The other two sources of pain are related to the central nervous system and visceral organs. These latter two sources of pain generation must always be ruled out in the evaluation process to ensure that the treatment approach is appropriate for the source of pain.

Somatic pain is described as deep and aching and is vague and hard to localize. The deeper the affected structure, the more widespread the distribution of the pain (Bogduk 1994). Nociceptors in the facet and sacroiliac joints are capable of referring pain down the leg (McKenzie and May 2004). The stronger the noxious stimulus, the more distal the pain travels. Neurogenic pain arises from pressure on nerve roots, which in turn causes further inflammation. Neurogenic pain is often severe and shooting in nature and felt in a narrow area of the leg, as opposed to somatic pain, which usually has a broad distribution of pain and achiness. All nerve root pain is felt in the leg, and often the leg pain is worse than the back pain. Motor and sensory abnormalities, if present, indicate significant inflammation and compression on the nerve root and should be observed closely by the clinician. Typically, inflammation of the L4 nerve root refers pain down the anterior aspect of the thigh, L5 refers pain down the lateral aspect of the leg, and S1 refers pain down the posterior aspect of the leg. This distribution can be variable among patients and should not be interpreted rigidly (McKenzie and May 2004). As noted earlier, the nociceptive source of leg pain can be from somatic and/or neurogenic sources; frequently, it is a combination of both.

ACTIVATION OF PAIN

Nociceptors are triggered by thermal, mechanical, and chemical stresses. In the rehabilitation environment, both the mechanical and chemical stressors must be treated to resolve pain and facilitate full return of function. Chemical stress occurs when a tissue is damaged or inflamed as a result of trauma or overuse. The result of such stress to a localized area triggers the release of chemicals including histamine, serotonin, substance P, and bradykinin. The local presence of these chemicals maintains the patient's perception of pain. This type of pain is treated with medication and modalities to reduce the chemical reaction of tissue damage. Chemical pain is experienced by the patient as constant pain but is most frequently observed in combination with mechanical pain.

Mechanical pain occurs when a mechanical force is applied to any tissue and that stress deforms the local nociceptors present within the tissue. Mechanical pain is intermittent and diminishes or totally resolves if the mechanical stress is removed. An example of this is placing a hyperextension force on a finger; by maintaining this position the nociceptive pain system is stimulated. When the force is released, the mechanical pain resolves. No chemical treatment will diminish pain arising from a mechanical deformation as no mechanical treatment will totally resolve pain arising from chemical stress. These simple principles are the basis for the McKenzie approach to treating any type of musculoskeletal pain with repeated movements (McKenzie and May 2004).

The degree of chemical and mechanical pain present with each individual injury must be determined during the subjective and objective examination and subsequent evaluation. Then, each component of pain must be treated accordingly. Table 75.1 gives some guidelines in determining the source of pain during examination and evaluation.

STAGES OF TISSUE HEALING

After the types of pain have been described, a review of the basic stages of healing and how the McKenzie approach may fit into treatment during these stages is warranted. The first stage is **inflammation** lasting a maximum of one week if treated promptly and correctly. Treatment principles during this phase are to minimize the inflammation by chemical means and eliminate mechanical stresses with proper body positioning and movements within pain-free range of motion. **Aggressive repeated movements applied during the inflammation stage may delay healing or prolong the inflammatory stage.**

The next stage is the **repair and healing stage,** which occurs during weeks two through four. The key in this phase is to apply gentle stresses to the soft tissues to facilitate repair of tissue. Imposed stresses should enable tissues to repair in correct orientation according to the functional stress lines and help to increase tensile strength of the healing tissues. During this stage, the induced movements should work into the edge of stiffness and pain, and the patient should be in control of the quantity of force delivered at the end range of movement. Caution should be taken to avoid overstressing the area and causing new inflammation, delaying recovery.

The final stage is **remodeling,** which occurs from the fifth week on. In this stage, it is important to apply regular stress sufficient to provide tension without damage so the soft tissues elongate and strengthen. Return to full range of motion in all directions of movement is the goal and should be present to achieve return to full function (McKenzie and May 2004). The principles of treatment for each stage are summarized in Table 75.2.

INTERVERTEBRAL DISC

The outer one-third of the annulus and a significant part of the disc end plate is innervated and may be a pain generator (Fields et al. 2014). Nerve endings found in the anterior and posterior longitudinal ligaments lie in close proximity to the intervertebral discs. Evidence exists that the intervertebral disc is mobile and, therefore, is a source of mechanically generated pain through two possible mechanisms. First, radial fissures that occur within the annular wall disrupt the normal load-bearing properties of the annulus and the weightbearing distribution becomes disproportionate and stress is shifted to the outer innervated lamellae.

The second, internal displacement of the disc material, has also been determined to be a potential source of pain. The position of the disc material is influenced by spinal postures and prolonged postural positions of flexion or extension, as originally described by Nachemson (1992) (Fig. 75.1). Such conditions cause disc material displacement according to direction. In both of these cases the pain that is caused results from uneven loading of the intervertebral disc, which may cause neurogenic pain from pressure on the nerve root (Bogduk 1997) (Fig. 75.2). A large volume of literature exists regarding disc function and mechanics; however, more discussion is beyond the scope of this text.

What is important to remember is that the disc is a mobile tissue, affected both by movement and sustained postures. This fundamental concept is the cornerstone of the McKenzie approach for treatment of spinal pain. The McKenzie system describes many types of mechanical back pain and hypothesizes that changing mechanical loads on the intervertebral disc will either increase or decrease pain, causing peripheralization or centralization of the neurogenic symptoms noted by the patient. Asymmetric loading of the disc will displace the nucleus pulposus (NP) to the area of least pressure. If the lumbar spine is flexed, the force is highest in the anterior aspect of the disc and thus the NP will be displaced in the opposite direction posteriorly within the disc. Many studies have supported this hypothesis and have shown that posterior displacement of the NP occurs with lumbar flexion and anterior displacement of the NP occurs with lumbar extension

TABLE 75.1	Key Factors of Chemical and Mechanical Types of Pain (McKenzie)	
Key Factors of Chemical Pain	**Key Factors of Mechanical Pain**	
Constant pain	Intermittent pain	
Pain appears shortly after injury	Repeated movements cause lasting reduction in pain, abolish and centralize pain	
Cardinal signs of inflammation may be present (swelling, redness, heat, tenderness)	Directional preference	
Lasting aggravation of pain by all repeated movements	One direction of movement will decrease pain, whereas the opposite direction will increase pain	
No movement found that reduces, abolishes, or centralizes pain	—	

TABLE 75.2	Treatment According to Stages of Healing	
Week 1 **Injury and Inflammation** ↓	**Weeks 2–4** **Repair and Healing** ↓	**Weeks 5+** **Remodeling** ↓
Minimize further mechanical deformation	Gentle tension and loading without lasting pain	Prevent contractures by increasing tensile load to tissue
Decrease inflammation	Work into edge of stiffness but no lasting pain cessation of exercise	Normal return to full range of motion
Relative rest	Patient in control of forces of pressure at end range	Overpressure applied to end range of repeated movements either by patient or therapist
Protected movements, with little to no stress	Progressive return to normal loads and tension	Return to full functional level with all activities

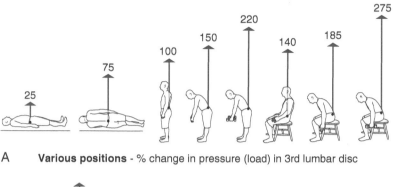

A   **Various positions** - % change in pressure (load) in 3rd lumbar disc

B   **Various exercises** - % change in pressure (load) in 3rd lumbar disc

Fig. 75.1   A, Relative change in the pressure (or load) in the third lumbar disc in various positions in living subjects. B, Relative change in the pressure (or load) in the third lumbar disc during various muscle strengthening exercises in living subjects.

Mechanical Assessment of Low Back Pain

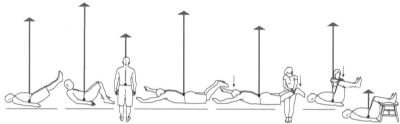

A   Anterior compression   B   Posterior compression   C   ↑Anterior compression

Fig. 75.2   Forces applied during asymmetric compression loading of the disc cause migration of the nucleus pulposus away from the load. They also create a vertical tension on the annulus, opposite the load. **A,** During anterior compression associated with our flexed lifestyles, these stresses are focused on the posterior annulus, frequently causing pain. **B,** In patients with a directional preference for extension, the posterior compression that occurs with extension loading may reverse the direction of these stresses, alleviating those lifestyle-related stresses on this posterior nucleo-annular complex. Pain then centralizes or abolishes. **C,** If the anterior asymmetrical loading forces create a sufficient pressure gradient across the disc to displace nuclear content significantly against the opposite annulus, a herniation could develop, as shown in this example of posterolateral herniation.

(Schnebel et al. 1988, Beattie et al. 1994, Fennell et al. 1996, Brault et al. 1997, Edmondstone et al. 2000). Authors consistently report that the aging NP becomes more fibrous over a lifetime and therefore demonstrates less predictable responses to repeated movements and may be displaced less easily in the older patient than in younger patients (Schnebel et al. 1988, Beattie et al. 1994).

In this section the term disc herniation is used as a nonspecific term to indicate disc material displacement, fissure, or disruption. The McKenzie approach uses repeated movements in the sagittal plane to evaluate and treat these disruptions. The McKenzie classification term for this is a *derangement*, which is detailed in the next section. A derangement can be labeled as reducible or irreducible based on the presence or absence of the

Centralization

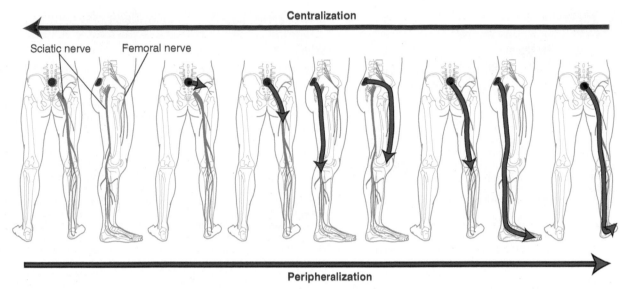

Sciatic nerve   Femoral nerve

Peripheralization

Fig. 75.3 Centralization is a rapid change of pain with maneuvers that result in peripheral or distal pain becoming more centralized (desirable). The converse (peripheralization of the pain) is not sought or desired.

hydrostatic mechanism within the disc wall. If the herniation is present in a disc where the outer wall is intact (hydrostatic mechanism intact), then it is reducible and repeated movements would correct the mechanical stresses on the disc. If the herniation is present in a disc where the outer wall is not intact (hydrostatic mechanism disrupted), then the derangement is irreducible and repeated movements will not improve the pain or symptoms (McKenzie and May 2004).

The direction of herniation is important because this directs the treatment approach. Fewer than 10% of derangements herniate directly laterally, requiring torsional or lateral forces to be a component of the treatment (Oeckler et al. 1992). One study found most cases of lumbar disc herniation to occur obliquely from the disc (Ebeling and Reulen, 1992). This suggests that most derangements occur partly in the sagittal plane, so lumbar flexion and extension are part of the mechanism of injury and the avenue for repeated movement treatment. Most derangements occur at the L4–L5 and L5–S1 levels (McKenzie and May 2004).

McKENZIE CLASSIFICATION OF SYNDROMES

The McKenzie classification consists of three different syndromes. Syndromes are groups of signs and symptoms that occur together and characterize a particular abnormality (Merriam-Webster 1999). The three syndromes are the derangement syndrome, dysfunction syndrome, and postural syndrome. Each syndrome has unique characteristics during a thorough history and physical examination. The physical examination consists of a series of loading maneuvers that impart stresses to the tissues of the spine, and each syndrome has unique responses to the loading tests. Correct identification of the syndromes will lead the clinician to the proper mechanical treatment.

Derangement Syndrome

The derangement syndrome is defined by McKenzie and May as follows: "Internal derangement causes a disturbance in the normal resting position of the affected surfaces. Internal displacement of articular tissue of whatever origin will cause pain to remain constant until such time as the displacement is reduced. Internal displacement of articular tissue obstructs movements" (McKenzie and May 2004). Derangement is the most common syndrome seen by the rehabilitation provider, and it relates to the presentation of internal intervertebral disc displacements. The clinical presentation of derangement syndrome may or may not include leg pain in addition to back pain. The patient's pain changes with induced directional movements as the forces change within the intervertebral disc because of varying positions of the spine. The pain may be present during the movement and at the end range of movement. Sagittal plane range of motion frequently is limited; however, as the derangement is reduced in response to treatment, the range of motion should improve and return to normal. McKenzie further breaks down the derangement syndrome into central symmetric, unilateral asymmetric symptoms to the knee, and unilateral asymmetric symptoms below the knee. Each of the subdivisions of the derangement syndrome has unique principles for intervention. The reader is directed to McKenzie and May's textbook for clarification of these subclassifications (McKenzie and May 2004).

The term centralization is associated with the derangement syndrome and is referred to extensively in the literature on disc herniations (Fig. 75.3). Centralization is the response to therapeutic loading strategies; pain is progressively abolished in a distal to proximal direction with each progressive abolition being retained over time until all symptoms are abolished. If distal or radicular pain is present, successful treatment results in the phenomenon of the pain moving from a widespread to a more central location and eventually being abolished (McKenzie and May 2004).

Dysfunction Syndrome

Dysfunction syndrome is characterized by pain caused by mechanical deformation of structurally impaired tissue and a limited range of motion in the affected direction. The patient reports pain only at the end range of available motion, and

TABLE 75.3	Characteristics and Descriptors of McKenzie's Syndromes (McKenzie)		
	Derangement	**Dysfunction**	**Postural**
Age	Usually 20–55	Usually older than 30 except following trauma or derangement	Usually younger than 30
Pain			
Constancy	Constant or intermittent	Intermittent	Intermittent
Location	Local and/or referred	Local (referred only with adherent nerve root)	Local
History	Gradual or sudden	Gradual	Gradual
Onset	Often related to prolonged positions or repetitive movements	History of trauma	Sedentary lifestyle
Reason			
Worse	Static/dynamic load at mid or end range	Static/dynamic loading at end range	Static loading at end range
Type of load	Worse AM and PM	No diurnal cycle	Worse end of day
Diurnal cycle			
Better	Opposite position of what causes pain	Positions that do not put shortened tissue at end range	Change of position and when active
Examination	Acute deformity may be present	Pain felt at end range of motion only	Movement does not produce pain
	Pain felt during movement	Pain stops shortly after removal of stretch	Range of motion is normal
	Pain changes location and/or intensity	Pain does not change location or intensity	Sustained end-range positions eventually produce local pain
	Pain centralizes or peripheralizes	Patient remains no better and no worse as a result	
	Patient remains better or worse as a result		
	Rapid changes in pain and range of motion		
Treatment	Correct the deformity	Repeated movements or stretches in the direction which produces end-range pain or limited motion	Correct posture
	Repeated movements performed in the direction that centralizes the pain		Education
	Correct posture	Correct posture	
	Education	Education	

when the mechanical load is released, the pain disappears. This syndrome is not common, and a few studies have reported it to be present in fewer than 20% of the patients with lumbar pain treated using the McKenzie approach (McKenzie and May 2004). The dysfunction syndrome may occur in the flexion, extension, or side gliding direction. The dysfunction is named for the direction that is limited, so if flexion is limited, then it would be labeled flexion dysfunction and vice versa for extension (McKenzie and May 2004).

Postural Syndrome

The postural syndrome is characterized by the presence of pain only when normal tissue is deformed over a prolonged period such as by sitting in a slouched posture. This syndrome is seldom seen in isolation, but if abnormal postural loading continues, this deformation of tissue may lead over time to derangement or dysfunction syndrome (McKenzie and May 2004).

Summary of Syndromes

In summary, the derangement syndrome is the most common syndrome and posterolateral derangement of the disc occurs most frequently. The treatment of a derangement is to mechanically load the compromised tissue in the opposite direction of the movement that increases the pain. In a posterolateral derangement, the treatment direction is extension of the lumbar spine. This concept may be why many clinicians associate McKenzie treatment only with lumbar extension. Further investigation of the McKenzie approach reveals there is much more than just interventions involving lumbar extension. The derangement syndrome can be compared to a meniscal tear in the knee joint. The tear influences the joint as a mechanical block limiting full function and altering the imposed mechanical forces through the knee, thereby changing the perception of

pain. The dysfunction syndrome can be compared to adhesive capsulitis of the glenohumeral joint. It is a soft tissue restriction that limits end-range motion and produces pain at end range. The treatment for a dysfunction is to repeatedly stretch into the direction of limitation. The postural syndrome is treated with postural correction exercises and patient education. See Table 75.3 for a review of McKenzie's syndromes.

McKENZIE EVALUATION

The evaluation process begins with a patient history/subjective portion and is followed by a physical movement examination. The aim of the McKenzie examination is to determine which positions and movements improve pain and function, thus directing the clinician toward the appropriate treatment strategy. The McKenzie examination process has a very specific pathway, and the key is to follow the same procedure for each patient for consistency and thoroughness in all areas of the examination.

Both the derangement and dysfunction syndromes present similarly during the subjective portion of the evaluation, and definitive conclusions regarding syndrome classification and appropriate treatment must be confirmed by movement testing. **A thorough mechanical physical examination is required to isolate the mechanical deficits and direct treatment properly.**

The goal of the physical examination is to confirm or refute clinical conclusions drawn initially from the subjective portion of the examination. The movement tests are used to expose the mechanical or nonmechanical nature of the injury and determine a directional preference. The reader is referred to the McKenzie text for details regarding testing procedures, positions, and varied responses (McKenzie and May 2004). The movement testing portion of the examination determines three things: (1) the baseline pain, (2) if pain is evident during the movement, and (3) if pain is evident at end range of the movement. On returning to the starting position of the movement,

TABLE 75.4	Physical Examination Using Movement Testing							
	DYSFUNCTION				**DERANGEMENT**			
Test	**Pain During**	**Centralize/ Peripheralize**	**End-Range Pain**	**ROM Response**	**Pain During**	**Centralize/ Peripheralize**	**End-Range Pain**	**ROM Response**
Posture correction	No	No effect	Not applicable	Not applicable	No effect	No effect	Not applicable	Not applicable
Repeated flex in stand (FIS)	No	No effect	Yes—with every repetition	No effect	Increase	Peripheralize	Yes	No effect
Repeated extension in stand (EIS)	No	No effect	No	No effect	Increase	Centralize	Yes	Increase extension
Repeated flexion in lying (FIL)	No	No effect	Yes—with every repetition	No effect	No	No effect	Yes	No effect
Repeated extension in lying (EIL)	No	No effect	No	No effect	Yes	Centralize	Yes	Increase extension

the clinician needs to know how the movement affected the baseline pain. When the patient has baseline pain, potential responses include:

1. Increase/decrease or no effect during loading (directional movement)
2. Centralize/peripheralize or no effect during or after loading
3. Pain abolished as a result of the loading
4. Better/worse or no effect after loading
5. End-range pain yes/no during loading
6. Mechanical response—increase/decrease of range of motion or no effect after loading
7. Pain response—worse/not worse or better/not better after loading

These responses will lead to the appropriate conclusion regarding syndrome classification, which then directs the treatment approach.

The following patient case illustrates the McKenzie examination and subsequent treatment process. The patient is an 18-year-old baseball catcher, currently unable to practice baseball (catching) for longer than 30 minutes. Batting is unaffected. He reports low-level aching into the lumbar region and buttocks with occasional tingling into the right posterior thigh and knee, which is intermittent but always increases after baseball practice. Playing baseball (catching), driving a car, sitting at school, and doing forward-bending activities make it worse, and walking/movement makes it better. He reports symptoms are getting worse. He reports a history of a lumbar contusion during football season, with pain resolution until attending a baseball catching camp six weeks earlier. This case presentation illustrates two possible presentations of low back–related signs and symptoms to demonstrate how a derangement and dysfunction may initially appear similar but display differences during the mechanical movement testing (Table 75.4).

Additional notes about the case patient's examination are as follows:

1. Trunk side gliding was not tested at this point because no limitations of range of motion were noted with this movement, and flexion and extension in the sagittal plane did not affect the pain.
2. Neurologic testing revealed no deficits in sensation, muscle strength, reflexes, or nerve tension tests.

Based on the physical examination chart (see Table 75.4), the patient could respond two ways. In the dysfunction columns, a flexion dysfunction is indicated by consistent end-range pain with repeated flexion demonstrated both in standing and in lying. The range of motion deficits associated with a dysfunction do not change quickly because repeated stress of the tight soft tissue over a few months' time is needed to make gains in motion. Repeated extension will have no effect on the tissue because it is putting slack on the tightened tissue rather than stress on the tissue as occurs with repeated flexion testing. The dysfunction syndrome is analogous to adhesive capsulitis of the shoulder and is painful only at end range of motion, and increasing the extensibility of tissue is a slow process.

The derangement columns reveal a unilateral asymmetric to the knee derangement. The key movement tests leading to this conclusion were repeated flexion in standing, which peripheralized and increased pain, and repeated extension in an unloaded position, which centralized the pain and improved range of motion into extension. A few bouts of repeated movements may change the range of motion losses present in a derangement, indicating that the derangement is being reduced. The reader may wonder why flexion in standing increased and peripheralized pain when flexion in an unloaded position did not in the derangement syndrome presentation in this athlete. When standing, the effects of gravity provide a greater cranial-to-caudal spinal force, as compared to flexion in an unloaded position, which eliminates the effects of gravity and forces occur in the caudal-to-cranial direction. In another apparent contradiction, in the derangement syndrome presentation, extension in standing may make the patient worse and extension in lying will centralize the pain. This is because when prone and performing extension, the line of force is assisted by gravity and almost perpendicular to the plane of the motion segments. The weight of the pelvis and abdomen also assists in applying an extension force to the lumbar vertebrae. It is important to have the athlete totally relax the buttock and lumbar muscles during the extension in lying movements to allow full lumbar extension and the mechanical benefits of this position. In standing extension, the line of force as assisted by gravity occurs in a cranial-to-caudal direction, and the patient is not able to fully relax the trunk musculature. Therefore, the mechanical forces exerted on the spine have far less extension mechanical benefits.

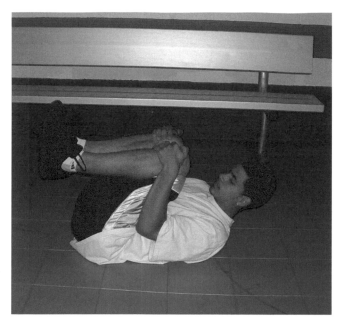

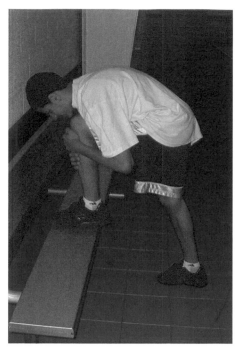

Fig. 75.4   Supine double knee to chest (flexion) stretch: Stretch force applied caudal to cranial to emphasize tension to the buttocks and lumbar region.

Fig. 75.5   Flexion in step standing: The leg to be placed up on the bench is opposite to the side of flexion dysfunction. As shown, the patient has a right-sided flexion limitation so the left foot is placed on the bench.

INTERVENTION

As can be seen in the evaluation section, it is essential to perform a detailed repeated movement testing process to expose the mechanical deficits and then direct intervention. The patient depicted in this case had signs and symptoms of both dysfunction and derangement during the subjective evaluation, and the differences were not exposed until the repeated movement testing. The appropriate treatment for the flexion dysfunction consists of stretching the soft tissue of the posterior lumbar region and the buttocks to restore normal elongation of these tissues. The treatment process consists of a minimum of daily stretching of the lumbar region and buttock musculature, and the direction of preference is lumbar flexion.

The various stretches may include:
1. Double knee to chest in supine lying (Fig. 75.4)
2. Step standing trunk flexion with involved side on ground and uninvolved leg on bench, in this case right leg on ground (Fig. 75.5)
3. Quadruped stretch using a bench to anchor the upper body to provide overpressure to and elongation of the trunk (Fig. 75.6); this type of stretch also can be done standing by anchoring hands on the fence at the baseball field (Fig. 75.7)
4. Lumbar extension following all flexion exercises to prevent development of a derangement (see next set of exercises)

The patient depicted in this case could easily have an alternative presentation, as noted in the derangement column of Table 75.4. This alternative classification is unilateral asymmetric above the knee derangement. This syndrome would be revealed with repeated trunk flexion, which would have increased and peripheralized the pain, whereas lumbar extension in an unloaded position would have decreased and centralized the pain. In a derangement presentation, the direction of preference for treatment is lumbar extension. Some of the exercises appropriate for this patient are:

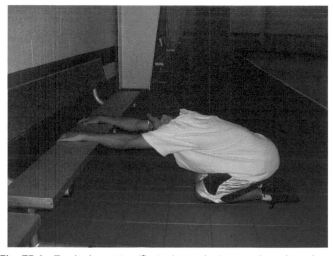

Fig. 75.6   Trunk elongation (flexion) stretch: Arms anchored overhead by grasping a bench, forward flex, and lean back to apply overpressure stretch to the soft tissues of the posterior trunk.

1. Prone press-ups without or with overpressure; note in the picture the overpressure is being applied by a belt, which is secured by another person (Fig. 75.8)
2. Standing lumbar extension using a baseball bat for overpressure (Fig. 75.9)
3. Standing lumbar extension using a wall to sag into (Fig. 75.10)

The dosing of all of these exercises is dependent on the acuity status of the patient and not discussed here because it is variable. The McKenzie textbook has an excellent section on this topic using a traffic-light analogy to guide decision making for the appropriate intensity of testing movements and treatment choices (McKenzie and May 2004). Other

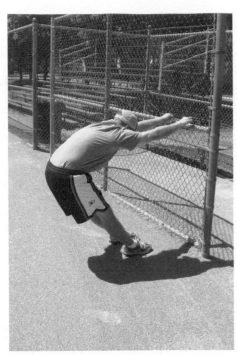

Fig. 75.7   Trunk elongation (flexion) stretch alternative: Arms anchored on a fence at the baseball field allows the athlete to stretch before or during performance of his sport.

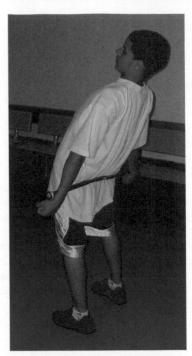

Fig. 75.9   Standing lumbar extension (loaded position) with overpressure: Note use of baseball bat by patient to apply overpressure. Place bat just inferior to the spinal level at which extension force is being applied.

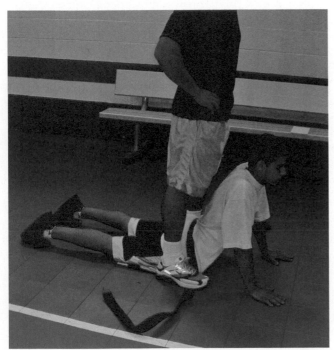

Fig. 75.8   Lumbar extension using prone press-ups (unloaded position): Note the overpressure applied by the belt, which is being secured by a teammate. Place belt just inferior to the spinal level at which extension force is being applied.

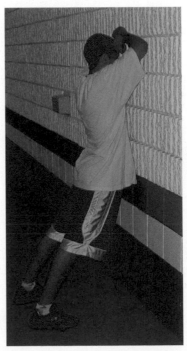

Fig. 75.10   Lumbar extension (loaded): In standing position, athlete uses a passive motion to allow trunk to lean into wall while feet remain stationary, toes 6 to 12 inches away from wall. This allows the lumbar spine to "sag" passively into extension while the trunk muscles remain relaxed.

exercises appropriate for this patient may exist, but those presented emphasize the importance of directional preference to abolish signs and symptoms and return to full function.

It should be emphasized that the direction of preference guides intervention until the patient's symptoms are abolished and stable, whether treating for a derangement or a dysfunction. When symptoms abate and are stable, the McKenzie approach emphasizes restoring full function and full range of motion in *all* directions and prevention of reoccurrence through patient education and overall conditioning.

The McKenzie approach is based on directional preference and repeated mechanical movements. Directional forces are applied either by the patient or an external device, such as a belt or a physical therapist's pressure during joint mobilization. Repeated movements are most often dynamic in nature, but some patients may respond best to static holding in certain mechanical positions. Patient education and postural restoration are key components of the McKenzie approach, as in most physical therapy approaches.

SUMMARY

Treatment of a patient with lumbar pain is multidimensional. The McKenzie approach is an efficient method for determining the treatment pathway and resolving the symptoms and functional limitations. The goal of the McKenzie technique is to determine treatment direction of preference for mechanical treatment and distinguish what mechanical syndrome exists, thus directing the treatment pathway to maximize efficiency and return to function. The case presentation demonstrates that a thorough mechanical or movement testing process is essential for exposing the mechanical deficits. As with other treatment philosophies, the McKenzie approach also utilizes patient education, general conditioning, neuromuscular training, and prevention techniques with the goal of minimizing the risk of recurrent injury.

REFERENCES

A complete reference list is available at https://expertconsult .inkling.com/.

Rehabilitation Following Lumbar Disc Surgery

Adriaan Louw, PT, MAppSc (Physio), CSMT

LUMBAR DISC SURGERY

Low back pain (LBP) is the most widely reported musculoskel-etal disorder in the world, and it is reported that 70% to 80% of all people will develop LBP during their lifetime (Deyo et al. 2006). Epidemiologic data show that the prevalence of LBP is not decreasing; it is still at epidemic proportions and is an increasingly debilitating and costly problem. With persistent pain and failed conservative management, patients with LBP may consider spinal surgery.

Spinal surgery is common in the United States. The likelihood of having back surgery in the United States is at least 40% higher than in any other country and more than five times higher than in the United Kingdom (Ostelo et al. 2008). Several studies have shown that lumbar surgery is more effective for leg pain (radicu-lopathy) than for LBP (Gibson et al. 2007, Ostelo et al. 2008). The primary surgical intervention for lumbar radiculopathy is lumbar laminectomy (full removal of the lamina) or lumbar laminotomy (partial removal of the lamina) with or without discectomy. The primary objective of a lumbar laminectomy or laminotomy with discectomy is to decompress the adjacent nerve root. The lami-nectomy or laminotomy allows the surgeon to access the inter-vertebral disc, which may partly be the cause of the nerve root compromise (Gibson et al. 2007, Ostelo et al. 2008).

Studies of lumbar disc surgery primarily for radiculopathy have shown that this surgical intervention has between a 60% and 90% success rate (Ostelo et al. 2008). These figures show that following lumbar disc surgery 10% to 40% of patients have a poor outcome, with resulting pain, loss of movement, and loss of function (Ostelo et al. 2003, Ostelo et al. 2008). Patients with continued pain and disability following lumbar discec-tomy often are referred to physical therapy for further treatment (Ostelo et al. 2008).

Studies measuring outcomes of lumbar discectomy have pro-vided a greater insight into the remaining disabilities after lum-bar discectomy and include back pain, leg pain, difficulty with walking tolerance, neurologic recovery (Fu et al. 2008), spinal instability resulting from decompressive surgery, and patient dissatisfaction (Atlas et al. 2005). It is these postoperative issues that physical therapists should aim to address with postopera-tive rehabilitation.

CURRENT BEST EVIDENCE: POSTDISCECTOMY REHABILITATION

With the increased cost of health care, third party payers are demanding more from providers. Enter the age of evidence-based medicine (EBM), which is defined by Sackett (1998) as "the conscientious, explicit and judicious use of current best evidence in making decisions about the care of the individual patient." The establishment of EBM led to a hierarchy of evi-dence. According to the hierarchy of EBM, systematic reviews of randomized controlled trials (RCT) or high-quality RCTs provide the highest form of evidence.

When developing a postoperative rehabilitation program for patients who have had lumbar discectomy, it is appropriate to start the process with a review of the highest forms of evidence. In 2014 a Cochrane review examined high-quality RCTs to determine the current best evidence for postdiscectomy reha-bilitation (Oosterhuis 2014). The review found the following:

- Low-quality evidence that a postoperative rehabilitation pro-gram consisting of exercise is more effective than no treat-ment for pain control at short-term follow-up.
- Low-quality evidence that postoperative exercise is benefi-cial in restoring function at short-term follow-up.
- 3% to 12% of patients in the postoperative programs (22 RCTs) suffered a reherniation, most times resulting in a sub-sequent reoperation.
- Low-quality evidence that high-intensity exercises are slight-ly more effective than low-intensity exercises for pain and disability at short-term follow-up.
- Low-quality evidence that there is no difference between supervised and home exercises for short-term pain relief or functional improvement.

The Cochrane review concluded that exercise programs starting 4 to 6 weeks after the operation led to a faster decrease in pain and disability in the short term.

The Cochrane review is important. For third party payers, it provides evidence that postoperative rehabilitation may be of short-term benefit for their clients, and for surgeons it shows that not only is postoperative rehabilitation effective in decreas-ing pain and disability in the short term, but also it does not lead to reoperations. Unfortunately, there is an "undercurrent" in the surgical community that rehabilitation is not only "not effec-tive" but also may actually make patients worse. This review, using the current best evidence, did not show any adverse reac-tions. Postoperative rehabilitation is a safe and effective means of decreasing pain and disability for patients who have had lum-bar disc surgery. Physical therapists, however, are left with sev-eral clinical questions:

- What is the exact content of the rehabilitation programs?
- Which exercises should be performed?
- Because clinical practice tends to be multimodal (includes manual therapy, education, modalities, and so forth), which other treatments should be used along with the exercise?
- How long should rehabilitation last?
- How frequent should rehabilitation sessions be?
- Which treatments may result in better long-term outcomes?

The Cochrane review highlights the need for continued research, heterogeneous studies, and answers to questions similar to these. Evidence-based medicine also has limitations. Many authors and researchers warn against relying on EBM alone. A major concern regarding EBM is the "mechanical" application of protocols without taking into regard the patient and his or her needs. Quantitative research focuses on the hierarchy of EBM. Qualitative research aims to investigate issues related to the needs of the patient—treating the patient as a human and not merely a subject in a research study. It is, however, proposed that a modern clinician should combine the best of both worlds—the research/evidence from the quantitative side of the equation and the experience and ability to interact and provide care to the patient on the qualitative side (Fig. 76.1). The reality is that many treatment approaches still lack evidence, yet clinically they may have benefit for the patient when used in an evidence-based framework. The postoperative rehabilitation description that follows can best be described as a combination of current best evidence for treating patients (Ostelo et al. 2008) who have had discectomy with evidence from treatments used for treating LBP and application of sound clinical reasoning.

THE POSTDISCECTOMY "PROTOCOL"

A good starting point for the development of a postoperative treatment plan for a patient who has had discectomy is to realize that every patient is different. Therapists should fight the urge to develop a "protocol." Each patient presents in physical therapy with many variables including type of surgery, pain rating, expectations, experiences, goals, psychosocial issues, and so on. This does not imply that therapists can include any or all treatments but should choose treatments carefully from a list of established guidelines based on the aforementioned section.

Subjective Evaluation: Although the goal of this chapter is to describe the treatment of a patient post discectomy, therapists should also carefully consider the evaluation. This is at the heart of the issue that every patient is different. The evaluation combines subjective and objective findings and is used in the development of an appropriate individualized treatment regimen for a particular patient. The subjective examination used for a patient after discectomy should not be much different from that for a typical patient with LBP, except for questions related to the surgery, precautions and limitations as set forth by the surgeon, information regarding postoperative visits, tests and interactions with the surgeon, and questions related to outcomes following the surgery (i.e., meet his or her expectations).

Outcomes Measures: It is highly recommended that therapists use outcomes measures, especially outcomes measures that have been validated in research. The outcomes measures provide reliable information regarding disability, prognosis, and even management options. In many cases third party payers insist that therapists use outcomes measures, and physicians also prefer progress notes that use outcomes measures. For patients who have had lumbar discectomy, therapists may consider the following:

- **The Oswestry Disability Index (ODI):** The ODI has been used extensively in measuring functional outcomes following lumbar discectomy (Gibson et al. 2007, Ostelo et al. 2008), and the ODI has been shown to be a valid and reliable measure of disability related to LBP (Vianin 2008).
- **The Roland Morris Disability Questionnaire (RMDQ):** The RMDQ is widely used to measure function related to spinal disorders and has been shown to be a reliable and valid method for measurement of self-perceived disability resulting from LBP (Nambi 2013).
- **Fear Avoidance Beliefs Questionnaire (FABQ):** The FABQ is a 16-item questionnaire that was designed to quantify fear and avoidance beliefs in individuals with LBP. The FABQ has two subscales, a seven-item scale to measure fear-avoidance beliefs about work and a four-item scale to measure fear-avoidance beliefs about physical activity. Higher scores represent an increase in fear-avoidance beliefs. The FABQ is a valid and reliable measure of fear-avoidance beliefs (Grotle et al. 2006).

Physical examination: The aim of the physical examination is to help establish the diagnosis, provide prognostication, guide treatment, screen for precautions/contraindications, and establish rapport with the patient. Care should be taken during the examination to develop a sequence of physical tests that do the following:

- Help the therapist establish a diagnosis. The physical examination is an extension of the subjective examination and helps the therapist validate his or her hypothesis as to the problems the patient has.
- Take into consideration safety and precautions. Care should be taken to use movement-based tests to aid in the decision making yet not exacerbate the patient's condition or violate any precautions or contraindications as set forth by the surgeon.
- Guide treatment. The physical tests for the patient having discectomy should aim to provide information that will help guide treatment, such as decreased motor control at the spinal level of the surgery. The therapist should use tests to examine the patient's ability to perform proper motor control at the affected level, which, if deficient, should be addressed during the treatment.

Based on the list of postoperative disabilities, current best evidence, and clinical experience, the following list of treatments may be seen as a starting point. Therapists should carefully review the list and choose treatments based on the patient's

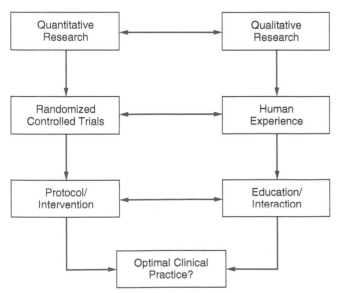

Fig. 76.1 Conceptual model of combining quantitative and qualitative research into clinical practice.

clinical presentation, surgeon's guidelines, their own clinical experience, and patient's goals.

- Education
- Exercise (spinal stabilization, range of motion, aquatic therapy, and cardiovascular)
- Walking program
- Manual therapy
- Neural tissue mobilization
- Modalities

EDUCATION

Education is therapy. Education has long been used to try to help alleviate the disability associated with LBP. In the orthopedic domain, there are a number of studies on the effect of education on pain and disability, with outcomes ranging from "excellent" to "poor." Unfortunately, most educational programs used in orthopedics use anatomic and biomechanical models for addressing pain, which not only have shown limited efficacy but may even increase patient fears and thus negatively affect their outcomes. Cognitive behavioral therapy (CBT), which aims to reassure patients and address fears related to movement, pathology, and function, has also been used to educate patients with LBP, although the outcomes of CBT are similar to those for non-CBT education, which shows limited efficacy when treating LBP.

Recent research, however, has evaluated the use of neuroscience education in decreasing pain and disability among patients with LBP. Although neuroscience education is aimed at reducing the fear associated with LBP surgery, it differs from CBT by focusing not on anatomic or biomechanical models but on neurophysiology and the processing/representation of pain. Studies that use neuroscience education have been shown to decrease fear and change a patient's perception of his or her pain. Additionally, neuroscience education has been shown to have an immediate effect on improvements in patients' attitudes about pain, improvements in pain cognition and physical performance, increased pain thresholds during physical tasks, improved outcomes of therapeutic exercises, and significant reduction in widespread brain activity characteristic of a pain experience. Furthermore, these neuroscience studies have shown results to extend beyond the short term and to be maintained at 1-year follow-up (Louw et al. 2011).

Therapists involved in treating patients who have had discectomy should spend time explaining issues related to the discectomy to the patient. Four broad categories are identified:

- *Diagnosis:* Patients want to know what is going on. A patient should receive information regarding the surgery in a nonthreatening way. A simple explanation of the surgical procedure and issues related to postoperative disability (e.g., why the leg is still numb) should be given.
- *Prognosis:* Patients want to know how long it will take for recovery. The therapist should provide information on the plan of care, especially time frames and goals. It may be as simple as explaining that therapy will consist of two visits per week for four weeks, at which time a certain disability (e.g., forward flexion) can be expected to improve by a certain amount.
- *Self-care:* Patients want to know what they can do to help themselves. The therapist should provide the patient with information regarding at-home instructions. This may include information on limiting sitting, a walking program, applica-

tion of heat or cold per surgeon guidelines, performing gentle stretches, and more. This is an important part in empowering patients and helping them develop coping strategies.

- *Rehabilitation:* Patients want to know what the clinician can do for them, and the therapist should provide a detailed description of the optimal treatment plan, including content, frequency, duration, and progress.

The primary objective of the educational session is to decrease unnecessary fear. Several studies have shown that fear is a major contributor in the development of persistent pain. Typically the four main issues described are conveyed to the patient during the first visit after completion of the evaluation. Additionally, therapists need to realize that as they embark on the "more physical" part of therapy (e.g., exercise, hands on, and so forth), they have opportunities to continually reinforce the educational messages. Finally, it is also important to realize the role of the acute care physical therapist. Patients encounter physical therapists in the immediate postoperative period, and although most interactions are brief during gait and transfer training in a typical 1- to 2-day hospitalization after surgery, these interactions can be used as effective means of providing high-quality education. Studies have shown that patients undergoing surgery have increased levels of fear and that educational strategies in or around the time of surgery by health care personnel are effective in decreasing fear. Several studies have also shown the effect of fear on LBP (Wertli 2014).

EXERCISE

The Cochrane review and several high-quality RCTs have shown that exercise is an effective means of treating patients with persistent disability following lumbar surgery (Dolan et al. 2000). In patients with chronic LBP (nonsurgical), there is also good evidence for the use of exercise for decreasing pain and disability. The exact content of the exercise program may consist of spinal stabilization exercises; cardiovascular exercises; general conditioning; and stretches of the lumbar spine, adjacent thoracic spine, and hip joints.

Spinal stabilization: Several RCTs have shown that a specific segmental spinal stabilization approach centered on retraining appropriate activation of the transversus abdominis (TA) and/or multifidus (MF) muscles is more effective than no treatment or multimodal treatment programs not explicitly focused on strengthening exercises (O'Sullivan et al. 1997). Specific segmental spinal stabilization focuses on two particular muscles—lumbar TA and MF—and their interaction through the thoracolumbar fascia plays a key role in segmental stabilization. The TA is the deepest of the abdominal muscles, and via its insertion into the lateral raphe posteriorly and the posterior lamina of the sheath of the rectus abdominis (RA) anteriorly, it exerts a compressive force on the abdominal contents and a pull on the thoracolumbar fascia. The lumbar MF contracting within the tensioned thoracolumbar fascia can be seen as a hydraulic effect leading to a stiffening of the lumbar spinal segments.

It is important to realize that spinal stabilization is motor control, well-defined by Hodges (Richardson et al. 2004): "Spinal stabilization is firing the right muscles at the right time, in the right sequence, for the right amount of time and disengaging at the appropriate time." Studies utilizing fine-wire needle EMG, diagnostic ultrasound (US), and magnetic resonance imaging (MRI) have been used to show that the TA and MF have unique characteristics that enable these muscles to provide stability (protection) to the spine mainly because of their mechanical/anatomic attachment to the spine and unique muscle properties (Okubo et al. 2010). With upper extremity or lower extremity use, the TA is active irrespective of the direction of the movement, implying a unique function. Additionally, during trunk motion (flexion and extension) the TA is active in both directions, compared to the prime movers, such as RA, external oblique (EO), internal oblique (IO), and/or erector spinae (ES), which activate during flexion or extension. This suggests that the TA performs a unique function not shared by the other abdominal muscles. Furthermore, both the TA and MF have high concentrations of slow-twitch fibers and higher levels of oxidative enzymes, which implies that they are uniquely designed to provide low-load, prolonged tonic contractions and underscores their ability to provide stability to the spine and not act as prime movers of the spine. For a complete and thorough review on stabilization, consult Richardson et al. (2004) and the section describing segmental spinal stabilization.

In patients with LBP, motor control and muscle property changes are observed in both TA and MF:

- Contraction of the TA is absent from the premovement period, failing to prepare the spine for the perturbation resulting from limb movement.
- In LBP, the TA begins to contract in a similar manner to other abdominal muscles that control direction-specific forces acting on the spine.
- In normal function, the TA contracts with longer-duration, continuous, low-level tonic contraction. In LBP, the TA contracts in distinct phasic bursts.
- In LBP, TA reaction time is affected by level of preparation, indicating a change in the central nervous system (CNS) control.
- Changes in control occur irrespective of specific pathology.
- Less activity is observed in the MF in subjects with LBP.
- Less activity is noted in the MF at unstable levels during concentric back activity, suggesting decreased muscular protection at the hypermobile level.
- The MF demonstrated greater fatigue rates in patients with LBP compared to normal control subjects.
- Biopsy studies of lumbar MF muscle conducted on patients with LBP undergoing lumbar surgery found selective atrophy of type I muscle fibers.
- Changes occur in internal structure of type I fibers without significant change in size.
- Using various imaging techniques such as computerized tomography (CT), MRI, and diagnostic US, LBP has been found to result in side-specific and level-specific atrophy (decreased cross-sectional area) (Fig. 76.2).
- Recovery of MF size is not spontaneous with pain relief.
- In LBP, the loss of automatic preparatory control of segmental spinal stiffness is corrected by normal functioning of the TA and MF.

How does all of this apply to spinal surgery? Several issues are related to discectomy and spinal stabilization:

- It could be argued that patients who undergo lumbar discectomy would most likely have had LBP prior to surgery, most likely during the early phases of seeking help through therapy, pain management, and self-care. Spinal stabilization research suggests that by the time surgery is performed, the patient most likely would have had significant decreased motor control (stability) in the lumbar spine (Gejo et al. 1999).

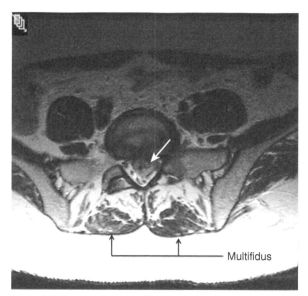

Fig. 76.2 T2-weighted image of central disc bulge (*arrow*) at L5/S1. Note the difference in the size and composition of the multifidus. In low back pain the multifidus has been shown to shut down side and level specifically and does not spontaneously return after surgery.

- Dysfunction in the TA and MF is irrespective of the specific tissue pathology. The issue is pain. This further supports the notion of dysfunction in the local stabilizing system after surgery (Gille et al. 2007).
- Return of motor control and muscle atrophy is not spontaneous after loss of pain. Even if the surgery resolves the pain, the stabilizing mechanism does not automatically "start up again." Patients should undergo a series of physical therapy visits after surgery to retrain motor control activity of the local stabilizing mechanisms.
- Studies have shown that fear of pain and catastrophizing also alter motor control. Several studies have shown that patients undergoing spinal surgery have high levels of anxiety and fear, which directly affects the spinal stabilizing system (Alodaibi et al. 2013). Patients need both spinal stabilization and education to address fear, thus the multimodal approach used in therapy.

The ability of the TA and MF to provide a low-level, bilateral tonic contraction should be evaluated in the patient who has had discectomy. Three tests are described by Richardson et al. (2004): the prone abdominal draw-in maneuver, segmental MF test, and leg-loading test. These are described in detail in the section on core stabilization training. When a dysfunction in the local stabilizing mechanism is found, therapists should work through a systematic process of retraining the local stabilizing mechanism:

- Retrain local muscles for control. Therapists can use biofeedback, palpation, verbal cues, or even diagnostic US to retrain the ability of the TA to contract. Focus should be on low load, tonic hold.
- Progress to weightbearing exercise. Once the patient demonstrates local stabilization control, therapists should progress to weightbearing exercise. This is a major shift from what has been taught traditionally in therapy. The basis for this is that during weight bearing, local one-joint, stabilizing muscles initiate better and faster compared to open kinetic chain exercises (Richardson et al. 2004). Additionally it is functional.

- During this phase, focus on slow, controlled movements.
- Focus on endurance. Progress the rehabilitation by increasing the contraction time of the TA.
- Because stabilization is a motor control activity, focus on repetition, constantly teaching the patient to engage the stabilizers while doing tasks, so that the contractions become automatic.
- Focus on functional tasks and positions.
- The final phase should focus on open kinetic chain exercises.

Range of motion exercises/stretches: Very little is known about the effect of treatments aimed at maintaining or increasing ROM of the adjacent joints to the surgical levels. Given the fact that numerous biomechanical studies have implicated the high incidence of adjacent joint problems (transitional syndrome) following surgery, clinicians should consider treatments aimed at increasing (borrowing) or at least maintaining ROM of the joints above and below the surgery site. This could be accomplished with exercises or manual therapy approaches. It is recommended that exercises be started with the patient supine. Several biomechanical studies have shown that supine positions, compared to sitting and standing, result in decreased disc pressure, which would be advisable for a patient recovering from disc surgery. Exercises that may be considered include:

- Single knee to chest: Stretches the hip joint and hamstrings, promotes hip flexion, and helps mobilize the proximal sciatic nerve without exposing the nerve to stretching.
- Double knee to chest: Stretches out the lower lumbar spine (erector spinae) and hips.
- Piriformis stretch: Mobilizes the hip joint and potentially alleviates continued irritation around the sciatic nerve.
- Lower trunk rotations: Provides gentle movement and circulation to the lumbar spine in a position that has little disc pressure.
- Hip flexor stretches: Tight hip flexors induce increased flexion and stretches encourage a more upright position.
- Hamstring stretches: Care is required with these exercises because nerves are extremely "blood thirsty" and do not respond well to stretch. Studies have shown that lengthening of a nerve more than 8% of its length is sufficient to slow down blood flow (Jou et al. 2000). Because most discectomies are performed for radiculopathy, therapists are advised to use static hamstring stretches only for patients with LBP and not leg pain. Patients with leg pain may respond better to neural tissue mobilization, which is discussed later.
- Pelvic tilts: Pelvic tilt exercises should not be viewed as stabilization (e.g., "Push your spine down against the bed and hold"). It has been established that a co-contraction of the TA and MF does not cause the spine to increase or decrease its lordosis. Pelvic tilt exercises should be seen as a novel, early, comfortable way of introducing movement to a patient after discectomy in a safe, clinical environment.

Additional considerations for basic, early comfortable exercises that therapists should carefully evaluate include the load on the spine (e.g., disc pressure is much higher in sitting), goals of the exercise, and precautions and limitations provided by the surgeon (e.g., lifting restrictions).

Aquatic therapy: Aquatic therapy should be viewed as an extension of exercise, the same exercises described before (stabilization and ROM) but in a different environment. There is evidence that aquatic therapy is beneficial in treating patients with chronic conditions such as chronic LBP and fibromyalgia. Aquatic therapy's benefits include the following:

- Pain control: A commonly held belief regarding spinal pain is that abnormal or repetitive loading of the spine is associated with trauma, degeneration, and pain. Aquatic therapy by virtue of its ability to "load the spine less" can be used to minimize load on the spine and thus decrease nociceptive input from the injured area, thus in essence alleviating pain. Because pain is such a potent inhibiting factor to motor control, patients may be able to initiate stabilization sooner as their pain is better controlled in the aquatic environment.
- Range of motion: With decreased pain (above) and increased buoyancy, patients may be inclined to move more freely and perform exercise more freely.
- Relaxation of paraspinal muscles: The studies on stabilization have shown that global muscles such as the ES muscles become more active when the TA and MF shut down. It could be argued that global muscles, with higher concentrations of fast-twitch fibers, may fatigue sooner and potentially become a source of pain. The heated water in an aquatic environment may be a mechanism (along with movement) for helping "overworked" muscles such as the ES to increase circulation, flush away byproducts of the increased muscle work, and thus alleviate pain.
- Stabilization: As described earlier, patients may be able to initiate stabilization exercises sooner as a result of the pain being better controlled in the aquatic environment.
- Neuroplasticity: Current pain science research using functional MRIs (fMRI) indicates that patients with LBP have poor cortical representations of their low back in their brain. The back becomes "smudged." Exercises/movements that are done in a safe, comfortable environment may be a powerful way of remapping that particular area in the brain. Comfortable, gentle exercises done in a novel and "less painful" environment (aquatic therapy) may allow the brain to learn healthy movement and help decrease the pain. For more information, see the section on chronic spinal pain.

Cardiovascular exercises: There is considerable evidence that cardiovascular exercise is beneficial in the treatment of patients with chronic pain, including LBP. Cardiovascular exercise works on many levels to benefit a patient who has had discectomy. A major system is the hypothalamus–pituitary–adrenal (HPA) axis. With a stress response (i.e., pain), failed surgery, or concerns regarding a job or family, the pituitary gland (via the HPA axis) dumps adrenaline into the bloodstream. Adrenaline causes the heart rate and blood pressure to elevate, leading to shallower breathing and blood getting "shunted" away from postural muscles. Adrenaline leads to muscle fatigue, poor oxygenation, muscle ischemia, and increased sensitivity of the peripheral nervous system. Adrenaline is a fast-acting substance and is supplemented by another stress chemical—cortisol (Geiss et al. 2005). Although there is a "normal" diurnal cortisol curve (e.g., peaks at mid- to late morning), constant stress (e.g., pain, failed surgery) leads to altered levels of cortisol. Altered cortisol levels for prolonged periods have been linked to memory changes, appetite changes, weight gain, poor concentration and focus, mood swings, increased tissue sensitivity, poor sleep, and alteration of the immune system. So how do cardiovascular exercises work?

- Cardiovascular exercises increase blood flow and oxygenation of the tired and fatigued muscles, thus alleviating ischemia.
- Memory improves.
- Appetite changes.

- Focus and concentration improve.
- Mood is affected.
- Cytokine signaling is altered, which decreases nerve sensitivity and improves the immune system.
- Deeper breathing engages the diaphragm and less accessory muscles and improves oxygenation of the blood.

WALKING PROGRAM

- The number-one activity recommended by surgeons following lumbar discectomy is walking. The primary reason provided by surgeons is the prevention of blood clots, but a walking program can be viewed as far more important in a patient who has had discectomy.
- A walking program will help keep blood flowing and decrease the possibility of developing blood clots.
- The walking program can fit in with a cardiovascular exercise program, which will increase blood flow and oxygenation to the musculoskeletal system, brain, and nervous system.
- The adult lumbar disc is avascular, and the disc cells depend on diffusion from blood vessels at the disc's margins to supply the nutrients essential for cellular activity and viability and to remove metabolic wastes such as lactic acid. Small nutrients such as oxygen and glucose are supplied to the disc's cells entirely by diffusion. It is suggested that exercise, and especially load-bearing exercise, may help (a little) with this diffusion process (sponge effect), which would make the reciprocal motion of the pelvis during the gait cycle a viable exercise to help facilitate this process.
- Neural mobilization. There is evidence that treadmill walking is beneficial for patients with degenerative lumbar spinal stenosis. Although the exact mechanism of why this may be helpful is not fully understood, one explanation is that walking helps provide much-needed movement and thus increased blood flow to the nervous system without putting undue stress on the nerves (e.g., stretches). Normal gait requires approximately 35 degrees of hip flexion, and a walking program aimed at helping "neural mobilization" could be seen as an easy way of improving the normal movement properties of the sciatic nerve.

MANUAL THERAPY

Manual therapy for a postoperative spine is a controversial topic, especially from the surgeon's perspective. First, manual therapy should not be considered as a first-choice treatment. A therapist who treats a patient who has had discectomy with manual therapy only and neglects to incorporate treatments suggested in this section and by the current best evidence is not practicing within the current best evidence or using sound clinical reasoning skills. Second, to date, few postoperative discectomy studies have been done on the use of manual therapy. The limited available evidence suggests patients may be able to tolerate manual therapy following lumbar spine surgery without adverse effects (Coulis and Lisi 2013). It could be argued that gentle, passive manual techniques provide effects similar to those of passive stretches and exercises, but therapists should be cautioned regarding the use of strong, end-range manual techniques on the surgical level in the acute and subacute phases. This does not mean that patients may not respond favorably to manual techniques months or years later. As stated before, there is a fair amount of research indicating increased stress on the levels

adjacent to the surgical level, potentially as a means to adjust to the changes in biomechanics of the patient's spine. A well-reasoning therapist may consider manual therapy techniques on adjacent regions such as the thoracic spine and/or hip joints as a means of "borrowing" movement from those areas and thus decreasing load on the surgical level. Care should be taken to evaluate the positioning of the patients in manual therapy procedures for these regions, and the loads occurring around the surgical level should be considered.

Neural Tissue Mobilization

Neural tissue mobilization is another controversial topic, primarily because of a lack of evidence of its use in this population. It is also important that therapists realize that neural tissue mobilization is relatively "new" compared to time-tested treatments such as exercise, modalities, and spinal manual therapy. To date, only one study has been published on the effect of neural tissue mobilization on patients who have had lumbar surgery. In an RCT of neural tissue mobilization following spinal surgery, Scrimshaw and Maher (2001) showed no added benefit when neural tissue was added to the postoperative programs, yet it can be argued that the heterogeneous nature of the patients (laminectomy, discectomy, and fusion) may have affected the outcome of the techniques. There is growing evidence as to the clinical use and efficacy of neural tissue mobilization techniques in other disorders (Ellis and Hing 2008). These studies showed that active and passive neural tissue mobilization may facilitate a faster return to work and recreational activities, increase the ROM associated with the neurodynamic test, decrease the need for surgery, and decrease pain. Finally, because discectomies are primarily performed for leg pain (radiculopathy), it is important also to note that there is emerging research showing the benefit of neural tissue mobilization in numerous orthopedic patient populations, including those with LBP with radiculopathy.

The case for adding neural tissue mobilization can also center on basic science research. Basic science research indicates that a normal, healthy nervous system requires certain physical properties to function properly and when these are violated (e.g., disc, scar tissue, swelling), the nervous system becomes a source of persistent dysfunction. Three physical properties have been identified:

Space: An easy way for clinicians to view the nervous system is to envision the delicate nerves, spinal cord, and meninges all traveling within containers or passageways. For nerves to properly function, they need to have the ability to "slide" and "glide" unhindered through different areas of the body. As nerves travel through the body, they encounter many surrounding tissues including muscle, bone, ligaments, and fascia. Numerous studies have shown that if the interface is injured or damaged, it may have repercussions for the adjacent neural tissues. When these spaces are compromised and nerves sustain unwanted pressure or irritation, it may lead to the onset of symptoms. All of the treatments described previously (stretches, ROM, unloading the spine, walking, etc.) can be viewed as a means of creating space for the nervous system.

Movement: Closely linked to the space requirements is the nervous system's ability to perform complex signaling processes during physiologic movement. For many years, medicine and physical therapy have been interested in the movement properties of joints, muscles, and even fascia while the nervous system's movement capabilities were apparently overlooked. Under normal conditions nerves move quite well. Early cadaver studies showed that the nervous system is extremely well designed to handle movement. It has also been shown that the spinal canal (the "container") can lengthen approximately 30% from spinal extension to spinal flexion. Although most of the original "movement studies" were performed on cadavers, newer research is using real-time US to show that nerves not only have longitudinal movement but also significant lateral movement capabilities. Furthermore, these US studies are showing that compared to normal populations, patients with pathology have decreased neural tissue movement. The concept of neural tissue movement disorders has led to the development of structured neurodynamic tests to assess the movement capabilities of a specific nerve branch. These tests are designed to identify physical dysfunction of the nervous system. After the development and refinement of these tests, clinicians began to use them in various forms of treatment, in essence trying to restore and maintain the normal anatomic and physiologic requirements of the nervous system.

Blood flow: Neural tissue is extremely "blood thirsty." The brain and spinal cord are estimated to account for only about 2% of the total body mass, yet they consume 20% to 25% of the available oxygen in the circulating blood (Lammert 2008). Additionally, it has been shown that if a nerve is "lengthened" more than 6% to 8% of its length, blood flow in the peripheral nerve slows. If the nerve is elongated approximately 15%, blood flow may be completely occluded. Adequate blood flow, nutrition, and movement (previous section) are therefore interdependent. If blood flow to neural tissue is interrupted, it can lead to a hypoxic state, which may in turn lead to an ischemic-based pain state. Ischemic pain is a class of nociceptive pain in which lack of movement, sustained posturing, or decreased circulation creates an acidic environment (lower pH), which has been linked to pain. Based on the enormous vascular needs of the nervous system, therapists should carefully evaluate stretches and/or positions of the spine that challenge the nervous system's demand for adequate blood flow. Exercise such as a walking program and cardiovascular exercise can be seen as a means of helping the patient restore or maintain adequate blood flow to the nervous system.

From the basic science literature, it seems clear that treatment techniques aimed at restoring movement, and thus blood flow, have the potential to decrease ischemic-based pain and maintain normal movement and function of the nervous system.

An important consideration when adding neural tissue mobilization to the treatment plan for a patient who has had discectomy is nerve sensitivity. Studies have shown that proinflammatory chemicals such as phospholipase A2 (PLA2), which is released in or around the intervertebral disc during a disc herniation, causes the nerve root to lose its protective myelin sheet (Piperno et al. 1997). Additionally, sustained pressure applied to a nerve may lead to demyelination. The demyelinization may in turn lead to "peripheral sensitization" where responses to mechanical, chemical, and/or thermal stimuli are exaggerated. Apart from antiseizure and membrane-stabilizing drugs, it is hypothesized that education (engaging the brain) and gentle, comfortable, nonthreatening movements such as neural mobilization may in fact decrease mechanosensitivity of the nerves. From a physiologic and pain science perspective, the addition of gentle neural tissue mobilization into the postoperative regimen along with the cardiovascular exercise, walking, aquatic therapy, and ROM exercises should be considered.

Additional Treatments

The previous list items are not necessarily the only treatment options a therapist may consider. It is hoped that therapists also develop an understanding that treatments that use modalities such as transcutaneous electrical nerve stimulation (TENS) or electrical stimulation may be valuable adjuncts to help ease pain, which in turn may help promote motor control. Additionally, short-term brace use to help ease pain may be a consideration. (The two key elements would seem to be sound clinical reasoning and consideration of precautions and contraindications related to the specific surgery.) Thus there is not a "protocol." Some patients may need more motor control training because they had a longer preoperative period with increased pain inhibition and atrophy but little to no pain after the operation to inhibit motor control. Other patients may present with increased LBP and the therapist may spend extra time and use various strategies to decrease pain, while others may have primarily leg pain and need lots of education to decrease their fear while the physical part may focus more on neural tissue mobilization, cardiovascular exercises, and a walking program.

Timing, Dosage, and Frequency

Little evidence is available for determining the immediate start of a postoperative program. A typical surgical patient revisits his or her surgeon two to three weeks after the surgery and, if the patient still experiences disability, he or she may then be referred to physical therapy. This practical/clinical scenario suggests that patients may not show up for rehabilitation until four weeks postoperatively. This fits with studies that show that rehabilitation started four to six weeks after surgery is effective in improving short-term disabilities (Dolan et al. 2000, Kjellby-Wendt and Styf 1998). Based on the research and clinical experience, it seems plausible that such a program may run two to three times a week for six to eight weeks (Dolan et al. 2000, Kjellby-Wendt and Styf 1998). Patients should also be instructed in a home exercise program, allowing them to become self-sufficient and able to manage their own well-being as they progress through formal rehabilitation toward discharge. It should once again be emphasized that good early postoperative information is important. The acute care therapist is in an ideal position to not only help ambulate and mobilize a patient postoperatively but also to provide information that can reassure the patient, decrease fear, and set appropriate goals.

REFERENCES

A complete reference list is available at https://expertconsult.inkling.com/.

FURTHER READING

Bogduk N. Management of chronic low back pain. *Med J Aust.* 2004;180:79–83.

Brox JI, Storheim K, Grotle M, et al. Systematic review of back schools, brief education, and fear-avoidance training for chronic low back pain. *Spine J.* 2008;8:948–958.

Buchbinder R, Jolley D, Wyatt M. Volvo award winner in clinical studies: effects of a media campaign on back pain beliefs and its potential influence on the management of low back pain in general practice. *Spine.* 2001;26:2535–2542.

Busch AJ, Barber KA, Overend TJ, et al. Exercise for treating fibromyalgia syndrome. *Cochrane Database Syst Rev.* 2007:CD003786.

Butler D, ed. *The Sensitive Nervous System.* Adelaide: Noigroup Publications; 2000.

Butler D, Moseley G, ed. *Explain Pain.* Adelaide: Noigroup; 2003.

Butler DS, ed. *The Sensitive Nervous System*. Adelaide: Noigroup Publications; 2000.

Cho DY, Lin HL, Lee WY, et al. Split-spinous process laminotomy and discectomy for degenerative lumbar spinal stenosis: a preliminary report. *J Neurosurg Spine*. 2007;6:229–239.

Cleland JA, Childs JD, Palmer JA, et al. Slump stretching in the management of non-radicular low back pain: a pilot clinical trial. *Man Ther*. 2006;11:279–286.

Cohen JE, Goel V, Frank JW, et al. Group education interventions for people with low back pain. An overview of the literature. *Spine*. 1994;19:1214–1222.

Coppieters MW, Alshami AM. Longitudinal excursion and strain in the median nerve during novel nerve gliding exercises for carpal tunnel syndrome. *J Orthop Res*. 2007;25:972–980.

Coppieters MW, Bartholomeeusen KE, Stappaerts KH. Incorporating nerve-gliding techniques in the conservative treatment of cubital tunnel syndrome. *J Manipulative Physiol Ther*. 2004;27:560–568.

Coppieters MW, Butler DS. Do "sliders" slide and "tensioners" tension? An analysis of neurodynamic techniques and considerations regarding their application. *Man Ther*. 2007. http://dx.doi.org/10.1016/j.math.2006.12.008.

Coppieters MW, Stappaerts KH, Wouters LL, et al. The immediate effects of a cervical lateral glide treatment technique in patients with neurogenic cervicobrachial pain. *J Orthop Sports Phys Ther*. 2003;33:369–378.

Costa F, Sassi M, Cardia A, et al. Degenerative lumbar spinal stenosis: analysis of results in a series of 374 patients treated with unilateral laminotomy for bilateral microdecompression. *J Neurosurg Spine*. 2007;7:579–586.

Devor M, Seltzer Z. Pathophysiology of damaged nerves in relation to chronic pain. In: Wall PD, Melzack R, eds. *Textbook of Pain*. 4th ed. Edinburgh: Churchill Livingstone; 1999.

Dilley A, Odeyinde S, Greening J, et al. Longitudinal sliding of the median nerve in patients with non-specific arm pain. *Man Ther*. 2007. http://dx.doi.org/10.1016/j.math.2007.07.004.

Dommisse GF. The blood supply of the spinal cord and the consequences of failure. In: Boyling J, Palastanga N, eds. *Grieve's Modern Manual Therapy*. 2nd ed. Edinburgh: Churchill Livingstone; 1994.

Dyck PJ, Lais AC, Giannini C, et al. Structural alterations of nerve during cuff compression. *Proc Natl Acad Sci*. 1990;87:9828–9832.

Engers A, Jellema P, Wensing M, et al. Individual patient education for low back pain. *Cochrane Database Syst Rev*. 2008:CD004057.

Ferreira ML, Ferreira PH, Latimer J, et al. Comparison of general exercise, motor control exercise and spinal manipulative therapy for chronic low back pain: a randomized trial. *Pain*. 2007;131:31–37.

Flor H. The functional organization of the brain in chronic pain. In: Sandkühler J, Bromm B, Gebhart GF, eds. *Progress in Brain Research*. vol. 129. Amsterdam: Elsevier; 2000.

Fokter SK, Yerby SA. Patient-based outcomes for the operative treatment of degenerative lumbar spinal stenosis. *Eur Spine J*. 2006;15:1661–1669.

Fritz JM, Irrgang JJ. A comparison of a modified Oswestry Low Back Pain Disability Questionnaire and the Quebec Back Pain Disability Scale. *Phys Ther*. 2001;81:776–788.

George SZ, Fritz JM, Bialosky JE, et al. The effect of a fear-avoidance-based physical therapy intervention for patients with acute low back pain: results of a randomized clinical trial. *Spine*. 2003;28:2551–2560.

Goldby LJ, Moore AP, Doust J, et al. A randomized controlled trial investigating the efficiency of musculoskeletal physiotherapy on chronic low back disorder. *Spine*. 2006;31:1083–1093.

Gross AR, Aker PD, Goldsmith CH, et al. Patient education for mechanical neck disorders. *Cochrane Database Syst Rev*. 2000:CD000962.

Guyer RD, Patterson M, Ohnmeiss DD. Failed back surgery syndrome: diagnostic evaluation. *J Am Acad Orthop Surg*. 2006;14:534–543.

Hides JA, Jull GA, Richardson CA. Long-term effects of specific stabilizing exercises for first-episode low back pain. *Spine*. 2001;26:E243–E248.

Hirsch MS, Liebert RM. The physical and psychological experience of pain: the effects of labeling and cold pressor temperature on three pain measures in college women. *Pain*. 1998;77:41–48.

Johnson RE, Jones GT, Wiles NJ, et al. Active exercise, education, and cognitive behavioral therapy for persistent disabling low back pain: a randomized controlled trial. *Spine*. 2007;32:1578–1585.

Koes BW, van Tulder MW, van der Windt WM, et al. The efficacy of back schools: a review of randomized clinical trials. *J Clin Epidemiol*. 1994;47:851–862.

Kornberg C, Lew P. The effect of stretching neural structures on grade one hamstring injuries. *J Orthop Sports Phys Ther*. 1989;10:481–487.

Liddle SD, Gracey JH, Baxter GD. Advice for the management of low back pain: a systematic review of randomised controlled trials. *Man Ther*. 2007;12:310–327.

Lundborg G, Rydevik B. Effects of stretching the tibial nerve of the rabbit. A preliminary study of the intraneural circulation and the barrier function of the perineurium. *J Bone Joint Surg Br*. 1973;55:390–401.

Lurie JD, Birkmeyer NJ, Weinstein JN. Rates of advanced spinal imaging and spine surgery. *Spine*. 2003;28:616–620.

McGregor AH, Burton AK, Sell P, et al. The development of an evidence-based patient booklet for patients undergoing lumbar discectomy and uninstrumented decompression. *Eur Spine J*. 2007;16:339–346.

McGregor AH, Dicken B, Jamrozik K. National audit of post-operative management in spinal surgery. *BMC Musculoskelet Disord*. 2006;7:47.

Melzack R. Pain and the neuromatrix in the brain. *J Dent Educ*. 2001;65:1378–1382.

Moseley GL. Evidence for a direct relationship between cognitive and physical change during an education intervention in people with chronic low back pain. *Eur J Pain*. 2004;8:39–45.

Moseley GL. Joining forces—combining cognition-targeted motor control training with group or individual pain physiology education: a successful treatment for chronic low back pain. *J Man Manip Therap*. 2003. in press.

Moseley GL. A pain neuromatrix approach to patients with chronic pain. *Man Ther*. 2003;8:130–140.

Moseley GL. Widespread brain activity during an abdominal task markedly reduced after pain physiology education: fMRI evaluation of a single patient with chronic low back pain. *Aust J Physiother*. 2005;51:49–52.

Moseley GL, Hodges PW, Nicholas MK. Evidence for a direct relationship between cognitive and physical change during an education intervention in people with chronic low back pain. *Eur J Pain*. 2004;8:39–45.

Moseley GL, Hodges PW, Nicholas MK. A randomized controlled trial of intensive neurophysiology education in chronic low back pain. *Clin J Pain*. 2004;20:324–330.

Moseley GL, Nicholas MK, Hodges PW. Does anticipation of back pain predispose to back trouble? *Brain*. 2004;127:2339–2347.

Moseley GL, Nicholas MK, Hodges PW. A randomized controlled trial of intensive neurophysiology education in chronic low back pain. *Clin J Pain*. 2004;20:324–330.

Moseley GL. Combined physiotherapy and education is efficacious for chronic low back pain. *Aust J Physiother*. 2002;48:297–302.

Ogata K, Naito M. Blood flow of peripheral nerve: effects of dissection, stretching and compression. *J Hand Surg [Am]*. 1986;11B:10–14.

Oliveira A, Gevirtz R, Hubbard D. A psycho-educational video used in the emergency department provides effective treatment for whiplash injuries. *Spine*. 2006;31:1652–1657.

Ostelo RW, de Vet HC, Waddell G, et al. Rehabilitation following first-time lumbar disc surgery: a systematic review within the framework of the Cochrane collaboration. *Spine*. 2003;28:209–218.

Ostelo RW, de Vet HC, Waddell G, et al. Rehabilitation after lumbar disc surgery. *Cochrane Database Syst Rev*. 2007:CD003007.

Poiraudeau S, Rannou F, Baron G, et al. Fear-avoidance beliefs about back pain in patients with subacute low back pain. *Pain*. 2006;124:305–311.

Richardson C, Jull GA, et al. *Therapeutic Exercise for Spinal Segmental Stabilization in Low Back Pain*. London: Churchill Livingstone; 1999.

Roland M, Morris R. A study of the natural history of back pain. Part I: development of a reliable and sensitive measure of disability in low-back pain. *Spine (Phila Pa 1976)*. 1983;8:141–144.

Rozmaryn LM, Dovelle S, Rothman ER, et al. Nerve and tendon gliding exercises and the conservative management of carpal tunnel syndrome. *J Hand Ther*. 1998;11:171–179.

Sackett DL, Rosenberg WMC, Muir JA, et al. Evidence based medicine: what it is and what it isn't. *Br Med J*. 1996;312:71–72.

Schofferman J, Reynolds J, Herzog R, et al. Failed back surgery: etiology and diagnostic evaluation. *Spine J*. 2003;3:400–403.

Shabat S, Arinzon Z, Folman Y, et al. Long-term outcome of decompressive surgery for lumbar spinal stenosis in octogenarians. *Eur Spine J*. 2008;17:193–198.

Shacklock M. *Clinical Neurodynamics*. Edinburgh: Elsevier; 2005.

Shacklock M. Improving application of neurodynamic (neural tension) testing and treatments: a message to researchers and clinicians. *Man Ther*. 2005;10:175–179.

Shaughnessy M, Caulfield B. A pilot study to investigate the effect of lumbar stabilisation exercise training on functional ability and quality of life in patients with chronic low back pain. *Int J Rehabil Res*. 2004;27:297–301.

Silagy C. Evidence vs experience. *Australian Doctor*. 1999.

Smith GC, Pell JP. Parachute use to prevent death and major trauma related to gravitational challenge: systematic review of randomised controlled trials. *BMJ*. 2003;327:1459–1461.

Stuge B, Veierod MB, Laerum E, et al. The efficacy of a treatment program focusing on specific stabilizing exercises for pelvic girdle pain after pregnancy: a two-year follow-up of a randomized clinical trial. *Spine (Phila Pa 1976)*. 2004;29:E197–E203.

Sweeney J, Harms A. Persistent mechanical allodynia following injury of the hand. Treatment through mobilization of the nervous system. *J Hand Ther.* 1996;9:328–338.

Thomas JS, France CR. Pain-related fear is associated with avoidance of spinal motion during recovery from low back pain. *Spine.* 2007;32:E460–E466.

Troup JDG. Biomechanics of the lumbar spinal canal. *Clin Biomech.* 1986;1:31–43.

Udermann BE, Spratt KF, Donelson RG, et al. Can a patient educational book change behavior and reduce pain in chronic low back pain patients? *Spine J.* 2004;4:425–435.

Waddell G. *The Back Pain Revolution.* 2nd ed. Edinburgh: Elsevier; 2004.

Waddell G, Burton AK. Concepts of rehabilitation for the management of low back pain. *Best Pract Res Clin Rheumatol.* 2005;19:655–670.

Waddell G, Newton M, Henderson I, et al. A fear-avoidance beliefs questionnaire (FABQ) and the role of fear avoidance beliefs in chronic low back pain and disability. *Pain.* 1993;52:157–168.

Weirich SD, Gelberman RH, Best SA, et al. Rehabilitation after subcutaneous transposition of the ulnar nerve: immediate versus delayed mobilization. *J Shoulder Elbow Surg.* 1998;7:244–249.

Woolf CJ, Mannion RJ. Neuropathic pain: aetiology, symptoms, mechanisms, and management. *Lancet.* 1999;353:1959–1964.

Wright TW, Glowczewskie Jr F, Cowin D, et al. Ulnar nerve excursion and strain at the elbow and wrist associated with upper extremity motion. *J Hand Surg [Am].* 2001;26:655–662.

Chronic Back Pain and Pain Science

Adriaan Louw, PT, MAppSc (Physio), CSMT | David S. Butler, BPHTY, MAppSc, EdD

INTRODUCTION

Current treatment of low back pain indicates that a classification-based approach may be of value in identifying patients who may benefit from particular interventions (Fritz et al. 2007). Epidemiologic data indicate that chronic, widespread, nonspecific musculoskeletal pain is on the rise, which results in a significant challenge to health care providers and adds to the ever-increasing costs of health care, especially in the area of chronic low back pain (CLBP) (Wall and Melzack 2005). Few treatment interventions are helpful for CLBP (Carville et al. 2008), which in turn adds to the frustration and challenge of treating these patients. One in five people in the United States has an ongoing (chronic) pain state, implying that approximately 65 to 70 million Americans have persistent pain (Wall and Melzack 2005).

Pain is complex and often poorly understood. The International Association on the Study of Pain (IASP) defines pain as follows:

An unpleasant sensory and emotional experience which follows actual or potential tissue damage or is described in terms of such damage.

This definition by the IASP of pain is important because it includes the fact that emotional pain is the same as physical pain. Additionally, the definition indicates that pain can be experienced with tissue injury or even potential injury or the threat of injury. However, a more recent definition of pain was provided by Moseley (2003) that not only includes the brain but also critical systems that protect the individual:

Pain is a multiple system output that is activated by an individual's specific neural signature. This neural signature is activated whenever the person perceives a threat.

CURRENT MODELS FOR MANAGING CHRONIC SPINAL PAIN

Potentially the biggest problem physical therapists face in treating patients with chronic pain is the fact that they use models that are inadequate to understand and explain pain (Butler 2000). Broader "bio-psycho-social" models are needed. The bio-psycho-social approach combines biology, psychology, and social interaction/awareness in treating a patient. The reality is that many physical therapists (based on their training) still tend to be heavily geared toward the biological part. A true bio-psycho-social approach consists of various models, held together with sound clinical reasoning (Fig. 77.1). Therapists should carefully evaluate these models of treating pain and determine which of these models they feel comfortable with and which ones they need additional information about:

Anatomy: Physical therapists cannot treat patients without knowing anatomy; however, anatomic models are limited in explaining pain, especially chronic, widespread pain.

Pathoanatomy: The extension of the anatomy model is the pathoanatomy model. Compared to showing a patient a healthy disc, a therapist shows a patient a "bad" disc, or knee, or foot. Although damaged tissue may result in pain and form a major component in acute, tissue-based pain states, it has limitations in explaining chronic pain. Many people have "bad" anatomy yet have no pain. Current data show up to 52% of adults have a bulging disc on magnetic resonance imaging without LBP (Jensen et al. 1994). Another example is spinal degeneration, which is a universal and common finding on any adult spine imaging study. If spinal degeneration from age 20 to age 80 were plotted on a graph, it would indicate a linear upward progression—with increased age comes increased spinal degeneration. However, the highest rates of LBP occur between ages 35 and 50. A quick view of the graphs would show little correlation between spinal degeneration (bad anatomy) and LBP incidence. Therapists need to have a good understanding of pathoanatomy including healing rates and phases of healing. Although tissues heal, many patients have persistent pain well beyond the "normal healing phase" for those tissues. Pathoanatomy models not only have limited effect in explaining pain to patients but also may actually make them worse. Images, posters, and spine models of "bad anatomy" may invoke fear instead of helping ease pain or discomfort.

Biomechanics: Another very common model used by therapists in explaining pain is the biomechanical model. Therapists correlate poor mechanics to pain. Although this is correct and obvious in an acute and subacute injury, it is less obvious in the more persistent, widespread pain states. As with pathoanatomy models, many people have "bad" mechanics and do not have pain. The three models (anatomy, pathoanatomy, and biomechanics) are the primary and most prevalent models used to train therapists in treating pain and disability. These models may have a valuable role to play in patients with acute, subacute, or even immediate postoperative pain but have a limited role in explaining pain to a patient with chronic pain (Fig. 77.2).

Onion-Skins Model: This model is another step in realizing that pain is not just purely nociceptive. Nociceptive injury refers to the stimulation of nerve endings in tissues supplied by the nervous system—for example, pinching or cutting skin. Pain in the onion-skins model is further enhanced by other factors that may influence the development and maintenance of a pain state, such as the patient's attitudes and beliefs; the suffering the patient is enduring because of this injury; his or her coping strategies (fighting it or passive coping strategies); and even social environment such as work, home, and family. More layers can obviously be added to the onion. The premise of the onion-skins model is that pain is not purely related to injury, but it is affected by numerous factors. A seemingly small injury that,

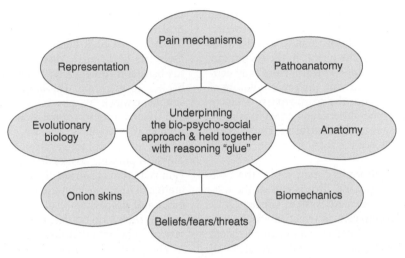

Fig. 77.1 Bio-psycho-social approach for managing spinal pain.

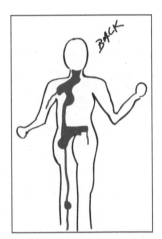

Fig. 77.2 Patient drawing of her low back pain. She presented in physical therapy with a primary complaint of low back pain for the past 3 years and a history of seeing many health care providers.

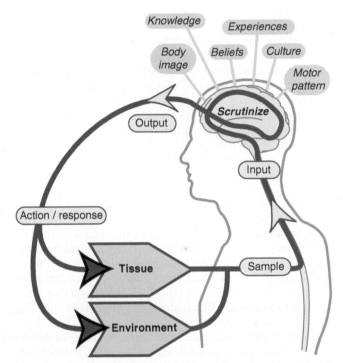

Fig. 77.3 Gifford pain mechanisms. The Mature Organism Model or Pain Mechanism Model. (Adapted from Gifford LS. Pain, the tissues and the nervous system. *Physiotherapy* 1998;84:27–33.)

according to the clinician's reasoning, "should have healed" now produces long-lasting pain. There may have been an injury, but the injury is heavily affected by other factors.

Pain Mechanism Model: The pain mechanism model provides a bigger picture of pain (Fig. 77.3). It allows therapists to "step back, out of the tissues" and view the pain through different processes—*input*-related processes, *processing* processes, and finally *output* processes.

Input processes describe three issues—tissue injury, environment, and input via the peripheral nervous system. Tissue injury has been described. The environment in which the injury occurs is also very important (e.g., hurting your back at home versus hurting your back at work are two completely different scenarios and may have significant clinical implications). Several studies regarding environment come to mind but none better than the "National Demolition Derby Driver" study in 2005 (Simotas and Shen 2005). Approximately 25% to 30% of the general population involved in a motor vehicle collision develop chronic pain (pain more than 1 year later). However, the Demolition Derby Driver study surveyed members of the National Demolition Derby Drivers Association and found interesting statistics: On average these drivers are involved in 30 career events and had an average of 52 car collisions per event (>1500 collisions),

yet only one of the 40 drivers reported having chronic neck pain more than 1 year after injury. This study is a powerful reminder of how the brain evaluates "threat," which is discussed in the neuromatrix (representation) model, but also reminds us how environment affects pain. Compare the demolition driver's fun event to an unexpected, stressful car accident experienced by a patient during a stressful time in his or her life. The third component to the input mechanism is the peripheral nervous system. With injury, the peripheral nervous system increases its resting membrane potentials, making it easier for the nervous system to "fire." This is normal and part of survival. A healthy way of viewing the nervous system is as an alarm system—there to warn of impending danger and there for survival. When you step on a rusted nail, there must be a system to tell you about it so you can act on it. In ideal situations, the nerves will become more sensitive (sending danger messages to the brain) and once the tissues heal or the threat is removed, the nerves calm to their typical resting level of excitement. Unfortunately, this does not happen in all patients. After injury, the nerves in the region stay at the heightened level of excitement. Several factors may contribute to this, including failed treatment, the representation of the injury, different explanations for the pain, anxiety/stress at work, and so on. Now the peripheral nervous system fires more easily and sends more messages to the central nervous system (Butler 2000). For more on this, see the section on The Sensitive Nervous System.

Regarding *processing,* with all the constant input, the CNS increases its sensitivity or "upregulates." This is part of the normal survival mechanism of the nervous system (Butler 2000, Woolf 2007). Patients may develop central sensitization. In central sensitization, the CNS may become the source of persistent pain with or without peripheral input (Butler 2000, Woolf 2007). The classic example is phantom limb pain. With injury and pain in a limb, the peripheral nerves upregulate and constantly barrage the CNS. Over time the CNS upregulates. On removal of the leg (amputation), the representation of the leg is still vivid in the brain and the patient may experience leg pain even though there is no leg present. Significant neuroplastic events occur in the brain in this scenario, which will be discussed in detail later. However, it is also suggested that more benign injuries such as neck pain following an MVC or LBP may lead to the development of an upregulated CNS. The disc has healed, but there is still pain. Additionally, because the CNS involves brain processing, environmental issues once again affect the processing of the patient's disorder and include experiences with back pain, expectations, and so on.

For *output mechanisms,* with all the "input and processing" the body (brain) will call on systems to defend the individual (Butler and Moseley 2003). These systems are often referred to as the homeostatic system and include the sympathetic nervous system, the parasympathetic nervous system, the motor system, language, the respiratory system, the pain system, and more. A good example of a dysfunctional "output" mechanism is complex regional pain syndrome (CRPS). It is believed that in CRPS the body draws on systems such as the sympathetic, circulatory, endocrine, pain, and more to protect the person.

A critical part of the pain mechanism model is determining which of these processes are dominant because LBP that is more input-dominant (tissue and peripheral nerve) responds relatively well to traditional therapy such as manual therapy exercises, whereas patients with processing and output-dominant mechanisms most likely will not. These patients need extensive neuroscience education, gentle movement, graded exposure, and even graded motor imagery.

Neuromatrix/Representational Model: The neuromatrix model takes on the brain or the representation of the injury in the brain (Melzack 2001, Moseley 2003). The neuromatrix model also refers to the fact that pain is processed all throughout the brain; there are no pain areas in the brain. When an injury occurs (e.g., LBP), areas in the brain are used to process incoming danger messages from the low back, but these areas have functions other than processing pain (e.g., memory, movement, sensation). As an example, a patient with a history of LBP and a back "giving out" frequently resulting in severe pain walks across a street and notices a shiny coin. As he bends over, he hears a terrible "crack" in the back. Does it hurt? Most therapists would answer "yes" because tissues were injured and resulted in pain. Now imagine

the same patient walking across a street, picking up a coin, and hearing the same "crack" in the back, but right as he hears the "crack" in the back he notices a speeding bus heading his way. Does the back hurt? Most therapists would now say no. But the back still (potentially) has tissue injury. Interesting changes happen in the brain. The brain is extremely complex, but in a simplistic way it "weighs the world"—evaluating the back sprain and tissue injury in comparison to the speeding bus. The brain decides if you will experience pain. Experiencing pain at that time is not helpful for survival. Basically the speeding bus wins. This is important. Tissues do not send pain messages to the brain. Pain is a brain construct. Tissues send danger messages and the brain can then interpret them and decide if the sum result of the input and processing results in pain. Again, many people have bad tissues but do not feel pain. Tissue injury may not be necessary or sufficient to produce pain.

The models presented here are not the only ones, but they may be considered as some of the main models used by rehabilitation professionals. Each therapist is urged to once again view his or her bio-psycho-social paradigm. When therapists use the anatomy, pathoanatomy, and biomechanical models, they still practice very "biologically." A greater understanding of the described models is needed (Butler 2000).

IMPORTANT ISSUES IN UNDERSTANDING PAIN

There have been many exciting discoveries and developments in the field of pain science and the general understanding of pain as it relates to the development and management of chronic LBP, enough to cover numerous chapters in books dedicated to pain science. Three key issues are discussed here:

- Nerve sensitivity
- The brain's processing of pain
- Output systems

The Sensitive Nervous System

Physical therapists have become much more familiar with the concept of neural tissue mobilization (Butler 2000). Neural tissue mobilization started with the premise that the nervous system is a physical tissue, and from an anatomic and physiologic perspective nerves require adequate space (container), movement, and blood supply (Butler 2000). This has led to the development of physical tests (neurodynamic tests such as straight leg raise, slump, and upper limb neurodynamic tests) that aim to examine the physical properties of the nervous system in dealing with its demand for space, movement, and blood flow (Butler 2000). For example, a straight leg raise examines the ability of the sciatic nerve to move freely through the surrounding tissues and whether the nerve has adequate blood supply to tolerate the movement. If a neurodynamic test reveals restricted movement (decreased ROM), a series of active and/ or passive neural tissue mobilization techniques would be used to restore the normal movement properties of the nervous system. The movement properties of nerves are still being studied extensively (Coppieters and Butler 2008).

An important shift has occurred in the understanding of nerve pain (Butler 2000). To develop a greater understanding of chronic spinal pain, therapists need to have a greater understanding of how nerves "become sensitive." To understand this, therapists need to understand the molecular targets of therapy—ion channels (Butler 2000, Wall and Melzack 2005). Ion channels are formed by proteins, based on the transcription from deoxyribonucleic acid (DNA) to messenger ribonucleic acid (mRNA). For a comprehensive discussion, the reader is referred to Wall and Melzack (2005). Following are seven key points regarding ion channels (from Butler 2001 with permission):

1. Ion channels are a collection of proteins shaped to form a channel, based on genetic coding (DNA). This channel is bound in the membrane of the neuron (axolemma). These channels are synthesized on ribosomes around the nucleus, all to a genetic instruction. Channels are transported in the axoplasm (nerve cytoplasm), and they are then inserted into the axolemma.

2. They essentially form a plug/channel in the axolemma with a hole through it. The hole can open or close; if it is open, ions flow through, based on the electrochemical gradient. This will cause a depolarization and then, secondary to other chemical events, the channel will usually shut.

3. Many different kinds of channels are expressed by genes. Some channels open to specific modalities such as stretch or temperature changes. Other channels open in response to changes in electrical potential or a neurotransmitter binding to it. Therapists may be interested in the fact that there are ion channels sensitive to temperature changes, circulating immune molecules, blood flow, pressure, stretch, and adrenaline (Fig. 77.4).

4. Most channels open for only a few milliseconds and thus allow equalization of the electrical gradient. Another class of ion channels (G protein) open for much longer, perhaps minutes, and instigate changes in the next neuron including second messenger activation and gene expression. These are sometimes referred to as "memory" channels.

5. Ion channels are continually changing. The half-life of an ion channel such as the Na+ channel may only be a few days. This allows a self-regulatory process that defines synaptic function. For example, in a stress situation the number of adrenosensitive channels could increase. Injury leads to upregulation or downregulation or even production of unique channels.

6. Ion channels are not distributed evenly in the peripheral nervous system. There are more channels at the cell body, axon hillock, dendrites, terminals, and the nodes of Ranvier. An area such as the axon hillock is a possible site for insertion of additional channels if needed.

7. Ion channel number, kind, and activity at any one time are fair representations of the sensitivity needed for best survival in society as computed for that individual. There is thus a plasticity in ion channel expression. In injury states the pattern of channel expression and insertion can change dramatically and receptor numbers in areas such as the amygdala, hippocampus, and dorsal root ganglia increase. In peripheral nerves, myelin normally resists channel insertion. However, after demyelination, the bared segment can acquire a high density of channels. This is thought to be the basis of abnormal impulse-generating sites in peripheral neurones. Said simply, they reflect the "need" of the individual.

The clinical application of ion channel research is that nerves can become increasingly sensitive to different types of stimuli (Fig. 77.5) (Butler 2000). Understanding how ion channels work provides a biological basis to explain why a patient may develop increased sensitivity to cold temperature, stress/anxiety, or fear. Additionally, it provides a general understanding of how the

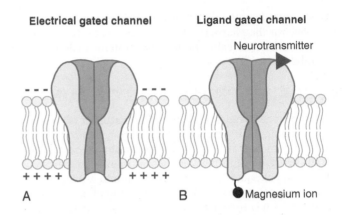

Fig. 77.4 Four different kinds of open ion channels. *A* is an electrically gated channel; *B* is a ligand gated channel, including a magnesium plug. Neurotransmitters "dock" into the protein, opening or closing the gate. *C* is a mechanically gated channel. The cytoskeleton may pull the channel open. *D* is a metabotrophic channel or G-protein gated channel. The receptor is separated from the ion channel, and G-protein activation is required to open the channel. (Adapted from Butler DS. *The Sensitive Nervous System.* Adelaide, South Australia: NOI Publications, 2000.)

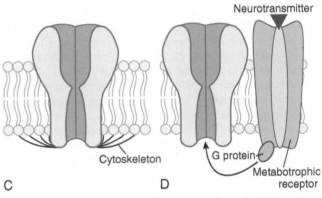

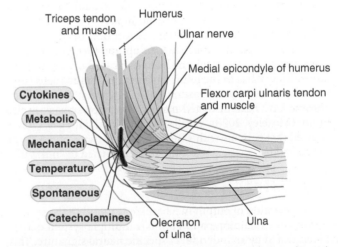

Fig. 77.5 The various stimuli known to activate an abnormal impulse-generating site in a peripheral nerve. (Adapted from Butler DS. *The Sensitive Nervous System.* Adelaide, South Australia: NOI Publications, 2000.)

nervous system in general "wakes up." This research is also the cornerstone for the pharmaceutical companies for the development of medicines to calm the nervous system, such as membrane stabilization drugs.

THE BRAIN'S PROCESSING OF PAIN

Noninvasive technologies such as functional MRI (fMRI) and positron emission tomography (PET) scans have provided scientists and clinicians with a great opportunity to explore how the brain processes information such as pain. The mantras of "no brain, no pain" and "use it or lose it" definitely apply here. It is all about representation. Our understanding of how the brain processes pain has increased considerably, and it is complex. The following is a summary of some key issues as they relate to mapping pain in the brain (Flor 2003):

- During a pain experience, the whole brain is active. This is a key issue. There are no pain areas in the brain. Pain uses areas that have functions other than pain. Although the pain experience is distributed, a basic common activation pattern exists but varies among people and in a chronic pain experience. Variation probably expresses our natural differences in pain experiences including experimental pain.
- The areas that are frequently "alight" are primary and secondary somatosensory cortices, in the limbic system, anterior cingulate (Butler and Moseley 2003), and insula cortex and subcortically, the thalamus, basal ganglia, and cerebellum. To date, more than 400 areas have been noted. It is the bilateral distributed recursive processing between these parts that must equal the experience of pain. This map in the brain is often referred to as a "neurotag" or neural signature (Fig. 77.6) (Butler and Moseley 2003).
- A noxious stimulation to either muscle or skin has a similar brain representation. Research data indicate that the brain runs the same pain map, regardless of the specific tissues injured. This implies that the brain runs basically the same map regardless of whether the disc or facet or sacroiliac joint is injured.
- "Emotional pain" uses similar areas as "physical pain." This fits with the IASP definition of pain. It also underscores the bio-psycho-social approach to management.
- An ignited representation can be easily modified, especially by cognitive factors. It is highly contextual. The representation can be elicited by anticipation of pain or illusions of pain. The representation can be modulated by cognitive mechanisms such as distraction, perception of unpleasantness, and anxiety. It can be "turned up" or "turned down."
- "Smudging" in the cortex has been measured in certain pain states. Body parts in the brain have neural images/maps (e.g., the lower back). Recent research has shown that patients with chronic LBP have distorted maps of their lower back in the brain (Moseley 2008). Similarly, Tsao and Hodges (2007) showed that patients with LBP have altered maps of the TA in the brain and, after exercise, the maps returned to "normal."

THE OUTPUT SYSTEMS

A brief description of output mechanism is found in the section on models of explaining pain. Pain is a multiple system output that is activated by an individual's specific neural signature. This neural signature is activated whenever the person perceives a threat. Output mechanisms refer to the different systems the body draws on to defend itself (Butler 2000, Butler and Moseley

A Typical Pain Neurotag

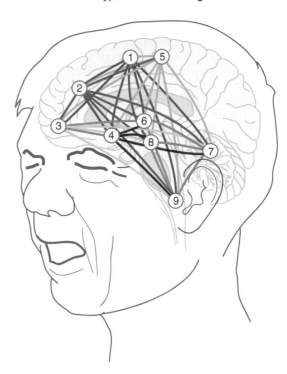

1) **Premotor/motor cortex:** organize and prepare movements
2) **Cingulate cortex:** concentration, focusing
3) **Prefrontal cortex:** problem solving, memory
4) **Amygdala:** fear, fear conditioning, addiction
5) **Sensory cortex:** sensory discrimination
6) **Hypothalamus/thalamus:** stress responses, autonomic regulation, motivation
7) **Cerebellum:** movement and cognition
8) **Hippocampus:** memory, spatial cognition, fear conditioning
9) **Spinal cord:** gating from the periphery

Fig. 77.6 A typical pain "neurotag" or neural signature, demonstrating common areas identified in the processing of pain.

2003). Pain is a threat, and in response to the threat, the body (brain) will call on various systems to defend itself. These systems include the sympathetic nervous system, parasympathetic nervous system, motor system, endocrine system, pain, respiratory system, immune system, and more. Some systems are fast acting (sympathetic, respiratory) when a threat occurs, whereas other systems are slower (parasympathetic, immune). These systems are designed to work in acute stress responses. When facing an acute stress situation (e.g., vicious dog), these systems activate and protect an individual (e.g., shunting blood to larger muscles to run or fight, increasing heart rate and respiration, increasing adrenaline levels). It is interesting to note that pain (as an output) will be downregulated in acute stress. When the stressor (dog) is removed, these systems return to normal levels—thus, it is called the homeostatic system. However, when these systems are turned on for weeks, months, or even years, there are long-lasting changes that not only have an effect on the patient but also show up clinically. Chronic pain, because it is long lasting, poorly diagnosed, associated with failed treatment, causes increased fear levels, and leads to social factors such as family and work-related issues, can be seen as a huge threat (dog) present in the patient's life for months or even years. In chronic pain these systems are turned on for long periods and linked to the following:

- Increased pain as a result of ion channel sensitization to adrenaline, ion channel sensitization to cytokines (immune molecules), central sensitization, and increased nerve sensitivity
- Shallow, fast breathing leading to fatigue of the accessory muscles and poor oxygenated blood contributing to ischemic, sensitive, and deconditioned tissues
- Dysfunction of the postural muscles and stabilizing muscles with blood being shunted to areas more needed for "survival"
- Cortisol levels becoming altered and leading to memory changes, appetite changes, mood swings, depression, altered immunity, sleep disturbance, and weight gain; tissues become more sensitive and deconditioned

The critical point is that therapists need to realize that patients with chronic pain have many of the aforementioned symptoms (fatigue, pain, sensitivity, etc.). Therapists' treatments should address these issues (e.g., poor posture), but as long as the threat (pain) is perceived these systems will remain activated. Exercises for posture may help a little or even "feel good," but no real changes will occur unless skillful delivery of hands-on, movement-based therapy is combined with neuroscience education that aims to decrease the threat (see next section on neuroscience education). Several studies utilizing neuroscience education in patients with CLBP have shown that patients move and exercise better following an educational (Louw et al. 2015a) session. It is hypothesized that neuroscience education helps patients understand their pain better, which de-threatens the issue and in essence calms the brain and nervous system.

CHRONIC PAIN: BEST EVIDENCE MANAGEMENT

Evidence-based medicine is the application of the best available treatment for the individual patient. A review of the current best evidence treatment for chronic pain, including spinal disorders, provides clinicians with guidelines.

1. Identify patients with "red flags." The first rule of medicine is "Do no harm." Clinicians should carefully screen patients to determine their appropriateness for treatment. This includes the patient with chronic pain. The same guidelines used for screening any or all patients apply to the patient with persistent pain. Patients with red flags should be referred for additional testing and medical management.
2. Educate the patient about the nature of the problem. Education has long been used to try to help alleviate the disability associated with LBP (Engers et al. 2008). In the orthopedic domain, there are a number of studies on the effect of education on pain and disability, with outcomes ranging from "excellent" to "poor." Most education programs used in orthopedics utilize anatomic and biomedical models for addressing pain (Butler and Moseley 2003, Moseley 2003, Moseley et al. 2004), which not only has shown limited efficacy but also may even increase patient fears and thus negatively affect their outcomes, as discussed in the section on models addressing pain (Butler and Moseley 2003). A suggested common shortcoming of biomechanical approaches is that they do not go deeply into neuroscience (Moseley 2002, Moseley 2003) or deal with psychosocial issues, which have been shown to be strong predictors of long-term disability and chronic pain. On the other end

of the educational spectrum is an approach of addressing some of the psychological issues related to LBP with cognitive behavioral therapy (CBT). CBT aims to reassure patients and address fears related to movement, pathology, and function. Systematic reviews of educational strategies for treating LBP have, however, shown that outcomes of CBT are similar to those for non-CBT education for LBP, demonstrating limited efficacy. Recent research has evaluated the use of neuroscience education in decreasing pain and disability among patients with LBP (Louw et al. 2015b). Although neuroscience education is aimed at reducing the fear associated with LBP, it differs from CBT by not focusing on anatomic or biomechanical models but rather on neurophysiology and the processing/representation of pain. Pain is a powerful motivating force that guides medical care and treatment-seeking behaviors in patients. Patients are interested in knowing more about pain, and studies have demonstrated that they are capable of understanding the neurophysiology of pain, although professionals usually underestimate patients' ability to understand the "complex" issues related to pain.

Studies that use neuroscience education have been shown to decrease fear and change a patient's perception of his or her pain. Additionally, neuroscience education has been shown to have an immediate effect on improvements in patients' attitudes about and relation to pain (Moseley 2003), improvements in pain cognition and physical performance, increased pain thresholds during physical tasks, improved outcomes of therapeutic exercises (Moseley 2002), and significant reduction in widespread brain activity characteristic of a pain experience. Furthermore, these neuroscience studies have shown results to extend beyond the short term and to be maintained at 1-year follow-up (Moseley 2002).

3. Provide prognostication. This may be one of the most difficult aspects of treatment. It is, however, imperative for the clinician to provide the patient with clear timelines regarding expected outcomes. Care should be taken to address pain. Outcome studies regarding pain ratings have shown that pain will decrease at typical 3-month, 6-month, and 1-year follow-up, yet the focus should be geared more toward function. A patient with chronic pain can expect to have significant functional increase, although there is pain. This is one of the mechanisms of "defocusing" the patient on the pain. The clinician should clearly explain to the patient his or her expectations regarding pain and function.
4. Promote self-care. A powerful management strategy for the patient with chronic pain is to teach strategies to help him or herself. This fosters greater independence and helps with the development of coping strategies—teaching the patient he or she is able to manage his or her own pain. This also creates less dependence on the health care provider. Self-help includes strategies such as the development of an aerobic exercise program, systematic application of stretches, use of modalities such as ice or heat, meditation, relaxation, breathing exercise, problem solving, time management, and more.
5. Get patients active and moving as early as possible and appropriately after injury. There are many reasons to get patients to move soon after injury and/or surgery. Obvious reasons include (from a biological perspective) blood flow, removal of irritant substances, and so on and (from a psychological aspect) coping strategies, empowerment, and

more. However, the mounting body of evidence regarding neuroplastic changes in the brain underscores the importance of early movement after surgery or injury. Recent studies utilizing fMRI and PET scans have shown that after an injury or immobilization of a body part (e.g., fingers) the representation of that area is altered in as little as 30 minutes. What is important about this is that when a body part is distorted (e.g., low back), it is linked to persistent pain. Studies using fMRI and PET scan further demonstrate that movement/exercise of the affected area changes the "neural signature" of the body part, which is associated with decreased pain and functional improvement. The neurobiology of this process is best described as a process whereby an injured area that loses its normal movement develops a "poorer" map in the brain—it becomes "smudged." By moving the body part, the map of that body part is "retrained" and the brain develops a healthy view of the injured area. This correlates to improvement. Movement after injury can be seen as homuncular refreshment—keeping the maps well defined and healthy after injury.

6. Decrease unnecessary fear related to movement, leisure, and work activities. Several factors are associated with the development and maintenance of a pain state. Epidemiologic data indicate that 6% of patients with LBP account for almost 50% of the expenditure associated with the management of LBP. With countries spending more and more money to treat LBP, scientists started investigating the factors associated with the development of CLBP. The list is exhaustive; however, many studies have focused on fear. Several authors believe that fear of pain, fear of injury, or fear of re-injury may be the most potent factor in the development of CLBP. This has led to the development of questionnaires to examine the level of fear a patient may have. The most commonly used "fear questionnaire" is the Fear Avoidance Belief Questionnaire. The FABQ is a valid and reliable measure of fear-avoidance (Grotle et al. 2006) beliefs. From a treatment perspective the clinician should aim to decrease fear. This is the essence of neuroscience education. It is believed that decreased fear will in essence "calm" the brain. The threat is less. Therapists should aim to develop a greater understanding (after the evaluation) as to what the patient is afraid of and address the issues. It may be an unrealistic expectation that a movement or exercise will injure tissue. Several studies using neuroscience education have shown improvement in movements such as straight leg raise and forward flexion after education sessions addressing fears (Louw et al. 2015a, Louw et al. 2015b).

7. Help the patient experience success. Unfortunately, a big focus of the evaluation is to determine "what a patient cannot do" and then treatment is aimed at restoring the functional deficit. It is recommended that clinicians also point out positive features, such as an efficient movement or muscle contraction. This also goes for the treatments. Encouragement is important. Patients with chronic pain have numerous psychological comorbidities such as depression, poor body image, and lack of self-confidence.

8. Perform a skilled physical examination, and communicate results to the patient. Numerous studies have shown that patients want to be physically examined. It is recommended that clinicians consider a skilled "low-tech" examination. This implies the evaluation is thorough yet more geared toward a global view of the physical test findings. Patients with chronic pain exhibit increased widespread sensitivity (hyperalgesia), which decreases the relevance of specific physical dysfunction. For example, in a patient with CLBP palpation of the L5 spinal level will most likely reveal increased sensitivity (pain) but so will L4, L3, and so forth. This does not imply that all the spinal levels are "injured." With the nervous system being so sensitive, any or all input sends danger signals to the brain. The relevance of pain on palpation on L5 becomes less. Carefully analyze the findings of the physical tests. Once the evaluation is complete, communicate the findings to the patient in a nonthreatening manner.

9. Make any treatment strategy as closely linked to evidence of the biological nature of the problem rather than syndrome or geography. Clinicians are encouraged to get away from syndromes and areas of pain. Low back pain only refers to the fact that the area of pain is not in the front and is below the shoulder blades. The geography (where the pain is) does not tell the patient anything about the underlying pathology or explain why treatments may be of benefit. Neither do syndromes. Failed back surgery syndrome (FBSS) only informs the patient he or she had spinal surgery that did not provide the desired results. There is growing evidence that the more patients understand the biology behind their pain, the better they understand the pathology and the proposed treatment plan. This is another cornerstone of neuroscience education—"biologizing" a patient's pain. The clinician should explain to the patient what happens on a biological level that causes the pain and what can be done. An example of this may be a patient who states that she gets arm pain when she becomes stressed. A neuroscience educational session will aim to explain to the patient that nerves have receptors or sensors and recent research has shown that some sensors are sensitive to "stress chemicals" such as adrenaline. When the patient gets stressed and these stress chemical levels increase, the nerves increase their level of excitement ("buzz" higher) and therefore are more likely to "fire" and send danger messages, which could be interpreted by the brain as pain. This may then be followed by a biological description of strategies to decrease stress and calm the nervous system.

10. Use any measures possible to reduce pain. With all the knowledge now available on the development of central sensitization, it seems imperative to decrease the constant barrage of danger messages to the CNS as soon as possible. With persistent input from the periphery, the CNS will upregulate, which may lead to long-lasting changes. Clinicians should use any and all means to decrease pain. This includes the use of medication, modalities, education, and hands-on treatment.

11. Minimize the number of treatments and contacts with medical personnel. The ideal scenario is for a patient with chronic pain to develop a greater understanding of his or her pain and develop a treatment plan focused on developing independence and an ability to help himself or herself. Therapists should aim to develop this independence through encouragement, home exercise programs, and education. The reality is that many patients most likely receive many unnecessary treatments by clinicians who have fostered a dependence on the medical practitioner rather than independence. Pain management is challenging. Even if a therapist anticipates a long process, he or she should con-

sider a series of treatments while having the patient continue with some of the home exercises and management strategies (e.g., breathing, meditation) and then perhaps have the patient return again a few weeks (or months) later, reassess, then work toward the next level of goals and strategies, and then again provide a short-term reprieve from therapy and so forth. This is more advisable than having a patient attend therapy indefinitely. For example, a patient may attend therapy for eight visits and be sent home with an HEP, walking program, and working on short-term goals, with a return to therapy in 6 to 8 weeks for a few sessions of reassessment, adjustment of the exercises and goals, and then again embark on a period of working on these at home.

12. Consider multidisciplinary management. The sad reality of chronic pain is that these patients have many comorbidities, long-lasting physical and emotional changes, and medication needs. This implies that patients may benefit from several health care providers including a physical therapist, psychologist, pain management physician, art therapist, dietician, and more. This does not mean that all patients need it. Clinicians should, based on their experience and evaluation, decide if a patient may need additional help. This needs to be discussed with the patient and his or her physician.

13. Manage identified and relevant physical dysfunctions. Patients present in physical therapy with various physical dysfunctions (e.g., stiff joints, muscles not recruiting). The important aspect is to determine if these are relevant. This may be more apparent in an acute tissue-based pain state but less obvious in the patient with chronic pain. Relevance relates to function. Correcting a dysfunction should help a patient function better. Therapists should manage these dysfunctions but always be aware of the larger picture of the patient's pain state.

14. Assess and assist recovery of general physical fitness. A vast body of evidence supports the use of aerobic exercise in the management of patients with chronic pain. Therapists should help patients develop a home exercise program that includes a large focus on aerobic exercise. The neurophysiologic mechanisms behind aerobic exercise include increasing blood flow and oxygenation of muscles and neural tissue, regulating stress chemicals such as adrenaline and cortisol, boosting the immune system, improving memory, decreasing sleep disturbance, providing distraction, and more.

15. Assess the effects on the patient's creative outlets. Therapists should embrace a holistic approach to management—embracing each patient's individualism, goals, strengths, and weaknesses and designing a treatment approach that will help the patient achieve his or her goals.

CONCLUSION

Pain is complex. Many patients suffer from long-lasting pain and more and more physical therapists will be called on to help these patients. Emerging pain science research validates the notion that a movement-based profession such as physical therapy is ideal to "take on pain" by virtue of its biological background, movement focus, hands-on methods, sheer numbers of therapists, psychology background, and utilization of exercise. Unfortunately, a big shortcoming is knowledge of pain. Physical therapists are well versed in biological models (anatomy, biomechanics, and pathoanatomy) but not models associated with pain. It is not only recommended that individual therapists familiarize themselves with pain science research but also that pain science research become a cornerstone of education in physical therapy. Physical therapists can then take their rightful place as the neuromusculoskeletal specialists they are and help patients with chronic pain.

REFERENCES

A complete reference list is available at https://expertconsult .inkling.com/.

FURTHER READING

Alshami AM, Cairns CW, Wylie BK, et al. Reliability and size of the measurement error when determining the cross-sectional area of the tibial nerve at the tarsal tunnel with ultrasonography. *Ultrasound Med Biol.* 2009;35:1098–1102.

Bernard AM, Wright SW. Chronic pain in the ED. *Am J Emerg Med.* 2004;22:444–447.

Bogduk N, Barnsley L. Back pain and neck pain: an evidence based review. *Pain.* An updated review. M. Max. Seattle: IASP Press; 1999.

Bonifazi M, Suman AL, Cambiaggi C, et al. Changes in salivary cortisol and corticosteroid receptor-alpha mRNA expression following a 3-week multidisciplinary treatment program in patients with fibromyalgia. *Psychoneuroendocrinology.* 2006;31:1076–1086.

Brox JI, Storheim K, Grotle M, et al. Systematic review of back schools, brief education, and fear-avoidance training for chronic low back pain. *Spine J.* 2008;8:948–958.

Butler D, ed. *Mobilisation of the Nervous System.* London: Churchill Livingstone; 1991.

Childs JD, Fritz JM, Flynn TW, et al. A clinical prediction rule to identify patients with low back pain most likely to benefit from spinal manipulation: a validation study. *Ann Intern Med.* 2004;141:920–928.

Cleland JA, Fritz JM, Childs JD. Psychometric properties of the Fear-Avoidance Beliefs Questionnaire and Tampa Scale of Kinesiophobia in patients with neck pain. *Am J Phys Med Rehabil.* 2008;87:109–117.

Cohen JE, Goel V, Frank JW, et al. Group education interventions for people with low back pain. An overview of the literature. *Spine.* 1994;19:1214–1222.

Coppieters MW, Hough AD, Dilley A. Different nerve-gliding exercises induce different magnitudes of median nerve longitudinal excursion: an in vivo study using dynamic ultrasound imaging. *J Orthop Sports Phys Ther.* 2009;39:164–171.

Devor M. Sodium channels and mechanisms of neuropathic pain. *J Pain.* 2006;7:S3–S12.

Deyo RA, Mirza SK, Martin BI. 2006 Back pain prevalence and visit rates: estimates from U.S. national surveys. *Spine.* 2002;31:2724–2727.

Flor H. The functional organization of the brain in chronic pain. *Prog Brain Res.* 2000;129:313–322.

Flynn T, Fritz J, Whitman J, et al. A clinical prediction rule for classifying patients with low back pain who demonstrate short-term improvement with spinal manipulation. *Spine.* 2002;27:2835–2843.

Fritz JM, George SZ, Delitto A. The role of fear-avoidance beliefs in acute low back pain: relationships with current and future disability and work status. *Pain.* 2001;94:7–15.

Fritz JM, Lindsay W, Matheson JW, et al. Is there a subgroup of patients with low back pain likely to benefit from mechanical traction? Results of a randomized clinical trial and subgrouping analysis. *Spine.* 2007;32:E793–E800.

Gifford LS. Pain, the tissues and the nervous system. *Physiotherapy.* 1998;84:27–33.

Gross AR, Aker PD, Goldsmith CH, et al. Patient education for mechanical neck disorders. *Cochrane Database Syst Rev.* 2000:CD000962.

Grotle M, Vollestad NK, Brox JI. Clinical course and impact of fear-avoidance beliefs in low back pain: prospective cohort study of acute and chronic low back pain: II. *Spine.* 2006;31:1038–1046.

Hefford C. McKenzie classification of mechanical spinal pain: profile of syndromes and directions of preference. *Man Ther.* 2008;13:75–81.

Heymans MW, van Tulder MW, Esmail R, et al. Back schools for nonspecific low back pain: a systematic review within the framework of the Cochrane Collaboration Back Review Group. *Spine.* 2005;30:2153–2163.

Hicks GE, Fritz JM, Delitto A, et al. Preliminary development of a clinical prediction rule for determining which patients with low back pain will respond to a stabilization exercise program. *Arch Phys Med Rehabil.* 2005;86:1753–1762.

Hirsch MS, Liebert RM. The physical and psychological experience of pain: the effects of labeling and cold pressor temperature on three pain measures in college women. *Pain*. 1998;77:41–48.

Johnson RE, Jones GT, Wiles NJ, et al. Active exercise, education, and cognitive behavioral therapy for persistent disabling low back pain: a randomized controlled trial. *Spine*. 2007;32:1578–1585.

Kendall NAS, Linton SJ, Main CJ, eds. *Guide to Assessing Psychosocial Yellow Flags in Acute Low Back Pain: Risk Factors for Long Term Disability and Work Loss*. Wellington: Accident Rehabilitation & Compensation Insurance Corporation of New Zealand and the National Health Committee; 1997.

Koes BW, van Tulder MW, van der Windt WM, et al. The efficacy of back schools: a review of randomized clinical trials. *J Clin Epidemiol*. 1994;47:851–862.

Liddle SD, Gracey JH, Baxter GD. Advice for the management of low back pain: a systematic review of randomised controlled trials. *Man Ther*. 2007;12:310–327.

Loeser JD. *Concepts of Pain*. In: Stanton-Hicks M, Boaz R, (eds), *Chronic Low Back Pain*. New York: Raven Press; 1982: p. 146.

Louw A, Louw Q, Crous LCC. Preoperative Education for Lumbar Surgery for Radiculopathy. *S Afr J Physiother*. 2009;65:3–8.

Louw A, Mintken P, Puentedura L. Neurophysiologic effects of neural mobilization maneuvers. In: Fernandez-De-Las-Penas C, Arendt-Nielsen L, Gerwin RD, eds. *Tension-Type and Cervicogenic Headache*. Boston: Jones and Bartlett; 2009: 231–245.

Magni G, Marchetti M, Moreschi C, et al. Chronic musculoskeletal pain and depressive symptoms in the national health and nutrition examination. 1. Epidemiologic follow up study. *Pain*. 1993;53:163.

Maier-Riehle B, Harter M. The effects of back schools—a meta-analysis. *Int J Rehabil Res*. 2001;24:199–206.

Masui T, Yukawa Y, Nakamura S, et al. Natural history of patients with lumbar disc herniation observed by magnetic resonance imaging for minimum 7 years. *J Spinal Disord Tech*. 2005;18:121–126.

Mortimer M, Ahlberg G. To seek or not to seek? Care-seeking behaviour among people with low-back pain. *Scand J Public Health*. 2003;31:194–203.

Moseley GL. Evidence for a direct relationship between cognitive and physical change during an education intervention in people with chronic low back pain. *Eur J Pain*. 2004;8:39–45.

Moseley GL. Graded motor imagery for pathologic pain: a randomized controlled trial. *Neurology*. 2006;67:2129–2134.

Moseley GL. Joining forces—combining cognition-targeted motor control training with group or individual pain physiology education: a successful treatment for chronic low back pain. *J Man Manip Therap*. 2003; in press.

Moseley GL. Widespread brain activity during an abdominal task markedly reduced after pain physiology education: fMRI evaluation of a single patient with chronic low back pain. *Aust J Physiother*. 2005;51:49–52.

Moseley GL, Hodges PW, Nicholas MK. A randomized controlled trial of intensive neurophysiology education in chronic low back pain. *Clin J Pain*. 2004;20:324–330.

Moseley L. Unraveling the barriers to reconceptualization of the problem in chronic pain: the actual and perceived ability of patients and health professionals to understand the neurophysiology. *J Pain*. 2003;4:184–189.

Nachemson AL. Newest knowledge of low back pain. A critical look. *Clin Orthop*. 1992:8–20.

Oliveira A, Gevirtz R, Hubbard D. A psycho-educational video used in the emergency department provides effective treatment for whiplash injuries. *Spine*. 2006;31:1652–1657.

Poiraudeau S, Rannou F, Baron G, et al. Fear-avoidance beliefs about back pain in patients with subacute low back pain. *Pain*. 2006;124:305–311.

Rooks DS, Gautam S, Romeling M, et al. Group exercise, education, and combination self-management in women with fibromyalgia: a randomized trial. *Arch Intern Med*. 2007;167:2192–2200.

Sackett DL. Evidence-based medicine. *Spine*. 1998;23:1085–1086.

Schmid AB, Brunner F, Luomajoki H, et al. Reliability of clinical tests to evaluate nerve function and mechanosensitivity of the upper limb peripheral nervous system. *BMC Musculoskelet Disord*. 2009;10:11.

Shacklock M, ed. *Clinical Neurodynamics*. London: Elsevier; 2005.

Spitzer WO, Skovron ML, Salmi LR. Scientific monograph of the Quebec task force on whiplash associated disorders: redefining whiplash and its management. *Spine*. 1995;20(Suppl): 10s–73s.

Udermann BE, Spratt KF, Donelson RG, et al. Can a patient educational book change behavior and reduce pain in chronic low back pain patients? *Spine J*. 2004;4:425–435.

Waddell G. *The Back Pain Revolution*. ed 2. Edinburgh: Elsevier; 2004.

Waddell G, Newton M, Henderson I, et al. A fear-avoidance beliefs questionnaire (FABQ) and the role of fear avoidance beliefs in chronic low back pain and disability. *Pain*. 1993;52:157–168.

Spinal Manipulation

Emilio "Louie" Puentedura, PT, DPT, GDMT, OCS, FAAOMPT

DEFINING SPINAL MANIPULATION

Spinal manipulation has a rich and diverse history. It has long been practiced by a wide variety of clinicians including physical therapists, physicians, osteopathic physicians, and chiropractors. There are many and varied definitions of the term *"spinal manipulation"*; however, the common denominator appears to be that it is considered a "manual therapy technique" applied to the spine. To some extent, the definitions used have depended on the practitioner applying the technique. The chiropractic profession has traditionally called it "spinal adjustment"; the osteopathic profession has used the term "high velocity low amplitude (HVLA) thrust manipulation"; and physical therapists have called it either "spinal manipulation" or "grade V spinal mobilization." Descriptions of the actual spinal manipulative techniques performed by the various professions have also been extremely diverse and often based on each profession's theoretic constructs and schemata. This confusion surrounding manipulation terminology led to a call for a more standardized nomenclature within the physical therapy profession, and in 2008, the American Academy of Orthopaedic Manual Physical Therapists (AAOMPT) formed a task force to develop a model for standardizing manipulation terminology in physical therapy practice (Mintken et al. 2008). The task force proposed that physical therapists use six characteristics when describing a manipulative technique (Table 78.1). The model proposed by the AAOMPT task force provides a step in the right direction toward improving accuracy and consistency in describing these interventions within the physical therapy profession. It may also serve as a bridge for improving descriptions of these interventions between the various professions.

Is there a difference between spinal manipulation and spinal mobilization? Manipulation of the spine is said to differ from mobilization because, theoretically, during a manipulation, the rate of vertebral joint displacement does not allow the patient to prevent joint movement (Maitland 1986). Mobilization of the spine involves cyclic, rhythmic, low-velocity (nonthrust) passive motion that can be stopped by the patient (Maitland 1986). Therefore, the speed of the technique (not necessarily the amount of force) is what differentiates manipulation from mobilization.

EVIDENCE FOR SPINAL MANIPULATIVE THERAPY

Until recently, much of the clinical research into the efficacy of spinal manipulative therapy for mechanical low back pain has provided equivocal results. At one time, there was a persistent myth within the medical community that "most people with low back pain will get better no matter what you do." This was based on clinical experience, where family physicians would note that nine out of ten patients with an acute episode of nonspecific low back pain would recover (no matter what treatment was administered) within a month or two. However, a British study involving 490 individuals consulting their general practitioner (family physician) with low back pain found that, although 92% of the subjects discontinued consultation within 3 months, only 20% had fully recovered within 12 months (Croft et al. 1998). Another similar study followed 323 patients with low back pain receiving physical therapy or chiropractic treatment. The study found that only 18% of patients reported no recurrence of symptoms over one year, and 58% sought additional health care (Skargren et al. 1998). These and similar studies effectively dispel the myth that low back pain is a self-limiting condition and indicate that it deserves early attention to avoid longer-term disability. There is now a common consensus among health care providers that (1) we can only diagnose definite pathology in about 15% of patients with low back pain; (2) there is limited relationship between physical pathology and associated pain and disability; (3) we continue to regard back pain as an injury, but most episodes occur spontaneously with normal everyday activities; (4) high-tech imaging (CT scans, MRI) tells us very little about simple low back pain, and indeed, it appears to contribute to the problem of unwanted and unnecessary surgical procedures; and (5) the exact pathoanatomic lesion remains resistant to traditional clinical triage in the majority of patients with low back pain.

Around the turn of the century, there was growing evidence for spinal manipulation but the conclusions were often conflicting. There were just as many randomized controlled trials in support of manipulation as there were against, and systematic reviews were evenly split on the evidence. Adding to the confusion, there were a variety of conclusions being drawn in national practice guidelines for the management of low back pain (Koes et al. 2001). A review of the research into spinal manipulative therapy for low back pain around the time finds that most studies had significant flaws in design methodology in that there was the incorrect assumption being made that subjects with low back pain were a homogenous sample group. An example is the United Kingdom back pain exercise and manipulation (UK BEAM) randomized trial on the effectiveness of physical treatments for back pain in primary care (UK BEAM et al. 2004). In this study, 1334 patients with low back pain were randomly assigned to four groups and received "best care" in general practice, "best care" plus exercise classes, "best care" plus spinal manipulation, and "best care" plus spinal manipulation followed by exercise classes. The outcome measure used in the study was the Roland Morris disability questionnaire at 3 and 12 months, compared to baseline. The results demonstrated all groups improved over time and the addition of manipulation and/or exercise provided only small to moderate benefits over "best care" at 3 months and only a small benefit over "best care" at 12 months. The big problem with this study (and many others

TABLE 78.1	**Describing Manipulative Techniques Using Six Characteristics**	
1	Rate of force application	A description of the rate at which the force should be applied
2	Location in range of available movement	A description of the point in range at which the motion is intended to occur (e.g., at the beginning, toward the middle, or at the end point of the *available* range of movement)
3	Direction of force	A description of the direction in which the therapist imparts the force
4	Target of force	A description of the location where the therapist intends to apply the force; this may be a specific spinal level or more generally across a particular region of the spine (e.g., lower lumbar)
5	Relative structural movement	A description of which structure (or region) is intended to remain stable and which structure (or region) is intended to move; the moving structure (or region) is described first and the stable segment second, separated by the word "on" (e.g., lower cervical spine on the upper thoracic spine)
6	Patient position	A description of the position of the patient (e.g., supine, left side lying, or prone)

(Adapted from Mintken PE, DeRosa C, Little T, Smith B: AAOMPT Clinical Guidelines: a model for standardizing manipulation terminology in physical therapy practice. JOSPT 2008;38(3):A1–A6.)

at the time) was that by using broad inclusion criteria (i.e., low back pain) it resulted in a heterogeneous sample that may have included many patients for whom no benefit with manipulation would have been expected, thus masking the intervention's true value (Childs and Flynn 2004). The take-home message was that low back pain does not equal low back pain, and this resonated with clinicians, who were well aware that certain patients with low back pain were more likely to benefit from a manipulative technique, whereas other patients would not.

A classification-based approach was soon proposed whereby patients with low back pain could be classified into more homogenous subgroups. Classification systems for patients with low back pain have been reported in the literature since the mid-1980s, with some systems designed to aid in prognosis, some designed to identify pathology, and others designed to determine the most appropriate treatment (Riddle 1998). A treatment-based classification approach was proposed by physical therapy researchers in 1995, with one subgroup defined as those more likely to respond to manipulation (Delitto et al. 1995); however, the criteria for membership of that low back pain subgroup had not been researched. This became the 1997 agenda for primary care research on low back pain: identifying the different varieties and subgroups of low back pain within the treatment-based classification system and determining the criteria for membership. In other words, the treatment-based classification approach would be a way of knowing ahead of time which patients would be helped by which particular treatment interventions. In addition to a classification system for patients with low back pain, significant strides have also been made toward developing a similar classification system for patients with neck pain (Childs et al. 2004).

CLINICAL PREDICTION RULES

A validation study for the clinical prediction rules (CPR) for patients with neck pain who respond favorably to thoracic manipulation was completed in 2010 (Cleland et al. 2010). One hundred and forty consecutive patients with neck pain, aged 18 to 60 years, who were referred to one of several physical therapy clinics throughout the United States, were randomly assigned to receive either thoracic spine thrust manipulation plus exercise or exercise alone for five treatment sessions over four weeks. Once subjects had been assigned to either of the two treatment groups, they were examined according to the CPR criteria to determine if they were positive or negative on the rule. Outcome measures assessed at baseline, one week, four weeks, and six months included neck disability index (NDI) and pain (NPRS). Results showed that all groups improved over time, and outcomes were not dependent upon the combination of the patient's treatment group and status of the rule. Using the CPR did not result in improved patient care as all of the patients who received thoracic manipulation had better outcomes than did those who didn't receive it, regardless of their status on the CPR. The authors concluded that patients with neck pain and no contraindications to manipulation should receive thoracic spine manipulation regardless of their clinical presentation (i.e., status on any CPR). This was a significant finding that would greatly change the landscape of spinal manipulation for low back pain. The next step required was to conduct a randomized controlled clinical trial to validate the rule.

The validation study was published in 2004 (Childs et al. 2004). In the study, 131 consecutive patients with low back pain, 18 to 60 years of age, were randomly assigned to receive manipulation plus exercise or exercise alone by a physical therapist for four weeks. Once allocated to the treatment groups, all subjects were examined according to the CPR criteria (symptom duration, symptom location, fear-avoidance beliefs, lumbar mobility, and hip rotation range of motion) and classified as being either positive (at least four out of five) or negative on the rule. Outcome measures were disability (ODI) and pain at one week, four weeks, and six months compared to baseline. There was a significant difference in outcomes between patients who were positive on the rule and received manipulation compared to patients who were negative on the rule and received manipulation, positive on the rule and received exercise only, or negative on the rule and received exercise only. A patient who was positive on the rule and received manipulation was found to have a 92% chance of a successful outcome, with an associated number needed to treat for benefit at 4 weeks of 1.9 (CI, 1.4 to 3.5) (Childs et al. 2004). This meant that only two patients who are positive on the rule need to be treated with manipulation to prevent one patient from failing to achieve a successful outcome. It is widely accepted that patients with persistent disability are at increased risk for chronic, disabling episodes of low back pain, and this study demonstrated that decision making based on the CPR may help prevent progression to chronic disability. In a follow-up analysis of the study, it was found that patients who were positive on the rule and completed the exercise intervention without manipulation were eight (95% CI: 1.1, 63.5) times more likely to experience a worsening in disability at the 1-week interval than patients who actually received manipulation (Childs et al. 2006). The authors noted that the risks associated with harm from lumbopelvic manipulation are almost negligible and concluded that the risk of not offering manipulation is real, and a more aggressive approach seems to be warranted (Childs et al. 2006).

A similar clinical prediction rule has been developed for patients with neck pain who respond to thoracic spine manipulation (Cleland et al. 2007a). Six clinical variables form the rule, including (1) symptom duration less than 30 days; (2) no symptoms distal to the shoulder; (3) looking up does not aggravate symptoms; (4) fear-avoidance beliefs physical activity score of 11 of less; (5) decreased T3–T5 kyphosis; and (6) cervical extension range less than 30 degrees. In the study, the pretest probability of dramatic success (based on the Global Rating of Change Scale) was 54%. The presence of four or more clinical predictors led to a positive likelihood of 12, which raised the post-test probability of dramatic success to 93% (Cleland et al. 2007a). However, the 95% confidence interval for the positive likelihood ranged from 2.3 to 70.8; therefore it was recommended that clinicians use the three or more rule, which still raised the post-test probability of dramatic success to 86% and had a smaller 95% confidence interval for the positive likelihood ratio of 5.5 (2.7–12.0) (Cleland et al. 2007a).

A validation study for the CPR for patients with neck pain who respond favorably to thoracic spine manipulation was reported in 2007 (Cleland et al. 2007b). Thirty subjects with neck pain were randomized to receive either thrust manipulation to the thoracic spine or nonthrust mobilization techniques to the thoracic spine followed by cervical spine active range of motion exercises. Follow-up was only for 48 hours (two visits), and results demonstrated significant improvements in Neck Disability Index scores, Numeric Pain Rating scores, and Global Rating of Change scores for the thrust manipulation group ($p < 0.01$) (Cleland et al. 2007b).

A CPR for patients with neck pain who respond dramatically to cervical spine manipulation was performed in 2012 (Puentedura et al. 2012). Eighty-two patients with a primary complaint of neck pain were studied. A clinical prediction rule was established consisting of four attributes including (1) symptom duration less than 38 days; (2) positive expectation that manipulation will help; (3) side-to-side difference in cervical rotation range of motion of 10 degrees or greater; and (4) pain with posteroanterior spring testing of the middle cervical spine.

THE AUDIBLE POP

For most practitioners of spinal manipulative therapy, the aim of the technique is to achieve joint cavitation that is accompanied by a "popping" or "cracking" sound (Gibbons and Tehan 2004). A 1995 review of the literature on the audible release associated with manipulation (Brodeur 1995) reported that *it is thought* that the audible release is caused by a cavitation process whereby a sudden decrease in intracapsular pressure causes dissolved gases in the synovial fluid to be released into the joint cavity. However, a clinical trial investigating the effect of manipulation on the size and density of cervical zygapophyseal joint spaces in 22 asymptomatic subjects using CT and plain-film radiography found no evidence of gas in the joint space or obvious increase in zygapophyseal joint space width immediately after the manipulation (Cascioli et al. 2003). A more recent 2015 study (Kawchuk et al. 2015) concluded that the mechanism of joint cracking or popping is related to cavity formation rather than bubble collapse.

A review of the literature to "critically discuss previous theories and research of spinal HVLAT manipulation, highlighting reported neurophysiologic effects that seem to be uniquely

associated with cavitation of synovial fluid" found that there appear to be two separate modes of action from zygapophyseal HVLAT manipulation: "mechanical" effects and "neurophysiologic" effects (Evans 2002). Evans (2002) also reported that the intra-articular "mechanical" effects of zygapophyseal HVLAT manipulation seem to be absolutely separate from and irrelevant to the occurrence of reported "neurophysiologic" effects, and although cavitation should not be an absolute requirement for the mechanical effects to occur, it may be a reliable indicator for successful joint gapping (Evans 2002). It is safe to say that currently we do not know how or why manipulation might work in patients with spinal pain. What we do know is that there are some patients with spinal pain who do benefit from manipulation and the development and validation of clinical prediction rules are helping us to determine, in advance, who those patients are.

Does the audible release matter? A secondary analysis of the CPR development study was conducted to determine the relationship between an audible pop with spinal manipulation and the improvement in pain and function noted in patients with low back pain (Flynn et al. 2006). Therapists recorded whether an audible pop was heard by the patient or therapist during the treatment interventions, and an audible pop was perceived in 59 (84%) of the patients. However, no differences were detected at baseline or at any follow-up period in the level of pain, the Oswestry score, or lumbopelvic range of motion based on whether a pop was achieved ($p > 0.05$). The results suggest that a perceived audible pop may not relate to improved outcomes from high-velocity thrust manipulation for patients with nonradicular low back pain at either an immediate or longer-term follow-up. Another study (Bialosky et al. 2010) similarly reported that hypoalgesia is associated with HVLAT manipulation, and it occurs independently of a perceived audible pop.

Is there any evidence for localization or specificity in manipulation? Spinal manipulative techniques are taught and then performed with a specific (sometimes biomechanical) intent. However, an evaluation study using accelerometers to locate the joints that produce an audible sound in response to manipulation (cavitation) during spinal manipulative techniques (SMTs) found that the accuracy and specificity of the manipulation was poor (Ross et al. 2004). In this particular study, 64 asymptomatic subjects received thoracic and lumbar spinal manipulative procedures from 28 clinicians (all were Canadian chiropractors with a range of clinical experience of 1 to 43 years). They found that for the lumbar spine, SMT was accurate "about half the time" (57/124), and in the thoracic spine, SMT appeared to be more accurate (29/54) (Ross et al. 2004). However, most of the procedures were associated with multiple cavitations and, in most cases, at least one cavitation emanated from the target joint. This may have skewed results toward greater accuracy.

SPINAL POSITIONING AND LOCKING

In both physical therapy and osteopathic manipulative techniques, *spinal locking* can be used to localize forces and achieve cavitation at a specific vertebral segment (Stoddard 1972, Downing 1985, Beal 1989, Kappler 1989, Nyberg 1993, Greenman 1996, Hartman 1997). This locking can be achieved by facet apposition, ligamentous myofascial tension, or a combination of both (Stoddard 1972, Downing 1985, Beal 1989, Nyberg 1993, Greenman 1996, Hartman 1997). This principle is used

TABLE 78.2	Coupled Motions in the Spine and Achieving Facet Apposition Locking	
Spinal Level	**Coupled Motion**	**Facet Apposition Locking**
0–C1 (atlanto-occipital)	Lateral flexion and rotation to **opposite** sides	Combine lateral flexion with **same** side rotation
C1–C2 (atlantoaxial)	Complex–primary rotation	Not applicable
C2–T4	Lateral flexion and rotation to **same** sides	Combine lateral flexion with **opposite** side rotation
T4–L5 with the spine in flexion	Lateral flexion and rotation to **same** sides	Combine lateral flexion with **opposite** side rotation
T4–L5 with the spine in neutral or extension	Lateral flexion and rotation to **opposite** sides	Combine lateral flexion with **same** side rotation

to position the spine in such a way as to localize the leverage or force moment to one joint without placing undue strain on adjacent segments. The osteopathic profession uses a nomenclature to classify spinal motion based on the coupling of side-bending and rotation movements (Gibbons and Tehan 2004). In type 1 movement, side-bending and rotation occur in *opposite* directions, whereas in type 2 movement, side-bending and rotation occur in the *same* direction. It is proposed that locking by facet apposition can be achieved when the spine is placed in a position *opposite* to that of normal coupling behavior. So, what is the normal coupling behavior?

CERVICAL SPINE

A systematic review of the literature on coupling behavior of the cervical spine found that, although there was 100% agreement in coupling direction in the lower cervical vertebral segments (C2–3 and lower), there was significant variation in coupling patterns reported in the upper cervical segments of occiput-C1 (during side flexion initiation) and C1–2 (Cook et al. 2006). They postulated that the dissimilarities may have been explained by factors such as differences in measurement devices, movement initiation, in vivo versus in vitro specimens, and anatomic variations. At the C1–C2 level, the type of coupled movement available at this segment is complex and has a predominant role in total cervical rotation. Up to 77% of total cervical rotation occurs at the atlantoaxial joint, with a mean rotation range of 40.5 degrees to either side (Penning and Wilmink 1987, Mimura et al. 1989, Iai et al. 1993, Guth 1995). The general consensus among manipulative therapists is that facet apposition locking does not apply at this level. At the C3–C7 levels, normal coupling behavior is type 2 (i.e., left side-bending coupled with left rotation and vice versa) and therefore facet locking can be achieved by producing type 1 movement (i.e., left side-bending coupled with right rotation and vice versa) (Cook et al. 2006). The principles of facet apposition locking that apply to the cervical spine are also used for thrust techniques to the cervicothoracic junction (C7–T4). This is achieved by introducing type 1 movements (side-bending with contralateral rotation).

THORACIC AND LUMBAR SPINE

The current research relating to coupled movements of side-bending and rotation in the thoracic and lumbar spine is inconsistent (Panjabi et al. 1989, Oxland et al. 1992, Steffen et al. 1997, Harrison et al. 1999, Plaugher and Burrow 1999, Feipel et al. 2001, Keller et al. 2003, Legaspi and Edmond 2007). There is some evidence that spinal posture and positioning alter coupling behavior in the thoracic and lumbar spine (Panjabi et al. 1989, Steffen et al. 1997, Harrison et al. 1999). Specifically, in the flexed position, the coupling of side-bending and rotation

is to the same side, and in the neutral/extended position, the coupling of side-bending and rotation occurs to the opposite sides. Although the research does not validate any single model for spinal positioning and locking in the thoracic and lumbar spine, many educators continue to find the model as shown in Table 78.2 useful for learning and motor skill acquisition with manipulative therapy techniques.

For neutral/extension positioning, if we use the model (Table 78.2), normal coupling behavior of side-bending and rotation is to the opposite side (type 1). Therefore, facet apposition locking can be achieved through side-bending and rotation to the same side (Fig. 78.1). For flexion positioning, normal coupling behavior of side-bending and rotation is to the same side (type 2); therefore, facet apposition locking can be achieved through side-bending and rotation to the opposite side (Fig. 78.2).

SAFETY AND MANIPULATIVE TECHNIQUES
Cervical Spine

Much attention has been given to the potential risks associated with the administration of thrust manipulation to the cervical spine (Di Fabio 1999, Mann and Refshauge 2001, Haldeman et al. 2002a and 2002b, Refshauge et al. 2002). Di Fabio (1999) completed a review of previously reported cases in which injuries were attributed to manipulation of the cervical spine. He found 177 published cases of injury reported in 116 articles published between 1925 and 1997. The most frequently reported injuries involved arterial dissection or spasm and lesions of the brain stem. Death occurred in 32 (18%) of the cases, and none of the serious irreversible events were attributed to manipulations performed by physical therapists (Kjellman et al. 2002). Studies have also shown that there are relatively high incidences of "side effects" to the application of manipulation (Bayerl et al. 1985, Powell et al. 1993, Assendelft et al. 1996, Leboeuf-Yde et al. 1997, Senstad et al. 1997, Adams and Sim 1998, Cagnie et al. 2004, Grier 2004, Hurwitz et al. 2004, Hurwitz et al. 2005, Dagenais and Moher 2006, Giles 2006, Haneline and Cooperstein 2006, Krippendorf 2006, Rosner 2006). These include local discomfort, headache, tiredness, and radiating discomfort. They are reported to be transient, lasting no longer than 24 hours. A study by Senstad et al. (1997) reviewed data from 4712 treatments on 1058 new patients by 102 Norwegian chiropractors and found that at least one reaction was reported by 55% of the patients some time during the course of a maximum of six treatments. The most common side effect was local discomfort and was experienced in 54% of the treatments (Senstad et al. 1997).

Cagnie et al. (2004) conducted a survey regarding adverse reactions associated with spinal manipulation in Belgium. Fifty-nine manipulative therapists (physiotherapists, osteopaths, and

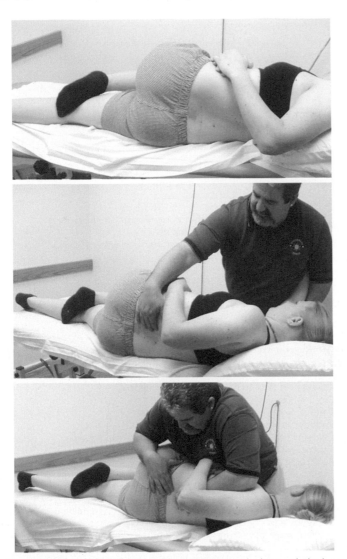

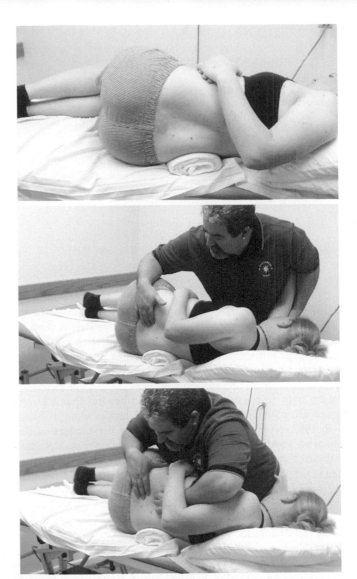

Fig. 78.1 Positioning to achieve facet apposition locking with the lumbar spine in neutral/extension. The patient is in right side lying with the lumbar and thoracic spine in neutral/extension. The extended position of the lower leg introduces left lateral flexion (*top plate*). The therapist palpates spinal segments as rotation (from the thorax down) is taken down to the appropriate lumbar level (*middle plate*). Rotation to the left is combined with lateral flexion to the left (same side to counter proposed opposite side coupling) (*lower plate*).

Fig. 78.2 Positioning to achieve facet apposition locking with the lumbar spine in flexion. The patient is in right side lying with the lumbar and thoracic spine in flexion. Knees and hips are flexed, and a rolled towel is placed under the right side to introduce right lateral flexion (*top plate*). The therapist palpates spinal segments as rotation (from the thorax down) is taken down to the appropriate lumbar level (*middle plate*). Rotation to the left is combined with lateral flexion to the right (opposite side to counter proposed same side coupling) (*lower plate*).

chiropractors) participated in the study. They asked 15 consecutive patients who received spinal manipulation as part of their initial treatment to complete a survey on any adverse reactions they felt within 48 hours of their treatment. A total of 639 questionnaires were analyzed and adverse reactions varied from headache (20%) and stiffness (19%) to dizziness (4%) and nausea (3%) (Cagnie et al. 2004). The majority of the patients (61%) reported that their adverse reactions began within four hours of their treatment, and 64% reported resolution of those symptoms within 24 hours. Predictors of experiencing an adverse reaction from spinal manipulation included gender (females more likely to experience side effects), previous history of headaches, fatigue, and a history of tobacco use.

Unfortunately, the authors did not clearly indicate which region of the spine (cervical, thoracic, or lumbar) was associated with what percentage of the overall side effects. In fact, it appears that the clinicians may have applied spinal manipulation

to two or more regions because the average number of manipulations per patient was two, with 28.5% receiving three or more manipulations during one session. Of the 930 recorded manipulations, 38.6% included the cervical spine, 25.7% the thoracic spine, 23.6% the lumbar spine, and 12.1% the sacroiliac joint.

It is extremely difficult to quantify the risk associated with cervical spine manipulation, and various estimates for a serious complication range between five and ten per ten million manipulations (Hurwitz et al. 1996). Many premanipulative screening procedures have been proposed to predict patients who may be at risk for serious injury from cervical mobilization/manipulation, with much of the attention focused on the vertebral artery (Rivett 1995, Grant 1996, Barker et al. 2000, Licht et al. 2000, Refshauge et al. 2002). There appears to be little evidence to support these decision-making schemes in their ability to accurately identify these patients (Bolton et al. 1989, Cote et al. 1996). The

TABLE 78.3	Causes of Complications From Spinal Manipulative Techniques	
Incorrect patient selection	Lack of a mechanical or clinical reasoning diagnosis	
	Lack of awareness of the possible complications	
	Inadequate palpation assessment	
	Inappropriate/inadequate progression through mobilization grades	
	Lack of patient consent	
Poor manipulative technique	Excessive force with technique	
	Excessive amplitude of movement	
	Excessive leverage of forces	
	Inappropriate combination of leverages	
	Incorrect plane of thrust	
	Poor patient positioning	
	Poor therapist positioning	
	Lack of patient feedback in the prethrust positioning	

TABLE 78.4	Contraindications for Spinal Manipulative Therapy	
Bony issues: Any pathology that may have led to bony compromise	Tumor (e.g., metastases)	
	Infection (e.g., tuberculosis, osteomyelitis)	
	Metabolic (e.g., osteomalacia, osteoporosis)	
	Congenital (e.g., dysplasia)	
	Iatrogenic (e.g., long-term corticosteroid medication)	
	Inflammatory (e.g., severe rheumatoid arthritis)	
	Traumatic (e.g., fracture)	
Neurologic issues	Cervical myelopathy	
	Cord compression	
	Cauda equina syndrome	
	Nerve root compression with increasing neurologic deficit	
Vascular issues	Diagnosed vertebrobasilar insufficiency	
	Aortic aneurysm	
	Bleeding diatheses (e.g., severe hemophilia)	
Lack of mechanical or clinical reasoning diagnosis		
Lack of patient consent		

lack of evidence for premanipulative screening has caused some authors to suggest that identifying patients at risk is virtually impossible (Haldeman et al. 1999, Haldeman et al. 2002b) and others to recommend that mobilization may be a safer alternative to manipulation. However, serious adverse events have also occurred following mobilization, and evidence suggests manipulation may have some value above and beyond that achieved by mobilization or other soft tissue techniques alone (Cassidy et al. 1992, Nilsson et al. 1997). Risks and benefits are associated with any therapeutic intervention; however, manipulative or thrust techniques are considered to be potentially more dangerous than nonthrust mobilization.

Lumbar Spine

What are the risks of spinal manipulation in the lumbar spine? Studies show that serious risks are minimal. Haldeman and Rubinstein (1992) completed a review of the literature and over a period of 77 years found 10 episodes of cauda equina syndrome following lumbar spinal manipulation. This equates to an estimated risk of less than one per 10 million manipulations. Shekelle et al. (1992) estimated the rate of occurrence of cauda equina syndrome as a complication of lumbar spinal manipulation to be of the order of less than one case per 100 million manipulations. Bronfort (1999) reported that overall serious complications of lumbar spinal manipulation seem to be rare.

An analysis of the possible causes of complications from spinal manipulative techniques can be seen in Table 78.3.

CONTRAINDICATIONS AND PRECAUTIONS

As with any therapeutic intervention, due consideration must be given to the risk–benefit ratio. That is, the benefit to the patient of providing the therapeutic intervention must outweigh any potential risk associated with the intervention. Clinicians should always be aware of contraindications and precautions for spinal manipulative therapy. Is there a difference between a contraindication and a precaution? A contraindication means a manipulative technique should not be used under any circumstances, whereas a precaution means that depending on the skill, experience, and training of the practitioner; the type of

TABLE 78.5	Precautions for Spinal Manipulative Therapy
Adverse reaction to previous manual therapy	
Disc herniation or prolapse	
Pregnancy	
Spondylolisthesis	
Psychological dependence on manipulative techniques	
Ligamentous laxity	
As a general rule, safety in manipulation is best provided by gradual progression of the strength of the technique (grades of mobilization) coupled with continual assessment and reassessment (Maitland 1986).	
How can we make manipulative techniques safer?	Receive appropriate clinician training. Take a thorough patient history. Perform a thorough physical examination. Use your clinical reasoning skills. Use graded mobilizations prior to the application of any manipulative procedure.

technique selected; the amount of leverage and force used; and the age, general health, and physical condition of the patient, it may not be the wisest choice to use a manipulative technique. Tables 78.4 and 78.5 provide some of the known and accepted contraindications and precautions for manipulative techniques and offer some advice on making manipulation safer.

SPINAL MANIPULATION TECHNIQUES

General Technique Versus Specific Intervertebral Level

General techniques include the following:
- Rotation and direct palpation
- Take up slack, ease back fractionally, then add very fast small-range movement.
- Presupposes that treatment has progressed through stages from gentle mobilization to stage when manipulation is thought necessary
- The movement is always small range at end of range (through 3 to 4 degrees).

- Movement should NEVER be large movement through a full range from the central position; to do so is to court disaster. Specific intervertebral level techniques include the following:
- Ligamentous locking of facet joints below the treatment level, keeping a firm but comfortable grip on the patient's upper body and hip; the patient must gain a sense of security from your handhold technique to fully relax
- Direction of the manipulative technique based on desired outcome
- Rotation to increase facet "opening" or "gapping"
- Lateral thrust to open up "gap" same side and close down opposite facet joint

- Longitudinal thrust to "distract" or apply sharp traction to same side facet joint
- Although there are specific positions to be achieved through a combination of rotation, lateral flexion, and extension, anatomic differences require "fine tuning" of the manipulative position; there is a definite "end feel" that one becomes accustomed to locating.

Descriptions of the more commonly performed manipulative techniques for the cervical, thoracic, and lumbar spines are provided in Rehabilitation Protocol 78.1.

REHABILITATION PROTOCOL 78.1 ● Spinal Manipulative Techniques

High-Velocity End-Range Rotation Thrust to Lumbopelvic Region, Pelvis on Lumbar Spine With Patient Supine (Anterior Innominate Technique)

Steps

- Patient lies supine
- Move patient's pelvis toward you.
- Move feet and shoulders in opposite direction to introduce left side-bending of the trunk.
- Place patient's left foot and ankle on top of the right ankle.
- Ask patient to clasp his or her fingers behind his or her neck, or ask patient to fold his or her arms across his or her chest (comfort for patient).

Method

- Rotate the patient's trunk to the right while maintaining left trunk side-bending (do not lose the side-bending).
- You can thread your hand through the patient's crossed arms to the treatment couch.
- Place the palm of your right hand directly over the ASIS.
- Make any necessary adjustments to achieve prethrust tension.

Thrust

- Against the ASIS in a curved plane toward the couch
- The left forearm, wrist, and hand over the patient's shoulder (or threaded through the patient's crossed arms) do not apply a thrust but act as stabilizers only

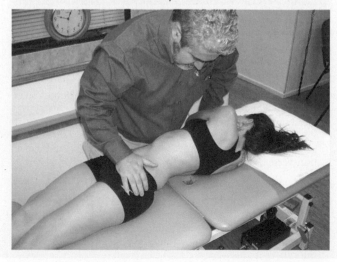

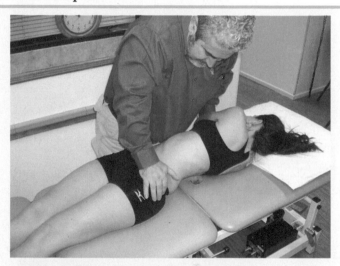

High-Velocity End-Range Rotation Thrust to Upper Lumbar Spine on Lower Lumbar Spine With Patient Side Lying (Side-Lying Rotation Technique or Rotation Gliding Thrust in Neutral Positioning)

Steps: (L rotation)

- Patient in right side lying
- Place the patient's right leg and spine in a straight line to achieve neutral/extension positioning.
- Flex the left hip to approx. 90 degrees.
- Left knee flexed and dorsum of left foot placed just behind the right knee
- Introduce left rotation of the upper body down to desired level.
- Avoid introducing any spine flexion.
- Take up axillary hold.

Method

- Stand close to the couch, feet spread and one leg behind the other.
- Maintain an upright posture facing the patient's upper body.
- Place the right forearm in the region between gluteus medius and maximus.
- Rotate the patient's pelvis and lumbar spine toward you until motion is palpated at the desired segment (pretension).
- Rotate the patient's upper body away from you until you sense tension at the desired segment.
- Roll the patient about 10 to 15 degrees toward you.

Continued

REHABILITATION PROTOCOL 78.1 ● Spinal Manipulative Techniques—cont'd

- Make any necessary adjustments to achieve prethrust tension.

Thrust

- With the forearm against the pelvis, the direction of force is down toward the couch by applying exaggerated pelvic rotation toward you
- The left arm against the patient's axillary region does not apply a thrust but acts as stabilizer only.

Thrust

- With the sternum or upper abdomen the thrust is down toward the couch and in a cephalad direction.
- Simultaneously apply a thrust with your left hand against the transverse processes in an upward and caudad direction.
- The hand contacting the transverse processes of T6 must actively participate in the generation of forces; it cannot remain passive and limp.

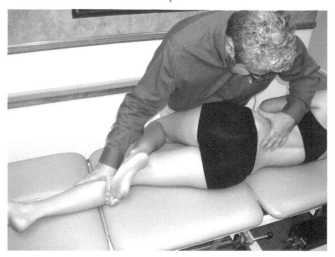

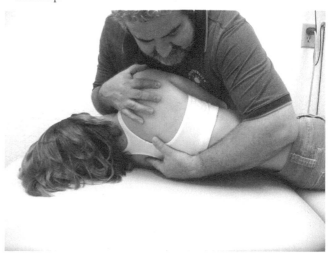

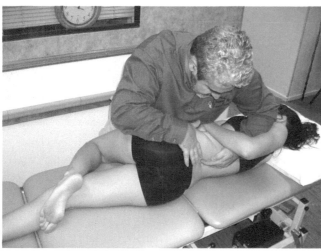

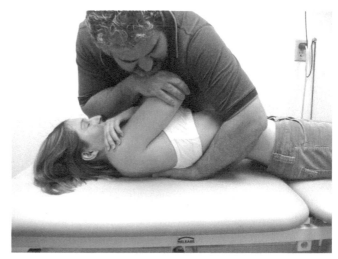

High-Velocity Mid-range Anterior-To-Posterior Thrust to Mid-Thoracic Spine With the Patient Supine Lying (Supine Anteroposterior Thrust or Flexion Gliding Technique)

Steps: (L hand under thorax)

- Patient in supine with arms crossed over chest
- Take hold of the patient's right shoulder and roll him or her toward you.
- Place your clenched left palm/fist against the transverse processes of T6.
- Roll the patient back into supine over your hand and place your right hand and forearm over the patient's crossed arms (hold at the elbows).

Method

- Flex and extend the patient's thorax over your left hand until you feel contact points directly over your left carpometacarpal (CMC) joint/thenar eminence and third middle phalanx.
- Apply pressure with your sternum or upper abdomen downward toward the couch.

High-Velocity Mid-range Posterior-to-Anterior Rotatory Thrust to Mid-Thoracic Spine With Patient Prone Lying (Prone Screw Technique or Rotation Gliding Technique)

Steps: (Rotation—short lever)

- Patient lies prone with arms hanging over the edge of the couch or placed along his or her body on the couch
- Head turned to either side (patient comfort)
- Place your contact points—hypothenar eminence/pisiform grip—on one transverse process (e.g., T5) on the left and the transverse process of the level below on the right (T6).

Method

- Stand to the left of the couch, feet spread and one leg behind the other.
- Maintain an upright posture facing the patient.
- This is a short lever technique and the velocity of the thrust is critical.
- Move your center of gravity directly over the patient and lean your body weight forward onto your arms and hypothenar eminences.

REHABILITATION PROTOCOL 78.1 ● **Spinal Manipulative Techniques—cont'd**

- Apply an additional force directed caudad with the left hand and cephalad with the right hand.

Thrust

- The direction is downward and cephalad against the transverse process of T5 with the right hand, while simultaneously applying a thrust downward and caudad against the transverse process of T6 with the left hand.

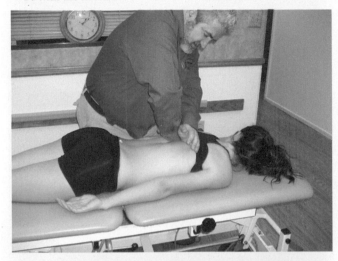

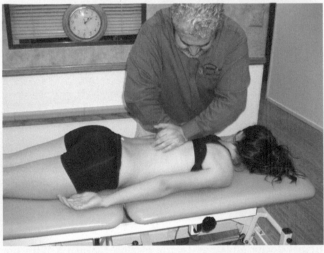

High-Velocity Midrange Extension-Distraction Mid-Thoracic on Lower Thoracic Spine With the Patient Seated (Seated Distraction Technique or Extension Gliding Technique)

Steps

- Patient sitting with arms crossed over chest
- Make sure he or she is well back on the couch.
- Stand directly behind the patient with your feet apart, knees bent slightly, and one leg behind the other.

Method

- Lean forward and place the thrusting part of your chest (and manipulation pillow) against the patient's spinous processes.
- Reach around and hold the patient's elbows.
- Introduce a backward (compressive) and upward force to the patient's folded arms.
- Maintain all holds and pressures, then bring the patient backward until your body weight is evenly distributed between both feet.

Thrust

- With your arms the direction is toward you and slightly upward.
- Simultaneously apply a thrust directly forward and upward against the spinous processes with your sternum (and manipulation pillow).

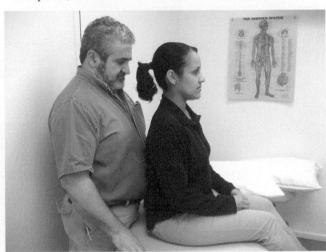

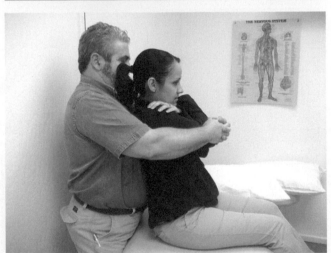

High-Velocity Mid-range Rotation C4 on C5 With the Patient Supine—Cradle Hold (Rotation Technique or Upslope Glide Technique)

Steps: (L rotation–R side upslope glide)

- Patient in supine with the neck in a neutral relaxed position on a pillow

Method

- Stand at the head of the couch, feet spread slightly.
- Contact point is the posterolateral aspect of the right articular pillar at the desired level
- Applicator is the lateral border of the proximal or middle phalanx

Cradle Hold

- The weight of the patient's head and neck is balanced between your left and right hands with cervical positioning controlled by converging pressure from both hands.
- Introduce primary leverage of rotation to the left and a small degree of secondary leverage of side-bending right while maintaining contact point on the posterolateral articular pillar.

Continued

REHABILITATION PROTOCOL 78.1 ● Spinal Manipulative Techniques—cont'd

Thrust

- The thrust is directed toward the patient's left eye.
- Simultaneously apply a slight, rapid increase of rotation of the head and neck to the left with no increase of side-bending to the right.

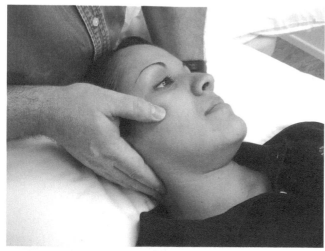

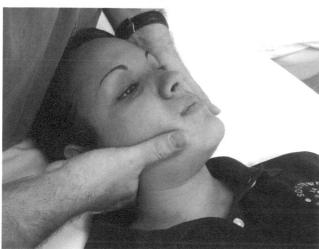

High-Velocity Midrange Rotation C4 on C5 With the Patient Supine—Chin Hold (Rotation Technique or Upslope Glide Technique)

Steps: (L rotation–R side upslope glide)

- Patient in supine with the neck in a neutral relaxed position on a pillow

Method

- Stand at the head of the couch, feet spread slightly.
- Contact point is the posterolateral aspect of the right articular pillar at the desired level
- Applicator is the lateral border of the proximal or middle phalanx

Chin Hold

- Your left forearm should be over or slightly anterior to the patient's ear.
- Use soft but firm hold over the chin.
- Step to the right and stand across the right corner of the couch.
- Introduce primary leverage of rotation to the left and a small degree of secondary leverage of side-bending right while maintaining contact point on the posterolateral articular pillar.

Thrust

- The thrust is directed toward the patient's left eye.
- Simultaneously apply a slight, rapid increase of rotation of the head and neck to the left with no increase of side-bending to the right.
- Avoid "pulling" on the chin with your left hand—both hands should work together in harmony.

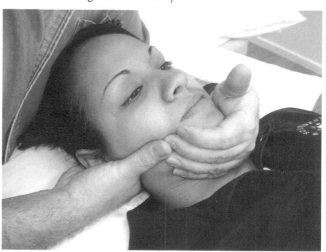

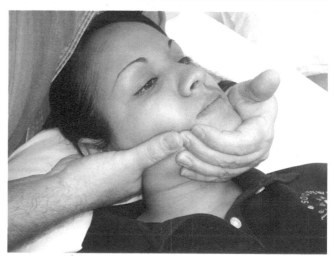

High-Velocity Midrange Lateral Flexion C4 on C5 With the Patient Supine—Cradle Hold (Lateral Flexion Technique or Downslope Glide Technique)

Steps: (L lateral flexion–L side downslope glide)

- Patient in supine with the neck in a neutral relaxed position on a pillow

Method

- Stand at the head of the couch, feet spread slightly.
- Contact point is the posterolateral aspect of the right articular pillar at the desired level
- Applicator is the lateral border of the proximal or middle phalanx

Cradle Hold

- The weight of the patient's head and neck is balanced between your left and right hands with cervical positioning controlled by converging pressure from both hands.
- Introduce primary leverage of side-bending to the left and a small degree of secondary leverage of rotation right while maintaining contact point on the posterolateral articular pillar.

REHABILITATION PROTOCOL 78.1 ● Spinal Manipulative Techniques—cont'd

Thrust

- The thrust is directed toward the patient's right axilla.
- Simultaneously apply a slight, rapid increase of side-bending of the head and neck to the left with no increase of rotation to the right.

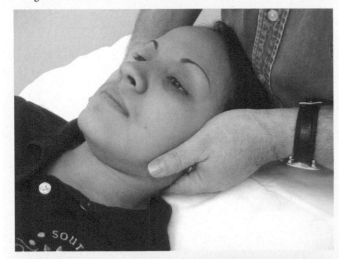

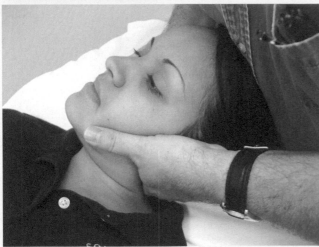

High-Velocity Midrange Lateral Flexion C4 on C5 With the Patient Supine—Chin Hold (Lateral Flexion Technique or Downslope Glide Technique)

Steps: (L lateral flexion–L side downslope glide)

- Patient in supine with the neck in a neutral relaxed position on a pillow

Method

- Stand at the head of the couch, feet spread slightly.
- Contact point is the posterolateral aspect of the right articular pillar at the desired level
- Applicator is the lateral border of the proximal or middle phalanx

Chin Hold

- Your left forearm should be over or slightly anterior to the patient's ear.
- Use soft but firm hold over the chin.
- Step to the left and stand across the left corner of the couch.
- Introduce primary leverage of side-bending to the left and a small degree of secondary leverage of rotation right while maintaining contact point on the posterolateral articular pillar.

Thrust

- The thrust is directed toward the patient's right axilla.
- Simultaneously apply a slight, rapid increase of side-bending of the head and neck to the left with no increase of rotation to the right.
- Avoid "pulling" on the chin with your right hand—both hands should work together in harmony.

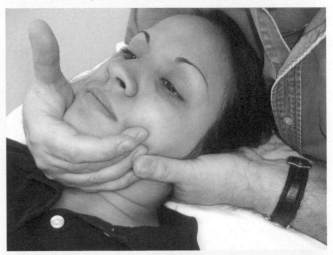

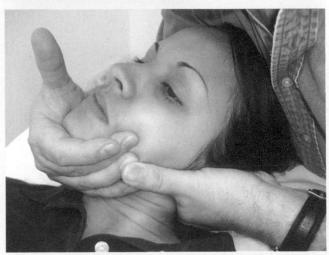

REFERENCES

A complete reference list is available at https://expertconsult .inkling.com/.

FURTHER READING

Childs JD, Fritz JM, et al. Proposal of a classification system for patients with neck pain. *J Orthop Sports Phys Ther.* 2004;34(11):686–696. discussion 697–700.

Stiell IG, Greenberg GH, et al. A study to develop clinical decision rules for the use of radiography in acute ankle injuries. *Ann Emerg Med.* 1992;21(4):384–390.

Stiell IG, Wells GA, et al. The Canadian C-spine rule for radiography in alert and stable trauma patients. *JAMA.* 2001;286(15):1841–1848.

Wainner RS, Fritz JM, et al. Reliability and diagnostic accuracy of the clinical examination and patient self-report measures for cervical radiculopathy. *Spine.* 2003;28(1):52–62.

Neurodynamics

Emilio "Louie" Puentedura, PT, DPT, GDMT, OCS, FAAOMPT

MANUAL THERAPY FOR THE NERVOUS SYSTEM

Maitland (1986) described manual therapy as the selective examination and evaluation of the effects of movement, position, and activities on the signs and symptoms of a neuromusculoskeletal disorder. The clinician is able to formulate a working hypothesis regarding the movement problem, which can be confirmed or denied following the careful reassessment during and after specific treatment applications. It is useful to think of the mechanics of the body's moving parts in terms of components comprising a chassis (skeletal framework), articulations (joints and supporting ligaments), motors (muscles and tendons), and electrical wiring (nervous system). Each of the components that makes up the neuromusculoskeletal system plays an important and interdependent role in its overall health and function.

Many of the early manual therapy systems placed a greater emphasis on the health and function of the articulations (joints); hence, "manual therapy" became synonymous with "passive joint mobilization" and "joint manipulation" (Butler 1991). Despite an underlying awareness of the interdependency of the components of the neuromusculoskeletal system, relatively little attention was paid to the physical health and movement of the nervous system. This changed dramatically following the published works of Gregory Grieve, Alf Breig, Geoffrey Maitland, Robert Elvey, and David Butler, whose collective works opened a new frontier in manual therapy—the hypothesis that the entire nervous system is a mechanical organ that could develop "adverse tension," or impaired mobility, which could then be treated with various movement therapies.

ADVERSE NEURAL TENSION VERSUS NEURODYNAMICS

Adverse neural tension can be defined as the abnormal physiologic and mechanical responses produced by nervous system structures when testing its normal range of movement and stretch capabilities (Butler 1991). A neural tension test is therefore designed to examine the physical (mechanical) abilities of the nervous system (Butler 2000). Using the term "tension" has significant limitations because it fails to take into account other aspects of nervous system function, such as movement, pressure, viscoelasticity, and physiology (Shacklock 1995a and 1995b, Shacklock 2005a and 2005b). Therefore, a more appropriate term is neurodynamic test (Shacklock 2005b).

The term "neurodynamics" refers to the mechanics and physiology of the nervous system within the musculoskeletal system and how these systems relate to each other (Shacklock 1995a). It allows for the consideration of movement-related neurophysiologic changes and the neuronal dynamics postulated to occur in the central nervous system during physical and mental activity (Butler 2002). A key tenet of this definition is that the nervous system is capable of movement and stretch and that there is a "normal" (and abnormal) response of the nervous system to movement and tension. Both Butler (2000) and Shacklock (2005b) advocated the transition to the term "neurodynamic" as opposed to "neural tension" because "neurodynamics" places less emphasis on stretching and tension and more emphasis on the nervous system, the "container" in which it lives, and the mechanisms that can alter the function of the nervous system. These other mechanisms include changes to intraneural blood flow (Ogata and Naito 1986), neural inflammation (Zochodne and Ho 1991), mechanosensitivity (Calvin et al. 1982, Nordin et al. 1984), and muscle responses (Hall et al. 1995, Hall et al. 1998, van der Heide et al. 2001).

Neurodynamic impairments should be conceptualized as any specific physical dysfunction (whether it be neural, muscular, or skeletal) that presumes to physically challenge the normal functioning of the nervous system. These impairments can arise from mechanical, chemical, and/or sensitivity changes anywhere in the neuromusculoskeletal system. Therefore, in neurodynamics, neural tissues may have a tension problem (mechanical), be hypersensitive (a problem of pathophysiology), or a combination of both (Shacklock 2005b). Instead of a length or "tension" problem, the primary mechanical fault within the nervous system may be one of reduced sliding (neural sliding dysfunction), or it could be a compression problem that relates to the tissues that form a mechanical interface to the nervous system. To further facilitate understanding for the rest of this chapter, some operational definitions are provided in Box 79.1.

NEUROPHYSIOLOGY IN NEURODYNAMICS

Initially, manual therapists were more interested in the mechanical aspects of neurodynamics (Breig 1978, Elvey 1979 and 1986, Butler 1991). Unfortunately, it has led to a very "mechanistic" view of the nervous system (Butler 2000). Most textbooks describe normal nerve mechanics related to various positions, postures, or movements; subsequent abnormal mechanics (pathomechanics); and finally movement-based treatment aimed at restoring normal nerve movement (Butler 1991 and 2000, Shacklock 2005b). However, increased knowledge in our understanding of nerve pain related to neurophysiologic changes and the processing within the brain of nerve movement (and pain) warrants some investigation and discussion.

Pathologies that affect peripheral nerves usually result in dysesthetic pain and/or nerve trunk pain (Asbury and Fields 1984). Dysesthetic pain (where light touch causes pain) often manifests as burning or tingling pain as a result of abnormal impulses from hyperexcitable afferent nerve fibers, which,

BOX 79.1 **DEFINITIONS OF TERMS: NEURODYNAMICS**

- **Neurodynamics:** The examination, evaluation, and treatment of the mechanics and physiology of the nervous system as they relate to each other and are integrated with musculoskeletal function.
- **Neurodynamic test:** A series of body movements that produces mechanical and physiologic events in the nervous system according to the movements of the test. A neurodynamic test aims to physically challenge or test the mechanics and/or physiology of a part of the nervous system.
- **Neurogenic pain:** Pain that is initiated or caused by a primary lesion, dysfunction, or transitory perturbation in the peripheral or central nervous system (Merskey and Bogduk 1994).
- **Sensitizing movements:** Movements that increase forces in the neural structures in addition to those movements used in the standard neurodynamic test. Sensitizing movements can be useful in loading or moving the nervous system beyond the effects of the standard neurodynamic test (i.e., strengthening the test). However, they also load and move musculoskeletal structures and are therefore not as helpful in determining the existence of a neurodynamic problem as a differentiating movement.
- **Differentiating movements:** Movements that emphasize or isolate the nervous system by producing movement in the neural structures in the area in question rather than moving the musculoskeletal structures in the same area. Differentiating movements place emphasis on the nervous system without affecting the other structures and are therefore used to help establish the existence of a neurodynamic problem.
- **Sliders:** Neurodynamic maneuvers performed to produce a sliding movement of neural structures relative to their adjacent tissues. Sliders involve application of movement/stress to the nervous system proximally while releasing movement/stress distally and then reversing the sequence.
- **Tensioners:** Neurodynamic maneuvers performed to produce an increase in tension (not stretch) in neural structures, which may improve neural viscoelastic and physiologic functions (help neural tissue cope better with increased tension). Tensioners are the opposite of sliders in that movement/stress is applied proximally and distally to the nervous system at the same time and then released.

because of injury, may become abnormal impulse generating sites (AIGS) (Devor et al. 1979, Asbury and Fields 1984, Woolf and Mannion 1999). AIGS may spontaneously fire as the result of mechanical or chemical stimuli (Butler 2000) such that dysesthetic pain may present as very bizarre patterns, from bursts of pain in response to a stimulus to pain that presents spontaneously with no apparent stimuli.

In contrast, nerve trunk pain commonly presents as deep, achy pain arising from nociceptors within the nervous tissue that are sensitized to mechanical or chemical stimuli (Asbury and Fields 1984, Kallakuri et al. 1998). Nerve trunk pain usually has a fairly straightforward stimulus-response relationship (Asbury and Fields 1984). These two types of pain can be evoked by a variety of chemical or mechanical stimuli and may lead to allodynia or hyperalgesia. Allodynia is a pain sensation that is evoked from stimuli that are not normally painful, whereas hyperalgesia is an exaggerated pain response to stimuli that would normally be painful (Asbury and Fields 1984, Woolf and Mannion 1999, Nee and Butler 2006).

NERVE SENSITIVITY

To understand nerve sensitivity, some knowledge of ion channels is required. Although the complexity of ion channel regulation

is not yet properly understood and research is based on animal studies, scientists and clinicians are using the information known about ion channels to improve patient care (Barry and Lynch 1991, Butler 2000). Ion channels are essentially proteins clumped together with an opening to allow ions to flow in/out of a membrane (Devor 2006). They are synthesized in the dorsal root ganglion (DRG) based on a genetic coding and are distributed along an axon to allow ions to flow in or out of the nerve to polarize or depolarize the membrane. Ion channels are not uniformly distributed along the axolemma with certain areas known to have higher concentrations of ion channels, such as the DRG, axon hillock, nodes of Ranvier, and areas where the axon has lost myelin (Fried et al. 1993, Devor 2006). Furthermore, there are countless types of ion channels, including channels that seem to respond to movement, pressure, blood flow, circulating adrenaline levels, and so on. From a survival perspective, this might seem logical as a means for the nervous system to become "sensitive" to various stimuli. However, the amount and type of ion channels found in the axolemma is in a constant state of change (Fried et al. 1993, Devor 2006). Research has shown that the half-life of some ion channels may be as short as two days (Barry and Lynch 1991), and ion channels that drop out of the membrane are not necessarily replaced by the same type. Ion channel deposition is directly affected by the environment in which the organism finds itself (Barry and Lynch 1991). For example, changes in temperature around an animal with experimentally removed myelin produce higher concentrations of "cold-sensing" channels in that area; animals in stressful environments produce higher concentrations of adrenosensitive channels, and animals that have joints with restricted movement cause upregulation of movement sensitive ion channels (Fried et al. 1993, Devor 2006). With higher concentrations of similar ion channels in an area, the chances for the nerve to depolarize and cause an action potential increase. In essence, the nerve may develop an AIGS. The nervous system can then become sensitive to various types of stimuli, such as temperature, movement, pressure, anxiety, stress, the immune system, and more (Butler 2000, Butler and Moseley 2003). The nervous system can therefore be viewed as an alarm system beautifully designed to protect the organism, and the amount and type of ion channels at any given time may be a fair representation of what the brain computes is needed for survival (Butler and Moseley 2003).

CENTRAL SENSITIVITY

Many clinicians are familiar with the term "central sensitivity." Central sensitivity is defined as a condition in which peripheral noxious input into the CNS leads to an increased excitability where the response to normal inputs is greatly enhanced (Woolf 2007). Repeated painful stimuli, such as easily excitable AIGS, may cause low-threshold neurons with large receptive fields to depolarize in response to stimuli that would normally be benign (Woolf 2007). It has been shown that injured neural tissue may alter its chemical makeup and reorganize synaptic contacts in the CNS such that innocuous stimuli are directed to cells that normally receive only noxious inputs (Woolf 2007). Hence, the CNS becomes "hyperexcitable" as a result of a combination of decreased inhibition and increased responsiveness (Woolf 2000). This is analogous to turning up the volume on the system such that innocuous stimuli begin to generate painful sensations, whereas noxious stimuli result in an exaggerated pain response. This process has been described as a change in both the software and the hardware of the CNS (Woolf 2000), and it could be argued that clinicians have the tools to affect both of these.

CLINICAL NEUROBIOMECHANICS

Neurobiomechanics is the study of the normal and pathologic ROM of the nervous system. Unfortunately, what we know is based on limited animal and cadaver research. This is an area in need of further research. For recent work, see Zoech et al. (1991), Szabo et al. (1994), Kleinrensink et al. (1995 and 2000), Wright et al. (2001), and Dilley et al. (2003).

A key issue in the understanding of neurobiomechanics is the concept of the nervous system as a continuous tissue tract. The system is continuous mechanically via its continuous connective tissue formats, electrically via conducted impulses, and chemically via its common neurotransmitters. The nervous system being a mechanical continuum is probably most relevant to the study of neurodynamics because it implies transmission of movement (sliding/gliding) and the development of tension (stretching) within and along the system. That is, wrist extension and elbow extension lengthen and move the median nerve distally within its neural pathway, and contralateral cervical lateral flexion adds a pull in the proximal direction. This has been demonstrated in cadaver studies in which the nerve roots are marked with paper markers or pins. When the shoulder is depressed and abducted in external rotation, the cervical nerve roots are pulled out of the vertebral foramen (Elvey 1979).

Another key concept in neurodynamics is that of the mechanical interface. The mechanical interface is defined as "that tissue or material adjacent to the nervous system that can move independently to the system" (Butler 1991). Mechanical interfaces are central to an understanding of neurodynamics because they represent the most likely sites for the development of movement/force transmission problems. Mechanical interfaces can be hard or bony (e.g., ulnar nerve at the cubital tunnel), ligamentous (ligament of Struthers in the forearm), joints (e.g., zygapophyseal joints), or muscular (e.g., supinator muscle in forearm). Mechanical interfaces can be normal, where movement and function are optimal and symptom free, or they can be pathologic, where something happens to restrict movement of the nervous system at the interface or compress the nervous tissue. Examples include osteophytes, extensive bruising, or swelling that could occupy space at the mechanical interface resulting in restricted ROM and independence of the nervous system and the interface. Numerous studies have shown that if the interface is injured or damaged, it may have repercussions for the adjacent neural tissues. Examples include the cubital tunnel (Coppieters et al. 2004), carpal tunnel (Novak et al. 1992, Nakamichi and Tachibana 1995, Rozmaryn et al. 1998, Greening et al. 1999), intervertebral foramen (de Peretti et al. 1989, Chang et al. 2006), and the spinal canal (Fritz et al. 1998, Chang et al. 2006). If this happens, ROM of the nervous system can be impaired, and this would presumably lead to the "abnormal mechanical response" in our definition of neurodynamics.

As the nervous system winds its way through its anatomic course, it is forced to stretch, slide (longitudinal or transverse), bend, and become compressed. Stretch is defined here as the elongation of the nerve relative to its starting length. However, nerves are not solid structures and stretch causes internal compression as a result of displacement of nerve tissue/fluid. The physiologic effects of stretch and compression include changes to intraneural blood flow, conduction, and axoplasmic transport. Studies have shown that if a peripheral nerve is held on an 8% stretch for 30 minutes, it will cause a 50% decrease in blood flow; an 8.8% stretch for one hour will cause a 70% decrease in blood flow; and a 15% stretch for 30 minutes will cause an 80% to 100% blockage in blood flow (Ogata and Naito 1986, Driscoll et al. 2002). Wall and others (1992) were able to demonstrate that a 6% stretch/strain of a peripheral nerve for one hour resulted in a 70% decrease in action potentials and a 12% stretch/strain for one hour caused complete conduction block. Of interest, other studies reported that from full wrist and elbow flexion to full wrist and elbow extension, the median nerve has to adapt to a nerve bed that becomes 20% longer (Millesi 1986, Zoech et al. 1991). Similar data have been provided with respect to the sciatic/tibial nerve (Beith et al. 1995). Research has demonstrated that flexion of the cervical spine leads to tension in the dura and spinal cord resulting in a cephalad movement of the cauda equina (Breig 1960 and 1978, Breig and Marions 1963, Breig and el-Nadi 1966, Breig et al. 1966, Breig and Troup 1979). This ultimately limits the available mobility of the sciatic nerve. Obviously, there must be some mechanical and physiologic adaptations within peripheral nerves to accommodate such significant changes in length and to cope with prolonged stretching or strain. The effects of compression have also been studied with as little as 20 to 30 mm Hg causing decreased venous blood flow and 80 mm Hg causing complete blockage of intraneural blood flow (Rydevik et al. 1981, Ogata and Naito 1986). Compression also has been shown to alter axonal transport (Dahlin et al. 1993) and action potential conduction (Fern and Harrison 1994).

Nerves move relative to their adjacent tissues, and this motion has been described as sliding or excursion (McLellan and Swash 1976, Wilgis and Murphy 1986). Excursion occurs both longitudinally and transversely. This sliding or excursion is considered an essential aspect of neural function because it serves to dissipate tension and distribute forces within the nervous system. Instead of stretching (and thereby developing tension) the nervous system can move longitudinally and/or transversely and distribute itself along the shortest course between fixed points; hence, it can equalize tension throughout the neural tract. An excellent example of transverse sliding or excursion can be seen at the wrist. Using real-time ultrasound imaging (RUSI) at the carpal tunnel, one can appreciate transverse sliding of the median nerve relative to the flexor tendons during performance of the upper limb neurodynamic test (Shacklock 2005b).

As joints move, there is nerve bed elongation (increase in length of the neural container) on the convex side of the joint and nerve bed shortening (decrease in length of the neural container) on the concave side of the joint. When there is nerve bed elongation, the nerve glides toward the joint that is moving; this is referred to as convergence. When there is nerve bed shortening, the nerve glides away from the joint that is moving; this is referred to as divergence. Dilley et al. (2003) used RUSI to examine the effects of elbow extension on the median nerve and found the magnitude of excursion for the median nerve in the mid-upper arm to be 10.4 mm distally toward the elbow and in the mid-forearm to be 3.0 mm proximally toward the elbow. With the elbow held in extension while applying wrist extension, they recorded excursion of the median nerve at the mid-upper arm 1.8 mm distally toward the elbow and in the mid-forearm 4.2 mm distally toward the wrist. It could be

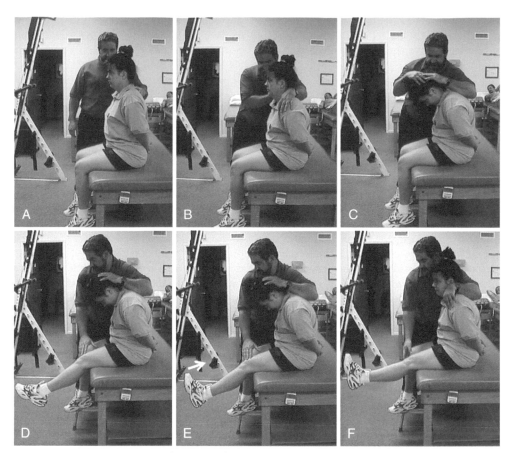

Fig. 79.1 Slump test. **A-F,** Stages 1-6.

argued that some degree of excursion must occur in the hand proximally toward the wrist also.

Studies have shown that the starting position and the sequencing of limb movement during neurodynamic tests affect the degree of excursion along the nerve. In the same study, Dilley and colleagues (2003) also examined the median nerve at the distal arm and mid-forearm using two different start positions—elbow in full extension and shoulder at 45 degrees or at 90 degrees of abduction—then performed wrist extension from neutral to 45 degrees. They found that greater excursion of the median nerve occurred when the shoulder was in a more slackened position (45 degrees of abduction). For the shoulder at 45 degrees abduction, excursion was 2.4 mm distally at the distal arm and 4.7 mm distally at the mid-forearm. For the shoulder at 90 degrees of abduction, excursion was 1.8 mm distally at the distal arm and 4.2 mm distally at the mid-forearm. The sequence of movements has also been shown to affect the distribution of symptoms in response to neurodynamic testing (Shacklock 1989, Zorn et al. 1995). These authors reported a greater likelihood of producing a response that is localized to the region that is moved first or more strongly. Tsai (1995) conducted a cadaveric study in which strain in the ulnar nerve at the elbow was measured during ulnar neurodynamic testing in three different sequences: proximal-to-distal, distal-to-proximal, and elbow-first sequence. The elbow-first sequence consistently produced 20% greater strain in the ulnar nerve at the elbow than the other two sequences. Therefore, it can be argued that greater strain in the nerves occurs at the site that is moved first—that is, the first component of a neurodynamic test or treatment technique.

THE BASE TESTS

Butler (1991) proposed a base test system for neurodynamic evaluation. It is a clinically intuitive system that evolved for ease of handling and to fulfill a perceived clinical demand. It is based on existing tests and the basic principles of neurodynamics already discussed, and in most clinical situations the tests are refined or adapted based on reasoned diagnoses and the clinical presentation of the patient. A positive neurodynamic test can be described as one that reproduces a familiar symptom, is changed by the movement of a body segment away from the site of symptoms, has side-to-side differences in the test response, or has differences from what is known to be normal in asymptomatic individuals (Nee and Butler 2006). However, a positive test does not allow the identification of a specific area of injury; it is merely suggestive of increased mechanosensitivity somewhere along the neural tissue tract (Nee and Butler 2006).

The base tests for the head, neck, and trunk (Figs. 79.1 through 79.4), the lower extremity, and the upper extremity (Figs. 79.2 through 79.5) are listed in Box 79.2. Each of the base tests includes attention to the major neural pathways and the major sensitizing movements. Active testing is recommended before passive testing. This allows gauging of the patient's ability and willingness to move and provides an approximate measure of the ROM likely to be encountered during the passive test. It also may decrease the patient's fears and anxieties about the test and symptoms likely to be elicited during the test. Finally, if the active movement

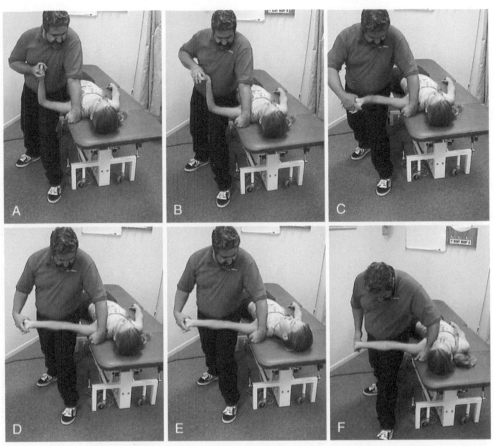

Fig. 79.2 The UNLT 1 (median) passive test. **A-F,** Stages 1-6.

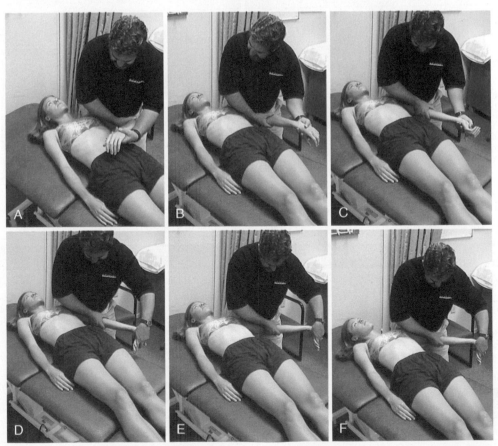

Fig. 79.3 The ULNT 2 (median) passive test. **A-F,** Stages 1-6.

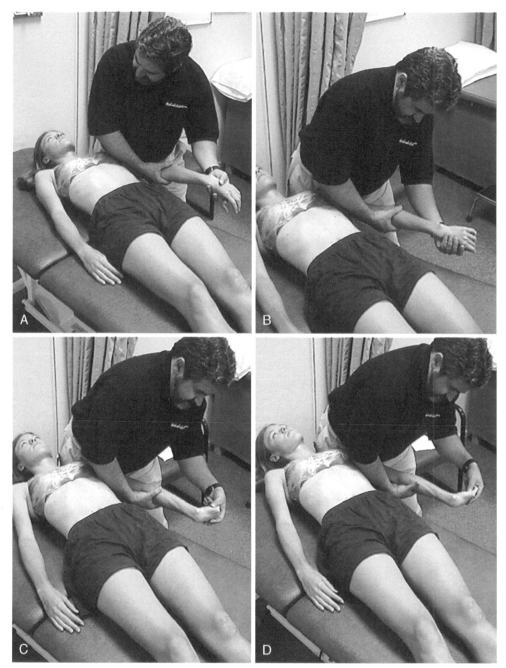

Fig. 79.4 The ULNT 2 (radial) passive test. A-D, Stages 1-4.

BOX 79.2 BASE TESTS IN NEURODYNAMICS

PASSIVE NECK FLEXION

Starting Position:

- Patient lies supine, arms by the side, no pillow if possible, and body straight.
- Therapist stands to one side of the patient's head and places his or her cephalad hand under the patient's occiput and the other hand overlying the chin.

Movement Sequence:

- Passive cervical flexion achieved through upper cervical (craniocervical) flexion followed by middle and lower cervical segments.

Structural Differentiation:

- Maintaining end-range passive neck flexion position and adding straight leg raise or perhaps an upper limb neurodynamic test (to draw the cervical cord and dura in a caudal direction) and note any changes in symptoms.

STRAIGHT LEG RAISE TEST

Starting Position:

- Patient lies supine, arms by the side, no pillow if possible, and body straight.
- Therapist faces patient and places one hand under the ankle and the other hand above the patella.

BOX 79.2 BASE TESTS IN NEURODYNAMICS—cont'd

Movement Sequence:

- Keeping the knee extended, therapist passively flexes the hip in the sagittal plane.
- Leg is taken short of, to, or into sensory or motor responses depending on prior reasoned hypotheses of pathobiological processes involved.

Sensitizing Movements:

- Adding ankle dorsiflexion and eversion (tibial component).
- Adding ankle plantarflexion and inversion (peroneal component).
- Hip adduction and/or internal rotation (sciatic component).
- Active or passive head and neck flexion (dural component).

SLUMP TEST

Starting Position:

- Patient sits with thighs supported, knees together, and arms comfortably behind back.
- Therapist stands beside and close to the patient, perhaps with one leg up on the treatment table.

Movement Sequence:

- Patient is asked to sag or slump; gentle hand pressure by therapist can guide the movement to obtain a bowing of the spine rather than hip flexion.
- Patient is asked to flex his or her head and neck forward in a chin-to-chest motion.
- Patient is asked to perform ankle dorsiflexion and then extend the knee actively as much as he or she is able to within symptom tolerance.

Structural Differentiation:

- Based on where the symptoms (if any) are located.
- If distal symptoms have developed (e.g., knee, posterior thigh), the head and neck are released from flexion and any change in the distal symptoms would constitute a positive structural differentiation.
- If proximal symptoms have developed (e.g., neck and upper back pain), the ankle is released from dorsiflexion and any change in the proximal symptoms would constitute a positive structural differentiation.

ULNT 1 (MEDIAN) PASSIVE TEST

Starting Position:

- Patient lies supine, arms by the side, and shoulder close to the edge of the examination table, no pillow if possible, and body straight.
- Therapist faces the patient's head and presses near hand on the table above the patient's shoulder in either a knuckles or fist position (avoiding downward or caudal pressure on the superior aspect of the patient's shoulder).
- With other hand, therapist holds patient's hand with the thumb extended to apply tension to the motor branch of the median nerve. Therapist's fingers wrap around the patient's fingers distal to the metacarpophalangeal joints.
- Patient's elbow is flexed at 90 degrees and supported on the therapist's near (front) thigh.

Movement Sequence:

- Glenohumeral abduction up to 90 to 110 degrees, if available, in the frontal plane.
- Wrist and finger extension and forearm supination.
- Glenohumeral external rotation to available range (generally stopped at 90 degrees if the patient is very mobile).
- Elbow extension should be done gently and with care not to cause any shoulder motion, especially adduction (which would ease off developing neurodynamic test).

Structural Differentiation:

- Based on where the symptoms (if any) are located.
- If distal symptoms have developed (e.g., forearm and wrist pain), the neck is moved into contralateral lateral flexion and any change in the distal symptoms would constitute a positive structural differentiation.

- If proximal symptoms have developed (e.g., neck and shoulder pain), the wrist is released from its extended position and any change in the proximal symptoms would constitute a positive structural differentiation.

ULNT 2 (MEDIAN) PASSIVE TEST

Starting Position:

- Patient lies supine on a slight diagonal with the shoulder just over the edge of the treatment table to allow for contact with the therapist's thigh.
- Therapist stands near the patient's shoulder and uses thigh to carefully depress the shoulder girdle.
- Therapist's right hand cradles the patient's left elbow and the left hand controls the patient's wrist and hand.
- Patient's arm is in approximately 10 degrees of abduction.

Movement Sequence:

- Elbow extension and then whole-arm external rotation.
- Wrist and finger extension.
- Glenohumeral abduction is then added if necessary.

Structural Differentiation:

- Based on where the symptoms (if any) are located.
- Same as for ULNT 1.

ULNT 2 (RADIAL) PASSIVE TEST

Starting Position:

- Patient lies supine on a slight diagonal with the shoulder just over the edge of the treatment table to allow for contact with the therapist's thigh.
- Therapist stands near the patient's shoulder and uses thigh to carefully depress the shoulder girdle.
- Therapist's right hand cradles the patient's left elbow and the left hand controls the patient's wrist and hand.
- Patient's arm is in approximately 10 degrees of abduction.

Movement Sequence:

- Elbow extension and then whole arm internal rotation.
- Wrist and finger flexion (may also add wrist ulnar deviation and thumb flexion).
- Glenohumeral abduction is then added if necessary.

Structural Differentiation:

- Based on where the symptoms (if any) are located.
- Same as for ULNT 1.

ULNT 3 (ULNAR) PASSIVE TEST

Starting Position:

- Patient lies supine, arms by the side, and shoulder close to the edge of the examination table, no pillow if possible, and body straight.
- Therapist faces the patient's head and presses near hand on the table above the patient's shoulder in either a knuckles or fist position (this time, applying a downward or caudal pressure on the superior aspect of the patient's shoulder to achieve shoulder girdle depression).
- With the other hand, the therapist holds the patient's hand palm against palm and the elbow starts in extension.

Movement Sequence:

- Wrist and fingers extended as the elbow is flexed.
- Forearm is then pronated and the shoulder taken into lateral rotation and abduction.
- Glenohumeral external rotation to available range (generally stopped at 90 degrees if the patient is very mobile)
- Elbow extension should be done gently and with care not to cause any shoulder motion, especially adduction (which would ease off developing neurodynamic test).

Structural Differentiation:

- Based on where the symptoms (if any) are located.
- Add in cervical contralateral lateral flexion or shoulder girdle depression.

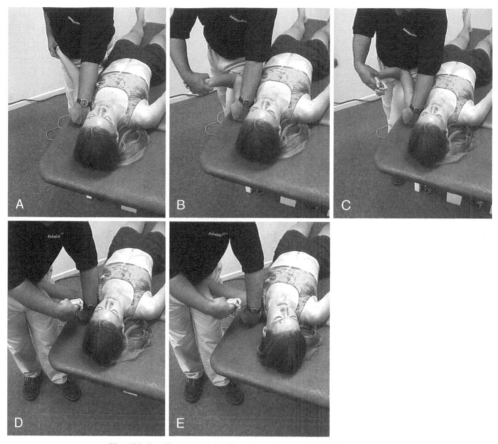

Fig. 79.5 The ULNT 3 (ulnar) passive test. **A-E**, Stages 1-5.

is found to be extremely sensitive, a reasoned decision may be made not to perform the tests passively to avoid symptom exacerbation. Some important handling issues with respect to performance of neurodynamic tests include the following:

- Only perform the testing if there is clinical rationale for doing so. Establish clinical reasoning categories prior to the test regarding pathobiology, likely specific dysfunctions to be found on examination, precautions, and sources of symptoms.
- Explain to patients exactly what you are going to do and what you want them to do. Patient comfort is vital for testing responses anywhere in their body.
- Test the less painful or nonpainful side first. If there is little difference between sides, perform the test on the left side first for consistency.
- Starting positions should be consistent, and any variations from normal practice should be noted/recorded (use of pillows, etc.).
- Note symptom responses including area and nature (type of response) with the addition of each component of the test.
- Watch for antalgic postures and other compensatory movements during the test (e.g., cervical movements or trapezius muscle activity).
- Test for symmetry between sides.
- Explain findings to the patient.
- Repeat the test gently a number of times before recording an actual measurement.

CLINICAL APPLICATION OF NEURODYNAMICS

An important consideration to always keep in mind is that healthy mechanics of the nervous system within the body enable pain-free posture and movement. In the presence of mechanical impairment (pathomechanics) of neural tissues (e.g., nerve entrapment), symptoms may be provoked during activities of daily living such as reaching to tie shoes, combing hair, or tucking in a shirt. The aim of using neurodynamic tests in assessment is to mechanically move neural tissues to gain an impression of their mobility and sensitivity to mechanical stresses. The purpose of treatment via these tests is to improve their mechanical and physiologic function (Butler 2000, Shacklock 2005b).

Mechanosensitivity is the chief mechanism that enables nerves to cause pain with movement. If a nerve is not mechanically sensitive, then it will not respond (cause pain) to mechanical forces applied to it. Mechanosensitivity can be defined as the ease with which impulses can be activated from a site in the nervous system when a mechanical force is applied. Normal nerves can be mechanosensitive (given sufficient force) and, therefore, respond to applied forces (Lindquist et al. 1973). This is a key fact to keep in mind when making judgments about whether the neural tissues are a problem. Responses to neurodynamic tests can be categorized as either normal or abnormal and relevant or irrelevant (Shacklock 2005b). Normal neurodynamic test responses are those that are in a normal location (relative to normative data), have a normal quality of symptoms, and show normal range of movement of the limb during the test.

Abnormal neurodynamic test responses are those that are in a different location than normal, have a different quality of symptoms, and/or range of movement of the limb is less than the uninvolved side. In most cases, there may be reproduction of the patient's symptoms. The next clinical question to consider is whether the test responses are relevant or irrelevant. Relevance, in this case, means that the test responses are causally related to the patient's current problem, and an irrelevant finding is a test response that is not causally related to the patient's current problem. Many times this can be elucidated by asking the patient, "Is that a familiar symptom to you?"

The symptoms evoked on a neurodynamic test can be inferred to be neurogenic (positive test in a clinical sense):

- If structural differentiation supports a neurogenic source
- If there are differences left to right and from known normal responses
- If the test reproduces the patient's symptoms or associated symptoms
- If there is support from other data such as history, area of symptoms, imaging tests, etc.

The greater the number of "ifs" present, the stronger the case for a clinically relevant test. Clinically, the information required from neurodynamic tests is symptom response, resistance encountered, and changes to symptom response and resistance encountered as each component of the test is added or subtracted. This information, along with the patient history, subjective and objective examination, and so on, should give the clinician the ability to provisionally diagnose the site of neuropathodynamics and then reassess after whatever treatment might be administered. It is important to realize that the treatment need not be a mobilizing technique for the nervous system because the clinician may decide to mobilize or treat the mechanical interface, or perhaps he or she may decide the problem is not peripheral neurogenic in nature but rather a "central processing enhancement" in which patient education/reassurance/discussion may be the treatment of choice. It is also important to remember that sensitivity to a neurodynamic test could be from a combination of primary (tissue-based) or secondary (CNS-based) processes (Butler 2000).

NEURODYNAMIC TREATMENT

Management of patients with a neurodynamic problem should focus on reducing mechanosensitivity and restoring normal movement to both the nervous tissue and its mechanical interface. Reassessment should be continual and should include clinical evaluation along with patient feedback. Patient education is paramount and should include a brief discussion of neurodynamics, the neurobiology of pain, and the continuity of the nervous system. Additionally, if there is a central sensitization component to the symptoms, this should also be addressed, along with any perceived or real fear of movement that the patient may have. This can reduce the threat value associated with their pain experience.

Next, it is useful to treat any impairment in non-neural tissues so as to reduce any mechanical forces the "container" may be placing on the nervous tissue. Interventions may include joint mobilization/manipulation, stretching, soft tissue work, and therapeutic exercise. Detailed discussion of these interventions is beyond the scope of this chapter. Any interventions should be followed by a reassessment of the provocative neurodynamic test to determine if change has occurred. If change has occurred, treatment may be discontinued for that day or specific neurodynamic interventions (either active or passive) may be added to the treatment.

It is also helpful to break neurodynamic interventions down into one of two approaches, "sliders" or "tensioners," each of which has its own indications and clinical usefulness (Nee and Butler 2006, Coppieters and Butler 2008). With a sliding or gliding technique, combined movements of at least two joints are alternated in such a way that one movement elongates the nerve bed while the other movement shortens the nerve bed. This results in a situation where the nerve is mobilized through a large degree of longitudinal excursion with a minimal amount of tension. These techniques should be unprovocative and may be more tolerable to patients than tensioning techniques. For example, abundant literature supports the use of cervical lateral glide mobilizations to effect changes in neck and/or arm symptoms (Vicenzino et al. 1998, Vicenzino et al. 1999a, Vicenzino et al. 1999b, Cowell and Phillips 2002, Coppieters et al. 2003, Cleland et al. 2005, Costello 2008, McClatchie et al. 2009, Young et al. 2009) because this intervention has been shown to produce immediate reductions in mechanosensitivity and pain in patients with lateral epicondylalgia (Vicenzino et al. 1996) and cervicobrachial pain (Elvey 1986, Cowell and Phillips 2002, Coppieters et al. 2003).

Elvey (1986) reported that gliding techniques were more effective than no intervention at reducing pain and disability in patients with cervicobrachial pain and was more effective than manual therapy directed at the shoulder and thoracic spine in reducing pain in these patients. Furthermore, the addition of neural gliding techniques to conservative management of patients with carpal tunnel syndrome reduced the need for surgery by 29.8% (Rozmaryn et al. 1998). An example of a passive slide mobilization for the median nerve includes positioning the patient's arm in 90 to 110 degrees of abduction with 90 degrees of shoulder external rotation with the elbow flexed to 90 degrees with wrist and finger extension and forearm supination. To then passively "slide" the median nerve, wrist extension is relaxed as the elbow is extended (distal slider) or the cervical spine is actively side bent to the ipsilateral side as the elbow is extended (proximal slider). This could also be given as an active technique performed by the patient at home.

With a tensioning technique, elongation of the nerve bed is obtained by moving one or several joints such that the "tension" within the nerve is elevated (Coppieters and Butler 2008). These techniques are, by nature, more stressful to the neural tissue and should be used with caution because they may irritate the patient who is mechanosensitive. They should not be static stretches and should always involve gentle oscillations into and out of resistance. These techniques are generally indicated for patients who experience symptoms as a result of impairments in the neural tissue's ability to elongate; hence, the goal is to restore the physical capabilities of the neural tissue to tolerate movement. The tension is increased to the point of a mild stretching sensation, or, in the case of patients who are not irritable, may be taken to the onset of mild symptoms at the end of the oscillation. Any of the active or passive neurodynamic tests can be used as "tensioners." Sets and repetitions should be determined by the irritability of the patients and the response (positive or negative) to the interventions. Starting with one to three sets of ten oscillations is useful, followed by a reassessment of the neurodynamic test to determine if the interventions had any effect. Finally, techniques aimed at non-neural structures can be combined with neurodynamic interventions, such as the cervical lateral glide technique while holding the arm in an upper limb neurodynamic test (ULNT) position (Vicenzino et al. 1998, Vicenzino et al. 1999b, Cowell and Phillips 2002, Coppieters et al. 2003, Cleland et al. 2005, Young et al. 2009).

SUMMARY

Clinicians should keep in mind the underlying principles of neurobiomechanics; that is, the nervous system is a continuous tract that is subject to slide, glide, bend, and stretch as it travels through its mechanical interface. Symptoms can arise as a result of intrinsic or extrinsic impairments anywhere along this tortuous course. Clinicians can render meaningful interventions that have a direct impact on the space, movement, and blood supply for the nervous system, in addition to producing beneficial neurophysiologic effects. Neurodynamic interventions (either passive or active) should involve smooth, controlled, gentle, large-amplitude movements. Sustained stretching is rarely indicated. Finally, neurodynamic interventions are but a small part of an overall patient-centered treatment approach that encompasses multiple interventions.

REFERENCES

A complete reference list is available at https://expertconsult .inkling.com/.

80

Spondylolisthesis

Andrew S.T. Porter, DO, FAAFP

DEFINITIONS

Spondylolysis is a defect of the pars interarticularis portion of the vertebra. The pars interarticularis is the area between the superior and inferior articulating processes of the vertebra (Figs. 80.1 and 80.2).

This defect of the vertebra can be the result of a broad range of etiologies, from stress fracture to a traumatic bony fracture. Wiltse (1969) and Beutler et al. (2003) reported an incidence of 6% to 7% for spondylolysis in the general population, and it is more commonly seen in males. Athletic activities that require repetitive hyperextension and rotation predispose athletes to develop pars defects. It is commonly seen with higher risk sports such as gymnastics (e.g., back walkovers), football (e.g., linemen blocking), track and field (e.g., pole vaulters and javelin throwers), butterfly swimming, and judo (Bono 2004).

When there is a bilateral spondylolysis, there can be slippage of one vertebral body relative to another and this results in a condition called spondylolisthesis. Most commonly spondylolisthesis occurs at the L5 vertebral body level followed by L4, then L3. There are different grades of spondylolisthesis and there are different types of spondylolisthesis, as described by Wiltse (1969):

Type 1: Congenital spondylolisthesis, characterized by the presence of dysplastic sacral facet joints allowing anterior translation of one vertebra relative to another

Type 2: Isthmic spondylolisthesis, caused by the development of a stress fracture of the pars interarticularis

Type 3: Degenerative spondylolisthesis, caused by intersegmental instability from facet arthropathy

Type 4: Traumatic spondylolisthesis, results from acute trauma to the facet or pars interarticularis

Type 5: Pathologic spondylolisthesis, results from any bone disorder that may destabilize the facet joint.

DIAGNOSIS

Patients with spondylolisthesis often present with low back pain localized to the paraspinal and gluteal region, restricted range of motion (ROM) of the lumbar spine, decrease in lumbar lordosis, and excessive hamstring tightness. Because spondylolisthesis can result in compression of the nerve root(s), patients can present with radicular pain with or without neurologic deficits. The classic Phalen-Dickson sign (i.e., a knee-flexed, hip-flexed gait) may be demonstrated in patients with spondylolisthesis (Phalen and Dickson 1961).

Palpation may identify a step-off over the spinous process, which may be indicative of spondylolisthesis, particularly over the L5–S1 level. Although this is not a definitive method for detection of spondylolisthesis (Collaer et al. 2006), a recent systematic review has found it to be an optimal test returning high specificity (87% to 100%) and moderate to high sensitivity (60% to 88%) values (Algami et al. 2015). In assessing lumbar ROM,

forward flexion is commonly diminished secondary to excessive hamstring tightness. Lumbar flexion typically does not increase symptoms, and in many cases, it provides relief. However, extension and rotation commonly cause discomfort for the patient. Common physical examination findings are pain that is localized to the pars interarticularis region on palpation and a positive stork test. The stork test is a one-legged hyperextension maneuver. The patient is asked to stand on one leg. Then, the clinician passively hyperextends and rotates the patient toward the weightbearing side. Reproduction of similar pain is a positive test and is suggestive of a spondylolysis and possible spondylolisthesis that needs further evaluation with imaging. Although this maneuver is most often described in association with spondylolysis and spondylolisthesis, it stresses other structures besides the pars interarticularis and can therefore be considered to be only suggestive of a pars interarticularis lesion within the context of the clinical picture (Fig. 80.3).

Most commonly plain radiographs are the initial imaging modality, with lateral and oblique views showing a break in the pars interarticularis ("neck of the Scottie dog"). This is indicative of spondylolysis (Fig. 80.4).

A computed tomography scan can be used to confirm the diagnosis because plain radiographs do not always demonstrate pars interarticularis fractures that are in fact present. Bone scans with single-photon emission computed tomography (SPECT) are necessary to tell if the pars interarticularis fracture is actively trying to heal indicated by focal uptake. Magnetic resonance

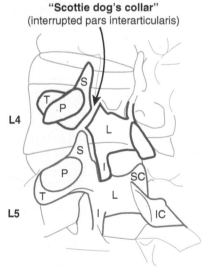

Fig. 80.1 Oblique view of lumbar spine showing spondylolysis. *I*, isthmus; *IC*, inferior articular process; *L*, lamina; *P*, pedicle; *S*, superior articular process; *T*, transverse process. (Micheli LS, Couzens GS. How I manage low back pain in athletes. *Phys Sports Med* 1993;21(3):182–194. Used with permission.)

imaging may also be used to confirm the diagnosis, although MRI does not always identify pars defects that are seen on SPECT. For example, as demonstrated by Masci et al. (2006), MRI identified only 80% of pars lesions seen on SPECT. Thus, CT, SPECT, and often MRI are helpful to determine the metabolic activity of the stress fracture, the potential for fracture healing, and the lesion acuity and to exclude other spinal pathology. Masci et al. (2006) have advocated the following guidelines for diagnosing a symptomatic pars lesion: nuclear imaging with SPECT followed by CT, with a limited role for plain radiography (Fig. 80.5).

If there is slippage of one vertebral body relative to another, the diagnosis of spondylolisthesis is made. Spondylolisthesis is generally diagnosed on the lateral plain radiographs, further defined on CT scan and SPECT bone scan, and classified by the percentage of displacement using the Meyerding system: Grade 1 (0%–25%), Grade 2 (25%–50%), Grade 3 (50%–75%), and Grade 4 (>75%) (Fig. 80.6).

TREATMENT

In general, treatment of spondylolisthesis should revolve around getting the patient back to preinjury activity level with injury prevention education also provided. The treatment and prevention continue to be further studied, with more evidence-based treatment methods being investigated.

Two-thirds of patients with grade 1 or grade 2 spondylolisthesis respond to nonoperative interventions that may include restricted activities, rehabilitation, and bracing (Pizzutillo and Hummer 1989). In grade 1 or 2 spondylolisthesis, treatment and management will most often involve activity restriction/modification, bracing/immobilization, an exercise program (avoiding extension, abdominal training, stabilization/endurance/motor control, muscle-length balancing), and education on biomechanics and movement patterns to avoid. With rehabilitation required for treatment, physical therapy is often recommended to reduce pain, restore ROM, and strengthen and stabilize the spine (Fritz et al. 1998). The use of braces for immobilization or restriction in ROM has been advocated by most authors (Standaert and Herring 2007, Herman et al. 2003, d'Hemecourt et al. 2000, Pizzutillo and Hummer 1989, Morita et al. 1995, Micheli and Couzens 1993, and Steiner and Micheli 1985). Bracing is thought to be beneficial for spondylolysis and spondylolisthesis, yet there are no controlled trials regarding the treatment of spondylolysis or spondylolisthesis. With respect to

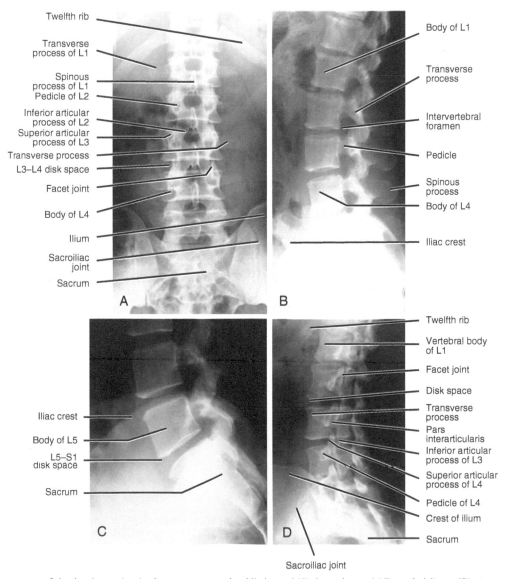

Fig. 80.2 Normal anatomy of the lumbar spine in the anteroposterior (*A*), lateral (*B*), lateral sacral (*C*), and oblique (*D*) views. (From Mettler F: Essentials of Radiology, ed. 2. Philadelphia, WB Saunders, 2005).

spondylolysis, clinical outcomes were good to excellent in 78% to 96% of patients when treated with antilordotic modified Boston brace for 6 months to 1 year and lordosis-maintaining brace for 6 months, respectively (Standaert and Herring 2000, Standaert et al. 2000).

Some form of bracing is recommended if the patient's symptoms are not improving with rest and activity modification,

but the specific type of bracing remains controversial. In one study, the rate of healing was 78% for unilateral and 8% for bilateral pars interarticularis defects when the athlete was treated with a lordotic brace (Standaert and Herring 2000, Standaert et al. 2000). Treatment may be required for 4 to 12 months, based on unilateral or bilateral involvement and response to bracing.

The decision to brace needs to be made on a case-by-case basis and needs to take into account if active healing is noted on SPECT bone scan. Overall, passive treatments such as activity restriction and bracing can help create an environment for potential healing of a pars interarticularis fracture.

Another key component in the treatment of spondylolisthesis is spine stabilization exercises. These exercises strengthen the muscles around the lumbar spine while maintaining a neutral spine position. Studies have suggested that core stabilization programs conditioning the multifidus and transversus abdominis muscles are effective in reducing pain and decreasing recurrence (O'Sullivan et al. 1997). Therapeutic spine stabilization exercises have been shown to be effective in treatment of chronic low back pain with concomitant spondylolysis or spondylolisthesis (Nelson et al. 1995, O'Sullivan et al. 1997, Spratt et al. 1993). O'Sullivan et al. (1997) reported the results of a randomized control trial comparing a specific exercise program with a program of general exercise (swimming, walking, gym exercises). The stabilization exercise group had less pain and functional disability following a 10-week treatment program than the general exercise group. This difference was maintained at a 30-month follow-up. Specific exercises proposed to address the abdominal muscles in an isolated manner involved a curl-up–type maneuver. One specific exercise was performed with the patient lying on his or her side and the upper body supported by the elbow to create a side-bending of the spine (Fig. 80.7, *A*). The patient would then lift the pelvis off the support surface to a position in line with the shoulders, eliminating the side-bending (Fig. 80.7, *B*).

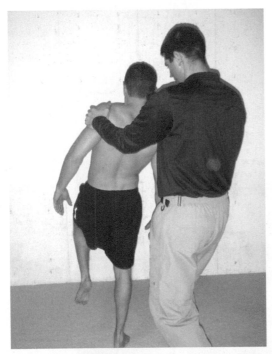

Fig. 80.3 To assess localized spondylolysis pain, a single-leg hyperextension "stork test" is performed. The patient stands on one leg and hyperextends and rotates the spine. Reproduction of the patient's pain complaint indicates a diagnosis of spondylolysis until proved otherwise.

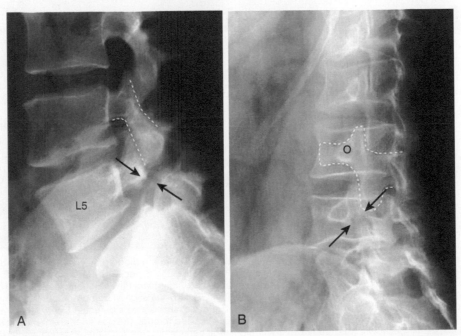

Fig. 80.4 Spondylolysis. On the lateral view of the lower lumbar spine (*A*), the normal contour of the posterior elements of L4 is outlined by the white dotted lines. At L5, lysis (fracture) of the posterior elements has occurred (*arrows*). On the oblique view (*B*), this is seen as a fracture through the "neck of the Scottie dog" (*arrows*). The normal outline for the L4 level is shown. (From Mettler F: Essentials of Radiology, ed. 2. Philadelphia, WB Saunders, 2005.)

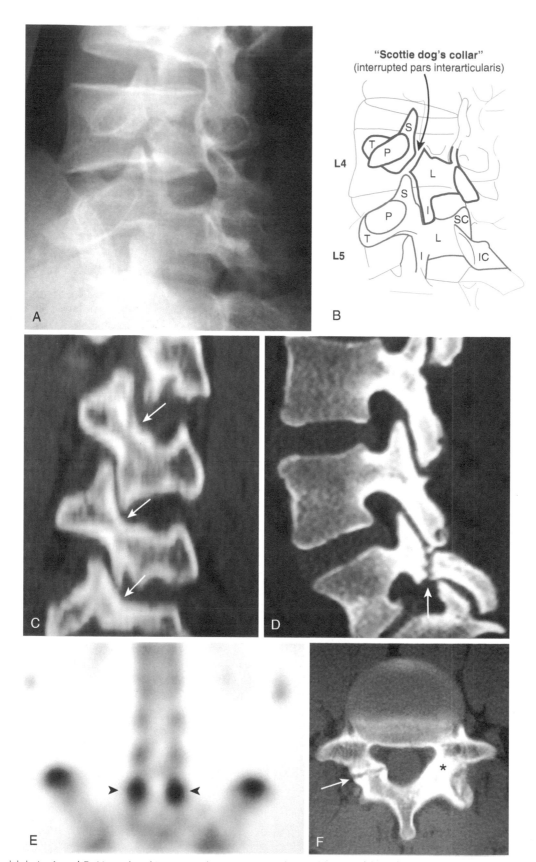

Fig. 80.5 Spondylolysis. **A and B,** Normal and interrupted pars interarticularis. Oblique radiograph (*A*) and corresponding line drawing (*B*) show an intact pars interarticularis at L5 and a pars defect with a collar around the "Scottie dog's" neck at L4 (*arrow* in part B). *P,* pedicle (the Scottie dog's eye); *T,* transverse process (nose); *S,* superior articulating facet (ear); *I,* inferior articulating facet (front leg); *L,* lamina (body); *IC,* contralateral inferior articulating facet (rear leg); *SC,* contralateral superior articulating facet (tail). **C,** Oblique sagittal computed tomography (CT) reconstruction in a normal patient. Note the intact pars interarticularis (*arrows*). **D,** Sagittal CT reformat shows a pars defect in L5 (*arrow*). **E,** Radionuclide bone scan of bilateral L5 pars defects. Coronal single-photon emission CT (SPECT) image obtained through the posterior elements shows increased tracer bilaterally at L5 (*arrowheads*). A CT scan (not shown) was needed to confirm bilateral defects because a unilateral defect with adaptive hypertrophy on the contralateral side could have similar bone scan findings. **F,** Axial CT image of unilateral spondylolysis. Note the spondylolysis on the right (*arrow*). Also note the sclerosis of the contralateral pars interarticularis (*asterisk*). This nonspecific finding may indicate that left-sided adaptive changes caused increased stress because of the right-sided pars defect or an impending left pars stress fracture. (From Manaster B: Musculoskeletal Imaging—The Requisites, ed. 3. Philadelphia, Elsevier, 2002.)

This exercise provides a challenge to the oblique abdominal muscles without imposing high compressive or shear loading forces on the lumbar spine. In addition, the horizontal side-support exercise challenges the quadratus lumborum muscle, which is an important spinal stabilizer. Nelson et al. (1995) also reported that 75% of 19 patients with spondylolisthesis reported good to excellent response in pain relief after an average of 18 sessions of trunk extensor and abdominal retraining. Diagonals are an example of a dynamic strength exercise for the trunk extensors and abdominal muscles (Fig. 80.8). These are performed by standing on all fours and then bringing the right hand together with the left knee. Then, the arm and leg are extended diagonally to a horizontal position. Finally, the exercise is repeated for the opposite diagonal (Baranto 2009), 10 repetitions in a three to five series.

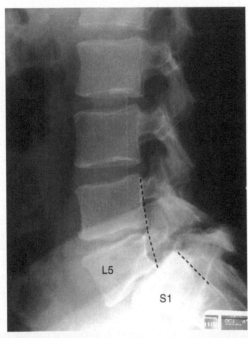

Fig. 80.6 Spondylolysis with resulting grade 2 spondylolisthesis. Degree of slippage is defined by looking at the relationship of the posterior portion of the vertebral bodies.

Sinaki et al. (1989) also reported that individuals with spondylolisthesis who performed specific trunk flexion exercise (abdominal strengthening and pelvic tilt, particularly of the multifidus and transversus abdominis muscles) achieved significant improvement in pain and ability to work. The abdominal muscles, particularly the transversus abdominis and oblique abdominals, and the multifidus muscle have been proposed to play an important role in stabilizing the spine by co-contracting in anticipation of an applied force. The multifidus muscle, because of its segmental attachments to the lumbar vertebrae, may be able to provide segmental control, particularly during lifting and rotational motions. Exercises targeting these muscle groups, therefore, may be desirable. A guideline for selected core exercises from Baranto (2009) includes a stability exercise program (stability with knee and underarm support, plank with unstable platform and with rotation, wheelbarrow, support on one arm—sideways, unstable—foot and underarm support, and stability with rotational element) and dynamic strength exercises (buttock lift, sit-ups with oblique abdominal muscles—unstable, sit-ups with fixed foot position and rotation, throwing sit-ups, sideways throwing, diagonals, and sideways pelvic tilt).

Lower extremity muscle tightness found in association with spondylolisthesis must also be addressed to allow for normal lumbar spine motion. The most common pattern of muscle tightness associated with spondylolisthesis involves tight hamstring muscles, which result in excessive posterior pelvic tilt and decreased lumbar lordosis, placing the back extensors at a mechanical disadvantage and making the spine less resilient to axial loads (Osterman et al. 1993). Treatment is primarily directed at stretching the hamstring muscles and strengthening the back extensors (lumbar erector spinae and quadratus lumborum).

Patient education plays an important role in the treatment of patients with spondylolisthesis. Education should focus on correcting poor posture while sitting or standing, faulty lifting, or sport-specific playing techniques and abnormal biomechanics. It is essential to avoid end-range movements of the lumbar spine to avoid positions that may overload the stabilizing structures of the spine. Patients should also be made aware that repetitive hyperextension and rotation can create potentially damaging forces in the lumbar spine, resulting in spondylolysis and eventually spondylolisthesis. Another vitally important educational component that

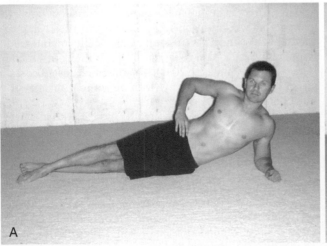 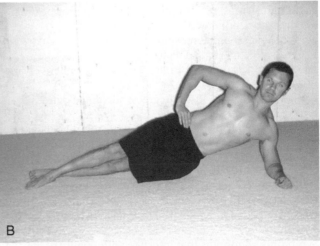

Fig. 80.7 One specific exercise proposed by O'Sullivan et al. (1997) was performed with the patient lying on the side and the upper body supported by the elbow to create a side-bending of the spine (A). The patient then lifts the pelvis off the support surface to a position in line with the shoulders, eliminating the side-bending (B).

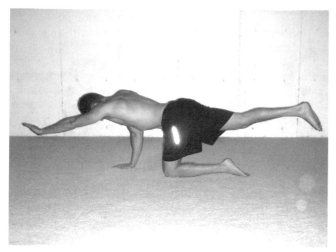

Fig. 80.8 Diagonals are one example of a dynamic strength exercise for the trunk extensors and abdominal muscles. Diagonals are performed by standing on all fours and then bringing the right hand together with the left knee. Then the arm and leg are extended diagonally to a horizontal position. Finally, repeat this exercise for opposite diagonal (Baranto 2009) for 10 repetitions in a three to five series.

needs to be stressed to patients is the importance of maintaining muscle strength and endurance in the muscles of the lumbar spine, particularly the lumbar erector spinae. The lumbar erector spinae are the primary source of extension torque for lifting. Fatigue can adversely affect the ability of the spinal muscles to respond to imposed loads, resulting in injury.

Most people with spondylolysis and low-grade spondylolisthesis (grade 1 or 2) respond to conservative treatment and successfully return to their particular sport or preinjury level of functioning. Occasionally, adolescent and young adult patients with isthmic spondylolisthesis evolve into candidates for pars repair or segmental lumbar fusion. Older adults with isthmic spondylolisthesis may become symptomatic with superimposed degenerative changes in the affected lumbar spine segment. The following are surgical recommendation guidelines for adults and children/adolescents with spondylolisthesis.

Surgical indications for a child or adolescent include the following (Amundson et al. 1999):

- Persistence or recurrence of symptoms in spite of aggressive conservative care for 1 year
- Tight hamstrings, persistently abnormal gait, or postural abnormalities unrelieved by physical therapy
- Sciatic scoliosis or lateral shift
- Progressive neurologic deficit
- Progressive slip beyond grade 2 spondylolisthesis even when asymptomatic
- A high slip angle (>40–50 degrees: slip angle defines degree of lumbosacral kyphosis)
- Psychological problems associated with spondylolisthesis

Surgical indications for an adult include the following (Amundson et al. 1999):

- Isthmic spondylolisthesis that becomes symptomatic as an adult
- Associated with progressive degenerative changes
- Degenerative spondylolisthesis associated with progressive symptoms
- Symptoms >4 months that interfere with quality of life

- Progressive neurologic deficits
- Progressive weakness
- Bowel/bladder dysfunction
- Sensory loss
- Reflex loss
- Limited walking tolerance (neurologic claudication)
- Associated segmental instability

Intractable pain after 1 year of appropriate treatment is the most common indication for surgery. At times, a patient will achieve acceptable symptomatic relief by conservative treatment but is unable to resume athletic activity without symptoms. For this instance, surgery may also be considered.

The traditional gold standard surgical treatment for spondylolisthesis is a posterior spinal fusion. For an L5 spondylolysis or low-grade (grade 1 to 2) L5–S1 slip, fusion from L5 to the sacrum is typically performed. In situ noninstrumented posterolateral fusion with autogenous iliac crest bone graft and cast immobilization have a very high success rate with minimal morbidity (Bradford and Hy 1994). Often, in the patient who is skeletally immature, the fusion rate with noninstrumented techniques is sufficiently high that the risk-to-benefit ratio for transpedicular instrumentation in the developing spine appears to be excessive. Fusion in skeletally mature teenagers, particularly in those with a high-grade (grade 3 or 4) spondylolisthesis, is more commonly performed with segmental pedicle screw instrumentation.

Bilateral posterolateral L4–S1 fusion, combined with cast reduction of the lumbosacral kyphosis (Bradford and Hy 1994) and pantaloon spica cast immobilization, is recommended for more severe slippage (grade 3 and beyond). Postoperative progression of slip has been reported in up to 30% of patients who have not been immobilized following posterior fusion. Outcomes are improved in patients immobilized for a minimum of 6 weeks postoperatively, in those with lesser degrees of slip, and those with a slip-angle measuring less than 55 degrees postoperatively. Lumbar decompression is rarely indicated in the immature patient with spondylolisthesis unless severe radiculopathy or bladder dysfunction is present preoperatively.

Direct repair of the pars interarticularis defect also may be performed. However, this is generally reserved for patients with minimal or no slip, for patients without chronic pars changes, and for patients with normal disc by MRI at the level of the spondylolysis. Repair may be performed by a tension band wiring technique, by a direct repair across the fracture with a screw, or with compression using a pedicle screw with a hook and rod.

Compared with patients who were treated nonoperatively, patients in whom degenerative spondylolisthesis and associated spinal stenosis were treated surgically maintained substantially greater pain relief and improvement in function for 4 years (Weinstein et al. 2009). Treatment consisted of standard decompressive laminectomy (with or without fusion) or usual nonoperative care.

In general, operative treatment is indicated to alleviate pain in patients not responding to conservative treatment and to prevent progression of the slip in those with severe slip (>50%) of the vertebrae (Fritz et al. 1998). With costs from surgery being high and inherent risks of surgical complications, further study into the efficacy of nonoperative treatment is warranted. A summary of the diagnosis and treatment for spondylolisthesis is recommended taking into account recommendations by Masci et al. (2006), Standaert (2005), and Lauerman et al. (2009) (Rehabilitation Protocol 80.1).

Christman and Li report (2016) in pediatric patients there is generally acceptable return to activity and sports. Pediatric patients treated with a direct pars repair for spondylolysis have good outcomes. Satisfactory outcomes have been demonstrated after fusion for low- and high-grade spondylolisthesis. Most surgeons allow return to noncontact sports by 6 months after surgical treatment. Return to contact and collision sports is controversial.

REHABILITATION PROTOCOL 80.1 ● Diagnosis and Treatment for Spondylolisthesis

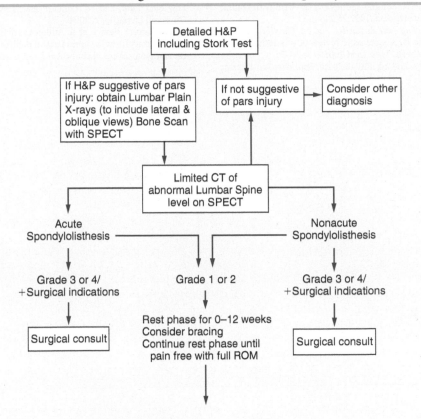

Weeks 12–16	Rehabilitation Phase
Acute Stage	ROM Low impact aerobic conditioning Neutral spine stabilization
Recovery Stage	ROM Aerobic conditioning Resistive strength training Progressive spinal stabilization Assess biomechanics and kinetic chain for activities.
Functional Stage	Aerobic conditioning Resistive strength training Dynamic, multiplanar spinal stabilization Sport-specific retraining
5–12 months	Return to play/full activity. Completed all of the above Nontender to palpation Full ROM and normal strength Appropriate aerobic fitness Adequate flexibility, spinal awareness, and mechanics Able to perform sport-specific/full activities without pain Grade 1: no activity restriction Grade 2: no participation in high-risk sports (e.g., gymnastics, football)

CT, computed tomography; *ROM,* range of motion; *SPECT,* single-photon emission computed tomography.

REFERENCES

A complete reference list is available at https://expertconsult .inkling.com/.

FURTHER READING

Congeni J, McCulloch J, Swanson K. Lumbar spondylolysis. A study of natural progression in athletes. *Am J Sports Med.* 1997;25:248–253.

Manaster B. *Musculoskeletal Imaging—the Requisites.* 2nd ed. Elsevier; 2002.

McNeeley M, Torrance G, Magee D. A systematic review of physiotherapy for spondylolysis and spondylolisthesis. *Man Ther.* 2003;8(2):80–91.

Mettler F. *Essentials of Radiology.* 2nd ed. Philadelphia: Saunders (an imprint of Elsevier); 2005.

Monteleone G. Spondylolysis and spondylolisthesis. In: Bracker M, ed. *The 5-minute Sports Medicine Consult.* Philadelphia: Williams & Wilkins , Lippincott; 2001:292–293.

Nadler SF, Malanga GA, Feinburg JH, et al. Relationship between hip muscle imbalance of pain in collegiate athletes: a prospective study. *Am J Phys Med Rehab.* 2001;80(8):572–577.

Richardson C, Hodges P, Hides J. *Therapeutic Exercise for Lumbopelvic Stabilization. A Motor Control Approach for the Treatment and Prevention of Low Back Pain.* 2nd ed. London: Harcourt Brace and Company Limited , Churchill Livingstone; 2004.

Sairyo K, Katoh S, Sasa T, et al. Athletes with unilateral spondylolysis are at risk of stress fracture at the contralateral pedicle and pars interarticularis: a clinical and biomechanical study. *Am J Sports Med.* 2005;33(4):583–590.

81

Lumbar Spine Microdiscectomy Surgical Rehabilitation

Cullen M. Nigrini, MSPT, MEd, PT, ATC, LAT | R. Matthew Camarillo, MD

Surgical versus nonoperative treatment for lumbar disc herniation is a well-studied topic with varying and contrasting opinions about the superiority, equivalence, or indifference of their long-term outcomes. Both options reduce symptoms and improve quality of life with acute and long-term results noted. Microdiscectomy to treat single-level lumbar disc herniation when conservative care fails has shown positive outcomes. It is reported that more than 250,000 elective surgeries take place in the United States annually for treatment of persistent symptoms of sciatica, and microdiscectomy remains one of the most common (Dewing et al. 2008).

Because this procedure is frequently done, there should be some consensus or guideline as to the rehabilitation following the surgery. Despite the prevalence of low back pain, specific guidelines for rehabilitation following microdiscectomy are scarce and represent a considerable gap in the literature.

A 2014 update of the Cochrane review for rehabilitation after lumbar disc surgery included 22 randomized controlled trials examining the effects of active rehabilitation for adults with first-time lumbar disc surgery (Oosterhuis et al. 2014). Overall, they found favor to include rehabilitation following microdiscectomy. The group found evidence that rehabilitative intervention 4 to 6 weeks following the procedure showed improved functional status and a faster return to work. When initiated 4 to 6 weeks postoperatively, exercise programs led to a faster decrease in pain and disability than no treatment. This decrease in pain and disability happened sooner in high-intensity programs, and there was no evidence that active programs increase the reoperation rate after first-time lumbar surgery.

Notably, the group did not find strong evidence to suggest initiating a program immediately following surgery. The group also concluded there was little clarity as to what should be included in a rehabilitation program or what activities should be limited postoperatively.

Although long-term outcomes between operative and nonoperative groups show little difference, young, active patients have a high success rate with regards to outcome measures, patient satisfaction, and return to work or military duty. Physical therapy and/or epidural injections are generally involved with conservative care and must prove ineffective prior to surgical intervention. Authors note single-level L5–S1 herniations fare significantly better than L4–L5 and multilevel injuries.

Intensive, progressive exercise programs coupled with education appear to reduce disability and improve function. Although the research supports exercise intervention, timing its initiation is less clear. Again the Cochrane review found evidence to begin exercise 4 to 6 weeks postoperatively. There is an emerging trend to initiate rehabilitation soon after surgery. Newsome et al. (2009) found immediate exercise (two hours postoperatively) to improve patient ability to become independently mobile and

obtain discharge from surgery and faster return to work times versus exercise initiated one day following the procedure.

Despite the evidence in support of early intervention, not all patients enter into a comprehensive outpatient rehabilitation program. Although several rehabilitation guidelines are available, there is much discrepancy as to postoperative instructions and what to include in a postoperative rehabilitation program. A UK study noted that only 23% of their survey respondents had guidelines or protocols for outpatient physical therapy (Williamson et al. 2007). Furthermore, sitting instructions range from "a few minutes maximum" to "30 minutes" or to simply increase gradually over a 6-week period. Some patients may immobilize to reduce stress when nonweight bearing may actually decrease healing. Current studies question the need to restrict activity postoperatively, theorizing this may encourage unhelpful thoughts and behaviors, ultimately slowing return to work and furthering disability.

Literature continues to work on a classification system for low back pain. Fritz, Cleland, and Childs (2007) reviewed this system with updated classification criteria for the four classification groups: manipulation, stabilization, specific exercise, and traction. This evidence-based move to guide conservative treatment for LBP is helpful and shows promising outcomes. With regards to postoperative care, clinicians can keep these global classifications in mind and integrate when appropriate. Postoperatively, stabilization and lumbar extension exercise are common inclusions to active rehabilitations. Although no classification groupings exist in the acute postoperative situation, all treatments should be considered and integrated when deemed appropriate.

Because a lumbar microdiscectomy can lead to acute relief and long-term improvement, patients may expect to return to prior levels of function. For the general population, pain relief, independent function with activities of daily living, and return to work are common patient goals and clinician objectives. Clinicians should focus rehabilitation techniques to help patients achieve these goals. With regards to low back injury, objective measures are in place to help clinicians gauge patient progress, pain levels, and functional status. Clinicians should incorporate these tools in a rehabilitation setting to create objective reports of patient progress.

The International Classification of Functioning (ICF) conceptual framework was used to determine objective measures for a study (Selkowitz et al. 2006) that divided groups and tests into primary or secondary outcome measures. Primary outcome measures can provide an assessment of the intervention, whereas secondary outcome measures are descriptive, informative, and hypothesis building. Table 81.1 summarizes the group's utilization of objective measures and lists additional options. The outcome measures listed help clinicians adhere to the Nagi framework categories using low back pain as the dysfunction. Impairments, functional limitations, and disability can all be objectively recorded and monitored to gauge patient progress. Integration of these objective data-gathering tools can not only aid researchers but also can allow clinicians to engage in evidence-based practice. Clinical decision-making skills, patient treatment options, and documentation can all benefit from these tools, and rehabilitation from microdiscectomy should include such measures.

Kulig et al. (2009) examined an intensive, progressive exercise program for patients after single-level lumbar microdiscectomy. The Oswestry Disability Index was used to assess ADLs. For assessing observed performance in activity, the 5-minute walk test, 50-foot walk test, and the repeated sit-to-stand test

were used. This article also highlighted a rehabilitation program that yielded positive results when implemented Table 81.2.

The University of Southern California created an educational and exercise protocol following lumbar microdiscectomy. Selkowitz used this protocol (Selkowitz et al. 2006) on 176 individuals in a study (Kulig et al. 2009). The group first provided a 60-minute one-on-one education session designed to help patients understand their back problem and how to care for it. This session took place 4 to 6 weeks postoperatively and was followed 2 to 3 days later by the 12-week "USC Spine Exercise Program" involving back extensor strength and endurance training in addition to mat and upright therapeutic exercises. This program was created to

TABLE 81.1	**Outcome Measures**	
Primary Outcome Measures **Participation (Disability)**	**Activity (Functional Limitations)**	**Body Functions and Structures/Physical (Impairments)**
Oswestry Disability Questionnaire Roland-Morris Disability Questionnaire (RM) SF-36 quality of life assessment Subjective Quality of Life Scale (SQOL)	50-foot walk test Repeated sit-to-stand test	Modified Sorenson test Pain Visual Analog Scales (VASs) Body diagram
Secondary Outcome Measures **Participation**	**Activity**	**Body Functions and Structures/Physical**
Fear Avoidance Belief Questionnaire (FABQ)	24-hour Physical Activity Scale (PAS) 5-minute walk test	Lower quarter neurologic screen Straight leg raising (SLR) Lower quarter flexibility Lumbar spine range of motion* Lumbar spine instability

*Lumbar range of motion measurements must consider postsurgical restrictions for patient safety.

TABLE 81.2	**Mat and Upright Therapeutic Exercise Program**
Exercise	**Training Goal**
ABDOMINAL PROGRESSION	
Level I Supine Alternating (Alt) UE Flexion	3 sets of 1-minute continuous motion 1 minute of rest between sets
Level 2 Supine Alt LE Extension	3 sets of 1-minute continuous motion 1 minute of rest between sets
Level 3 Supine Alt UE Flexion & LE Extension	3 sets of 1-minute continuous motion 1 minute of rest between sets
Level 4 Supine Leg Ext Unsupported	3 sets of 1-minute continuous motion 2 minutes of rest between sets
Level 5 Supine Leg Ext Unsupported w/Alt Arms	3 sets of 1-minute continuous motion 2 minutes of rest between sets
Level 6 With 1# and 3# Weights	3 sets of 1-minute continuous motion 2 minutes of rest between sets
Level 7 With 2# and 5# Weights	3 sets of 1-minute continuous motion 2 minutes of rest between sets
QUADRUPED PROGRESSION	
Level 1 Alt Arm Raises	10 repetitions with 10-second hold per extremity raise No resting time
Level 2 Alt Leg Ext	10 repetitions with 10-second hold per extremity raise No resting time
Level 3 Alt Arm and Leg Raises	10 repetitions with 10-second hold per extremity raise No resting time
Level 4 Prone Plank on Knees	6 repetitions with 30-second hold per repetition 30 seconds rest between repetitions
Level 5 Prone Plank on Forefoot	6 repetitions with a 30-second hold per repetition 30 seconds rest between repetitions
Level 6 Prone Plank w/Alt Leg Lift	6 repetitions with a 30-second hold per repetition 30 seconds rest between repetitions
Level 7 Prone Plank w/Alt Leg Lift w/3#	6 repetitions with a 30-second hold per repetition 30 seconds rest between repetitions
Level 8 Prone Plank w/Alt Leg Lift w/5#	6 repetitions with a 30-second hold per repetition 30 seconds rest between repetitions

Continued

TABLE 81.2	Mat and Upright Therapeutic Exercise Program—cont'd
Exercise	**Training Goal**

SQUAT/LUNGE PROGRESSION

Exercise	Training Goal
Level 1	3 sets of 20 repetitions
Wall Squat to 45 Degrees Knee Flexion	5-second hold per rep. 2 minutes rest between sets
Level 2	3 sets of 20 repetitions
Free Standing Squats to 90 Degrees Hip Flexion	2 minutes of rest between sets
Level 3	3 sets of 20 repetitions
Forward Lunges	2 minutes of rest between sets
Level 4	3 sets of 2 cycles
Lunges Series	2 minutes of rest between sets
Level 5	3 sets of 3 cycles
Lunge Series	2 minutes of rest between sets

Recreated from Selkowitz DM, Kulig K, Poppert EM, Flanagan SP, Matthews ND, Beneck GJ, et al.: Physical Therapy Clinical Research Network (PTClinResNet). The immediate and long-term effects of exercise and patient education on physical, functional, and quality-of-life outcome measures after single-level lumbar microdiscectomy: a randomized controlled trial protocol. BMC Musculoskeletal Disorders 2006;7(70).

REHABILITATION PROTOCOL 81.1 ● Trunk Strengthening and Endurance Program Using the Backstrong Apparatus

Phase	Goals	Week	Training Level	Sets	Reps	Hold Time	Rest Length/ Reps	Rest Length Sets
Teaching	1. Correct Technique	1	2 Levels < Submax Test Level	1	4	30	30	NA
	2. Identification of Starting Training Level	2	2 Levels < Submax Test Level	1	4	30	30	NA
Strength I	I. Level 6 for 20 seconds	3	2 Levels < Max Test Level	2	3	30	30	60
		4	2 Levels < Max Test Level	3	3	30	30	60
Endurance I	I. Submax Level for 90 seconds	5	2 Levels < Max Test Level	1	6–8	Max	Max*	NA
		6	2 Levels < Max Test Level	1	8–10	Max*	Max*	NA
		7	2 Levels < Max Test Level	1	8–10	Max*	Max*	NA
Strength II	I. Level 6 for 20 seconds	8	1 Level < Max Test Level	4	5	30	30	60
		9	1 Level < Max Test Level	5	5	30	30	60
Endurance II	I. Level 6 for 180 seconds	10	1 Level < Max Test Level	2	4	Max*	Max*	180
		11	1 Level < Max Test Level	2	5	Max*	Max*	180
		12	1 Level < Max Test Level	2	6	Max*	Max*	180

*Up to 90 seconds.

target trunk muscle performance impairments seen postoperatively to help decrease pain and functional limitations.

The endurance program was designed to be goal oriented, performance based, and periodized. The extension portion goal is to hold the Sorensen test position ("prone/horizontal body position with spine and lower extremity joints in neutral position, arms crossed at the chest, lower extremities and pelvis supported with the upper trunk unsupported against gravity") for 180 seconds. The group used the Backstrong Spinal Rehabilitation apparatus (Backstrong LLC, Brea, CA), a variable-angle Roman chair to train progressively to Level 6 or 0 degrees relative to the horizontal. The angle begins at 75 degrees (Level 1) and decreases to Level 6 (60, 45, 30, 15, and 0 degrees). The mat

and upright program can be used concomitantly, and an outline of the protocols is given in Rehabilitation Protocol 81.1. If the Backstrong apparatus is readily available, this protocol can be considered a viable option for rehabilitation once cleared by the clinician for outpatient rehabilitation.

Communication with the surgeon is critical for patient care. If the treating physician has given precautions or guidelines to follow, these must be adhered to. If the rehabilitation specialist is given the ability to use his or her professional judgment, early intervention appears to be the best strategy.

Rehabilitation Protocol 81.2 illustrates a protocol that can be initiated prior to or immediately following surgery. These protocols show a multivariate approach to rehabilitation following microdiscectomy with patient goals to include pain reduction and return to work and ADLs. Athletes, particularly elite athletes, represent the other end of the spectrum. It is likely that this patient's ultimate goal is full return to sport. These sport-specific physical demands can be expectedly greater than those placed on the general population. It is thus reasonable to assume a successful rehabilitation should include objective return-to-play criteria or progression to a high-level function prior to release to sport.

REHABILITATION PROTOCOL 81.2 ● Single-Level Lumbar Microdiscectomy Protocol

Preoperative

- Introduction of neutral spine, neutral pelvis, and transverse abdominal contraction.
- Inform patient of the nature of the rehabilitation following microdiscectomy.
  - Expected outcome.
  - Timeline.
  - Precautions/contraindications.
- Bending strategies to maintain neutral spine lumbar-pelvic/hip dissociation.
  - Neutral spine/pelvis in seated position.
  - Oswestry Disability Questionnaire.
  - SF-36 quality of life assessment.
  - Pain Visual Analog Scales (VASs).

Postoperative

Days 1–6
Goals

- Initiate walking sessions, 1 to 3 per day as tolerated.
- Become independent with bed mobility, sit-to-stand, and toileting by day 2.
- Discharge from 12 to 48 hours postoperatively.
- Protection of wound.
  - Limit bending and lifting until wound is healed.
- Pain management with medications as per MD and cryotherapy.

Exercises

- Walking progression 5 to 10 minutes on level surface with minimal assisted device.
- Administer 50-foot walk, VAS, and repeated sit-to-stand.

Weeks 1–3

- It is critical to adhere to and honor the surgeon's specific guidelines with regards to activity levels, lifting/bending restrictions, and wound care.

Precautions

- Avoid deep trunk flexion, high-velocity movement, Valsalva, prolonged sitting.

Goals

- Increase walking tolerance to 30 minutes without pain.
- No symptoms into the lower extremity.
- Wound protection and complete closure.
- Pain management.
- Administer Oswestry, SF-36, and VASs.

Exercises

- Prone press-ups to tolerance from slight flexion to neutral.
- Prolonged prone extension 30 seconds to 2 minutes with pillow/cushion under stomach.
- Focus on increasing endurance and ability of muscles to contract without increasing pain.
  - Treadmill with arms supported.
  - Initial goal of 5 minutes; progress as tolerated to 30 minutes.
  - Aquatic therapy once MD clears for wound submerge.
  - Progress as tolerated.
  - Cryotherapy post-treatment and PRN for pain.
  - Modalities as indicated for pain.
  - Review bed mobility, sit-to-stand, utilization of upper extremity.

- Transverse abdominal setting: Ensure patient is able to contract musculature and maintain neutral pelvis. Clinician can utilize manual/verbal feedback and cues, diagnostic ultrasound if possible. Use clinical skills and patient performance to determine progression to the next level of exercise. Work patient in a variety of positions including:
  - Supine.
  - Prone.
  - Quadruped (if tolerated).
  - Seated (if tolerated and >5 feet).
  - Standing.
- Supine gluteal progression.
- Upper-body ergometer for cardiovascular.
- Supported quarter wall slides/isometrics as tolerated.
- Introduce pain-free hip abductor strengthening/isometrics.

Weeks 3–8
Goals

- Return to work (modified or light duty) and activities of daily living (ADLs).
- Adhere to surgeon guidelines for upper extremity lifting and activity.
- Patient able to walk on level surfaces without restriction.
- Oswestry, VAS, and SF-36 score improvement at week 8 or with re-evaluation.

Exercises

- Advance transverse abdominal exercises in all positions.
- Advance glute/bridging exercises.
- Advance hip abductor strengthening.
- Initiate nonimpact lower-extremity involved cardiovascular exercise.
- Pool workouts.
- Treadmill.
- Elliptical.
- Stationary bike.
- Initiate Watkins protocol for athlete or patient with high-level goals.

Weeks 8–12
Goals

- Patient has returned to full work duty.
- Objective measures have improved.
- Release to activity based on achievement of goals and MD clearance.
- Athlete is continuing to work with Watkins protocol.
- Return to play is based on the Watkins criteria:
  - Achieving the proper level of the stabilization program.
  - Good aerobic conditioning.
  - Performing sports-specific exercises.
  - Returning slowly to sport.
  - Continuing stabilization exercise once returned to sport.

Exercises

- Patient will initiate return to jogging protocol if desired and as per MD.
- Patient will initiate resistance training if desired and as per MD.
- Patient will continue with transverse abdominal/core stabilization progression.
- Patient will continue to advance cardiovascular status.
- Continue to increase exercise with total body and functional positions.

REFERENCES

A complete reference list is available at https://expertconsult .inkling.com/.

FURTHER READING

Chin KR, Tomlinson DT, Auerbach JD, et al. Success of lumbar microdiscectomy in patients with modic changes and low-back pain: a prospective pilot study. *J Spinal Disord Tech*. 2008;21(2):139–144.

Choi G, Raiturker PP, Kim MJ, et al. The effect of early isolated lumbar extension exercise program for patients with herniated disc undergoing lumbar discectomy. *Neurosurgery*. 2005;57(4):764–772.

Chou R, Quaseem A, Snow V, et al. Diagnosis and treatment of low back pain: a joint clinical practice guideline from the American College of Physicians and the American Pain Society. *Ann Intern Med*. 2007;147(7):478–491.

Fairbank JC, Pynsent PB. The Oswestry Disability Index. *Spine*. 2000;25(22):2940–2952.

Ostelo RWJG, de Vet HCW, Waddell G, et al. [Review] Rehabilitation after lumbar disc surgery. Cochrane Database of Systematic Reviews. *Spine*. 2009;34(17):1839–1848.

Roland MO, Morris RW. A study of the natural history of back pain. Part 1: development of a reliable and sensitive measure of disability in low back pain. *Spine*. 1983;8:141–144.

Ronnberg K, Lind B, Zoega B, et al. Patients' satisfaction with provided care/information and expectations on clinical outcome after lumbar disc herniation surgery. *Spine*. 2007;32(2):256–261.

Watkins RG, Williams LA, Watkins RG. Microdiscopic lumbar discectomy results for 60 cases in professional and Olympic athletes. *Spine J*. 2003;3:100–105.

Weinstein JN, Tostesson TD, Lurie JD, et al. Surgical vs nonoperative treatment of lumbar disk herniation. The spine patient outcomes research trial (SPORT): a randomized trial. *JAMA*. 2000;296(20):2441–2450.

SECTION 8

Special Topics

Running Injuries: Etiology and Recovery-Based Treatment

Allan Besselink, PT, DPT, Dip MDT | Bridget Clark, PT, MSPT, DPT

An estimated 38 million runners are in the United States, of which 10.5 million are running at least twice a week. Participation in running events (such as a 5K, 10K, or marathon) has increased dramatically in the past 10 years. For example, the number of marathon finishers in the United States has increased from 143,000 in 1980 to 425,000 in 2008. Many health benefits are associated with running, including weight loss, decreased blood pressure, increased bone density, and a decreased risk of both cardiovascular disease and diabetes.

However, running also displays a trend toward increased injury rates. Current literature indicates various injury rates. Koplan et al. (1982) reported that **60% of all runners will sustain an injury within any given year that is severe enough to force them to alter their training.** It has also been reported that **the yearly incidence injury rate for runners training for a marathon is as high as 90%.** Given that the average runner will have 800 to 2000 footstrikes per mile, the opportunity for injury to occur is significant. Running injuries are not limited to any one joint or anatomic region (Table 82.1), although a large percentage of injuries tend to occur at the knee.

Data indicate that running has become a significant health care issue. The number of participants is growing, and a large percentage of those participants will become injured. This suggests a need to better understand the causes of running injuries. Health care providers can then not only provide effective means of treatment should an injury occur but also provide effective injury prevention programs.

GAIT: WALKING AND RUNNING

The gait cycle has been defined by Thordarson (1997) as the period from initial contact of one foot until the initial contact of that same foot. A brief review of the gait cycle will provide some background on the nature of mechanical loading and the neuromuscular requirements of both walking and running.

Running Mechanics

The walking gait cycle consists of two phases, stance and swing. The stance phase begins with initial contact, the moment when the foot contacts the ground. During initial contact, the loading response commences as forces are controlled eccentrically. Midstance starts as the contralateral limb toes off and enters swing phase. Once the center of gravity is directly over the stance foot, terminal stance begins. As the contralateral foot contacts the ground, preswing begins. Stance phase can also be viewed in terms of functional components—the absorption of forces on loading, followed by the propulsion of the body

forward. During the swing phase of gait, initial swing begins at toe-off and continues until the knee reaches a maximal knee flexion of approximately 60 degrees. Midswing follows and continues until the lower leg/shank is perpendicular to the ground. Terminal swing then proceeds until initial contact is made.

The running gait cycle (Fig. 82.1) is also divided into a stance phase and a swing phase. The stance phase may involve an initial foot contact that takes place as a heel strike, midfoot strike, or forefoot strike. Initial foot contact exists on a continuum with increasing gait speed, progressing from heel strike in walking to forefoot strike in sprinting. The percentage of the gait cycle spent in the stance phase varies depending on gait speed—60% with walking, 40% with running, and just 22% with world class sprinters. The walking gait cycle is distinct in that it involves a period of double limb support in which both of the feet are on the ground. The running gait cycle is distinct in that it involves a period of double float in which both of the feet are off the ground. The progression from walking gait to running gait is a continuum—from double limb support in walking to double float period in running.

At a certain walking speed, there is a transition from walking to running gait which occurs in order to maintain biomechanical, metabolic, and aerobic efficiency (Fig. 82.2). The speed at which this transition occurs varies between individuals, although it tends to be at or near a velocity of 12:00 per mile (5.0 mph) for most. This becomes an important issue when 70% of the running population runs at a pace of 10:00 per mile or slower. Though fast walking and slow jogging have a similar cardiovascular response, slow jogging creates ground reaction forces and loading rates as much as 65% greater than fast walking (Table 82.2). The progression from walking to running involves certain requirements from the body including the ability to tolerate increased mechanical loads (i.e., ground reaction

TABLE 82.1	Incidence of Injuries by Body Area	
Anatomic Region	**Percentage of Injuries**
Knee	7.2–50.0
Shin, Achilles tendon, calf, heel	9–32.0
Foot and toes	5.7–39.0
Hamstring, quadriceps	3.4–38.0

Data from van Gent RN, Siem D, van Middelkoop M, van Os AG, Bierma-Zeinstra SM, Koes BW: Incidence and determinants of lower extremity running injuries in long distance runners: A systematic review. Br J Sports Med 2007;41:469–480.

forces) and the strength not only to progress the body forward concentrically but also to eccentrically control the stance leg. Running and sprinting require more power and range of motion at the hip, knee, and ankle as speed is increased.

During the running gait cycle, the initial functional task of the stance leg is absorption—to eccentrically decelerate and stabilize the limb—before concentrically activating the lower limb for propulsion. The initial phase of stance involves absorbing the ground reaction forces. For walking and slow running up to 3.0m/s^{-1} (6.7 mph, or 8:57/mile), there are two notable peaks in ground reaction forces: the impact peak and the thrust maximum. This two-peaked configuration of the ground reaction curve is consistent in the literature for heel-strike runners. The impact peak occurs during the first 15% to 25% of stance phase. For faster running speeds involving a midfoot or forefoot

strike, there is no initial impact peak but usually a single peak, the thrust maximum, and this occurs during the first 40% to 50% of the stance phase.

Ground reaction forces appear to increase linearly up to a gait speed of 60% of maximum speed (average of 4.0m/s^{-1}), but at higher speeds, ground reaction forces appear to stay at approximately 2.5 to 2.8 times body weight (Table 82.2). It is also noteworthy that during running, athletes that heel strike upon initial contact have a higher initial peak in vertical ground reaction force than midfoot strikers. There is a strong relationship between impact peak and loading rate. The loading rate associated with running has been found to be positively correlated with running velocity, finding an average rate of 77 BW/s^{-1} (body weight) at slower speeds of 3.0m/s^{-1}, increasing to 113 BW/s^{-1} at faster speeds of 5.0 m/s^{-1}.

Normal Running Gait Cycle

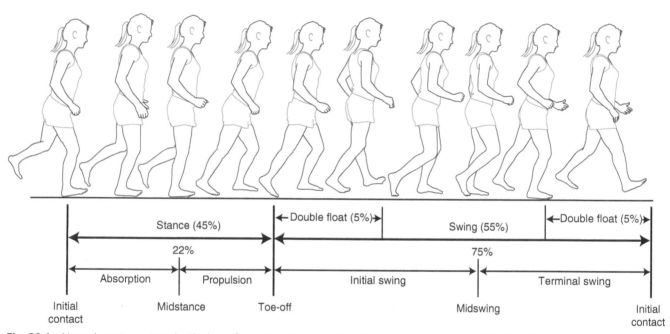

Fig. 82.1   Normal running gait cycle. (Redrawn from Mann RA, Coughlin MJ: Surgery of the Foot and Ankle, 6th ed. St. Louis, Mosby, 1993.)

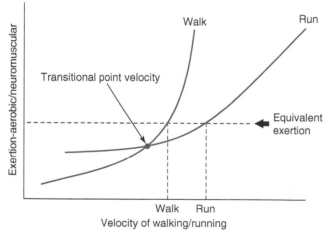

Fig. 82.2   Transition from walking to running. (Redrawn from Besselink A: RunSmart: A Comprehensive Approach to Injury-Free Running, Morrisville, Lulu Press, 2008.)

TABLE 82.2	Ground Reaction Forces Associated With Walking and Running at Various Speeds		
Running Speed		**Pace (Per Mile)**	**Vertical Ground Reaction Force (Body Weight)**
1.5 m/s^{-1} (3.4 mph) (walk)		17:53/mile	1.1–1.5
2.5 to 3.0 m/s^{-1} (5.6–6.7 mph) (slow jog)		8:56–10:44/mile	2.5
5.0 to 8 m/s^{-1} (11.2–17.9 mph) (run)		3:21–5:22/mile, or 0:50–1:20/quarter	2.5–2.88

Data adapted from Keller TS, Weisberger AM, Ray JL, Hasan SS, Shiavi RG, Spengler DM: Relationship between vertical ground reaction force and speed during walking, slow jogging, and running. Clin Biomech 1996;11: 253–259 and Munro CF, Miller DI, Fuglevand AJ: Ground reaction forces in running: A reexamination. J Biomech 1987;20: 147–155.

For a runner who has a heel strike, these forces transmit directly through the heel and, therefore, are attenuated by the heel fat pad, pronation of the foot, and primarily passive, more than active, mechanisms in the lower extremity. However, for a runner with a midfoot or forefoot strike, these forces are primarily attenuated by the eccentric activation of the gastrocnemius/soleus complex, the quadriceps, and to a lesser degree, the pronation of the foot. The anterior and posterior calf muscles, quadriceps, hip extensors, and hamstrings all work eccentrically during the stance phase. Of note is the function of the quadriceps, which is the primary shock absorber, absorbing 3.5 times as much energy as it produces. After the initial ground reaction forces are attenuated, the foot supinates during the propulsion phase to provide a more rigid lever for push off. Winter (1983) noted that the gastrocnemius generates the primary propulsive force during the propulsion phase of running and produces forces between 800 and 1500 W, compared to 150 W for slow walking and 500 W for fast walking.

The primary purpose of the swing phase is to return the leg back to the stance phase as efficiently as possible. Flexion of the knee shortens the swing limb, effectively reducing the length of the swinging pendulum. The hip flexors (including rectus femoris), hamstrings, and ankle dorsiflexors are active both concentrically and eccentrically during the swing phase. There is a small vertical and horizontal translation of the whole body with running. The center of gravity will lower with an increasing velocity of gait. Arm swing is important for balance and for reciprocal running movement, as posterior arm swing corresponds with and assists the propulsive phase of the contralateral limb. The posterior deltoid muscle is very active during posterior arm swing.

Causes of Running Injuries

With the high incidence of running injuries, the suspected factors contributing to injury have been researched for decades. There are virtually as many perceived causes of injury as there are injured runners. A review of the scientific literature would reveal a plethora of perceived causes of and contributing factors to running injury, including but not limited to gender, age, asymmetries and malalignment, leg-length discrepancy, flat feet, high arches, mileage per week, speed work, shoe wear, flexibility (too much or too little), running surfaces (too hard or too soft), gait deviations, history of prior injuries, "muscle imbalances," training programs, running experience, orthotics, and others.

Review of the current scientific research does in fact yield a definitive answer. ***One primary factor has been directly associated with the onset of running injury—training or errors in training***. James et al. (1978) noted that the primary etiology in two-thirds of all causes of injury can be directly related to "training error." Lysholm and Wiklander (1987) reported that training errors alone, or in combination with other factors, were implicated in injuries in 72% of runners. **Simply stated, training error is most often an issue of "too much, too soon,"** the importance of which is explained later.

Contrary to the commonly held beliefs of the medical and running communities, there is not any specific correlation between anatomic malalignment or variations in the lower extremity and any specific pathologic entities or predisposition to any "overuse" syndromes. In fact, Reid (1992) noted that "normal variations in the human body abound, and only a few percent of the population are actually good examples of 'normal.' ... Furthermore, all of these variations are found in world class athletes and seem to produce little adverse effect on their ability to perform their sports. ... [T]he corollary of this enormous variation of body build among enthusiastic amateur and the professional athletes is that there is a poor correlation of specific malalignments with specific conditions." Table 82.3 summarizes the sport sciences literature regarding the factors that have been noted to have a direct association with running injury and those that either have no direct association or do not presently have scientific evidence to support an association with running injuries.

Training error is the only factor that consistently displays a cause–effect relationship with running injuries. Reid (1992) has gone so far as to state that "*every running injury should be viewed as a failure of training technique*, even if other contributing factors are subsequently identified." In addition, running distance of more than 25 to 40 miles per week, previous competition in running events, and a history of prior injury have been found to be strongly associated with running injuries.

There are two types of injuries: traumatic and overuse. A **traumatic injury** occurs when a single force applied to the tissues exceeds the critical limit of the tissues, such as a collision in football that results in a fractured leg or an ankle sprain while trail running. **Overuse injuries** occur when repetitive forces are applied to the tissues without allowing the tissues to recover.

Under-Recovery Not Overuse

For years, the health care community has pointed to the "overuse" running injury, but if "overuse" were the problem, then there would be a preset threshold at which point *all* runners would get injured—and this simply is not the case. Physiologic causes of running injuries can be explained by Wolfe's law. The body aims to attain homeostasis at the cellular level. As a **stimulus** is applied to tissues (including bone, tendon, muscle, ligament,

TABLE 82.3	Evidence-Based Factors Associated and Not Associated With Running Injuries	
Factors Having a Direct Association With Injury	Factors That Do Not Have Evidence for Association With Injury	Factors Known to Not Have a Direct Association With Injury
"Training error" (most often too much, too soon)	Warmup and stretching exercises	Gender
	Body height	Age
	Malalignment	Body mass index
Running distance	Muscular imbalance	Running on hard surfaces
	Decreased range of motion	Running hills
History of prior injury	Running frequency	Participation in other sports
	Level of performance (current skill level)	Time of year
Previous competition in running events	Stability of running shoes	Time of day
	Running on one side of the road	
	Orthotics	

Data from van Mechelen W: Running injuries. A review of the epidemiological literature. Sports Med 1992;14:320–335.

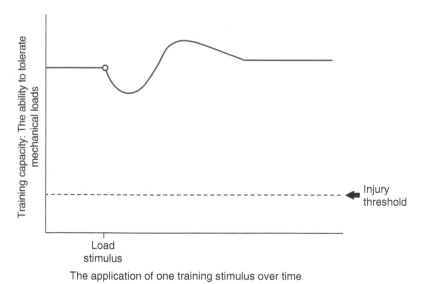

Fig. 82.3 Training stimulus and response. This depicts the body's ability to recover from and adapt to a single training stimulus. (Graph originally published in *UltraRunning* magazine, April 2010.)

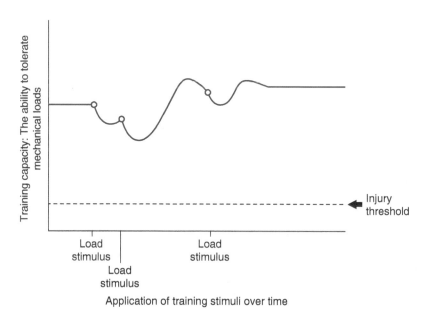

Fig. 82.4 Repeated training stimuli and responses, given appropriate and sufficient recovery. This depicts the body's ability to recover from and adapt to repeated training stimuli successfully. (Graph originally published in *UltraRunning* magazine, April 2010.)

and collagen-based tissues), a cellular response is triggered and, over time and with sufficient **recovery**, an **adaptation** occurs. This adaptation could be greater tissue integrity, strength, or similar mechanical response. Tissues adapt to mechanical loading if given an environment in which to do so and sufficient metabolic capacity to allow this to occur (Fig. 82.3). This has been shown repeatedly with studies on astronauts and deep sea divers, two populations that face altered repeated and/or sustained mechanical loads. *There is a precise balance between stimulus and response*—or, for the athlete, the application of a training stimulus and the recovery and adaptation to this stimulus. With this in mind, *"overuse" injuries should be more accurately described as "under-recovery" injuries because, given appropriate time for recovery, adaptation to the stimulus will take place successfully.*

Fig. 82.3 illustrates the body's ability to recover from and adapt to a single training stimulus. Figs. 82.4 and 82.5 display the effect of several training stimuli, Fig. 82.4 with appropriate and sufficient recovery and Fig. 82.5 with insufficient recovery and poor training adaptation. **Injuries occur when the rate of application of training stimulus exceeds the rate of recovery and adaptation.**

The rate of recurrence of running injuries is as high as 70%. There is little scientific evidence to relate any specific biomechanical factors to the onset of these injuries, yet upward of 70% of running injuries have been found to be related to training errors alone. It becomes imperative for the clinician to understand the relationship between training stimulus and training recovery and adaptation, keeping in mind that the human body is well adapted to respond to the demands required for running. Assessment and

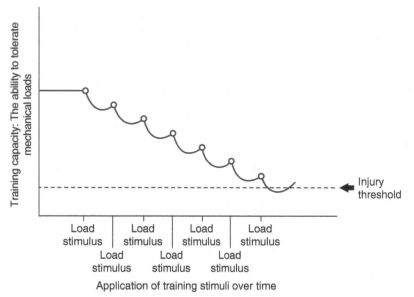

Fig. 82.5 Repeated training stimuli and responses, given insufficient recovery and poor training adaptation. This depicts the body's inability to recover from and adapt to repeated training stimuli when insufficient recovery time and poor training adaptations occur. (Graph originally published in *UltraRunning* magazine, April 2010.)

treatment should focus on the training error that disrupted the normal adaptation process. Using this information, the clinician can create an environment that promotes healing and builds the capacity to tolerate the demands of running.

A Problem: Our Perception of Running Injuries

Run training and the assessment and treatment of running-related injuries are at a crossroads. Assessment and treatment efforts have focused on biomechanical malalignments and the like, yet we now have 30+ years of sports science research that indicate that the primary issue related to the onset of running injuries is training error. Although the scientific evidence exists, the application of it has been absent or misguided clinically. Perceptually, there has been a quantum leap between perceived causes and treatments, a leap that is simply unsubstantiated in the scientific literature. With this in mind, it becomes readily apparent that health care providers need to understand training demands to effectively and optimally address the problems of the injured runner. Instead of simply being a case of "overuse," most running injuries will in fact be an issue of "under-recovery" or impaired adaptation. **It is the body's inability to adapt to the imposed demands of training that is most commonly an error in the training program**. Simply put, if training is the problem, then training is the solution.

Assessment must focus *not* on the isolation of the perceived specific biomechanical malalignment but on the (1) understanding of the mechanical dynamics leading to injury and (2) dynamics of the training program. Treatment then focuses on a graded "return-to-training" progression, given the basic rules of tissue repair and remodeling.

Mechanical Assessment

Subjective

A thorough examination should begin with a review of the patient's prior running program. We have compiled a list of characteristic traits of the run training program that typically contribute to factors related to **overuse/under-recovery** (Table 82.4). This assists the clinician's understanding of the athlete's current capacity to tolerate mechanical loading. The intent and rationale for each question has also been provided.

Objective

Care of the athlete has many approaches. Establishing a mechanical cause and effect is integral in effectively diagnosing and treating the athletic population. A reliable and valid assessment and clinical reasoning process—for the injured runner and the orthopedic patient in general—would entail some form of mechanical evaluation. The primary goal of any assessment process is to utilize reliable and valid procedures; however, review of the scientific literature to date indicates that many currently used assessment procedures—including palpation-based methods of assessment—are not only unreliable but also have questionable validity in the clinical reasoning process. Research does, however, support the use of provocation- and movement-based testing procedures.

The McKenzie method of Mechanical Diagnosis and Therapy, or MDT™ (The McKenzie Institute, Syracuse, NY), forms the basis of the mechanical assessment and is presented here because it is a comprehensive classification and treatment system that has scientific research to support not only its assessment process but also its classification algorithm. Although MDT™ initially gained widespread international acceptance for the treatment of spinal pain, its principles also are readily applied to the extremities. *Three primary aspects are unique to the McKenzie method™: mechanical assessment, self-treatment, and prevention* (Table 82.5). Although a complete description of the McKenzie method™ is not within the scope of this chapter, further resources can be found in the reference list at the end of this chapter.

The mechanical therapist seeks to understand the effect of a systematic progression of mechanical forces and loading

TABLE 82.4	Run Training History	

Running Experience

1. Have you been involved in any other sport or fitness activities, and if so, for how long?
2. How long have you been a runner?
3. Have you had any previous running injuries? If so, where and when?

Current Training Program

1. How many days per week do you run?
2. How many miles do you run per week?
3. What is your average running pace (minutes/mile)?
4. What was your longest run in the month prior to injury?
5. Do you recall any change in your running program that occurred just prior to the onset of your injury?
6. Are you training with a group or individually? Are you using a published program or a coach?
7. What is the longest run that you have done since you noted the injury? How long ago was this done?
8. Do you compete in races? If so, what distance(s)? Are you currently training for a particular event?
9. Do you do interval training (speed work) in your training program? If so, what and how often?
10. Do you do strength and/or plyometric training as part of your training program? If so, what exercises are you doing? Typical number of sets and repetitions? Light, moderate, or heavy resistance? Number of days per week?
11. Is there anything else you would like to tell me about your running program?

Intent/Rationale of Question

General level of conditioning and tissue "health" and current loading capacity

More experienced runners tend toward lower injury risk

Injury risk increases if history of a prior running injury

Intent/Rationale of Question

Number of recovery days per week

Most programs emphasize "more is better"; injury risk tends to increase at 25 to 40 miles per week.

Running mechanics change with running pace.

The rate of progression of the total volume of training and loading capacity

Injured runners most typically have some type of sudden change in the volume of their training; the rate of application of training stimuli exceeds the rate of adaptation to training.

Access to the program itself can be valuable for further analysis by the clinician (see #5).

Allows the clinician to better understand where to resume running when the athlete is ready (i.e., longer break = more gradual resumption of training)

Injury risk is higher in those who have competed in the past. If they are currently training for an event, it may affect their rate of progression and return to running, along with their overall goal setting.

Is the athlete doing any run training activities that are building power and loading capacity?

Strength and plyometric training (high load, low repetitions) build greater loading capacity and power output.

It is common that the athlete will have an inherent "sense" of the factors that contributed to the injury. Ask him or her!

TABLE 82.5	Basic Concepts of Mechanical Diagnosis and Therapy™	
Mechanical Assessment	1. Establish a relationship between symptom response and mechanical loading (typically via repeated test movements).	
	2. Systematically apply progressive mechanical loading strategies.	
	3. Use reliable classification system that leads naturally to treatment and patient self-care.	
Self-treatment	1. Provide patients with the necessary knowledge and tools to treat themselves.	
	2. Decrease reliance on clinician.	
	3. Empower patient to become self-responsible.	
Prevention	1. Provide patients with the knowledge of what to do if problem reoccurs.	
	2. Develop patient understanding of cause of problem to know how to prevent problems in the future.	

strategies (and the symptomatic and functional responses to these strategies) to diagnose and treat conditions of the musculoskeletal system. Mechanical loading strategies include the use of static sustained positions and dynamic repeated movements. This helps to establish a cause and effect between mechanical loading and symptom response. The MDT™ classification uses a well-defined algorithm and provides a reproducible means of separating patients with apparently similar presentations into definable subgroups (syndromes) to determine appropriate treatment interventions. It is not so much a

"treatment technique" as it is a "process of thinking." Research has shown the initial MDT™ assessment procedures to be as reliable as costly diagnostic imaging (i.e., magnetic resonance imaging [MRI]) to determine the source of the problem. The assessment process quickly establishes **responders** and **nonresponders** with classification guiding the treatment intervention.

MDT™ fits well within a sports medicine paradigm given that training will involve many hours of repetitive mechanical loading. Add to this axial loading (i.e., that which occurs with ground reaction forces) and you have the potential for mechanical disorders related to **sustained positioning** and/or **repetitive mechanical loading** while running. The mechanical assessment process is clinical reasoning based on sound mechanical principles.

Other sport-specific functional mechanical tests can be used to allow the clinician to further assess the athlete's dynamic eccentric loading capacity and neuromuscular control. Running injuries are typically a problem of eccentric loading and weight bearing; thus functional mechanical tests should incorporate similar types of loading, including strength and plyometric testing. The functional tests can be simple and are again directly related to treatment. For example, **knee hops** (hopping motions using ankles and knees) and **ankle hops** (hopping motions with the knee locked) can be used with a graded progression of loading. The progression would be two-legged hops (for vertical), to one-legged hops (for vertical), to two-legged hops (for horizontal), to one-legged hops (for horizontal). Reproduction of concordant symptoms (or lack thereof) is key. This uses the principle of **"hurt, not harm"** in which loading may reproduce the symptoms during the activity, but the symptoms are not increasing and do not remain worse afterward, indicating that the affected tissues are being loaded appropriately.

Gait assessment is also considered a functional mechanical test and serves two primary purposes. It is a benchmark for the athlete's current movement pattern and provides the foundation for running form development. It also provides insight into the athlete's ability to tolerate eccentric loading and, combined with his or her running/injury history, provides a more complete understanding of the potential training factors related to the onset of the injury.

Treatment

As mentioned earlier, if training is the primary problem with most running injuries, then training needs to be a primary element in the rehabilitation of injury and return to normal sport activity. Effective treatment means that health care providers must become familiar with the functional elements of training recovery and adaptation, running form, the principles of run training, and mechanical loading strategies. **Because running injuries are a problem of eccentric mechanical loading and weight bearing, the solution to these injuries must incorporate aspects of both as part of the "periodized rehabilitation" of the athlete.** Much as periodization is used in the appropriate timing and integration of training sessions into the overall scope of the training plan, the same is true during the injury recovery timeline. This is no different from an optimized run training program with injury prevention and optimal performance in mind.

A general runner-friendly overview of the assessment and treatment progression is described in *RunSmart: A Comprehensive Approach to Injury-Free Running* by Allan Besselink (2008).

EDUCATION

Education of the patient is a critical element in the effective treatment of the injured runner. MDT™ uniquely emphasizes education and active patient involvement in the management of his or her treatment, which minimizes the number of visits to the clinic. Ultimately, most patients can successfully treat themselves when provided with the necessary knowledge and tools. Active approaches to care enhance patient self-responsibility, and education and empowerment of the individual become integral to effectively dealing with injury and the further goal of injury prevention. By learning how to self-treat the current problem, patients gain hands-on knowledge on how to minimize the risk of recurrence and to rapidly deal with recurrences.

The goal of the assessment process is to establish movements, positions, and exercises that will allow the patient to self-treat if an injury responds successfully to a certain direction of movement. **Self-care strategies** can be used so that the athlete can be applying mechanical loads to the affected tissues on a regular and consistent basis to promote reduction of the mechanical problem (directional preference) or to stimulate tissue repair and remodeling. The athlete needs to be aware of how to apply safe and appropriate mechanical loads and how (and when) to progress them. By doing so, the athlete can be applying the right forces at the right frequency, far more effectively than a two- or three-times-per week clinical treatment approach. In this way, the practitioner becomes the "guide" and the patient takes an active role in implementing the prescribed treatment with increasing independence. This refines the role of the clinician in the health care spectrum—to one of problem solver, educator, and mentor.

As the patient recovers from injury and returns to running, the physical therapist thoroughly reviews the progression back to running to prevent re-injury (see Table 82.4). Runners, like most athletes, are eager to return to athletic training and competition. Because running injuries are generally training related, it is imperative that athletes understand how to modify their training to foster injury recovery and tissue repair, how to prepare their body to accept the increasing mechanical loads with running, and how to optimize their performance. Most runners are under the mindset that "more is better." Because research clearly dictates otherwise for runners, it is imperative to educate the patient.

Progression of the program is based on appropriate symptomatic, functional, and mechanical responses to loading. Based on this loading response, the athlete is given the green light to progress the functional loading within his or her training program. Having knowledge of this allows the athlete to progress steadily within the timeline and limits of normal tissue repair and under his or her own control.

BUILDING CAPACITY
Strength and Plyometric Training for Runners

Strengthening is often a key component in recovery for a runner. The important eccentric role of the stance leg has been discussed previously. The posterior calf muscles also function eccentrically and concentrically during gait as the primary propulsive force. The practitioner should evaluate the athlete's ability to tolerate both concentric and eccentric loading of these muscles via mechanical and functional assessment strategies.

Strengthening should be performed as appropriate to weakened tissues not only to build the capacity for mechanical loading but also to provide a neuromuscular stimulus. Clinicians often incorrectly think of strengthening in one way for all endurance athletes, which is typically three sets of 10 to 20 repetitions of moderate weight to gain "muscular endurance." Strength training should be considered more as a means of altering the neuromuscular and tissue integrity because the intent is to increase loading capacity and improve tissue architecture, not "endurance." Muscular and collagenous tissues require tensile loading to increase their strength and improve their architecture. **This can be accomplished only by applying a high load with few repetitions**—again, given the "hurt not harm" rules of mechanical loading. This provides the necessary stimulus and thus the intended cellular response. There is little difference in strength gains between one set and multiple sets of the same exercise. **Multiple sets, however, do require a significantly greater recovery effort,** which is not the intent of the exercises in the first place. This can initially be implemented on a 2 days on, 1 day off cycle to foster the necessary training adaptations. Strength training will also have a positive effect on running performance.

The same rationale holds for progressive lower extremity plyometrics, which will also benefit the running athlete because this builds capacity and tolerance for eccentric loading specifically. Plyometric training activities can be similar to the functional mechanical tests used in the assessment process. It is important to remember that eccentric loading does impose greater demands on recovery and adaptation. Both means of building capacity require an appropriate "dosage" to provide high load yet few repetitions. The goal is to simply apply a stimulus to cause the tissues to adapt to higher tensile tissue loads.

Interval Training and Return to Running

Interval training provides a number of key benefits in the recovery process. In most cases, gait quality (running form) improves as the athlete runs faster (as opposed to slower).

A faster running pace entails a gradual transition toward the more desired midfoot strike pattern. A midfoot strike requires greater active neuromuscular control mechanisms compared to the passive mechanisms found with a heel strike initial contact. Faster speeds also require more joint ROM and power. **There is minimal difference in ground reaction forces with increased speed of running.** Finally, faster running speeds build muscular power, which is essential for running both faster and longer.

Overwhelming data suggest that runners incorporate interval or speed training in both their return to training program and their normal run training program. Interval training, much like strength training, has a positive effect on running performance. **Building power is key to being able to tolerate more frequent loads and longer runs, contrary to the belief of the average runner or coach that "more is better." The strongest predictor of a race performance at one distance, such as a marathon, is the race performance at a significantly shorter distance, such as a 10K.** Interval training also allows the clinician to provide a graded "dosage" of good quality running and mechanical loading with appropriate recovery. It is essential to progress slowly with purposeful increments, again using the patient's understanding of loading responses as a guideline ("hurt, not harm").

Research indicates that an athlete can maintain his or her aerobic capacity for up to 4 weeks before significant decline is demonstrated. If injury prevents return of weightbearing activities for an extended time, weight-altering activities such as deep-water running and unloaded treadmill ambulation may be considered. However, because running injuries are typically a problem of weight bearing, activities must focus on fostering the necessary adaptations to weight bearing as soon as possible. Tissues benefit from mechanical loading, and most injuries tolerate loading in a "hurt, not harm" format. This significantly limits the role of aqua jogging and "unloading" for running injuries because deep-water running may be just 10% of body weight. If the injured athlete can tolerate normal daily weight bearing, then walking or brisk walking is more functional for improving tolerance to load and a faster return to activity than aqua jogging.

Interval training is an integral first step in the return to running program based on these loading characteristics. When the athlete is able to tolerate eccentric loading without increasing symptoms that remain worse afterward (following the "hurt,

not harm" guideline) and has initiated a program of strength and plyometric training, in most cases, the athlete is ready to return to running.

It is recommended to begin the returning running athlete with 1 minute of running (brisk pace, relative to the particular individual) alternating with 1 minute of walking, for a total of 20 minutes. The run pace is deemed appropriate if it takes the athlete the full 1 minute of walking to recover from the previous bout of activity. *This activity can be increased as indicated until the patient can perform 1 minute of running, alternating with 1 minute of walking, for a total of 30 minutes.* Once the athlete can achieve this, he or she is ready to resume continuous running, typically for 20 minutes total. In our experience, the ability to successfully tolerate 30 minutes of alternating a 1-minute walk with a 1-minute run provides a clinically relevant and predictable prognostic indicator of return to continuous running.

PRINCIPLES OF OPTIMAL RUN TRAINING

The training plan is essential to review, discuss, and modify if necessary as an integral part of the treatment plan. The following training principles should assist the clinician in making good recommendations for the running athlete (Table 82.6).

TABLE 82.6	Optimal Training Principles for Runners
Principles	**Intent/Rationale**
1. A runner requires at least 2 days of recovery per week.	The time is required to foster training adaptations.
2. Incorporate at least 1 day of strength and plyometric training per week (high load, low repetition, e.g., one set of 10 reps).	To foster training adaptations and increase loading capacity
3. 1–2 days of interval training per week, depending on the total number of run days per week	Interval training provides a small dosage of quality work, which has favorable effects on running mechanics, loading capacity, and power output.
4. Plan of progression should be on a biweekly basis.	It takes about 10 to 14 days for the body to adapt to the current level of training load. At this time, training volume and load can be progressed.
5. Progress the longest run according to the following guidelines: If running less than 30 minutes, increase longest run by no more than 5 minutes every other week. If running 30–60 minutes, increase longest run by no more than 10 minutes every other week. If running >60 minutes, increase longest run by no more than 20 minutes every other week.	This accommodates the normal time factor for rate of adaptation to training.

Adapted from Besselink A: RunSmart: a comprehensive approach to injury-free running, Raleigh, NC, 2008, Lulu Publishing.

- The clinician should promote recovery-centered training by first determining which days are recovery days. These are the most important days because this is the time in which the body is adapting to the loads that have been placed on it.
- There should be at least 1 day of strength and plyometric training per week. This is done with specific parameters to build the loading capacity necessary for running.
- Interval work is also recommended for the runner to both build power and improve running form. The length of the interval would vary based on the individual's goals but should include an appropriate warmup and cool-down.

Evidence suggests that an arbitrary 10% increase in weekly mileage is not effective at reducing running-related injuries because 7 days may not be long enough for the body to adapt to increased repeated loading. Because of this and **evidence to support that recovery from an increased run distance takes 10 to 14 days, we recommend a progression of loading based on the current level of training adaptations** (Table 82.6). Table 82.6 is not a comprehensive list, but it does include the primary elements of an optimal and effective training program.

Much like any other sport, improving running biomechanics will help improve efficiency over the long term. The feedback of a professional coach can be exceedingly useful in improving a person's running mechanics. At the time of this publication, a number of running philosophies are targeted at this subject, including Chi Running,™ POSE Method,™ RunSmart,™ and Evolution™ running, among many others. Most propose similar premises regarding running form but use different cues and strategies to attain it and varying levels of training-related information to support it. Running injuries are not simply a "running form error"; education regarding recovery-based training is critical to developing an optimal and safe training program.

SUMMARY

Lessons learned from running injuries have a significant impact on our perception of the role of rehabilitation and self-care strategies on all orthopedic and musculoskeletal conditions. It is imperative to look to the training program for both the cause and the solution for running injuries. Patients need to play the most important role in their recovery for successful recovery and prevention of injury re-occurrence. Education may be the most valuable treatment the clinician can provide.

REHABILITATION PROTOCOL 82.1 ● **Runner's Guide for Return to Running After Absence From Training of 4 Weeks or More (Nonsurgical)**

Week Schedule

1. Walk 30 min, alternating 1 min normal and 1 min fast.
2. Walk 30 min, alternating 1.5 min normal and 1.5 min fast. If doing well, jog easily instead of walking fast.
3. Alternate walking 1 min and jogging 2 min × 7. The next day, run easy 5 min and walk 1 min × 3.
4. Alternate walking 1 min and jogging 3 min × 7. The next day, run 5 min and walk 1 min × 4.
5. Run continuously 20 min. The next day, run 5 min and walk 1 min × 5.
6. Run continuously 20 min. The next day, run 10 min and walk 1 min × 3.
7. Run continuously 20 min 1 day and 35 min the next.
8. Run continuously 20 min 1 day and 40 min the next.
9. If doing well, resume a training schedule, increasing the duration, intensity, and frequency appropriately. The key is to avoid reinjury.

From James SL, Bates BT, Oslering LR. Injuries to Runners. *Am J Sports Med* 1978;6:40.

REHABILITATION PROTOCOL 82.2 ● **Return to Running Program: Postsurgical**

Purpose: This program is intended for those individuals who have been off running for an extended period because of an injury or surgery. Please discuss with your therapist specific modifications to this program depending on the circumstances leading up to your return to running.

Guidelines: The following guidelines need to be followed to ensure an optimal outcome of the progressive running program.

1. For the first 4 weeks, run every other day for the time allotted. If allowed, it is okay to cross-train with other forms of cardio activities (e.g., elliptical trainer, stationary bike) after your run or on specified "off" days.
2. Complete warmup and cool-down exercises as prescribed.
3. Run up to, but not into, the "pain zone."
4. Use ice as needed (10 minutes) to decrease postexercise tissue irritation.
5. Do not progress to next allotted time if symptoms occur while running or if limping.

6. Do not forget to do prescribed strength training exercises on "off" days.

Warmup: A 5- to 10-minute period of light cardiovascular activity (e.g., bike, walking, elliptical trainer) is needed to sufficiently warm up the tissues for running or stretching. Your physical therapist will provide you with a list of appropriate stretches. They should be done in a controlled, low-load, prolonged manner that does NOT cause pain. For static stretching, hold the position for 30 seconds and repeat three times. For dynamic stretching, follow the instructions provided by your physical therapist.

Cool-down: Complete your stretching/strengthening program as recommended by your physical therapist or continue with additional cross-training activities. Ice as needed following runs for mild pain/soreness (10 minutes).

Continued

REHABILITATION PROTOCOL 82.2 ● **Return to Running Program: Postsurgical—cont'd**

ACTUAL DAY

Week #1	5 minutes	OFF/CT	5 minutes	OFF/CT	7.5 minutes	OFF/CT	7.5 minutes
Week #2	OFF/CT	10 minutes	OFF/CT	10 minutes	OFF/CT	12.5 minutes	OFF/CT
Week #3	12.5 minutes	OFF/CT	15 minutes	OFF/CT	15 minutes	OFF/CT	17.5 minutes
Week #4	OFF/CT	17.5 minutes	OFF/CT	20 minutes	OFF/CT	20 minutes	OFF/CT
Week #5	10 minutes	20 minutes	OFF/CT	10 minutes	20 minutes	OFF/CT	15 minutes
Week #6	20 minutes	OFF/CT	15 minutes	25 minutes	OFF/CT	15 minutes	25 minutes
Week #7	OFF/CT	15 minutes	25 minutes	OFF/CT	20 minutes	25 minutes	OFF/CT
Week #8	20 minutes	25 minutes	OFF/CT	20 minutes	30 minutes	OFF/CT	*

CT = cross-training

*After reaching 30 minutes of continuous running, begin to estimate the mileage completed in that time and progress distance by a total of 10% to 15% per week.

Example: 30 minutes @ 7:30 min/mile pace = 4.0 miles

4.0 miles × 10% = 0.4 miles

4.0 miles × 15% = 0.6 miles

Therefore, increase each training run by 0.4 to 0.6 miles.

Used with permission from Scott Miller, PT, MS, SCS, CSCS, from Agility Physical Therapy & Sports Performance, LLC. Portage, MI.

REHABILITATION PROTOCOL 82.3 ● **Return to Running Program: Poststress Fracture**

Purpose: This program is intended for those individuals who have been off running for an extended period because of an injury or surgery. Please discuss with your therapist specific modifications to this program depending on the circumstances leading up to your return to running.

Guidelines: The following guidelines need to be followed to ensure an optimal outcome of the progressive running program.

1. For the first 4 weeks, run every other day for the time allotted. If allowed, it is okay to cross-train with other forms of cardio activities (e.g., elliptical trainer, stationary bike) after the run or on specified "off" days.

2. Complete warmup and cool-down exercises as prescribed.
3. Run up to, but not into, the "pain zone."
4. Use ice as needed (10 minutes) to decrease postexercise tissue irritation.
5. Do not progress to next allotted time if symptoms occur while running or if limping.
6. Do not forget prescribed strength training exercises on "off" days.

Seven-Week Schedule for Returning from Injury

Week	Monday	Tuesday	Wednesday	Thursday	Friday	Saturday	Sunday
1	Walk 10 min, Run 5 min, Walk 5 min, Run 5 min	Run in water or other training	Run in water or other training	Walk 5 min, Run 5 min, Walk 5 min, Run 5 min, Walk 5 min, Run 5 min	Run in water or other training	Run in water or other training	Walk 3 min, Run 7 min, Walk 3 min, Run 7 min, Walk 3 min, Run 7 min
2	Run in water or other training	Walk 2 min, Run 8 min, Walk 2 min, Run 8 min, Walk 2 min, Run 8 min	Run in water or other training	Run 10 min, Walk 2 min, Run 10 min, Walk 2 min, Run 10 min	Run in water or other training	Run 12 min, Walk 2 min, Run 12 min, Walk 2 min, Run 10 min	Run in water or other training
3	Run 15 min, Walk 2 min, Run 15 min	Run in water or other training	Run 20 min, Walk 2 min, Run 10 min	Run in water or other training	Run 25 min	Run in water or other training	Run 30 min
4	Run in water or other training	Run 25 min	Run 30 min	Run in water or other training	Run 25 min	Run 35 min	Run in water or other training
5	Run 30 min	Run 35 min	Run in water or other training	Run 30 min plus 6 × 100-m strideouts	Run 30 min	Run 40 min	Run in water or other raining

REHABILITATION PROTOCOL 82.3 ■ Return to Running Program: Poststress Fracture—cont'd

Week	Monday	Tuesday	Wednesday	Thursday	Friday	Saturday	Sunday
6	Tempo run (15-min warmup, 15 min @ 15-km race pace)	Run 30 min	Run 45 min	Run in water or other training	Run 40 min plus 6 × 100-m strideouts	Run 30 min	Run 50 min
7	Run in water or other training	Run 35 min	Tempo run (15 min warmup, 20 min @ 15-km race pace)	Run 35 min	Run in water or other training	Run 40 min plus 6 × 100-m strideouts	Run 55 min

From http://pfitzinger.com/labreports/stressfracture.shtml.

Cooldown: Complete the stretching/strengthening program as recommended by the physical therapist or continue with additional cross-training activities. Ice as needed following runs for mild pain/soreness (10 minutes).

Used with permission from Scott Miller, PT, MS, SCS, CSCS, from Agility Physical Therapy & Sports Performance, LLC. Portage, MI.

REFERENCES

A complete reference list is available at https://expertconsult.inkling.com/.

FURTHER READING

Abelin T, Vader JP, Marti B, et al. On the epidemiology of running injuries. The 1984 Bern Grand-Prix study. *Am J Sports Med.* 1988;16(3):285–294.

Alfredson H, Pietilä T, Jonsson P, et al. Heavy-load eccentric calf muscle training for the treatment of chronic Achilles tendinosis. *Am J Sports Med.* 1998;26(3):360–366.

Arem AJ, Madden JW. Effects of stress on healing wounds: I. intermittent noncyclical tension. *J Surg Res.* 1976;20(2):93–102.

Arem AJ, Madden JW. Is there a Wolff's law for connective tissue? *Surg Forum.* 1974;25(0).

Besselink A. 1994 WalkSmart: implications of a graded high-intensity walking program. *Phys Ther.* 1994;74(5).

Brushøj C, Larsen K, Albrecht-Beste E, et al. Prevention of overuse injuries by a concurrent exercise program in subjects exposed to an increase in training load: a randomized controlled trial of 1020 army recruits. *Am J Sports Med.* 2008;36(4):663–670.

Buist I, Bredeweg SW, van Mechelen W, et al. No effect of a graded training program on the number of running-related injuries in novice runners: a randomized controlled trial. *Am J Sports Med.* 2008;36(1):33–39.

Cavanagh PR. *Biomechanics of Distance Running.* Champaign, IL: Human Kinetics; 1990.

Cavanagh PR, Lafortune MA. Ground reaction forces in distance running. *J Biomech.* 1980;13:397–406.

Clare HA, Adams R, Maher CG. Reliability of McKenzie classification of patients with cervical or lumbar pain. *J Manipulative Physiol Ther.* 2005;28(2):122–127.

Cole GK, Nigg BM, Van Den Bogert AJ, et al. Lower extremity joint loading during impact in running. *Clin Biomech (Bristol, Avon).* 1996;11(4):181–193.

Donelson R, April C, Medcalf R, et al. A prospective study of centralization of lumbar and referred pain. A predictor of symptomatic discs and anular competence. *Spine.* 1997;22(10):1115–1122.

Donelson R, Silva G, Murphy K. Centralization phenomenon. Its usefulness in evaluating and treating referred pain. *Spine.* 1990;15(3):211–213.

Evans P. The healing process at cellular level: a review. *Physiotherapy.* 1980;66(8):256–259.

Fredericson M, Misra AK. Epidemiology and aetiology of marathon running injuries. *Sports Med.* 2007;37(4):437–439.

Hefford C. McKenzie classification of mechanical spinal pain: profile of syndromes and directions of preference. *Man Ther.* 2008;13(1):75–81.

Hinrichs R. Upper extremity function in distance running. In: Cavanagh PR, ed. *Biomechanics of Distance Running.* Champaign, IL: Human Kinetics; 1990:107–134.

Hreljac A. Impact and overuse injuries in runners. *Med Sci Sports Exerc.* 2004;36(5):845–849.

Hreljac A, Marshall RN, Hume P. Evaluation of lower extremity overuse injury potential in runners. *Med Sci Sports Exerc.* 2000;32(9):1635–1641.

Jacobs SJ, Berson BL. Injuries to runners: a study of entrants to a 10,000 meter race. *Am J Sports Med.* 1986;14(2):151–155.

James SL, Jones DC. Biomechanical aspects of distance running injuries. In: Cavanagh PR, ed. *Biomechanics of Distance Running.* Champaign, IL: Human Kinetics; 1990:249–270.

Johnson ST, Golden GM, Mercer JA, et al. Ground-reaction forces during form skipping and running. *J Sports Rehab.* 2005;14:338–345.

Jung A. The impact of resistance training on distance running performance. *Sports Med.* 2003;33(7):539–552.

Keller TS, Weisberger AM, Ray JL, et al. Relationship between vertical ground reaction force and speed during walking, slow jogging, and running. *Clin Biomech (Bristol, Avon).* 1996;11(5):253–259.

Kessler MA, Glaser C, Tittel S, et al. Recovery of the menisci and articular cartilage of runners after cessation of exercise: additional aspects of in vivo investigation based on 3-dimensional magnetic resonance imaging. *Am J Sports Med.* 2008;36(5):966–970.

Knechtle B, Wirth A, Knechtle P, et al. Personal best marathon performance is associated with performance in a 24-h run and not anthropometry or training volume. *Br J Sports Med.* 2009;43(11):836–839.

McKenzie R. *The Cervical and Thoracic Spine: Mechanical Diagnosis and Therapy.* Waikanae: Spinal Publications; 1990.

McKenzie R, May S. *The Human Extremities: Mechanical Diagnosis and Therapy.* Waikanae: Spinal Publications; 2000.

McKenzie R. *The Lumbar Spine: Mechanical Diagnosis and Therapy.* Waikanae: Spinal Publications; 1981.

McQuade KJ. A case-control study of running injuries: comparison of patterns of runners with and without running injuries. *J Orthop Sports Phys Ther.* 1986;8(2):81–84.

Miller DI. Ground reaction forces in distance running. In: Cavanagh PR, ed. *Biomechanics of Distance Running.* Champaign: Human Kinetics; 1990:203–224.

Munro CF, Miller DI, Fuglevand AJ. Ground reaction forces in running: a reexamination. *J Biomech.* 1987;20(2):147–155.

Nigg BM, Bahlsen HA, Luethi SM, et al. The influence of running velocity and midsole hardness on external impact forces in heel-toe running. *J Biomech.* 1987;20(10):951–959.

Novacheck T. The biomechanics of running. *Gait Posture.* 1998;7(1):77–95.

Paavolainen L, Häkkinen K, Hämäläinen I, et al. Explosive-strength training improves 5-km running time by improving running economy and muscle power. *J Appl Physiol.* 1999;86(5):1527–1533.

Pratt D. Mechanisms of shock attenuation via the lower extremity during running. *Clin Biomech (Bristol, Avon).* 1989;4(1):51–57.

van Gent RN, Siem D, van Middelkoop M, et al. Incidence and determinants of lower extremity running injuries in long distance runners: a systematic review. *Br J Sports Med.* 2007;41(8):469–480.

van Mechelen W. Running injuries. A review of the epidemiological literature. *Sports Med.* 1992;14(5):320–335.

Yamamoto LK. The effects of resistance training on endurance distance running performance among highly trained runners: a systematic review. *J Strength Cond Res.* 2008;22(6):2036–2044.

Running Injuries: Shoes, Orthotics, and Return-to-Running Program

Scott T. Miller, PT, MS, SCS, CSCS | Janice K. Loudon, PT, Phd, SCS, ATC, CSCS

BIOMECHANICAL AND ANATOMIC FACTORS

No specific anatomic or biomechanical variation necessarily correlates with a specific condition or injury, but lower-quarter biomechanics do play an important role (Table 83.1). The most important aspect of the examination is to evaluate the entire lower extremity and not just concentrate on the area of injury (Table 83.2). The lower extremity functions as a kinetic chain and disruption at any given area can affect function throughout.

The running stride is divided into an active and passive absorption phase and a generation phase (see Fig. 83.1, *A*). The purpose of the **active absorption phase** is initially to decelerate the rapidly forward-swinging recovery leg with eccentric hamstring activity, first absorbing and then transferring the energy to the extending hip, placing the hamstrings under considerable stress. **Passive absorption** begins at footstrike with absorption of the shock of ground reaction force resulting in a force 2.5 to 3 times body weight (BW) and up to 10 times BW running downhill. This initial shock is attenuated by the surface, the shoe, and the heel pad but not to a great extent. Subsequently, the ground reaction force is actively absorbed by muscles and tendons as it increases to midsupport with a relative shortening of the extremity. This is accomplished by hip and knee flexion, ankle dorsiflexion, and subtalar pronation accompanied by eccentric contraction of the hip abductors, quadriceps, and gastroc–soleus muscles along with stretching of the quadriceps and patellar tendon, Achilles tendon, and plantar fascia. At this point, the ground reaction force with running may be as much as five times BW. The stretched tendons absorb energy, store it as potential energy, and then return 90% of it later in the generation or propulsive phase as kinetic energy, with the remaining 10% creating heat in the tendon.

During the **generation phase** in the second half of support, there is a relative lengthening of the extremity with concentric muscle contraction and joint extension, with return of stored potential energy as kinetic energy from the tendons significantly assisting the now concentrically contracting muscles. Peak forces maximize at the sites of chronic injury (Scott and Winter 1990). Forces in the patellofemoral joint estimated at 7 to 11.1 times BW, 4.7 to 6.9 times BW in the patellar tendon, 6 to 8 times BW in the Achilles tendon, and 1.3 to 2.9 times BW in the plantar fascia predispose the tissues to potential injury from repetitive overuse—particularly if combined with even a minor anatomic or functional variation.

Examination of the entire lower extremity thus becomes essential (Fig. 83.1, *B*) when the extremity is viewed as a kinetic chain whose normal function is dependent on the proper sequential function of each segment. Therefore, concentrating on only the area of complaint may overlook the underlying cause of the problem (e.g., anterior knee pain related to compensatory foot pronation and imbalances in proximal stabilizers).

The examination evaluates the following (Fig. 83.2):
- Bilateral lower extremity length
- Extremity alignment in the frontal and sagittal planes
- Hip motion
- Core and lower-quarter muscle strength and flexibility
- Gluteus maximus and medius recruitment patterns
- Extensor mechanism dynamics
- Leg-heel alignment
- Heel-forefoot alignment
- First ray alignment
- Mobility of first ray, subtalar, and midtarsal joints
- Shoe inspection
- Dynamic evaluation of slow-motion videotaped running gait

A basic two-dimensional video analysis of the runner's gait can be accomplished with an inexpensive camcorder setup or utilizing more advanced video management software (Dartfish) with multiple high-speed camcorders in the office.

SHOES

It is evident that the etiology of overuse running injuries is a multifactorial problem and successful management often relies on sound decision making by the clinician. One key factor is the consideration of matching the appropriate footwear to an individual's foot classification, including alignment, mobility, and biomechanical factors related to running. Clinically, footwear recommendations are a necessary complement to the various treatment approaches for running injuries.

To provide appropriate recommendations on running footwear, having a basic understanding of how the shoe is constructed is important. The key features of a running shoe include the outsole, midsole, and upper. The outsole is the bottom of the shoe and is generally made from carbon or blown rubber. The midsole is the shock-absorbing layer between the outsole and the "upper" part of the shoe. This midsole is the most important part of a running shoe because the construction and materials used will affect the levels of both cushioning and stability in the shoe. The amount of cushioning in the shoe is generally proportionate to the shoe's heel height. The two types of cushioning generally found in running shoes are ethylene vinyl acetate (EVA) and polyurethane (PU). Increased stability in a shoe is accomplished through the incorporation of a heavier density EVA or PU in combination with the existing cushioning materials. This type of construction is referred to as a **dual-density midsole.** Finally, the "upper" is the soft body of the shoe that encloses the foot and is usually made of a combination of materials, from lightweight, durable synthetic mesh to heavier materials such as leather. The materials and construction of the

TABLE 83.1	Common Running Mechanics Faults	
Biomechanical Fault	**Contributing Factor(s)**
Increase vertical excursion	Overstriding; weak core muscles
Horizontal sway/tilt	Scoliosis; leg-length difference; pelvic obliquity; weak gluteus medius
Forward trunk lean	Tight hip flexors; SI joint pain
Arm swing crosses midline	Excessive pelvic rotation; scoliosis; leg-length difference; weak abdominals
Asymmetric pelvic rotation	Hypomobile SI joint; leg-length difference, lumbar spine dysfunction
Excessive lateral pelvic tilt	*Contralateral drops:* Weak hip abductors on reference limb
	Ipsilateral drops: Compensation for shortened limb
Increase AP pelvic tilt between foot contact and midstance	Weak gluteal and abdominal muscles
Increase AP pelvic tilt during propulsion	Tight hip flexors; lack of hip extension
Increase lumbar extension	Tight hip flexors; weak abdominal muscles
Decreased hip flexion	Weak hip flexors; tight hamstrings; hip dysfunction (OA, labrum)
Excessive hip internal rotation	Weak hip ER; femoral anteversion; excessive lumbar rotation
Excessive hip external rotation (ER)	Femoral retroversion; tight ER; limited dorsiflexors
Genu valgum	Weak gluteus medius; excessive pronation; excessive lumbar motion
Genu varum	Tight iliotibial band; rigid foot
Forefoot striker	Tight Achilles tendon/calf; hallux rigidus
Heel whip	Tibial torsion; tight lateral hamstring; genu valgum
Foot abduction	Limited dorsiflexion; tight hip; tight foot evertors

AP, anteroposterior; SI, sacroiliac; OA, osteoarthritis; ER, external rotation

TABLE 83.2	Objective Examination of the Running Athlete

STANDING
- Walking gait
- Navicular drop test
- Calcaneal position
- Soleus length
- Tibial varum/torsion
- Genu varum/valgum
- Pelvic obliquity
- Lumbar spine range of motion
- Single-leg stance (30 sec)
- Single-leg squat (5 reps)

PRONE
- Calcaneal inversion/eversion
- Rearfoot position
- First ray position
- Great toe extension
- Hip joint rotation
- Quadriceps length
- Dorsiflexion range of motion
- Callus pattern

SUPINE
- Leg length
- Hamstring length
- Hip flexor length
- Hip rotation
- Patellar position/mobility
- Midfoot mobility
- Midtarsal mobility

SIDE LYING
- Iliotibial band length
- Gluteus medius strength

SITTING
- Hip flexor strength

upper provide stability, comfort, and a snug fit. Features to consider in the upper include the last (the shape of the shoe), the toe box (the front of the shoe), the heel counter (the part holding the heel, which can vary in stiffness for increased stability), and the Achilles notch (a groove in the heel piece to protect the tendon from irritation). Running footwear can be divided into four primary categories related to their overall cushioning and stability properties (Table 83.3): (1) light cushion, (2) straight last cushion, (3) stability, and (4) motion control.

A *light cushion running shoe* (Fig. 83.3, *A*) is best for a true supinatory foot or for someone who is an underpronator. This foot type is generally fairly rigid in nature with pes cavus presentation; thus it does not absorb shock during the initial contact phase of running. A light cushion running shoe is not a very substantial shoe and is constructed of single-density material for the midsole with minimal arch support. This shoe is extremely flexible through the arch to allow the foot as much motion as possible. In general, a light cushion shoe will break down quickly (typically less than 400 miles/643 km).

A *straight last cushion running shoe* (Fig. 83.3, *B*) is a newer category shoe, described as a hybrid shoe that is a transition between a light cushion and stability (described next) shoe. This type of shoe is best for someone who is an underpronator but still presents with some of the forefoot and/or rearfoot alignment concerns (e.g., forefoot varus or calcaneal varus). This foot type is generally somewhat rigid but more accurately does not have the necessary motion available at the subtalar joint to accommodate for the positional faults (e.g., uncompensated forefoot varus). This unique shoe still uses the single-density cushioning material for the midsole, while providing more inherent stability based on the geometry of the shoe (straight last construction) versus implementing a dual-density midsole or stability system commonly seen in the stability shoes. Clinically, this shoe provides a more stable platform for the foot and/or foot orthosis to function without the extrinsic influence of the shoe, which may or may not be desirable.

A *stability running shoe* (Fig. 83.3, *C*) is best for someone who is a mild to moderate overpronator. This type of shoe generally has enough mobility in the subtalar joint to assist in shock absorption during stance phase. This shoe encompasses some additional stability through the midsole with some type of added stability feature like a dual-density material found in most brands or the Graphite Rollbar system found exclusively in the New Balance shoes. A stability shoe does allow for some flexibility through the midfoot, but it has enough rigidity to provide pronation control.

RUNNER ENCOUNTER SHEET

Name _____   Date _____

Age _____ Sex _____ Weight _____ Height _____

1. Describe how your injury occurred and where you are hurting.
_____
_____
_____
_____

2. How long ago did you notice your first symptoms?
_____
_____

3. Pain is present
_____ At all times
_____ During running
_____ During walking
_____ After running
_____ At rest

4. If pain during running starts:
_____ Midrun
_____ Late run
_____ After run
_____ Start of run

5. Pain is _____ improving _____ worsening _____ unchanged

6. Present running mileage
_____ miles per day
_____ miles per week

7. How many days a week do you run? _____

8. Mileage before injury
_____ miles per day
_____ miles per week

9. What surface do you run on?
_____ Grass   _____ Indoor track
_____ Concrete _____ Hills
_____ Asphalt   _____ Street with slope or pitch
_____ Cinder   _____ Other

10. Have you recently
_____ Increased your distance   _____ Increased hill running   _____ Increased workout intensity
_____ Gained significant weight   _____ Changed shoes   _____ Started interval training
_____ Changed surfaces

11. Do you stretch
_____ Before run
_____ After run

12. List and describe other running injuries in the past year
_____
_____

13. Describe pain
_____ Burning   _____ Sharp
_____ Aching   _____ Dull
_____ Cramping   _____ Pins and needles

14. On a scale of 1 to 10 (10 worst pain you've ever had)
rate your pain _____   _____ at rest _____ during activity

15. How many miles do you run on each pair of shoes before changing? (approximate)

16. Do your shoes wear out in more than one area _____ ?
_____ inner toe
_____ outer toe
_____ inner heel
_____ outer heel
_____ other Describe _____

Other notes:

Fig. 83.1 Runner's encounter form.

RUNNER EXAM SHEET

Standing exam

Increased Q angle _____

Genu valgum _____

Genu varum _____

Normal knee align _____

Tibial torsion _____

Foot pronation _____

　　(pes planus) _____

Foot supination _____

　　(pes cavus) _____

Pelvic obliquity _____

Scoliosis _____

Obesity _____

Sitting exam

Patellar maltracking _____

Patellar crepitance _____

Motor strength _____

Hip extension _____

　　flexion _____

Knee flexion _____

　　extension _____

Ankle _____

　　inversion _____

　　eversion _____

DF _____

PF _____

Muscle imbalance(s) _____

_____

_____

Forefoot alignment _____

Hindfoot alignment _____

Supine exam

Leg length

discrepancy of _____

shorter leg is L or R _____

ROM

Hip _____

Knee _____

Ankle _____

Subtalar _____

INFLEXIBILITY

Hip _____

Hamstring _____

Quad _____

Iliotibial band (Ober s) _____

Meniscal

Pathology _____

Patellofemoral _____

Gait assessment

Antalgic gait _____

Pronator _____ Supinator _____

Areas of point tenderness

_____

_____

_____

Shoes

___ new ___ very worn

Type of shoe _____

Wear pattern

___ medial toe box

___ lateral toe box

___ medial hindfoot

___ lateral hindfoot

Assymetric arm motion _____

Excessive pelvic tilt _____

neutral _____

Miscellaneous

Pathology _____

_____

_____

Knee effusion _____

Ligament _____

Exam knee _____

Generalized _____

Ligamentous _____

Laxity _____

Forefoot alignment _____

Hindfoot alignment _____

Excess callosities _____

_____

_____

_____

_____

_____

_____

_____

_____

Fig. 83.2 Runner's examination sheet.

Finally, a *motion control shoe* (Fig. 83.3, *D*) is designed for the moderate to severe overpronator. This foot type generally has the same forefoot and rearfoot alignment concerns, but by stark contrast to the more rigid foot, it has an excessive amount of subtalar and/or midtarsal joint motion available. A foot type that can compensate for a forefoot or calcaneal varus can present dynamically as an overpronator (at midsupport) or as a late pronator (at take-off). This causes the foot to roll inward, placing excessive stress on soft tissue structures proximal to the foot, including the lower leg, knee, hip, and back. Motion control shoes are straight lasted, have a very broad base for support, and are constructed of either a dual-density midsole or a Graphite Rollbar system. This shoe is very rigid through the midsole, much more than the stability shoe, to provide maximum pronation control.

When making footwear recommendations, several factors that can influence the type of shoe ideal for each individual runner must be considered. It is imperative that the individual's foot type matches the shoe by evaluating whether the runner has a flexible or rigid foot type. Next, consider whether the runner has an overall neutral, varus, or valgus alignment. A clinically challenging foot to manage is in the runner who has a forefoot varus combined with a rigid foot type. Furthermore, overstabilizing the foot can be just as detrimental to the soft tissue structures of the lower extremity as understabilizing the foot. Finally, for an individual who has significantly different foot types (e.g., left foot = supinatory foot; right foot = overpronator), the best clinical decision may be to understabilize the foot (e.g., straight-last cushion shoe) and selectively increase the stability with a customized foot orthosis.

TABLE 83.3	Classifications and Characteristics of Running Shoe Types

LIGHT CUSHION SHOE
- Indication: Supinatory foot
- Traditional cushion shoe typically more of a curve last shape
- Central or peripheral slip last construction
- Midsole materials (EVA or PU) dependent on body weight but usually lean to lighter-weight EVA
- Single-density midsole
- Very flexible through the midfoot
- Midsole cushioning units (rearfoot and forefoot)

STRAIGHT LAST CUSHION SHOE
- Indication: Neutral to supinatory foot that is unstable
- Newer transition shoe that bridges the gap between a traditional cushion and stability mostly by the geometry of the shoe
- Straight last shoe
- Midsole materials (EVA or PU) dependent on body weight but usually lean to lighter-weight EVA
- Single-density midsole
- Midsole cushioning units (rearfoot and forefoot)
- May utilize stability pillars (e.g., Brooks Dyad series) with less flexibility noted through the midfoot as compared to a traditional cushion shoe
- Firmer heel counter

STABILITY SHOE
- Indications: Neutral to mild overpronator
- Semi-curved last shape
- Combination or peripheral last construction
- Midsole materials (EVA or PU) dependent on body weight
- Firmness of medial midsole or stabilization device dependent on range of stability shoe. Lower-end stability shoes may not have a stabilization device.
- Some flexibility through the midfoot and firm heel counter

MOTION CONTROL SHOE
- Indications: Moderate to severe overpronator
- Straighter last shape
- Board or combination last construction*
- Midsole materials (EVA or PU) dependent on body weight
- Firmer medial midsole or stabilization device
- Reinforced and/or extended heel counter
- Will sometimes use higher medial side versus lateral side (wedge) for increased early motion control

COMMON LAST TYPES

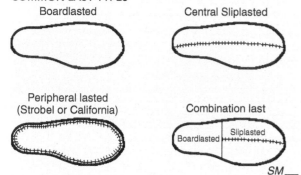

Boardlasted   Central Sliplasted

Peripheral lasted (Strobel or California)   Combination last

Boardlasted   Sliplasted

SM___

*Board last construction primarily used with older running shoes and basketball shoes. Combination last primarily used now in newer running shoes.
Source: Gazelle Sports, Grand Rapids, MI, and Agility Physical Therapy & Sports Performance, Portage, MI.

Other factors to take into consideration include
- the type of foot striker (e.g., midfoot vs. forefoot)
- distance or race training for (5K vs. marathon)
- body weight (e.g., heavier vs. lighter runner)
- selecting a training shoe vs. racing shoe
- width of foot (e.g., selecting the shoe manufacturer that traditionally has a wider toe box)
- whether or not a foot orthosis will be used in the shoe
- history of running injuries

Much emphasis has been placed on the role of shoes in shock absorption at footstrike, and shoes are of some benefit but provide little, if any, force attenuation when the forces are maximal at midsupport or during push-off. This does not mean shoes are of no importance in protecting the runner, but perhaps realizing their limitations is critical in injury management. For example, if a runner has been identified as having a late-pronation problem dynamically, in most cases, a customized foot orthosis with posting extending medially into the forefoot may be indicated. The overall goal with any shoe or shoe–orthosis combination is to provide the optimal biomechanical balance from the foot proximally to the pelvis.

Inspection of a runner's shoes that have been worn a while for excessive wear or distortion, including the midsole, heel wedge, heel counters, or midfoot, can provide useful information.

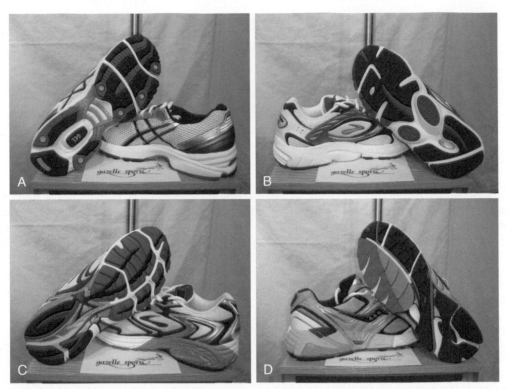

Fig. 83.3 Running shoe categories. Light cushion (*A*), straight last cushion (*B*), stability (*C*), and motion control (*D*).

PATTERNS OF WEAR FOR RUNNING SHOES

A typical wear pattern for running shoes reveals breakdown of the outer sole laterally at the heel to midfoot region, with the pattern of wear extending down the center to the toe. Noted concerns regarding wear pattern would include the following:

- Excessive wear extending through the outer sole into the midsole
- Fissures or "wrinkles" noted in the midsole when the shoe is *not* under load
- Distortion or excessive torque through the midfoot of the shoe
- Heel counter over-run medially (severe compensatory pronation) or laterally (cavus foot)

A shoe that still "looks good" may have lost many of its protective qualities, with most midsole material lasting approximately 300 to 400 miles. Shoes that have exceeded their "life expectancy" are commonly a source of injury and need to be replaced.

ORTHOTICS

The use of a foot orthosis (commonly referred to as an "orthotic") to address lower extremity overuse running injuries by controlling foot abnormalities has been recommended by various health care professionals for years. Despite the disagreement in the literature as to what type of foot orthosis is superior (e.g., rigid vs. semiflexible; full-length), successful treatment with the use of orthotics is dependent on careful evaluation of the runner and formulation of a properly fitted device. Several advantages and disadvantages of each device need to be factored into the decision-making process. The normal foot functions most efficiently when no deformities are present that predispose it to injury or exacerbation of existing injuries. However, in many cases, when a lower limb overuse

injury is present, lower extremity extrinsic or primary foot abnormalities are present. An orthosis can be used to control abnormal compensatory movements of the foot by "bringing the floor to the foot." This will allow the foot to function more efficiently in a subtalar joint neutral position and provide the necessary support so that the foot does not have to move abnormally.

When making a clinical decision regarding the type of device to use, it is important to have an understanding of how the device is to function. There are basically two types of orthoses:

- A *biomechanical orthosis* is a hard device (Fig. 83.4, *A*) or semi-flexible device (Fig. 83.4, *B*) capable of controlling movement-related pathology by attempting to guide the foot into functioning at or near subtalar joint neutral. This device consists of a shell (or module) that is either rigid or flexible with noncompressible posting (wedges) that is angled in degrees on the medial or lateral side of the foot that will address both forefoot and rearfoot deformities. The rigid-style shell is fabricated from carbon graphite, acrylic Rohadur, or (polyethylene) hard plastic. The control acquired is high, whereas shock absorption is sacrificed somewhat. The flexible shell is fabricated from thermoplastic, rubber, or leather and is the preferred device for the more active or sports-specific patient. The semi-rigid device takes advantage of various types of materials that provide both shock absorption and motion control under increased loading, while retaining their original shape. The rigid devices take the opposite approach and are designed to firmly restrain foot motion and alter its position with nonyielding materials. Both the rigid and flexible shells are molded from a neutral cast and allow control for most overuse symptoms.
- *An accommodative orthosis* is a device that does not attempt to establish foot function around the subtalar neutral position but instead allows the foot to compensate. These devices are designed for patients who are deemed to be poor candidates for biomechanical control as a result of congenital

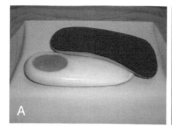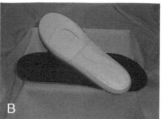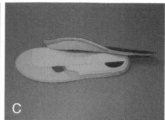

Fig. 83.4 Biomechanical orthoses. Rigid, sulcus-length device (*A*), semi-flexible, full-length device (*B*), and semi-flexible, full-length device with rearfoot to forefoot medial posting (*C*).

malformations, restricted motions in the foot or leg, neuro-muscular dysfunctions, insensitive feet, illness, or physiologic old age. The materials used to fabricate the shell will yield to foot forces rather than resist them. Compressible wedges are used to conservatively bias the foot into a more varus or valgus position depending on the desired direction.

When specifically dealing with runners, a semi-flexible, full-length device using extrinsic posting on a neutral shell (Fig. 83.4, *C*) is recommended for several clinical reasons. First, the functions of the foot during the gait cycle are adaptation, shock absorption, rigid support for leverage, and torque conversion. More specifically, at footstrike, the foot acts as a shock absorber to the impact forces and then adapts to the uneven surfaces. If the prescribed device is rigid (e.g., carbon fiber), this rigidity creates the potential for decreased shock absorption by the device attenuated through the soft tissue structures and less ability for the foot to adapt to the surface. Furthermore, at take-off, the foot has to return to a rigid lever to transmit the explosive force from the lower extremity to the running surface. If primary abnormalities of the foot are related to the forefoot (e.g., forefoot varus), consideration needs to be given to correcting this alignment issue with a full-length device to assist in the transition back to a rigid foot from a supple foot. Finally, most researchers will concur that the use of orthotic therapy is both a "science and an art." There are advantages to using extrinsically posted, neutral module devices (versus intrinsically designed modules) such as ease of modifications or adjustments. With extrinsically posted devices, different types and density of materials can be selected for support and posting. For example, felt, cork, and EVA are common supportive or posting materials used for this type of orthosis. There is also variability in the stiffness (durometer) rating of such materials as EVA depending on the desired function of the material or the weight of the patient.

Regardless of the clinician's philosophy regarding orthotic therapy or the type of orthosis that is used, the goal is to create biomechanical balance at the foot that will subsequently influence the proximal kinetic chain the patient will wear. A device that is uncomfortable or painful is undesirable and will be detrimental to the overall rehabilitation process.

Foot orthotics should be considered for any lower extremity overuse syndrome related to runners, not just the obvious diagnoses of plantar fasciitis or medial tibial stress syndrome. Often a trial with a less expensive over-the-counter (OTC) insert to see whether there is a benefit may be a reasonable approach before prescribing a more expensive custom orthosis. A semi-custom foot orthotic can be fabricated by attaching different density materials to the underside of the OTC device. This may be a cost-effective solution, especially for younger,

still-growing runners, to achieve the desired outcome. When prescribing a custom foot orthotic, it is mandatory to understand and fulfill the fabricator's requests for measurements and cast molds. Selecting an orthotics laboratory that has the same philosophical approach to managing foot biomechanics is critical. A poorly fabricated orthotic is a waste of the patient's time and money.

MEDICATIONS

Medications such as aspirin, acetaminophen, and nonsteroidal anti-inflammatory drugs (NSAIDs) are useful in reducing minor pain and inflammation, but they do not substitute for ceasing the abusive activity or taking steps to correct the offending condition. The use of narcotics or the injection of analgesics to continue running cannot be condoned. Excessive or prolonged use of NSAIDs can have significant side effects, even at the recommended reduced dose when purchased over the counter.

The literature cautions against indiscriminate use of oral or injectable steroids. One condition in which steroid injection may have reasonable success is acute iliotibial band friction syndrome with injection deep to the iliotibial band over the prominence of the lateral femoral condyle. Injection directly into tendons should be avoided and should be administered with caution into the peritendinous tissues.

Cortisone should NEVER be injected in or around the Achilles tendon or posterior tibial tendon. This will result in weakening and probable rupture of the tendon.

SURGERY

An earnest, conservative rehabilitation program is generally effective for most running-related conditions. Surgery should be considered only after failure of a conservative program. However, this does not mean an unnecessary delay for well-indicated surgery, but many serious runners can be impetuous in electing surgery as an anticipated "quick fix." The indications for surgery are the same as for any athletically active person. If surgery is elected, all the options should be explained in detail and, with some conditions, the patient should be cautioned that in spite of well-planned and executed surgery, there may not be good odds for return to running.

PHYSICAL THERAPY AND REHABILITATION

The treatment of runners must be a coordinated effort on the part of the physician, physical therapist, athletic trainer, coach, parent, and runner. The goal of a rehabilitation program for

TABLE 83.4	Running Injuries and Treatment Strategy		
Syndrome	**Contributing Factors**	**Movement Error**	**Treatment Strategy**
Anterior knee pain	Laterally tilted patella Weak quadriceps Tight lateral structures Excessive hip internal rotation Rearfoot pronation Weak core/hip muscles	Increased hip adduction and IR Dynamic knee valgus Inactive foot/ankle in propulsion	Quadriceps strengthening Hip/core strengthening Running re-training Patellar taping
Iliotibial band syndrome	Adducted gait Ilium anteriorly rotated Weak hip abductors and ER Functional leg-length discrepancy Genu varum Limited great toe extension	Excessive femoral rotation Overstriding	Strengthen hip ER Soft tissue massage Superior tibiofibular joint mobilization Cross-train
Exercise-related leg pain	More common in females Higher BMI Leg-length discrepancy Training error	Increased tibial shock Overstriding Increased heel strike	Retraining for softer landing STJ mobilization/manipulation Calf stretching Hip strengthening Taping Orthotics
Achilles tendinopathy	Facilitated segment L5/S1 Heel height change in shoes Training/surface errors (hills) Joint mechanics: anterior talus, plantarflexed cuboid	Overstriding-forefoot strike Excessive vertical displacement Abnormal pronation Propulsive whip Poor ankle rocker	Heel lift Slow return to running Core stability Dural stretches Taping Orthotics Strengthen: ant tib, soleus, eccentric heel raises, FHL
Plantar fasciitis	Hallux limitus Forefoot varus Subtalar varus Abnormal pronation Tight calf Improper shoe wear Tight hamstrings	Strike control Soft strike Active heel rise retraining Excessive hip IR Medial position of knee	Arch taping Orthotics Night splint STJ mobilization/manipulation Calf stretching FHL strengthening
Proximal hamstring strain	Neuromuscular timing (gluteal mm. vs. hamstrings) Neural restriction Proximal adhesions Eccentric overload Pelvic malalignment SI hypo/hypermobility L5 radiculopathy	Overstriding Unilateral strike variance	Eccentric hamstring loading Slump stretching Gluteal strengthening Core stability Hip ROM Soft tissue massage Kinesio tape

IR, internal rotation; ER, external rotation; STJ, subtalar joint; FHL, flexor hallucis longus; BMI, body mass index; SI, sacroiliac

runners after injury or surgery is restoration of flexibility, ROM, muscle strength, balance, motor control, and endurance of the entire lower extremity with return to uninterrupted running.

As a general rule, closed chain exercise including concentric and eccentric muscle activity is preferable for runners. Although a good starting point in some cases, isolated, concentric, open chain exercises may induce strength changes in ROM not present during running and create the potential for muscle imbalance. Specific rehabilitation regimens for a given condition are covered in several different sections in this book specific to the condition. Overall, the goal is to develop a functionally based exercise program that will correct any imbalances in the neuromusculoskeletal system. See Table 83.4 for an overview of running injuries and corresponding treatment strategies.

Stretching for flexibility (Figs. 83.5 and 83.6) should be an integral part not only of a rehabilitation program but also of the daily training program (see each section). Although important for all runners regardless of age, stretching becomes even more significant with aging as tendons become less extensible and joints tend to lose flexibility. Furthermore, isolated tightness can cause muscle inhibition, as described by Janda (1983).

One example is the concept of lower cross syndrome, which is the reciprocal inhibition of the gluteus maximus resulting from iliopsoas tightness. This is a common presentation with runners who have recalcitrant hamstring strains or chronic low back pain. If the iliopsoas tightness is not corrected, the likelihood of retraining the proper gluteus maximus firing pattern is reduced.

The vague complaint of the extremity "not feeling right" may be a result of muscle imbalance secondary to either weakness or contracture. It is imperative to evaluate both the flexibility and endurance strength to determine potential risk factors. For example, regardless of the cause, runners presenting with hamstring and gastrocnemius–soleus muscle contractures or weakness resulting in recurrent or chronic muscle/tendon strains can develop alterations in stride, predisposing tissues to excessive stress.

A functional rehabilitation program should be designed to simulate, as closely as possible, the normal muscle and joint function of running. Often, so much emphasis is placed on the injured area that the rest of the body is ignored. It is critical to think above and below the affected area (e.g., diagnosis of iliotibial band friction syndrome, evaluation of the foot and hip). Total body fitness and cross-training techniques, such as

RUNNER'S FLEXIBILITY PROGRAM

If indicated, each stretch is to be done _____ times per day, _____ repetitions of each exercise. *Hold all stretches for 30 seconds.*

1. BACK STRETCH

Lie on your back with both knees bent. Pull one or both knees up to your chest and hold.

2. HIP ABDUCTOR STRETCH

Stand with your feet together. Move your hips sideways, while your torso moves in the opposite direction. You will feel a stretch on the outside of your hip. Place your hands on your hips or grasp a stationary object for support.

3. ILIOTIBIAL BAND STRETCH

Cross one leg over in front of the other leg. Bend the knee of the back leg slightly. Move your hips sideways toward the side with the bent knee. You will feel a stretch on the outside of the bent knee.

4. HAMSTRING STRETCH

Sit on the floor with your legs straight in front of you. Reach for your toes until you feel a stretch in the back of your thighs. Tip at your hips and keep your back neutral.

5. QUAD STRETCH

Stand facing a stationary object for support. Bend one knee as far as possible, reach back, and grasp the foot. Pull the heel toward your buttocks until you feel a stretch in the front of the thigh. *Do not arch back or twist your knee.*

6. HEEL CORD STRETCH

Stand facing a stationary object with your feet apart (one in front of the other) and your toes turned in slightly. Slightly roll your back foot to the outside, place your hands on the object, and lean forward until you feel a stretch in the calf of your leg. *Do not bend your knees or allow your heels to come off the floor.*

7. SOLEUS STRETCH

Assume the same position as in number 6. Place one foot in front of the other foot and bend both knees. Lean forward, keeping the heel of the front foot on the ground. You should feel a stretch in the lower calf of the front leg.

Fig. 83.5   Runner's flexibility program.

running in water with an AquaJogger® (Excel Sports Science, Inc., Springfield, OR), can be beneficial in maintaining overall cardiovascular and muscular endurance while tissue healing takes place.

Once the runner is ready to return to running after missing training, the following guidelines may be helpful. If left to their own judgment, most will return too quickly, resulting in either delayed recovery or re-injury.

RETURN-TO-RUNNING ALGORITHM 2 (MILLER'S RECOMMENDATIONS)

The following return-to-running programs should be considered a "guide" for return to running after a significant absence from training of 4 weeks or more as a result of injury or surgery. The four different return-to-running programs are designed to meet the needs of the individual runner and the type of injury involved.

- Return to running after missed training (0 to 4 weeks)
- Return to running after missed training (4 weeks or more/nonsurgical) (Rehabilitation Protocol 83.1)
- Return to running after missed training (6 weeks or more/postsurgical) (Rehabilitation Protocol 83.2)
- Return to running after missed training (poststress fracture) (Rehabilitation Protocol 83.3)

The purpose of any return-to-running program is to condition the musculoskeletal system; it is not intended to be a significant aerobic conditioning program, which can be accomplished with low or no-impact cross-training. Generally, the running pace should be no faster than 7 minutes per mile and the walking should be done briskly. The program is based on time, not distance. Rest days should be scheduled every 7 to 10 days or as indicated. The schedule can be varied to meet individual situations. If need be, the runner may hold at a given level longer, drop back a level, or, in some instances, skip a level if progressing well. Generally, if the runner's "original symptoms" return during a workout, then the runner should be instructed to return to the previous "successful" workout before trying to advance any further. Discomfort may be experienced, but it should be transient and not accumulate or create any gait deviations (e.g., limping).

ILIOTIBIAL BAND STRETCHING PROGRAM

If indicated, each stretch is to be done _____ times per day, _____ repetitions of each exercise. *Hold all stretches for 30 seconds.*

1. HIP ABDUCTOR STRETCH
Stand with legs straight, feet together. Bend at waist toward side opposite leg to be stretched. Unaffected knee may be bent.

2. ILIOTIBIAL BAND STRETCH
Stand with knees straight; cross leg to be stretched behind other as far as possible. Stretch to side of leg in front.

3. ILIOTIBIAL BAND STRETCH
Same stance as exercise number 2. Slightly bend back knee. Move trunk toward unaffected side and hips toward affected side. Stretch will be felt along outside of bent knee.

4. ILIOTIBIAL BAND/HAMSTRING STRETCH
Stand with knees straight. Cross legs so that affected knee rests against back of unaffected leg. Turn trunk away from affected side as far as possible, reaching and attempting to touch heel of affected leg.

5. ILIOTIBIAL BAND STRETCH
Lie on unaffected side with your back a few inches from table edge. Bend unaffected hip to maintain balance. Straighten affected knee and place leg over edge of table so leg hangs straight. Let gravity pull leg down, causing the stretch.

6. ILIOTIBIAL BAND STRETCH
Lie on affected side with knee locked and leg in a straight line with trunk; bend upper knee with your hands placed directly under shoulders to bear the weight of the trunk. Push up, extending your arms as far as possible. Affected leg must be kept straight to get maximum stretch in hip.

Fig. 83.6 Iliotibial band (ITB) stretching program. (Modified from Lutter LD. Form used in Physical Therapy Department at St. Anthony Orthopaedic Clinic and University of Minnesota, St. Paul, MN.)

SUMMARY

It is important to incorporate general strength training, specific prescribed rehabilitation exercises (e.g., neuromuscular re-education), and/or stretching program with the return-to-running program. A comprehensive evaluation of the individual plays a vital role in the appropriate management and successful outcomes. This requires looking proximal and distal to the affected area or joint. Performing some type of videotaped gait analysis (Table 83.5) is critical in being able to accurately determine running form aberrances (e.g., heavy slapping asymmetric heel strike) and prescribe the necessary footwear changes or the need for a customized foot orthotic. Finally, a functional exercise program and appropriate return-to-running progression will provide the individual with the greatest opportunity for a successful return and to accomplish their personal goals.

REHABILITATION PROTOCOL 83.1 ■ **Runner's Guide for Return to Running After Absence From Training of 4 Weeks or More (Nonsurgical)**

Week Schedule

1. Walk 30 min, alternating 1 min normal and 1 min fast.
2. Walk 30 min, alternating 1.5 min normal and 1.5 min fast. If doing well, jog easily instead of walking fast.
3. Alternate walking 1 min and jogging 2 min × 7. The next day, run easy 5 min and walk 1 min × 3.
4. Alternate walking 1 min and jogging 3 min × 7. The next day, run 5 min and walk 1 min × 4.
5. Run continuously 20 min. The next day, run 5 min and walk 1 min × 5.
6. Run continuously 20 min. The next day, run 10 min and walk 1 min × 3.
7. Run continuously 20 min 1 day and 35 min the next.
8. Run continuously 20 min 1 day and 40 min the next.
9. If doing well, resume a training schedule, increasing the duration, intensity, and frequency appropriately. The key is to avoid re-injury.

REHABILITATION PROTOCOL 83.2 ● Return-to-Running Program: Postsurgical

Purpose: This program is intended for those individuals who have been off running for an extended period because of an injury or surgery. Please discuss with your therapist specific modifications to this program depending on the circumstances leading up to your return to running.

Guidelines: The following guidelines need to be followed to ensure an optimal outcome of the progressive running program.

1. For the first 4 weeks, run every other day for the time allotted. If allowed, it is okay to cross-train with other forms of cardio activities (e.g., elliptical trainer, stationary bike) after your run or on specified "off" days.
2. Complete warmup and cool-down exercises as prescribed.
3. Run up to, but not into, the "pain zone."
4. Use ice as needed (10 minutes) to decrease postexercise tissue irritation.
5. Do not progress to next allotted time if symptoms occur while running or if limping.
6. Do not forget to do prescribed strength training exercises on "off" days.

Warmup: A 5- to 10-minute period of light cardiovascular activity (e.g., bike, walking, elliptical trainer) is needed to sufficiently warm up the tissues for running or stretching. Your physical therapist will provide you with a list of appropriate stretches. They should be done in a controlled, low-load, prolonged manner that does NOT cause pain. For static stretching, hold the position for 30 seconds and repeat three times. For dynamic stretching, follow the instructions provided by your physical therapist.

Cool-down: Complete your stretching/strengthening program as recommended by your physical therapist or continue with additional cross-training activities. Ice as needed following runs for mild pain/soreness (10 minutes).

ACTUAL DAY

Week #1	5 minutes	OFF/CT	5 minutes	OFF/CT	7.5 minutes	OFF/CT	7.5 minutes
Week #2	OFF/CT	10 minutes	OFF/CT	10 minutes	OFF/CT	12.5 minutes	OFF/CT
Week #3	12.5 minutes	OFF/CT	15 minutes	OFF/CT	15 minutes	OFF/CT	17.5 minutes
Week #4	OFF/CT	17.5 minutes	OFF/CT	20 minutes	OFF/CT	20 minutes	OFF/CT
Week #5	10 minutes	20 minutes	OFF/CT	10 minutes	20 minutes	OFF/CT	15 minutes
Week #6	20 minutes	OFF/CT	15 minutes	25 minutes	OFF/CT	15 minutes	25 minutes
Week #7	OFF/CT	15 minutes	25 minutes	OFF/CT	20 minutes	25 minutes	OFF/CT
Week #8	20 minutes	25 minutes	OFF/CT	20 minutes	30 minutes	OFF/CT	*

CT, cross-training.
*After reaching 30 minutes of continuous running, begin to estimate the mileage completed in that time and progress distance by a total of 10% to 15% per week.
Example: 30 minutes @ 7:30 min/mile pace = 4.0 miles
4.0 miles × 10% = 0.4 miles
4.0 miles × 15% = 0.6 miles
Therefore, increase each training run by 0.4 to 0.6 miles.

Used with permission from Scott Miller, PT, MS, SCS, CSCS, from Agility Physical Therapy & Sports Performance, LLC. Portage, MI.

REHABILITATION PROTOCOL 83.3 ● Return-to-Running Program: Poststress Fracture

Purpose: This program is intended for those individuals who have been off running for an extended period because of an injury or surgery. Please discuss with your therapist specific modifications to this program depending on the circumstances leading up to your return to running.

Guidelines: The following guidelines need to be followed to ensure an optimal outcome of the progressive running program.

1. For the first 4 weeks, run every other day for the time allotted. If allowed, it is okay to cross-train with other forms of cardio activities (e.g., elliptical trainer, stationary bike) after your run or on specified "off" days.
2. Complete warmup and cool-down exercises as prescribed.
3. Run up to, but not into, the "pain zone."

4. Use ice as needed (10 minutes) to decrease postexercise tissue irritation.
5. Do not progress to next allotted time if symptoms occur while running or if limping.
6. Do not forget to do prescribed strength training exercises on "off" days.

Cool-down: Complete the stretching/strengthening program as recommended by the physical therapist or continue with additional cross-training activities. Ice as needed following runs for mild pain/soreness (10 minutes).

Seven-Week Schedule for Returning From Injury

Week	Monday	Tuesday	Wednesday	Thursday	Friday	Saturday	Sunday
1	Walk 10 min, Run 5 min, Walk 5 min, Run 5 min	Run in water or other training	Run in water or other training	Walk 5 min, Run 5 min, Walk 5 min, Run 5 min, Walk 5 min, Run 5 min	Run in water or other training	Run in water or other training	Walk 3 min, Run 7 min, Walk 3 min, Run 7 min, Walk 3 min, Run 7 min
2	Run in water or other training	Walk 2 min, Run 8 min, Walk 2 min, Run 8 min, Walk 2 min, Run 8 min	Run in water or other training	Run 10 min, Walk 2 min, Run 10 min, Walk 2 min, Run 10 min	Run in water or other training	Run 12 min, Walk 2 min, Run 12 min, Walk 2 min, Run 10 min	Run in water or other training
3	Run 15 min, Walk 2 min, Run 15 min	Run in water or other training	Run 20 min, Walk 2 min, Run 10 min	Run in water or other training	Run 25 min	Run in water or other training	Run 30 min
4	Run in water or other training	Run 25 min	Run 30 min	Run in water or other training	Run 25 min	Run 35 min	Run in water or other training
5	Run 30 min	Run 35 min	Run in water or other training	Run 30 min plus 6 × 100-m strideouts	Run 30 min	Run 40 min	Run in water or other raining
6	Tempo run (15-min warmup, 15 min @ 15-km race pace)	Run 30 min	Run 45 min	Run in water or other training	Run 40 min plus 6 × 100-m strideouts	Run 30 min	Run 50 min
7	Run in water or other training	Run 35 min	Tempo run (15 min warmup, 20 min @ 15-km race pace)	Run 35 min	Run in water or other training	Run 40 min plus 6 × 100-m strideouts	Run 55 min

Used with permission from Scott Miller, PT, MS, SCS, CSCS, from Agility Physical Therapy & Sports Performance, LLC, Portage, MI.

TABLE 83.5	Video Running Analysis Form (Gait Laboratory)

SAGITTAL
- Trunk lean
- Elbow bend (80–100 deg)
- Hands (relaxed)
- **Pelvis (anterior/posterior tilt)**
- Hip extension (20–30 deg)
- Hip flexion (30 deg)
- **Stride (length, symmetry)**
- Metatarsophalangeal extension (70 deg)
- Presence/absence of normal lumbar lordosis flat back

ANTERIOR
- Head position (tilt, rotated)
- Shoulders/arm (high, low, level)
- Arm swing (cross midline)
- Femoral rotation (internal, external)
- Knee alignment (varus, valgus)
- Tibial rotation
- **Foot strike (heel, mid, forefoot)**
- Foot abduction

POSTERIOR
- Head motion
- **Horizontal sway/tilt of trunk**
- Excessive lateral pelvic tilt
- Thoracic spine (excessive rotation)
- Lumbar spine (flex, extend, rotated, side bent)
- **Pelvis (level, tilt)**
- Subtalar joint position
- Slapping

REFERENCES

A complete reference list is available at https://expertconsult .inkling.com/.

FURTHER READING

American Physical Rehabilitation Network. 2000. When the feet hit the ground . . . everything changes. Program outline and prepared notes—a basic manual Sylvania, OH.

American Physical Rehabilitation Network. 1994. When the feet hit the ground . . . take the next step. Program outline and prepared notes—an advanced manual Sylvania, OH.

Bates BT, Osternig L, Mason B. Foot orthotic devices to modify selected aspects of lower extremity mechanics. *Am J Sports Med.* 1979;7:338.

Burke ER. *Precision Heart Rate Training.* 1st ed. Champaign, IL: Human Kinetics; 1998.

Cavanaugh PR. *An evaluation of the effects of orthotics force distribution and rearfoot movement during running;* 1978. Paper presented at meeting of American Orthopedic Society for Sports Medicine Lake Placid.

Collona P. Fabrication of a custom molded orthotic using an intrinsic posting technique for a forefoot varus deformity. *Phys Ther Forum.* 1989;8:3.

Cosca DD, Navazio F. Common problems in endurance athletes. *Am Fam Physician.* 2007;76:237–244.

Fadale PD, Wiggins ME. Corticosteroid injections: their use and abuse. *J Am Acad Orthop Surg.* 1994;2:133–140.

Fredericson M, Mirsa AK. Epidemiology and aetiology of marathon running injuries. *Sports Med.* 2007;37:437–439.

Fredericson M. Common injuries in runners. Diagnosis, rehabilitation and prevention. *Sports Med.* 1996;21:49–72.

Gill E. Orthotics. *Runner's World.* 1985:55–57. Feb.

Gross ML, Napoli RC. Treatment of lower extremity injuries with orthotic shoe inserts. An overview. *Sports Med.* 1993;15:66.

Gross ML, Davlin LB, Evanski PM. Effectiveness of orthotic shoe inserts in the long-distance runner. *Am J Sports Med.* 1991;19:409.

Hart LE. Exercise and soft tissue injury. *Baillieres Clin Rheumatol.* 1994;8:137–148.

Hreljac A. Impact and overuse injuries in runners. *Med Sci Sports Exerc.* 2004;36:845–849.

Hunter S, Dolan M, Davis M. *Foot Orthotics in Therapy and Sports.* Champaign, IL: Human Kinetics; 1996.

Itay S. Clinical and functional status following lateral ankle sprains: Follow-up of 90 young adults treated conservatively. *Orthop Rev.* 1982;11:73.

James SL. Running injuries of the knee. *Instr Course Lect.* 1998;47:82.

James SL, Bates BT, Osternig LR. Injuries to runners. *Am J Sports Med.* 1978;6:40–50.

Jull G, Janda V. Muscles and motor control in low back pain: assessment and management. In: Twomey L, Taylor JR, eds. *Physical Therapy of the Low Back.* New York: Churchill Livingstone; 1987.

Knobloch K, Yoon U, Vogt PM. Acute and overuse injuries correlated to hours of training in master running athletes. *Foot Ankle Int.* 2008;29:671–676.

Leadbetter WB. Cell-matrix response in tendon injury. *Clin Sports Med.* 1992;11:533–578.

Lysholm J, Wiklander J. Injuries in runners. *Am J Sports Med.* 1987;15:168–171.

MacLean CL, Davis IS, Hamill J. Short- and long-term influences of a custom foot orthotic intervention on lower extremity dynamics. *Clin J Sport Med.* 2008;18:338.

McNicol K, Taunton JE, Clement DB. Iliotibial tract friction syndrome in athletes. *Can J Appl Sport Sci.* 1981;6:76.

Messier SP, Pittala KA. Etiological factors associated with selected running injuries. *Med Sci Sports Exerc.* 1988;20:501–505.

Michaud TC, Nawoczenski DA. The influence of two different types of foot orthoses on first metatarsophalangeal joint kinematics during gait in a single subject. *J Manipulative Physiol Ther.* 2006;29:60.

Nigg BM, Nurse MA, Stefanyshyn DJ. Shoe inserts and orthotics for sport and physical activities. *Med Sci Sports Exerc Suppl.* 1999;31:S421–S428.

Novachek TF. Running injuries: a biomechanical approach. *Instr Course Lect.* 1998;47:397–406.

Novachek TF, Trost JP. Running: injury mechanisms and training strategies. Instructional videotape. St. O'Tolle ML: Prevention and treatment of injuries to runners. *Med Sci Sports Exercise.* 1992;(Suppl 9):S360–S363.

Paul M. *Gillette Children's Specialty Healthcare Foundation;* 1997.

Rogers MM, LeVeau BF. Effectiveness of foot orthotic devices used to modify pronation in runners. *J Orthop Sports Phys Ther.* 1982;4:86.

Rolf C. Overuse injuries of the lower extremity in runners. *Scand J Med Sci Sports.* 1995;5:181–190.

Satterthwaite P, Norton R, Larmer P, et al. Risk factors for injuries and other health problems sustained in a marathon. *Br J Sports Med.* 1999;33:22–26.

Saxena A, Haddad J. The effect of foot orthoses on patellofemoral pain syndrome. *J Am Podiatr Med Assoc.* 2003;93:264.

Subotnick SI. The flat foot. *Phys Sports Med.* 1981;9:85.

Subotnick SI, Newell SG. *Podiatric Sports Medicine.* Kisko, NY: Futura: Mt; 1975.

Taunton JE, Ryan MB, Clement DB, et al. A retrospective case-control analysis of 2002 running injuries. *Br J Sports Med.* 2002;36:95–101.

vanMechelen W. Running injuries. A review of the epidemiological literature. *Sports Med.* 1992;14:320–335.

Wen DY. Risk factors for overuse injuries in runners. *Curr Sports Med Rep.* 2007;6:307–313.

Williams JGP. The foot and chondromalacia—a case of biomechanical uncertainty. *J Orthop Sports Phys Ther.* 1980;2:50.

84

Tendinopathy

Robert C. Manske, PT, DPT, MEd, SCS, ATC, CSCS

The treatment of overuse tendon pathology has undergone a tremendous change in the past several years. Overuse injuries account for up to 50% of all sports maladies (Herring and Nilson 1987, Khan and Cook 2003). Traditionally, treatments have focused on anti-inflammatory strategies, which are often to no avail. No longer is it accepted that most tendon problems occur as an inflammatory overuse process. Increased knowledge about the histologic responses, histopathologic analysis, and differences in tendon pathologies requires further clarification of language used when discussing tendon injuries. The latest conventional wisdom is that the process of tendinopathy is any pathology involving tendons, which can be broken down into several different classifications. Because of this there has been a shift to changing the general descriptor to use the term *"tendinopathy"* to include the condition of tendon pain and pathologic changes. See Box 84.1 for a list of features that distinguish tendinosis tissue from normal healthy tendon. A tendinopathy therefore can include tendon injuries such as paratenonitis, tendonitis, and tendinosis.

Tendons are covered by a loose areolar connective tissue known as paratenon. This specialized tissue is like an elastic sleeve around the tendon that allows the tendon to slide and move easier against adjacent tissues. The term "paratenonitis" describes an inflammation of only the paratenon, regardless of whether the paratenon is lined by synovium. This tendon injury is caused by repetitive loading and overuse due to the space-limiting factor involved with a swollen inflamed tendon sheath. A paratenonitis can include separate pathologies including that of peritendinitis, tenosynovitis, and tenovaginitis. Signs of symptoms of paratenonitis include pain, swelling, warmth, and crepitus that is caused by the tendon adhering to the surrounding structures. The term "tendonitis" was historically used in an indiscriminate manner to describe literally all tendon pathology. The suffix "-itis" is used to denote inflammation. A tendonitis is an injury to the tendon involving partial or complete tearing vascular disruption, acute inflammatory, and repair response. A true tendonitis is caused by a recent increase in activity level in which overuse or excessive tendon strain occurs. It may progress to degeneration if chronic. Numerous histopathologic studies have determined that in the case of chronic tendon injuries, the process undergone in many cases is degenerative in nature rather than inflammatory, showing minimal to no inflammation present in tissues (Alfredson and Lorentzon 2003, Almekinders and Temple 1998, Astrom and Rausiing 1995, Cook and Purdam 2009, Fredberg 2004, Gabel 1999, Hashimoto et al. 2003, Khan and Maffulli 1998, Maffulli et al. 2003b, Movin et al. 1997). Therefore, a tendinosis is a tendon that has undergone intratendinous degeneration that is noninflammatory in nature. Tendons that undergo degenerative processes and are of particular concern to the surgeon and physical therapist include the Achilles (Maffulli et al. 2003a), patellar (Crossley et al. 2007, Cook

et al. 2001), high hamstring (Fredericson et al. 2005), gluteus medius (Lequesne et al. 2008), rotator cuff (Lewis 2009), and common wrist extensor/flexor tendons (Bissest et al. 2005).

Recently a newly developed three-stage continuum model of tendinopathy has been proposed (Cook and Vicenzino 2009, McCreesh 2013, Joseph 2015). Three overlapping stages are described in this disease progression: reactive tendinopathy, tendon disrepair, and degenerative tendinopathy. Reactive tendinopathy occurs in response to an acute overload and may be described as a noninflammatory proliferative response to acute injury. Tendon disrepair is the second stage and includes a failure of healing response. Neovascularity and neuronal ingrowth represent the unsuccessful reparative process. Degenerative tendinopathy, the third stage, is thought to be irreversible and includes hypocellularity, pooling of proteoglycan, and disorganized collagen tissue.

Any form of tendon pain can cause lasting disability for any patient, but this can be especially frustrating for active individuals and athletes. These problem tendons can be treated both medically and with rehabilitation. Medical treatments include oral and topical medications and medications via injections and shock-wave therapy. Oral medications can be a first line of defense against tendinopathies but are not typically effective for chronic tendinopathy lasting more than 6 to 12 months.

MEDICAL METHODS OF TREATMENT
Anti-Inflammatory Agents

Although NSAIDs are a common treatment method for acute tendinopathy (Salminen and Kihlström 1987, Abramson 1990, Green et al. 2002), little evidence exists supporting this as a treatment with any strength in chronic cases, especially those lasting more than 6 to 12 months (Green et al. 2002, McLauchlan and Handoll 2001). Almekinders and Temple (1998) performed a thorough review of the literature and found only nine true randomized, placebo-controlled trials utilizing NSAIDs as a treatment form. In several of these studies there appeared to be an analgesic effect of NSAIDs. There is some concern that use of NSAIDs could weaken tendon tensile strength (Magra and Maffulli 2008). Animal models have demonstrated impaired healing related to NSAID administration (Dimmen et al. 2009, Chechik et al. 2014, Connizzo 2014, Zhang et al. 2014). Decreased tendon strength and a blunting of discomfort may give the athlete a false sense of security that could lead to disastrous results if the tendon ruptures as a result of supraphysiologic loads placed on it during functional activities.

Corticosteroids

Corticosteroid injections into or around tendons are fraught with hazard. Tendon rupture is always a concern following direct corticosteroid injections into the tendon, especially if repeated (Andres and Murrell 2009, Clark et al. 1995, Lambert et al. 1995, Jones 1985, Kleinman and Gross 1983, Ford and DeBender 1979). However, if inflammation lies in the paratenon, injection into the sheath may be useful (Richie and Briner 2003, Alvarez-Nemegyei and Canoso 2004). Skjong and colleagues (2012) have suggested that an inflammatory response in tissues surrounding the degenerative tendon may also be responsible for some of the pain associated with this condition and injections in these tissues may explain an analgesic response. Injections for epicondylitis have been shown to provide some short-term relief (Stahl and Kaufman 1997, Hay et al. 1999, Schmidt et al. 2002, Assendelft et al. 1996, Canton and Marks 2003). Evidence appears to be a toss-up with regard to treatment of shoulder impingement and rotator cuff disease as some authors approve (Akgun et al. 2004, Blair et al. 1996), whereas others report no differences when compared to a control treatment (Alvarez et al. 2005, Koester 2007).

It may be safe to treat an injected tendon early on as if it were a partial tendon tear. Curwin (2007) suggested that tensile forces should be reduced for 10 to 14 days following tendon injection and treatment should progress as if it were an acute condition (i.e., rest, ice, and modalities) followed by progressive incremental loads to the tissue starting at about 2 weeks.

Topical Glyceryl Trinitrate Patches

In several level I randomized controlled clinical trials, topical glyceryl trinitrate patches were compared to control patches for Achilles, wrist extensor, and supraspinatus tendinopathies (Paoloni et al. 2003, 2004, 2005). In each of these studies the patients received patches that released 1.25 mg of glyceryl trinitrate every 24 hours. Patients in the control group received a sham patch. Both patch applicators and patients were blinded to which patches were medicated and which were not. **All of the studies demonstrated a significant amount of pain relief and improved function for those with the medicated patches.** In each of these studies patches were not used exclusively because patients performed other treatments that included stretching and eccentric strengthening, which could have played a role in the demonstrated changes.

Extracorporeal Shock Wave Therapy

Extracorporeal shock wave therapy (ESWT) is a recently developed treatment for tendinopathy. A series of low-energy shock waves are applied directly to the area of painful tendon. Although the evidence for how ESWT works is still debatable, some believe that it may cause nerve degeneration, whereas others think it causes tenocytes to release growth factors in response to the pulsing shock waves. The ideal use of ESWT is

still emerging. Trials using ESWT for tendinopathies are widely varied in regards to duration, intensity, frequency of treatments, and timing of treatment in regard to chronicity. The most favorable outcomes for use of ESWT have been seen in randomized controlled trials of its use in patients with calcific tendinitis of the rotator cuff (Harniman et al. 2004, Cosentino et al. 2003, Loew et al. 1999, Wang 2003).

Modalities

Physical therapy modalities such as low-intensity laser and methods of therapeutic ultrasound have been advocated. At this point there are no high-quality studies that demonstrate low-level laser (Basford 1995) or ultrasound (Robertson and Baker 2001, Speed 2001, van der Windt et al. 1999, Warden et al. 2008) as useful tools in treating chronic tendon conditions. Phonophoresis, which is a form of ultrasound in which a topical medication is driven into the superficial layers of the skin, has been recommended for lateral epicondylitis and calcific tendinitis of the shoulder by some (Trudel et al. 2004, Gimblett et al. 1999) but not by others (Klaiman et al. 1998, Penderghest et al. 1998). Because of the huge variation of parameters that can be modified when using modalities such as these, it is hard to determine if they are beneficial. The evidence is not strong at this point. That by no means indicates that these modalities are not beneficial—it simply suggests that studies have not yet determined which methods and parameters are best. There is a huge need for high-level, randomized, controlled studies using therapeutic modalities for treatments of these chronic conditions.

Sclerotherapy

Sclerotherapy uses an injectable chemical into blood vessels near the tendinopathy. During the process of tendinosis, a condition called neovascularization occurs. This appears to be the body's response to try to facilitate small blood vessel proliferation at the site of pathology. Small nerves also travel in close proximity to these newly formed vessels, thus being a potential cause of tendinosis pain. Injecting chemicals into these vessels not only may sclerose the vessels but also sclerose the pain-generating nerve fibers that are in the local proximity. Some limited evidence suggests that sclerotherapy may be beneficial in those with patellar or Achilles tendinopathies (Hoksrud et al. 2006, Ohberg and Alfredson 2002), tennis elbow (Zeisig and Ohberg 2006), and shoulder impingement (Alfredson et al. 2006).

PHYSICAL THERAPY

Because rest can be described as a catabolic process for tendons (Cook and Vicenzino 2009), physical therapy and therapeutic exercise can be beneficial for patients suffering from tendon pain. Cryotherapy seems to be a treatment of choice for acute cases. Cryotherapy decreases capillary blood flow, preserves deep tendon oxygenation saturation, and facilitates venous capillary outflow (Rees et al. 2009). This more than likely provides some form of beneficial analgesia.

Eccentric exercise has been discussed as a treatment method for tendinopathy for more than 25 years. Exercise dosage using eccentric protocols varies greatly. Exact intensity, speed, load, and frequency are still being determined and may depend on the acuteness of the condition and the location. Dosage required for the patellar tendon may be different for that of the lateral epicondyle, which may even be different from that of the Achilles tendon. Regardless of anatomic location, eccentric tendon loading and exercise volume should progress as dictated by the amount of pain generated during the exercise. Curwin (2007) describes the training load being based on the number of repetitions performed and amount of pain perceived. In this program the athlete performs both concentric and eccentric components of the exercise. The eccentric portion is done at a slightly faster rate than the eccentric portion. An attempt should be made to elicit pain and discomfort between 20 and 30 reps. If there is no discomfort after 30 repetitions, the stimulus is too low and should be increased. Three sets of 10 repetitions are the optimal number presently thought to be conducive to tendon repair. Lorenz (2010) described progressing the patient to sets of 8 repetitions once he or she has been able to safely achieve four sets of 15 repetitions without symptoms. Additionally, three to four sessions per week may be advocated versus the daily routine advised by others.

It has not been until the last 15 years that significant evidence has proved this to be true. The exact role of eccentric exercise is not yet completely clear. There is proof that following eccentric exercise tendon structure is improved and neovascularization is decreased (Kongsgaard et al. 2005, Ohberg and Alfredson 2004). Multiple studies have demonstrated a positive effect with the use of eccentric exercise on the Achilles tendon (Stanish et al. 1986, Cook et al. 2000, Niesen-Vertommen et al. 1992, Mafi et al. 2001, Alfredson et al. 1998, Silbernagel et al. 2001, Roos et al. 2004, Shalabi et al. 2004, Ohberg et al. 2004, Ohberg and Alfredson 2004), the patellar tendon (Cannell et al. 2001, Purdam et al. 2004, Stasinopoulos and Stasinopoulos 2004), and lateral epicondylitis (Martinex-Silvestrini et al. 2005, Svernlov and Adolfsson 2001, Schmid et al. 2002).

Two of the areas that have the largest amount of evidence demonstrating effectiveness are the patellar and Achilles tendons. To perform eccentric loading of the *patellar tendon,* from an upright position the patient stands with both extremities on a slanted board (Fig. 84.1, *A*). All the weight is then transferred to the involved extremity, and the muscle is loaded eccentrically as the patient lowers him or herself to about 90 degrees of knee flexion unilaterally on the involved lower extremity (Fig. 84.1, *B*). Once on the bottom position, the patient bears weight bilaterally again to return to the starting position.

Heavy slow resistance training (HSRT) has been shown to be successful in the treatment of patellar tendinopathy (Zwerver et al. 2011, Kongsgaard et al. 2010). HSRT is similar to traditional squats except they are done over the course of 3 seconds. Types of lifts used for HSRT can include squats, leg presses, or hack squats performed up to three times per week. Four sets of increasing loads are used for HSRT. Week 1 to 15 repetition maximum (RM); week 2 to 3, 12 RM; week 4 to 5, 10 RM; week 6 to 8, 8 RM; week 9 to 12, 6 RM. A progression of this routine will result in a greater resistance and lower amount of repetitions.

A technique similar to single-leg squats is used for the *Achilles tendon.* From a bilateral weightbearing position with forefeet on the edge of a step, the patient plantar flexes the feet to the end of available range (Fig. 84.2, *A*). The patient then shifts all of the weight onto the involved side only and loads the gastrocnemius and soleus eccentrically as he or she lowers into dorsiflexion. This is done with the knee fully extended (Fig. 84.2, *B*) and with

Patellar Tendon Exercises

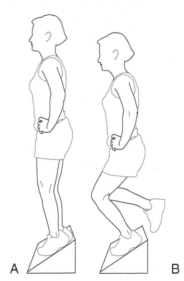

Fig. 84.1 Eccentric exercises for patellar tendinopathy. A, Start of exercise with both knees extended. B, End of exercise with uninvolved leg lifted while involved stance knee flexed.

Eccentric Achilles Tendon Loading Exercises

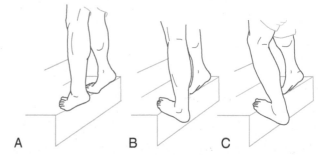

Fig. 84.2 Eccentric exercises for Achilles tendinopathy. A, Starting position with both knees extended and ankles plantarflexed. B, Mid position with knee extended and ankle dorsiflexed. C, Ending position with knee flexed and ankle plantarflexed.

the knee flexed (Fig. 84.2, *C*). Silbernagel et al. (2001) described a three-phased program. The initial phase is considered a warmup phase designed to increase blood flow, ankle range of motion, and tissue compliance. Movements include ankle dorsiflexion and plantarflexion and toe extension and flexion. Three sets of 20 seconds of gastrocnemius and soleus stretching are performed. Other warmup exercises include toe and heel walking, single-leg balance, and heel raise three times per day for 2 weeks. Phase 2 lasts only 2 weeks and includes a progression to single-leg toe raises. Weeks 4 to 12 constitute Phase 3, which introduces plyometric exercises of quick rebounding toe raises 20 to 100 reps three times per day. These exercises may elicit pain during or after the activity to a level of up to 5/10. Pain and stiffness should not increase the day after. If this does occur the exercise volume and intensity should be reduced by returning to the prior phase.

REFERENCES

A complete reference list is available at https://expertconsult .inkling.com/.

FURTHER READING

Curwin, Stanish. In: Curwin S, Stanish WD, eds. *Tendinitis: Its Etiology and Treatment*. Lexington, KY: Collamore Press; 1984:189.

Khan KM, Cook JL, Kannus P, et al. Time to abandon the "tendinitis" myth. *BMJ*. 2002;324(7338):626–627.

Maffulli N, Khan KM, Puddu G. Overuse tendon conditions: time to change a confusing terminology. *Arthroscopy*. 1998;14:840–843.

Worrell TW, Perrin DH. Hamstring muscle injury: the influence of strength, flexibility, warm-up, and fatigue. *J Orthop Sports Phys Ther*. 1992;16: 12–18.

Note: Pages followed by *b*, *t*, or *f* refer to boxes, tables, or figures, respectively